CARDIOMYOPATHIES – FROM BASIC RESEARCH TO CLINICAL MANAGEMENT

Edited by **Josef Veselka**

Cardiomyopathies – From Basic Research to Clinical Management
Edited by Josef Veselka

Published by InTech
Janeza Trdine 9, 51000 Rijeka, Croatia

Publishing Process Manager Ivona Lovric

Technical Editor Teodora Smiljanic

Cover Designer InTech Design Team

Additional hard copies can be obtained from orders@intechopen.com

Cardiomyopathies – From Basic Research to Clinical Management, Edited by Josef Veselka
p. cm.
978-953-307-834-2

Meet the editor

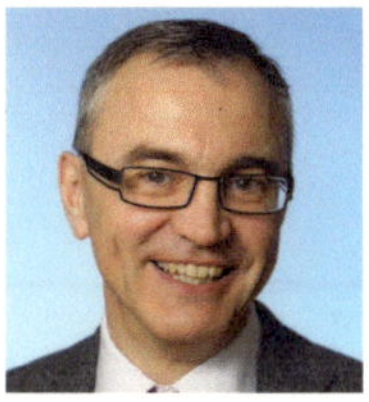

Dr Josef Veselka, PhD attended medical school at Charles University, Prague, Czech Republic, and graduated in 1989. He is a Professor of Medicine and Chief of Department of Cardiology at the 2nd Faculty of Medicine, Charles University and University Hospital Motol, Prague. His main areas of expertise and interest are cardiomyopathies and interventional cardiology, and he is one of the pioneers and leaders in the field of structural and coronary interventions. Dr Veselka has published more than 250 scientific papers, edited 5 monographs and textbooks and is a member of several editorial boards of medical journals.

Contents

Preface

Cardiomyopathy means "heart (cardio) muscle (myo) disease (pathy)". Currently, cardiomyopathies are defined as myocardial disorders in which the heart muscle is structurally and/or functionally abnormal in the absence of coronary artery disease, hypertension, valvular heart disease or congenital heart disease sufficient to cause the observed myocardial abnormalities. Usually, cardiomyopathies are classified into three major groups: dilated, hypertrophic and restrictive. However, this book also deals with some specific issues of Takotsubo cardiomyopathy, Chagas' heart disease and the heart dysfunctions that accompany some metabolic diseases. The unique feature of this book is that it incorporates chapters covering both basic research and clinical management.

Dilated cardiomyopathy is characterized by left ventricular dilation and systolic dysfunction. It is probably the most common form of heart muscle disease, comprising approximately 60% of all cardiomyopathies identified. The underlying aetiologies are viral infection, cardiac toxins (including alcohol), metabolic disorders and genetic causes, which might represent 30%-40% of all causes of dilated cardiomyopathies. The disorder is clinically very heterogeneous and some affected individuals suffer from progressive left ventricular dysfunction with clinical signs of heart failure and malignant arrhythmias. Although many causative genes of dilated cardiomyopathy have been identified, there is still a lack of data regarding correct genotype-phenotype interpretations. Therefore, determining the prognosis of each patient with familial dilated cardiomyopathy is still an important goal for the future. Moreover, therapeutic approaches better than just the symptomatic relief of heart failure or the implantation of a cardioverter-defibrillator are badly needed.

Hypertrophic cardiomyopathy is probably the most common inherited cardiac disorder, with an estimated prevalence of 1 in 500 individuals. The clinical course varies significantly. Some patients remain asymptomatic throughout their whole lives, whereas some have severe symptoms of heart failure or angina pectoris; others die suddenly, even in the absence of previous symptoms. The annual mortality rate varies in different studies and it has been reported to be about 1% in unselected populations. Also, in the field of hypertrophic cardiomyopathy, advances in genetics have enabled genetic-based diagnoses. However, similar to dilated cardiomyopathy, there is an absence of studies resulting in the knowledge of reliable genotype-phenotype correlations. Moreover, although costs of sequencing and mutational analyses have decreased considerably, the price of testing remains in the thousands of Euros (dollars). In addition, discovering the genetic heterogeneity and the number of so far unidentified causative genes and "private" mutations remain a persistent challenge. On the other hand, there have been important developments in the field of prevention of sudden cardiac death with the introduction of risk stratification and subsequent defibrillator implantation. Similar to dilated cardiomyopathy, we can expect further improvements in genetic testing that should mainly focus on "healthy" genetic carriers.

Restrictive cardiomyopathy is the least common type of cardiomyopathy, which is characterized not by morphological criteria but by increased myocardial stiffness leading to high ventricular filling pressures. Restrictive haemodynamics was described in many conditions, but the archetype and most common of these diseases is cardiac amyloidosis. Unfortunately, symptomatic cardiac amyloidosis is associated with an unfavourable prognosis and attention should next be focused on the earliest establishment of its diagnosis. This seems to be the only way of improving the prognosis of these patients.

Readers of this book will also find several chapters that specifically deal with Takotsubo cardiomyopathy. Interestingly, although almost two decades have passed since the introduction of this diagnosis, the rich literature on this confusing syndrome has contained little that definitively clarifies the fundamental aspects of this type of cardiomyopathy. It seems that improving our understanding of the pathophysiologic mechanisms of Takotsubo cardiomyopathy in the future is essential, as it could result in its better prevention and treatment.

Very interesting chapters review Chagas' heart disease. It is estimated that approximately 10 million patients suffer from this disease, which is still the third largest parasitic burden globally, after malaria and schistosomiasis. Although Chagas' heart disease occurs mainly in South America, there is an increasing number of patients being diagnosed in non-endemic areas worldwide, and this disease has become a global public health issue.

Although significant advances have been made in most fields dealing with the understanding and therapy of cardiomyopathies, much work still remains to be done. Generally, research efforts will be focused more on genetic and pathophysiological principles of cardiomyopathies in order to prevent the development of the phenotype and major adverse clinical events.

It was impossible to meet all our goals or cover all the problems found regarding cardiomyopathies in this book. However, we believe that this book will be able to provide both researchers and clinicians alike with modern information that will aid in their work.

Josef Veselka, MD, PhD
Professor of Medicine, Head of Department of Cardiology,
2nd Faculty of Medicine, Charles University, University Hospital Motol, Prague,
Czech Republic

Part 1

Classification, Evaluation and Management of Cardiomyopathies

1

Classification and Definitions of Cardiomyopathies

Bhulan Kumar Singh[1], Krishna Kolappa Pillai[1], Kanchan Kohli[2] and Syed Ehtaishamul Haque[1]
[1]*Department of Pharmacology, Faculty of Pharmacy, Hamdard University, New Delhi*
[2]*Department of Pharmaceutics, Faculty of Pharmacy, Hamdard University, New Delhi, India*

1. Introduction

Cardiomyopathies are an important and heterogeneous group of diseases. The awareness and knowledge of these diseases in both the public and medical communities historically has been impaired by persistent confusion surrounding definitions and nomenclature. Classification schemes, of which there have been many, (Thiene et al., 2000, 2004; Richardson et al., 1996) are potentially useful in drawing relationships and distinctions between complex disease states for the purpose of promoting greater understanding; indeed, the precise language used to describe these diseases are profoundly important.

Cardiomyopathies are diseases of the heart muscle, characterized by abnormality in chamber size and wall thickness, or functional contractile dysfunctions mainly systolic or diastolic dysfunction in the absence of coronary artery disease, hypertension, valvular disease, or congenital heart disease (Elliott et al., 2008). These diseases are classified as either primary or secondary. Primary cardiomyopathies consist of disorders solely or predominantly confined to the heart muscle, which have genetic, non-genetic, or acquired causes. Secondary cardiomyopathies are disorders that have myocardial damage as a result of systemic or multiorgan disease (Maron et al., 2006). Cardiomyopathies are classified traditionally according to morphological and functional criteria into four categories: dilated cardiomyopathy (DCM), hypertrophic cardiomyopathy (HCM), restrictive cardiomyopathy (RCM) and arrhythmogenic right ventricular cardiomyopathy/dysplasia (ARVC/D). These cardiomyopathies can be primary myocardial disorders or develop as a secondary consequence of a variety of conditions, including myocardial ischemia, inflammation, infection, increased myocardial pressure or volume load and toxic agents.

The definitions of cardiomyopathies presented here are in concert with the molecular era of cardiovascular disease and have direct clinical applications and implications for cardiac diagnosis. However, the classification of cardiomyopathies presented herein is not intended to provide precise methodologies or strategies for clinical diagnosis. Rather, the classification of cardiomyopathies represents a scientific presentation that offers new perspectives to aid in understanding this complex and heterogeneous group of diseases and basic disease mechanisms.

2. Definition

The term cardiomyopathy was used for the first time in 1957. Over the next 25 years, a number of definitions for cardiomyopathies were advanced. Indeed, in the original 1980 WHO classification, cardiomyopathies were defined only as "heart muscle diseases of unknown cause," reflecting a general lack of available information about basic disease mechanisms. In 1968, the WHO defined cardiomyopathies as "diseases of different and often unknown etiology in which the dominant feature is cardiomegaly and heart failure." The final WHO classification published in 1995 proposed "diseases of myocardium associated with cardiac dysfunction" and included for the first time ARVC/D, as well as primary RCM.

The American Heart Association (AHA) expert consensus panel proposed definition of cardiomyopathies is as follows: "Cardiomyopathies are a heterogeneous group of diseases of the myocardium associated with mechanical and/or electrical dysfunction, which usually (but not invariably) exhibit inappropriate ventricular hypertrophy or dilatation, due to a variety of etiologies that frequently are genetic. Cardiomyopathies are either confined to the heart or are part of generalized systemic disorders, and often lead to cardiovascular death or progressive heart failure–related disability." This definition of cardiomyopathies, similar to that reported by the European Society of Cardiology (ESC), under the auspices of the Working Group on Myocardial and Pericardial Diseases, excludes myocardial involvement secondary to coronary artery disease, systemic hypertension, and valvular and congenital heart disease.

3. Classifications of cardiomyopathies

Cardiac diseases can have an external cause, such as coronary artery disease, valve disease or hypertension, or may involve cardiomyopathies, in which the heart muscle itself is abnormal (i.e. an intrinsic cause of the disease is present in the heart muscle). The distinction between different classes of cardiac diseases are an important one to make, as cardiac diseases with similar phenotypes can have a diverse origin and may need different types of management. However, classification of cardiomyopathies is difficult, as the origin or pathophysiology is not always understood. Furthermore, at present there is no consensus on how to classify cardiomyopathies (e.g., based on origin, physiology or treatment) among clinicians.

In order to promote a uniform nomenclature and well-defined clinical patient groups, recent knowledge on underlying causes and pathophysiology of cardiomyopathies has been implemented in a cardiomyopathy classification system both on behalf of the American Heart Association (AHA) and of the European Society of Cardiology (ESC).

The AHA divided cardiomyopathies into 2 major groups based on predominant organ involvement. Primary cardiomyopathies (genetic, nongenetic, acquired) are those solely or predominantly confined to heart muscle and are relatively few in number (Fig. 1). Secondary cardiomyopathies show pathological myocardial involvement as part of a large number and variety of generalized systemic (multiorgan) disorders (Table 1). The frequency and degree of secondary myocardial involvement vary considerably among these diseases, some of which are exceedingly uncommon and for which the evidence of myocardial pathology may be sparse and reported in only a few patients. Because many cardiomyopathies may predominantly involve the heart but are not necessarily confined to that organ, some of the distinctions between primary and secondary cardiomyopathy are necessarily arbitrary and inevitably rely on judgment about the clinical importance and consequences of the myocardial process (Maron, 2008; Maron et al., 2006).

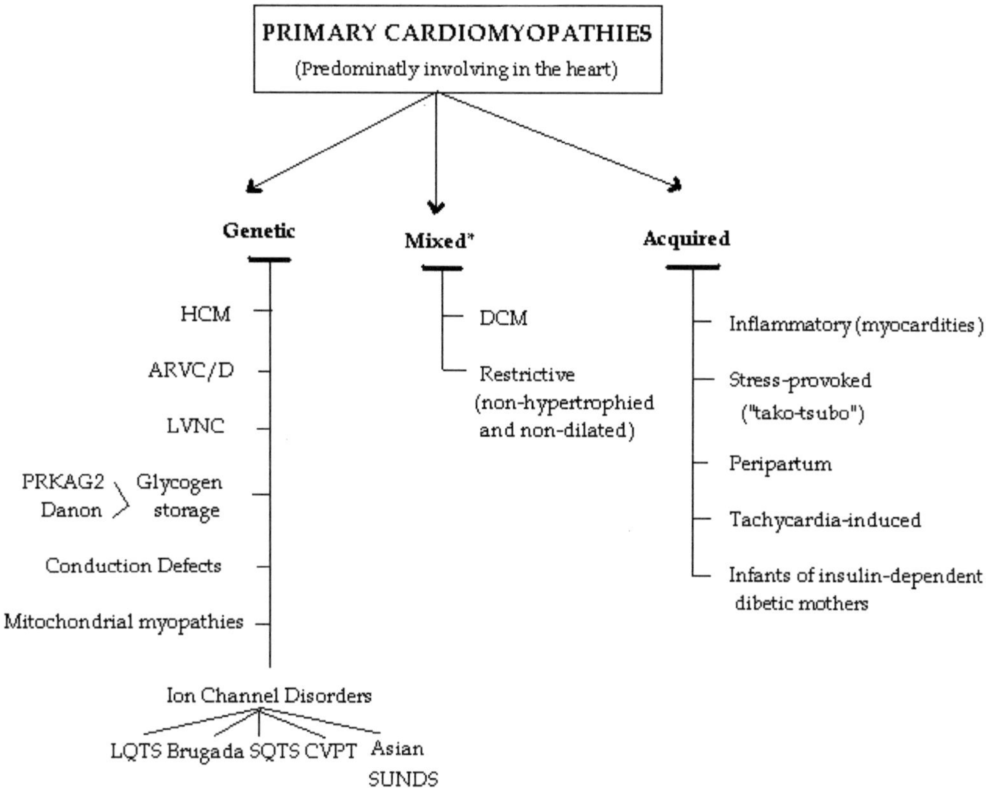

Fig. 1. Classification model for Primary cardiomyopathies (disease processes solely or predominantly involves the myocardium). The conditions have been segregated according to their genetic or nongenetic etiologies. *Predominantly nongenetic; familial disease with a genetic origin has been reported in a minority of cases. ARVC/D indicates arrhythmogenic right ventricular cardiomyopathy/dysplasia; CPVT, catecholaminergic polymorphic ventricular tachycardia; DCM, dilated cardiomyopathy; HCM, hypertrophic cardiomyopathy; LQTS, long QT syndrome; LVNC, left ventricular noncompaction; SQTS, short QT syndrome; and SUNDS, sudden unexplained nocturnal death syndrome.

Infiltrative[*]	
	Amyloidosis (primary, familial autosomal dominant[†], senile, secondary forms)
	Gaucher disease[†]
	Hurler's disease[†]
	Hunter's disease[†]
Storage[‡]	
	Hemochromatosis
	Fabry's disease[†]
	Glycogen storage disease[†] (type II, Pompe)
	Niemann-Pick disease[†]
Toxicity	
	Drugs, heavy metals, chemical agents
Endomyocardial	
	Endomyocardial fibrosis
	Hypereosinophilic syndrome (Löeffler's endocarditis)
Inflammatory (granulomatous)	
	Sarcoidosis
Endocrine	
	Diabetes mellitus[†]
	Hyperthyroidism
	Hypothyroidism
	Hyperparathyroidism
	Pheochromocytoma
	Acromegaly
Cardiofacial	
	Noonan syndrome[†]
	Lentiginosis[†]
Neuromuscular/neurological	
	Friedreich's ataxia[†]
	Duchenne-Becker muscular dystrophy[†]
	Emery-Dreifuss muscular dystrophy[†]
	Myotonic dystrophy[†]
	Neurofibromatosis[†]
	Tuberous sclerosis[†]
Nutritional deficiencies	
	Beriberi (thiamine), pallagra, scurvy, selenium, carnitine, kwashiorkor
Autoimmune/collagen	
	Systemic lupus erythematosis
	Dermatomyositis
	Rheumatoid arthritis
	Scleroderma
	Polyarteritis nodosa
Electrolyte imbalance	
Consequence of cancer therapy	
	Anthracyclines: doxorubicin (adriamycin), daunorubicin
	Cyclophosphamide
	Radiation

[*]Accumulation of abnormal substances between myocytes (i.e., extracellular).
[†]Genetic (familial) origin.
[‡]Accumulation of abnormal substances within myocytes (i.e., intracellular).

Table 1. Important secondary cardiomyopathies

The ESC guidelines are more clinically orientated, which is appealing as this circumvents the complex pathophysiology of cardiomyopathies, which is not always comprehended upon presentation of the patient. According to the ESC guidelines cardiomyopathies are grouped into specific morphological and functional phenotypes; each phenotype is then sub-classified into familial and non-familial forms (Fig. 2). In this context, familial refers to the occurrence, in more than one family member, of either the same disorder or a phenotype that is (or could be) caused by the same genetic mutation and not to acquired cardiac or systemic diseases in which the clinical phenotype is influenced by genetic polymorphism. Most familial cardiomyopathies are monogenic disorders (i.e., the gene defect is sufficient by itself to cause the trait). A monogenic cardiomyopathy can be sporadic when the causative mutation is de novo, i.e. has occurred in an individual for the first time within the family (or at the germinal level in one of the parents). In this classification system, patients with identified de novo mutations are assigned to the familial category as their disorder can be subsequently transmitted to their offspring (Elliott et al., 2008). Non-familial cardiomyopathies are clinically defined by the presence of a cardiomyopathy in the index patient and the absence of disease in other family members (based on pedigree analysis and clinical evaluation). They are subdivided into idiopathic (no identifiable cause) and acquired cardiomyopathies in which ventricular dysfunction is a complication of the disorder rather than an intrinsic feature of the disease (Elliott et al., 2008).

Therefore, on the basis of all these considerations, cardiomyopathies can be most effectively classified as primary: genetic, mixed (genetic and nongenetic), acquired; and secondary.

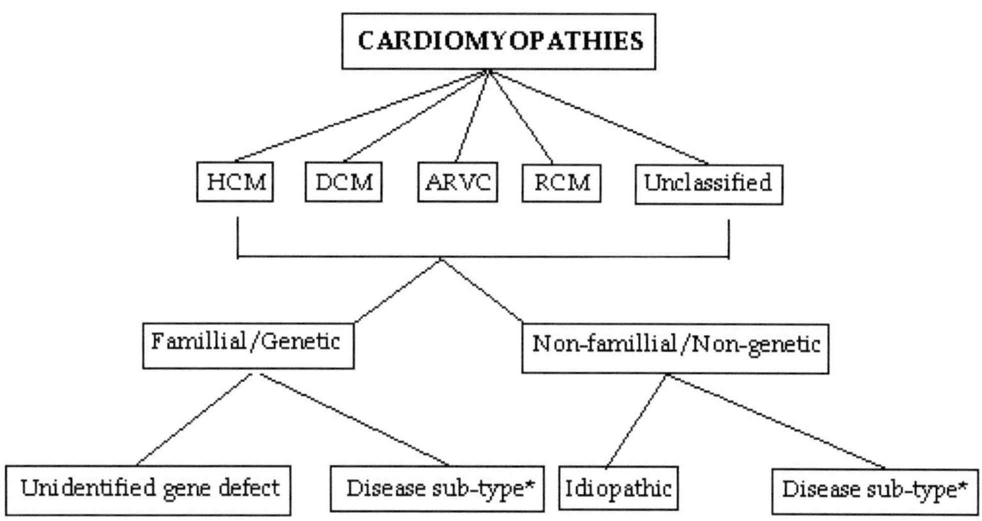

Fig. 2. Summery of proposed classification. HCM, hypertrophic cardiomyopathy; DCM, dilated cardiomyopathy; ARVC, arrhythmogenic right ventricular cardiomyopathy; RCM, restrictive cardiomyopathy (*see table 2).

	HCM	DCM	ARVC	RCM	Unclassified
Famillial	Familial, unknown gene Sarcomeric protein mutations β-myosin heavy chain Cardiac myosin binding protein C Cardiac troponin I Troponin T α-tropomyosin Essential myosin light chain Regulatory myosin light chain Cardiac actin α-myosin heavy chain Titin Troponin C Muscle LIM protein Glycogen storage disease (e.g. Pompe; PRKAG2, Forbes', Danon) Lysosomal storage diseases (e.g. Anderson–Fabry, Hurler's) Disorders of fatty acid metabolism Carnitine deficiency Phosphorylase B kinase deficiency Mitochondrial cytopathies Syndromic HCM Noonan's syndrome LEOPARD syndrome Friedreich's ataxia Beckwith–Wiedermann syndrome Swyer's syndrome Other Phospholamban promoter Familial amyloid	Familial, unknown gene Sarcomeric protein mutations (see HCM) Z-band Muscle LIM protein TCAP Cytoskeletal genes Dystrophin Desmin Metavinculin Sarcoglycan complex CRYAB Epicardin Nuclear membrane Lamin A/C Emerin Mildly dilated CM Intercalated disc protein mutations (see ARVC) Mitochondrial cytopathy	Familial, unknown gene Intercalated disc protein mutations Plakoglobin Desmoplakin Plakophilin 2 Desmoglein 2 Desmocollin 2 Cardiac ryanodine receptor (RyR2) Transforming growth factor-β3 (TGFβ3)	Familial, unknown gene Sarcomeric protein mutations Troponin I (RCM +/– HCM) Essential light chain of myosin Familial amyloidosis Transthyretin (RCM + neuropathy) Apolipoprotein (RCM + nephropathy) Desminopathy Pseuxanthoma elasticum Haemochromatosis Anderson–Fabry disease Glycogen storage disease	Left ventricular non-compaction Barth syndrome Lamin A/C ZASP α-dystrobrevin
Non-familial	Obesity Infants of diabetic mothers Athletic training Amyloid (AL/prealbumin)	Myocarditis (infective/toxic/immune) Kawasaki disease Eosinophilic (Churg Strauss syndrome) Viral persistence Drugs Pregnancy Endocrine Nutritional – thiamine, carnitine, selenium, hypophosphataemia, hypocalcaemia Alcohol Tachycardiomyopathy	Inflammation	Amyloid (AL/prealbumin) Scleroderma Endomyocardial fibrosis Hypereosinophilic syndrome Idiopathic Chromosomal cause Drugs (serotonin, methysergide, ergotamine, mercurial agents, busulfan) Carcinoid heart disease Metastatic cancers Radiation Drugs (anthracyclines)	Tako Tsubo cardiomyopathy

ARVC, arrhythmogenic right ventricular cardiomyopathy; DCM, dilated cardiomyopathy; HCM, hypertrophic cardiomyopathy; RCM, restrictive cardiomyopathy.

Table 2. Examples of different diseases that cause cardiomyopathies

3.1. Primary cardiomyopathies
3.1.1 Genetic
3.1.1.1 Hypertrophic cardiomyopathy

HCM is a condition of the heart in which a part of the myocardium or the muscle of the heart is enlarged without any obvious reasons. It is very common and affects people of all ages. HCM is a clinically heterogeneous but relatively common autosomal dominant genetic heart disease (1:500 of the general population for the disease phenotype recognized by echocardiography) that probably is the most frequently occurring cardiomyopathy (Maron, 2002). It is the most common cause of sudden cardiac death in the young (including trained athletes) and is an important substrate for heart failure disability at any age.

HCM is characterized morphologically and defined by a hypertrophied, nondilated left ventricle (LV) in the absence of another systemic or cardiac disease that is capable of producing the magnitude of wall thickening evident (e.g., systemic hypertension, aortic valve stenosis). Clinical diagnosis is customarily made with 2 dimensional echocardiography (or alternatively with cardiac magnetic resonance imaging) by detection of otherwise unexplained LV wall thickening, usually in the presence of a small LV cavity, after suspicion is raised by the clinical profile or as part of family screening (Maron et al., 2006).

When LV wall thickness is mild, differential diagnosis with physiological athlete's heart may arise. Furthermore, individuals harboring a genetic defect for HCM do not necessarily express clinical markers of their disease such as LV hypertrophy on echocardiogram, ECG abnormalities, or symptoms at all times during life, and ECG alterations can precede the appearance of hypertrophy. Indeed, virtually any LV wall thickness, even when within normal limits, is consistent with the presence of an HCM-causing mutant gene, and diagnosis can be made by laboratory DNA analysis. Furthermore, recognition of LV hypertrophy may be age related with its initial appearance delayed well into adulthood (adult morphological conversion). Most HCM patients have the propensity to develop dynamic obstruction to LV outflow under resting or physiologically provocable conditions, produced by systolic anterior motion of the mitral valve with ventricular septal contact (Maron et al., 2006).

HCM is caused by a variety of mutations encoding contractile proteins of the cardiac sarcomere. Currently, 11 mutant genes are associated with HCM, most commonly β-myosin heavy chain (the first identified) and myosin binding protein C (Barry et al., 2008; Lowey, 2002). The other 9 genes appear to account for far fewer cases of HCM and include troponin T and I, regulatory and essential myosin light chains, titin, α-tropomyosin, α-actin, α-myosin heavy chain, and muscle LIM protein (Barry et al., 2008; Selvetella & Lembo, 2005). This genetic diversity is compounded by considerable intragenic heterogeneity, with >400 individual mutations now identified. These most commonly are missense mutations but include insertions, deletions, and splice (split-site) mutations encoding truncated sarcomeric proteins (Maron et al., 2006). The characteristic diversity of the HCM phenotype is attributable to the disease causing mutations and probably to the influence of modifier genes and environmental factors.

In addition, nonsarcomeric protein mutations in 2 genes involved in cardiac metabolism have recently been reported to be responsible for primary cardiac glycogen storage diseases in older children and adults with a clinical presentation mimicking (or indistinguishable from) that of sarcomeric HCM. One of these conditions involves the gene encoding the γ-2-regulatory subunit of the AMP-activated protein kinase (PRKAG2), associated with variable degrees of LV hypertrophy and ventricular pre-excitation. The other involves the gene encoding lysosome-associated membrane protein-2 (LAMP-2), resulting in Danon-type storage disease (Maron et al., 2006). Clinical manifestations are limited largely to the heart, usually with massive degrees of LV hypertrophy and ventricular pre-excitation. These disorders are now part of a subgroup of previously described infiltrative forms of LV hypertrophy such as Pompe disease, a glycogen storage disease caused by α-1,4 glycosidase (acid maltase deficiency) in infants, and Fabry's disease, an X-linked recessive disorder of glycosphingolipid metabolism caused by a deficiency of the lysosomal enzyme α-galactosidase A, resulting in intracellular accumulation of glycosphingolipids. Undoubtedly, many other mutations causing cardiac hypertrophy by disrupting sarcomere, metabolic, and other genes remain to be identified (Elliott et al., 2008).

A number of other diseases associated with LV hypertrophy involve prominent thickening of the LV wall, occurring mostly in infants and children ≤4 years of age, which may resemble or mimic typical HCM caused by sarcomere protein mutations. These cardiomyopathies include secondary forms such as Noonan syndrome, an autosomal dominant cardiofacial condition associated with a variety of cardiac defects (most commonly, dysplastic pulmonary valve stenosis and atrial septal defect) resulting from mutations in PTPN11, a gene encoding the nonreceptor protein tyrosine phosphatase SHP-2 genes. At present, the causes of most cases of pediatric cardiomyopathies are unknown (Maron et al., 2006).

Other diseases in this category are mitochondrial myopathies resulting from mutations encoding mitochondrial DNA (including Kearns-Sayre syndrome) or mitochondrial proteins associated with ATP electron transport chain enzyme defects that alter mitochondrial morphology. Also included in these considerations are metabolic myopathies representing ATP production and utilization defects involving abnormalities of fatty acid oxidation (acyl CoA dehydrogenase deficiencies) and carnitine deficiency, as well as infiltrative myopathies, i.e., glycogen storage diseases (type II; autosomal recessive Pompe disease), Hunter's and Hurler's diseases, and the transient and nonfamilial cardiomyopathy as part of generalized organomegaly, recognized in infants of insulin-dependent diabetic mothers. In older patients, a number of systemic diseases have been associated with hypertrophic forms of cardiomyopathy; these include Friedreich's ataxia, pheochromocytoma, neurofibromatosis, lentiginosis, and tuberous sclerosis.

3.1.1.2 Arrhythmogenic right ventricular cardiomyopathy/dysplasia

ARVC/D is predominantly a genetically determined heart muscle disorder that is characterized pathologically by fibrofatty replacement of the right ventricular (RV) myocardium (Basso et al., 2009). In the early stage of the disease, structural changes may be absent or subtle and confined to a localized region of the RV, typically the inflow tract, outflow tract, or apex of the RV, the "triangle of dysplasia." Progression to more diffuse RV disease and left ventricular (LV) involvement, typically affecting the posterior lateral wall, is common (Marcus et al., 2010).

ARVC/D is a familial disease in at least 50% of cases and is typically transmitted as an autosomal dominant trait with variable penetrance. On the basis of clinical studies and data obtained from pre-participation screening for sport activity, the estimated prevalence of the disease in the general population ranges from 1 in 1000 to 1 in 5000 (Nava et al., 2000).

ARVC/D has a broad clinical spectrum, usually presenting clinically with ventricular tachyarrhythmias (e.g., monomorphic ventricular tachycardia). Noninvasive clinical diagnosis may be confounding, without an easily obtained single test or finding that is definitively diagnostic, and generally requires an integrated assessment of electrical, functional, and anatomic abnormalities. Diagnosis often requires a high index of suspicion, frequently triggered by presentation with arrhythmias, syncope, or cardiac arrest, as well as global or segmental chamber dilatation or wall motion abnormalities (Marcus et al., 2010).

Noninvasive tests used to diagnose ARVC/D, in addition to personal and family history, include 12-lead ECG, echocardiography, right ventricular angiography, cardiac magnetic resonance imaging, and computerized tomography. Endomyocardial biopsy from the right ventricular free wall is a sensitive diagnostic marker when fibrofatty infiltration is associated with surviving strands of myocytes. ECGs most commonly show abnormal repolarization with T-wave inversion in leads V_1 through V_3 and small-amplitude potentials at the end of the QRS complex (epsilon wave); Brugada syndrome–like right bundle-branch block and right precordial ST-segment elevation accompanied by polymorphic ventricular tachycardia also have been reported in a small subpopulation of ARVC/D patients (Basso et al., 2009; Protonotarios et al., 2011).

ARVC/D shows autosomal dominant inheritance, albeit often with incomplete penetrance. Autosomal dominant ARVC/D has been mapped to 8 chromosomal loci, with mutations identified thus far in 4 genes: the cardiac ryanodine receptor RyR2, which is also responsible for familial catecholaminergic polymorphic ventricular tachycardia (CPVT); desmoplakin; plakophillin-2; and mutations altering regulatory sequences of the transforming growth factor-β gene, which has a role in inflammation. Two recessive forms have been described in conjunction with palmoplantar keratoderma and woolly hair (Naxos disease) and with Carvajal syndrome, caused by mutations in junctional plakoglobin and desmoplakin, respectively. Although the function of desmosomal proteins to anchor intermediate filaments to desmosomes implicates ARVC/D as a primary structural abnormality, there is also a link to ion channel dysfunction (Maron et al., 2006).

3.1.1.3 Left ventricular noncompaction

Noncompaction of ventricular myocardium is a recently recognized congenital cardiomyopathy characterized by a distinctive ("spongy") morphological appearance of the LV myocardium. Noncompaction involves predominantly the distal (apical) portion of the LV chamber with deep intertrabecular recesses (sinusoids) in communication with the ventricular cavity, resulting from an arrest in the normal embryogenesis (Freedom et al., 2005). LV noncompaction (LVNC) may be an isolated finding or may be associated with other congenital heart anomalies such as complex cyanotic congenital heart disease.

Diagnosis is made with 2-dimensional echocardiography, cardiac magnetic resonance imaging, or LV angiography (Chin et al., 1990). The natural history of LVNC is largely unresolved but includes LV systolic dysfunction and heart failure (and some cases of heart transplantation), thromboemboli, arrhythmias, sudden death, and diverse forms of remodeling. Both familial and nonfamilial cases have been described. In the isolated form of LVNC, ZASP (Z-line) and mitochondrial mutations, and X-linked inheritance resulting from mutations in the G4.5 gene encoding tafazzin (including association with Barth syndrome in neonates) have been reported. Noncompaction associated with congenital heart disease has been shown to result from mutations in the α-dystrobrevin gene and transcription factor NKX2.5 (Monserrat Iglesias, 2008).

3.1.1.4 Conduction system disease

Lenegre disease, also called as progressive cardiac conduction defect. It is characterized by primary progressive development of cardiac conduction defects in the His-Purkinje system, leading to widening of the QRS complex, long pauses, and bradycardia that may trigger syncope. Phenotypically sick sinus syndrome is similar to progressive cardiac conduction defect. Familial occurrence of both syndromes has been reported with an autosomal dominant pattern of inheritance. An ion channelopathy, in the form of SCN5A mutations, is thought to contribute to these conduction system defects. Wolff-Parkinson-White syndrome is familial in some cases, but information about the genetic causes is unavailable.

3.1.1.5 Ion channelopathies

There is a growing list of uncommon inherited and congenital arrhythmia disorders caused by mutations in genes encoding defective ionic channel proteins, governing cell membrane transit of sodium and potassium ions (Aleong et al., 2007). These ion channel disorders include LQTS, short-QT syndrome (SQTS), Brugada syndrome, and CPVT. Nocturnal sudden unexplained death syndrome in young Southeast Asian males and Brugada syndrome are based on similar clinical and genetic profiles. A small proportion (5% to 10%) of sudden infant deaths also may be linked to ion channelopathies, including LQTS, SQTS, and Brugada syndrome (Modell & Lehmann, 2006). Clinical diagnosis of the ion channelopathies often can be made by identification of the disease phenotype on standard 12-lead ECG. Some of these cases had previously been classified as idiopathic ventricular fibrillation, a description that persists for a syndrome in which mechanistic understanding is lacking (Aleong et al., 2007; Kass, 2005).

3.1.1.5.1 Long-QT syndrome

This is the most common condition of the ion channelopathies. It is characterized by prolongation of ventricular repolarization and QT interval (corrected for heart rate) on the standard 12-lead ECG, a specific form of polymorphic ventricular tachycardia (torsade des pointes), and a risk for syncope and sudden cardiac death. Phenotypic expression (on the ECG) varies considerably, and ~25% to 50% of affected family members may show borderline or even normal QT intervals.

Two patterns of inheritance have been described in LQTS: a rare autosomal recessive disease associated with deafness (Jervell and Lange-Nielsen syndrome), which is caused by 2 genes that encode for the slowly activating delayed rectifier potassium channel (KCNQ1 and KCNE1 (minK)), and the much more common autosomal dominant disease unassociated with deafness (Romano-Ward syndrome), which is caused by mutations in 8 different genes. These include KCNQ1 (KvLQT1, LQT1), KCNH2 (HERG, LQT2), SCN5A (Na1.5, LQT3), ANKB (LQT4), KCNE1 (minK, LQT5), KCNE2 (MiRP1, LQT6), KCNJ2 (Kir2.1, LQT7, Andersen's syndrome), and CACNA1C (Ca1.2, LQT8, Timothy syndrome). Of the 8 genes, 6 encode for cardiac potassium channels, 1 for the sodium channel (SCN5A, LQT3), and 1 for the protein ankyrin, which is involved in anchoring ion channels to the cellular membrane (ANKB) (Maron et al., 2006).

3.1.1.5.2 Brugada syndrome

This syndrome is a relatively new clinical entity associated with sudden cardiac death in young people. First described in 1992, the syndrome is identified by a distinctive ECG pattern consisting of right bundle-branch block and coved ST-segment elevation in the anterior pre-cordial leads (V_1 through V_3). The characteristic ECG pattern is often concealed and may be unmasked with the administration of sodium channel blockers, including ajmaline, flecainide, procainamide, and pilsicainide. Familial autosomal dominant and sporadic forms have been linked to mutations in an α-subunit of the cardiac sodium channel gene SCN5A (the same gene responsible for LQT3) in 20% of patients. Another locus has been reported on the short arm of chromosome 3, but no gene has been identified. Sudden unexplained nocturnal death syndrome, found predominantly in young Southeast Asian males (i.e., those from Thailand, Japan, the Philippines, and Cambodia), is a disorder causing sudden death during sleep as a result of ventricular tachycardia/fibrillation. Some cases of sudden unexplained nocturnal death syndrome resulting from SCN5A gene mutations and Brugada syndrome have been shown to be phenotypically, genetically, and functionally the same disorder (Antzelevitch et al., 2005; Krittayaphong et al., 2003).

3.1.1.5.3 Catecholaminergic polymorphic ventricular tachycardia

CPVT is characterized by syncope, sudden death, polymorphic ventricular tachycardia triggered by vigorous physical exertion or acute emotion (usually in children and adolescents), a normal resting ECG, and the absence of structural cardiac disease. Family history of 1 or multiple sudden cardiac deaths are evident in 30% of cases. The resting ECG is unremarkable, except for sinus bradycardia and prominent U waves in some patients. The most typical arrhythmia of CPVT is bidirectional ventricular tachycardia presenting with an alternating QRS axis. The autosomal dominant form of the disease has been linked to the RyR2 gene encoding for the cardiac ryanodine receptor, a large protein that forms the Ca^{2+} release channel in the sarcoplasmic reticulum that is essential for regulation of excitation-contraction coupling and $[Ca^{2+}]i$ levels. An autosomal recessive form has been linked to CASQ2, a gene that encodes for calsequestrin, a protein that serves as a major Ca^{2+}-binding protein in the terminal cisternae of the sarcoplasmic reticulum. Calsequestrin is bound to the ryanodine receptor and participates in the control of excitation-contraction coupling (Wilde et al., 2008).

3.1.1.5.4 Short-QT syndrome

First described in 2000, the SQTS is characterized by a short QT interval (<330 ms) on an ECG and a high incidence of sudden cardiac death resulting from ventricular tachycardia/fibrillation. Another distinctive ECG feature of SQTS is the appearance of tall peaked T waves similar to those encountered with hyperkalemia. The syndrome has been linked to gain-of-function mutations in KCNH2 (HERG, SQT1), KCNQ1 (KvLQT1, SQT2), and KCNJ2 (Kir2.1, SQT3), causing an increase in the intensity of I_{kr}, I_{ks} and I_{kl}, respectively (Gaita et al., 2003; Schimpf et al., 2005).

3.1.1.5.5 Idiopathic ventricular fibrillation

A subgroup of patients with sudden death appears in the literature with the designation of idiopathic ventricular fibrillation. However, it is likely that idiopathic ventricular fibrillation is not an independent disease entity but rather a conglomeration of conditions with normal gross and microscopic findings in which arrhythmic risk undoubtedly derives from molecular abnormalities, most likely ion channel mutations. At present, insufficient data are available to permit the classification of idiopathic ventricular fibrillation as a distinct cardiomyopathy (Chen et al., 1998).

3.1.2 Mixed (genetic and nongenetic)

3.1.2.1 Dilated cardiomyopathy

DCM is the most common cardiomyopathy worldwide and has many causes. It is a heart muscle disorder defined by the presence of a dilated and poorly functioning left or both ventricles. It can be primary (genetic, mixed or predominantly familial non-genetic, or acquired) or secondary (e.g., infiltrative or autoimmune). This disease can be diagnosed in association with recognized cardiovascular disease; however, to qualify as DCM, the extent of myocardial dysfunction cannot be explained exclusively by abnormal loading conditions (hypertension, valve disease) or ischaemic heart disease (Elliott et al., 2008; Jefferies & Towbin, 2010). A large number of cardiac and systemic diseases can cause systolic impairment and left ventricular dilatation, but in the majority of patients no identifiable cause is found hence the term "idiopathic" dilated cardiomyopathy (IDC). There are experimental and clinical data in animals and humans suggesting that genetic, viral, and immune factors contribute to the pathophysiology of IDC (Elliott, 2000). DCM is associated with sudden cardiac death and heart failure, resulting in a large cost burden because of the very high rate of hospital admission and the potential need for heart transplantation.

DCM is characterized mainly by left ventricular systolic (or diastolic in some case) dysfunction (abnormality of contraction), with an associated increase in mass and volume. Right ventricular dilation and dysfunction can also develop but are not needed for diagnosis. Prevalence in the general population remains undefined. This disorder develops at any age, in either sex, and in people of any ethnic origin (Rosamond et al., 2008; Towbin et al., 2006). In adults, DCM arises more commonly in men than in women. In children, the yearly incidence is 0.57 cases per 100000 per year overall, but is higher in boys than in girls (0.66 vs. 0.47 cases per 100000, $P<0.006$), in black people than in white people (0.98 vs. 0.46 cases per 100000, $P<0.001$), and in babies younger than 1 year than in children (4.40 vs. 0.34 cases per 100000, $P<0.001$). Two thirds of children are thought to have idiopathic disease (Towbin et al., 2006). In adults, the prevalence is 1 in 2500 individuals, with an incidence of 7 per 100000 per year (but it could be underdiagnosed). In many cases, the disease is inherited, and is called familial dilated cardiomyopathy (FDC). The familial type might account for 20-48% of all cases (Taylor et al., 2006). To achieve improved care and outcomes in children and adults, a broadened understanding of the causes of these disorders are needed.

In this disease, the left ventricle is dilated, and more spherical than usual with raised wall stress and depressed systolic function. Mitral regurgitation, thromboembolic events and ventricular arrhythmias can also develop. Occasionally, other rhythm disturbances such as atrioventricular block, supraventricular tachycardia with or without pre-excitation including Wolf-Parkinson-White syndrome and atrial fibrillation develop. In the most severe cases, affected individuals present with signs and symptoms of HF–diaphoresis, breathlessness at rest or with exertion, orthopnoea, exercise intolerance, early onset fatigue, abdominal pain, and pallor. Cachexia and peripheral oedema typically arise late in the course of the disease. Young children often have poor appetite and cachexia, similar to adults. Sinus tachycardia, gallop rhythm, jugular-venous distention, pallor, cool hands and feet, hepatomegaly, and a murmur that is consistent with mitral regurgitation are common findings at physical examination (Jefferies & Towbin, 2010; Luk et al., 2009). Additionally, peripheral oedema and ascites are late signs in children. DCM can occur in a number of X-linked diseases such as Becker's and Duchenne's muscular dystrophies. It may also occur in patients with mitochondrial DNA mutations and inherited metabolic disorders. Thus when taking a family history, specific attention should be given to a history of muscular dystrophy, features of mitochondrial disease (for example, familial diabetes, deafness, epilepsy, maternal inheritance), and signs and symptoms of other inherited metabolic diseases (Elliott, 2000)

About 20-48% of DCM have been reported as familial, although with incomplete and age-dependent penetrance, and linked to a diverse group of >20 loci and genes ((Taylor et al., 2006)). Although genetically heterogeneous, the predominant mode of inheritance for DCM is autosomal dominant, with X-linked autosomal recessive and mitochondrial inheritance less frequent. Several of the mutant genes linked to autosomal dominant DCM encode the same contractile sarcomeric proteins that are responsible for HCM, including α-cardiac actin; α-tropomyosin; cardiac troponin T, I, and C; β- and α-myosin heavy chain; and myosin binding protein C. Z-disc protein-encoding genes, including muscle LIM protein, α-actinin-2, ZASP, and titin, also have been identified.

DCM is also caused by a number of mutations in other genes encoding cytoskeletal/sarcolemmal, nuclear envelope, sarcomere, and transcriptional coactivator proteins. The most common of these probably is the lamin A/C gene, also associated with conduction system disease, which encodes a nuclear envelope intermediate filament protein. Mutations in this gene also cause Emery-Dreifuss muscular dystrophy. The X-linked gene responsible for Emery-Dreifuss muscular dystrophy, emerin (another nuclear lamin protein), also causes similar clinical features. Other DCM genes of this type include desmin, caveolin, and β- and α-sarcoglycan, as well as the mitochondrial respiratory chain gene. X-linked DCM is caused by the Duchenne muscular dystrophy (dystrophin) gene, whereas G4.5 (tafazzin), a mitochondrial protein of unknown function, causes Barth syndrome, which is an X-linked cardioskeletal myopathy in infants (Maron et al., 2006).

3.1.2.2 Restrictive cardiomyopathy

RCM is defined as heart-muscle disease that results in impaired ventricular filling, with normal or decreased diastolic volume of either or both ventricles. Systolic function usually remains normal, at least early in the disease, and wall thickness may be normal or increased, depending on the underlying cause (Kushwaha et al., 1997).

The exact prevalence of RCM is unknown but it is probably the least common type of cardiomyopathy. RCM may be idiopathic, familial, or result from various systemic disorders, in particular, amyloidosis, sarcoidosis, carcinoid heart disease, scleroderma and anthracycline toxicity. Familial RCM is often characterized by autosomal dominant inheritance, which in some families is caused by mutations in the troponin I gene; in others, familial RCM is associated with conduction defects, caused by mutations in the desmin gene (usually associated with skeletal myopathy) (Fitzpatrick et al., 1990). Rarely, familial disease can be associated with autosomal recessive inheritance (such as haemochromatosis caused by mutations in the HFE gene, or glycogen storage disease), or with X-linked inheritance (such as Anderson–Fabry disease) (Elliott et al., 2008).

RCM can also be caused by endocardial pathology (fibrosis, fibroelastosis, and thrombosis) that impairs diastolic function. These disorders can be sub-classified according to the presence of eosinophilia into endomyocardial diseases with hypereosinophilia (e.g., hypereosinophilic syndromes (HES)) and endomyocardial disease without hypereosinophilia (e.g., endomyocardial fibrosis (EMF)) (Fauci et al., 1982). Parasitic infections, drugs such as methysergide, and inflammatory and nutritional factors have been implicated in acquired forms of EMF. Fibrous endocardial lesions of the right and/or left ventricular inflow tract cause incompetence of the atrioventricular valves (Kushwaha et al., 1997). Isolated left ventricular involvement results in pulmonary congestion and predominant right ventricular involvement leads to right heart failure.

3.1.3 Acquired

3.1.3.1 Myocarditis (inflammatory cardiomyopathy)

Myocarditis is an acute or a chronic inflammatory process affecting the myocardium produced by a wide variety of toxins and drugs (e.g., cocaine, interleukin 2) or infectious agents, most commonly including viral (e.g., coxsackievirus, adenovirus, parvovirus, HIV), bacterial (e.g., diphtheria, meningococcus, psittacosis, streptococcus), rickettsial (e.g., typhus, Rocky Mountain spotted fever), fungal (e.g., aspergillosis, candidiasis), and parasitic (Chagas disease, toxoplasmosis), as well as Whipple disease (intestinal lipodystrophy), giant cell myocarditis, and hypersensitivity reactions to drugs such as antibiotics, sulfonamides, anticonvulsants, and anti-inflammatories. Endocardial fibroelastosis is a DCM in infants and children that is a consequence of viral myocarditis in utero (mumps) (Maron et al., 2006).

Myocarditis typically evolves through active, healing, and healed stages. It is characterized progressively by inflammatory cell infiltrates leading to interstitial edema and focal myocyte necrosis and ultimately replacement fibrosis (Calabrese & Thiene, 2003). These pathological processes create an electrically unstable substrate predisposing to the development of ventricular tachyarrhythmias. In some instances, an episode of viral myocarditis (frequently subclinical) can trigger an autoimmune reaction that causes immunologic damage to the myocardium or cytoskeletal disruption, culminating in DCM with LV dysfunction. Evidence for the evolution of myocarditis to DCM comes from several sources, including animal models, the finding of inflammatory infiltrates and persistence of viral RNA in endomyocardial biopsies from patients with DCM, and the natural history of patients with selected conditions such as Chagas disease. The list of agents responsible for inflammatory myocarditis overlaps with that of the infectious origin of DCM, thereby underscoring the potential interrelationship between the 2 conditions (Cooper, 2009).

Myocarditis can be diagnosed by established histopathological, histochemical, or molecular criteria, but it is challenging to identify clinically. Suspicion may be raised by chest pain, exertional dyspnea, fatigue, syncope, palpitations, ventricular tachyarrhythmias, and conduction abnormalities or by acute congestive heart failure or cardiogenic shock associated with LV dilatation and/or segmental wall motion abnormalities and ST-T changes on ECG. When myocarditis is suspected from the clinical profile, an endomyocardial biopsy may resolve an otherwise ambiguous situation by virtue of diagnostic inflammatory (leukocyte) infiltrate and necrosis (i.e., the Dallas criteria) but also is limited by insensitivity and false-negative histological results. The diagnostic yield of myocardial biopsies can be enhanced substantially by molecular analysis with DNA-RNA extraction and polymerase chain reaction amplification of the viral genome. In addition to the inflammatory process, viral genome encoded proteases appear to disrupt the cytoskeletal sarcomeric linkages of cardiomyocytes (Calabrese & Thiene, 2003; Parrillo, 2001).

3.1.3.2 Stress ("Tako-Tsubo") cardiomyopathy

Stress cardiomyopathy, first reported in Japan as "takotsubo," is a recently described clinical entity characterized by acute but rapidly reversible LV systolic dysfunction in the absence of atherosclerotic coronary artery disease, triggered by profound psychological stress (Sealove et al., 2008; Sharkey et al., 2005). This distinctive form of ventricular stunning typically affects older women and preferentially involves the distal portion of the LV chamber ("apical ballooning"), with the basal LV hypercontractile. Although presentation often mimics ST-segment–elevation myocardial infarction, outcome is favorable with appropriate medical therapy.

3.2 Secondary cardiomyopathies

The most important secondary cardiomyopathies are provided in the Table 1. This list, however, is not intended to represent an exhaustive and complete tabulation of the vast number of systemic conditions reported to involve the myocardium. Rather, it is limited to the most common of these diseases most consistently associated with a cardiomyopathy.

4. References

Aleong, R.G., Milan, D.J. & Ellinor, P.T. (2007). The diagnosis and treatment of cardiac ion channelopathies: congenital long QT syndrome and Brugada syndrome. *Current Treateatment Options in Cardiovascular Medicine*, Vol. 9, No. 5, (October 2007), pp. 364-371, ISSN 1092-8464

Antzelevitch, C., Brugada, P., Borggrefe, M., Brugada, J., Brugada, R., Corrado, D., Gussak, I., LeMarec, H., Nademanee, K., Perez Riera, A.R., Shimizu, W., Schulze-Bahr, E., Tan, H. & Wilde, A. (2005). Brugada syndrome: report of the second consensus conference: endorsed by the Heart Rhythm Society and the European Heart Rhythm Association. *Circulation*, Vol. 111, No. 5, (January 17, 2005), pp. 659-670, ISSN 0009-7322

Barry, S.P., Davidson, S.M. & Townsend, P.A. (2008). Molecular regulation of cardiac hypertrophy. *The International Journal of Biochemistry and Cell Biology*, Vol. 40, No. 10, (February 26, 2008), pp. 2023-2039, ISSN 1357-2725

Basso, C., Corrado, D., Marcus, F.I., Nava, A. & Thiene G. (2009). Arrhythmogenic right ventricular cardiomyopathy. *Lancet*, Vol. 373, No. 9671, (April 11, 2009), pp. 1289-1300 ISSN 0140-6736

Calabrese, F. & Thiene, G. (2003). Myocarditis and inflammatory cardiomyopathy: microbiological and molecular biological aspects. *Cardiovascular Research.*, Vol. 60, No. 1, (October 2003), pp. 11-25, ISSN 0008-6363

Chen, Q., Kirsch, G.E., Zhang, D., Brugada, R., Brugada, J., Brugada, P., Potenza, D., Moya, A., Borggrefe, M., Breithardt, G., Ortiz-Lopez, R., Wang, Z., Antzelevitch, C.,

O'Brien, R.E., Schulze-Bahr, E., Keating, M.T., Towbin, J.A. & Wang, Q. (1998). Genetic basis and molecular mechanism for idiopathic ventricular fibrillation. *Nature*, Vol. 392, No. 6673, (March 19, 1998), pp. 293-296, ISSN 0028-0836

Chin, T.K., Perloff, J.K., Williams, R.G., Jue, K. & Mohrmann, R. (1990). Isolated noncompaction of left ventricular myocardium. A study of eight cases. *Circulation*, Vol. 82, No. 2, (August 1990), pp. 507-513, ISSN 0009-7322

Cooper, L.T. Jr. (2009). Myocarditis. *The New England Journal of Medicine*, Vol. 360, No. 15, (April 9, 2009), pp. 1526-1538, ISSN 0028-4793

Elliott, P. (2000). Cardiomyopathy. Diagnosis and management of dilated cardiomyopathy. *Heart*, Vol. 84, No. 1, (July 2000), pp. 106-112, ISSN 1355-6037

Elliott, P., Andersson, B., Arbustini, E., Bilinska, Z., Cecchi, F., Charron, P., Dubourg, O., Kühl, U., Maisch, B., McKenna, W.J., Monserrat, L., Pankuweit, S., Rapezzi, C., Seferovic, P., Tavazzi, L. & Keren, A. (2008). Classification of the cardiomyopathies: a position statement from the European Society Of Cardiology Working Group on Myocardial and Pericardial Diseases. *European Heart Journal*, Vol. 29, No. 2, (January 2008), pp. 270-276, ISSN 0195-668x

Fauci, A.S., Harley, J.B., Roberts, W.C., Ferrans, V.J., Gralnick, H.R. & Bjornson, B.H. (1982). The idiopathic hypereosinophilic syndrome: clinical, pathophysiologic, and therapeutic considerations. *Annals of Internal Medicine*, Vol. 97, No. 1, (July 1982), pp. 78-92, ISSN 0003-4819

Fitzpatrick, A.P., Shapiro, L.M., Rickards, A.F. & Poole-Wilson, P.A. (1990). Familial restrictive cardiomyopathy with atrioventricular block and skeletal myopathy. *British Heart Journal*, Vol. 63, No. 2, (February 1990), pp. 114-118, ISSN 0007-0769

Freedom, R.M., Yoo, S.J., Perrin, D., Taylor, G., Petersen, S. & Anderson, R.H. (2005). The morphological spectrum of ventricular noncompaction. *Cardiology in the Young*, Vol. 15, No. 4, (August 2005), pp. 345-364, ISSN 1047-9511

Jefferies, J.L. & Towbin, J.A. (2010). Dilated cardiomyopathy. *Lancet*, Vol. 375, No. 9716, (Febuary 27, 2010), pp. 752-762, ISSN 0140-6736

Gaita, F., Giustetto, C., Bianchi, F., Wolpert, C., Schimpf, R., Riccardi, R., Grossi, S., Richiardi, E. & Borggrefe, M. (2003). Short QT Syndrome: a familial cause of sudden death. *Circulation*, Vol. 108, No. 8, (August 18, 2003), pp. 965-970, ISSN 0009-7322

Kass, R.S. (2005). The channelopathies: novel insights into molecular and genetic mechanisms of human disease. *The Journal of Clinical Investigation*, Vol. 115, No. 8, (August), pp. 1986-1989, ISSN 0021-9738

Krittayaphong, R., Veerakul, G., Nademanee, K. & Kangkagate, C. (2003). Heart rate variability in patients with Brugada syndrome in Thailand. *European Heart Journal*, Vol. 24, No. 19, (October 2003), pp. 1771-1778, ISSN 0195-668x

Kushwaha, S.S., Fallon, J.T. & Fuster, V. (1997). Restrictive cardiomyopathy. *The New England Journal of Medicine*, Vol. 336, No. 4, (January 23, 1997), pp. 267-276, ISSN 0028-4793

Lowey, S. (2002). Functional consequences of mutations in the myosin heavy chain at sites implicated in familial hypertrophic cardiomyopathy. *Trends in Cardiovascular Medicine*, Vol. 12, No., 8, (November 2002), pp. 348-354, ISSN 1050-1738

Marcus, F.I., McKenna, W.J., Sherrill, D., Basso, C., Bauce, B., Bluemke, D.A., Calkins, H., Corrado, D., Cox, M.G., Daubert, J.P., Fontaine, G., Gear, K., Hauer, R., Nava, A., Picard, M.H., Protonotarios, N., Saffitz, J.E., Sanborn, D.M., Steinberg, J.S., Tandri,

H., Thiene, G., Towbin, J.A., Tsatsopoulou, A., Wichter, T. & Zareba, W. (2010). Diagnosis of arrhythmogenic right ventricular cardiomyopathy/dysplasia: proposed modification of the task force criteria. *Circulation*, Vol. 121, No. 13, (February 19, 2010), pp. 1533-1541, ISSN 0009-7322

Maron, B.J. (2002). Cardiology patient pages. Hypertrophic cardiomyopathy. *Circulation*, Vol. 106, No. 19, (November 2002), pp. 2419-2421, ISSN 0009-7322

Maron, B.J. (2008). The 2006 American Heart Association classification of cardiomyopathies is the gold standard. *Circulation Heart Failure*, Vol. 1, No. 1, (May 2008), pp. 72 75, ISSN 1941-3289

Maron, B.J., Towbin, J.A., Thiene, G., Antzelevitch, C., Corrado, D., Arnett, D., Moss, A.J., Seidman, C.E. & Young, J.B. (2006). Contemporary definitions and classification of the cardiomyopathies: an American Heart Association Scientific Statement from the Council on Clinical Cardiology, Heart Failure and Transplantation Committee; Quality of Care and Outcomes Research and Functional Genomics and Translational Biology Interdisciplinary Working Groups; and Council on Epidemiology and Prevention. *Circulation*, Vol. 113, No. 14, (March 27, 2006), pp. 1807-1816. ISSN 0009-7322

Modell, S.M. & Lehmann, M.H. (2006).The long QT syndrome family of cardiac ion channelopathies: a HuGE review. *Genetics in Medicine*, Vol. 8, No. 3, (March 2006), pp. 143-155, ISSN 1098-3600

Monserrat Iglesias, L. (2008). Left ventricular noncompaction: a disease in search of a definition. *Revista Espanola de Cardiologia*, Vol. 61, No. 2, (February 2008), pp. 112-115, ISSN 0300-8932

Nava, A., Bauce, B., Basso, C., Muriago, M., Rampazzo, A., Villanova, C., Daliento, L., Buja, G., Corrado, D., Danieli, G.A. & Thiene, G. (2000). Clinical profile and long-term follow-up of 37 families with arrhythmogenic right ventricular cardiomyopathy. *Journal of the American College of Cardiology*, Vol. 36, No. 7, (December 2000), pp. 2226-2233, ISSN 0735-1097

Parrillo, J.E. (2001). Inflammatory cardiomyopathy (myocarditis): which patients should be treated with anti-inflammatory therapy? *Circulation*, Vol. 104, No. 1, (July 3, 2001), pp. 4-6, ISSN 0009-7322

Protonotarios, N., Anastasakis, A., Antoniades, L., Chlouverakis, G., Syrris, P., Basso, C., Asimaki, A., Theopistou, A., Stefanadis, C., Thiene, G., McKenna, W.J. & Tsatsopoulou, A. (2011). Arrhythmogenic right ventricular cardiomyopathy/dysplasia on the basis of the revised diagnostic criteria in affected families with desmosomal mutations. *European Heart Journal*, Vol. 32, No. 9, (Febuary 22, 2011), pp. 1097-1104, ISSN 0195-668x

Richardson, P., McKenna, W., Bristow, M., Maisch, B., Mautner, B., O'Connell, J., Olsen, E., Thiene, G. & Goodwin, J. (1996). Report of the 1995 World Health Organization/International Society and Federation of Cardiology Task Force on the Definition and Classification of Cardiomyopathies. *Circulation*, Vol. 93, No. 5, (March 1, 1996), pp. 841-842, ISSN 0009-7322

Rosamond, W., Flegal, K., Furie, K., Go, A., Greenlund, K., Haase, N., Hailpern, S.M., Ho, M., Howard, V., Kissela, B., Kittner, S., Lloyd-Jones, D., McDermott, M., Meigs, J., Moy, C., Nichol, G., O'Donnell, C., Roger, V., Sorlie, P., Steinberger, J., Thom, T., Wilson, M. & Hong, Y. (2008). Heart disease and stroke statistics-2008 update: a report from the American Heart Association Statistics Committee and Stroke Statistics Subcommittee. *Circulation*, Vol. 117, No. 4, (January 29, 2008), pp. e25-e146, ISSN0009-7322

Schimpf, R., Wolpert, C., Gaita, F., Giustetto, C. & Borggrefe, M. (2005). Short QT syndrome. *Cardiovascular Research*, Vol. 67, No. 3, (August 15, 2005). pp. 357-366, ISSN 0008-6363

Sealove, B.A., Tiyyagura, S. & Fuster, V. (2008). Takotsubo cardiomyopathy. *Journal of General Internal Medicine*, Vol. 23, No. 11, (August 2008), pp. 1904-1908, ISSN 0884-8734

Selvetella, G. & Lembo, G. (2005). Mechanisms of cardiac hypertrophy. *Heart Failure Clinics*, Vol. 1, No. 2, (July 2005), pp. 263-273, ISSN 1551-7136

Sharkey, S.W., Lesser, J.R., Zenovich, A.G., Maron, M.S., Lindberg, J., Longe, T.F. & Maron, B.J. (2005). Acute and reversible cardiomyopathy provoked by stress in women from the United States. *Circulation*, Vol. 111, No. 4, (Febuary 1, 2005), pp. 472-479, ISSN 0009-7322

Taylor, M.R., Carniel, E. & Mestroni, L. (2006). Cardiomyopathy, familial dilated. *Orphanet Journal of Rare Diseases*, Vol. 1, (July13, 2006), pp. 27, ISSN 1750-1172

Thiene, G., Angelini, A., Basso, C., Calabrese, F. & Valente, M. (2000). The new definition and classification of cardiomyopathies. *Advances in Clinical Pathology*, Vol. 4, No. 2, (April, 2000), pp. 53-57, ISSN 1125-5552

Thiene, G., Corrado, D. & Basso, C. (2004). Cardiomyopathies: is it time for a molecular classification? *European Heart Journal*, Vol. 25, No. 20, (October 2004), 1772-1775, ISSN 0195-668x

Towbin, J.A., Lowe, A.M., Colan, S.D., Sleeper, L.A., Orav, E.J., Clunie, S., Messere, J., Cox, G.F., Lurie, P.R., Hsu, D., Canter, C., Wilkinson, J.D. & Lipshultz, S.E. (2006). Incidence, causes, and outcomes of dilated cardiomyopathy in children. *The Journal of the American Medical Association*, Vol. 296, No. 15, (October 18, 2006), pp. 1867-1876, ISSN 0098-7484

Wilde, A.A., Bhuiyan, Z.A., Crotti, L., Facchini, M., De Ferrari, G.M., Paul, T., Ferrandi, C., Koolbergen, D.R., Odero, A. & Schwartz, P.J. (2008). Left cardiac sympathetic denervation for catecholaminergic polymorphic ventricular tachycardia. *The New England Journal of Medicine*, Vol. 358, No. 19, (May 8, 2008), pp. 2024-2029, ISSN 0028-4793

2

Management of Hypertrophic Obstructive Cardiomyopathy with a Focus on Alcohol Septal Ablation

Josef Veselka
Department of Cardiology, 2nd Medical School, Charles University, University Hospital Motol, Prague
Czech Republic

1. Introduction

Hypertrophic cardiomyopathy (HCM) is a complex cardiac disease with unique pathophysiological characteristics and a great diversity of morphological, functional, and clinical features. HCM is defined as primary myocardial hypertrophy in the absence of aortic valve disease or significant hypertension (Elliott, 2008)

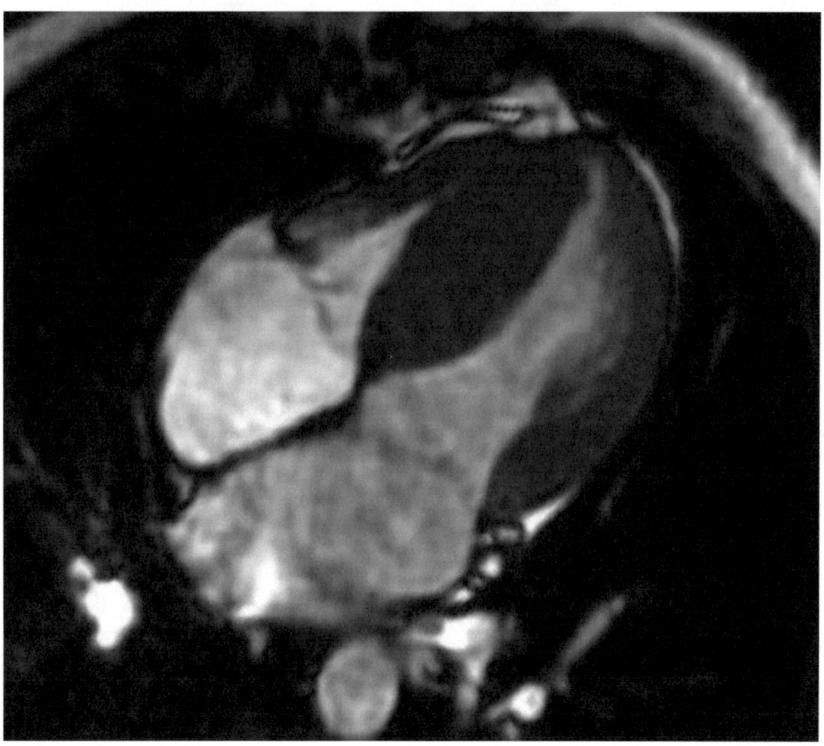

Fig. 1. Magnetic resonance imaging; hypertrophic left and right ventricle.

Several observations suggest that the prevalence of HCM is globally 1 in 500 (Maron, 1994). The condition therefore seems to be a common genetic malformation of the heart. The clinical course varies markedly. Some patients remain asymptomatic throughout their whole lives, some have severe symptomatology of heart failure or angina pectoris, while others die suddenly even in the absence of previous symptoms. The annual mortality rate varies in different studies. In unselected populations, it has been reported to be about 1% (Elliott, 2008). These observations suggest that a substantial proportion of patients with HCM has a more favourable course than previously believed. Two thirds of patients with HCM display evidence of obstruction in the left ventricular outflow tract (hypertrophic obstructive cardiomyopathy, HOCM), that is negatively associated with prognosis of the patients.

During the last decade, technological developments in non-surgical treatment have provided new therapeutic options for patients with this disease. Recent changes have also generated considerable questions about the optimal management of HOCM and the role of percutaneous alcohol septal ablation (ASA) (Veselka, 2007).

With respect to various clinical courses, it seems to be impossible to define precise guidelines for management. As in many diseases, it is often necessary to individualise therapy.

2. Drug therapy of patients with hypertrophic obstructive cardiomyopathy

Drug therapy is used as the initial measure for controlling cardiac symptoms that has resulted in functional limitation. Beta-blockers and verapamil have traditionally been administered on an empirical basis, relying on the patient´s subjective perception of benefit. Drug selection is based on preferences of individual physicians. Most favour beta-blockers over verapamil for use in initial treatment, although it is not of critical importance which drug is used first.

There is no evidence that beta-blockers or verapamil protect patients with HOCM from sudden death. On the other hand, they are able to relieve symptoms in the majority of patients. Whether these drugs should be used prophylactically to delay disease progression and improve prognosis in asymptomatic patients has been a subject of debate for many years. The effectiveness of a prophylactic treatment has not been tested prospectively because study populations are small and traditional endpoints are infrequent (death, clinical deterioration). Accordingly, we reserve medical therapy only for symptomatic patients.

3. Surgery to relieve the left ventricular obstruction

The group of patients who have both a large outflow gradient and severe symptoms and also do not respond to medical treatment are the best candidates for surgery. Based on outstanding experience of several surgical centres worldwide, myectomy has become the primary therapeutic option for patients with severe symptoms and marked functional disability (McCully, 1996). Surgical reduction of the outflow gradient is achieved by removing a small amount of muscle (5 to 10 g) from the basal septum. Recently, some surgeons have performed more extended myectomies and reconstruction of the subvalvular mitral apparatus. In these cases, the septal myectomy deeply extends into the left ventricular cavity. Subsequently, both papillary muscles are mobilised and all hypertrophied muscular trabeculae are also resected. Mitral valve replacement has also been used as an alternative therapy in selected patients, but the role of this operation remains unsettled.

Surgery substantially reduces the basal outflow gradient in more than 90% of patients and provides large improvements in objective measures of symptoms and functional status.

However, the procedure requires extracorporeal circulation and great surgical experience. Mortality rates less than 2% are achieved only in heart centres with extensive surgical experience and numerous performed procedures. The effect of surgery on survival is not known. Accordingly, surgery is not performed in asymptomatic or mildly symptomatic patients.

4. Cardiac pacing to relieve the left ventricular obstruction

The role of cardiac pacing in reducing the left ventricular outflow gradient in HOCM was first reported more than 40 years ago (Gilgenkrantz, 1968). At the same time, it had been noticed that patients who developed left bundle branch block after septal myectomy had a better functional outcome. Sporadic reports over the years have culminated in the interest of cardiac pacing in the 1990s´.

In the early 1990s, several observational studies reported that dual-chamber pacing with shortened A-V delay was associated with both substantial decrease in the outflow gradient and symptomatic improvement of patients unresponsive to drug treatment. However, the mechanisms by which pacing might reduce outflow gradient was not understood. Later, three more carefully controlled and randomised studies found the effects of cardiac pacing to be less favourable (Linde, 1999; Maron, 1999; Nishimura, 1997). These studies were randomised, double-blind and crossover. Subjective symptomatic improvement was reported with similar frequency by patients after three months pacing and after the same period without pacing. Objective measurements of exercise capacity (for example maximal oxygen consumption) with and without pacing did not differ significantly. These findings suggested that a placebo effect might play an important role in the symptomatic improvement reported by the paced patients. Currently, cardiac pacing cannot be regarded as a primary treatment for patients with HOCM, although a modest reduction in outflow gradient is achieved in a number of paced patients. Probably a small subset of patients could profit from pacing, but this effect is inconsistent and usually only modest. Therefore, further randomized, controlled trials should be undertaken to resolve the uncertainties surrounding the utility and efficacy of cardiac pacing in patients with HOCM.

5. Alcohol septal ablation to relieve the left ventricular obstruction

The idea of inducing a septal infarction by catheter techniques was suggested by the observation that myocardial function of selected areas of the left ventricle can be suppressed by balloon occlusion of the supplying artery during angioplasty. The outflow pressure gradient in HOCM decreased significantly when the first septal artery was temporarily occluded by an angioplasty balloon catheter (Sigwart, 1982). This concept was also supported by observations that the outflow pressure gradient decreased after anterior myocardial infarction in HOCM patients.

Sigwart published his experience with "non-surgical myocardial reduction" of three patients with HOCM in 1995 (Sigwart, 1995). However, at the same time, other centres in Germany also started with the same interventional procedure (Kuhn, 2010). Since then, several modifications of the original technique have been described. The majority of authors prefer an echocardiography-guided anatomical approach for identifying the target septal branch (Veselka, 2007), where the target septal branch is detected using myocardial contrast echocardiography (MCE). Estimation of the size of the septal vascular territory with MCE is accurate and safe. Using MCE, it is possible to delineate the perfusion bed of the septal perforators and predict the infarct size that follows the alcohol injection.

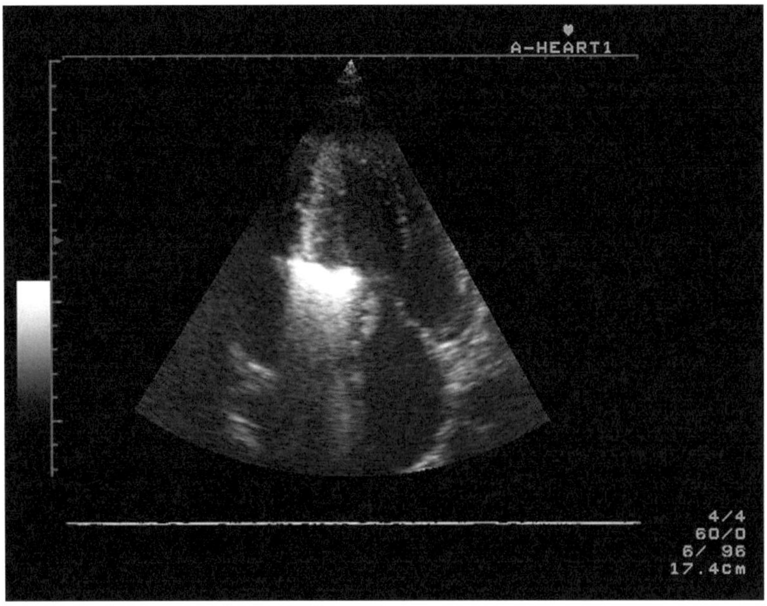

Fig. 2. Transthoracic echocardiography, apical 4-chamber view with optimal opacification of the basal interventricular septum by echocontrast medium.

Recently, we have proposed the use of real-time myocardial contrast echocardiography with very low mechanical index that allows better delineation of the target area than conventional contrast echocardiography (Veselka, 2009).

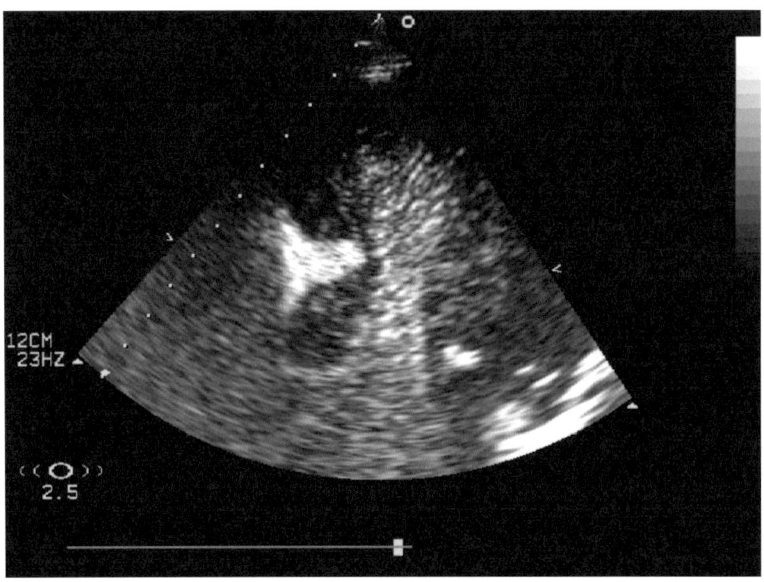

Fig. 3. Transthoracic echocardiography, apical 4-chamber view with real time myocardial contrast echocardiography utilizing power modulation and intracoronary injection of small amount of echocontrast agent.

There is a significant correlation between MCE septal area and reduction of ouflow gradient. In general, a higher biomarker level (extent of necrosis) was detected with larger sections of the infarcted septum. However, since alcohol injection is directed mainly to the portion of the septum causing the obstruction, many patients have a small defect with a large reduction of outflow gradient. Additionally, it has been found that MCE in 5 to 10% of cases shows contrast within myocardium away from the septal target area, indicating threatening misplacement of the myocardial necrosis. Accordingly, necrotisation of myocardium distant from the septal target area as a source of potentially fatal complications can be avoided by this approach. The introduction of echocardiographic guidance of ASA led to an improvement in haemodynamic results, despite a decrease in the infarcted septal area estimated by the maximal creatine kinase rise.

5.1 Indication

Accepted patient selection criteria for ASA were as follows: (1) anatomical findings of marked septal hypertrophy that projects from the LVOT; (2) dynamic obstruction of LVOT; (3) unresponsiveness to the medical therapy. There were no sufficient data available to confirm exact haemodynamic (pressure gradient > 50 mmHg), anatomical (septum thickness > 18 mm) or clinical (dyspnoea with NYHA class III or IV) criteria that resulted in a certain relaxation of indications in clinical practice. Patients with moderate symptoms were treated if they had high gradients and additional findings, such as recurrent exercise-induced syncope, markedly abnormal blood pressure response at exercise, paroxysmal atrial fibrillation or extremely high pressure gradient after provocative manoeuvres (Valsalva manoeuvre or use of nitrates). It is a very important question in clinical practice whether the increased risk of sudden cardiac death associated with LVOT obstruction justifies the use of ASA in slightly symptomatic or completely asymptomatic patients. At present, there are no sufficient data to answer this question. However, a relatively low risk of sudden death in asymptomatic patients with obstruction and none of the recognised risk factors for sudden death (1.ventricular tachycardia, 2. abnormal exercise blood pressure response, 3. family history of premature death, 4. unexplained syncope, 5. severe left ventricular hypertrophy in any myocardial segment > 30 mm) suggests that aggressive interventions are unjustified in this group. The situation in asymptomatic patients with obstruction and additional risk factors is less clear. The approach must be individualised. It seems to be reasonable to implant an AV-sequential implantable cardioverter-defibrillator (ICD) to try atrio-ventricular sequential pacing to reduce obstruction for 6 months, and then to perform ASA if needed. Nevertheless, ASA as the primary treatment is still unjustified in this group of patients, given potential mortality and morbidity associated with this procedure. Patient preference should, of course, be considered in such discussion and surgical myectomy should be mentioned as the gold standard in most western countries.

5.2 Alcohol septal ablation procedure

We usually recommend the following course of ASA procedure. A temporary pacemaker is placed in the apex of the right ventricle in everyone except patients who already have a permanent dual-chamber pacemaker in place. However, fluctuation of the pacing threshold has to be anticipated if the lead is directed towards the septum, i.e., with the tip in proximity to the ablation lesion. A multipurpose catheter is advanced through the aortic valve into the apex of the left ventricle and intraventricular gradient is measured by a pull-back technique. A 6 or 7F guiding catheter is then engaged into the ostium of the left coronary artery. Initial angiography is performed to localise the origin of septal arteries. Over-the-wire balloon catheter is introduced over a coronary wire into one of the major and proximal septal perforators and inflated. Contrast medium is injected through the central balloon lumen to delineate the area supplied by the septal branch and to ensure that balloon inflation prevents spillage into the left anterior descending artery. Contrast myocardial echocardiography is performed to delineate the area to be infarcted (Figures 1 and 2) and to exclude contrast (and subsequently alcohol) deposition in remote myocardial regions like the left ventricular posterior wall or papillary muscles. The optimal septal branch is identified by opacification of the area in the basal septum that is adjacent to the zone of maximal acceleration of the outflow jet and includes the point of coaptation between the septum and anterior mitral leaflet. Usually, the target septal branch originates from the proximal segment of the left anterior descending artery. However, in exceptional cases, it originates from diagonal or intermediate branches of the left coronary artery. Depending on the septal artery size and septal thickness, 1 to 2 ml of absolute ethanol are very slowly (2 to 3 minutes) instilled through the lumen of the inflated balloon catheter and left in place for 5 minutes. After balloon deflation and removal, angiography is done to confirm the patency of the left anterior descending artery and occlusion of the target septal branch. Measurement of intraventricular gradient is usually performed by a multipurpose catheter and guiding catheter and/or Doppler echocardiography. The gradient should decrease at least to one half.

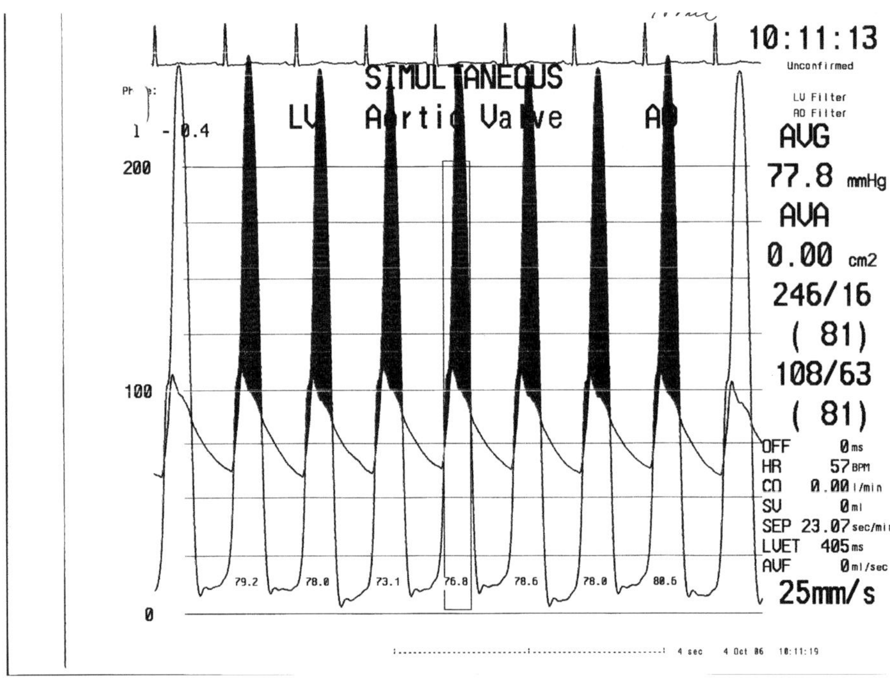

Fig. 4. Pressure gradient between left ventricle and aorta before ASA.

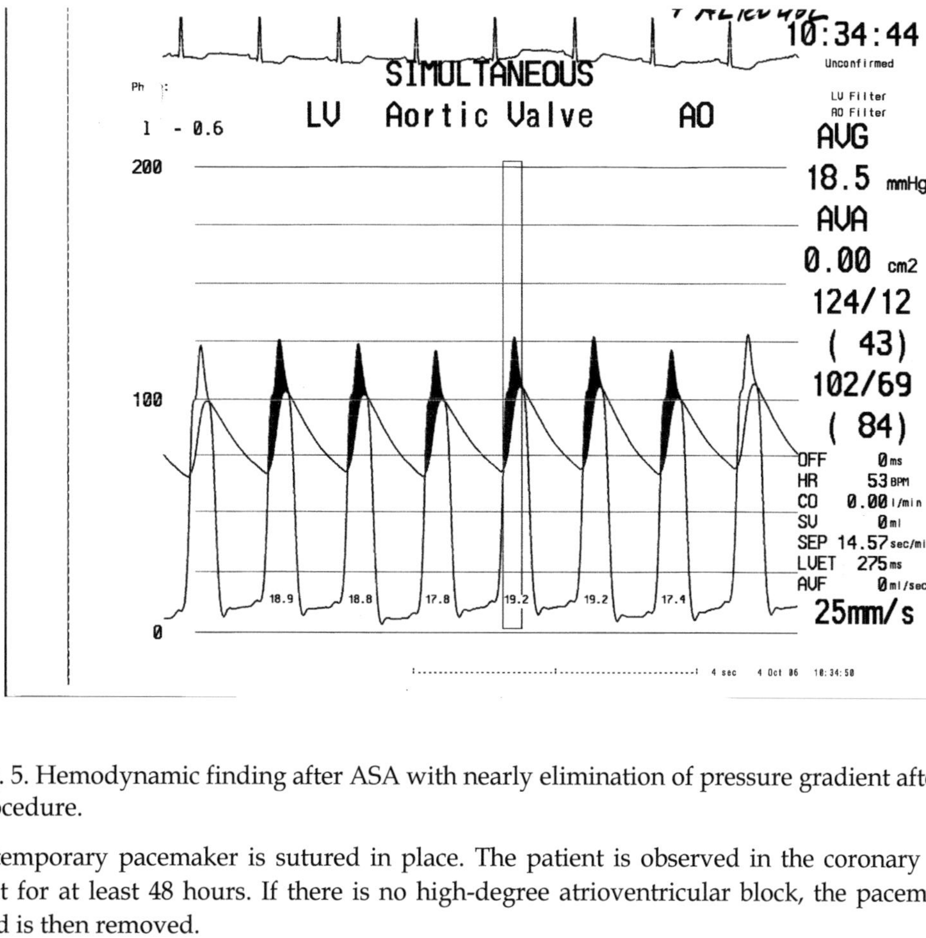

Fig. 5. Hemodynamic finding after ASA with nearly elimination of pressure gradient after procedure.

A temporary pacemaker is sutured in place. The patient is observed in the coronary care unit for at least 48 hours. If there is no high-degree atrioventricular block, the pacemaker lead is then removed.

5.3 Complications

In-hospital death, the most significant complication of ASA, is rare. Nevertheless, it ranges in the literature from 1 to 4%. However, some observations suggest that in skilled hands, the mortality rate is close to zero.

Historically, the incidence of complete heart block following ASA has ranged from 0 to 40% with a mean value of 8 to 18% (Veselka, 2007). However, the original technique of ASA has undergone several modifications and lower occurrence of post-procedural complete heart block has been reported (Veselka, 2010). The most important trend in the continuously developing ASA technique involves the lowering of the alcohol dose (1 to 2 ml) injected in very small fractions (0.1 to 0.3 ml) (Veselka, 2005). Subsequent small infarctions are sufficient in reducing obstruction to a similar extent as larger infarctions induced by a higher dose of alcohol. Moreover, it seems to be likely that a low dose of alcohol is associated with lower incidence of major post-procedural conduction disturbances and improved prognosis (Kuhn, 2008).

The selection of appropriate patients for this procedure appears to be as important as the procedural ASA technique itself. Only highly symptomatic patients without the left bundle branch block should be treated by ASA because of high incidence of right bundle branch block following ASA. Unfortunately, the resulting complete heart block can occur with no previous symptoms within hours or days after the procedure. Therefore, based on our clinical experience, patients after uncomplicated ASA should be observed in the coronary care unit for at least 2 or 3 days and consequent telemetric monitoring should be considered for at least 1 week.

To improve the risk stratification of complete heart block occurrence, Faber et al. proposed a scoring system based on baseline ECG, heart rate profile, severity of obstruction, peri-interventional enzyme kinetics, and peri-interventional conduction problems that might discriminate patients with a high risk for permanent pacemaker dependency from those with a stable atrioventricular conduction after ASA (Faber, 2007).

Sustained ventricular tachycardia has been rarely reported following ASA and only few reports have described it as an early post-procedural complication (Veselka, 2010). There is the hypothesis that the early post-procedural period can be compared to the same period after acute myocardial infarction, and the development of sustained ventricular arrhythmias after the ASA is not as rare as was thought before. It seems to be likely that a lower dose of alcohol with the minimising of the resulting necrosis (scar) is unable to entirely eliminate either occurrence of ventricular arrhythmias that are dependent on disorganised cellular architecture of myocardium or serious conduction abnormalities.

Still, some uncertainty persists regarding the ICD indication for the prevention of sudden death in patients with post-procedural sustained ventricular arrhythmias, and no data are available regarding their predictive power. Nevertheless, based on both our clinical experience (and lack of scientific evidence), we do not consider early post-procedural ventricular arrhythmias to be a sufficient justification per se for an ICD implantation.

A serious complication of ASA is a leakage of ethanol from the target septal branch into the left anterior descending artery. This potentially fatal complication is avoided by the use of a slightly over-sized angioplasty balloon catheter and a very careful septal branch angiography that precedes alcohol ablation. Additionally, the slow administration of alcohol per fractions and septal branch occlusion for 5 minutes after the last alcohol injection ensure the safe course of the procedure.

Theoretically, the potential risk of ventricular septal rupture following ASA should be considered. Surprisingly, this serious complication is probably very rare, although it is possible that it is underreported in the literature.

5.4 Results

ASA has not been subjected to many randomised clinical trials. However, observational data from European and US centres over a 16-year follow-up are consistent, attributing a number of favourable effects to ASA that generally parallel that of surgery, including gradual and progressive reduction in outflow gradient over 3 to 12 months and alleviation of symptoms.

The most important finding after ASA is an impressive symptomatic improvement during both short- and long-term follow-up that is consistently reported by all groups dealing with

ASA. The mean functional class improved very significantly from NYHA 2.5-3 to 1.2-1.6. Similarly, objective measurements showed an increase in exercise capacity and peak oxygen consumption.

During ASA, an acute LVOT gradient reduction is followed by a significant LVOT gradient increase during the early post-procedural period and a continuous LVOT gradient decrease during the follow-up. The rapid post-procedural LVOT gradient decrease is probably associated mainly with stunning, myocardial necrosis and the change in the left ventricular ejection dynamics. The later pressure gradient decrease is caused by scarring and thinning of the basal septum, resulting in left ventricular remodelling (Veselka, 2004).

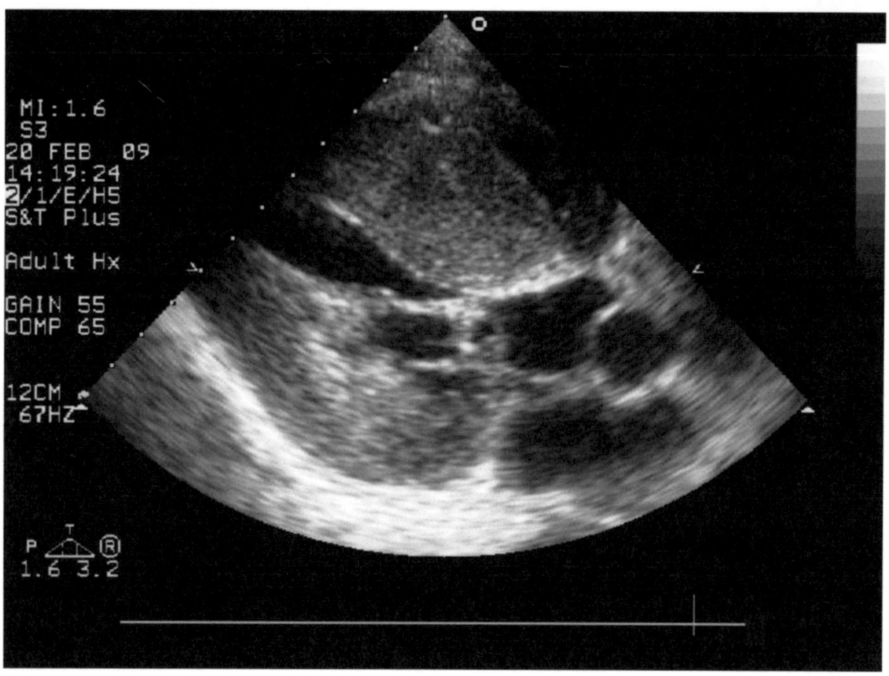

Fig. 6. Transthoracic echocardiography, parasternal long axis view with impressive finding of subaortic obstruction.

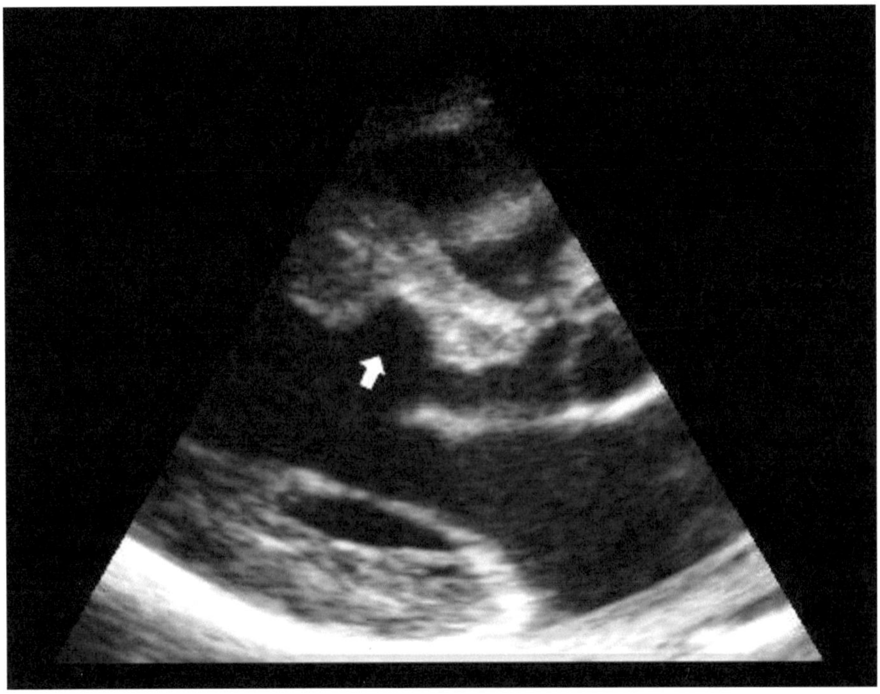

Fig. 7. Transthoracic echocardiography, parasternal long axis view with thinning of the basal interventricular septum (arrow) three months following ASA.

This haemodynamic course characterised by "down-up-down" changes in pressure gradient occurs in the majority of patients and is called the "biphasic" response. In most trials, the resting LVOT pressure gradient is reduced from 60 to 70 mmHg at baseline to 10 to 20 mmHg at mid- or long-term follow-up.

6. Conclusion

At present, there is not a single therapy that should be applied to all patients with severely symptomatic HOCM unresponsive to medical management. There are benefits and disadvantages of both surgical myectomy and ASA. Septal myectomy requires specialised tertiary referral centres and is a more complex procedure than ASA. Furthermore, there is no cardio-thoracic surgical centre in our country that would be able to perform this procedure routinely. On the other hand, there are no sufficient data concerning the long-term follow-up of patients after ASA.

Further investigation is required to be able to identify the best responders for cardiac pacing, ASA and surgical myectomy and compare the results for the available methods. Mainly, a randomised study comparing myectomy and ASA would be needed. However, low incidence of end points would require extremely high number of participants and, therefore, such a study will probably not be performed.

Currently, a decision concerning the best therapy of patients with HOCM must be individualised to each patient depending on their wishes and expectations, way of life, age and haemodynamics. Centres of excellence are able to perform both ASA and myectomy very safely and effectively. Therefore, choice of the final therapy should be tailored for the individual patient treated in a particular centre.

7. References

Elliott P, Anderson B, Arbustini E, et al. *Classification of the cardiomyopathies: a position statement from the European Society of Cardiology working group on myocardial and pericardial diseases*. Eur Heart J 2008;29:270–6.

Faber L, Welge D, Fassbender D, Schmidt HK, Horstkotte D, Seggewiss H. *One-year follow-up of percutaneous septal ablation for symptomatic hypertrophic obstructive cardiomyopathy in 312 patients: predictors of hemodynamic and clinical response.* Clin Res Cardiol 2007;96:864-873.

Gilgenkrantz J, Cherrier F, Petitier H, Dodinot B, Houplon M, Legoux J. *Cardiomyopathie obstructive du ventricle gauche avec block auriculo-ventriculaire complet. Considerations therapeutiques*. Arch Mal Coeur 1968;61:439-53.

Kuhn H, Lawrenz T, Lieder F, Leuner C, Strunk-Mueller C, Obergassel L, Bartelsmeier M, Stellbrink C. *Survival after transcoronary ablation of septal hypertrophy in hypertrophic obstructive cardiomyopathy (TASH): a 10year experience*. Clin Res Cardiol 2008;97:243-34.

Kuhn HJ. *The history of alcohol septal ablation*. Cardiovasc Revasc Med 2010;11:260-261.

Linde C, Gadler F, Kappenberger L, et al. *Placebo effect of pacemaker implantation in obstructive hypertrophic cardiomyopathy*. Am J Cardiol 1999;83:903-7.

Maron BJ, Gardin JM, Flack JM, Kurosaki TT, Bild TE. *Prevalence of hypertrophic cardiomyopathy in general population of young adults: echocardiographic analysis of 4111 subjects in the CARDIA study*. Circulation 1995;92:785-9.

Maron BJ, Nishimura RA, McKenna WJ, et al. *Assessment of permanent dual-chamber pacing as a treatment for drug-refractory symptomatic patients with obstructive hypertrophic cardiomyopathy. A randomized, double-blind, crossover study (M-PATHY)*. Circulation 1999;99:2927-2933.

McCully RB, Nishimura RA, Tajik AJ, et al. *Extent of clinical improvement after surgical treatment of hypertrophic obstructive cardiomyopathy*. Circulation 1996;94:467-71.

Nishimura RA, Trusty J, Hayes DL, et al. *Dual-chamber pacing for hypertrophic cardiomyopathy: a randomised, double-blind, crossover trial*. J Am Coll Cardiol 1997;435-441.

Sigwart U, Grbie M, Essinger A, Rivier JL. *L´effet aigu d´une occlusion coronarienne par ballonet de la dilatation transluminale*. Schweiz Med Wochenschr 1982;45:1631.

Sigwart U. *Non-surgical myocardial reduction of hypertrophic obstructive cardiomyopathy*. Lancet 1995;346:211-4.

Veselka J, Duchoňová R, Procházková Š, Homolová I, Páleníčková J, Zemánek D, Pernišová Z, Tesař D. *The biphasic course of changes of left ventricular outflow gradient after alcohol septal ablation for hypertrophic obstructive cardiomyopathy*. Kardiol Pol 2004;60:133-5.

Veselka J, Duchoňová R, Procházková Š, Páleníčková J, Sorajja P, Tesař D. *Effects of varying ethanol dosing in percutaneous septal ablation for obstructive hypertrophic cardiomyopathy on early hemodynamic ganges*. Am J Cardiol 2005;95:675-8.

Veselka J. *Alcohol septal ablation for hypertrophic obstructive cardiomyopathy: a review of the literature*. Med Sci Monit 2007;13:RA62-8.

Veselka J, Zemánek D, Fiedler J, Šváb P. *Real-time myocardial contrast echocardiography for echo-guided alcohol septal ablation*. Arch Med Sci 2009;5:271-272.

Veselka J, Zemánek D, Tomašov P, Homolová S, Adlová R, Tesař D. *Complications of low-dose echo-guided alcohol septal ablation*. Catheter Cardiovasc Interv 2010;75:546-550.

3

Hypertrophic Cardiomyopathy in Infants and Children

Luis E. Alday and Eduardo Moreyra
Divisions of Cardiology, Hospital Aeronáutico and Sanatorio Allende, Córdoba Argentina

1. Introduction

The definition and classification of the cardiomyopathies has been traditionally a complex and quite variable subject. In 2006, the American Heart Association issued a scientific statement elaborated by a task force of experts that contemplated the important development of molecular genetics in recent years, to explain the etiology of the diseases of cardiac muscle, or cardiomyopathies, previously considered idiopathic (B.J. Maron et al., 2006a). The document stated that "Cardiomyopathies are an heterogeneous group of myocardial diseases associated with mechanical and/or electrical dysfunction that usually, but not always, exhibit inappropriate ventricular hypertrophy or dilation, and are originated by a variety of causes, frequently genetic. Cardiomyopathies involve just the heart or are part of systemic disorders that often lead to cardiovascular death or heart failure related disability". Myocardial damage secondary to coronary atherosclerosis, heart valve disease, congenital heart disease, and systemic hypertension, is excluded from this definition. Primary or metastatic cardiac tumors and diseases primarily affecting the endocardium with minimal or absent myocardial damage neither are included. The document also discourages the use of the classical terminologies hypertrophic, dilated, and restrictive cardiomyopathies because they have overlapping features and often mutate from one type to another during the course of the disease. Cardiomyopathies are then classified into 2 groups, *primary* when there is only heart involvement, and *secondary* if the heart is affected by systemic diseases with multiorganic involvement. (Table 1) *Primary cardiomyopathies* are divided into *genetic, acquired,* and *mixed* (genetic and acquired).

GENETIC	MIXED	ACQUIRED
Hypertrophic	Dilated	Inflammatory
Arrhythmogenic Right Ventricular	Restrictive	Tako-tsubo
Noncompaction		Peripartum
Glycogen Storage		Tachycardia-induced
Mitochondrial		Infants of diabetic mothers
Conduction Defects		
Ion Channelopathies		

Table 1. Classification of the primary cardiomyopathies (modified from B.J. Maron, et al., 2006a).

A salient feature of this classification is the inclusion of *ion channelopathies* caused by gene coding mutations of Na, K, and Ca channels. These channelopathies may result in deadly ventricular arrhythmias and can only be identified by molecular genetic studies since no structural cardiac damage is objectified. The Brugada syndrome, the long and short QT syndromes, the cathecolaminergic polymorphic ventricular tachycardia, and the unexplained nocturnal sudden death in Southeastern Asian youngsters belong to the channelopathies. Some conduction disorders are also included in the classification.

In contrast with the American Heart Association point of view, the European Society of Cardiology issued a report in the year 2008 with an updated definition and classification of the cardiomyopathies (Elliot et al., 2008). (Table 2) It was there stated that "Cardiomyopathies are structural and functional myocardial diseases in the absence of systemic hypertension, coronary atherosclerosis, valvulopathies, or congenital heart disease sufficient to explain the observed abnormality". Therefore, *hypertrophic cardiomyopathy* was defined as "Increased ventricular thickness or mass in the absence of loading conditions sufficient to cause the observed abnormality". This definition better reflects the terminology used in pediatrics (Elliot et al., 2008; Franklin et al., 1999). With regard to the classification, it was based on the identification of phenotypes according to their structural and functional features recognizing the following cardiomyopathies: *hypertrophic, dilated, restrictive, arrhythmogenic right ventricular, and unclassified* (Colan et al., 2007). Every phenotype could be *familial* or *non-familial* emphasizing the role of genetics in some cardiomyopathies and orienting the etiologic diagnosis. The differentiation between primary and secondary cardiomyopathy is then abandoned. *Left ventricular non-compaction* and the *takotsubo cardiomyopathy* are included in the group of unclassified cardiomyopathies. The European Society of Cardiology experts do not believe that *channelopathies* and *conduction disorders* should be considered as cardiomyopathies. In our opinion, the European Society of Cardiology classification is more user-friendly for general physicians.

CARDIOMYOPATHIES				
HCM	DCM	ARVC	RCM	Unclassified

FAMILIAL/	GENETIC	NON-FAMILIAL/	NON-GENETIC
Unidentified gene defect	Disease sub-type	Idiopathic	Disease sub-type

HCM: hypertrophic cardiomyopathy, DCM: dilated cardiomyopathy, ARVC: arrhythmogenic right ventricular cardiomyopathy, RCM: restrictive cardiomyopathy.

Table 2. European Society of Cardiology classification of primary cardiomyopathies (modified from Elliot, et al., 2008).

2. Classification

Though hypertrophic cardiomyopathy was first recognized by Liouville in France in 1869, (Liouville, 1869, as cited in Marian, 2007), it was not until the 1950's that was rediscovered in Britain by Brock and Teare (Brock & Fleming, 1956; Teare, 1958). Initial reports emphasized the presence of left ventricular outflow tract obstruction until it was realized that this could be absent (B. J. Maron et al, 2009). Since then, two main types of hypertrophic cardiomyopathy were distinguished, with or without obstruction. Nowadays, we know that hypertrophic cardiomyopathy, is the most frequent monogenic disorder in cardiology and the commonest cause of sudden death in youngsters in either form of presentation (J. Seidman & C. Seidman, 2001).

Regardless of the presence or absence of obstruction, hypertrophic cardiomyopathy is classified into two main groups, *familial* and *non-familial.* (Table 3) The latter comprises 4 subgroups: hypertrophic cardiomyopathy associated with *obesity, infants born to diabetic mothers, athlete's heart,* and *amyloidosis.* This chapter will mainly address the *familial forms* of hypertrophic cardiomyopathy also composed of 4 subgroups: *sarcomeric,* and 3 others in association with *malformation syndromes, inborn errors of metabolism,* and *neuromuscular disorders* (Elliot et al., 2008). The sarcomeric forms are the most frequent and have an autosomal dominant inheritance. They are caused by missence mutations of genes encoding the contractile proteins of the sarcomere. A mutation involves the change of a DNA base for another resulting in the replacement of an aminoacid in a polypeptide for another. Though readable, the meaning (sense) of the genetic message is changed. Considerable genetic and phenotypic heterogeneity is found in hypertrophic cardiomyopathy. In other words, different gene mutations may cause similar phenotypes or on the contrary, the same gene may result in dissimilar ones. The presence of modifying genes, like that encoding angiotensin II, environmental influences, gender, and associated conditions might explain some of these dissimilarities (Alcalai et al., 2008). About 20 genes carrying a great number of mutations have already been identified in hypertrophic cardiomyopathy (Kim et al., 2011). (Table 4) However, just 3 of them, beta-myosin heavy chain (*MYH7*), myosin binding protein C (*MYBPC3*), and troponin T (*TNNT2*) are responsible for almost 75% of the cases, thence, the remaining are rare. The genes involved in pediatric hypertrophic cardiomyopathy have a similar frequency and distribution as in adult patients (Kaski et al., 2009).

FAMILIAL	NON-FAMILIAL.
Sarcomeric	Associated with obesity
Associated with malformation syndromes	Infants born to diabetic mothers
Associated with inborn errors of metabolism	Athlete's heart
Associated with neuromuscular disorders	Amyloidosis

Table 3. Classification of the hypertrophic cardiomyopathies (modified from Elliot et al., 2008).

It has been suggested that the genotype might have an influence in the prognosis in hypertrophic cardiomyopathy. Patients with *MYH7* mutation would have more severe ventricular hypertrophy and present earlier in life, those with *TNNT2* would have less left ventricular hypertrophy but higher risk of sudden death, and late onset of the disease and favorable prognosis would be found in patients with *MYBPC3* mutation (Moolman et al., 1997; Niimura et al., 1998; Watkins et al., 1992). Nevertheless, a more recent study showed that regardless of the gene mutation, patients with a positive molecular genetic study, had a higher risk of cardiovascular death, stroke, worse functional class, diastolic and systolic left ventricular dysfunction, and that the long term outcome was worse for patients carrying more than one mutation. (Bos et al., 2009) The latter finding was not corroborated in children. (Kaski et al., 2009).

GENE	PROTEINS	GENE	PROTEINS
MYH7	β-Myosin heavy chain	**TTN**	Titin
MYH6	α-Myosin heavy chain	**LBD3**	LIM binding domain 3
MYBPC3	Cardiac myosin binding protein C	**CSRP3**	Muscle LIM protein
TNNT2	Cardiac troponin T	**TCAP**	Telethonin
TNNI3	Cardiac troponin I	**VCL**	Vinculin/metavinculin
TNNC1	Cardiac troponin C	**ACTN2**	α-Actinin 2
TPM1	α-Tropomyosin	**MYOZ2**	Myozenin 2
MYL3	Myosin essential light chain	**JPH2**	Junctophillin-2
MYL2	Myosin regulatory light chain	**PLN**	Phospholamban
ACTC	α-Cardiac actin		

Table 4. Susceptibility genes in hypertrophic cardiomyopathy (modified from Bos et al., 2009 & Kim et al., 2011).

3. Prevalence

The estimated prevalence of hypertrophic cardiomyopathy in the adult population as assessed by echocardiographic screening is 1:500 (B.J. Maron et al., 1995a). However, in pediatrics, the observed prevalence is much lower because hypertrophic cardiomyopathy usually has late gene expression. Large population registries from Australia and the US show a prevalence varying between 0.47 and 1.24:100,000 inhabitants and an occurrence of nearly 25% among all types of cardiomyopathies (Lipschultz et al., 2003; Nugent et al., 2003). In our institution, the incidence of hypertrophic cardiomyopathy was 1.1% for all children with heart disease attending the Division of Cardiology of the Children's Hospital (Bruno et al., 2002).

4. Pathology

4.1 Macroscopic findings

The gross anatomy generally shows severe left ventricular hypertrophy and small cavity size. (Fig. 1) The hypertrophy mainly involves the ventricular septum, and for this reason, one of the early denominations of the disease was *asymmetric septal hypertrophy* (Henry et al., 1973). Notwithstanding, hypertrophy may occur symmetrically or affect other segments like the posterior wall, and the apical or middle sections of the left ventricle (Falicov & Resnekov, 1977; Louie & Maron, 1987; Minami et al., 2011; Yamaguchi et al., 1979). Midventricular obstructive hypertrophic cardiomyopathy is more frequent in Asians with a prevalence of around 10% in tertiary centers and carries a higher risk for adverse events (B.J. Maron et al., 2003a; Minami et al., 2011). Patients with apical involvement are less commonly genotype positive than those with the more frequent variants of the disease but the affected genes are usually the same frequently found in the other patients (*MYBPC3 and MYH7*) (Gruner et al., 2011). In infants and children, the right ventricle can also be involved (Biagini et al., 2005).Almost 5% of patients with hypertrophic cardiomyopathy evolve to end stage dilated cardiomyopathy with

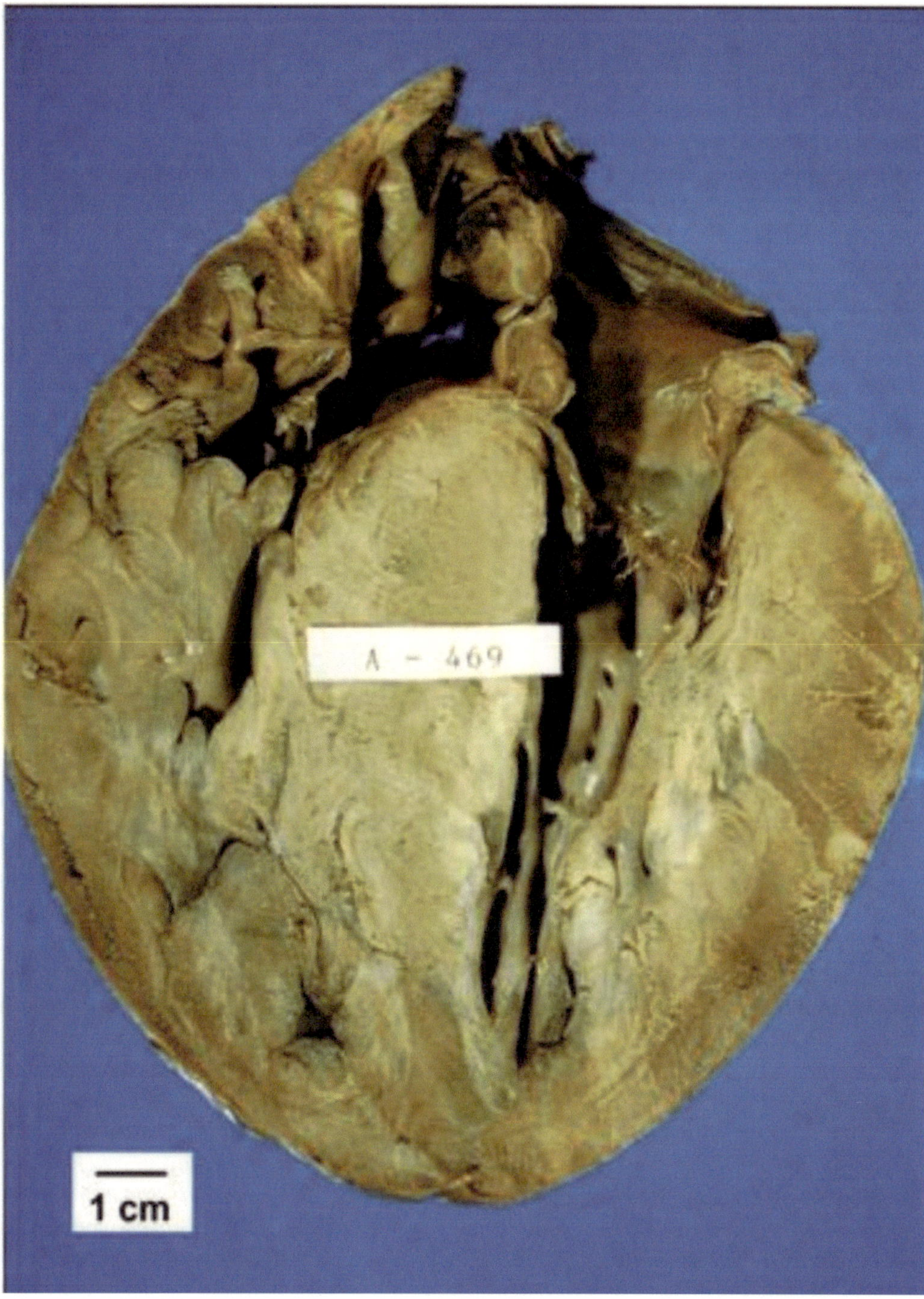

Fig. 1. Longitudinal section of the heart of a 9 year-old boy, who died suddenly during ordinary activities, with predominant hypertrophy of the septum but also showing increased thickness of the free wall of both ventricles. During life, obstruction of both the left and right ventricular outflow tracts was present.

extensive fibrosis, myocardial wall thinning and cavity dilation (Harris et al., 2006). The left atrium is enlarged as a consequence of the elevated left ventricular end diastolic pressure caused by diastolic dysfunction and mitral regurgitation secondary to left ventricular outflow tract obstruction or associated mitral valve anomalies (Klues et al., 1992). The physiopathology of mitral insufficiency in hypertrophic obstructive cardiomyopathy was initially attributed to the Venturi effect produced by systolic flow acceleration in the left ventricular outflow tract dragging the anterior mitral valve leaflet towards the ventricular septum causing both obstruction and insufficiency (Grigg et al., 1992; Panza et al., 1992; Shah et al., 1969 & 1971). A subsequent echocardiographic and Doppler study suggested instead, that the mitral valve leaflets are protruding into a narrow left ventricular outflow tract at the onset of ejection causing that rapid forward flow becomes the dominant force that pushes the leaflets toward the septum being the immediate cause of obstruction. After the onset of obstruction the leaflets are forced against the septum by the pressure difference across the orifice. The raising gradient leads to a smaller orifice and a higher gradient (Sherrid et al., 1993). The systolic anterior motion of the mitral leaflets precludes the proper sealing of the mitral orifice generating mild to moderate mitral regurgitation (M. Maron et al., 2011). The mitral valve in these patients shows alterations in size and shape which are thought to be primary abnormalities of the disease. The main changes are elongation and increase of the leaflet area usually not symmetrical. The size of the left ventricular outflow, the hyperdynamic contraction and the alterations of the mitral valve are the causes of the obstruction.

4.2 Microscopy

The distinct feature of the microscopic examination of the myocardium is hypertrophy and marked disarray (greater than 5% of the myocardial tissue) of individual and grouped myocardiocytes (myofibers) that instead of being normally aligned are interspersed in different directions forming whorls around areas of fibrosis. Cells and fibers lose their normal parallelism and can even be found almost perpendicular to each other. (Fig. 2) The disarray also includes the intracellular myofibrils. Other findings include increased connective tissue leading to interstitial fibrosis and thickening of the microvascular coronary artery walls with luminal reduction resulting in ischemia and fibrosis (Ferrans et al., 1972). Fibrosis and scar replacement of necrosed cells is more evident in areas with greater hypertrophy. Initially, it was postulated that the mechanism for the disarray and hypertrophy was caused by the increased effort of the myocytes to compensate the inefficient contractility of the affected sarcomere proteins. This would activate the insulin and tissue growth factors and angiotensin II resulting in the myocardial changes (J. Seidman & C. Seidman, 2001). Further experimental animal investigations and studies of hypertrophic cardiomyopathy mutations in man, by the same authors, found instead that the mutated sarcomeres had in fact increased function. It was then hypothesized that they would activate signals for hypertrophic remodeling. Abnormalities in calcium signaling were encountered leading to necrosis and replacement fibrosis producing diastolic dysfunction, a main feature of hypertrophic cardiomyopathy (C. Seidman & J. Seidman, 2011). An investigation by the same group, also found that a profibrotic marker like serum procollagen is significantly higher in patients with full blown hypertrophic cardiomyopathy and mutation carriers, with a still not developed phenotype, than in controls, pointing to increase collagen synthesis and fibrosis. Late gadolinium enhancement studies are positive when hypertrophy is already present (Ho et al., 2010). The myocardial disarray, interstitial fibrosis, and ischemia are also the substrate for the occurrence of arrhythmias.

4.3 Phenocopies

Patients with nonsarcomeric hypertrophic cardiomyopathy are considered to be phenocopies (Table 5), and might have the same pathologic findings as has been reported in some *malformation syndromes* or *neuromuscular disorders* like *Noonan's syndrome* and *Friedreich's ataxia* (Burch et al., 1992; Kawai et al., 2000). However, this is not the case for inborn *errors of metabolism* like *glycogen storage disease* where the gross anatomy resembles hypertrophic cardiomyopathy but microscopic examination shows the glycogen deposits in the myocytes without disarray. (Fig. 3) It should be noted that the present definition of phenocopy, according to the Webster's New World Medical Dictionary in its second acception is: "A person who has an environmental condition that mimics a condition that is produced by a gene". Since the examples just mentioned are genetic in origin, the term phenocopy could be inappropriate but is how these entities have been named for a long time.

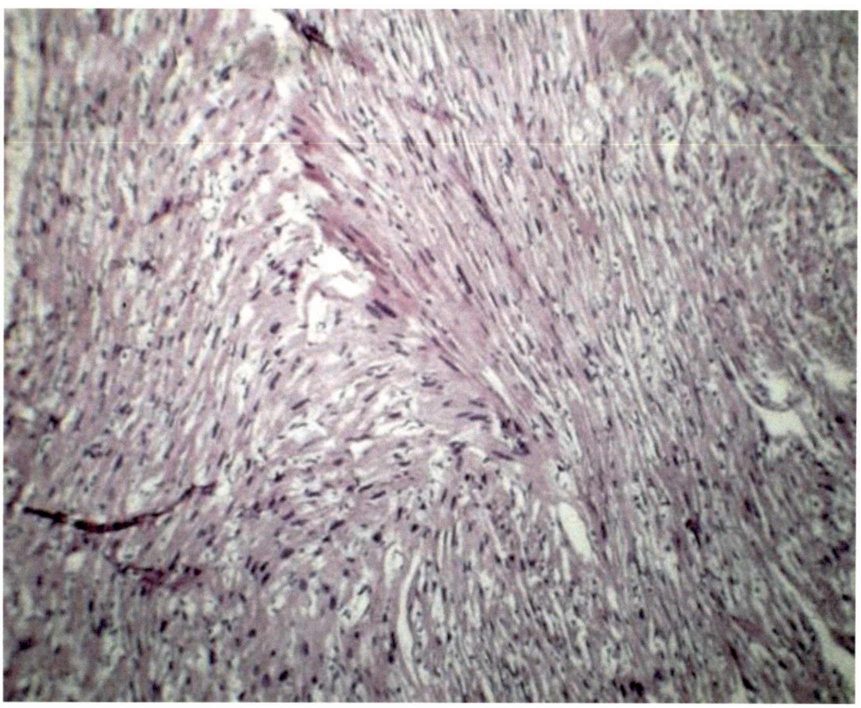

Fig. 2. Microscopic view of the myocardium with the typical disarray of hypertrophic cardiomyopathy in an infant who died in congestive heart failure. Myofibers have lost the usual parallel disposition and describe whorls around areas of fibrosis. The disarray is present in the myofibers, among myocytes and in the myofibrils within the myocytes.

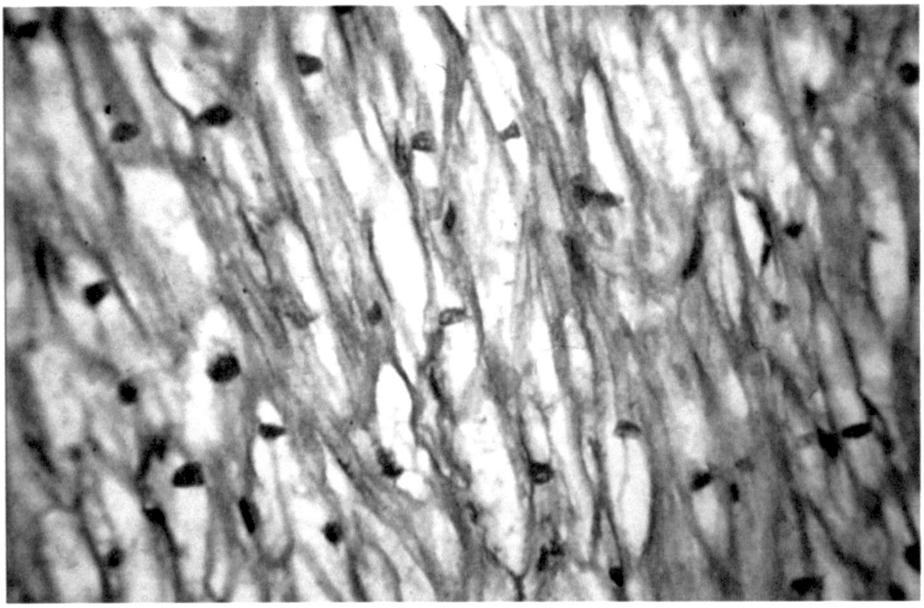

Fig. 3. Typical lacework appearance of the myocardium in a patient with type II Pompe's disease. There is normal alignment of the vacuolated myocardial fibers with glycogen storage.

GENE	PROTEIN	SYNDROME
TAZ	Tafazzin (G4.5)	Barth syndrome/LVNC
DTNA	α-dystrobrevin	Barth syndrome/LVNC
LAMP2	Lysosome-associated membrane protein 2	Danon's syndrome/WPW
GLA	α-galactosidase	Fabry's disease
AGL	Amylo-1,6-glucosidase	Forbes disease
FXN	Frataxin	Friedreich's ataxia
PTPN11	Protein tyrosine phosphatase. nonreceptor type 11, SHP-2	Noonan's syndrome, LEOPARD syndrome
RAF1	V-RAF-1 murine leukemia viral oncogene homolog 1	Noonan's syndrome, LEOPARD syndrome
KRAS	v-Ki-ras2 Kirsten rat sarcoma viral oncogene homolog	Noonan's syndrome
SOS1	Son of sevenless homolog 1	Noonan's syndrome
GAA	α-1,4-glucosidase deficiency	Pompe's disease
PRKAG2	AMP-activated protein kinase	WPW/HCM

LVNC: left ventricular noncompaction, WPW: Wolff-Parkinson-White, HCM: hypertrophic cardiomyopathy.

Table 5. Genes involved in the production of phenocopies (modified from Bos et al., 2009).

5. Clinical findings

Aside from the genetic and phenotypic heterogeneity already mentioned in hypertrophic cardiomyopathy, the age, form of presentation, and outcome, are also quite diverse. The age of the patient at presentation is a determinant of prognosis (Colan et al., 2007). Newborn and infants are more likely to be referred for congestive heart failure while older children are usually asymptomatic at the time of diagnosis and the consultation is requested because of the presence of a heart murmur, cardiomegaly casually detected on a chest x-ray, or electrocardiographic abnormalities (Bruno et al., 2002). Initially, asymptomatic patients may go on without symptoms for a long period of time until they begin experiencing fatigue and dyspnea, and less frequently, palpitations, chest pain, and syncope or sudden death which might be the first symptom ever. Another cause of referral is the investigation of cardiac involvement in patients with conditions known to be associated with hypertrophic cardiomyopathy like the *malformation syndromes, inborn errors of metabolism* or *neuromuscular disorders*. However, in other circumstances, the associated disease may have been unnoticed and the cardiomyopathy is discovered first. The presence of physical findings suggesting an association then prompts referral to the geneticist (Alday & Moreyra, 1984). With regard to the physical examination itself, in hypertrophic obstructive cardiomyopathy, the peripheral pulses may rise and descend rapidly. When considerable cardiac enlargement is present, a precordial bulge and outward displacement of the point of maximal impulse are usually found. A double apical impulse caused by a 4th heart sound is often noted. A harsh, blowing systolic murmur with varying intensity, related to the degree of obstruction and mitral regurgitation, can be listened along the left sternal border and at the apex. A distinctive feature of these murmurs is the variability seen with maneuvers that increase or reduce the obstruction intensifying or decreasing their intensity (Moreyra et al, 1972). (Fig. 4) Patients with non obstructive hypertrophic cardiomyopathy may also have ejection systolic murmurs along the left sternal border though softer than when there is left ventricular outflow obstruction. An ambulatory electrocardiographic study performed in infants, children and adolescents with hypertrophic cardiomyopathy concluded that arrhythmias occur rarely before adolescence. However, from then on, prevalence of nonsustained ventricular tachycardia is as high as 18%. It is also worth mentioning that absence of arrhythmias is not synonymous of low risk for sudden death (McKenna et al., 1988). Supraventricular and ventricular tachycardias may be equally found. Atrial fibrillation may occur in end-stage dilated hypertrophic cardiomyopathy (Harris et al., 2006). Very rarely, patients with hypertrophic cardiomyopathy have associated Wolff-Parkinson-White syndrome (Bockowski et al., 2007). The development of high rate supraventricular tachycardias is poorly tolerated in these patients with left ventricular diastolic dysfunction. This might lead to syncope and sudden death which are the most feared complications of hypertrophic cardiomyopathy. Several mechanisms have been reported as a cause of syncope like tachyarrhythmias, left ventricular outflow tract obstruction, systemic hypotension, and 3rd degree AV block. Sudden unexpected death may be the first and only symptom in hypertrophic cardiomyopathy and this is the most frequent cause of death in young athletes during competition. However, sudden death also occurs during usual activities, at rest, or during sleep time. The estimated rate of sudden death in children is 3% per year, a similar figure to that found in adults cared for in tertiary centers (Bruno & al., 2002; B.J. Maron et al., 1982; McKenna & Deanfield, 1984). Heart failure in this disease is usually provoked by diastolic dysfunction secondary to left ventricular hypertrophy, myocyte disarray and fibrosis. The presence of outflow obstruction is an additional factor leading to heart failure. In 3 to 5 % of patients the end stage is reached and systolic failure associated with left ventricular wall thinning and increased ventricular volume become a serious indication of poor prognosis (Biagini et al., 2005 & Harris et al., 2006).

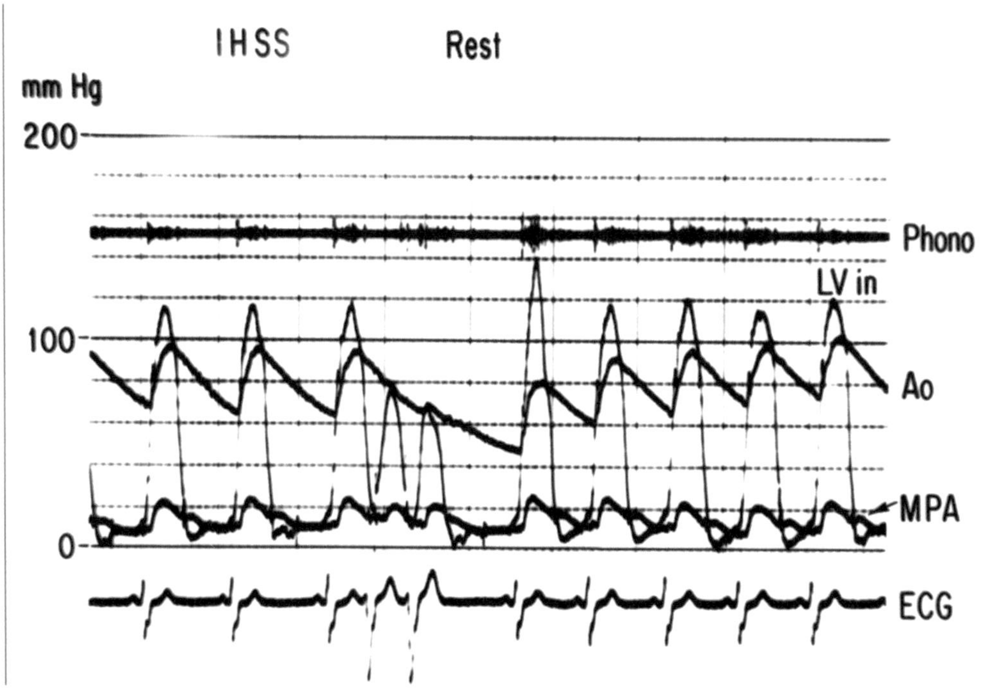

Fig. 4. Simultaneous hemodynamic recordings of the left ventricular inflow (LV in), aorta (Ao) and main pulmonary artery (MPA). An electrocardiogram (ECG) and a phonocardiogram (phono) were also recorded. There is a small basal gradient between the left ventricular inflow and the aorta which increases in a post-extrasystolic beat together with the intensity of the systolic murmur shown in the phonocardiogram, as a consequence of the stronger contraction following the post-extrasystolic pause. (IHSS: idiopathic hypertrophic subaortic stenosis).

6. Laboratory studies

6.1 Radiology

The chest x-ray is usually normal in early stages of the disease but following the pubertal growth spurt shows cardiomegaly at the expense of the left sided chambers (B.J. Maron et al., 1986). (Fig. 5) The same is true for patients evolving to end-stage hypertrophic cardiomyopathy (Biagini et al., 2005). Finally, infants with severe heart failure nearly always have considerable cardiac enlargement at presentation. Pulmonary venous hypertension secondary to elevation of the left ventricular end diastolic pressure is reflected by the well known resultant pulmonary vascular changes.

6.2 Electrocardiography and allied techniques

The electrocardiogram is usually abnormal in almost all patients with hypertrophic cardiomyopathy. (Panza & Maron, 1989) The electrocardiographic abnormality, even a slight one, may precede the echocardiographic findings showing left ventricular hypertrophy in family members carrying the genotype of probands with hypertrophic cardiomyopathy. Therefore, this should be kept on mind when screening relatives of hypertrophic cardiomyopathy patients (Gregor et al., 1989). Left atrial enlargement and left ventricular hypertrophy by voltage criteria usually associated with ST-T abnormalities are seen. (Fig. 6) Younger patients may have combined ventricular or isolated right ventricular hypertrophy with a rightwards QRS axis. (Fig. 7) Another frequent finding is the presence of pathological deep and narrow Q waves. An R + S sum higher than 10 mV on the limb leads of the electrocardiogram has been recently proposed as a risk factor for sudden death in children with hypertrophic cardiomyopathy (Ostman-Smith et al., 2005). (Fig. 8) An electrocardiographic Wolff-Parkinson-White pattern or syndrome is very rare in patients with sarcomeric hypertrophic cardiomyopathy. However, it has been described in mutations of genes like those encoding AMP-activated protein kinase (*PRKAG2*) and lysosome associated membrane protein 2 (*LAMP2*) producing *glycogen storage disease* and *Danon disease* respectively. Both of them recognized as phenocopies of hypertrophic cardiomyopathy (Alday et al., 2010). Ambulatory electrocardiography and exercise testing are used for arrhythmia detection and risk stratification in older children with hypertrophic cardiomyopathy. The presence of nonsustained ventricular tachycardia by Holter monitoring or an abnormal blood pressure response to exercise are considered risk factors for sudden death (Elliot et al., 2000).

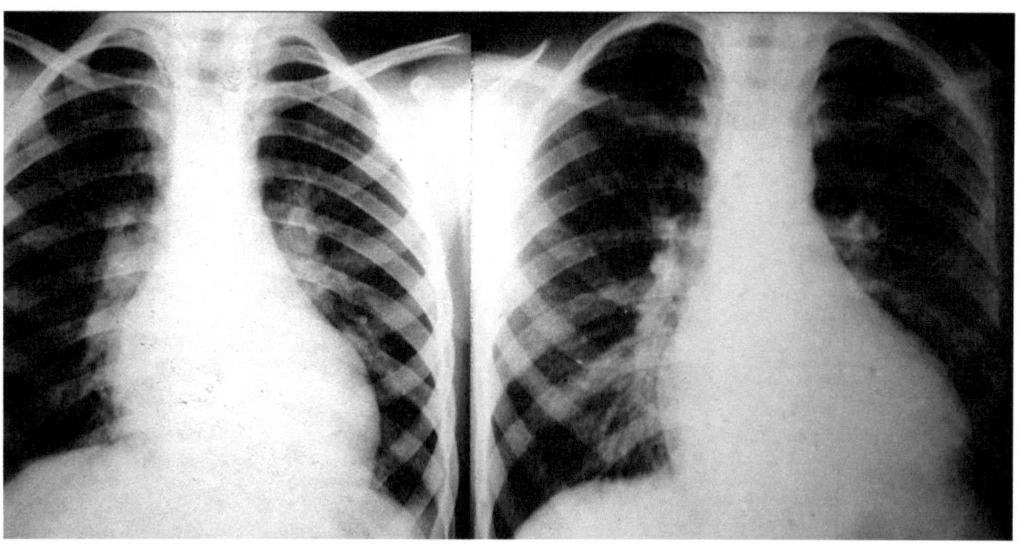

Fig. 5. Chest x-rays of a boy at 11 and 13 years of age showing great increase in the heart size coincident with pubertal growth spurt.

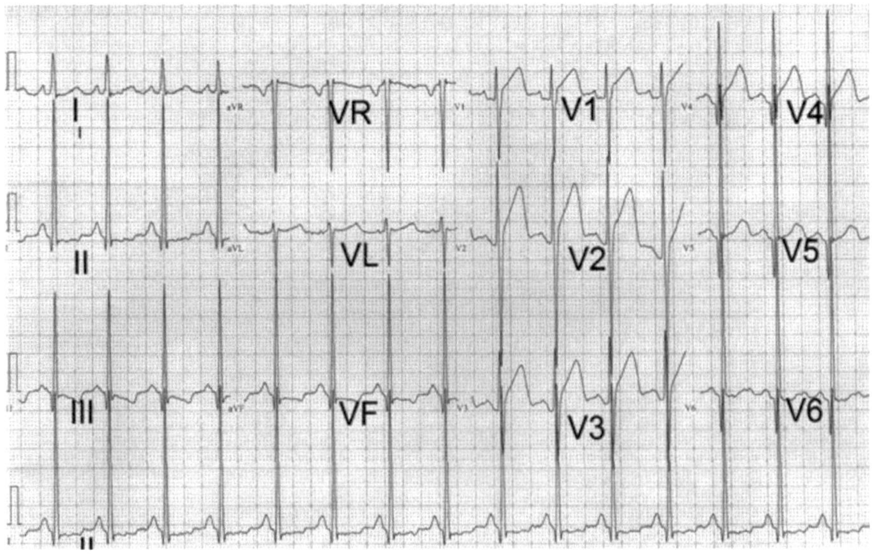

Fig. 6. Electrocardiogram of a 16 year-old male patient showing increased R wave voltages and secondary ST-T changes indicating severe left ventricular hypertrophy.

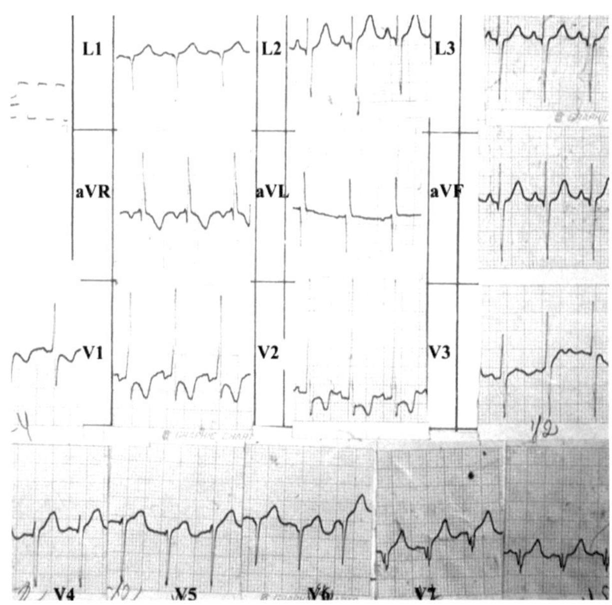

Fig. 7. Electrocardiogram belonging to a 4 year-old boy with a QRS axis of -120° with Q waves in leads II, III and aVF. There are signs of combined ventricular hypertrophy, loss of R wave voltage from V4 to V8 with appearance of QS complexes in V6 and pathological Q waves in V7 and V8.

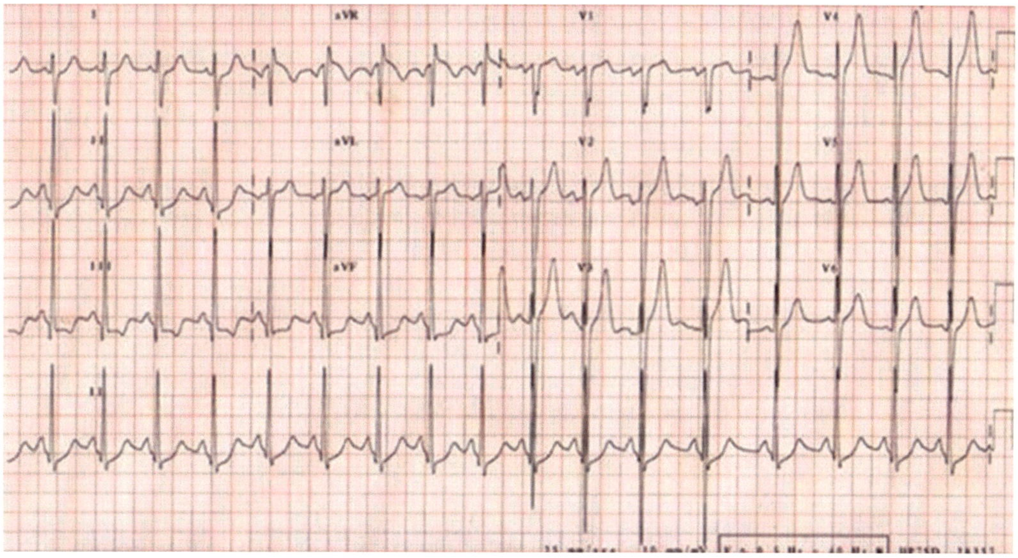

Fig. 8. Electrocardiogram of a 14 year-old male patient with a vertical QRS axis (+120º) and voltage criteria for left ventricular hypertrophy. A limb lead voltage sum > 10 mV is considered a risk factor for sudden death in children.

6.3 Echocardiography

Echocardiography associated with color flow Doppler is the most effective test for the diagnosis of hypertrophic cardiomyopathy (B.J. Maron et al., 2003a). It allows detection of the disease, follow-up of progression, and risk stratification for sudden death (B.J. Maron et al., 1986, Ostman-Smith et al., 2005). The wall thickness echocardiographic criteria for the diagnosis of hypertrophic cardiomyopathy was set at greater than 2 SD above the mean for the body surface area of the population for a localized or general myocardial hypertrophy (Grenier et al., 2000). When in the absence of pulmonary valve stenosis the right ventricular wall thickness exceeds 4 mm the right ventricle is considered to be involved too (Nugent et al., 2005). Left ventricular hypertrophy is most frequently asymmetric with greater involvement of the interventricular septum than the rest of the walls, though it can also be concentric. (Fig. 9 - 11) More rarely, it is localized in the anterior wall, the apex, or in the mid left ventricle (M. Maron et al., 2009, Minami et al., 2011). The mid ventricular obstruction may lead to the development of an apical left ventricular aneurysm. (Fig. 12) In younger children the right ventricle may also be affected (Biagini et al., 2005). As a consequence of mitral insufficiency and/or diastolic dysfunction, there is left atrial enlargement. The systolic anterior movement of the mitral valve contacting the ventricular septum that causes left ventricular outflow tract obstruction in patients with hypertrophic obstructive cardiomyopathy is readily seen (B.J. Maron et al., 2003). Color flow mapping allows detection of the site of obstruction. (Fig. 13) The gradient across the outflow tract is estimated by continuous wave Doppler that also allows assessment of the mitral regurgitation severity. (Fig. 14) Transesophageal echocardiography is more sensitive than transthoracic studies for evaluation of primary mitral valve anomalies producing mitral incompetence (Kuhl & Hanrath, 2004). The presence of left ventricular outflow tract obstruction is now considered a risk factor for adverse events in hypertrophic cardiomyopathy (M. Maron et al., 2003). Furthermore, we now know that almost 70% of patients with hypertrophic cardiomyopathy have gradients across the left ventricular outflow considering the obstruction caused by exercise, when studied with stress echo. Actually, it should be performed in all patients with no significant gradient at rest (M. Maron et al., 2006). Estimation of diastolic dysfunction in hypertrophic cardiomyopathy is performed by studying the pulmonary vein and transmitral Doppler flow tracings but since they depend on loading conditions are not reliable to predict adverse outcomes in children with hypertrophic cardiomyopathy (McMahon et al., 2004). Tissue Doppler velocities measurements at the mitral annulus level are more sensitive in detecting diastolic dysfunction allowing early diagnosis in hypertrophic cardiomyopathy genetic carriers before they develop hypertrophy (Nagheb et al., 2003). (Fig. 15) Tissue Doppler studies can also predict adverse events like death, ventricular tachycardia, cardiac arrest, and exercise intolerance in affected children with the disease (McMahon et al., 2004).

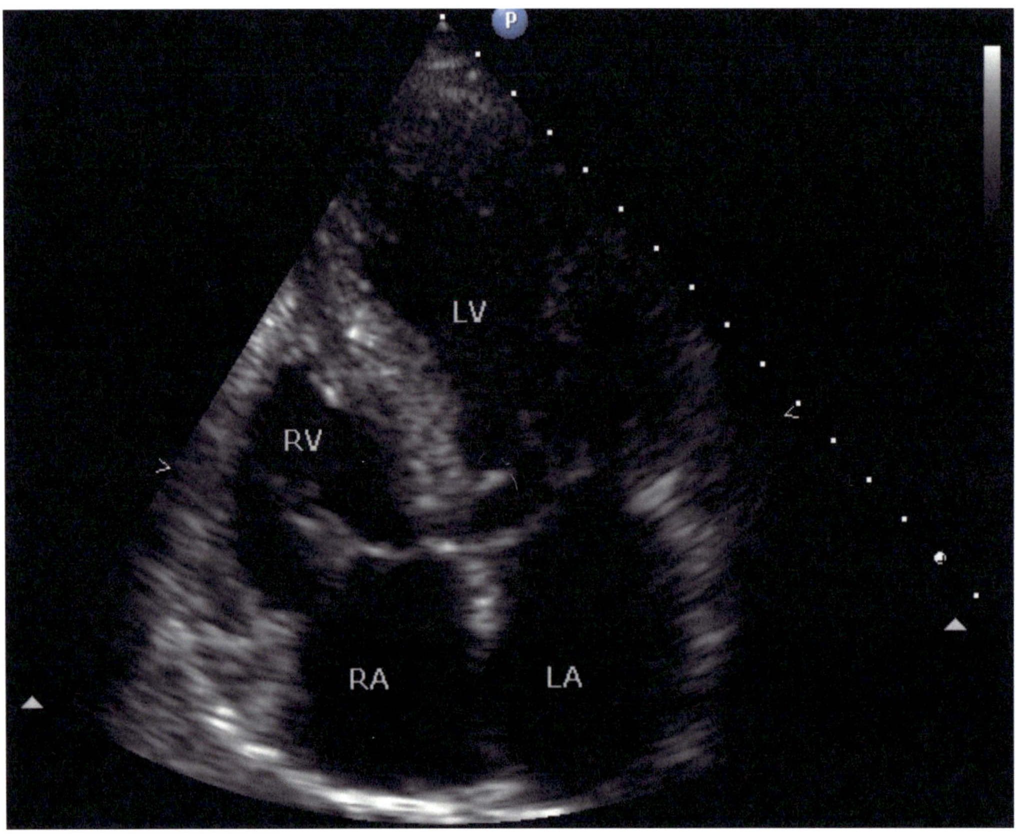

Fig. 9. Four-chamber bidimensional echocardiographic view of a 16 year-old asymptomatic male patient with hypertrophic cardiomyopathy with asymmetric septal hypertrophy. The septum and the posterior wall measure 21 mm and 9.5 mm respectively.

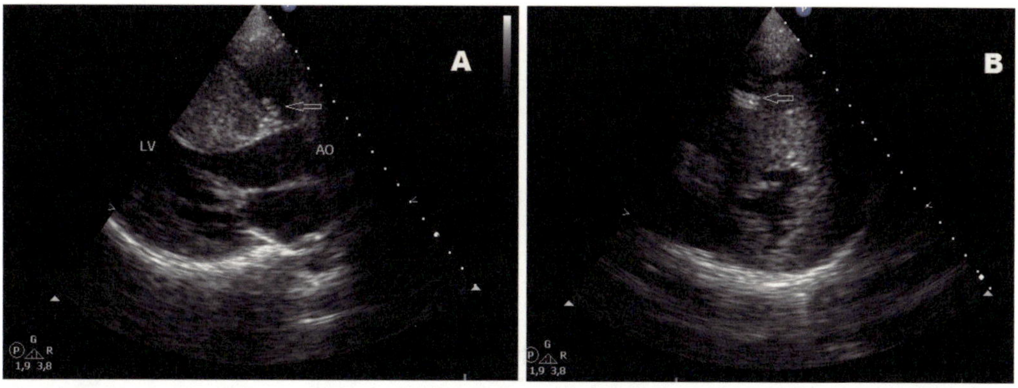

Fig. 10. Bidimensional echocardiogram showing long (A) and short (B) axis parasternal views of the left ventricle of a 22 year-old female followed since early childhood with severe asymmetrical hypertrophy of the septum measuring 31 mm in diameter. There is convexity toward the left ventricular cavity. The mitral leaflets initiate an anterior motion to provoke mitral septal contact and the resultant left ventricular outflow tract obstruction. The left atrium is mildly enlarged. The tip of a catheter for DDD pacing is seen in the right ventricular cavity (arrows).

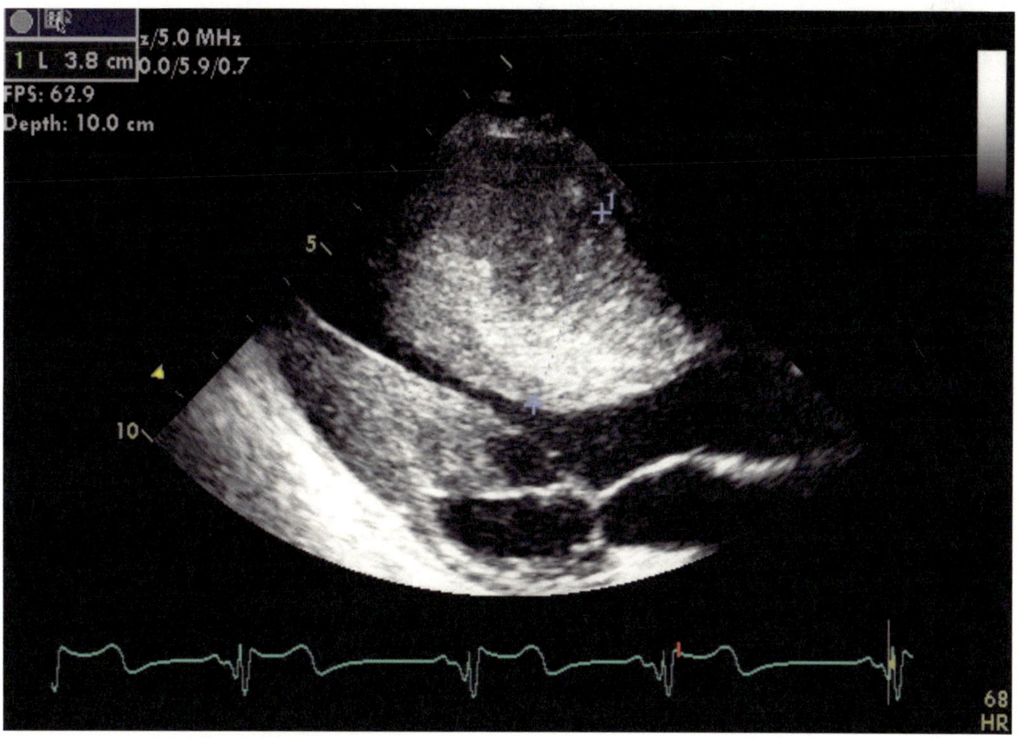

Fig. 11. Bidimensional echocardiographic long axis view with massive septal hypertrophy (38 mm) in a girl with a strong family history (2 siblings). Courtesy Dr Ricardo Pignatelli, Texas Children's Hospital.

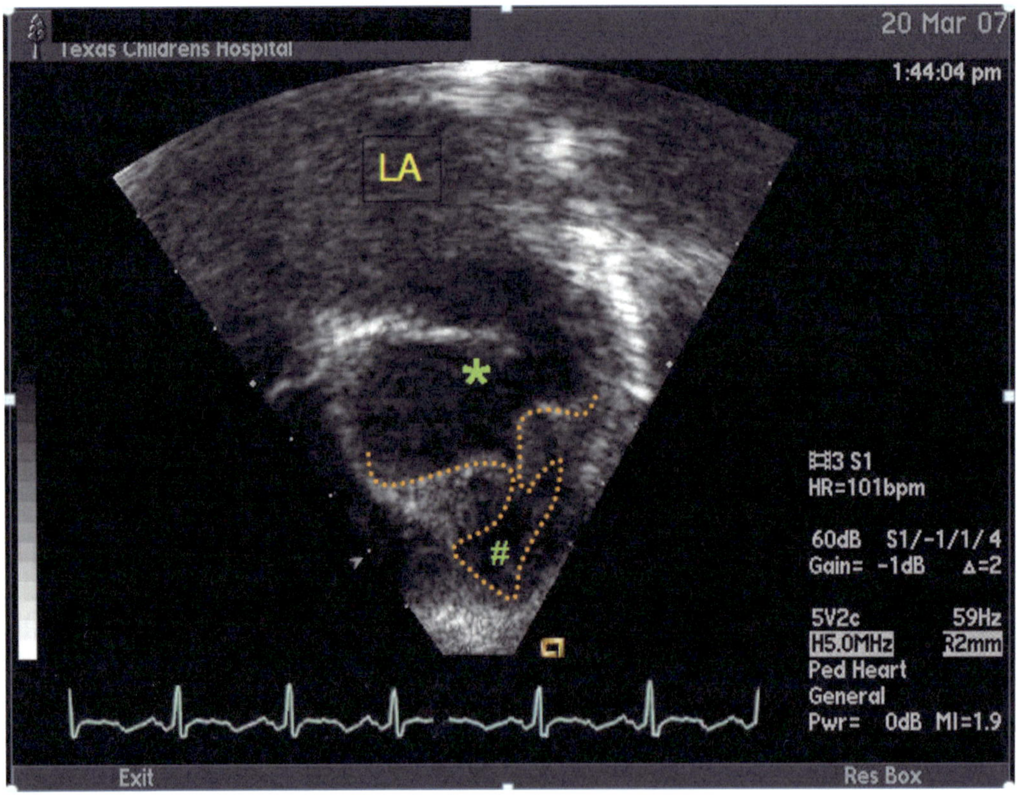

Fig. 12. Bidimensional echocardiographic view of a patient with midventricular obstruction. The left ventricle has an upper inflow (*) and a lower apical chamber (#) as a result of the obstruction. Courtesy Dr Ricardo Pignatelli, Texas Children's Hospital.

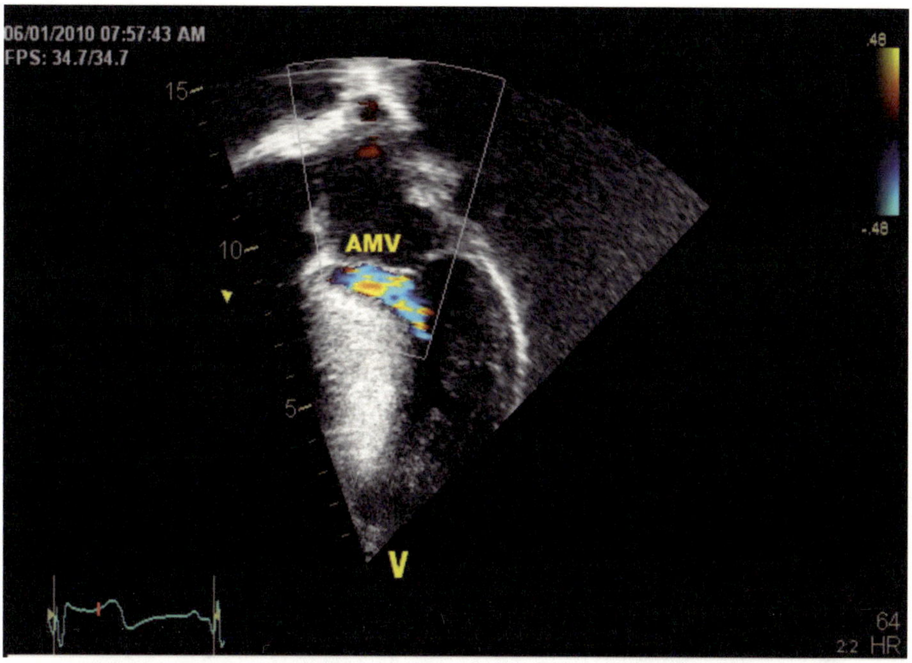

Fig. 13. Echocardiographic 4-chamber view of asymmetric septal hypertrophy with left ventricular outflow tract flow acceleration (arrow) by color Doppler. (AMV: anterior mitral valve). Courtesy Dr Ricardo Pignatelli, Texas Children's Hospital.

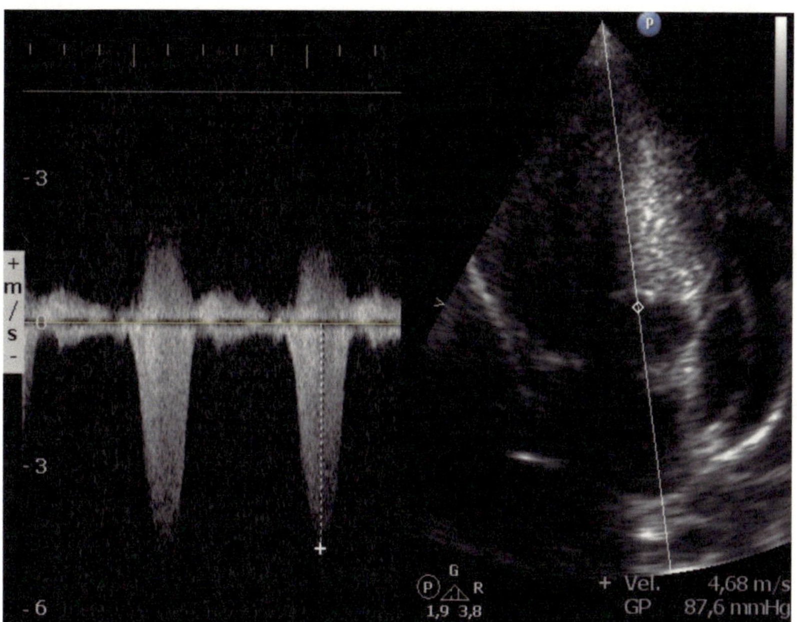

Fig. 14. Continuous wave Doppler showing a severe gradient (87.6 mmHg) across the left ventricular outflow tract in the same patient shown on figure 10.

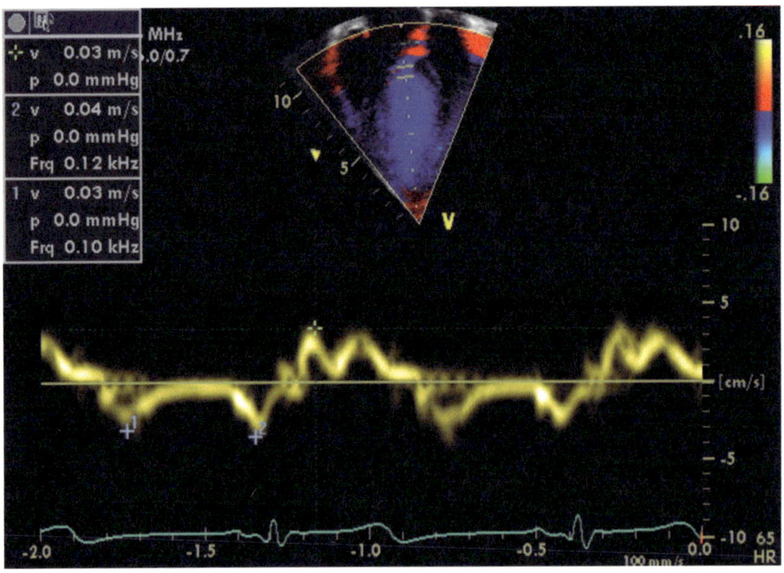

Fig. 15. Decreased Doppler tissue septal velocities (<5cm/second) in a patient with massive hypertrophic cardiomyopathy. Courtesy Dr Ricardo Pignatelli, Texas Children's Hospital.

6.4 Computed tomography and magnetic resonance imaging

Cardiac computed tomography and magnetic resonance imaging yield superior anatomic data than echocardiography since they allow better definition of the anterolateral wall and tip of the left ventricle and the right ventricle. However, these procedures are more costly and the former exposes the patient to radiation (M. Maron et al., 2009). (Fig. 16) Nevertheless, they are very useful when thoracic deformities prevent satisfactory cardiac visualization by transthoracic echocardiography. Cardiovascular magnetic resonance has also demonstrated that mitral leaflet elongation is present in hypertrophic cardiomyopathy independently of other phenotypic variants indicating that the mitral abnormalities are primary, thus, their important role in the pathophysiology of the left ventricular outflow obstruction (M. Maron, et al.; 2011). On the other hand, gadolinium magnetic resonance imaging late enhancement allows detection of the amount of myocardial fibrosis and is a predictor of systolic dysfunction (M. Maron et al., 2008). A more recent study reports that is also effective for prognostication of adverse outcomes and which patients might require a cardioverter-defibrillator (Fig. 17) (Bruder et al., 2010).

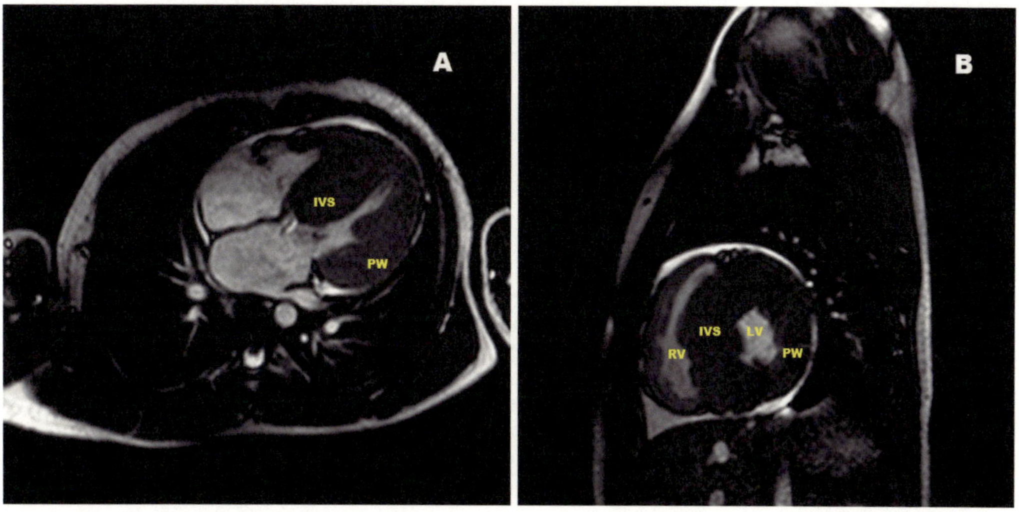

Fig. 16. A. Long axis view of a cardiac magnetic resonance image of a 5 year-old asymptomatic boy with severe hypertrophic cardiomyopathy. **B:** Magnetic resonance imaging of a short axis projection of the heart of a 3 year-old boy with severe heart failure. (IVS: interventricular septum, LV: left ventricle, PW: posterior wall, RV: right ventricle). Courtesy Dr Ricardo Pignatelli, Texas Children's Hospital.

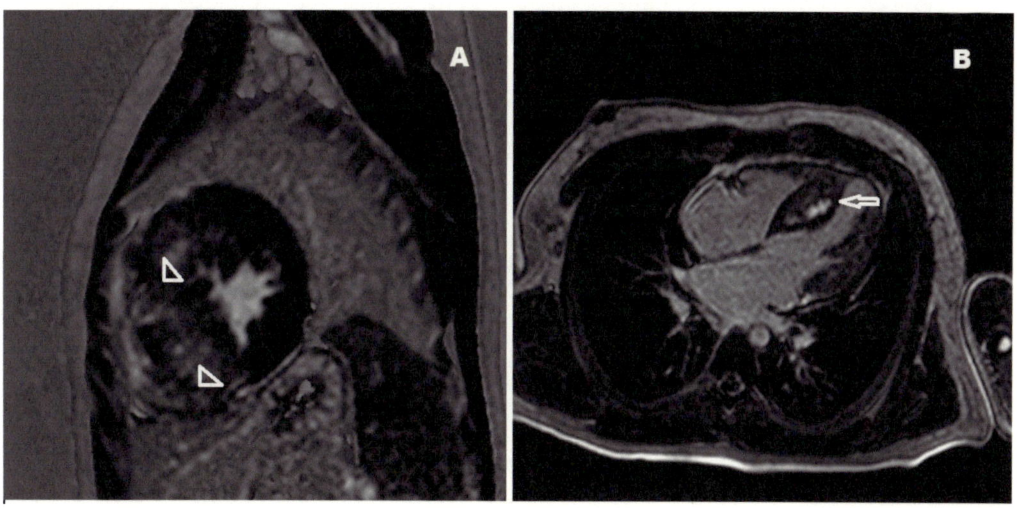

Fig. 17. **A.**Cardiac magnetic resonance image of the heart of a patient with positive delayed gadolinium enhancement indicating a diffuse pattern of fibrosis (arrowheads). **B:** Long axis view of a cardiac magnetic resonance image of the heart of a 9 year-old boy with a localized delayed gadolinium enhancement image in the interventricular septum (arrow). Courtesy Dr Ricardo Pignatelli, Texas Children's Hospital.

6.5 Cardiac catheterization and cineangiocardiography

We owe to cardiac catheterization and cineangiocardiography the initial understanding of the physiopathology of hypertrophic cardiomyopathy shortly after its rediscovery about half a century ago (Braunwald et al., 1964; Wigle, Auger & Marquis, 1967). These techniques were then considered the gold standard for the diagnosis of hypertrophic obstructive cardiomyopathy. (Fig. 18) With the advent of the just discussed noninvasive imaging techniques like Doppler-echocardiography, computed tomography, and magnetic resonance imaging, this invasive procedure is no longer necessary for diagnostic purposes. Nowadays, this method is only used before planned surgical treatment or percutaneous interventions for septal reduction.

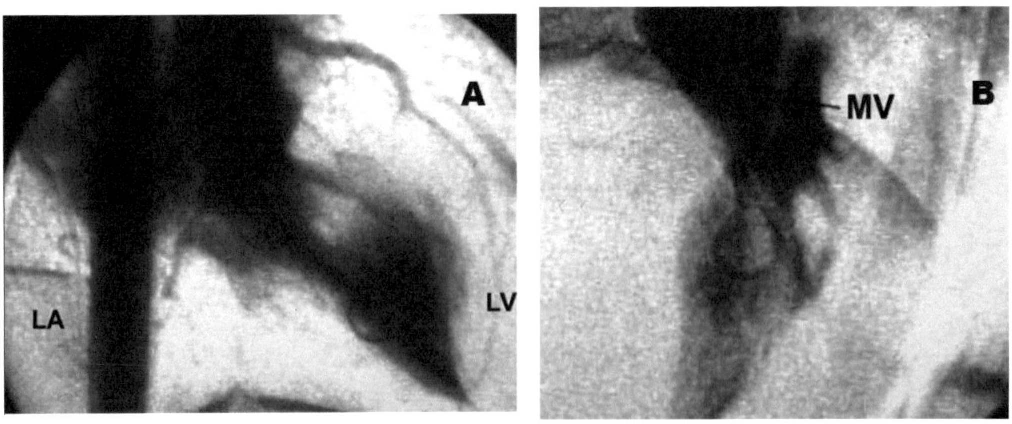

Fig. 18. A. Left ventricular cineangiocardiogram in the right anterior oblique projection showing a hypertrophied chamber with subaortic obstruction and moderate mitral insufficiency with left atrial enlargement. B. In the left anterior oblique view the anterior mitral valve can be seen contacting the septum. LV: left ventricle; LA: left atrium; MV: mitral valve.

7. Complications

7.1 Sudden death and congestive heart failure

The main complications in children with hypertrophic cardiomyopathy are syncope and sudden unexpected death. The latter may be the first and only manifestation of the disease and is considered to be secondary to ventricular tachycardia and fibrillation caused by myocardial fibrosis and ischemia (Basso et al., 2000; B.J. Maron et al., 2000b). Sudden death occurs more often in older children with hypertrophic cardiomyopathy either during strenuous sport activities or at rest but is infrequent in infants (B.J. Maron et al., 2003a) who are more prone to present and die with congestive heart failure specially in secondary forms (Bruno et al., 2002).

7.2 Arrhythmias

Supraventricular and nonsustained ventricular tachycardias, were found in almost a third of pediatric and adolescent patients with hypertrophic cardiomyopathy studied by ambulatory electrocardiography (McKenna, et al., 1988). However, their outcome after a mean follow-up of 3 years was rather benign. In a study from our group, a quarter of the patients had symptomatic atrial or ventricular tachycardia. Three out of 7 died suddenly during follow-up (Bruno et al., 2002). Rarely, 3rd degree atrioventricular block is found in children with hypertrophic cardiomyopathy. They could present with near syncope or syncopal attacks as the 1st manifestation of the disease (Rosen et al., 1997).

7.3 Evolving phenotype

Children with hypertrophic cardiomyopathy may evolve to dilated or restrictive cardiomyopathy phenotypes in 5% of the cases. In both circumstances they have a dimmer prognosis and become candidates for heart transplantation (Biagini et al., 2005; Denfield et al., 1997; Shirani et al., 1993).

7.4 Infectious endocarditis

Bacterial endocarditis is an uncommon complication in hypertrophic cardiomyopathy though can occur affecting the left ventricular aspect of the anterior mitral valve leaflet, especially in the presence of obstruction (Aoun et al., 1994; Morgan-Hughes & Motwani, 2002). Antibiotic prophylaxis for infectious endocarditis is then recommended.

7.5 Stroke

Ischemic stroke is somewhat frequent and a cause of death in adult hypertrophic cardiomyopathy but has not been mentioned in children (B.J. Maron et al., 2000a).

8. Differential diagnosis

The most important differential diagnosis is with the athlete's heart and is sometimes somewhat difficult to make. Highly trained competitive athletes may have electrocardiographic abnormalities that resemble those of hypertrophic cardiomyopathy. As in this situation, the left ventricle is hypertrophied but the wall thickness as determined by echocardiography does not exceed 15 mm in diameter and the hypertrophy is symmetrical. The left ventricular cavity is dilated and the ejection fraction is normal while hypertrophic cardiomyopathy is frequently accompanied by unusual distribution of hypertrophy, the left ventricle is smaller in size (<4.5 cm) and the ejection fraction is higher than normal. Furthermore, left ventricular diastolic function is normal in young athletes but is always impaired in hypertrophic cardiomyopathy (B.J. Maron, Spirito & Pelliccia, 1995b). Tissue Doppler studies has also been very useful to distinguish those patients in the "grey zone" (Cardim et al., 2003). When still in doubt regarding the diagnosis, cessation of physical activities usually results in regression of the left ventricular mass in a few weeks' time (B.J. Maron et al.., 1993). Genetic screening might be useful when they are positive for a mutation which occurs in up to 70% of patients with hypertrophic cardiomyopathy. On the contrary, a negative test does not exclude the possibility of a mutation still not discovered.

9. Phenocopies and associations

A recent large epidemiologic study of the pediatric population with hypertrophic cardiomyopathy established that almost a quarter of patients with unexplained left ventricular hypertrophy do not have a sarcomeric etiology (Colan et al., 2007). These variants are called phenocopies and are listed in Table 5. They are classified as *malformation syndromes, inborn errors of metabolism, and neuromuscular disorders* and each group numbers about one third of the total.

9.1 Malformation syndromes

9.1.1 Noonan's and LEOPARD syndromes

The most common *malformation syndromes* associated with hypertrophic cardiomyopathy included in the European Society of Cardiology classification of familial hypertrophic cardiomyopathy, are Noonan's syndrome and its allelic variant LEOPARD syndrome, acronym for lentiginosis, electrocardiographic anomalies, ocular hypertelorism, pulmonic stenosis, abnormal male genitalia, retardation of growth, and deafness. The prevalence of Noonan,s syndrome, initially described as the Turner phenotype with normal karyotype (Noonan, 1968), is estimated in 1:2,000 births (Nora et al., 1974). (Fig. 19) It is inherited as an autosomic dominant form and nearly 80% have congenital heart disease, most frequently pulmonic valve and arterial stenoses, and atrial and ventricular septal defects. The introduction of echocardiography as a diagnostic tool, allowed the recognition of an association with hypertrophic cardiomyopathy in almost a quarter of patients (Nora et al., (1975). In the Australian epidemiologic study of childhood cardiomyopathies, 28% of 80 patients with hypertrophic cardiomyopathy had Noonan's syndrome (Nugent et al., 2005). These patients presented earlier and had more frequent biventricular involvement. However, they did not find greater adverse events rate than in sarcomeric hypertrophic cardiomyopathy. In about 40-50% of patients a mutation of protein tyrosine phosphatase nonreceptor type 11 (*PTPN11)* is found (Type 1 Noonan's syndrome), but this is present in 90% of LEOPARD patients (Sznajer et al., 2007; Tartaglia et al., 2001). This gene controls a series of developmental processes, among them the genesis of semilunar valves. The mutation is then mainly present in patients with heart defects but not in those with hypertrophic cardiomyopathy.

9.1.2 Related conditions

Some related genetic conditions to Noonan's syndrome like the Costello syndrome, the cardiofaciocutaneous syndrome, and palmo-plantar hyperkeratosis with woolly hair may also be associated with hypertrophic cardiomyopathy (Peirone et al., 2005, Roberts et al., 2006).

9.2 Inborn errors of metabolism

9.2.1 Pompe's disease

Pompe's disease or type II glycogen storage disease is an autosomal recessive inherited disorder caused by absence of the acid alpha-glucosidase enzyme (*GAA*) preventing the normal degradation of glycogen in the cardiac myocyte (Hers, 1963). There is an infantile type with massive cardiac enlargement as seen in hypertrophic cardiomyopathy with obstruction leading to congestive heart failure and early death (Ehlers et al., 1962). A typical electrocardiogram is shown in Fig. 20. Late onset Pompe's disease with a better outcome has also been described (Winkle et al., 2005). Enzyme replacement therapy is now available for treatment of *GAA* deficiency.

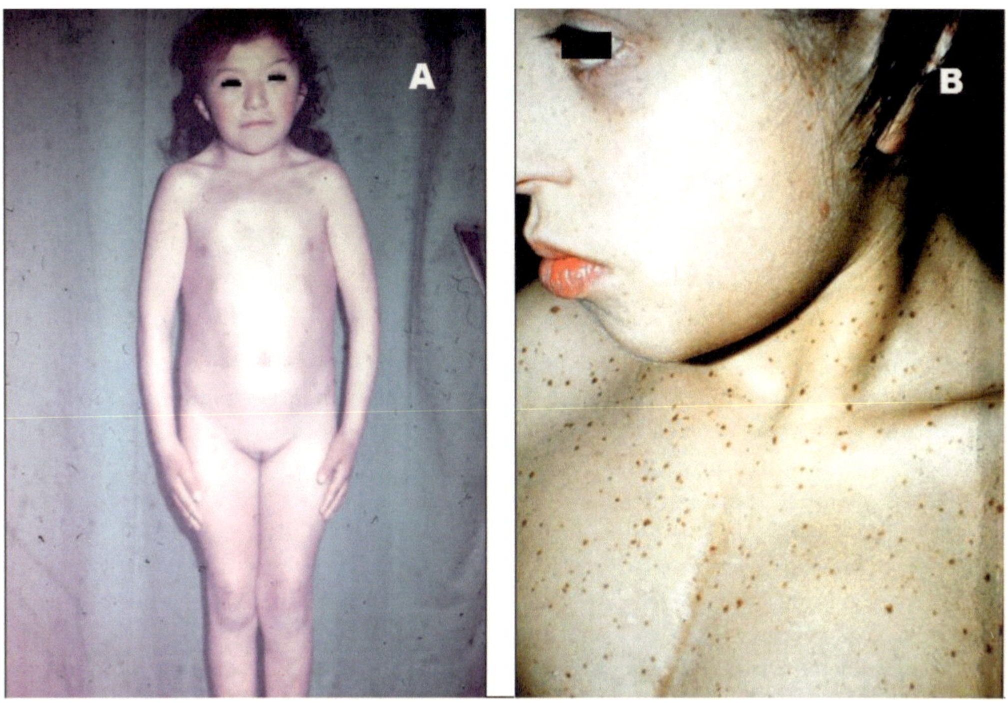

Fig. 19. **A.** Phenotype of a 10-year-old girl with Noonan's syndrome and hypertrophic cardiomyopathy. There is short stature, peculiar face, eyelid ptosis with downward slant, ocular and mammillar hypertelorism, low set ears, pterigium colli, and a prominent chest. **B.** Ten-year-old girl with LEOPARD syndrome. The multiple lentigines and hypertrophic obstructive cardiomyopathy became apparent long after she had been operated on for severe pulmonary valve stenosis when she was 6-month old (Reproduced with permission from *Am Heart J*, 1984; Vol.108, pp. 996-1000).

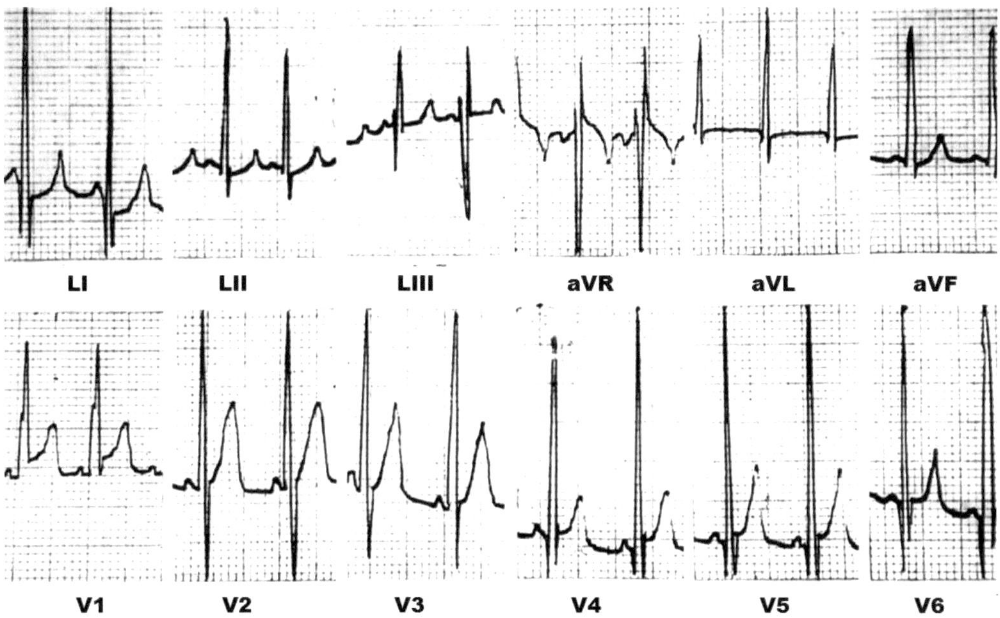

Fig. 20. Typical electrocardiogram of an infant with Pompe's disease. There is short atrioventricular conduction and biventricular hypertrophy with large voltages and no repolarization abnormalities.

9.2.2 Other glycogen storage diseases

A genetic study of 75 patients with hypertrophic cardiomyopathy found that 3 out of 35 patients with negative sarcomere protein mutations had genetical defects in lysosome-associated membrane protein 2 (*LAMP2*) responsible for the X-linked disorder Danon's disease/Wolff-Parkinson-White in 2 of the 3, and in AMP-activated protein kinase gamma 2 (*PRKAG2*) in the remaining, causing Wolff-Parkinson-White/hypertrophic cardiomyopathy (Arad et al., 2005). Both conditions produce glycogen storage and might wrongly be considered as sarcomeric hypertrophic cardiomyopathies. The presence of preexcitation should point to the correct diagnosis. Type IIIa and IV glycogen storage diseases are very rare conditions caused by deficiencies in debrancher and branching enzymes respectively. These patients have muscular hypotonia with elevated creatine kinase and heart and liver involvement. There is heterogenous severity of the disease and the hypertrophic cardiomyopathy is concentric. The inheritance is autosomal recessive (Kishnani et al., 2010). (Fig. 21)

9.2.3 Fabry's disease

Fabry's disease, an X-linked disorder characterized by intracellular accumulation of glycosphingolipids caused by deficiency of the lysosomal enzyme alpha-galactoside A (*GLA*) may result in late onset hypertrophic cardiomyopathy, therefore it is rare in children. The reported prevalences in adult males and females with hypertrophic cardiomyopathy are 7.5 and 12% respectively (Chimenti et al., 2004; Sachdev et al., 2002). Enzyme replacement therapy for these patients is available (Eng et al., 2001).

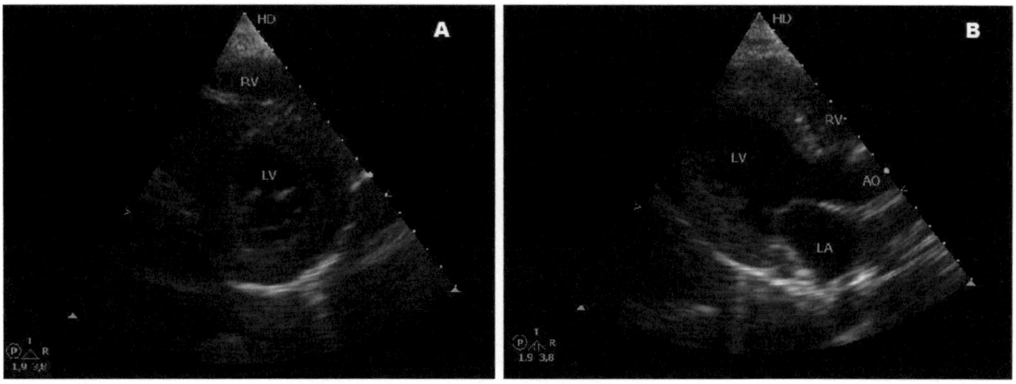

Fig. 21. Short and long axis parasternal echocardiographic views of the heart of a 19-year-old female with type III glycogen storage disease with concentric hypertrophic cardiomyopathy.

9.3 Neuromuscular disorders

Friedreich's ataxia is an autosomic recessive hereditary disorder with spinocerebellar degeneration and frequently associated with hypertrophic cardiomyopathy (Gottdiener et al., 1982). A mutation of the frataxin gene (*FXN*) alters the energy production through mitochondrial iron dysmetabolism resulting in mitochondrial damage producing muscle fiber fibrosis (Michael et al., 2006). The cardiomyopathy may precede the neurological manifestations (Alday & Moreyra, 1984).

9.4 Association with congenital heart disease

Not infrequently, hypertrophic cardiomyopathy and congenital heart disease are associated in children (Somerville & Becu, 1978). In most circumstances the defects are not severe. Ventricular and atrial septal defects and pulmonary valve stenosis have been reported, the last two mainly in patients with Noonan's and LEOPARD syndromes (Bruno et al., 2002; Tikanoja et al., 1999). However, associations with severe conditions like tetralogy of Fallot and atrioventricular septal defect have also been found (Alday et al., 1985; Eidem et al., 2000). (Fig. 22)

9.5 Association with left ventricular noncompaction

Left ventricular noncompaction belongs to the category of unclassified cardiomyopathies . It is characterized by the presence of prominent myocardial trabeculations and sinusoid tracts mainly in the left ventricle. (Fig. 23) Affected patients frequently develop a dilated cardiomyopathy with heart failure, arrhythmias, and systemic thromboembolism. Recent molecular studies have shown that mutations of genes producing phenocopies like Barth syndrome, or even dilated and hypertrophic cardiomyopathies, are present in patients with left ventricular noncompaction. We recently reported a family with overlapping phenotypes for left ventricular noncompaction, hypertrophic cardiomyopathy, and Wolff- Parkinson-White syndrome. We could not obtain genetic molecular studies but on the basis of features shared with affected patients suspected a mutation of either *PRKG2 and LAMP-2* which cause hypertrophic cardiomyopathy with Wolff-Parkinson-White syndrome or Danon's disease respectively (Alday et al., 2010).

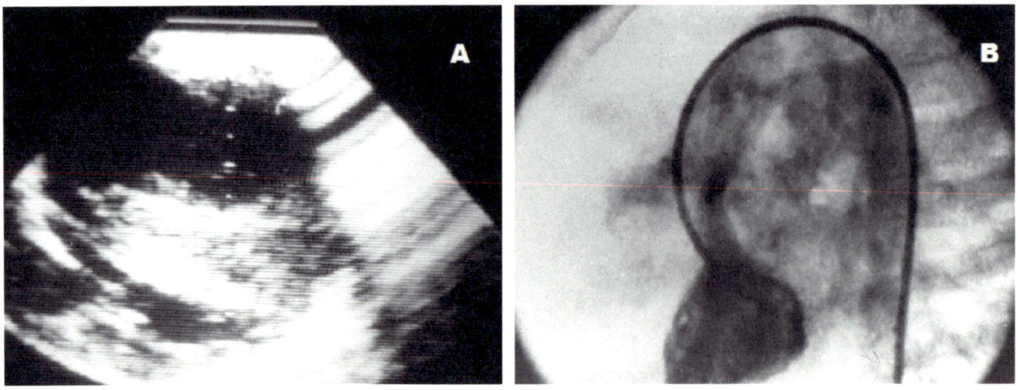

Fig. 22. Two dimensional echocardiogram (A) and left ventricular cineangiography (B) in a patient with tetralogy of Fallot six months after a right modified Blalock-Taussig shunt showing severe ventricular septal hypertrophy, a hypoplastic left ventricle and a dilated aorta overriding a ventricular septal defect.

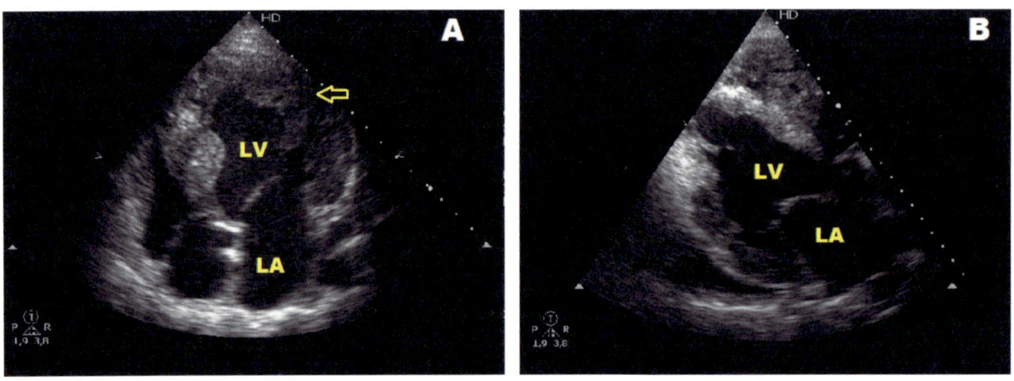

Fig. 23. A and B. Echocardiographic four-chamber view of two sisters followed since infancy showing hypertrophic cardiomyopathy and associated left ventricular noncompaction. The arrow in A points deep sinusoid tracts. LV: left ventricle, LA: left atrium.

10. Treatment

The treatment of hypertrophic cardiomyopathy aims to improve the quality of life alleviating symptoms and to stratify the risk for sudden death to prevent it from happening. Several algorrhythms have been proposed, a slightly modified one is shown in Fig. 24 (Berger et al., 2009). These authors emphasize the existing difficulties to implement prospective controlled randomized trials to define the benefits of different treatment options for this population, therefore most current therapies are empirical or the result of consensus. In older children intensive physical exercise is contraindicated. The disease presenting early has a severe prognosis this being the reason for indicating medical treatment even in asymptomatic children (Bruno et al., 2002). Patients who are symptomatic should receive pharmacological treatment with adrenergic beta blockers which do not decrease the basal outflow gradient but are able to prevent its accentuation in situations of exacerbated inotropism of the heart.

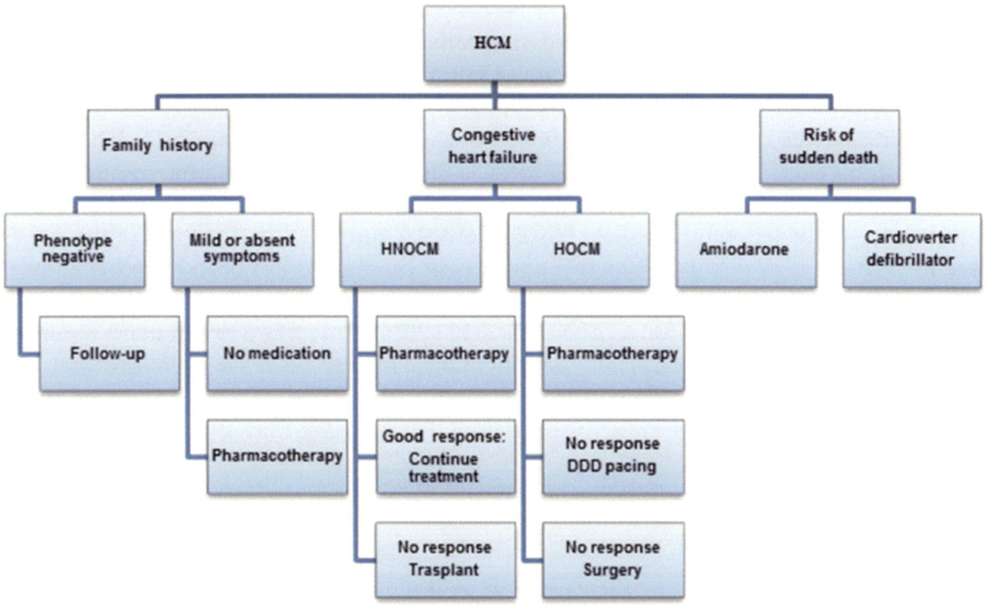

Fig. 24. Algorithm for the treatment of hypertrophic cardiomyopathy (Modified from Berger, et al. (2009) *Cardiol Young,* Vol.19, pp. 66-73).

Beta blockers also have anti-ischemic properties which increase ventricular filling by decreasing the heart rate. In these patients, calcium channel blockers like verapamil can be an alternative to beta blockers. It is not recommended to use them together. In patients with severe gradients and pulmonary hypertension are not advised because of the danger of precipitating acute pulmonary edema. If there is no improvement, disopyramide, which is an antiarrhythmic drug with negative inotropic effects, is able to decrease basal gradients. The combination of disopyramide and beta blockers has been used succesfully in adults but there is no reported experience in children (Sherrid et al., (2005). For very symptomatic smaller children, in spite of full medical treatment, permanent DDD pacing with short atrioventricular interval to favor the consistent capture of the right ventricle has been used to lower the left ventricular outflow tract obstruction by changing the pattern of left ventricular activation (Alday et al., 1998 & Fananapazir et al., 1992). DDD pacing is a reasonable alternative to surgery in symptomatic children despite pharmacological treatment if they are still too young for surgery, taking into account that the approach to an extended septal myectomy is just the aortic valve with a small annulus at this age. A very recent study has also shown progressive relief of symptoms and gradient reduction at long term follow-up (Galve et al., 2010). However, as with other types of treatment, DDD pacing does not protect against the possibility of sudden arrhythmic death (Bruno et al., 2002). The gold standard for the treatment of hypertrophic obstructive cardiomyopathy is still the surgical septal myomectomy (B.J. Maron et al., 2003a; Stone et al., 1993). In experienced centers the mortality is very low and the abolition of the gradient is instantaneous and persistent. The remaining obstruction is usually negligible. These excellent hemodynamic results are associated with improvement of symptoms. The results have been followed for many years and the need for repeat procedures is rare. It should be remembered that the child has to be old enough to permit the transaortic approach to the septum (Berger et al.,

2009). For this reason, reoperation might be necessary in children 14-year-old or younger (Minakata et al., 2005). With regard to catheter septal ablation with alcohol or radiofrequency the 2003 Expert Consensus Document on Hypertrophic Cardiomyopathy, addressing alcohol septal ablation, states that until the long-term effects of the myocardial scar are known, the procedure is not advised in children (Jensen et al., 2011; B.J. Maron et al., 2003a; Sigwart 1995) In patients with symptomatic hypertrophic nonobstructive cardiomyopathy, calcium antagonists like verapamil could be used to improve the diastolic performance of the left ventricle. Beta blockers are also indicated in this form of the disease. Recently the use of perhexiline which is a metabolic modulator has been introduced for the treatment of patients with this phenotype with improvement of the diastolic performance of the left ventricle and of symptoms (Abozguia et al.; 2010). This was a preliminary report that has still to be supported by further investigations. Infants with heart failure and older children with evolution to a dilated cardiomyopathy should be treated with drugs usually employed for treatment of systolic heart failure. These cases may eventually need heart transplantation (Shirani et al., 1993).

11. Prevention

Risk stratification of sudden death in infants and children differs from what is done in adults. In children, cardiac death occurs infrequently and non sudden cardiac death is as common as sudden arrhythmic death. The main risk factors for sudden death in children with hypertrophic cardiomyopathy are, according to Maron et al., previous cardiac arrest, syncope, or sustained ventricular tachycardia, family history of sudden death, frequent repetitive non sustained ventricular tachycardia, abnormal blood pressure response to exercise, end-stage hypertrophic cardiomyopathy, and massive left ventricular hypertrophy (B.J. Maron et al., 2003b). Other criteria for death prognostication proposed more recently, specifically in children, take into account the electrocardiographic voltage and echocardiographic parameters like the septal thickness and the left ventricular wall/left ventricular diastolic dimension ratio (Ostman-Smith et al., 2005). For non-sudden cardiac death, massive left ventricular hypertrophy and abnormal blood pressure response to exercise are considered significant risk factors for mortality (Decker et al., 2009). Sudden cardiac death due to hypertrophic cardiomyopathy occurs mostly in adolescence and early adulthood and very infrequently before 10 years of age. These cases are due to ventricular tachycardia or ventricular fibrillation. In fact, hypertrophic cardiomyopathy is the most common cause of sudden death in the young including athletes (J. Seidman & C. Seidman, 2001). This is the reason why the diagnosis of hypertrophic cardiomyopathy at this age is a strong indication to discontinue the practice of competitive sports. At this time it seems that to establish a prognosis by the knowledge of the specific disease causing mutation is not reasonable for the individual patient. Implantable cardioverter defibrillators are effective to prevent arrhythmic sudden death but in infants and children are indicated mainly in secondary prevention (B.J. Maron, et al., 2000b; Epstein, A.; et al., 2008). The cardioverter defibrillator implantation is plagued with complications in children, this being the reason for the reluctance of its use in primary prevention (Berul et al., 2008). In a nonrandomized controlled trial amiodarone was at one time reported to improve survival in hypertrophic cardiomyopathy associated with ventricular tachycardia (McKenna et al., 1985). However, the frequent toxic effects of amiodarone might counteract its benefits (Berger et al., 2009). It then could be concluded that the properly functioning cardioverter defibrillator is nowadays the only effective treatment for the prevention of sudden arrhythmic death (B.J. Maron, et al., 2000b).

12. Screening strategies

It is well known that hypertrophic cardiomyopathy is a genetic disease of the sarcomeric proteins with great heterogeneity of genetic basis and fenotypic expression which does not only involve these structures but also include abnormalities of the connective tissue, mitral valve, and intramural coronary arteries. The genetic defect may be influenced by modifiers genes and unknown enviromental factors. The strategy for clinical screening for hypertrophic cardiomyopathy with 12 lead electrocardiogram and echocardiogram in non affected family members including < 12 year-old children, is optional, unless there is history of early death due to hypertrophic cardiomyopathy or other serious complications in the family, or is an athlete in training, or evidence of incipient left ventricular hypertrophy, or onset of suspicious symptoms. In family members 12 to 18 years of age, clinical follow-up should be performed every 12 to 18 months and from then on every 5 years. The period of screening should be extended to adulthood since we now know that certain mutant genes can provoke a disease of rather late onset (B.J. Maron et al., 2004).

13. Conclusion

Great strides have been made since the rediscovery of hypertrophic cardiomyopathy in the late 50's last century. Important advances in the understanding of the genetics and physiopathology of the disease have occurred as well as development of superb imaging technologies. Treatment is tailored according to the phenotype and stage of the disease. The very important differences between adult and childhood hypertrophic cardiomyopathy have been underlined in this chapter hoping that will help physicians in decision making when dealing with these patients.

14. Aknowledgement

We thank Professor Ricardo Pignatelli from Texas Children's Hospital for providing us with excellent images from his personal archives and helpful advice.

We also thank Mr. Alfredo Benito from Photographic Resources for helping us with the artwork, and Dr. Ana Grassani for her assistance in the preparation of the manuscript.

Finally, we thank our patients for trusting us for many years.

15. References

[1] Abozguia, K.; Elliott, P.; McKenna, W.; et al. (2010). Metabolic modulator perhexiline corrects energy deficiency and improves exercise capacity in symptomatic hypertrophic cardiomyopathy. *Circulation*, Vol.122, pp. 1562-9.

[2] Alcalai, R.; Seidmann, J. & Seidman, C. (2008). Genetic basis of hypertrophic cardiomyopathy from bench to the clinic. *Cardiovasc Electrophysiol*, Vol.19, pp. 104-110.

[3] Alday, L.; Moreyra, E. (1984). Secondary hypertrophic cardiomyopathy in infancy and childhood. *Am Heart J*, Vol.108, pp. 996-1000.

[4] Alday, L.; Moreyra, E.; Juaneda, E.; et al. (1985). Hypertrophic cardiomyopathy in a child with tetralogy of Fallot. *J Cardiovasc Ultrasonography,* Vol.4, pp. 87-90.
[5] Alday, L.; Bruno, E.; Moreyra, E.; et al. (1998). Mid term results of dual-chamber pacing in children with hypertrophic obstructive cardiomyopathy. *Echocardiography,* Vol.15, pp. 289-295.
[6] Alday, L.; Moreyra, E.; Bruno, E.; et al. (2010). Left ventricular noncompaction associated with hypertrophic cardiomyopathy and Wolff-Parkinson-White syndrome. *Health,* Vol.2, pp. 200-3.
[7] Aoun, N.; Fernandes, L.; Succi, E.; et al. (1994). Beta-hemolytic streptococcus endocarditis in an adolescent with hypertrophic cardiomyopathy. *Arq Bras Cardiol,* Vol.63, pp. 211-3.
[8] Arad, M.; Maron, B.; Gorham, J.; et al. (2005). Glycogen storage diseases presenting as hypertrophic cardiomyopathy. *N Eng J Med,* Vol.352, pp. 362-72.
[9] Basso, C.; Thiene, G.; Corrado, D.; et al. (2000). Hypertrophic cardiomyopathy and sudden death in the young: pathologic evidence of myocardial ischemia. *Hum Pathol,* Vol.31, pp. 988-98.
[10] Berger, S.; Dhala, A. & Dearani J. (2009). State-of-the-art management of hypertrophic cardiomyopathy in children. *Cardiol Young,* Vol.19 (suppl 2), pp. 66-73.
[11] Berul, C.; Van Hare, G., Kertesz, N.; et al. (2008). Results of a multicenter retrospective implantable cardioverter-defibrillator registry of pediatric and congenital heart disease patients. *J Am Coll Cardiol* Vol.51, 1685-91.
[12] Biagini, E.; Coccolo, F.; Ferlito, M.; et al. (2005) Dilated-hypokinetic evolution of hypertrophic cardiomyopathy. Prevalence, incidence, risk factors, and prognostic implications in pediatric and adult patients. *J Am Coll Cardiol, Vol.* 46: 1543-50.
[13] Bobkowski, W.; Sobieszczańska, M.; Turska-Kmieć, A.; et al. (2007). Mutation of the MYH7 gene in a child with hypertrophic cardiomyopathy and Wolff-Parkinson-White syndrome. *J Appl Genet,* Vol.48, pp. 185-8.
[14] Bos, J.; Towbin, J. & Ackerman, M. (2009). Diagnostic, prognostic, and therapeutic implications of genetic testing for hypertrophic cardiomyopathy. *J Am Coll Cardiol,* Vol.54, pp. 201-11.
[15] Braunwald, E.; Lambrew, C.; Rockoff, S.; et al. (1964). Idiopathic hypertrophic subaortic stenosis. I. A description of the disease based upon an analysis of 64 patients. *Circulation,* Vol.30 (suppl. IV), pp. 3-119.
[16] Brock, R. & Fleming, P. (1956). Aortic subvalvar stenosis. *Guys Hosp Rep,* Vol.105: pp. 391-408.
[17] Bruder, O.; Wagner, A.; Jensen, C.; et al. (2010). Myocardial scar visualized by cardiovascular magnetic resonance imaging predicts major adverse events in patients with hypertrophic cardiomyopathy. *J Am Coll Cardiol,* Vol,56, pp. 875-87.
[18] Bruno, E.; Maisuls, H.; Juaneda, E.; et al. (2002). Clinical features of hypertrophic cardiomyopathy in the young. *Cardiol Young,* Vol.12, pp. 147-52.
[19] Burch, M.; Mann, J.; Sharland, M.; et al. (1992). Myocardial disarray in Noonan syndrome. *Br Heart J,* Vol.68, pp. 586-8.
[20] Cardim, N.; Oliveira, A.; Longo, S.; et al. (2003). Doppler tissue imaging: regional myocardial function in hypertrophic cardiomyopathy and in athlete's heart. *J Am Soc Echocardiogr,* Vol.16, pp. 223-32.

[21] Chimenti, C.; Pieroni, M.; Morgante, E.; et al. (2004). Prevalence of Fabry disease in female patients with late-onset hypertrophic cardiomyopathy. *Circulation,* Vol.110, pp. 1047-53.

[22] Colan, S.; Lipshultz, S.; Lowe, A.; et al. (2007). Epidemiology and cause-specific outcome of hypertrophic cardiomyopathy in children. Findings from the Pediatric Cardiomyopathy Registry. *Circulation,* Vol.115, pp. 773-81.

[23] Denfield, S.; Rosenthal, G.; Gajarski, R.; et al. (1997). Restrictive cardiomyopathies in childhood. Etiologies and natural histories. *Tex Heart Inst J,* Vol.24, pp.38-44.

[24] Decker, J.; Rossano, J.; O'Brian Smith, E.; et al. (2009). Risk factors and mode of death in isolated hypertrophic cardiomyopathy in children. *J Am Coll Cardiol,* Vol.54, pp. 250-4.

[25] Ehlers, J.; Hagstrom, J.; Lukas, D.; et al. (1962). Glycogen storage disease of the myocardium with obstruction to left ventricular outflow. *Circulation,* Vol.25, pp.96-109.

[26] Eidem, B. ; Jones, C. & Cetta, F. (2000). Unusual association of hypertrophic cardiomyopathy with complete atrioventricular canal defect and Down syndrome. *Tex Heart Inst J,* Vol.27, pp. 289-91.

[27] Elliott, P.; Poloniecki, J.; Dickie, S.; et al. (2000). Sudden death in hypertrophic cardiomyopathy: identification of high risk patients. *J Am Coll Cardiol,* Vol.36, pp. 2212-8.

[28] Elliott, P.; Andersson, B.; Arbustini, E.; et al. (2008). Classification of the cardiomyopathies: a position statement from the European Society of Cardiology Working Group on Myocardial and Pericardial Diseases. *Eur Heart J,* Vol .29(2), pp. 270-6.

[29] Eng, C.; Guffon, N.; Wilcox, W.; et al. (2001). Safety and efficacy of recombinant human alpha-galactosidase. A replacement therapy in Fabry's disease. *N Eng J Med,* Vol.345, pp. 9-16.

[30] Epstein, A.; Dimarco, J.; Ellenbogen, K.; et al. (2008). ACC/AHA/HRS 2008 guidelines for device-based therapy of cardiac rhythm abnormalities. *Heart Rhythm,* Vol.5, pp. e1-62.

[31] Falicov, R.; Resnekov, L. (1977). Mid ventricular obstruction in hypertrophic obstructive cardiomyopathy. New diagnostic and therapeutic challenge. *Brit Heart J,* Vol.39, pp. 701-5.

[32] Fananapazir, L.; Cannon, R.; Tripodi, D.; et al. (1992). Impact of dual chamber permanent pacing in patients with obstructive hypertrophic cardiomyopathy with symptoms refractory to verapamil and beta adrenergic blocker therapy. *Circulation,* Vol.85, pp. 2149-61.

[33] Ferrans, V.; Morrow, A.; Roberts, W. (1972). Myocardial ultrastructure in idiopathic hypertrophic subaortic stenosis: a study of operatively excised left ventricular outflow tract muscle in 14 patients. *Circulation,* Vol.45, pp. 769-92

[34] Franklin, R., Anderson, R., Elliot, M., et al. (1999). The European pediatric cardiac code. *Cardiol Young,* Vol.9, pp. 633-57.

[35] Galve, E.; Sambola, A.; Saldaña, G.; et al. (2010). Late benefits of dual-chamber pacing in obstructive hypertrophic cardiomyopathy: a 10-year follow-up study. *Heart,* Vol .96, pp. 352-6.

[36] Gottdiener, J.; Hawley, R.; Maron, B.; et al. (1982). Characteristics of the cardiac hypertrophy in Friedreich's ataxia. *Am Heart J*, Vol.103, pp. 525-31.
[37] Gregor, P.; Widimsky, P.; Cenenka, V; et al. (1989). Electrocardiographic changes can precede the development of myocardial hypertrophy in the setting of hypertrophic cardiomyopathy. *Int J Cardiol*, Vol.23, pp. 335-41.
[38] Grenier, M.; Osganian, S.; Cox, G.; et al. (2000). Design and implementation of the North American Pediatric Cardiomyopathy Registry. *Am Heart J*, Vol.139, pp. 586-95.
[39] Grigg, L.; Wigle, E.; Williams, W.; et al. (1992). Transesophageal Doppler echocardiography in obstructive hypertrophic cardiomyopathy: classification of pathophysiology and importance in intraoperative decision making. *J Am Coll Cardiol*, Vol.20, pp. 42-52.
[40] Gruner, C.; Care, M.; Siminovitch, K.; et al. (2011). Sarcomere protein gene mutations in patients with apical hypertrophic cardiomyopathy. *Circ Cardiovasc Genet*, Vol.4, pp. 288-95.
[41] Harris, K.; Spirito, P.; Maron, M.; et al. (2006). Prevalence, clinical profile, and significance of left ventricular remodeling in the end-stage phase of hypertrophic cardiomyopathy. *Circulation*, Vol.114, pp. 216-25.
[42] Henry,W. ; Clark, C. & Epstein, S. (1973). Asymmetric septal hypertrophy (ASH): a unifyimg link in the IHSS disease spectrum. Observations regarding its pathogenesis, pathophysiology, and course. *Circulation*, Vol.47, pp. 827-32.
[43] Hers, H. (1963). Alpha-glucosidase deficiency in generalizad glycogen storage disease (Pompe's disease). *Biochem J*, Vol.86, pp. 11-6.
[44] Ho, C.; Lopez, B.; Coelho-Filho, O; et al. (2010). Myocardial fibrosis as an early manifestation of hyprtrophic cardiomyopathy. *New Eng J Med*, Vol.363, pp. 552-63.
[45] Jensen, M.; Almaas, V.; Jacobsson, L.; et al. (2011) Long-term outcome of percutaneous transluminal septal myocardial ablation in hypertrophic obstructive cardiomyopathy. A Scandinavian multicenter study. *Circ Cardiovasc Interv*, Vol.4, pp. 256-265.
[46] Kaski, J.; Syrris, P.; Esteban, M.; et al. (2009). Prevalence of sarcomere protein gene mutations in preadolescent children with hypertrophic cardiomyopathy. *Circ Cardiovasc Genet*, Vol.2, pp. 436-41.
[47] Kawai, C.; Kato, S.; Takashima, M.; et al. (2000). Heart disease in Friedreich's ataxia: observation of a case for half a century. *Jpn Circ J*, Vol.64, pp. 229-36.
[48] Kim, L.; Devereux, R. & Basson, C. (2011). Impact of genetic insight into Mendelian disease on cardiovascular clinical practice. *Circulation*, Vol.123, pp. 544-50.
[49] Kishnani, P.; Austin, S.; Arn, P.; et al. (2010) Glycogen storage disease type III diagnosis and management guidelines. *Genet Med*, Vol.12, pp.446-63.
[50] Klues, H.; Maron, B.; Dollar, A.; et al. (1992) Diversity of structural mitral valve alterations in hypertrophyc cardiomyopathy. *Circulation*, Vol.85, pp. 1651-60.
[51] Kuhl, H. & Hanrath P. (2004). The impact of transesophageal echocardiography on daily clinical practice. *Eur J Echocardiogr*, Vol.5, pp. 455-68.
[52] Lipshultz, S.; Sleeper, L.; Towbin, J.; et al. (2003). The incidence of pediatric cardiomyopathy in two regions of the United States. *New Eng J Med*, Vol.348, pp. 1647-55.
[53] Louie, E. & Maron, B. (1987). Apical hypertrophic cardiomyopathy: clinical and two dimensional echocardiographic assessment. *Ann Intern Med*, Vol.106, pp. 663-70.

[54] Marian A.J. (2007). Hypertrophic cardiomyopathy, in *Cardiovascular genetics and genomics for the cardiologist,* Dzau & Liew, pp. 30-54, Blackwell Futura ISBN: 978-1-4051-3394-4, Malden, Massachusetts.

[55] Maron, B. ; Roberts, W.; & Epstein, S. (1982). Sudden death in hypertrophic cardiomyopathy : a profile of 78 patients. *Circulation,* Vol.65, pp. 1388-94.

[56] Maron, B.; Spirito, P.; Wesley, Y.; et al. (1986). Development and progression of left ventricular hypertrophy in children with hypertrophic cardiomyopathy. *New Engl J Med,* Vol.315, pp. 610-4.

[57] Maron, B.; Pelliccia, A.; Spataro, A.; et al. (1993). Reduction in left ventricular wall thickness after decondinioning in highly trained Olimpic athletes. *Br Heart J,* Vol.69; pp. 125-128.

[58] Maron, B.; Gardin, J.; Flack, J.; et al. (1995a). Prevalence of hypertrophic cardiomyopathy in a general population of young adults: echocardiographic analysis of 4111 subjects in the CARDIA Study Coronary Artery Risk Development in (Young) Adults. *Circulation,* Vol.92, pp. 785-89.

[59] Maron, B.; Pelliccia, A. & Spirito, P. (1995b). Cardiac disease in young trained athletes: insights into methods for distinguishing athlete's heart from structural heart disease with particular emphasis on hypertrophic cardiomyopathy. *Circulation,* Vol.91, pp. 1596-1601.

[60] Maron, B.; Olivotto, I.; Spirito, P.; et al. (2000a). Epidemiology of hypertrophic cardiomyopathy-related death: revisited in a large non-referral-based patient population. *Circulation,* Vol.102, pp. 858-64.

[61] Maron, B.; Shen, W-K.; Links, M.; et al. (2000b). Efficacy of implantable cardioverter-defibrillators for the prevention of sudden death in patients with hypertrophic cardiomyopathy. *N Engl J Med,* Vol.342, pp. 365-73.

[62] Maron, B., McKenna, W., Danielson, G., et al. (2003a). American College of Cardiology/European Society of Cardiology clinical expert consensus document on hypertrophic cardiomyopathy. *J Am Coll Cardiol,* Vol.42, pp. 1687-713.

[63] Maron, B.; Estes, N., III; Maron, M.; et al. (2003b). Primary prevention of sudden death as a novel treatment strategy in hypertrophic cardiomyopathy. *Circulation,* Vol.107, pp. 2872-75.

[64] Maron, B.; Seidman, J. & Seidman, C. (2004). Proposal for contemporary screening strategies in families with hypertrophic cardiomyopathy. *J Am Coll Cardiol,* Vol.44, pp. 2125-32.

[65] Maron, B., Towbin, J., Thiene, G., et al. (2006). Contemporary definitions and classification of the cardiomyopathies. *Circulation,* Vol.113, pp. 1807-16.

[66] Maron, B.; Maron, M.; Wigle, E.; et al. (2009). The 50-year history, controversy, and clinical implications of left ventricular outflow tract obstruction in hypertrophic cardiomyopathy. *J Am Coll Cardiol,* Vol. 54 (3), pp. 191-200.

[67] Maron, M.; Olivotto, J.; Bettochi, S.; et al. (2003). Effect of left ventricular outflow tract obstruction on clinical outcome in hypertrophic obstructive cardiomyopathy. *New Eng J Med,* Vol.348, pp. 295-303.

[68] Maron, M.; Olivotto, I.; Zenovich, A.; et al. (2006). Hypertrophic cardiomyopathy is predominantly a disease of left ventricular outflow tract obstruction. *Circulation,* Vol.114, pp. 2232-9.

[69] Maron, M.; Appelbaum, E.; Harrigan, C.; et al. (2008). Clinical profile and significance of delayed enhancement in hypertrophic cardiomyopathy. *Circ Heart Fail,* Vol.1, pp. 184-91.

[70] Maron, M.; Maron, B.; Harrigan, C.; et al. (2009). Hypertrophic cardiomyopathy phenotype revisited after 50 years with cardiovascular magnetic resonance. *J Am Coll Cardiol*, Vol.54, pp. 220-8.

[71] Maron, M.; Olivotto, I.; Harrigan, C.; et al. (2011). Mitral valve abnormalities identified by cardiovascular magnetic resonance represent a primary phenotypic expression of hypertrophic cardiomyopathy. *Circulation,* Vol.124, pp. 40-7.

[72] McKenna, W. & Deanfield, J. (1984). Hypertrophic cardiomyopathy. An important cause of sudden death. *Arch Dis Childhood,* Vol.59, pp. 971-75.

[73] McKenna, W.; Oakley, C.; Krikler D.; et al. (1985). Improved survival with amiodarone in patients with hypertrophic cardiomyopathy and ventricular tachycardia. *Br Heart J,* Vol.53, pp. 412-6.

[74] McKenna, W.; Franklin, R.; Nihoyannopoulos, P.; et al. (1988). Arrhythmia and prognosis in infants, children and adolescents with hypertrophic cardiomyopathy. *J Am Coll Cardiol,* Vol.11, pp. 147-53.

[75] McMahon, C.; Nagueh, S.; Pignatelli, R.; et al. (2004). Characterization of left ventricular diastolic function by tissue Doppler imaging and clinical status in children with hypertrophic cardiomyopathy. *Circulation,* Vol.109, pp. 1756-62.

[76] Michael, S.; Petrocine, S.; Qian, J.; et al. (2006). Iron and iron-responding proteins in the cardiomyopathy of Friedreich's ataxia. *Cerebellum,* Vol.5, pp. 257-67.

[77] Minakata K.; Dearani J.; O'Leary, P,; et al. (2005). Septal myectomy for obstructive hypertrophic cardiomyopathy in pediatric patients: early and late results. *Ann Thorac Surg,* Vol.80, pp. 1424-30.

[78] Minami, Y.; Kajimoto, K.; Terajima, Y.; et al. (2011). Clinical implications of midventricular obstruction in patients with hypertrophic cardiomyopathy. *J Am Coll Cardiol,* Vol.57, pp. 2346-55.

[79] Moolman, J.; Corfield, V.; Posen, B.; et al. (1997). Sudden death due to troponin T mutations. *J Am Coll Cardiol,* Vol.29, pp. 549-55.

[80] Moreyra, E.; Buteler, B.; Madoery, R.; et al. (1972) Drugs and maneuvers in the diagnosis of muscular subaortic stenosis. *Am Heart J,* Vol.83, pp. 431-3.

[81] Morgan-Hughes, G. & Motwani, J. (2002). Mitral valve endocarditis in hypertrophic cardiomyopathy: case report and literature review. *Heart,* Vol.87, pp. e8.

[82] Nagueh, S.; McFalls, J.; Meyer, D.; et al. (2003). Tissue Doppler imaging predicts the development of hypertrophic cardiomyopathy in subjects with subclinical disease. *Circulation,* Vol.108, pp. 395-8.

[83] Noonan, J. (1968). Hypertelorysm with Turner phenotype: a new syndrome with associated congenital heart disease. *Am J Dis Child,* Vol.116, pp. 373-80.

[84] Nora, J.; Nora, A.; Sinha, A.; et al. (1974). The Ulrich-Noonan syndrome (Turner phenotype). *Am J Dis Child,* Vol.127, pp. 48-55.

[85] Nora, J.; Lortscher, R. & Spangler, R. (1975). Echocardiographic studies of left ventricular disease in Ulrich-Noonan syndrome. *Am J Dis Child,* Vol.129, pp. 1417-20.

[86] Nugent, A.; Daubeney, P.; Chondros, P.; et al. (2003). The epidemiology of childhood cardiomyopathy in Australia. *New Eng J Med,* Vol.348, pp. 1703-5.

[87] Nugent, A.; Daubeney, P.; Chondros, P.; et al. (2005). Clinical features and outcomes of childhood hypertrophic cardiomyopathy. Results from a national population-based study. *Circulation,* Vol.112, pp. 1332-8.
[88] Niimura, H.; Bachinski, L.; Sangwatanaroj, S.; et al. (1998). Mutations in the gene for cardiac myosin-binding protein C and late-onset familial hypertrophic cardiomyopathy. *N Eng J Med,* Vol.338, pp. 1248-57.
[89] Ostman-Smith, I.; Wettrell, G.; Keeton, B.; et al. (2005). Echocardiographic and electrocardiographic identification of those children with hypertrophic cardiomyopathy who should be considered at high-risk of dying suddenly. *Cardiol Young,* Vol.15, pp. 632-42.
[90] Panza, J. & Maron, B. (1989). Relation of electrocardiographic abnormalities to evolving left ventricular hypertrophy in hypertrophic cardiomyopathy during childhood. *Am J Cardiol,* Vol.63, pp. 1258-65.
[91] Panza, J.; Maris, T. & Maron, B. (1992). Development and determinants of dynamic obstruction to left ventricular outflow in young patients with hypertrophic cardiomyopathy. *Circulation,* Vol.85, pp. 1398-405.
[92] Peirone, A.; Bruno, E.; Rossi, N.; et al. (2005). Woolly hair and palmoplantar hyperkeratosis may present with hypertrophic cardiomyopathy. *Pediatr Cardiol,* Vol.26, pp. 470-2.
[93] Roberts, A.; Allanson, J.; Jadico, S.; et al. (2006). The cardiofaciocutaneous syndrome. *J Med Genet,* Vol.43, pp. 833-842.
[94] Rosen, K.; Cameron, R.; Bigham, P. (1997). Hypertrophic cardiomyopathy presenting with 3rd-degree atrioventricular block. *Texas Heart J,* Vol.24, pp. 372-5.
[95] Sachdev, B.; Takenaka, T.; Teraguchi, H.; et al. (2002). Prevalence of Anderson-Fabry disease in male patients with late onset hypertrophic cardiomyopathy. *Circulation,* Vol.105, pp. 1407-11.
[96] Seidman, J. & Seidman, C. (2001). The genetic basis for cardiomyopathy: from mutation identification to mechanistic paradigms. *Cell,* Vol.104, pp. 557-67.
[97] Seidman, C. & Seidman, J. (2011). Identifying sarcomere gene mutations in hypertrophic cardiomyopathy. *Circ Res.* Vol.108, pp. 743-50.
[98] Shah, P.; Gramiak, R. & Kramer, D. (1969). Ultrasound localization of left ventricular outflow obstruction in hypertrophic obstructive cardiomyopathy. *Circulation,* Vol.40, pp. 3-11.
[99] Shah, P.; Gramiak, R.; Adelman, A.; et al. (1971). Role of echocardiography in diagnostic and hemodynamic assessment of hypertrophic subaortic stenosis. *Circulation,* Vol.44, pp. 891-8.
[100] Sherrid, M.; Chu, C.; Delia, E.; et al. (1993). An echocardiographic study of the fluid mechanics of obstruction in hypertrophic cardiomyopathy. *J Am Coll Cardiol,* Vol.22, pp. 816-25.
[101] Sherrid, M.; Barac, I.; McKenna, W.; et al. (2005). Multicenter study of the efficacy and safety of disopyramide in obstructive hypertrophic cardiomyopathy. *J Am Coll Cardiol,* Vol.45, pp. 1251-8.
[102] Shirani, J.; Maron, B.; Cannon, R.; et al. (1993). Clinicopathologic features of hypertrophic cardiomyopathy managed by cardiac transplantation. *Am J Cardio,* Vol.72, pp.434-40.

[103] Sigwart, U. (1995). Non-surgical myocardial reduction for hypertrophic obstructive cardiomyopathy. *Lancet,* Vol.346, pp. 211-4.
[104] Somerville, J. & Becu, L. (1978). Congenital heart disease associated with hypertrophic cardiomyopathy. *Br Heart J,* Vol.40, pp. 1034-39.
[105] Sznajer, Y.; Keren, B.; Baumann, C.; et al. (2007). The spectrum of cardiac anomalies in Noonan syndrome as a result of mutations in the *PTPN11* gene. *Pediatrics,* Vol.119, pp. e1325-31.
[106] Tartaglia, M.; Mehler, E.; Goldberg, R.; et al. (2001). Mutations in PTPN11, encoding the protein tyrosine phosphatase SHP-2, cause Noonan syndrome. *Nat Genet,* Vol.29, pp. 465-8.
[107] Teare, D. (1958). Asymmetrical hypertrophy of the heart in young adults. *Br Heart J,* Vol.20, pp. 1-8.
[108] Tikanoja, T.; Jaaskelainen, P.; Laakso, M.; et al. (1999). Simultaneous hypertrophic cardiomyopathy and ventricular septal defect in children. *Am J Cardiol,* Vol.84, pp. 485-6.
[109] Watkins, H.; Rosenzweig, A.; Hwang, D.; et al. (2009). Characteristic and prognostic implications of myosin missense mutations in familial hypertrophic cardiomyopathy. *N Eng J Med,* Vol.326, pp. 1108-14.
[110] Wigle, E.; Auger, P. & Marquis, Y. (1967). Muscular subaortic stenosis. The direct relation between the intraventricular pressure difference and the left ventricular ejection time. *Circulation,* Vol.36, pp. 36-44.
[111] Winkel, L.; Hagemans, M.; van Doorn, P.; et al. (2005). The natural course of non-classic Pompe's disease; a review of 225 published cases. *J Neurol,* Vol.252, pp. 875-84.
[112] Yamaguchi, H.; Ishimura, T.; Nishiyama, S.; et al. (1979). Hypertrophic nonobstructive cardiomyopathy with giant negative T waves (apical hypertrophy): ventriculographic and echocardiographic features in 30 patients. *Am J Cardiol,* Vol.44, pp. 401-12.

4

Quality of Life in Dilated Cardiomyopathy with Refractory Chronic Heart Failure Undergoing Devices Implantation

Elisabete Nave Leal[1], José Luís Pais Ribeiro[2] and Mário Martins Oliveira[3]
[1]Polytechnic Institute of Lisbon /School of Health Technology of Lisbon
[2]University of Porto/Faculty of Psychology and Educational Sciences
[3]Lisbon Central Hospital Center, Santa Marta Hospital
Portugal

1. Introduction

Heart failure is the final stage of most of cardiac diseases. It is a complex syndrome in which the patients should have the following features: symptoms of heart failure, typically shortness of breath at rest or during exertion, and/or fatigue; signs of fluid retention such as pulmonary congestion or ankle swelling; and objective evidence of an abnormality of the structure or function of the heart at rest. This progressive syndrome as a high incidence and prevalence and poor prognosis: four-year mortality is around 50% with 40% of the patients admitted to hospital dying or readmitted within a year (European Society of Cardiology, 2008). With ageing, many patients will develop chronic heart failure, which, because of its symptoms, patient's awareness of their risk of dying, and the effects of therapy, together with frequent hospitalizations, has considerable impact on patient's health-related quality of life.

In the actual field of management, implantable devices have an important role for select patients. According to the European Society of Cardiology guidelines for the diagnosis and treatment of acute and chronic heart failure (2008), cardiac resynchronization therapy with defibrillator function is recommended to reduce morbidity and mortality in patients in New York Heart Association III-IV class who are symptomatic despite optimal medical therapy, and who have a reduced ejection fraction (left ventricular ejection fraction ≤35%) and QRS prolongation (QRS width ≥120 ms) and implantable cardioverter-defibrillator is recommended for primary prevention of sudden death to reduce mortality in patients with ventricular dysfunction due to prior myocardial infarction or non-ischemic cardiomyopathy with a left ventricular ejection fraction ≤35% in New York Heart Association functional class II or III, receiving optimal medical therapy, and who have reasonable expectation of survival with good functional status for more than one year.

The effect of these therapies in the quality of life in general and regarding the type of therapeutic response in particular is a field under investigation.

The aim of this study was to evaluate the impact of cardiac resynchronization therapy and implantable cardioverter-defibrillator in the quality of life of patients with chronic heart failure refractory to optimal pharmacological therapy in the first six months after device implantation.

2. Method

2.1 Participants

From ninety-six patients with chronic heart failure refractory to optimal pharmacological therapy in consecutive sequential analysis, fifty-two underwent implantation of cardiac resynchronization therapy system combined with implantable cardioverter-defibrillator and forty-four systems with implantable cardioverter-defibrillator alone for primary prevention of sudden death.

In the cardiac resynchronization therapy group, age was 64,2±8,9 (37-78) years with 35 males and 17 females, left ventricular ejection fraction was 24,6±5,4 (11-35)% and 94% in class III of the New York Heart Association classification. The etiology was mostly idiopathic (46,2%) or ischemic (34,6%).

In the implantable cardioverter-defibrillator group, age was 61,1±12,6 (25-83) years with 38 males and 6 females, left ventricular ejection fraction was 26,1±5,4 (15-37)% and 82,9% in class II of New York Heart Association classification. The etiology was mostly ischemic (75%) (Figure 1).

	Characteristics	Cardiac Resyncrhronization Therapy	Implantable Cardioverter-Defibrillator
Age	M	64,2	61,1
	DP	8,9	12,6
Gender	Male	67,3%	86,4%
	Female	32,7%	13,6%
Left Ventricular Ejection Fraction	M	24,6%	26,1%
	DP	5,4	5,4
New York Heart Association Classification	Class I	0%	0%
	Class II	4,0%	82,9%
	Class III	94%	17,1%
	Class IV	2%	0%
Etiology of Chronic Heart Failure	Ischemic	34,6%	75,0%
	Hypertensive	7,7%	0%
	Valvular	7,7%	2,3%
	Idiopathic	46,2%	20,5%
	Other	3,8%	2,3%

Fig. 1. Population Characteristics

2.2 Instruments and procedure

Patients were assessed at admission, immediately before the intervention, and in the outpatient clinic within 6 months. We considered functionality by the New York Heart Association classification, left ventricular ejection fraction and the quality of life Kansas City Cardiomyophathy Questionnaire.

The Kansas City Cardiomyopathy Questionnaire (Green et al., 2000) validated for the portuguese population (Nave-Leal et al., 2010) is composed of twenty three items divided into five domains: physical limitation, symptoms, quality of life, self-efficacy and social interference. The physical limitation domain measures the extent to which congestive heart failure symptoms have limited some of the patient's physical activities over the previous two weeks. The symptom domain assesses the number of times that congestive heart failure symptoms such as fatigue, dyspnea or limb edema have occurred in the previous two weeks and whether there have been changes in symptoms during the same period. The self-efficacy domain measures the patient's knowledge of how to avoid worsening of symptoms and of what to do if this occurs. The quality of life domain evaluates patients' perception of their enjoyment of life and of their sense of discouragement due to their heart failure, while the social interference domain assesses how congestive heart failure affects the patient's lifestyle. To facilitate interpretability, two summary scores were developed: the first, the functional status score, combines the physical limitation and symptom domains, and the second, the clinical summary score, combines the functional status score with the quality of life and social interference domains (Figure 2).

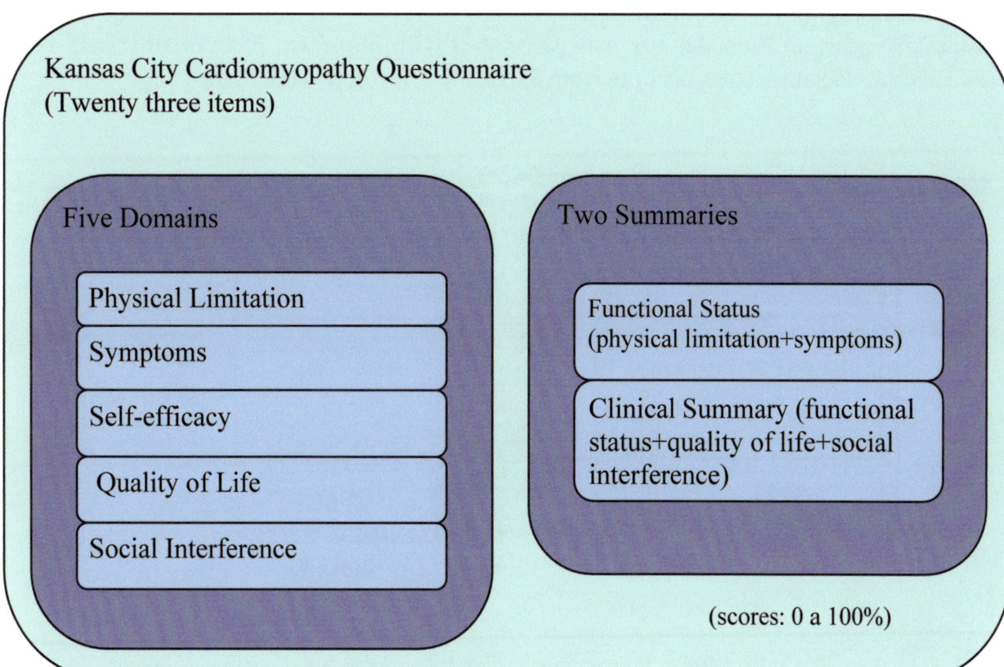

Fig. 2. Domains and Summaries of the Kansas City Cardiomyopathy Questionnaire

His psychometrics proprieties shows that it's a good instrument regarding fidelity, validity, sensitive to clinical change and specific to measure quality of life in a population with chronic heart failure.

The New York Heart Association classification (The Criteria Committee of the New York Heart Association, 1994 cited by European Society of Cardiology, 2008) measures the functional capacity based on the severity of symptoms and limitation of physical activity and is the most widely used measure to assess functionality of cardiac patients. Class I is defined as the absence of limitations on the exercise usually does not cause fatigue, dyspnoea or palpitations; Class II is characterized by a slight limitation of physical activity, being comfortable at rest but ordinary physical activity causes fatigue, palpitations or dyspnea; Class III is defined by a marked limitation of physical activity, being comfortable at rest but in a less intense activity that usually causes symptoms of heart failure, class IV is characterized by an inability to perform any physical activity without discomfort, where the symptoms of heart failure are present.

The left ventricular ejection fraction calculated by echocardiography in a percentage below 35% is indicative of poor prognosis.

3. Results

During the first six months of follow-up post-implant there was no detection of sustained ventricular tachyarrhythmias.

3.1 Cardiac resynchronization therapy

Cardiac resynchronization therapy was associated with improved functionality with New York Heart Association classification, from 3,0±0,2 to 2,1±0,5, $\rho<0.05$ (Figure 3).

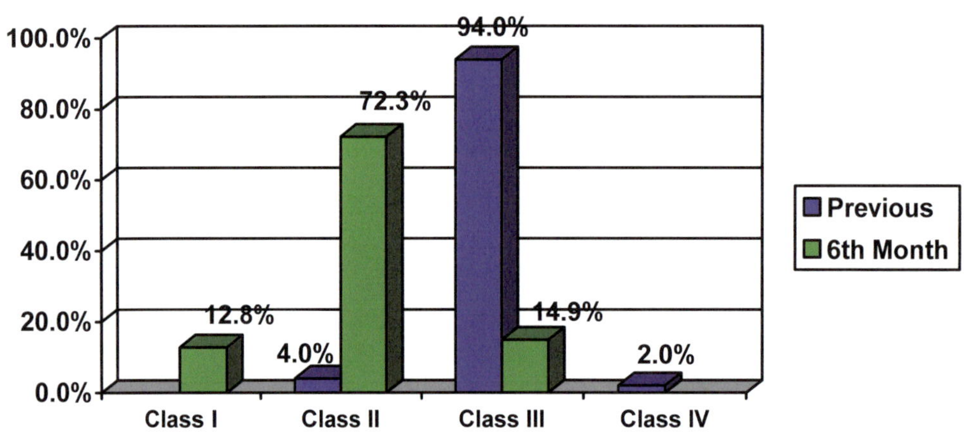

Fig. 3. Functionality at 6th Month Follow-up in Cardiac Resynchronization Therapy

This therapy improved left ventricular ejection fraction, from 24,6±6,4% to 35,5±11,9%, $\rho<0.05$ (Figure 4).

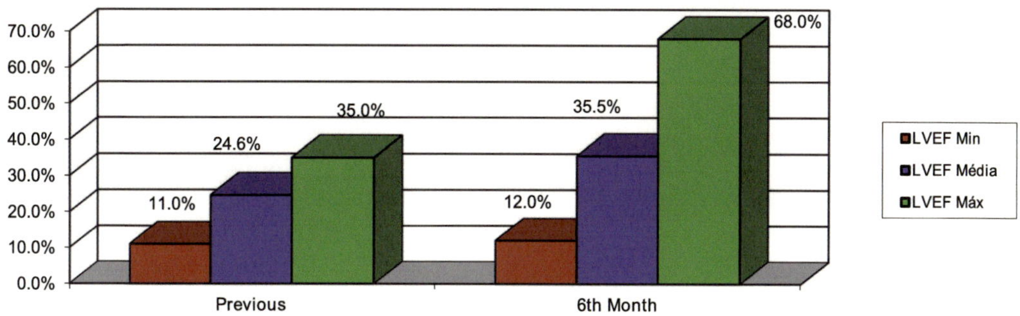

Fig. 4. Left Ventricular Ejection Fraction (LVEF) at 6th Month Follow-up in Cardiac Resynchronization Therapy

Cardiac resynchronization therapy improved quality of life in the various fields and sums assessed except for the self-efficacy domain, high before this therapy (from 81,6±28,9 to 88,1±24,1, non significant): physical limitation domain from 52,3±26,7 to 83,1±23,6; symptoms domain from 55,6±27,6 to 80,1±22,3; quality of life domain from 37,4±30,1 to 75,9±28,6; social interference domain from 57,8±30,9 to 84,6±25,9; functional status sum from 55,7±25,6 to 82,7±20,7 and clinical summary sum from 53,1±25,7 to 81,1±22,1,$\rho<0.05$ (Figure 5).

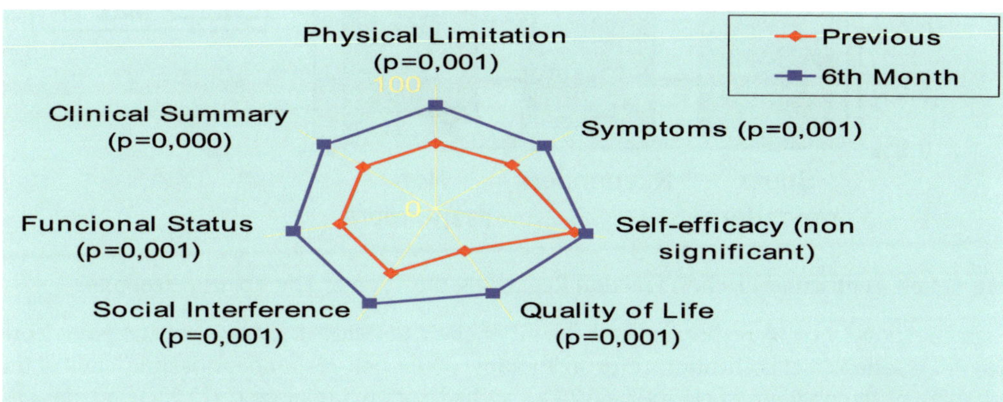

Fig. 5. Quality of Life at 6th Month Follow-up in Cardiac Resynchronization Therapy

We have stratified some of these patients regarding the type of therapeutic response: thirty four patients responded to this therapeutic and nine did not respond to cardiac resynchronization therapy.

Fifteen patients have a left ventricular ejection fraction superior to 45% post cardiac resynchronization therapy and were classified as super-responders, nineteen patients have a sustained improvement in functional class and an increase in left ventricular ejection fraction of 15% and were classified as responders and nine patients have no clinical or left ventricular ejection fraction improvement and were classified as non-responders.

The age and the etiology was identical (65,1±8,2 years between 48-75 years, 63,2±11,1 years between 37-78 and 62,8±6,1 years between 55-71 years for super-responders, responders e non-responders respectively and etiology mainly idiopathic with the majority of the cases

followed by ischemic etiology according to the results described for the whole group submitted to cardiac resynchronization therapy) but the gender was different with super-responders being in majority women (53,3% female and 46,7% male) and responders and non responders being in majority men (84,2% male and 15,8% female and 77,8% men and 22,2% female for responders and non-responders respectively).
Super-responders had a left ventricular ejection fraction prior to cardiac resynchronization therapy average superior to 25% (29,5±4,5) while responders and non responders presented a left ventricular ejection fraction prior to cardiac resynchronization therapy average inferior to 25% (22,6±6,2 and 23,9±6,5) (Figure 6).

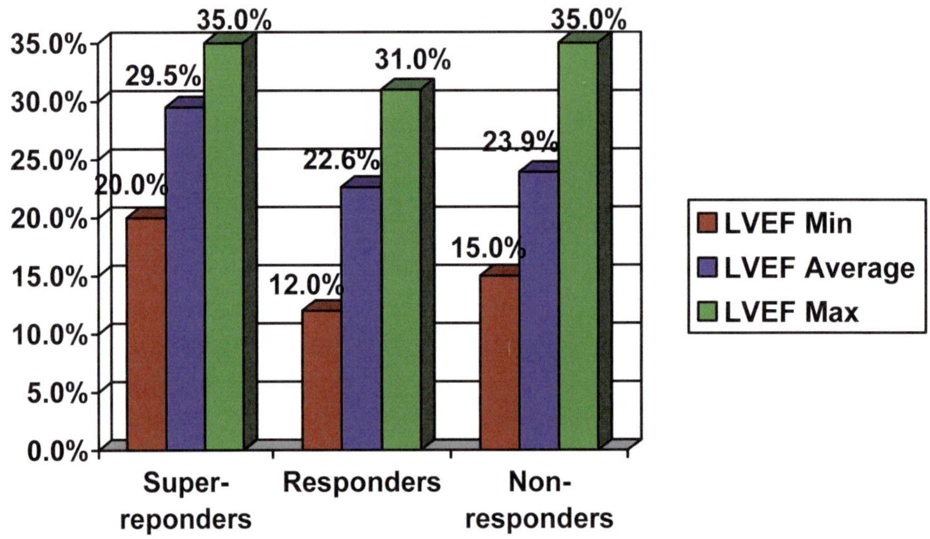

Fig. 6. Left Ventricular Ejection Fraction Regarding the Type of Therapeutic Response

Super responders and responder had the all of their patients in class III of the New York Heart Association classification prior to therapy while non-responders despite having the majority of the patients in class III (66,7%) also had patients in class II (22,2%) and class IV (11,1%) of the New York Heart Association classification prior to therapy (Figure 7).
Non responders presented a low quality of life before this therapy and have not perceived any improvement on their quality of life (physical limitation domain from 25,2±21,9 to 59,1±37,4; symptoms domain from 46,5±33,3 to 63,6±28,2; self-efficacy domain from 95,8±7,3 to 97,59±7,1; quality of life domain from 20,8±27,4 to 52,1±35,1; social interference domain from 37,5±31,5 to 63,8±36,8; functional status sum from 38,1±28,9 to 63,8±30,4 and clinical summary sum from 34,8±28,4 to 60,1±32,2) (Figure 8).
Super-responders and responders started with a better perception of their quality of life and identify improvement in quality of life in all dimensions and sums,p≤0,05 except for the auto-efficacy dimension in responders where there was no statistical significant change (physical limitation domain from 51,8±24,6 to 90,4,1±13,7; symptoms domain from 53,9±27,6 to 84,5±21,8; self-efficacy domain from 76,2±34,3 to 95,7±11,6; quality of life domain from 38,7±31,6 to 85,1±24,5; social interference domain from 55,8±27,1 to 85,7±28,9; functional status sum from 55,3±22,6 to 87,7±17,4 and clinical summary sum from 52,6±23,4 to

60,1±32,2 for super responders and physical limitation domain from 63,1±23,7 to 89,1±15,3; symptoms domain from 60,1±25,7 to 82,4±20,9; self-efficacy domain from 76,9±33,1 to 83,3±26,8; quality of life domain from 39,8±27,4 to 75,1±27,6; social interference domain from 63,9±31,7 to 90,2±18,3; functional status sum from 62,6±23,8 to 86,6±15,7 and clinical summary sum from 59,2±23,7 to 84,9±17,8 for responders) (Figure 9 and Figure 10).

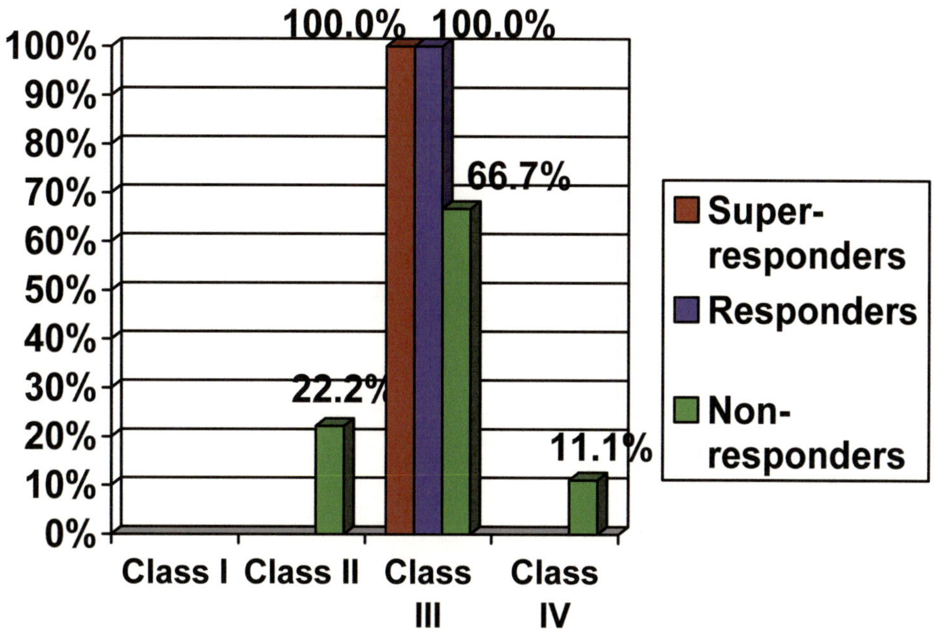

Fig. 7. New York Heart Association Classification Regarding the Type of Therapeutic Response

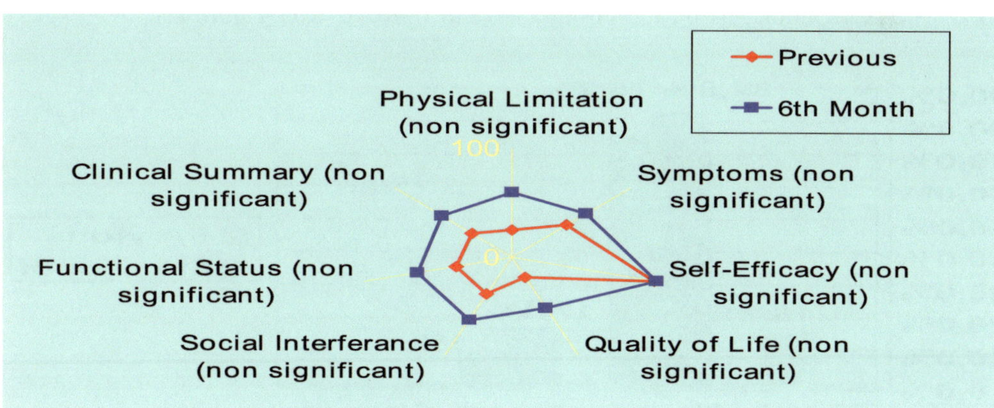

Fig. 8. Quality of Life in Non-responders

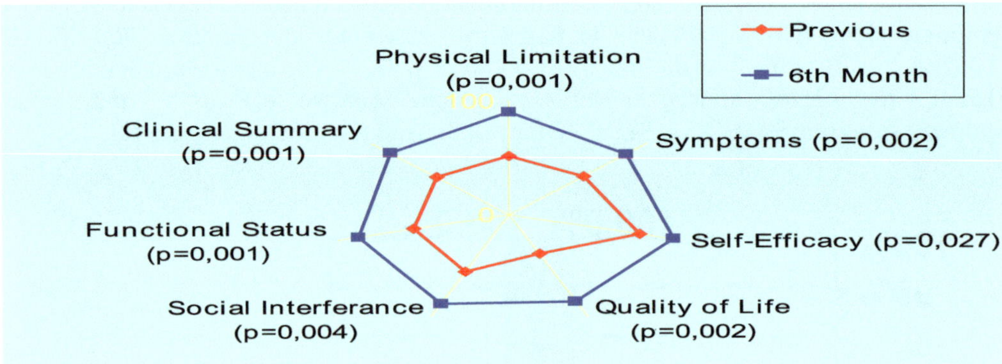

Fig. 9. Quality of Life in Super-responders

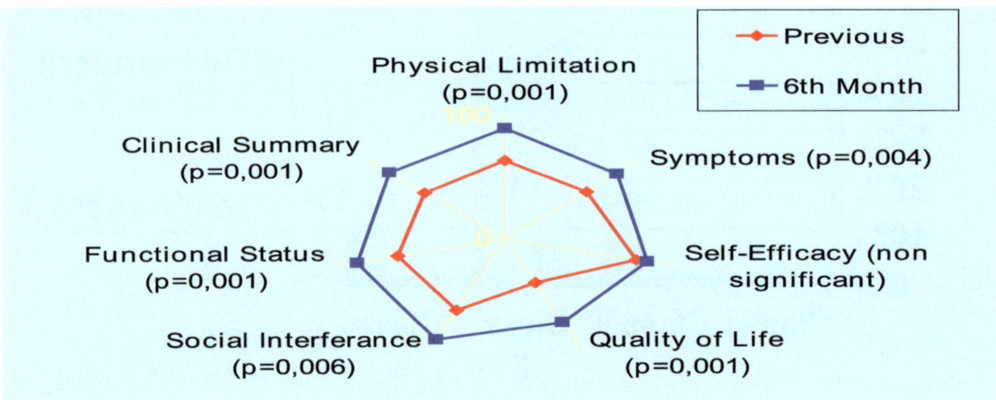

Fig. 10. Quality of Life in Responders

3.2 Implantable cardioverter-defibrillator

Implantable cardioverter defibrillator was associated with improved functionality with New York Heart Association classification from 2,1±0,3 to 1,9±0,5 $\rho<0.05$ (Figure 11).

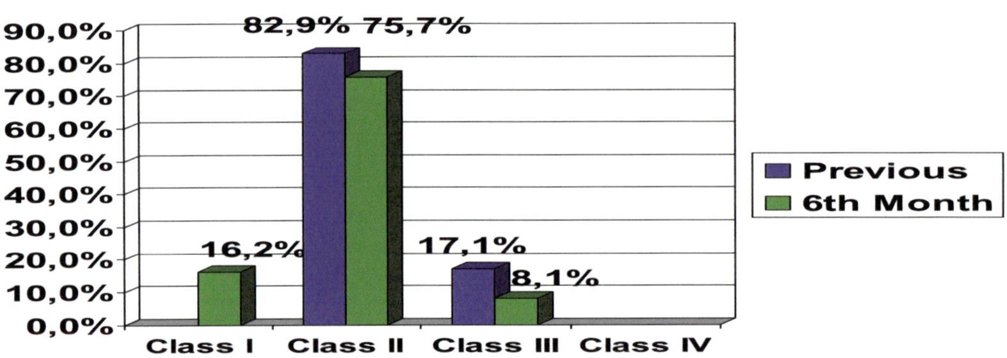

Fig. 11. Functionality at 6th Month Follow-up in Implantable Cardioverter Defibrillator

This device was not associated with improvement in left ventricular ejection fraction (from 26,1±5,4 to 26,4±5,9), where changes were no significant (Figure 12).

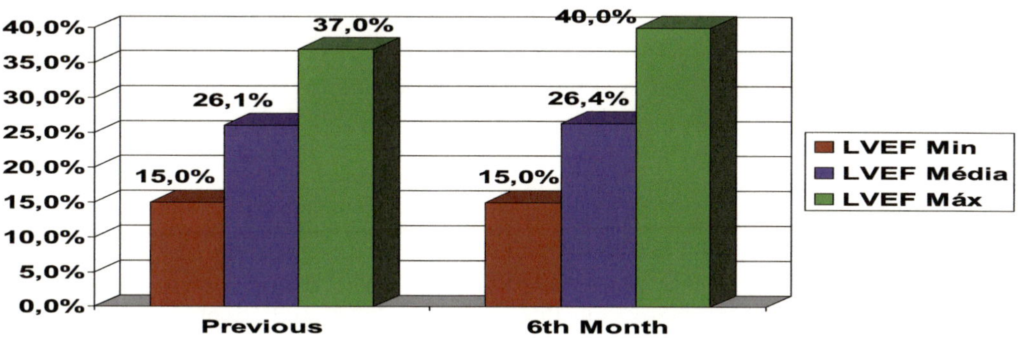

Fig. 12. Left Ventricular Ejection Fraction (LVEF) at 6th Month Follow-up in Implantable Cardioverter Defibrillator

Implantable cardioverter-defibrillator improved quality of life only in social interference domain from 73,9±34,4 to 82,7±27,5, quality of life domain from 54,3±32,1 to 71,1±28,1 and clinical summary sum from 72,4±24,1 to 78,4±25,1,$\rho<0.05$. In the physical limitation domain (from 76,2±24,5 to 80,4±26,1), symptoms domain (from 73,6±24,7 to 78,1±24,6), self-efficacy domain (from 80,3±26,2 to 83,6±25,1) and functional status sum (from 76,2±23,1 to 80,4±23,9), changes were no significant (Figure 13). Initial scores in every dimension and sum were high before the implantation of this device.

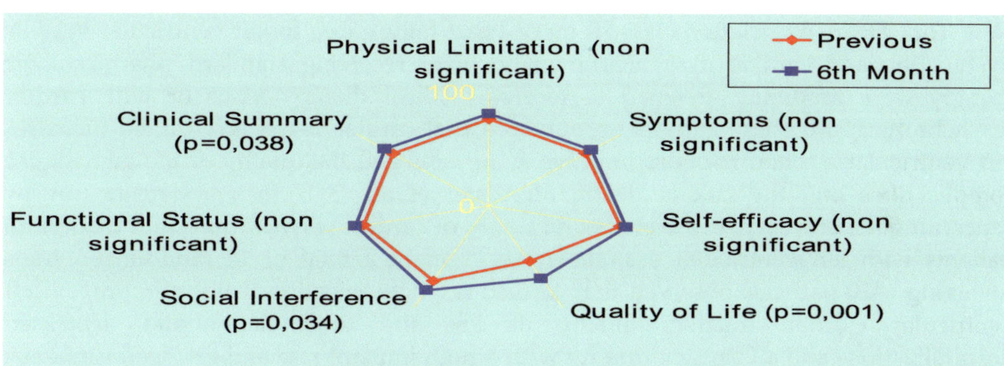

Fig. 13. Quality of Life at 6th Month Follow-up in Implantable Cardioverter Defibrillator

4. Discussion

In this study the cardiac resynchronization therapy combined with implantable cardioverter-defibrillator improved left ventricular function, functionality and quality of life at six months follow-up. According to the European Cardiac Society, 2008 the survival advantage of cardiac resynchronization therapy with implantable cardioverter-defibrillator has not been adequately addressed. However due to the documented effectiveness of implantable cardioverter-defibrillator therapy in the prevention of sudden cardiac death, the use of cardiac resynchronization therapy associated to implantable cardioverter-defibrillator is commonly preferred in clinical practice in patients satisfying cardiac resynchronization therapy criteria including an expectation of survival with good functional status for more than one year. Lousano et al., 2005 in the VENTAK CHF/CONTAK CD study followed 490 heart failure patients with indication for an implantable cardioverter-defibrillator compared antitachycardia pacing efficacy in patients with or without cardiac resynchronization therapy. These authors encountered that the efficacy of biventricular antitachycardia pacing in heart failure patients is significantly better in those with cardiac resynchronization therapy than in those without.

Other studies have identified the benefits of this therapy in mortality and morbidity of patients with heart failure. Bristow et al., 2004 in the COMPANION study analysed the effect of the cardiac resynchronization therapy in mortality and hospitalization among patients with advanced chronic heart failure and intraventricular conduction delays. 1520 patients in New York Heart Association class III or IV due to ischemic or non-ischemic cardiomyopathies and a QRS interval of at least 120 ms were randomly assigned in three groups to receive optimal pharmacologic therapy (diuretics, angiotensin-converting-enzyme inhibitors, beta-blockers and spironolactone) alone or in combination with cardiac resynchronization therapy with either a pacemaker or a pacemaker-defibrillator. These authors encountered that cardiac resynchronization therapy decreases the combined risk of death from any cause or first hospitalization and, when combined with an implantable defibrillator, significantly reduces mortality. Cleland et al., 2005 in the CARE-HF study analyzed the effects of cardiac resynchronization therapy on morbidity and mortality among patients with heart failure due to left ventricular systolic dysfunction and cardiac dyssynchrony. 813 patients with New York Heart Association class III or IV heart failure due to left ventricular systolic dysfunction and cardiac dyssynchrony who were receiving standard pharmacologic therapy were randomly assigned to receive medical therapy alone or with cardiac resynchronization. These authors encountered that cardiac resynchronization increases left ventricular ejection fraction, improve symptoms and the quality of life and reduce complications and the risk of death. McAlister et al., 2007 in a systematic review concerning the efficacy, effectiveness and safety of cardiac resynchronization therapy in patients with left ventricular systolic dysfunction in a total of 14 randomized trials involving 4420 patients, observed that cardiac resynchronization therapy improved left ventricular ejection fraction, quality of life and functionality and decreased hospitalizations and all cause mortality with a high implant rate and low lead problems during eleven months follow-up. They conclude that this therapy reduces morbidity and mortality in patients with left ventricular systolic dysfunction, prolonged QRS duration and New York Heart Association class III and IV symptoms when combined with optimal pharmacotherapy. About the sustained effect of this therapy Sutton et al., 2006 in the MIRACLE study followed 228 patients submitted to cardiac resynchronization therapy during twelve months post-implantation to determine whether reverse left ventricular remodeling and symptomatic benefit from this therapy were sustained at one year and if so, in what proportion. These authors encountered that reverse left ventricular remodeling and symptom benefit are sustained at twelve months in patients with New York Heart Association class III/IV heart failure but occur to a lesser degree in patients with ischemic versus non-ischemic etiology, according to them most likely owing to the inexorable progression of ischemic disease.

Despite the good results achieved with cardiac resynchronization therapy according to Santos et al., 2006 one third of the patients do not benefit from it. In our study, from forty-three patients, eight did not respond to this therapy. This group identified a low quality of live before implantation and did not perceive any improvement after cardiac resynchronization therapy. Also in this non-responding group we had patients in class II to IV of the New York Heart Association classification before intervention. Interestingly the super-responders were majority women and have a left ventricular ejection fraction prior to implantation superior to 25%. The response to this therapy was associated to improvement of quality of life perceived by the patients and a New York Heart Association class III classification before implantation. There are few studies regarding the predictors of response to this therapy. Quiao et al., 2011 in a study with seventy-six consecutive patients submitted to cardiac resynchronization therapy divided in to super-responders, responders and non-responders conclude that patients with a smaller left ventricle would have a better chance to become super-responders. Santos et al., 2006 in twenty-three consecutive patients with heart failure refractory to medical therapy who underwent cardiac resynchronization therapy studied regarding the type of response before and six months after the procedure evaluating clinical, electrocardiographic and echocardiography characteristics concluded that left ventricular dyssynchrony can be quantified by tissue Doppler imaging using QS (max-min) and values greater than 60 ms can identify responders to this therapy. This actual field under investigation requires more studies to determine the reasons for a percentage of these patients do not respond to cardiac resynchronization therapy including personal characteristics of the patients.

In this study implantable cardioverter-defibrillator alone was associated with improvement of functionality and quality of life already high in baseline due to the majority of the patients being in class II of the New York Heart Association classification. When looking to the various dimensions concerning the quality of life we stated that this improvement is observed in social and quality of life domains with this patients referring improvement of the perception of their enjoyment of life and of their sense of discouragement due to their heart failure and how congestive heart failure affects the patient's lifestyle at six month follow-up, emphasizing the necessity of looking to all dimensions evaluated in quality of life and not only the overall score to characterize the evolution of patients to clinical interventions. It is known the effect of this device on improving survival, however remains unclear the effect of this treatment in quality of life. Bardy et al., 2005 in the SCD-HeFT study concerning the effect of amiodarone or a conservatively programmed, shock-only implantable cardioverter-defibrillator in reducing the risk of death in patients with mild-to-moderate congestive heart failure, followed 2521 patients in class II or III with chronic stable heart failure due to ischemic or non-ischemic causes and left ventricular ejection fraction ≤35% randomized for receiving amiodarone, implantable cardioverter-defibrillator or placebo. These authors encountered that in patients with mild-to-moderate congestive heart failure, conservatively programmed, shock-only implantable cardioverter-defibrillator significantly reduces risk of death while amiodarone shown no benefit compared with placebo; implantable cardioverter-defibrillator therapy had significant benefit in patients with New York Heart

Association class II but no significant effect in patients with class III; amiodarone had no benefit in patients with New York Heart Association class II and showed a significant reduction in survival in patients with class III compared to placebo. Noyes et al., 2009 in the MADIT-II study followed 938 patients randomized to receive an implantable cardioverter-defibrillator or medical therapy alone during thirty six months. These authors encountered that development of congestive heart failure and shocks among patients and their negative effect on quality of life may partially explain the lack of quality of life benefit from this therapy. Probst et al., 2011 have studied the psychological impact of implantable cardioverter-defibrillator on Brugada syndrome patients. 190 patients were divided in three groups: symptomatic implanted patients, asymptomatic implanted patients and asymptomatic patients without implantable cardioverter-defibrillator and were evaluated regarding the quality of life. These authors concluded that whatever the group, Brugada patients have a good quality of life with no difference between implanted and non-implanted patients. Despites the difficulties in their social and professional life regarding the tolerance of this device, patients considered implantation of cardioverter-defibrillator reassuring.

5. Conclusion

In a selected population with severe chronic heart failure, cardiac resynchronization therapy was associated with improvement in all domains of quality of life, functional class and left ventricular function. Regarding the type of response to this therapy, patients with positive clinical response and reverse remodeling, obtained a favorable impact in all dimensions of quality of life, while the group without response showed no improvement, with some differences between the responding and the non-responding patients like gender, perceived quality of life and the New York Heart association classification prior to implantation of the device that needs further investigation.

Implantable cardioverter-defibrillator benefits were restricted to the social dimension of quality of life and perception of life satisfaction, indicating that this intervention as no unfavorable impact in quality of life in the first six months after the implantation of this device in patients without detection of sustained ventricular tachyarrhythmias

6. Acknowledgements

The authors are grateful to the following bodies and staff of Hospital de Santa Marta: the Administrative Board; the Ethics Committee; cardiologists and cardiopneumologists of the arrhythmology clinic; and cardiologists of the heart failure clinic.

7. References

Bardy, G., Lee, K., Mark, D., Poole, J., Packer, D., Boineau, R., Domansky, M., Troutman, C., Anderson, J., Johnson, G., McNulty, S., Clapp-Channing, N., Davidson-Ray, L., Fraulo, E., Fishbein, D., Luceri, R., & Ip, J. (2005). Amiodarone or an implantable cardioverter-defibrillator for congestive heart failure.*The New England Journal of Medicine,* Vol.352,pp. 225-237

Bristow, M., Saxon, L., Boehmer, J., Krueger, S., Kass, D., De Marco, T., Carson, P., DiCarlo, L., DeMets, D., White, B., DeVries, D., & Feldman, A. (2004). Cardiac-Resynchronization Therapy with or without an Implantable Defibrillator in Advanced Chronic Heart Failure. *The New England Journal of Medicine,* Vol.350, No.21 (May 2004),pp. 2140-2150

Cleland, J., Daubert, J., Erdmam, E., Fremantle, N., Gras, D., Kappenberger, L., & Tavazzi, L. (2005). The Effect of Cardiac Resynchronization on Morbidity and Mortality in Heart Failure. *The New England Journal of Medicine,* Vol.325, No.15 (April 2005),pp. 1539-1549

European Society of Cardiology (2008). ESC Guidelines for the diagnosis and treatment of acute and chronic heart failure *2008. European Heart Journal,* vol. 29,pp. 2388-2442

Green, C., Porter, C., Bresnahan, D., & Spertus, J. (2000) Development and Evaluation of the Kansas City Cardiomyopathy Questionnaire: A New Health Status Measure for Heart Failure. *Journal of the American College of Cardiology,* Vol.35, No.5,pp. 1245-1255

Lousano, I., Higgins, S., Villa, J., Niazi, I., Toquero, J., Yong, P., Madrid, A., & Pulpón, L. (2005) Antitachycardia Pacing Efficacy Significantly Improves With Cardiac Resynchronization Therapy. *Revista Espanhola de Cardiology,* Vol.58, No.10,pp. 1148-1154

McAlister, F., Ezekowitz, J., Hooton, N., Vandermeer, B., Spooner, C., Dryden, D., Page, R., Hlatky, M., & Rowe, B. (2007). Cardiac Resynchronization Therapy for Patients with Left Ventricular Systolic Dysfunction: A Systematic Review. *Journal of the American Medical Association,* Vol.297, No.22,pp. 2502-2514

Nave-Leal, E., Pais-Ribeiro, J., Oliveira, M., Nogueira da Silva, J. Soares, R, Fragata, J. & Ferreira, R. (2010). Psychometric Properties of the Portuguese Version of the Kansas City Cardiomyopathy Questionnaire in Dilated Cardiomyopathy with Congestive Heart Failure. *Revista Portuguesa de Cardiologia,* Vol.29, No.3,pp. 353-372

Noyes, K., Corona, E., Veazie, P., Dick, A., Zhao, H., & Moss, A. (2009). Examination of the Effect of Implantable Cardioverter-Defibrillators on Health Related Quality of Life: Based on Results from the Multicenter Automatic Defibrillator Trial-II. *American Journal of Cardiovascular Drugs,* Vol.9, No.6,pp. 393-400

Probst, V., Plassard-Kerdon-Cuf, D., Mansourati, J., Mabo, P., Sacher, F., Fruchet, C., Babuty, D., Lande, G., Guyomarc´h, B., & Le Marec, H. (2011). The Psychological Impact of Implantable Cardioverter Defibrillator Implantation on Brugada Syndrome Patients. *Europace,* Vol.13, No.7,pp. 1034-1039

Quiao, Q., Ding, L., Hua, W., Chen, K., Wang, F., & Zhang, S. (2011). Potencial Predictors of Non-response to Cardiac Resynchronization Therapy. *Chinese Medical Journal,* Vol.124, No.9 (May 2011),pp. 1338-1441

Santos, J., Parreira, L., Madeira, J., Seixo, F., Mendes, L., Lopes, C., Venâncio, J., Lourenço, J., Caetano, F., Inês, L., & Mendes, M. (2006). Predictors of Response to Cardiac Resynchronization Therapy: Importance of Left Ventricular

Dyssynchrony. *Revista Portuguesa de Cardiologia*, Vol.25, No.6 (June 2006),pp. 569-581

Sutton, M., Plappert, T., Hilpisch, B., Abraham, W., Hayes, D., & Chinchoy, E. (2006). Sustained Reverse Left Ventricular Structural Remodling with Cardiac Resynchronization at One Year in Function of Etiology. *Circulation*, Vol.113,pp. 266-272

5

Peripartum Cardiomyopathy: A Systematic Review

Viviana Aursulesei and Mihai Dan Datcu
University of Medicine and Pharmacy "Gr. T. Popa", Iasi
Romania

1. Introduction

Peripartum cardiomyopathy (PPCM) is a rare but potentially life-threatening condition that occurs in previously healthy women during the last month of pregnancy and up to 5-6 months postpartum. The etiology and pathophysiology remain uncertain, although recent observations strongly suggest the specific role of prolactin cleavage secondary to unbalanced peri/postpartum oxidative stress. PPCM is a diagnosis of exclusion, as it shares many clinical characteristics with other forms of systolic heart failure secondary to cardiomyopathy. The heart failure management requires a multidisciplinary approach during pregnancy, considering the possible adverse effects on the fetus. After delivery, the treatment is in accordance with the current guidelines of heart failure. Some novel therapies, such as prolactin blockade, are proposed to either prevent or treat the patients with PPCM. A critical individual counseling concerning the risks of subsequent pregnancy must be considered. Because of its rare incidence, geographical differences, and heterogeneous presentation, PPCM continues to be incompletely characterized and understood. For all these reasons, PPCM remains a challenge in clinical practice, so future epidemiological trials and national registries are needed to learn more about the disease.

2. Historical perspective, definition, nomenclature

Peripartum cardiomyopathy has been described since the 19th century. In 1849, Ritchie was the first to establish a relationship between heart failure and puerperium (Ritchie, 1849). After 20 years, Virchow and Porak reported autopsy evidence of myocardial degeneration in females who died in the puerperium (Porak, 1880).

However, PPCM was not recognized as a distinctive form of cardiomyopathy until 1937, when Gouley et al. described the clinical and pathological features of seven pregnant women. The patients had severe or fatal heart failure associated with a dilated cardiomyopathy in the later months of pregnancy, which persisted after delivery, and autopsy findings of enlarged hearts with focal areas of fibrosis and necrosis, but no ischemic lesions. The authors remarked these features as atypical compared with those of other forms of myocardial failure and proposed that this heart failure was related to pregnancy and puerperium, directly or indirectly (Gouley et al., 1937). Since then, there were many reports on this form of cardiomyopathy. In 1965, Walsh et al. was the first to propose the specific

period for the diagnosis, and highlighted that other conditions, which may be revealed by pregnancy, labor or postpartum period, must be excluded (Walsh et al., 1965).
In 1971, Demakis et al. described the natural history of 27 pregnant females who presented with cardiomegaly and congestive heart failure and defined the condition *peripartum cardiomyopathy* (Demakis et al., 1971). The investigators established 3 original diagnostic criteria, which were subsequently confirmed by the National Heart Lung and Blood Institute [NHLBI] and the Office of Rare Diseases of the National Institutes of Health [NIH] Workshop, and completed with an echocardiographic criterion (Pearson et al., 2000). The new definition based on the presence of 4 criteria is summarized in Table 1.

Classic criteria (Demakis et al., 1971)
1. The development of heart failure in the last month of pregnancy or within the first 5 months postpartum
2. The absence of an identifiable cause for heart failure
3. The absence of recognizable heart disease prior to the last month of pregnancy
Additional criterion (NHLBI & the Office of Rare Disease of NIH, 1997)
4. Left ventricular systolic dysfunction demonstrated by classic echocardiographic criteria (depressed ejection fraction or shortening fraction)

Table 1. Original definition of peripartum cardiomyopathy

In 1999, Hibbard et al. proposed a more precise echocardiographic criterion that parallels those for detecting idiopathic dilated cardiomyopathy (Hibbard et al., 1999) (Table 2). The new definition has been widely accepted and has improved the diagnosis of both ventricular dysfunction and PPCM. The original definition states that PPCM must develop during the last month of pregnancy or within 5 months after delivery. However, several reports described females who presented with clear PPCM symptoms earlier during pregnancy (Alvarez, 2001; Brown, 1992; Forssell, 1994; Rizeq, 1994; Yahagi, 1994). In 2005, Elkayam et al. provided the largest retrospective database, challenging the classic criteria when they found that clinical course and outcome of females with pregnancy-associated cardiomyopathy diagnosed earlier than the last gestational month are similar to those of females with traditional PPCM. The authors concluded that these two conditions might represent a continuum of a spectrum of the same disease (Elkayam et al., 2005). Since then, several definitions have been proposed (Table 2).
In 2010, the experts considered the modification of the first criterion might be necessary. This definition specifically excludes females who develop cardiomyopathy early in their pregnancy and emphasizes that not all cases of PPCM present with LV dilation. In addition, it is recommended that other conditions which may be exacerbated and associated with heart failure in the puerperium, are excluded before the diagnosis of PPCM is considered. However, in clinical practice, it remains difficult to distinguish females with preexisting asymptomatic cardiomyopathy, progressing during pregnancy and labor, from actual PPCM females (Sliwa et al., 2010a).
Ever since the early descriptions of PPCM, the condition has been defined by several confusing names, such as post-partum heart failure, post-partum myocarditis, Meadow's syndrome, idiopathic myocardial degeneration associated with pregnancy, Zaria syndrome, toxic post-partum heart disease, or recently, postpartal heart disease, post-partum cardiomyopathy or peripartum cardiomyopathy.

Hibbard et al., 1999	NHLBI definition and a strict ecocardiographic criterion of left ventricular (LV) dysfunction: 1. ejection fraction < 45% or fractional shortening < 30% 2. end-diastolic dimension > 2.7cm/m^2
American Heart Association [AHA] Scientific Statement on contemporary definitions and classifications of the cardiomyopathies (Maron et al., 2006)	A rare and dilated acquired primary cardiomyopathy associated with LV dysfunction and heart failure
European Society of Cardiology [ESC] on the classification of cardiomyopathies (Dickstein et al., 2008)	A non-familial, non-genetic form of dilated cardiomyopathy associated with pregnancy
Heart Failure Association of the ESC Working Group on PPCM (Sliwa et al., 2010a)	An idiopathic cardiomyopathy presenting with heart failure secondary to LV systolic dysfunction *towards the end of pregnancy or in the months following delivery*, where no other cause of heart failure is found. It is a diagnosis of exclusion. The LV may not be dilated but the ejection fraction is nearly always reduced below 45%

Table 2. Definitions of peripartum cardiomyopathy

Peripartum cardiomyopathy is the preferred term because it highlights the overall chronological spectrum of the disease (Abboud et al., 2007). Another accepted term is *pregnancy-associated cardiomyopathy* or *early peripartum cardiomyopathy*, used for those females with cardiomyopathy developing heart failure before the last month of pregnancy or at least five months after delivery (Ntobeko et al., 2009). These cases may be subclinical dilated cardiomyopathies presenting the first symptoms in early pregnancy, or viral myocarditis, both distinct entities from PPCM (Pyatt & Dubey, 2011).

3. Epidemiology

Good data about incidence are unavailable because so few population-based registries exist. Most studies have been performed in South Africa, Haiti, and USA, but PPCM was also reported in Caucasian, Japanese, Chinese, Indian, and Korean women. Until recently, only small prospective studies reporting the experience of single centers were available to estimate the incidence of the disease (Desai et al., 1995; Fett et al., 2002, 2005a; Pyatt & Dubey, 2011). Only two large retrospective population-based studies have been conducted in USA to identify cases of PPCM. Mielniczuk et al. reported an estimated incidence of 1:3189 live births, with a trend toward an increase over the study period (1 case/2289 live births for the years 2000-2002), probably related to increasing maternal age and rates of multiple births or to increasing recognition and diagnosis of the disease (Mielniczuk et al., 2006). The second study was performed by Brar et al., who reported an incidence of 1:4025 live births (Brar et al., 2007). The estimates are almost similar for Japan and Australia. PPCM is sporadic in Europe in the white women (Bahloul et al., 2009; Ramaraj & Sorell, 2009). The estimated in-hospital mortality due to PPCM in USA is 1.36% in more recent reports, less than in older series, perhaps due in part to high utilization of modern heart failure therapy (Mielniczuk et al., 2006). These more recent data from the United States suggest a significant difference in the incidence between certain ethnic groups. The lowest observed incidence is reported in Hispanics and the highest in African-Americans (Brar et al., 2007). Outside the United States, the most comprehensive data come from the Peripartum Cardiomyopathy Project in Haiti, which estimates the incidence of PPCM as high as 1case/299 live births (Fett et al., 2005a). The data have been confirmed by Gentry et al., who noted an incidence of 1 case/1000 live births in South Africa (Gentry et al, 2010). In fact, in the absence of a multicentric trial, the incidence varies widely between African countries. For example, in Tunisia the reported incidence is very low unlike Nigeria where older studies have reported 1 case/100 live births (Bahloul et al., 2009).

On the basis of several reports series of PPCM, varying genetic pools and diverse environmental factors have been proposed as risk factors in different areas. Although not clearly delineated, there are several suggested risk factors for development and recurrence of PPCM (Bahloul et al., 2009; Demakis et al., 1971; Fett et al., 2005a; Fisher et al., 2008; Murali & Baldisseri, 2005; Moioli et al., 2010; Nkoua et al., 1991; Ntusi & Mayosi, 2009; Pearson et al., 2000; Sliwa 2006a, 2006b):

- African race - appears to be the strongest risk factor, possibly due to a greater incidence of arterial hypertension in this group. Brar et al. reported the incidence of PPCM in African-American women to be 2.9-fold higher than in whites, and 7-fold than in Hispanics (Brar et al., 2007). Recently, Elkayam has shown that PPCM in USA is not limited to African women (Elkayam et al., 2005). It remains unclear whether race represents an independent risk factor.
- advanced maternal age - the disease generally occurs over the age of 30 years;
- multiparity - 71% of cases occur after ≥ 3 pregnancies compared with 8% in primigravidas (Demakis, 1971, as cited in Ntusi, 2009);
- twin pregnancies - which are observed in 8-13% of cases compared with 1-2% rate noted among healthy women;
- gestational hypertension - with an incidence of approximately 43%, substantially higher than the 8% to 10% incidence in the overall pregnant population. It is important to note that pregnancy-related hypertensive disorders should be considered as distinct entities from PPCM, and not included in the spectrum of PPCM. The complete recovery of LV function in pregnancy-related hypertensive disorders is the rule, whereas persistent cardiac dysfunction is frequent in PPCM patients.
- prolonged use of tocolytics refers to the use of terbutaline, salbutamol, ritodrine, isoxsuprine, magnesium sulfate etc for a period of at least four weeks (Bassett, 1985 as cited in Ntusi, 2009). The association with left ventricular dysfunction seems to be unique to pregnancy, as the same drugs do not determine similar complications in non-pregnant patients, even at high doses.
- certain cultural practices performed during the puerperium which are frequently related with high incidence of PPCM, such as consuming lake salt or rock salt known as "kanwa" (to promote the flow of breast milk), or heating of the body on a clay bed with a fire beneath to keep warm (Moioli et al., 2010; Murali & Baldisseri, 2005);
- socio-economic level is discussed as a risk factor, and can be summarized in a stereotyped profile: "poor African female, with malnutrition and multiparity, making strenuous and sustained physical effort during pregnancy" (Bahloul et al., 2009).

Main concerns

What is the true incidence? Physicians still do not know how often PPCM occurs. Despite being a rare disease in many geographic areas of the world, PPCM remains an important cause of morbidity and mortality in pregnant females.
Who is at risk? There are several cardiac factors that may play a causative role. Regardless of the documented risk factor, the association with PPCM is not clearly explained.

Implications for research

Collaborative, multicenter, prospective, population-based, well-conducted trials are required for adequate diagnosis of this condition.

4. Etiology and pathogenesis

Despite extensive research into its underlying etiology and pathogenesis, it is not clear exactly how PPCM occurs (Ntusi et al., 2009).
Previously, PPCM was generally considered a form of idiopathic dilated cardiomyopathy that was unmasked by the hemodynamic stress of pregnancy (Cunningham et al., 1986). In this case, one would expect PPCM to present during the second trimester coincident with the maximum hemodynamic load of pregnancy. However, it more commonly presents later in pregnancy or postpartum. Moreover, 30% of patients with PPCM experience complete recovery, with partial recovery in many cases, in contrast to rare recovery in idiopathic dilated cardiomyopathy (Fett et al., 2002). Finally, epidemiological data show that PPCM is diagnosed in young women during the peripartum period, whereas idiopathic dilated cardiomyopathy is more common in older patients (Pearson et al., 2000). Although the two conditions have similar clinical presentations and hemodynamic features, there are also significant differences in histological characteristics.
It is now accepted that PPCM is a distinct entity, rather than a clinically silent underlying cardiomyopathy exacerbated by the hemodynamic changes during pregnancy (Robson et al., 1989).
The pathogenetic mechanisms of PPCM have been difficult to study as its incidence is too low to allow meaningful evaluations, and the suitable animal models to study the disease are rare. Several hypotheses have been proposed (Figure 1), but at the present time, two hypotheses are foremost: pregnancy associated hormonal changes, specifically the role of prolactin, and viral infection.

4.1 Excessive prolactin production

Pregnancy is a physiological state associated with enhanced oxidative stress related to high metabolic turnover and elevated tissue oxygen requirements. In order to protect the heart, an efficient antioxidant defense mechanism counteracts the oxidative stress. The total antioxidant capacity increases in the last trimester with a peak early postpartum (Toescu et al., 2002).
Prolactin has been suggested as a potential mechanism in the development of PPCM (Kothari, 1997). Experimental data in a mouse model of PPCM demonstrates the activation of STAT3 pathway by 23-kDa prolactin to be necessary (Hilfiker-Kleiner et al., 2007a). STAT3 is a cardiac tissue-specific DNA-binding protein, activator of transcription-3 that promotes myocardial angiogenesis and cardiomyocyte hypertrophy. In addition,

STAT3 protects the heart from pregnancy-induced oxidative stress in part by up-regulation of a powerful reactive oxygen species, scavenging mitochondrial enzyme named manganese superoxide dismutase (MnSOD) (Negoro et al., 2001). Reduced levels of STAT3 lead to an unbalanced peri/postpartum oxidative stress, a potent stimulus for the activation of prolactin-cleaving protease catehpsin D in cardiomyocytes. The result is cleavage of the nursing hormone prolactin into an antiangiogenic, proapoptotic, and proinflammatory 16-kDa subfragment (Roberg & Ollinger, 1998). Interestingly, prolactin is a hormone with opposing cardiovascular effects, depending on the circulating form. The full-length 23-kDa prolactin had no adverse effects on the heart (Hilfiker-Kleiner et al., 2007a). In contrast, high expression of 16-kDa fragment destroys the cardiac microvasculature, reduces in vivo cardiac function, promotes ventricular dilatation. The same fragment inhibits vascular endothelial growth factor-induced proliferation of endothelial cells and migration, induces apoptosis, dissociation of capillary structures, impairs nitric oxide-mediated vasorelaxation, and cardiomyocyte function (Hilfiker-Kleiner et al., 2008). Prolactin production is not limited to pituitary gland, various other cell types, such as fibroblasts, being able to produce it (Nagafuchi et al., 1999). PPCM is often associated with a high degree of cardiac fibrosis mediated by locally produced prolactin, which enhances the circulating pituitary 16-kDa prolactin damaging cardiac effects.

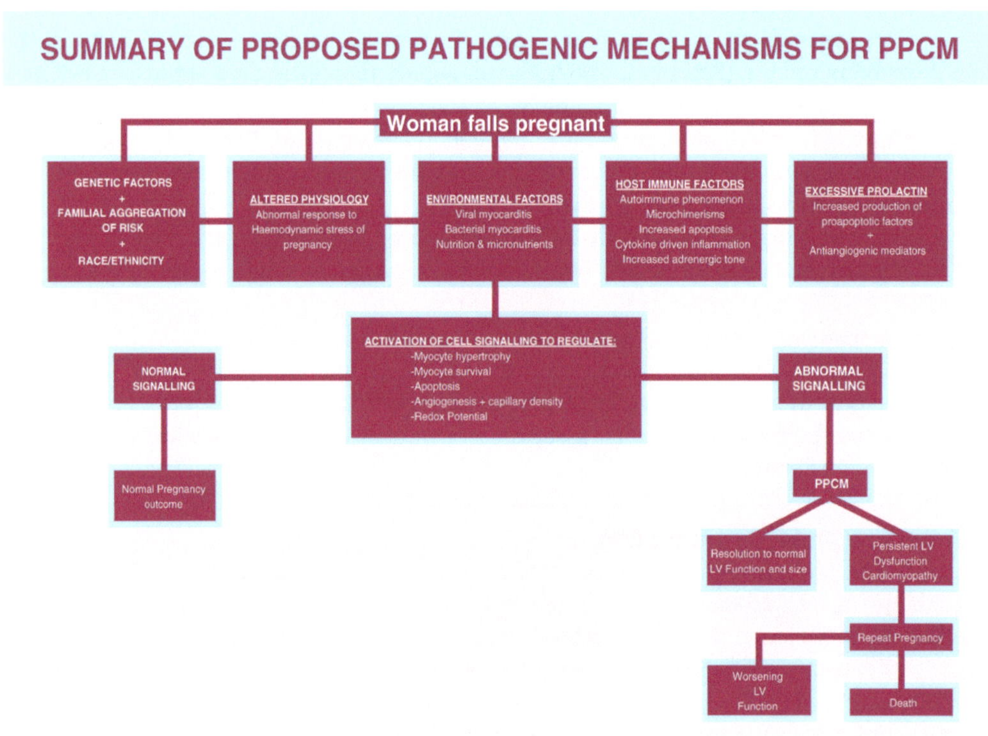

Fig. 1. Summary of proposed pathogenic mechanisms for PPCM (from Ntusi, N.B.A. & Mayosi, B.M. Aetiology and risk factors of peripartum cardiomyopathy: A systematic review. *Int J Cardiol*, Vol.131, No.2 (Jan 2009), pp. 168-179, with permission from Elsevier)

There is more evidence linking findings from experimental models to human PPCM. Patients with acute PPCM have increased serum levels of oxidized low-density lipoprotein indicative for enhanced oxidative stress, activated cathepsin D, and 16-kDa prolactin compared with pregnancy matched healthy controls (Hilfiker-Kleiner et al., 2007a). It is therefore likely that activation of this cascade plays a key functional role in human PPCM. PPCM patients have also significantly elevated pro-apoptotic serum markers (e.g. soluble death receptor sFas/Apo-1) with predictive power of impaired functional status and mortality (Sliwa et al., 2006b). In explanted terminally failing hearts from PPCM patients, low STAT3 protein levels are displayed, suggesting the role of this signaling pathway in the pathogenesis (Hilfiker-Kleiner et al., 2007a) (Figure 2).

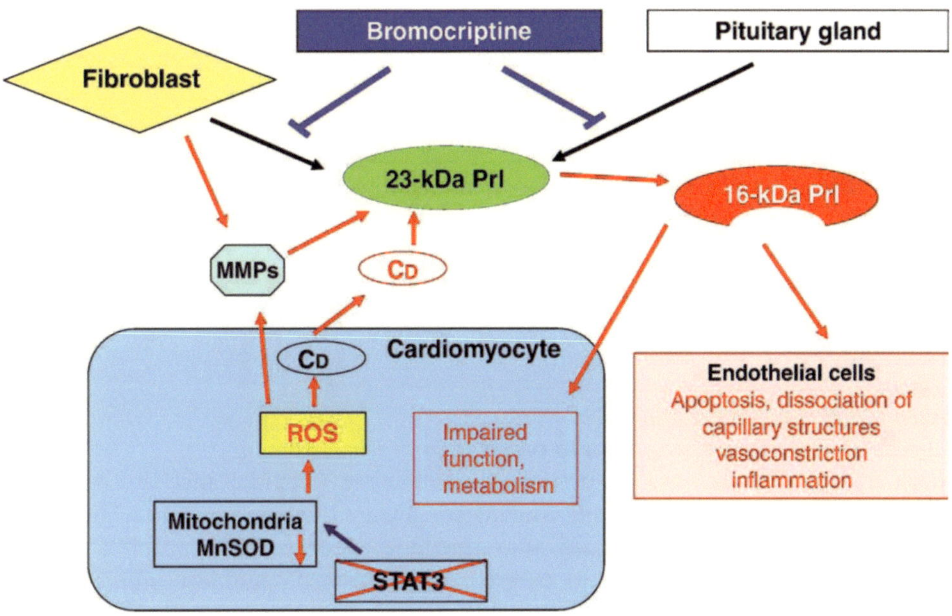

Fig. 2. Schematic mechanism for the development of PPCM (from Hilfiker-Kleiner, D., Sliwa, K. & Drexler, H. (2008). Peripartum Cardiomyopathy: Recent Insights in its Pathophysiology. *Trends Cardiovasc Med,* Vol.18, No.5 (July 2008), pp. 173–179; with permission from Elsevier)

Consistent with the idea of prolactin involvement, blockade by bromocriptine, a dopamine D2 receptor agonist, was tested. Bromocriptine eliminates the substrate for the generation of 16-kDa prolactin, and prevents the onset of disease in the mouse model of PPCM (Hilfiker-Kleiner et al., 2007a) (Figure 2). Several reports suggest that bromocriptine may have beneficial effects when added to the standard therapy of heart failure in women with acute onset of PPCM (Habedank et al., 2008; Hilfiker-Kleiner et al., 2007b; Sliwa et al., 2010b). However, at present, bromocriptine is not recommended until results of ongoing controlled randomized trials will provide information for the actual benefit of this therapy concept in patients with PPCM.

4.2 Viral myocarditis

The relationship between pregnancy and viral myocarditis was established in 1968 in pregnant mice (Farber & Glasgow, 1970). Myocarditis as a cause of PPCM in humans was first suggested by Gouley et al., who corroborated infection with enlarged hearts with focal areas of fibrosis and necrosis (Gouley et al., 1937). Since then, several investigators have suggested myocarditis as a cause of PPCM (Cenac, 2003 as cited in Ntusi, 2009; Melvin, 1982; O'Connell, 1986). The prevalence of viruses detected in endomyocardial biopsies varies considerably between the different studies, ranging from less than 10% (Rizeq et al., 1994) to 78% (Midei et al., 1990), with a similar incidence in controls, suggesting no specific role for viral infection in the etiology of PPCM. It is worth noting that the molecular pathological study of endomyocardial biopsies within a cohort with PPCM found a high prevalence of viral genomes (parvovirus B19, human cytomegalovirus and herpes virus 6, Epstein-Barr virus) as well as inflammatory changes consistent with myocarditis (30.7%) (Bultmann et al., 2005). Other investigation suggests that viral infection increases the severity of myocardial damage in postpartum mice in comparison with non-pregnant control subjects (Lyden & Huber, 1984, as cited in Ramaraj & Sorrell, 2009). It is possible that the postviral immune response to be directed inappropriately against native cardiac tissue proteins leading to LV systolic dysfunction in the presence of the characteristic hemodynamic changes during pregnancy. Given the imunosuppressed state of pregnancy, it is logical that pregnant women are more susceptible to infection or viral reactivation (Pearson et al., 2000). At the present time, the exact role of viral infection or reactivation is far from conclusive. No convincing data exist that myocarditis is the primary etiology of PPCM. Further studies using newer technologies such as PCR are needed for detecting actively replicating viruses and myocardial viral load in PPCM (Ntusi et al, 2009) and confirming a pathogenic role.

4.3 Other putative hypotheses

4.3.1 Abnormal immune response to pregnancy

Abnormal immune response to pregnancy is another potential mechanism, probably generated by the decreased immunity during pregnancy (Cruz et al., 2010). The abnormal immune response may be produced after previous exposure immunization from prior pregnancy, or previous exposure to paternal major histocompatibility antigens. A local tissue inflammatory response is induced, followed by releasing of cytokines and a nonspecific innocent bystander myotoxicity and myocarditis (Pearson et al., 2000). Circulating auto-antibodies to selected cardiac tissue proteins were reported by several studies in more than 50% of PPCM patients (Sliwa, 2000, 2006a; Sundstrom, 2002, as cited in Cruz, 2010). Auto-antibodies are associated with increased levels of cytokines (tumor necrosis factor-α, interleukin-6, soluble Fas receptors), and are correlated with dilation of LV and systolic dysfunction (Sliwa et al., 2006b). The circulating auto-antibodies are formed against proteins released after delivery (e.g. actin, myosin), when the degeneration of the uterus occurs, and may cross-react with "target-proteins" found in the maternal myocardium (Freedman, 2004; Jahns, R., 2004). It was reported that in all patients with PPCM, irrespective of geographic location, auto-antibodies against cardiac myosin are non-selectively increased immunoglobulins G (class G and subclasses G1, G2, G3) (Warraich et al., 2005). Other studies have reported the phenomenon called chimerism, when fetal cells of hematopoietic origin reside in maternal serum, but remain undetected because of the weak immunogenicity of paternal haploytpe or maternal altered immunity (Ansari, 2002, as cited in Ramaraj & Sorrell, 2009). If fetal cells lodge in maternal myocardium during pregnancy, it is possible to be recognized as non-self while postpartum immune recovery, and an abnormal immune response is triggered (Pearson et al., 2000). At the present time, it is unclear if all these data contribute directly to myocardial injury in PPCM, or should be considered as a consequence of the disease.

4.3.2 Citokine-mediated inflammation

Citokine-mediated inflammation is a basic pathophysiological mechanism in heart failure. The vasodepressor pro-inflammatory cytokines, like tumor necrosis factor-α, interleukin-6 and 1, interpheron-γ, expressed at high concentrations result in LV systolic dysfunction and remodeling, fetal gene expression, and cardiomyopathy. Increased levels of the same cytokines, and of hs-C-reactive protein have been reported in the serum of patients with PPCM (Fett, 2004; Sliwa, 2006b). It is still unclear if a true causal link between cytokines and PPCM does exist. If cytokines are involved in the pathogenesis of PPCM, these would prove useful targets for immunomodulatory therapy.

4.3.3 Increased myocyte apoptosis

Increased myocyte apoptosis represents an imbalance between cellular elimination and cellular regeneration. Experimental data suggest that terminally differentiated cardiac myocytes undergo apoptosis as the final common pathway in many cardiomyopathies (Narula, 2000; Wencker, 2003). Transgenic mice develop PPCM when cardiac-specific α-subunit of Gq is over-expressed (Hayakawa, 2003, as cited in Hilfiker-Kleiner, 2008). The Gq subunit is discussed to be responsible for coupling several cell surface receptors to intracellular signaling pathways involved in cardiomyocyte hypertrophy and apoptosis.

The inhibition of caspases, the proteases that mediate apoptosis, has been demonstrated to improve LV systolic function and reduce the mortality in pregnant Gαq mice. Recently, the proapoptotic gene Nix or Bnip3 have been demonstrated to play a key role in peripartum cardiac apoptosis and heart failure (Diwan, 2008, as cited in Hilfiker-Kleiner, 2008). Thus, experimental models, as well as indirect evidence in humans (increased plasma levels of key-proteins like Fas and Fas ligand), provides evidence for a role of apoptosis (Sliwa et al., 2006a). On the other side, the role of cardiomyocyte loss as a general key mechanism seems unlikely, since complete recovery of cardiac function has been observed in PPCM patients. Further studies are needed to evaluate the prevalence and exact role of apoptosis in PPCM patients, as well as the therapeutic value to prevent cardiomyopathy decompensation.

4.3.4 Abnormal response to hemodynamic stress

Abnormal response to hemodynamic stressis a hypothesis that suggests the exaggerated decrease in systolic function of LV in the presence of the cardiovascular changes in pregnancy (Ntusi et al., 2009). The normal hemodynamic changes during pregnancy result in a physiological transient and reversible hypertrophy and enlargement of the LV to meet the needs of the fetus and mother (Geva, 1997, as cited in Ntusi, 2009). These changes normally maintain up to 2-3 weeks postpartum and may persist until the 12th week after delivery. In patients with PPCM, LV anatomy may return to normal, but the contractile reserve is persistently decreased when assessed by dobutamine stress echocardiography (Lampert et al., 1997). Until now, there are no convincing data to support this hypothesis.

4.3.5 Genetic susceptibility

Genetic susceptibilitywas first suggested in the 1960s (Pierce at al., 1963). Since that time, several other documented cases with familial clustering of PPCM, as well as familial reports with familial PPCM and idiopathic dilated cardiomyopathy have been published, suggesting the contribution of genetics (Sliwa et al., 2010a). It is not clearly documented whether these cases meet the criterion of absence of an identifiable cause of heart failure, or whether an inherited idiopathic dilated cardiomyopathy becomes symptomatic because of the hemodynamic changes during pregnancy and after delivery. Also, the very high incidence in certain geographic regions or communities is strongly suggestive for environmental factors role. A genetic mutation cannot be excluded, but genetic testing is not usually performed in PPCM. Secondly, experimental studies have reported a genetic susceptibility to viral myocarditis in animals deficient in transforming growth factor-β, as well as the potential role of the defective STATE3 gene, or gene polymorphism of MnSOD (Hilfiker-Kleiner, 2008; Horwitz, 2007; Kim, 2005; Kühl 2005b; Lang 2008). Recently, van Spaendonck-Zwarts et al. investigated the occurrence of PPCM in 90 families with idiopathic dilated cardiomyopathy. The authors suggested that a subset of PPCM could be an initial manifestation of the disease, when a mutation in the gene encoding cardiac troponin C was identified (van Spaendonck-Zwarts et al., 2010). In another study from the USA, Morales et al. confirmed PPCM in 5 cases with gene mutations. The involved genes encoded myosin heavy chain 7 (MYH7), sodium channel, voltage-gated, type V, α-subunit (SCN5A), and presenilin 2 (PSEN2) in 3 cases with familial disease and myosin heavy chain 6 (MYH6), cardiac troponin T2 (TNNT2) in 2 with sporadic disease (Morales et al., 2010). Both reports have important implications, suggesting the necessity for the cardiologic screening in first-degree family members of PPCM patients without recovery of LV function and dimensions. In addition, reproductive risk counseling about PPCM or pregnancy-associated cardiomyopathy is appropriate for first-degree family members of patients with idiopathic dilated cardiomyopathy in the context of a genetic evaluation (Hershberger et al., 2009).

4.3.6 Malnutrition

Malnutrition was thought to be involved because of increased incidence of PPCM in communities with low socio-economic level (Hull, 1937, as cited in Ntusi, 2009; Walsh, 1965). For example, selenium deficiency has been reported in Sahel region of Africa (Cenac et al., 1992) but not in Haiti, and excessive consumption of salt in Nigeria (Ntusi et al., 2009). However, malnutrition it is not a key factor because many cases of PPCM are reported in well-nourished cohorts.

4.3.7 Abnormal hormonal regulation

Abnormal hormonal regulation although proposed in the 1930s, cannot be affirmed (Musser, 1938, as cited in Ntusi, 2009). Estrogens and relaxin were believed to play a role in PPCM, due to the cardiovascular effects, but no convincing evidence has been documented.

4.3.8 Increased adrenergic tone

Increased adrenergic tone secondary to physical or emotional stress has been proposed to cause "myocardial stunning" and transient cardiac dysfunction, fluid overload, decreased colloid osmotic pressure (Wittstein et al., 2005). Considering the evidence for the role of β1-

adrenergic receptor antibodies, it is possible to contribute to cardiac muscle dysfunction (Jahns R., 2004; Freedman, 2004).

4.3.9 Vascular disease

Vascular disease with subsequent myocardial ischemia has also been suggested, but morphology and function of coronary arteries were unaffected in PPCM patients (Koide, 1972; Lampert, 1995, as cited in Cruz, 2010).

4.3.10 Other possible mechanisms

Other possible mechanisms postulate the role of cardiac nitric oxide synthase, cardiac dystrophin, immature dendritic cells, toll-like receptors etc (Ramaraj & Sorell, 2009).

Main concern
What causes PPCM? Contributing factors and specific mechanisms remain unclear. Although various hypotheses have been proposed, so far no cause has been clearly identified. It is likely that PPCM is a heterogenous disorder, with a multifactorial etiology and complex biopathological processes.
Implications for research
Further studies are needed to elucidate this difficult condition. "The challenge will be to devise a study with sufficient power to give valid results" (Fett, 2010).

5. Diagnosis

5.1 Clinical presentation

Patients with PPCM present with classical signs and symptoms of systolic heart failure due to other cardiomyopathies. The most common symptoms are dyspnea and fatigue (90%), tachycardia (62%), and peripheral edema (60%) (Elkayam et al., 2005). Other symptoms like persistent nocturnal dry cough, orthopnea, paroxysmal nocturnal dyspnea are frequently reported (Moioli et al., 2010). NYHA class III or IV functional status seem to be the most common initial presentation (Desai et al., 1995). Other non-specific signs and symptoms include dizziness, non-specific praecordial pain (50%), abdominal discomfort, palpitations, most frequently due to tachycardia or supraventricular tachiarryhtmias (Bertrand, 1977; de Beus, 2003; Weinblatt, 1995). Complex ventricular arrhythmias and cardiac arrest have also been reported (Diao et al., 2004). Some case series describe unusual presentations such as acute cyanosis (Cole et al., 2001), multiple thromboembolic events (Carlson et al., 2000) or liver failure (Fussell et al., 2005). Systemic and pulmonary embolic episodes are found during the clinical course of PPCM more frequently than in patients with other forms of cardiomyopathy (Bennani, 2003; Box, 2004; Helms & Kittner, 2005; Jha, 2005; Lasinska-Kowara, 2001). Sudden dyspnea, pleuritic pain, and hemoptysis suggest an episode of pulmonary embolism.

Regarding the physical signs in PPCM, a high incidence of the third heart sound (92%) and displaced apical impulse (72%) are reported (Desai et al., 1996). New murmurs consistent with mitral and tricuspid regurgitation are present in almost 50% of PPCM patients (Fadouach et al., 1994). Sinus tachycardia is the rule of cardiac exam. In the later stages, signs of pulmonary hypertension, including a loud or split second heart sound and pulmonary crackles, are common. Elevated jugular venous pressure and hepatomegaly associated with edema are present as signs of congestive heart failure. Blood pressure may be normal or increased (when gestational hypertension is associated). In the later stages, postural hypotension can occur (Sliwa et al., 2010a). A latent form of PPCM without overt clinical symptoms has been reported (Elkayam et al., 2005).

The clinical diagnosis still represents a challenge because symptoms of early heart failure such as dyspnea, fatigue, palpitations, pedal edema, can appear in normal late pregnancy and after delivery. Therefore, in many cases, patients and their physicians may consider the symptoms to be normal.

There are some important clues for making the diagnosis. Clinical exam remains essential because a persistent sinus tachycardia, third heart sound, basal pulmonary crackles, and elevated jugular venous pressure are abnormal for pregnancy state and heart failure may be considered. Secondly, the diagnosis should be considered whenever women experience unexplained heart failure symptoms and signs during the last month of pregnancy or within 5 months following delivery, in accordance with PPCM definition. It is important to note that 78% of PPCM cases develop heart failure symptoms in the first 4 months after delivery, and only 9% of patients present in the last month of pregnancy (Lampert et al., 1995). It is possible that some patients to present later in postpartum because their symptoms are not initially recognized as heart failure (Sliwa et al., 2010a). Interestingly, Fett et al. reported clinically normal postpartum in Haitian women with asymptomatic echocardiographic systolic dysfunction, who either developed dilated cardiomyopathy or completely recovered LV function (Fett et al., 2005b). These cases may represent a latent phase of PPCM before the development of dilated cardiomyopathy later in life or subclinical dilated cardiomyopathy presenting in early pregnancy or a viral myocarditis, distinct conditions from true PPCM (Fett, 2008; Pyatt &Dubey, 2011). Thirdly, the rapid onset of heart failure symptoms in the peripartum period may also distinguish this clinical entity and requires further investigations.

In conclusion, there are no specific criteria for differentiating symptoms of early heart failure from normal late pregnancy, so it is imperative to maintain a high index of suspicion in conjunction with timing of symptoms to identify the patients with PPCM.

5.2 Investigation of peripartum cardiomyopathy

Blood tests should be done in all patients, although none of these can help in screening or positive diagnosis of PPCM. Initial laboratory assessment should include complete blood count and biochemical parameters. The thyroid function, a septic screen, and viral serology should also be performed in order to exclude other causes of cardiomyopathy and heart failure (Pyatt &Dubey, 2011). Molecular markers of an inflammatory process are found in most of the patients. It was reported that 90% of the patients with PPCM had high levels of plasma C-reactive protein, positively related with LV dimensions and inversely with LV ejection fraction (Fett, 2005a; Sliwa, 2006b). Cardiac markers, such as troponin T determined early after the onset of PPCM, are suggested to have prognostic significance. Only B-type natriuretic peptide (BNP) and N-terminal pro-BNP (NT-proBNP), commonly increased in patients with PPCM, are recommended by the Heart Failure Association of the ESC Working Group on PPCM to be determined (Sliwa et al., 2010a). Measurement of natriuretic peptides can be also helpful for risk stratification and volume status assessment. Increased levels in pregnancy have been related with systolic dysfunction, increased LV filling pressures and LV hypertrophy, acute myocardial infarction (Hameed, 2009; Garrison, 2005).

Genetic testing is not recommended as a routine, but only for research purposes (Sliwa et al., 2010a).

Electrocardiogram is seldom normal in patients with heart failure caused by PPCM, but it is mostly non-specific. Sinus rhythm or sinus tachycardia are usually present, atrial fibrillation or ventricular tachycardia may occur, particularly if LV systolic dysfunction becomes chronic (Diao, 2004; Duran, 2008). An intraventricular block pattern or prolonged PR and QRS are seldom reported. LV hypertrophy pattern, Q waves in the anteroseptal leads, ST-T abnormalities largely vary in incidence between studies (Brown, 1998; O'Connell, 1986, as cited in Moioli, 2010). Negative T waves can be of ischemic origin in 50% of cases (Bertrand, 1975, as cited in Bahloul, 2009).

Chest X-ray should be part of the initial assessment of all patients with PPCM and clinical heart failure. Radiological findings can be cardiomegaly, pulmonary congestion/edema, and pleural effusion.

Echocardiography is the most widely used imaging method, which provides valuable, reproducible diagnostic and prognostic information. The technique is not diagnostic for PPCM, but is important to exclude other causes of heart failure. Hibbard et al. proposed precise echocardiographic criteria that should be applied (**Table 2**). Several studies highlighted the strong relation between LV end-diastolic diameter > 60 mm, or ejection fraction < 30% and the recovery of LV function (Duran, 2008; Elkayam, 2005). Another important finding may be the presence of LV thrombus, particularly when LV function is severely depressed. It is important to note that LV dilatation is not always present (Kane, 2001; Sliwa, 2000). It is strongly recommended to monitor the evolution under treatment before patient's discharge, at 6 weeks, 6 months, and annually (Sliwa et al., 2010a).

Cardiac magnetic resonance imaging (MRI) is widely used in other forms of cardiomyopathy for assessment of cardiac structure and function as a reference technique. Also it has a high ability to detect myocardial fibrosis as a consequence of myocarditis, using delayed contrast enhancement technique with gadolinium. In PPCM, cardiac MRI provides more accurate quantification of chamber volumes and ventricular function, and is more sensitive in detecting LV thrombus than echocardiography (Mouquet, 2008; Srichai, 2006). At the present time, there are four case series with PPCM assessed by cardiac MRI (Caballero-Borrego, 2008; Kawano, 2008; Leurent, 2009; Mouquet, 2008). In only two of these studies the technique revealed myocardial inflammation. Baruteau et al. consider that all these MRI results are not in contradiction, but underline the complex pathogenesis of PPCM. Cardiac MRI can distinguish two forms of PPCM, inflammatory and non-inflammatory, according to the presence or absence of late gadolinium enhancement. Therefore, cardiac MRI can be helpful at initial presentation to conduct further etiologic investigations (Baruteau et al., 2010). The interest for the technique is also suggested by the ability to differentiate PPCM from other forms of cardiomyopathy, like Tako-Tsubo or ischemic cardiomyopathy. The technique might be a useful method for guiding biopsy to the abnormal area (Leurent et al., 2009), and for prognostic stratification (Kawano et al., 2008). In his comment, Fett supports cardiac MRI for PPCM which is not responding to conventional therapy as long as late gadolinium enhancement is more likely to be present in these cases (Fett, 2009). In other words, cardiac MRI could guide the immunosuppressive therapy in the inflammatory forms of PPCM, as this option of treatment has successfully been tested in "myocarditis-like" PPCM (Ntusi et al., 2009). Further larger prospective studies are needed to evaluate these findings, and the real diagnostic contribution of MRI in PPCM. The Heart Failure Association of the ESSC Working Group on PPCM recommends cardiac MRI to be performed at 6 and 12 months for a better assessment of cardiac functional changes (Sliwa et al., 2010a). It remains the problem of using gadolinium during pregnancy, not recommended by the European Society of Radiology until after delivery, unless absolutely necessary (Webb et al., 2005).

Invasive evaluation including cardiac catheterization and coronary angiography are not routinely indicated, as no specific findings are present, and coronary arteries are usually normal in PPCM.

Endomyocardial biopsy is not routinely recommended in PPCM for multiple reasons. Its role is controversial because a specific microscopic pattern for PPCM does not exist, even though a "myocarditis-like" form is frequently found (Fett, 2006a; Zimmermann, 2005). In addition, the technique is not widely available, is invasive, and has a relatively high complication rate.

Considering all these data, PPCM should be suspected whenever the patient experiences symptoms and signs of heart failure during peripartum period. A careful history and physical exam should be performed to identify heart failure due to other cardiac or non-cardiac entities. The differential diagnosis of PPCM should include all the pre-existing clinical conditions, either unrecognized, such as congenital heart disease, or unmasked by pregnancy, such as sporadic and familial idiopathic dilated cardiomyopathies, HIV/AIDS cardiomyopathy, valvular heart disease, particularly rheumatic mitral valve disease. Other non-cardiac conditions (collagen vascular disease, sexually transmitted disease, thyroid disorders) and precipitating factors (current use of alcohol, tobacco, illicit drugs, sodium intake, other therapies) may be also considered. A useful clue for diagnosis is the onset of symptoms, most frequently in postpartum for PPCM unlike the other clinical conditions, which usually present by the 2nd trimester. Pregnancy-associated myocardial infarction, venous thromboembolism, hypertensive heart disease must be also included in the diagnostic approach. Timely diagnosis of PPCM is critical for best outcomes of survival and recovery. Very recently, Fett proposed a screening tool for early diagnosis of PPCM. The test is a focused medical history for PPCM screening, looking for the most common early signs and symptoms of heart failure during last month of pregnancy (Fett, 2011). The author proposes 6 clinical categories, easy to quantify, which are included in a self-scoring system (Table 3). A score ≥ 5 has always been associated with LV systolic dysfunction. A score > 4 suggests the need for further investigation. In this case, a blood BNP test and an echocardiography are recommended. If the score is < 4 the patient should be monitored for BNP and C-reactive protein levels. If increased levels, echocardiography should be performed. The author emphasizes that this test is not diagnostic for PPCM, but encourages an expanded use, because it may be a useful tool for early recognition of the new onset heart failure.

In conclusion, the diagnostic work-up should focus on precise echocardiographic identification of new LV systolic dysfunction, peptide natriuretic measurement (Murali, 2005; Pearson, 2000), and ruling out other causes of heart failure. Additional investigations should be based on clinical suspicion. PPCM remains a *diagnosis of exclusion*. Early detection is critically important to the patient with PPCM, because delayed diagnosis may be associated with increased morbidity and mortality (Fett, 2008; Fussell, 2005; Pearson, 2000; Sliwa, 2006a).

Sign/symptom	Characterstics	Scoring
Orthopnea (difficulty breathing when lying flat)	None	0
	Need to elevate head	1
	Need to elevate $\geq 45^0$	2
Dyspnea (shortness of breath on exertion)	None	0
	Climbing 8 or more steps	1
	Walking on level	2
Unexplained cough	None	0
	At night	1
	Day and night	2
Swelling lower extremities	None	0
	Below knee	1
	Above and below knee	2
Excessive weight gain (during last month of pregnancy)	< 2 pounds/week	0
	2-4 pounds/week	1
	> 4 pounds per week	2
Palpitations (sensation of irregular heart beats)	None	0
	When lying down at night	1
	Day and night, any position	2

Table 3. Self-test for early diagnosis of heart failure in PPCM (adapted from Fett JD, 2011).

Main concerns

How to optimize the diagnosis? Early involvement of a cardiologist is needed for a timely diagnosis. The rapid onset of heart failure symptoms in the peripartum period may distinguish this difficult entity, only if other causes of cardiomyopathy are excluded. A screening clinical self-test for early recognition of PPCM is now proposed. Cardiac MRI is also suggested to have a great diagnostic and prognostic potential.

What's next in PPCM investigation?

A multicentre registry systematically using these tools may be considered for a better diagnostic approach.

6. Management of peripartum cardiomyopathy

When considering treatment during the peripartum period, a multidisciplinary approach is needed. Involvement of a maternal-fetal medical team, including a cardiologist, obstetrician, anesthetist, intensivist, and neonatologist is imperative as earliest as possible after the diagnosis. The type of monitoring and care should be individualized to minimize maternal and fetal morbidity and mortality.

6.1 General management of peripartum cardiomyopathy

The medical treatment is generally similar to that for other forms of non-ischemic dilated cardiomyopathy, with some possible exceptions because of the risks of certain drugs on the fetus and newborn. The aims of medical treatment should be to reduce cardiac afterload and preload, while increasing myocardial contractility, to prevent complications, particularly thromboembolism, cardiac arrhythmia, progressive heart failure, and to improve long-term prognosis. Current therapeutic options consist of conventional supportive treatment for acute and chronic heart failure.

6.1.1 Management of acute heart failure

The principles of treatment in PPCM are no different than those applying to acute heart failure from other etiologies (Dickstein et al., 2008). A careful bedside clinical assessment may be helpful to identify the hemodynamic profile. Acute heart failure is usually manifested by worsening pulmonary congestion to pulmonary edema and hypoxemia, peripheral congestion with large weight gain, or low output status indicated by signs of hypoperfusion. All patients should be hospitalized and closely monitored.

Oxygen therapy should be promptly administered in order to relieve symptoms, while achieving an arterial oxygen saturation of ≥ 95%. Non-invasive ventilation with a positive end-expiratory pressure of 5-7.5 cm H_2O should be used when necessary. Extracorporeal membrane oxygenation to treat severe pulmonary edema shortly after delivery has been reported to be useful (Yang et al., 2007).

Patients with significant volume overload but adequate perfusion are treated with *intravenous diuretics*, with an initial bolus of furosemide 20-40 mg i.v. Particular potential adverse effects of diuretics were reported during pregnancy, such as pancreatitis, decreased carbohydrate tolerance (Lindheimer & Katz, 1973) bleeding, and hyponatremia in newborns (Ferrero et al., 2003).

Intravenous nitrates may be added when diuretics are inadequate in controlling symptoms. Nitroglycerin starting at 10-20 up to 200 μg/min is safe when systolic blood pressure is > 110 mmHg. Nitroprusside may be used in certain cases, but theoretically, accumulation of its catabolites thiocyanate and cyanide may be harmful to the fetus (Egan et al., 2009). Nesiritide is insufficiently studied in human pregnancy (Cruz et al., 2010).

Inotropic agents can be used without unnecessary delay in patients with low output status or those with persistent congestion despite diuretic and/or vasodilatator therapy. Dobutamine or levosimendan are strongly recommended when needed. Small studies with levosimendan suggest persistent hemodynamic improvement attributable to production of an active long half-life metabolite (OR-1896), and no safety concern, but breast-feeding should be avoided (Benezet-Mazuecos & de la Hera, 2008; De Luca, 2006).

Mechanical ventricular support and cardiac transplantation are needed in patients dependent on inotropic agents, or intra-aortic balloon pump counterpulsation, despite optimal medical strategy. Surgical support with ventricular assist devices may be considered in appropriately selected patients as a bridge to recovery or to cardiac transplantation. Heart Failure Association of the ESC Working Group on PPCM recommends an individualized discussion between experts in such cases, as the optimal strategy in PPCM is not known (Sliwa et al., 2010a). If the type of ventricular assist devices is discussed, two prosthetic ventricles - BiVADs and CardioWest TAH, depending on body surface area, heart size and presence of multiorgan failure were proposed (Zimmerman et al., 2010). Complications may occur with ventricular assist devices, such as a high incidence of thrombotic events (Potapov et al., 2008). Recovery of myocardial function can occur in approximately 15% of patients with PPCM on ventricular assist device support (Murali et al., 2005). If the clinical improvement does not occur, cardiac transplantation should be considered. Since 1987, when Aravot et al. reported their first experience (Aravot, 1987, as cited in Abboud, 2007), several case series were treated by heart transplantation with mixed results. In 1994, Keogh et al. demonstrated no difference in survival rates for cardiac transplantation in women with dilated cardiomyopathy, irrespective of etiology, but higher rates of early rejection in PPCM were noted (Keogh, 1994, as cited in Zimmerman, 2010). Other authors supported the hypothesis of an overactive immunological response in "myocarditis-like" PPCM, which predisposes to recurrent severe rejection, and subsequent development of fatal transplant-associated complications. A recent prospective study demonstrated that survival and freedom from cardiac allograft vasculopathy in PPCM was similar to that of women with other indications for heart transplantation (Rasmusson et al., 2007). At the present time, based on available data, 0-11% PPCM patients undergo heart transplantation, with a similar outcome compared with other etiologies of heart failure (Sliwa et al., 2010a). Generally, heart transplantation in PPCM is associated with survival rates similar to that in patients with idiopathic dilated cardiomyopathy (88% at 2 years, and 78% at 5 years) (Murali et al., 2005).Very recently, a long term survey on 8 patients with PPCM (mean post-transplant survival 7.1 years) has shown that cardiac transplantation alone can be a successful option (Zimmerman et al., 2010).

6.1.2 Management of stable heart failure

There are no clinical trials to support any particular treatment regimen for PPCM. After delivery, the patient should be treated according to the current guidelines for heart failure (Pearson, 2000; Sliwa, 2010a). During pregnancy and lactation, the management approach must consider the welfare of the fetus along with that of the mother, so several restrictions to these guidelines will be applied.

Dietary restrictions and lifestyle changes are essential and complementary to pharmacological therapy. Fluid restriction to ≤ 2 liters per day and salt restriction (2-4 g per day) are advisable for volume overload control, particularly when NYHA class III and IV symptoms occur. Daily monitoring for edema and weight loss is clinically useful (Oakley et al., 2003). Smoking and alcohol cessation is strongly recommended. Strict bed rest was the standard in the past, still not recommended, except the patients with severe symptoms. Regular modest exercise may be resumed after relief of symptoms (Pyatt &Dubey, 2011; Sliwa 2006a). Since many of pharmacological agents are secreted in the breast milk, breast-feeding is not advised in patients with PPCM (Sliwa et al., 2010a).

Diuretics should be used cautiously because of decreasing placental perfusion with aggressive administration (Egan, 2007; Sliwa 2006a). After delivery, diuretics are safe to reduce preload, and relieve symptoms of pulmonary congestion and volume overload (Amos, 2006; Oakley, 2003). Loop diuretics, such as furosemide, are most frequently used and safer during hospitalization. Thiazide diuretics may be added, if loop diuretics are insufficient, or used in mild cases (Oakley, 2003; Sliwa 2010a). Possible increase of risk of births defects or fetal thrombocytopenia, were reported (Cruz et al., 2010). On experimental studies, spironolactone is reported to have antiandrogenic effects during late pregnancy, but it can be safely added in postpartum period (Pyatt &Dubey, 2011). Eplerenone should be also avoided during pregnancy, as its effects on human fetus are insufficiently studied (Muldowney et al., 2009).

Angiotensin-converting enzyme inhibitors (ACEI) and *angiotensin-II receptor blockers* (ARB) are contraindicated, because of severe fetal toxicity in the 2nd and 3rd trimester of pregnancy, particularly on kidney, resulting in oligohydramnios, fetal renal failure, and neonatal death, but also hypocalvaria, limb contractions, hypoplastic lungs (Cruz et al., 2010). After delivery, or in postpartum onset PPCM, ACEI and ARB are efficient agents to reduce the afterload, and are strongly recommended, as it has been demonstrated to improve survival in all patients with systolic heart failure. It is also recommended the patient counseling about the teratogenic potential of these drugs, with a recurrent pregnancy (Cruz et al., 2010). Some of ACEI, such as captopril and enalapril, are safe during breast-feeding (Ghuman et al., 2009).

Hydralazine and long-acting nitrates are considered safe and useful to reduce preload. The combination can replace ACEI/ARB during pregnancy, or if there is drug intolerance, and may be added to standard therapy in symptomatic patients (Moioli et al., 2010). The agents are reported to be especially effective and further increase survival among African-American patients with NYAH II and III class heart failure (Hunt et al., 2009). The combination is also compatible with breast-feeding.

β-blockers have not been tested in PPCM, but have been safely used in pregnancy-induced hypertension. *β1-selective blockers* are preferred, as *β2*-blockade is theoretically reported to have anti-tocolytic effect (Ghuman et al., 2009). The benefit of these drugs to maternal survival usually outweighs the potential risk to the fetus and newborn. The risks consist of growth retardation, resulting in low-birth-weight newborns, hypoglicemia and bradycardia. Therefore, care should be given when these drugs are used in late pregnancy. β-blockers are recommended for all patients with PPCM, unless contraindicated, as these drugs improve symptoms, ejection fraction, and long term prognosis, reduce the risk of arrhythmia and sudden death. Because transient worsening of heart failure may appear with initiation of therapy, patients should be stable, with minimal evidence of volume overload, and doses should be titrated cautiously. Although carvedilol has been shown to improve overall survival in dilated cardiomyopathy, no safety information related to its use during pregnancy are available. Therefore, use of metoprolol is preferred under careful monitoring, as the drug is also compatible with breast-feeding (Abboud, 2007; Cruz, 2010).

Antiarrhythmic drugs, although well tolerated, should be used only in the acute setting, because their safety for fetus cannot be guaranteed. β-blockers are often adequate for treating supraventricular arrhythmias, also in chronic use. Sotalol or amiodarone may be needed, but, considering their systemic side effects during chronic use, are not recommended. Calcium channel blockers, because of their negative inotrop effects, are also not recommended. Ventricular arrhythmias may be frequently life-threatening, and should be managed aggressively. Class I and class II antiarrhythmic agents are not recommended, because the drugs are poorly tolerated and have proarrhythmic effect. Digoxin is safe during pregnancy, even if it crosses the placental barrier. Careful monitoring of serum levels is recommended, because of the narrow therapeutic-to-toxic window. A digoxinemia of ≤ 1-1.2 ng/dl and early use of the drug in symptomatic women with ACEI/ARB contraindications are recommended (Cruz et al., 2010). Digoxin is also secreted in breast milk, but no adverse effect has been described in newborns (Moioli et al., 2010). In appropriate patients, electrical cardioversion may be necessary, after transesophageal echocardiography rules out the presence of a left atrial thrombus.

Antithrombotic therapy is recommended as pregnancy and puerperium are prothrombotic states. In addition, LV dysfunction (particularly ejection fraction < 35%), severely dilated cavities, and mural thrombus, history of venous thromboembolism and atrial fibrillation are associated with an increased risk of thromboembolic events. A recent study of 182 women with PPCM demonstrated an incidence of 2.2% for thromboembolic complications (Goland et al., 2009). VKA antagonists are contraindicated prior to delivery, because of their risk of fetal and neonatal cerebral hemorrhage, and central nervous system anomalies for warfarin. Heparins are considered necessary and preferred, as they do not cross the placental barrier, and are found in breast milk in significant amount. Low-weight molecular heparins are preferred, as they have a lower risk of premature maternal osteoporosis and thrombocytopenia. Also, low-weight heparins have a short half-life, so they can be discontinued at least 12 hours prior to delivery, to prevent maternal hemorrhage, and resumed 12-24 hours after delivery. Currently, low-weight heparins are safely used in weight-adjusted doses. A strictly adaptation using anti-Xa monitoring is necessary in women at extremes of body weight, or with renal disease. Fondaparinux cannot be used during pregnancy, as there are no consistent data. In 5-7 days postpartum, heparin can be replaced with VKA antagonists, even to breast-feeding mothers (Torbicki et al., 2008).

Cardiac resynchronization therapy and implantable cardioverter/defibrillators have individualized indication, otherwise very difficult to decide in the context of the natural history of PPCM and lack of specific data. The main concern is the usefulness of such methods in patients who may not need them, if ventricular function will recover. For this reason, the indication is advisable when LV ejection fraction < 35% persists after 6 months following presentation. Patients with recurrent symptomatic ventricular arrhythmias may be candidates for an implantable defibrillator. If NYHA III and IV heart failure symptoms and a QRS duration > 120 ms are present, cardiac resynchronization may be required (Sliwa et al., 2010a).

Novel therapies are emerging, but the available data are inconsistent and limited.

Immune modulatory therapy in PPCM is not clear, although an immune pathogenesis has been postulated. The beneficial effects of intravenous immunoglobulin therapy have been inconsistently demonstrated by several studies. Likewise, immunosuppressive drugs, such as azathioprine, cyclosporine or steroids, have shown mixed results. For all these reasons, a multicenter prospective clinical trial in PPCM is needed to support use of such agents. Some studies suggested that immunosuppressive drugs might be helpful in patients with active biopsy proven lymphocytic myocarditis, only after active viral infection is excluded (Sliwa, 2006a; Zimmerman, 2005). Also, recent studies demonstrate the role of cardiotrophic viruses in some cases of idiopathic dilated cardiomyopathy (Kűhl, 2005a, 2005b), but only one study had demonstrated viral genomic material in endomyocardial biopsy from patients with PPCM (Bultmann et al., 2005). At the present time, the role of immunosuppressive therapy in women with negative biopsies remains unknown. It is important to note that current therapies with ACEI, ARB (Godsel et al., 2003), and β blockers (Pauschinger et al., 2005) may have an additional effect on controlling the overactive immune system in PPCM. Also, immunomodulatory therapy acting on inflammatory cytokine TNF-α may be beneficial. Pentoxifyline, a xanthine agent known to inhibit the production of TNF-α and to prevent apoptosis, has been studied in PPCM. In a prospective study of 59 women with PPCM, 30 treated with pentoxifyline 400 mg three times a day in addition to standard therapy of heart failure, a significant improvement of LV function > 10%, and end-diastolic dimensions, a reduction of mortality rate, and greater increase in functional status, compared with the control group were found (Sliwa et al., 2002).

Bromocriptine therapy

Considering the observations that strongly suggest prolactin cleavage as a specific mechanism for the development of PPCM, specific inhibition of its secretion with bromocriptine, a dopamine D2 receptor agonist, is promising. Thus, bromocriptine might represent a novel specific therapeutic approach to either prevent or treat patients with acute PPCM (Hilfiker-Kleiner et al., 2008). Several case reports demonstrated recovery of LV function after treatment with bromocriptine (Elkayam & Goland, 2010; Habedank, 2008; Hilfiker-Kleiner, 2007b; Jahns, B.G., 2008; Meyer, 2010). Very recently, Sliwa et al. reported the results of a prospective, single-center, randomized, proof-of-concept pilot study of women with newly diagnosed PPCM receiving standard therapy with or without bromocriptine for 8 weeks. The addition of bromocriptine appeared to significantly improve LV function (27% at baseline, to 58% at 6 months, p=0.012), and a composite clinical outcome (Sliwa et al., 2010b). Analyzing these data together, Fett remarked that important details of studies design must be corrected for appropriate results. The author proposes some essential conditions to conduct further trials. Patients included in such trials may be best to have serum cathepsin-D activation, positive test for serum 16-kDa prolactin, and very important, to accept lactation suppression while assuring alternative newborn nutrition (Fett, 2010). Also, Fett suggests that bromocriptine treatment should be limited to those patients with LV ejection fraction < 35%, because of poor prognosis with standard therapy in this category. Concerning the safety of bromocriptine in early postpartum women, there are several reports of myocardial infarction (Hopp et al., 1996), while adding adequate anticoagulant therapy, thromboembolism is not reported in such patients (Meyer, 2010; Sliwa, 2010b). Secondly, there are many reports on myocardial infarction in early postpartum independent from bromocriptine administration (Hilfiker-Kleiner et al., 2008).

The results of these studies may represent breakthroughs in the understanding of PPCM pathogenesis, and in the development of a new specific therapy for this clinical entity. But, at the present time, a large, prospective, multicenter, randomized trial is needed to allow bromocriptine extensive use. Such a trial is on-going in Haiti and South Africa (Pyatt & Dubey, 2011).

Other proposed therapies are based on the potential of several agents, such as calcium channel antagonists, statins, interferon-β, monoclonal antibodies, or methods (immunoadsorbtion, apheresis) to influence pro-inflammatory cytokines in acute myocarditis (Ramaraj & Sorrell, 2009).

Main concern

How to treat better? The current medical strategies are not always safe enough for maternal prognostic. There is no clear evidence for the beneficial effect of standard therapy on the recovery of cardiac function in patients with PPCM. As the cause of PPCM is still unknown, no specific therapy has been established to treat this condition.

Implications for research

As the excessive prolactin hypothesis seems to be specific for PPCM, a specific therapeutic intervention using bromocriptine should be tested in an extensive, controlled manner.

6.2 Specific management of peripartum cardiomyopathy

In addition to treatment of heart failure, an obstetrical plan for close monitoring must be developed when PPCM is diagnosed during pregnancy. A collaborative approach, including the obstetrician, cardiologist, anesthesiologist, and neonatologist is essential to optimal care. Serial clinical assessment should be scheduled during late pregnancy. Antenatal testing, such as non-stress test and amniotic fluid index, or biophysical profile is also recommended (Cruz et al., 2010). A baseline ultrasound scan is best to be performed during pregnancy for monitoring the fetus (Sliwa et al, 2010a). If patient is stable, responsive to medical therapy, the pregnancy should be allowed to go to term. The medical team should discuss the delivery mode, primarily considering the mother's benefit. Spontaneous vaginal delivery is preferred in stable women with healthy fetus. For patients with newly diagnosed PPCM before delivery, labor should be induced, or a cesarean section must be planned if mothers are critically ill, or LV function is deteriorating rapidly, or with obstetrical indication (Murali, 2005). After delivery, strict maintenance of fluid status is recommended, using diuretic therapy to prevent volume overload, as fluids are resorbed into the intravascular space (Cruz et al., 2010). Continuous invasive maternal monitoring, including an arterial line and pulmonary catheter, for adequate assessment of patient's hemodynamic status and guide management, as well as continuous fetal cardiotocography are strongly recommended (de Beus et al., 2003). Antenatal medication may be administered, except heparin which should be discontinued at least 12 hours prior to delivery, and resumed 12-24 hours after delivery, with obstetrician and anesthesiologist's permission. Continuous analgesia and anesthesia are needed to minimize further cardiac stress and pain relief, and should be performed with careful specialized monitoring. Epidural analgesia is preferred during labor, as it stabilizes cardiac output through a sympathectomy-induced afterload reduction (Sliwa et al., 2010a). Continuous spinal anesthesia, with epidural analgesia are recommended for cesarean section, as the hemodynamic stability may be more easily maintained (Murali et al., 2005). If general anesthesia is required, drugs with myocardial depressant effect should be avoided, and induction and maintenance with a high-dose opioid technique is preferred. The second stage of labor can cause maximum hemodynamic and oxidative cardiac stress, so these periods must be shortened using a vacuum device or low forceps. A single dose of intramuscular oxytocin can optimally manage the third stage of labor; ergometrine is forbidden (Oakley et al., 2003).Breastfeeding should be avoided in patients with PPCM, although several drugs have been tested and are safe.

7. Prognosis

7.1 Predictive factors and follow–up

Very few studies have been done to assess the long-term survival and recovery outcomes in PPCM. Although PPCM is a form of dilated cardiomyopathy, a characteristic feature is that a higher rate of spontaneous recovery of LV function occurs. A subset of women with PPCM, despite using an optimal medical treatment, follows a rapid and irreversible course, associated with persistent LV dysfunction, severe heart failure, or premature death.

Whitehead et al. reported that in USA 30-50% of patients return to normal within 6 months post partum (Whitehead et al., 2003), while a single centre prospective study, conducted in South Africa, described only a 23% recovering rate of LV function, despite optimal therapy with ACEI and β blockers (Sliwa et al., 2006b). The same author reported a 32% 6-month mortality rate in case series from South Africa (Sliwa et al., 2000). In another study, in Haitian women, with a mean follow-up period of 5 years, the rate of recovery was 31.5%, while mortality rate was 15 %. An important finding of this study was that the recovery to normal LV function can occur later, after 2-3 years after diagnosis, so it is not limited to the first 6-12 months (Fett et al., 2005a). A recent study describes similar rates of LV function recovery and survival in women from USA, Haiti, and South Africa, probably related to improvements in medical therapy, and to the aggressive use of cardioverters in the non-American studied population (Modi et al., 2009). Analyzing *the predictive factors* for long-term prognostic, Duran et al. concluded NYHA functional class, QRS duration, and LV parameters at the time of diagnosis were important predictors. Initial cut-off values of ≤ 5.5 cm for LV end-systolic diameter, and > 27% for LV ejection fraction were identified to predict complete recovery of LV function, while QRS duration on electrocardiogram ≥ 120 ms was a predictor for mortality (Duran et al., 2008). Reviewing 182 patients with PPCM for major adverse events and death, Goland et al. also demonstrated that in all cases there was a strong relation with severe LV dysfunction, non-Caucasian race, and a delayed diagnosis (Goland et al., 2009). These findings complete previous observations about the relation between the severity and persistence of LV dysfunction and the incidence of morbidity and mortality. A LV ejection fraction > 30% at the time of diagnosis might be a predictor for recovery (Elkayam et al., 2005). LV end-diastolic diameter ≥ 6 cm and fractional shortening ≤ 20% are proposed as risks factors for long-term prognosis, as are correlated with a more than threefold higher risk of progressing to persistent LV dysfunction later on (Chapa, 2005; Wittin, 1997). Recently, Baruteau et al. discussed the potential significance of cardiac MRI in prognostic stratification, by assessing LV size, function, and contractile reserve, as well as prognostic MRI factors identified in myocarditis for "myocarditis-like" forms of PPCM (end-diastolic volume, septal localization, and total amount of late gadolinium enhancement at initial time) (Baruteau et al., 2010). Other authors propose immunological mediators and markers of apoptosis to predict outcome. Elevated C-reactive protein and Fas/APO-1 were reported to be related to decreased LV function and mortality (Sliwa et al., 2006b). These perspectives remain to be evaluated by further studies.

In summary, the prognosis varies according to geographical region, and probably, the most important predictor remains the recovery of LV systolic function.

Follow-up of patients with PPCM is similar with that for other forms of cardiomyopathy and LV systolic dysfunction. Patients should be monitored regularly to assess clinical course, complications, LV systolic dysfunction and dimensions, and the response to treatment. Considering that the recovery interval is not restricted to the first 6-12 months postpartum, it is strongly recommended to continue treatment and follow-up for a long period of time to achieve best results (Fett, 2009). However, the optimal period remains unknown. At the present time, echocardiography is the most important tool for serial assessment. In the first several weeks after diagnosis, an echocardiogram should be performed to assess the level of LV function. After that, it should be repeated at about every 6-12 months until recovery is confirmed, or a plateau is reached (Sliwa et al., 2006a). Dobutamine stress echocardiography may be performed to assess the potential for LV function recovery, by measuring the inotropic contractile reserve (Dorbala et al., 2005). The technique is useful especially when LV systolic function is normal, and the contractile reserve remains decreased (Lampert et al., 1997).

7.2 Subsequent pregnancies, risk of relapse

One of the most important issues in PPCM is the safety of subsequent pregnancies. Even after the full recovery of LV function, the risk of relapse might be present.

In Haitian women, Fett et al. described a rate of recurrence of 53% with subsequent pregnancy. In a retrospective study in USA, it was observed that subsequent pregnancy was associated with the recurrence of heart failure, regardless the previous LV function. However, in women who had a normal LV function, the rate of heart failure was 21% compared with 44% in women who had altered function. Also, all deaths occurred in the last group. Furthermore, recovery of LV function was more frequent in patient with an ejection fraction > 30% at diagnosis of disease (Elkayam et al., 2001). Another retrospective study confirmed a better prognosis for subsequent pregnancy in women who had a higher ejection fraction at diagnosis. However, no relation between ejection fraction and worsening clinical symptoms was found in 29% of patients. Also, a baseline ejection fraction of ≤ 25% at index pregnancy was associated with a higher rate of cardiac transplant (Habli et al., 2008). According to these data, it is especially important to provide the most appropriate information about a potential relapse with subsequent pregnancy. LV systolic function seems to be the key prognostic factor when counseling women with PPCM about the further risks. Individual planning might be done after an echocardiogram was performed:

- if LV ejection fraction is < 25% at diagnosis or incompletely recovered, the advice should be against further pregnancy (Sliwa et al., 2010a);
- even if LV function is normal, the patients ought to have stress-echocardiography:
    - women with an abnormal LV inotropic response to dobutamine have a moderate risk of relapse and pregnancy is not recommended;
    - women with complete recovery on both echocardiography and dobutamine stress test can be informed about the low rate of complications. In this group, despite a 35% rate of risk of recurrence, pregnancy can be completed in almost all cases (Pyatt & Durbey, 2011).

In postpartum period, it is imperative to give contraceptive counseling and educate the patients about the existent alternatives. Women who had PPCM should avoid pregnancy, best until LV function has recovered. The combined oral contraceptives, containing estrogens and progestins are contraindicated, as estrogens increase the thromboembolic risk. Progesterone contraception alone is permitted (Thorne et al., 2006). Barrier methods are not recommended as they have a high rate of failure. Intrauterine systems are the most efficient and safe methods of contraception. Sterilization methods, including vasectomy, tubal ligation, and insertion of intratubal stents may be considered (Sliwa et al., 2010a).

At the present time, no protocols for decision-making when counseling women with PPCM about risks of subsequent pregnancies are established. For this reason, it is advisable that every women who experienced PPCM, to be considered at risk, and to be closely monitored by the medical team, in a high-risk obstetrical center.

Main concern

What is the course and prognosis of the disease? With the sparse knowledge in this field, the individual outcome is difficult to predict.

Implications for research

Novel diagnostic strategies, based on improved understanding of pathophysiology and molecular basis of PPCM, should be developed to enhance both diagnostic and prognostic utility. Collecting data from the children born to affected women should be an important priority.

8. Conclusions and future directions

Since its original description, peripartum cardiomyopathy remains a challenge for both diagnosis and treatment. Although several advances have been made to further the knowledge, the condition is still considered a cardiomyopathy of unknown cause. In terms of future research, a better understanding of its molecular basis and fundamental underlying mechanisms, including potential genetic contribution and life-style aspects, is needed. From a clinical perspective, the ability to identify patients at risk to develop the disease is mandatory. Despite current definition, PPCM can remain undiagnosed until it's too late, as some important issues, such as, its rarity in developed countries, the heterogenity of studied populations, and the lack of adherence to diagnostic guidelines, are not resolved. Collaborative, multicentre prospective, well-conducted, population-based trials are required for the development of national and international health policies on prevention, early diagnosis and management, and standard therapeutic control. The Peripartum Cardiomyopathy Netwotk is a NIH-funded North America ongoing trial conducted in order to address some of unresolved issues, as long as the Haitian PPCM Registry is the only existing population-based registry in the world (Fett, 2005a, 2010). Novel diagnostic strategies and biomarkers are potential candidates that should be validated in large clinical trials. Cardiac MRI and prolactin production might provide valuable diagnostic and prognostic information. Also, it would be ideal to have some specific therapeutic strategies. The most realistic candidate seems to be bromocriptine, although potential new treatments, including immune-modulatory therapy, apheresis, and antiviral agents might have a decisive role. Considering all these data, it is important for clinicians to be aware of this condition, so that unnecessary delays in diagnosis can be avoided, and appropriate therapy can be prescribed in a timely fashion. With current technology, clinicians and researchers are now connected, and new bases for multidisciplinary collaboration might be developed.

9. References

Abboud, J., Murad, Y., Chen-Scarabelli, C., Saravolatz, L., & Scarabelli, T.M. (2007).
Peripartum cardiomyopathy: A comprehensive review. *Int J Cardiol,* Vol.118, No.3, (Jun 2007), pp. 295-303, ISSN 0167-5273

Alvarez Navascues, R., Marin, R., Testa, A., Pañeda, F., & Alvarez-Grande, J. (2001). Preeclampsia and peripartum cardiomyopathy: infrequent association. *Nefrologia,* Vol.21, No.1, (Jan-Feb 2001), pp. 84-87, ISSN 0211-6995

Amos, A.M., Jaber, W.A. & Russell, S.D. (2006). Improved outcomes in peripartum cardiomyopathy with contemporary. *Am Heart J,* Vol.152, No.3 (Sep 2006), pp. 509-513, ISSN 0002-8703

Bahloul, M., Ben Ahmed, M.N., Laaroussi, L., Chtara, K., Kallel H., Dammak, H., Ksibi, H., Samet, M., Chelly, H., Hamida, C.B., Chaari, A., Amouri, H., Rekik, N. & Bouaziz, M. (2009). Myocardiopathie du péripartum: incidence, physiopathologie, manifestations cliniques, prise en charge thérapeutique et prognostic. *Annales Françaises d'Anesthésie et de Réanimation,* Vol.28, No.1 (Jan 2009), pp 44-60, ISSN 0750-7658

Baruteau, A.E., Leurent, G., Martins, R.P., Thebault, C., Treguer, F., Leclercq, C., Daubert, J.C. & Mabo, P. (2010). Peripartum cardiomyopathy in the era of cardiac magnetic resonance imaging: First results and perspectives. *Int J Cardiol,* Vol.144, No.1, (Sep 2010), pp 143-145, ISSN 0167-5273

Benezet-Mazuecos, J. & de la Hera, J. (2008). Peripartum cardiomyopathy: A new successful setting for levosimendan. *Int J Cardiol,* Vol.123, No.3 (Jan 2008), pp. 346-347, ISSN 0167-5273

Bennani, S.L., Loubaris, M., Lahlou, I., Haddour, N., Badidi, M., Bouhouch, R., Cherti, M. & Arharbi, M. (2003) Postpartum cardiomyopathy revealed by acute lower limb ischemia. *Ann Cardiol Angeiol (Paris)*, Vol.52, No.6 (Dec 2003), pp. 382–385, ISSN 0003-3928

Bertrand, E., Langlois, J., Renambot, J., Chauvet, L. & Ekra, A. (1977). La myocardiopathie du post-partum : à propos de 25 cas. *Arch Mal Coeur Vaiss*, Vol.70, No.2 (Feb 1977), pp 169–178, ISSN 0003-9683

Box, L.C., Hanak, V. & Arciniegas, J.G. (2004). Dual coronary emboli in peripartum cardiomyopathy. *Tex Heart Inst J*, Vol.31, No.4 (Oct-Dec 2004), pp. 442-444, ISSN 0730-2347

Brar, S.S., Khan, S.S., Sandhu, G.K., Jorgensen, M.B., Parkih, N., Hsu, J.W.Y & Shen, A.Y.J. (2007). Incidence, mortality, and racial differences in peripartum cardiomyopathy. *Am J Cardiol*, Vol.100, No.2 (Jul 2007), pp. 302-304, ISSN 0002-9149

Brown, G., O'Leary, M., Douglas, I. & Herkes, R. (1992). Perioperative management of a case of severe peripartum cardiomyopathy. *Anaesth Intensive Care*, Vol.20, No.1 (Feb 1992), pp. 80-83, ISSN 0310-057X

Bultmann, B.D., Klingel, K., Nabauer, M., Wallwiener, D. & Kandolf, R. (2005). High prevalence of viral genomes and inflammation in peripartum cardiomyopathy. *Am J Obstet Gynecol*, Vol.193, No.2 (Aug 2005), pp. 363-365, ISSN 0002-9378

Caballero-Borrego, J., Garcia-Pinilla, J.M., Rueda-Calle, E. & de Teresa-Galvan, E. (2008). Evidence of gadolinium late-enhancement on cardiac magnetic resonance imaging in a patient with peripartum cardiomyopathy. *Rev Esp Cardiol*, Vol.61, No.2 (Feb 2008), pp. 215-222, ISSN 0300-8932

Carlson, K.M., Browning, J.E., Eggleston, M.K. & Gherman, R.R. (2000). "Peripartum cardiomyopathy presenting as lower extremity arterial thromboembolism. A case report," *Journal of Reproductive Medicine for the Obstetrician and Gynecologist*, Vol.45, No.4 (Apr 2000), pp. 351–353, ISSN 0024-7758

Cenac, A., Simonoff, M., Moretto, P. & Djibo, A. (1992). A low plasma selenium is a risk factor for peripartum cardiomyopathy. A comparative study in Sahelian Africa. *Int J Cardiol*, Vol.36, No. (Jul 1992), pp. 57-59, ISSN 0167-5273

Chapa, J.B., Heiburger, H.B., Weinert, L., Decara, J., Lang, R.M. & Hibbard, J.U. (2005). Prognostic value of echocardiography in peripartum cardiomyopathy. *Obstet Gynecol*, Vol.105, No.6 (Jun 2005), pp. 1303–1308, ISSN 0961-2033

Cole, W.C., Mehta, J.B., Roy, T.M. & Downs, C.J. (2001). "Peripartum cardiomyopathy: echocardiogram to predict prognosis," *Tennessee Medicine*, Vol.94, No.4 (Apr 2001), pp. 135–138, ISSN 1088-6222

Cruz, M.O., Briller, J. & Hibbard, J.U. (2010). Update on Peripartum Cardiomyopathy. *Obstet Gynecol Clin N Am*, Vol.37, No.2 (Jun 2010), pp. 283-303, ISSN 0889-8545

Cunningham, F.G., Pritchard, J.A., Hankins, G.D., Anderson, P.L., Lucas, M.J. & Armstrong, K.F. (1986). Peripartum heart failure: idiopathic cardiomyopathy or compounding cardiovascular events? *Obstet Gynecol*, Vol.67, No.2 (Feb 1986), pp. 157-168, ISSN 0300-8835

de Beus, E., van Mook, W.N., Ramsay, G., Stappers, J.L. & van der Putten, H.W. (2003). Peripartum cardiomyopathy: a condition intensivists should be aware of. *Int Care Med*, Vol.29, No.2 (Feb 2003), pp. 167-174, ISSN 0342-4642

De Luca, L., Colucci, W.S., Nieminen, M.S., Massie, B.M. & Gheorghiade, M. (2006). Evidence-based use of levosimendan in different clinical settings. *Eur Heart J*, Vol.27, No.16 (Aug 2006), pp.1908–1920, ISSN 0195-668x

Demakis, J.G., Rahimtoola, S.H., Sutton, G.C., Meadows, W.R., Szanto, P.B., Tobin, J.R. & Gunnar, R.M. (1971). Natural course of peripartum cardiomyopathy. *Circulation*, Vol.44, No.5 (May 1971), pp. 1053-1061, ISSN 0025-619

Desai, D., Moodley, J. & Naidoo, D. (1995). Peripartum cardiomyopathy: experiences at King Edward VIII Hospital, Durban, South Africa and a review of the literature. *Trop Doct*, Vol.25, No.3 (Jul 1995), pp. 118-123, ISSN 0049-4755

Diao, M., Diop, I.B., Kane, A., Camara, S., Sarr, M., Ba, S.A. & Diouf, S.M. (2004). Electrocardiographic recording of long duration (Holter) of 24 hours during idiopathic cardiomyopathy of the peripartum. *Arch Mal Coeur Vaiss*, Vol.97, No.1 (Jan 2004), pp. 25–30, ISSN 0003-9683

Dickstein, K., Cohen-Solal, A., Filippatos, G., McMurray, J.J.V., Ponikowski, P., Poole-Wilson P.A., Strömberg A., van Veldhuisen D.J., Atar D., Hoes A.W., Keren A., Mebazaa A., Nieminen M., Silvia Giuliana Priori S.G. & Swedberg K. (2008). ESC guidelines for the diagnosis and treatment of acute and chronic heart failure 2008: the Task Force for the diagnosis and treatment of acute and chronic heart failure 2008 of the ESC. *Eur J Heart Fail*, Vol.10, No.10 (Oct 2008), pp. 933-989, ISSN 1388-9842

Dorbala, S., Brozena, S., Logsetty, G., Galatro, K., Homel, P., Ren, JF. & Chaudhry, FA. (2005). Risk stratification of women with peripartum cardiomyopathy at initial presentation: a dobutamine stress echocardiography study. *J Am Soc Echocardiogr*, Vol.18, No.1 (Jan 2005), pp. 45–48, ISSN 0003-2999

Duran, N., Gunes, H., Duran, I., Biteker, M. & Ozkan, M. (2008). Predictors of prognosis in patients with peripartum cardiomyopathy. *Int J Gynaecol Obstet*, Vol.101, No.2 (May 2008), pp. 137–140, ISSN 0020-7292

Egan, R.J., Bisanzom M.C. & Hutson, H.R. (2009). Emergency department evaluation and management of peripartum cardiomyopathy. *J Emerg Med*, Vol.36, No.2 (Feb 2009), pp. 141-147, ISSN 0736-4679

Elkayam, U., Tummala, P.P., Rao, K., Akhter, M.W., Karaalp, I.S., Wani, O.M., Hameed, A., Gviazda, I. & Shotan A. (2001). Maternal and fetal outcomes of subsequent pregnancies in women with peripartum cardiomyopathy. *N Engl J Med*, Vol.344, No.21 (May 2001), pp. 1567–1571, ISSN 0028-4793

Elkayam, U., Akhter, M.W., Singh, H., Khan, S., Bitar, F., Hameed, A. & Shotan, A. (2005). Pregnancy-associated cardiomyopathy: clinical characteristics and a comparison between early and late presentation. *Circulation*, Vol.111, No.6 (Apr 2005), pp. 2050-2055, ISSN 0025-619

Elkayam, U. & Goland, S. (2010). Bromocriptine for the treatment of peripartum cardiomyopathy. *Circulation*, Vol.121, No.13 (Apr 2010), pp. 1463–1464, ISSN 0025-619

Fadouach, S., Matar, N., Meziane, M., Tahiri, A. & Chraibi, N. (1994). Syndrome de Meadows : cardiomyopathie du pèripartum. *Rev Fr Gynecol Obstet*, Vol.89, No.6 (Jun 1994), pp. 335–336, ISSN 1941-2797

Farber, P.A. & Glasgow, L.A. (1970). Viral myocarditis during pregnancy: encephalomyocarditis virus infection in mice. *Am Heart J*, Vol.80, No.1 (Jul 1970), pp. 96-102, ISSN 0002-870

Ferrero, S., Colombo, B.M., Fenini, F., Abbamonte, L.H. & Arena, E. (2003) Peripartum cardiomyopathy. A review. *Minerva Ginecol*, Vol.55, No.2 (Apr 2003), pp. 151-158, ISSN 0026-4784

Fett, J.D., Carraway, R.D., Dowell, D.L., King, M.E. & Pierre, R. (2002). Peripartum cardiomyopathy in the Hospital Albert Schweitzer District of Haiti. *Am J Obstet Gynecol*, Vol.186, No.5 (May 2002), pp. 1005-1010, ISSN 0002-9378

Fett, J.D., Christie, L.G., Carraway, R.D. & Murphy, J.G. (2005a). Five-year prospective study of the incidence and prognosis of peripartum cardiomyopathy at a single institution. *Mayo Clin Proc*, Vol.80, No.12 (Dec 2005), pp. 1602-1606, ISSN 0025-6196

Fett, J.D., Christie, L.G., Carraway, R.D., Ansari, A.A., Sundstrom, J.B. & Murphy, J.G. (2005b). Unrecognized peripartum cardiomyopathy in Haitian women. *Int J Gynaecol Obstet*, Vol.90, No.2 (Aug 2005), pp. 161-166, ISSN 0020-7292

Fett, J.D. (2006a). Inflammation and virus in dilated cardiomyopathy as indicated by endomyocardial biopsy. *Int J Cardiol*, Vol.112, No.1 (Sep 2006), pp. 125-126, ISSN 0167-5273

Fett JD, Christie LG, Murphy JG. (2006b). Brief communication: Outcomes of subsequent pregnancy after peripartum cardiomyopathy: a case series from Haiti. *Ann Intern Med*, Vol.145, No.1 (Jul 2006), pp. 30-34, ISSN 0003-4819

Fett, J.D. (2008). "Understanding peripartum cardiomyopathy, 2008". *Int. J. Cardiol*, Vol.130, No.1 (Oct 2008), pp. 1-2, ISSN 0167-5273

Fett, J.D. (2009). The role of MRI in peripartum cardiomyopathy. *Int J Cardiol*, Vol.137, No.2 (Oct 2009), pp. 185-186, ISSN 0167-5273

Fett, J.D. (2010). What's next in peripartum cardiomyopathy investigation? *Expert Rev Cardiovasc Ther*, Vol.8, No.6 (Jun 2010), pp. 743-746, ISSN 1477-9072

Fett, J.D. (March 2011). "Validation of a self-test for early diagnosis of heart failure in peripartum cardiomyopathy". *Crit Paths Cardiol*, Vol.10, No.1 (Mar 2011), pp. 44-45, ISSN 1535-282X

Fisher, S.D., Etherington, A., Schwartz, D.B. & Pearson, G.D. (2008). Peripartum cardiomyopathy: An update. *Progr Ped Cardiol*, Vol.25, No.1 (Apr 2008), pp. 79-84, ISSN 1058-9813

Forssell, G., Laska, J., Olofsson, C. Olsson, M. & Mogensen, L. (1994). Peripartum cardiomyopathy: three cases. *J Intern Med*, Vol.235, No.4 (May 1994), pp. 493-496, ISSN 0954-6820

Freedman, N.J. & Lefkowitz, R.J. (2004). Anti-b1-adrenergic receptor antibodies and heart failure: causation, not just correlation. *J Clin Invest*, Vol.113, No.10 (May 2004), pp. 1379-1382, ISSN 0021-9738

Fussell, K.M., Awad, J.A. & Ware, L.B. (2005). "Case of fulminant hepatic failure due to unrecognized peripartum cardiomyopathy". *Crit. Care Med*, Vol.33, No.4 (Apr 2005), pp. 891-893, ISSN 1529-7535

Garrison, E., Hibbard, J.U., Studee, L., Fontana, D., Klibatrick, S. & Briller, J. (2005). Brain natriuretic peptide as a marker for heart disease in pregnancy. *Am J Obstet Gynecol*, Vol.193, No.6 Suppl (Dec 2005), pp. S83, ISSN 0002-9378

Gentry, M.B., Dias, J.K., Luis, A., .Patel, R., Thornton J. & Reed, G.L. (2010). African-American women have a higher risk for developing peripartum cardiomyopathy. *J Am Coll Cardiol*, Vol.55, No.7 (Feb 2010), pp. 654-659, ISSN 0301-4711

Ghuman, N., Rheiner, J., Tendler, B.E. & White, W.B. (2009). Hypertension in the postpartum woman: clinical update for the hypertension specialist. *J Clin Hypertens (Greenwich)*, Vol.11, No.12 (Dec 2009), pp. 726–733, ISSN 1524-6175

Glück, B., Schmidtke, M., Merkle, I., Stelzner, A. & Gemsa, D. (2001). Persistent expression of cytokines in the chronic stage of CVB3-induced myocarditis in NMRI mice. *J Mol Cell Cardiol*, Vol.33, No.9 (Sep 2001), pp. 1615-1626, ISSN 0022-2828

Godsel, L.M., Leon, J.S. & Engman, D.M. (2003). Angiotensin converting enzyme inhibitors and angiotensin II receptor antagonists in experimental myocarditis. *Curr Pharm Des*, Vol.9, No.9 (2003), pp. 723–735, ISSN 1381-6128

Goland, S., Modi, K., Bitar, F., Janmohamed, M., Mirocha, J.M., Czer, L.S., Illum, S., Hatamizadeh, P. & Elkayam, U. (2009). Clinical profile and predictors of complications in peripartum cardiomyopathy. *J Card Fail*, Vol.15, No.8 (Oct 2009), pp. 645–650, ISSN 0091-2700

Gouley, B.A., McMillan, T.M. & Bellet, S. (1937). Idiopathic myocardial degeneration associated with pregnancy and especially the puerperium. *Am J Med Sci*, Vol.194 (1937), pp. 185-189, ISSN 0002-9629

Habedank, D., Kuhnle, Y., Elgeti, T., Dudenhausen, J.W., Haverkamp, W. & Dietz, R. (2008). Recovery from peripartum cardiomyopathy after treatment with bromocriptine. *Eur J Heart Fail*, Vol.10, No.11 (Nov 2008), pp. 1149-1151, ISSN 1388-9842

Habli, M., O'Brien, T., Nowack, E., Khoury, S., Barton, J.R. & Sibai, B. (2008). Peripartum cardiomyopathy: prognostic factors for long-term maternal outcome. *Am J Obstet Gynecol*, Vol.199, No.4 (Oct 2008), pp. 415.e1–5, ISSN 0025-6196

Hameed, A.B., Chan, K., Ghamsary, M. & Elkayam, U. (2009). Longitudinal changes in the B-type natriuretic peptide levels in normal pregnancy and post partum. *Clin Cardiol*, Vol.32, No.8 (Aug 2009), pp. E60–E62, ISSN 0160-9289

Helms, A.K., & Kittner, S.J. (2005). Pregnancy and stroke. *CNS Spectr*, Vol.10, No.7 (Jul 2005), pp. 580–587, ISSN 1092-8529

Hershberger, R.E., Lindenfeld, J., Mestroni, L., Seidman, C.E., Taylor, M.R. & Towbin, J.A. (2009). Genetic evaluation of cardiomyopathy: a Heart Failure Society of America practice guideline. *J Card Fail*, Vol. 15, No.2 (Mar 2009), pp. 83-97, ISSN 0091-2700

Hibbard, J.U., Lindheimer, M., Lang, R.M. (1999). A modified definition for peripartum cardiomyopathy and prognosis based on echocardiography. *Obstet Gynecol*, Vol.94, No.2 (Aug 1999), pp. 311–316, ISSN 0029-7844

Hilfiker-Kleiner, D., Kaminski, K., Podewski, E., Bonda, T., Schaefer, A., Sliwa, K., Forster, O., Quint, A., Landmesser, U., Doerries, C., Luchtefeld, M., Poli, V., Schneider, M.D., Balligand, J.L., Desjardins, F., Ansari, A., Struman, I., Nguyen, N.Q., Zschemisch, N.H., Klein, G., Heusch, G., Schulz, R., Hilfiker, A. & Drexler, H. (2007a). A cathepsin D-cleaved 16 kDa form of prolactin mediates postpartum cardiomyopathy. *Cell*, Vol.128, No.3, (Feb 2007), pp. 589-600, ISSN 0092-8674

Hilfiker-Kleiner, D., Meyer, G.P., Schieffer, E., Goldmann, B., Podewski, E., Struman, I., Fischer, P. & Drexler, H. (2007b). Recovery from postpartum cardiomyopathy in 2 patients by blocking prolactin release with bromocriptine. *J Am Coll Cardiol*, Vol.50, No.24 (Dec 2007), pp. 2354-2355, ISSN 0735-1097

Hilfiker-Kleiner, D., Sliwa, K. & Drexler, H. (2008). Peripartum Cardiomyopathy: Recent Insights in its Pathophysiology. *Trends Cardiovasc Med*, Vol.18, No.5 (July 2008), pp. 173–179, ISSN 1050-1738

Hopp, L., Haider, B. & Iffy, L. (1996). Myocardial infarction postpartum in patients taking bromocriptine for the prevention of breast engorgement. *Int J Cardiol*, Vol.57, No.3 (Dec 1996), pp. 227–232, ISSN 0167-5273

Horwitz, M.S., Knudsen, M., Fine, C., Fine, C. & Sarvetnick, N. (2007). Transforming growth factor-beta inhibits cocksackievirus mediated autoimmune myocarditis. *Viral Immunol*, Vol.19, No.4 (Jan 2007), pp. 722–733, ISSN 0882-8245

Hu, C.L., Li, Y.B., Zou, Y.G., Zhang, J.M., Chen, J.B., Liu, J., Tang, Y.H., Tang, Q.Z. & Huang, C.X. (2007). Troponin T measurement can predict persistent left ventricular dysfunction in peripartum cardiomyopathy. *Heart*, Vol.93, No.4 (Apr 2007), pp. 488–490, ISSN 1355-6037

Hunt, S.A., Abraham, W.T., Chin, M.H., Feldman, A.M., Francis, G.S., Ganiats, T.G., Jessup, M., Konstam, M.A., Mancini, D.M., Michl, K., Oates, J.A., Rahko, P.S., Silver, M.A., Stevenson, L.W. & Yancy, C.W. (2009). 2009 Focused update incorporated into the ACC/AHA 2005 guidelines for the diagnosis and management of heart failure in adults: a report of the American College of Cardiology Foundation/ American Heart Association Task Force on Practice Guidelines. *Circulation*, Vol.119, No.14 (Apr 2009), pp. e391–479, ISSN 0006-3363

Jahns, R., Boivin, V., Hein, L., . Triebel, S., Angermann, C.E., Ertl, G. & Lohse, M.J. (2004). Direct evidence for a b1-adrenergic receptor directed autoimmune attack as a cause of idiopathic dilated cardiomyopathy. *J Clin Invest*, Vol.113, No.10 (May 2004), pp. 1419-1429, ISSN 0021-9738

Jahns, B.G., Stein, W., Hilfiker-Kleiner, D., Pieske, B. & Emons, G. (2008). Peripartum cardiomyopathy–a new treatment option by inhibition of prolactin secretion. *Am J Obstet Gynecol*, Vol.199, No.4 (Oct 2008), pp. e5–e6, ISSN 0002-9378

Jha, P., Jha, S. & Millane, T.A. (2005). Peripartum cardiomyopathy complicated by pulmonary embolism and pulmonary hypertension. *Eur J Obstet Gynecol Reprod Biol*, Vol.123, No.1 (Nov 2005), pp. 121–123, ISSN 0301-2115

Kane, A., Dia, A.A., Diouf, A., Dia, D., Diop, I.B., Moreau, J.C., Faye, E.O., Sarr, M., Ba, S.A., Diadhiou, F. & Diouf, S.M. (2001). La myocardiopathie idiopathique du péripartum: étude prospective échocardiographique. *Ann Cardiol Angeiol*, Vol.50, No.6 (Oct 2001), pp. 305–311, ISSN 0003-3928

Kawano, H., Tsuneto, A., Koide, Y., Tasaki, H,. Sueyoshi, E., Sakamoto, I. & Hayashi, T. (2008). Magnetic resonance imaging in a patient with peripartum cardiomyopathy. *Intern Med*, Vol.47, No.2 (Jan 2008), pp. 97–102, ISSN 1444-0903

Kim, Y.J., Park, H.S., Park, M.H., Suh, S.H. & Pang, M.G. (2005). Oxidative stress-related gene polymorphism and the risk of preeclampsia. *Eur J Obst. Gyn. Reprod. Biol.*, Vol.119, No.1 (Mar 2005), pp. 42–46, ISSN 1360-9947

Kothari, S.S. (1997). Aetiopathogenesis of peripartum cardiomyopathy: prolactin–selenium interaction? *Int J Cardiol*, Vol.60, No.1 (*June* 1997), pp. 111–114, ISSN 0167-5273

Kühl, U., Pauschinger, M., Noutsias, M., Seeberg, B., Bock, T., Lassner, D., Poller, W., Kandolf, R. & Schultheiss, H.P. (2005a). High prevalence of viral genomes and multiple viral infections in the myocardium of adults with "idiopathic" left ventricular dysfunction. *Circulation*, Vol.111, No.7 (Feb 2005), pp. 887-893, ISSN 0009-7322

Kűhl, U., Pauschinger, M., Seeberg, B., Lassner, D., Noutsias, M., Poller, W. & Schultheiss, H.P. (2005b). Viral persistence in the myocardium is associated with progressive cardiac dysfunction. *Circulation*, Vol.112, No.13 (Sep 2005), pp. 1965–1970, ISSN 0009-7322

Lampert, M.B. & Lang, R.M. (1995). Peripartum cardiomyopathy. *Am Heart J*, Vol.130, No.4 (Oct 1995), pp. 860–870, ISSN 0002-8703

Lampert, M.B., Weinert, L., Hibbard, J., Korcarz, C., Lindheimer, M. & Lang, R.M. (1997). Contractile reserve in patients with peripartum cardiomyopathy and recovered left ventricular function. *Am J Obstet Gynecol*, Vol.176, No.1 (Jan 1997), pp. 189-195, ISSN 0002-9378

Lang, C., Sauter, M., Szalay, G., Racchi, G., Grassi, G., Rainaldi, G., Mercatanti, A., Lang, F., Kandolf, R. & Klingel, K. (2008). Connective tissue growth factor: a crucial cytokine-mediating cardiac fibrosis in ongoing enterovirus myocarditis. *J Mol Med*, Vol.86, No.1 (Jan 2008), pp. 49-60, ISSN 0946-2716

Lasinska-Kowara, M., Dudziak, M. & Suchorzewska, J. (2001). "Two cases of postpartum cardiomyopathy initially misdiagnosed for pulmonary embolism". *Can J Anaesth*, Vol.48, No.8 (Sep 2001), pp. 773–777, ISSN 0832-610X

Leurent, G., Baruteau, A.E., Larralde, A., Ollivier, R., Schleich, J.M., Boulmier, D., Bedossa, M., Langella, B. & Le Breton, H. (2009). Contribution of cardiac MRI in the comprehension of peripartum cardiomyopathy pathogenesis. *Int J Cardiol*, Vol.132, No.3 (Mar 2009), pp. e91–93, ISSN 0301-471

Lindheimer, M.D. & Katz, A.I. (1973). Sodium and diuretics in pregnancy. *N Engl J Med*, Vol.288, No.17 (Apr 1973), pp. 891–894, ISSN 0028-4793

Maron, B.J., Towbin, J.A., Thiene, G., Antzelevitch, C., Corrado, D., Arnett, D., Moss, A.J., Seidman, C.E. & Young, J.B. (2006). Contemporary definitions and classification of the cardiomyopathies: an American Heart Association Scientific Statement from the Council on Clinical Cardiology, Heart Failure and Transplantation Committee; Quality of Care and Outcomes Research and Functional Genomics and Translational Biology Interdisciplinary Working Groups; and Council on Epidemiology and Prevention. *Circulation*, Vol.113, No.14 (Apr 2006), pp. 1807-1816, ISSN 0009-7322

Meyer, G.P., Labidi, S., Podewski, E., Sliwa, K., Drexler, H. & Hilfiker-Kleiner, D. (2010). Bromocriptine treatment associated with recovery from peripartum cardiomyopathy in siblings: two case reports. *J Med Case Rep*, Vol.4, No.4 (Mar 2010), pp. 80, ISSN 1752-1947

Midei, M., DeMent, S., Feldman, A., Hutchins, G.M. & Baughman, K.L. (1990). Peripartum myocarditis and cardiomyopathy. *Circulation*, Vol. 81, No. 3 (Mar 1990), pp. 922-928, ISSN 0009-7322

Mielniczuk, L.M., Williams, K., Davis, D.R., Tang, A.S., Lemery, R., Green, M.S., Gollob, M.H., Haddad, H. & Birnie, D.H. (2006). Frequency of peripartum cardiomyopathy. *Am J Cardiol*, Vol.97, No.12 (Jun 2006), pp. 1765-1768, ISSN 0002-9149

Modi, K.A., Illum, S., Jariatul, K., Caldito, G. & Reddy, P.C. (2009). Poor outcome of indigent patients with peripartum cardiomyopathy in the United States. *Am J Obstet Gynecol*, Vol.201, No.2 (Aug 2009), pp. 171.e1–5, ISSN 0002-9378

Moioli, M., Menada, M.V., Bentivoglio, G. & Ferrero, S. (2010). Peripartum cardiomyopathy. *Arch Gynecol Obstet*, Vol. 281, No. 2 (Feb 2010), pp. 183-188, ISSN 0932-0067

Morales, A., Painter, T, Li, R., Siegfried, J.D., Li, D., Norton, N. & Hershberger, R.E. (2010). Rare variant mutations in pregnancy-associated or peripartum cardiomyopathy. *Circulation*, Vol.121, No.20 (May 2010), pp. 2176–2182, ISSN 0009-7322

Mouquet, F., Lions, C., de Groote, P., Bouabdallaoui, N., Willoteaux, S., Dagorn, J., Deruelle, P., Lamblin, N., Bauters, C. & Beregi, J.P. (2008). Characterisation of peripartum cardiomyopathy by cardiac magnetic resonance imaging. *Eur Radiol*, Vol.18, No.12 (Dec 2008), pp.:2765–2769, ISSN 0033-8419

Muldowney, J.A. III., Schoenhard, J.A. & Benge, C.D. (2009). The clinical pharmacology of eplerenone. *Expert Opin Drug Metab Toxicol*, Vol.5, No.4 (Apr 2009), pp. 425-432, ISSN 1742-5255

Murali, S. & Baldisseri, M.R. (2005). Peripartum cardiomyopathy. *Crit Care Med*, Vol.33, No.10 (Suppl) (Oct 2005), pp. S340-S346, ISSN 0090-3493

Nagafuchi, H., Suzuki, N., Kaneko, A., Asai, T. & Sakane, T. (1999). Prolactin locally produced by synovium infiltrating T lymphocytes induces excessive synovial cell functions in patients with rheumatoid arthritis. *J Rheumatol*, Vol.26, No.9 (Sep 1999), pp. 1890–1900, ISSN 0315-162x

Narula, J., Kolodgie, F.D. & Virmani, R. (2000). Apoptosis and cardiomyopathy. *Curr Opin Cardiol*, Vol.15, No.3 (May 2000), pp. 183-188, ISSN 0268-4705

Negoro, S., Kunisada, K., Fujio, Y., Funamoto, M., Darville, M.I., Eizirik, D.L., Osugi, T., Izumi, M., Oshima, Y., Nakaoka, Y., Hirota, H., Kishimoto, T. & Yamauchi-Takihara, K. (2001). Activation of signal transducer and activator of transcription 3 protects cardiomyocytes from hypoxia/reoxygenation-induced oxidative stress through the upregulation of manganese superoxide dismutase. *Circulation*, Vol.104, No.9 (Aug 2001), pp. 979-981, ISSN 1524-4539

Nkoua, J.L., Kimbaly-Kaky, G., Onkani, A.H., Kandosi, S. & Bouramoue, C. (1991). La myocardiopathie du post-partum. À propos de 24 cas. *Cardiol Trop*, Vol. 17, No. 67 (1991), pp. 105-110, ISSN 1995-1892

Ntusi, N.B.A. & Mayosi, B.M. Aetiology and risk factors of peripartum cardiomyopathy: A systematic review. *Int J Cardiology*, Vol.131, No.2 (Jan 2009), pp. 168-179, ISSN 0167-5273

Oakley, C., Child, A., Iung, B., Presbitero, P., Tornos, P., Klein, W., Garcia, M.A.A., Blomstrom-Lundqvist, C., de Backer, G., Dargie, H., Deckers, J., Flather, M., Hradec, J., Mazzotta, G., Oto, A., Parkhomenko, A., Silber, S., Torbicki, A., Trappe, H.J., Dean, V., & Poumeyrol-Jumeau, D. (2003). Expert consensus document on management of cardiovascular diseases during pregnancy.Task force on the management of cardiovascular diseases during pregnancy of the European society of cardiology. *Eur Heart J*, Vol.24, No.8 (Apr 2003), pp. 761-781, ISSN 0195-668x

Pauschinger, M., Rutschow, W., Chandrasekharan, K., Westermann, D., Weitz, A., Peter, S.L,, Zeichhardt, H., Poller, W., Noutsias, M., Li, J., Schultheiss, H.P. & Tschope, C. (2005). Carvedilol improves left ventricular function in murine coxsackievirus-induced active myocarditis associated with reduced myocardial interleukin-1beta and MMP-8 expression and a modulated immune response. *Eur J Heart Fail*, Vol.7, No.4 (Jun 2005), pp. 444–452, ISSN 1388-9842

Pearson, G.D., Veille, J.C., Rahimtoola, S., Hsia, J., Oakley, C.M., Hosenpud, J.D., Ansari, A. & Baughman, K.L. (2000). Peripartum cardiomyopathy. National Heart Lung and Blood Institute and Office of Rare Diseases (National Institutes of Health)

workshop recommendations and review. *JAMA*, Vol.283, No.9 (Mar 2000), pp. 1183-1888, ISSN 0098-7484

Pierce, J.A., Price, B.O. & Joyce, J.W. (1963). Familial occurrence of postpartal heart failure. *Arch Intern Med*, Vol.111, No.5 (May 1963), pp. 151-155, ISSN 0003-9926

Porak C. (1880). De l'influence reciproque de la grossesse et des maladies du Couer, thesis, Paris, 1880

Potapov, E.V., Loforte, A., Weng, Y., Jurmann, M., Pasic, M., Drews, T., Loebe, M., Hennig, E., Krabatsch, T., Koster, A., Lehmkuhl, H.B. &, Hetzer, R. (2008). Experience with over 1000 implanted ventricular assist devices. *J Card Surg*, Vol.23, No.3 (May-Jun 2008), pp. 185–194, ISSN 0886-0440

Pyatt, R.J. & Dubey, G. (2011). Peripartum cardiomyopathy: current understanding, comprehensive management review and new developments. *Postgrad Med J*, Vol.87, No.1023 (Jan 2011), pp. 34-39, ISSN 1560-5876

Ramaraj, R. & Sorrell, V.L. (2009). Peripartum cardiomyopathy: causes, diagnosis, and treatment. *Clev Clin J Med*, Vol.76, No.5 (May 2009), pp. 289-296, ISSN 0891-1150

Rasmusson, K.D., Stehlik, J., Brown, R.N., Renlund, D.G., Wagoner, L.E., Torre-Amione, G., Folsom, J.W., Silber, D.H. & Kirklin, J.K. (2007). Longterm outcomes of cardiac transplantation for peri-partum cardiomyopathy: a multiinstitutional analysis. *J Heart Lung Transplant*, Vol.26, No.11 (Nov 2007), pp. 1097–1104, ISSN 1053-2498

Ritchie, C. (1849). Clinical contribution to the pathology, diagnosis and treatment of certain chronic diseases in the heart. *Edinburgh Med Surg*, Vol.2, pp. 333, ISSN 0003-2999

Rizeq, M.N., Rickenbache, P.R., Fowler, M.B. & Billingham ,M.E. (1994). Incidence of myocarditis in peripartum cardiomyopathy. *Am J Cardiol*, Vol.74, No.5 (Sep 1994), pp. 474-477, ISSN 0002-9149

Roberg, K. & Ollinger, K. (1998). Oxidative stress causes relocation of the lysosomal enzyme cathepsin D with ensuing apoptosis in neonatal rat cardiomyocytes. *Am J Pathol*, Vol.152, No.1 (May 1998), pp. 1151-1156, ISSN 0002-9440

Robson, S.C., Hunter, S., Boys, R.J. & Dunlop, W. (1989). Serial study of factors influencing changes in cardiac output during human pregnancy. *Am J Physiol Heart Circ Physiol*, Vol.256, No.4 (Apr 1989), pp. 1060-1065, ISSN 0363-6135

Sliwa, K., Skudicky, D., Bergemann, A., Cand,y G., Puren, A. & Sareli, P. (2000). Peripartum cardiomyopathy: analysis of clinical outcome, left ventricular function, plasma levels of cytokines and Fas/APO-1. *J Am Coll Cardiol*, Vol.35, No.3 (Mar 2000), pp. 701–705, ISSN :0735-1097

Sliwa, K., Skukicky, D., Candy, G., Bergemann, A., Hopley, M. & Sareli, P. (2002). The addition of pentoxifylline to conventional therapy improves outcome in patients with peripartum cardiomyopathy. *Eur J Heart Fail*, Vol.4, No.3 (Jun 2002), pp. 305–309, ISSN 1388-9842

Sliwa, K., Fett, J. & Elkayam, U. (2006a). Peripartum cardiomyopathy. *Lancet*, Vol.368, No.9536 (Aug 2006), pp. 687-693, ISSN 0140-6736

Sliwa, K., Forster, O., Libhaber, E., Fett, J.D., Sundstrom, J.B., Hilfiker-Kleiner, D. & Ansari, A.A. (2006b). Peripartum cardiomyopathy: inflammatory markers as predictors of outcome in 100 prospectively studied patients. *Eur Heart J*, Vol.27, No.4 (Feb 2006), pp. 441–446, ISSN 0195-668X

Sliwa, K., Hilfiker-Kleiner, D., Petrie, M.C., Mebazaa, A., Pieske, B., Buchmann, E., Regitz-Zagrosek, V., Schaufelberger, M., Tavazzi, L,, van Veldhuisen, D.J., Watkins, H.,

Shah, A.J., Seferovic, P.M., Elkayam, U., Pankuweit, S., Papp, Z., Mouquet, F. & McMurray, J.J. (2010a). Current state of knowledge on aetiology, diagnosis, management, and therapy of peripartum cardiomyopathy: a position statement from the Heart Failure Association of the European Society of Cardiology Working Group on peripartum cardiomyopathy. *Eur J Heart Fail*, Vol.12, No.8 (Aug 2010), pp. 767-778, ISSN 1388-9842

Sliwa, K., Blauwet, L., Tibazarwa, K. Libhaber, E., Smedema, J.P., Becker, A., McMurray, J., Yamac, H., Labidi, S., Struman, I. & Hilfiker-Kleiner, D. (2010b). Evaluation of bromocriptine in the treatment of acute severe peripartum cardiomyopathy. A proof-of-concept pilot study. *Circulation*, Vol.121, No.13 (Mar 2010), pp. 1465-1473, ISSN 1524-4539

Srichai, M.B., Junor, C., Rodriguez, L.L., Stillman, A.E., Grimm, R.A., Lieber, M.L., Weaver, J.A., Smedira, N.G. & White, R.D. (2006). Clinical, imaging, and pathological characteristics of left ventricular thrombus: a comparison of contrast-enhanced magnetic resonance imaging, transthoracic echocardiography, and transesophageal echocardiography with surgical or pathological validation. *Am Heart J*, Vol.152, No.1 (Jul 2006), pp. 75–84, ISSN 0002-8703

Thorne, S., MacGregor, A. & Nelson-Piercy, C. (2006). Risks of contraception and pregnancy in heart disease. *Heart*, Vol.92, No.10 (Oct 2006), pp. 1520–1525, ISSN 1355-6037

Toescu, V., Nuttall, S.L., Martin, U., Kendall, M.J. & Dunne, F. (2002). Oxidative stress and normal pregnancy. *Clin Endocrinol (Oxf)*, Vol. 57, No. 5 (Nov 2002), pp. 609-613, ISSN 0300-0664

Torbicki, A., Perrier, A., Konstandinides, S., Galiè, N., Pruszczyk, P., Bengel, F., Brady, A.J, Ferreira, D., Janssens, U., Klepetko, W., Mayer, E., Remy-Jardin, M. & Bassand, J.P. (2008). Guidelines on the diagnosis and management of acute pulmonary embolism. The Task Force for the Diagnosis and Management of Acute Pulmonary Embolism of the European Society of Cardiology. *Eur Heart J*, Vol.29, No.18 (Sep 2008), pp. 2276-2315, ISSN 0195-668x

van Spaendonck-Zwarts, K., van Tintelen, J., van Veldhuisen, D.J., van der Werf, R., Jongbloed, J.D., Paulus, W.J., Dooijes, D. & van den Berg, M.P. (2010). Peripartum cardiomyopathy as part of familial dilated cardiomyopathy. *Circulation*, Vol.121, No.20 (May 2010), pp. 2169–2175, ISSN 0009-7322

Walsh, J.J., Burch, C.E., Black, W.C., Ferrans, V.J. & Hibbs, R.G. (1965). Idiopathic myocardiopathy of the peripartum. *Circulation*, Vol.32 (Jul 1965), pp. 19-31, ISSN 0009-7322

Warraich, R.S., Sliwa, K., Damasceno, A., Carraway, R., Sundrom, B., Arif, G., Essop, R., Ansari, A., Fett, J. & Yacoub, M. (2005). Impact of pregnancy-related heart failure on humoral immunity: clinical relevance of G3-subclass immunoglobulins in peripartum cardiomyopathy. *Am Heart J*, Vol.150, No.2 (Aug 2005), pp. 263-269, ISSN 0002-870

Webb, J.A., Thomsen, H.S. & Morcos, S.K. (2005). The use of iodinated and gadolinium contrast media during pregnancy and lactation. *Eur Radiol*, Vol.15, No.6 (Jun 2005), pp. 1234–1240, ISSN 0033-8419

Weinblatt, M., Singer, M.A. & Iqbal, I. (1995). Peripartum cardiomyopathy: a case report and review of literature. *Primary Care Update for Ob Gyns*, Vol.2, No.2 (Mar-Apr 1995), pp 59–62, ISSN 1068-607X V

Wencker, D., Chandra, M., Nguyen, K., Miao, W., Garantziotis, S., Factor, S.M., Shirani, J., Armstrong, R.C. & Kitsis, R.N. (2003). A mechanistic role for cardiac myocyte apoptosis in heart failure. *J Clin Invest*, Vol.111, No.10 (May 2003), pp. 1497-1504, ISSN 0895-4356

Whitehead, S.J., Berg, C.J. & Chang J. (2003). Pregnancy related mortality due to cardiomyopathy: United States, 1991-1997. *Obstet Gynecol*, Vol.102, No.6 (Dec 2003), pp. 1326-1331, ISSN 0029-7844

Wittstein, I.S., Thiemann, D.R., Lima, J.A.C., Baughman, K.L., Schulman, S.P., Gerstenblith, G., Wu, K.C., Rade, J.J., Bivalacqua, T.J. & Champion, H.C. (2005). Neurohumoral features of myocardial stunning due to sudden emotional stress. *N Engl J Med*, Vol. 352, No.6 (Feb 2005), pp. 539-548, ISSN 0028-4793

Yahagi, N., Kumon, K. & Nakatani, T. (1994). Peripartum cardiomyopathy and tachycardia followed by multiple organ failure. *Anesth Analg*, Vol.79, No.3 (Sep 1994), pp. 581-582, ISSN 0003-2999

Yang, H.S., Hong, Y.S., Rim, S.J. & Yu, S.H. (2007). Extracorporeal membrane oxygenation in a patient with peripartum cardiomyopathy. *Ann Thorac Surg*, Vol.84, No.1 (Jul 2007), pp. 262-264, ISSN 0003-4975

Zimmermann, O., Kochs, M., Zwaka, T.P., Kaya, Z., Lepper, P.M., Bienek-Ziolkowski, M., Hoher, M., Hombach, V. & Torzewski, J. (2005). Myocardial biopsy based classification and treatment in patients with dilated cardiomyopathy. *Int J Cardiol*, Vol.104, No.1 (Sep 2005), pp. 92-100, ISSN 0167-5273

Zimmerman, H., Bose, R., Smith, R. & Copeland, J.G. Treatment of Peripartum Cardiomyopathy With Mechanical Assist Devices and Cardiac Transplantation. *Ann Thorac Surg*, Vol. 89, No.4 (Apr 2010), pp. 1211-1217, ISSN 0003-4975.

6

Cardiomyopathy Detection from Electrocardiogram Features

Mirela Ovreiu and Dan Simon
Cleveland Clinic Foundation, Cleveland State University
United States

1. Introduction

Cardiomyopathy refers to diseases of the heart muscle that becomes enlarged, thick, or rigid. These changes affect the electrical stability of the myocardial cells, which predisposes the heart to failure or arrhythmias. Cardiomyopathy in its two common forms, dilated and hypertrophic, implies enlargement of the atria. Therefore, computer intelligence techniques are proposed for the recognition and classification of P wave features for cardiomyopathy diagnosis. The technique that we propose is a neuro-fuzzy network. The neuro-fuzzy classifier will be trained with innovative evolutionary algorithms, which have recently been shown to be efficient global optimizers.

Cardiomyopathy is a significant clinical problem which is mainly generated by volume/diastolic overload. To accommodate the increased blood volume, the heart chambers may stretch or dilate. Valvular regurgitation and congestive heart failure are two conditions that contribute to chamber dilation.

Cardiomyopathy is generally diagnosed by an electrocardiographic (ECG) investigation. In the current standards published by the American Heart Association, chamber hypertrophy or enlargement is a separate diagnostic category which can be detected with ECG analysis (Masson, Hancock, & Gettes, 2007). Although many algorithms have been implemented for ECG analysis, the proposed research is unique in several ways.

- We propose the development of **non-invasive** and **automatic cardiomyopathy diagnosis**, which has not been reported in the literature.
- We propose the development of algorithms for **P wave analysis**, which have not been reported in the literature.
- We propose the use of **5-lead ECG data**, which is more readily available than 12-lead data.
- We propose the use of a powerful **neuro-fuzzy architecture** for ECG analysis, which has not been reported in the literature.
- We propose neuro-fuzzy ECG classifier optimization using **evolutionary algorithms**, which has not been reported in the literature.

Our preliminary studies of postoperative cardiovascular patients reveal our hypothesis: the ECG presents different electrical activity for patients with cardiomyopathy, compared with patients who do not have cardiomyopathy. This working hypothesis indicates that an automated method that selects the best ECG parameters to include in a cardiomyopathy diagnosis algorithm will be extremely valuable. Although such a method will not be fool-proof or 100% correct, and thus cannot replace medical doctors, it will help physicians diagnose or prognose life threatening conditions such as stroke or ventricular or atrial fibrillation. This will expedite the initiation of medical treatment as appropriate to minimize the risk of these conditions, or to prevent their onsets.

Although it has long been suggested that cardiomyopathy is reflected in modification of ECG characteristics, statistics-based attempts to classify cardiomyopathy from the ECG have been underwhelming (Macfarlane, 2006; Magdic, Saul, 1997). Motivated by the universal approximation theorem for neuro-fuzzy networks discussed in the chapter, we hypothesize that earlier limitations may be overcome by a neuro-fuzzy classification model.

Cardiovascular diseases are the major cause of death in the western world, resulting in more than 800,000 deaths per year in the United States alone (American Heart Association, 2009). One in five Americans has some form of cardiovascular disease (Olson, 2004).

Cardiomyopathy is a significant clinical problem which is mainly generated by volume/diastolic overload. To accommodate the increased volume of blood, the heart chambers may stretch or dilate. Valvular regurgitation and congestive heart failure are two conditions that contribute to chamber dilation.

Cardiomyopathy is generally diagnosed by an echocardiograph investigation. For an echocardiography the patient has to be referred to a cardiologist or an echocardiographic investigation. But the electrocardiographic (ECG) investigation is always part of a cardiologic work-up.

The ECG represents the recording of the deflection of ionic current across myocardial cell membranes and throughout the extracellular space of the different tissues of the thoracic cavity. The ECG, in competition to many other techniques, retains an important role in diagnosis and prognosis of cardiovascular diseases.

It has been suggested that cardiomyopathy is reflected in modification of ECG characteristics such as P wave morphology. Previous statistics-based attempts to classify the cardiomyopathy from ECG have been underwhelming (Macfarlane, 2006; Magdic, Saul, 1997), but we hypothesize that these limitations can be overcome using a hybrid neuro-fuzzy classification model. To test this hypothesis and direct the results to patient care, we follow these directions. First we design a neuro-fuzzy model to diagnose cardiomyopathy. Then we train the network using an aquired clinical database of ECG signals.

Neuro-fuzzy systems can be trained with derivative-based methods like gradient descent (Chen, Linkens, 2001; Linkens, Chen, 1999) or with evolutionary algorithms such as genetic algorithms and swarm intelligence (Kennedy, Eberhart, & Shi, 2001). Evolutionary algorithms have the advantage of not requiring derivative information, and have less likelihood of getting stuck in a local optimum. Hence we use a new biologically motivated optimization algorithm called biogeography-based optimization (BBO) (Simon, 2008) to train the neuro-fuzzy ECG classification network. We also incorporate opposition-based learning in the BBO algorithm (Ergezer, Simon, & Du, 2009) for better classification.

2. Background

2.1 Cardiomyopathy

The term "cardiomyopathy" defines a group of diseases primarily affecting the cardiac muscle by weakening it or changing its structure. Cardiomyopathy can be acquired or inherited, and in many cases its cause is unknown. Hypertrophic cardiomyopathy is inherited and is supposed to be a result of defects of genes that regulate heart muscle growth. Abnormal cardiac enlargement can be due to an increase in length or diameter of existing cardiac muscle cells (Olson, 2004). Cardiomyopathy, through electrical instability of myocardial cells, is associated with cardiac conduction abnormalities that can degenerate to arrhythmia or heart failure (Dische, 1972).

Cardiomyopathies, especially hypertrophic, are considered a common cause of sudden cardiac death in young adults and children (Ingles, Semsarian, 2007; Bar-Cohen, Silka, 2008). The Chagas and idiopathic dilated etiologies of cardiomyopathy led to Pereira et al.'s study in adults (Pereira et al., 2010); after 40 months, almost half of the cases studied (113 out of 284) registered deaths (104) or heart transplants (9).

The ECG records the deflection of ionic current across myocardial cell membranes and through the extracellular space of the thoracic cavity tissues. The history of cardiomyopathy research reveals the evolution of the analysis of ECG correlations. Due to the left ventricle's critical role, initial studies were focused only on the ECG features of the hypertrophic left ventricle (Sox, Garber, Littenberg, 1989). The QRS and T waves, as the reflections of ventricular depolarization and repolarization respectively, were analyzed (Ziegler, 1970). In the study by Sox et al., citing the Framingham Study, the left ventricular hypertrophy (LVH) was defined by a prolonged ventricular activation period of 0.05 s, tall R waves, depressed ST segments, and inverted T waves (Sox, Garber, Littenberg, 1989). Ziegler was the first to analyze T waves related to LVH; he presented different patterns of the QRS and T configurations into left or right precordial limb leads (Ziegler, 1970). The P wave portrays atrial electrical activity, so changes in the atrial action potential and substrate are reflected in P wave timing or morphology (Chandy, 2004). Bahl et al. presented the P wave changes associated with the type and stage of the disease (Bahl, 1972). Analyzing the four chamber enlargements, Johnson et al. presented P wave changes for enlarged left and right atria (Johnson, Horan, & Flowers, 1977).

The atria, characterized by thin walls, respond to volume and pressure overload due to dilatation. Moreover, the enlargement of the associated ventricle is recognized as the cause of the enlargement of the atrium (Macfarlane, 2006; Magdic, Saul, 1997). The right atrium enlargement is recognized by the increased amplitude of the P wave (0.25 mV) while left atrial abnormality is reflected by the lengthened P wave duration (>120 ms) as well as a notched P wave.

The American Heart Association, American College of Cardiology Foundation, and the Heart Rhythm Society, recently concluded on standards to be used when interpreting ECG data related to cardiomyopathy (Hancock et al., 2009). In left ventricular hypertrophy, the P wave shape is mentioned as a criterion. In right ventricular hypertrophy (LVH), a P wave amplitude larger than 0.25 mV in lead II is presented as a threshold. Left atrial abnormality implies a prolongation of the total atrial activation time (>120 ms), widely notched P wave, and possible changes in P wave area. The right atrial abnormality list includes a larger amplitude of the P wave (> 0.25 mV) and a prolongation of the P wave in patients after cardiac surgery, which is the case for the patients in our proposed research.

Our proposed algorithm presents the advantage of compatibility with the clinical Cardio-Vascular Intensive Care Unit (CVICU) setting since it is designed to analyze P wave parameters from a 5-lead ECG, versus the laboratory 12-lead ECG. P wave delineation is made automatically on the ECG signal using wavelet transforms. The P wave features obtained by the wavelets are then processed by a neuro-fuzzy system. Neuro-fuzzy systems are combinations of fuzzy systems and artificial neural networks. Such combined systems have the advantage that they can learn faster and more accurately than an individual artificial neural network or fuzzy logic system. A benefit over artificial neural networks is that the rules that describe the system are explicit, thus permitting easy interpretation and validation.

Considering the frequent association of cardiomyopathy and atrial fibrillation, a future application of this successful classification process is the inclusion of the results in an automatic prediction algorithm for atrial fibrillation (AF). AF is a threatening arrhythmia that is encountered in 25% of post-cardiovascular surgical patients in the CVICU of the Cleveland Clinic.

Cardiomyopathy diagnosis will be performed by a multivariate, neuro-fuzzy classification model that uses P wave parameters to generate a cardiomyopathy classification index. Artificial Neural Networks are universal approximators (Buckley, Hayashi, 1995), and there has also been extensive work to prove that neuro-fuzzy systems can approximate any continuous function to any desired degree of accuracy (Feuring, Lippe, 1999). Alvisi et al. (Alvisi et al., 2006) have studied the performances of fuzzy logic and Artificial Neural Networks, revealing the weaknesses and strengths of each of the methods. The strengths can be emphasized, and some of the weaknesses can be attenuated, by combining the techniques into a hybrid neuro-fuzzy model. **The universal approximation theorem is the reason that a neuro-fuzzy system may be able to overcome the limitations of previous statistics-based methods for ECG analysis.**

2.2 Neuro-fuzzy networks

Consider a multi-input, single-output fuzzy logic system. Our discussion can be easily generalized to multiple output systems, but restricting our discussion to single-output systems simplifies the notation considerably. In addition, the ECG classification system that we consider in this paper is single-output. The ith rule R_i of the fuzzy system can be written as follows (Chen, Linkens, 2001).

$$\begin{aligned} R_i : \text{If } x_1 \text{ is } A_{i1} \text{ and } \ldots \text{ and } x_m \text{ is } A_{im} \text{ then} \\ y = z_i(x), \qquad (i = 1, \cdots, p). \end{aligned} \tag{1}$$

The inputs x_i and the output y are linguistic variables, A_{ij} are fuzzy sets, and $z_i(x)$ is a function of the input $x = [x_1 \ \ldots \ x_m]^T$. The output function $z_i(x)$ typically takes one of the following forms: (1) singleton, (2) fuzzy set, (3) linear function. If the fuzzy system uses center average defuzzification, product inference, and singleton fuzzification, then $z_i(x) = z_i$ (a singleton) and the fuzzy system output can be written as

$$y = \frac{\sum_{i=1}^{p} z_i \prod_{j=1}^{m} \mu_{ij}(x_j)}{\sum_{i=1}^{p} \prod_{j=1}^{m} \mu_{ij}(x_j)} \tag{2}$$

where $\mu_{ij}(x_{ij})$ denotes the degree of membership of x_j in R_i. As in many neuro-fuzzy networks, we use a Gaussian form for μ_{ij}:

$$\mu_{ij}(x_j) = \exp\left(\frac{-(x_j - c_{ij})^2}{\sigma_{ij}^2}\right) \tag{3}$$

where c_{ij} is the jth element of the center of the ith rule, and σ_{ij} is its standard deviation. In this case, Eq. (2) becomes

$$y = \frac{w}{\sum_{i=1}^{p} m_i(x)} \tag{4}$$

$$w = \sum_{i=1}^{p} z_i m_i(x) \tag{5}$$

$$m_i(x) = exp[-(x - c_i)^T P^{-2}(x - c_i)] \tag{6}$$

where $c_i = [c_{i1} \cdots c_{im}]^T$ and $P = \text{diag}(\sigma_1, \cdots, \sigma_m)$. Eq. (5) is in the form of a radial basis function, which is a type of neural network (Chen, Linkens, 2001). The system of Eqs. (5) and (6) is therefore called a neuro-fuzzy system. It can be depicted as shown in Figure 1.

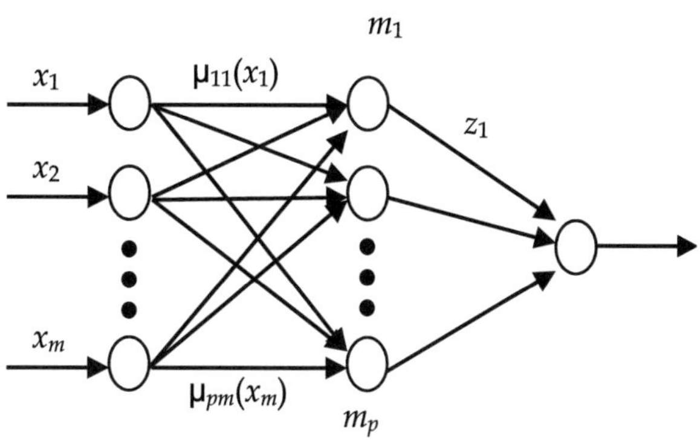

Fig. 1. Multi-input single-output neuro-fuzzy system architecture

The neuro-fuzzy system in Figure 1 is a function of the pxm elements of the membership centers c_{ij}, the pxm elements of the membership standard deviations σ_{ij}, and the p elements of the singleton outputs z_i. There are thus $p(2m+1)$ parameters that define the neuro-fuzzy system. For a given neuro-fuzzy system architecture and a given training set of input/output data, the neuro-fuzzy system parameters can be optimized with respect to these $p(2m+1)$ parameters.

2.3 Biogeography-Based Optimization (BBO)

Biogeography-based optimization (BBO) is a recently-developed population-based evolutionary optimization algorithm (Simon, 2008). As its name implies, BBO is motivated by biogeography, which is the study of the distribution of species over time and space (Whittaker, 1998). BBO has demonstrated good performance on various benchmark functions (Lomolino, Riddle, & Brown, 2009; Simon, 2008). It has also been successfully applied to several real-world optimization problems, including sensor selection (Simon, 2008), power system optimization (Rarick et al., 2009), groundwater detection (Kundra, Kaur, & Panchal, 2009), and satellite image classification (Panchal et al., 2009).

Given an optimization problem and a population of candidate solutions (individuals), a biogeography-based optimization (BBO) solution with high fitness is likely to share its features with other solutions, and a solution with low fitness is unlikely to share its features. Conversely, a solution with high fitness is unlikely to accept features from other solutions, while a solution low fitness is likely to accept features. Solution feature sharing, which is called immigration and emigration, tends to improve the solutions and thus evolve a good solution to the problem.

In biogeography-based optimization (BBO), each individual solution has its own immigration rate λ_i and emigration rate μ_i. A good solution has relatively high μ and low λ, while the converse is true for a poor solution. The immigration rate and the emigration rate are functions of the fitness of the solution. They are often calculated as

$$\begin{aligned} \lambda_i &= f_i/n \\ \mu_i &= 1 - \lambda_i \end{aligned} \quad (7)$$

where n is the population size and f_i is the fitness rank of the ith individual (the most fit individual has a rank $f_i = 1$). The immigration rates λ_i are interpreted by the BBO algorithm as immigration probabilities. The emigration rates μ_i are proportional to fitness and so are used in a roulette-wheel type of algorithm to determine the emigrating solution in case immigration is selected for a solution.

Although the migration rates in Eq. (1) are linear with respect to fitness rank as originally proposed in earlier study (Simon, 2008), more natural migration rates which are sigmoid with respect to fitness rank generally seem to give better optimization performance (Lomolino, Riddle, & Brown, 2009). However, in this paper we retain the original linear migration rates for the simplicity reason.

As with other evolutionary algorithms, mutation is typically implemented to increase exploration, and elitism is often implemented to retain highly fit solutions. The standard BBO algorithm is shown in Figure 2.

```
For each solution Hi
   For each solution feature s
      Select solution Hi with probability proportional to λi
      If solution Hi is selected then
         Select Hj with probability proportional to μj
         If Hj is selected then
            Hi(s) ← Hj(s)
         end
      end
   next solution feature
   Probabilistically mutate Hi
next solution
```

Fig. 2. One generation of the standard BBO algorithm.

2.4 Oppositional BBO

Opposition-based learning (OBL) has been introduced as a method that can be used by Evolutionary Algorithms (EAs) to accelerate convergence speed by comparing the fitness of an individual to its opposite and retaining the fitter one in the population (Rahnamayan, Tizhoosh, & Salama, 2007; Tizhoosh, 2005). The "opposite" of an individual is defined as the reflection of that individual's features across the midpoint of the search space. Opposition-based differential evolution (ODE) (Rahnamayan, Tizhoosh, & Salama, 2008.) was the first application of OBL to Evolutionary Algorithms (EAs). OBL was first incorporated in BBO in earlier research study (Ergezer, Simon, & Du, 2009) and was shown to improve BBO by a significant amount on standard optimization benchmarks.

Given an Evolutionary Algorithm (EA) population member x, there are at least three different types of oppositional points that can be defined. These oppositional points are referred to as the opposite x_o, the quasi-opposite x_q, and the quasi-reflected-opposite x_r. Figure 3 illustrates these points for an arbitrary x in a one-dimensional domain. The point c is the center of the domain, x_o the reflection of x across c, x_q is a randomly generated point from a uniform distribution between c and x_o, and x_r is a randomly generated point from a uniform distribution between x and c.

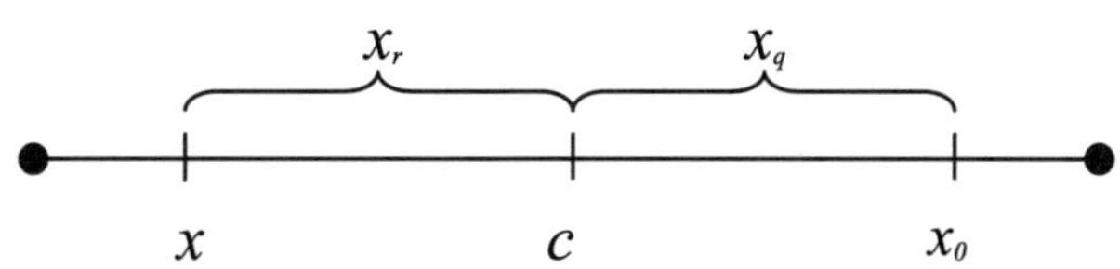

Fig. 3. Illustration of an arbitrary EA individual x, its opposite x_o, its quasi-opposite x_q, and its quasi-reflected-opposite x_r, in a one-dimensional domain.

OBL is essentially a more intelligent way of implementing exploration instead of generating random mutations. Another way of viewing OBL is from the perspective of social revolutions in human society. Society often progresses on the basis of a few individuals who embrace philosophies that are not just random, but that are deliberately contrary to accepted norms. Given that an EA individual is described by the vector x, and that the solution to the optimization problem is uniformly distributed in the search domain, it is shown in Rahnamayan' study (Rahnamayan, Tizhoosh, Salama, 2007) that x_q is probably closer to the solution than x or x_0. Further, it is presented in our earlier publication (Ergezer, Simon, & Du, 2009) that x_r is probably closer to the solution than x_q. These results are nonintuitive, but results related to random numbers are often nonintuitive, and the OBL results are derived not only analytically by also using simulation.

In this paper we use oppositional BBO (OBBO) to train the neuro-fuzzy ECG classification network. Suppose that the population size is N. OBBO works by generating a population of N opposite individuals which are the opposite of the current population. Then, given the entire $2N$ individuals comprised of both the original and the opposite populations, the best N individuals are retained for the next population. However, this does not occur at each generation. Instead it occurs randomly with a probability of J_r at each generation. J_r is called the jump rate. Based on (Rahnamayan, Tizhoosh, & Salama, 2006) we use $J_r = 0.3$ in this paper.

In order to increase the likelihood of improvement at each generation we implement OBBO as follows. At each generation, we save the original population of N individuals before creating a population of N new individuals via migration. We then create an opposite population of N additional individuals if indicated by the jump rate. Of the total $2N$ or $3N$ individuals, we finally select the best N for the next generation. Note that this approach guarantees that the best individual in each generation is at least as good as that of the previous generation. This is similar to a ($\mu+\lambda$) evolutionary strategy (Du, Simon, & Ergezer, 2009), whose parameters are not to be confused with the μ and λ migration parameters in BBO. The resulting OBBO algorithm is summarized in Figure 4.

```
H^(1) ← H (make a copy of the population H)
For each solution H_i ∈ H^(1) (i = 1, …, N)
   For each solution feature s
      Select solution H_i with probability proportional to λ_i
      If solution H_i is selected then
         Select H_j with probability proportional to μ_j
         If H_j is selected then
            H_i(s) ← H_j^(1)
         end
      end
   next solution feature
   Probabilistically mutate H_i
next solution
if rand(0,1) < J_r then
   Use H to create an N-member opposite population H^(2)
else
   H^(2) = ∅
end
Copy the best N individuals from {H, H^(1), H^(2)} to H
```

Fig. 4. One generation of oppositional BBO (OBBO).

3. ECG data

In preparation for the testing of a cardiomyopathy diagnosis model, a database of long-duration ECG signals was collected. The database includes signals from 55 subjects, 18 of them with cardiomyopathy. Not all subjects experienced chronic or paroxysmal atrial fibrillation. The cardiomyopathy group contained 10 males and 8 females with a mean age of 54 (range 23–88) years. The control group contained 22 males and 15 females with a mean age of 60 (range 27–77) yrs. The inclusion criteria were the same for both groups: no chronic or paroxystic atrial fibrillation and no perioperative pacing.

ECG parameters describing P wave morphology were computed for each minute of data recording for all 55 patients in the training data set. This set of ECG parameter values constitutes the input component of the training data set for neuro-fuzzy model development. For additional details of ECG parameter computation algorithms see (Bashour et al., 2004; Visinescu et al., 2004; Visinescu, 2005; Visinescu et al., 2006; Ovreiu et al., 2008)

The P wave from the electrocardiogram reflects the electrical activity of the atria and may indicate the existence of irregularities in electrical conduction. Using a previously developed P wave detection method, the starting, ending, and maximum points of the P wave were determined (Visinescu, 2005). The average P wave morphology parameters were computed once per minute. The P wave morphology parameters included the following:

a. Duration
b. Amplitude
c. A shape parameter which represents monophasicity or biphasicity
d. Inflection point, which is the duration of the P wave between the onset and the peak points
e. Energy ratio, defined as the fraction between the right atrial excitation energy and the total atrial excitation energy.

Initial investigation revealed that the monophasicity / biphasicity parameter did not vary appreciably between cardiomyopathy and control patients. We therefore discarded the monophasicity / biphasicity parameter from our data set. Differences between the remaining P wave morphology parameters for cardiomyopathy and control patients in the training database are presented in Figure 5. Based on the standard deviation bars, there is apparently important information included in these parameters. Their usefulness in identifying the patients with cardiomyopathy is determined by the proposed neuro-fuzzy model as discussed in the following section.

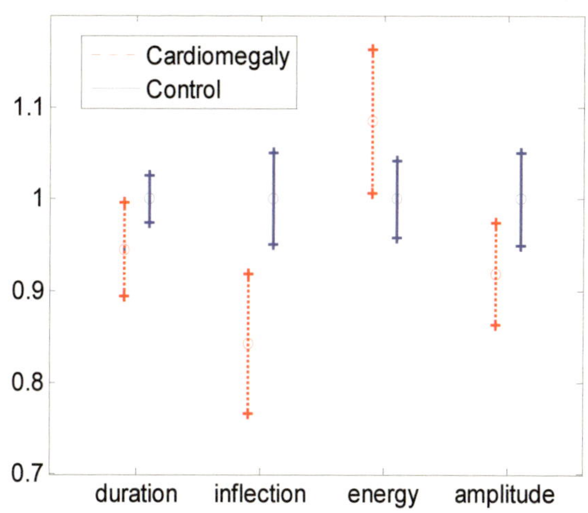

Fig. 5. P wave characteristics of cardiomyopathy and control patients. Data are normalized to the mean values of the control patients. Error bars show one standard deviation.

4. Experimental results

4.1 Problem setup

Cardiomyopathy diagnosis is performed by a multivariate, neuro-fuzzy classification model that uses current values of ECG P wave parameters to generate a cardiomyopathy classification index. The initial model is a multi-input single-output fuzzy inference system with a three-layer architecture (Figure 1). The fuzzification layer takes crisp parameter values and determines their memberships in linguistic categories (low, medium, high, etc.).

Each of these fuzzy variables are then input to each node of the fuzzy rule layer (i.e., the middle layer shown in Figure 1). The model output, which is the cardiomyopathy classification index, is the weighted average of the output rules.

Since we have four inputs (see Figure 5), we have $m = 4$ in Figure 1. The number of middle-layer neurons is equal to p and should be chosen as a tradeoff between good training performance and good generalization. If p is too small then training performance will be poor because we will not have enough degrees of freedom in the neuro-fuzzy network. If p is too large then test performance will be poor because the training algorithm will tend to "memorize" the training inputs rather than obtaining a good generalization for test data.

The output y shown in Eq. (4) is chosen to be +1 for cardiomyopathy patients and –1 for control patients. The ECG database is used for training and the output of the neuro-fuzzy system is compared to the known classification of the ECG patient. The RMS training error is defined as

$$E = \sqrt{\frac{1}{N}\sum_{i=1}^{N}(d_i - y_i)^2} \tag{8}$$

where N is the number of training inputs, d_i is the desired output of the ith training datum (+1 or –1), and y_i is the corresponding neuro-fuzzy output. In order to determine the best value of p (the number of middle-layer neurons) we run 10 Monte Carlo simulations with various values for p and compare training and testing errors. The BBO parameters that we use are as follows:

- Population size = 200
- Mutation rate = 2% per solution feature
- Generation limit = 50

Mutation is implemented by randomly generating a new parameter from a uniform distribution between the minimum and maximum parameter bounds. The parameter bounds that we use are as follows:

- Output singletons $z_i \in [-10, +10]$
- Membership centroids $c_{ij} \in [0, \pi]$
- Membership standard deviations $\sigma_{ij} \in [0.01, 5]$

We use ECG data from 55 test subjects as described in Section 3, which includes 37 control patients and 18 cardiomyopathy patients. We randomly divide the patients into approximately equal numbers of training patients and test patients. We therefore have 9 cardiomyopathy patients and 19 control patients for training the network, and 9 cardiomyopathy patients and 18 control patients for testing the network. We randomly choose 200 ECG data points from a 700-minute time interval for each patient for both training and testing. Therefore, we have 200×(9+19) = 5600 data points for training, and 200×(9+18) = 5400 data points for testing.

4.2 Parameter tuning and results

Table 1 shows the minimum training error attained as specified in Eq. (2) for various numbers of middle-layer neurons, along with the resulting correct classification rate for training and testing. An ECG data point is classified as cardiomyopathy if the neuro-fuzzy output $y > 0$, and control if the neuro-fuzzy output $y < 0$. The quantity of primary interest is the correct classification rate for the test data, and Table 1 shows that this is attained with 3 middle-layer neurons. Fewer neurons gives too few degrees of freedom, and more neurons results in a tendency of the neuro-fuzzy system to overfit the training data and hence not provide adequate generalization for the test data.

p	Training Error		Train CCR (%)		Test CCR (%)	
	Best	Mean	Best	Mean	Best	Mean
2	0.85	0.88	76	72	66	58
3	**0.77**	**0.84**	**82**	**77**	**75**	**62**
4	0.78	0.83	84	77	65	55
5	0.78	0.83	82	76	63	58

Table 1. Training error and correct classification rate (CCR) for training and testing as a function of the number of middle layer neurons p.

Next we implement OBBO to explore the effect of OBL on classification performance. Table 2 shows results for three different OBL options: standard BBO, OBBO using quasi-opposition (Q-BBO), and OBBO using quasi-reflected opposition (R-BBO). We use the same population size, mutation rate, and generation limit as discussed earlier. We use 3 middle-layer neurons as indicated by Table 1. Table 2 shows that OBBO using quasi-opposition provides the best neuro-fuzzy classification performance when test performance is used as the criterion.

Note that the numbers in Tables 1 and 2 do not match exactly because they are the results of different sets of Monte Carlo simulations. In future work we will use a more extensive set of simulations in order to obtain results with a smaller margin of error.

	Training Error		Train CCR (%)		Test CCR (%)	
	Best	Mean	Best	Mean	Best	Mean
BBO	0.77	0.86	84	76	66	58
Q-BBO	**0.83**	**0.86**	**79**	**74**	**69**	**62**
R-BBO	0.80	0.85	81	75	65	60

Table 2. Training error and correct classification rate (CCR) for training and testing for alternative implementations oppositional BBO.

After settling on Q-BBO with 3 middle-layer neurons, we explore the effect of mutation rate on Q-BBO performance. Table 3 shows neuro-fuzzy results for various mutation rates. We use the same population size and generation limit as before. Table 3 shows that mutation rate does not have a strong effect on neuro-fuzzy system results, but based on test data performance, a low mutation rate generally gives better results than a high mutation rate.

Mutation rate (%)	Training Error		Train CCR (%)		Test CCR (%)	
	Best	Mean	Best	Mean	Best	Mean
0.1	**0.79**	**0.85**	**81**	**76**	**71**	**61**
0.2	**0.82**	**0.86**	**80**	**75**	**72**	**59**
0.5	**0.77**	**0.85**	**82**	**76**	**69**	**62**
1.0	0.80	0.85	80	74	67	57
2.0	0.83	0.86	79	74	69	62
5.0	0.82	0.87	81	74	68	58
10.0	0.80	0.87	78	73	65	59

Table 3. Training error and correct classification rate (CCR) for different mutation rates using Q-BBO.

Figure 6 shows the progress for a typical Q-BBO training simulation. Note that the minimum training error in the top plot is monotonically nonincreasing due to the inherent elitism of the algorithm (see Figure 3). However, the average cost in the top plot, along with the success rates in the bottom plot, sometimes increases and sometimes decreases from one generation to the next. The results shown in Figure 6 also indicate that better results might be obtained if the generation limit were increased. However, care must be taken when increasing the generation limit. As the generation count increases, the training error will continue to decrease but the test error will eventually begin to increase due to overtraining (Tetko, Livingstone,& Luik, 1995).

The Q-BBO training run illustrated in Figure 6 resulted in the following neuro-fuzzy parameters:

$$c = \begin{bmatrix} 0.513 & 0.116 & 0.981 & 0.065 \\ 0.316 & 0.930 & 0.138 & 0.214 \\ 0.899 & 0.235 & 0.041 & 0.613 \end{bmatrix} \tag{9}$$

$$\sigma = \begin{bmatrix} 1.119 & 0.409 & 0.133 & 0.101 \\ 0.326 & 0.805 & 1.963 & 1.529 \\ 1.825 & 0.356 & 0.858 & 0.438 \end{bmatrix} \tag{10}$$

$$z = [1.641 \quad -0.967 \quad 0.779]. \tag{11}$$

Recall that we used a c range of $[0, \pi]$, but from Eq. (3) the highest membership centroid was less than 1 after Q-BBO training. This indicates that we could decrease the c range in order to get better resolution during training.

Similarly, recall that we used a σ range of [0.01, 5], but from Eq. (4) the highest standard deviation was less than 2 after Q-BBO training. This indicates that we could decrease the σ range in order to get better resolution during training.

Finally, recall that we used an output singleton z range of [–10, +10], but from Eq. (5) the output singletons were between –1 and 2 after Q-BBO training. This indicates that we could decrease the z range in order to get better resolution during training.

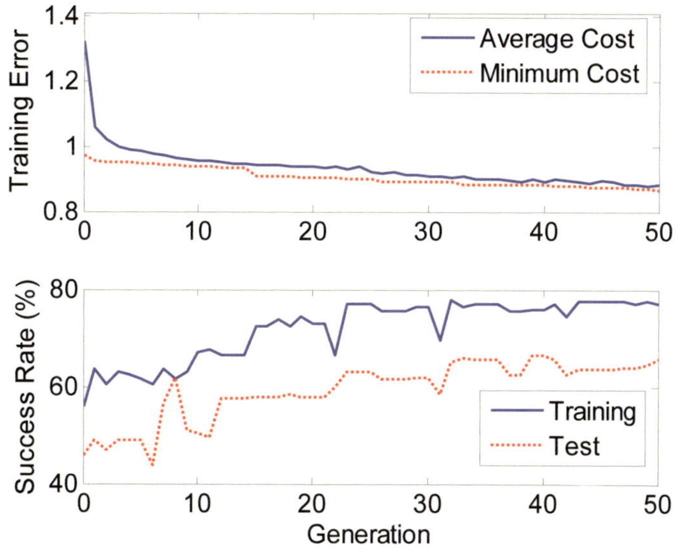

Fig. 6. Typical Q-BBO training results.

4.3 Clustering and pruning

The appropriate number of clusters in the neuro-fuzzy system is equivalent to the number of middle-layer neurons p shown in Figure 1. Determination of the optimal number of fuzzy rules is equivalent to finding a suitable number of clusters for the given data set. This can also be performed using fuzzy c-means clustering (Chen, Linkens, 2001; Linkens, Chen, 1999). Clustering is itself a multiobjective optimization problem that maximizes compactness within clusters, maximizes separation between clusters, and maximizes neuro-fuzzy system performance.

In the previous section we solved for cluster count using a direct approach involving manual tuning (see Table 1). However, we could also solve for cluster count by observing the output singletons z_i after training, discarding those that are significantly smaller than the others, and then retraining the network. This is a type of pruning. For example, when using BBO to train the neuro-fuzzy system with 5 middle-layer neurons, a typical result for the output singletons after convergence is

$$z = [1.766 \quad 1.880 \quad -1.712 \quad 0.392 \quad -1.542].$$

It is seen that the magnitude of z_4 (0.392) is smaller by a factor of 4 than any of the other elements of z. This indicates that the corresponding fuzzy rule might be able to be safely removed from the neuro-fuzzy system without sacrificing performance. Retuning should then be performed because the neuro-fuzzy parameters will need to be adjusted to compensate for the network size reduction.

Another way to check if we are using too many middle-layer neurons is by looking at the distance between fuzzy membership function centers. If, after training, two membership function centers are very close to each other, that indicates that those two fuzzy sets could be combined. For example, the matrix of fuzzy centroids after a typical training run with 5 middle-layer neurons (i.e., 5 fuzzy membership sets) is given by

$$c = \begin{bmatrix} 0.5587 & 0.0046 & 0.9480 & 0.6628 \\ 0.4908 & 0.3719 & 0.4274 & 0.2847 \\ 0.5534 & 0.9005 & 0.9880 & 0.2659 \\ 0.9839 & 0.7428 & 0.3904 & 0.2067 \\ 0.9992 & 0.6061 & 0.2754 & 0.2185 \end{bmatrix}.$$

Each row of c corresponds to a fuzzy set centroid, and each column of c corresponds to one dimension of the input data. A cursory look at the c matrix shows that rows 4 and 5 are similar to each other. A matrix of Euclidean distances between centroids (i.e., between columns of c) can be derived as

$$\Delta c = \begin{bmatrix} 0 & 0.7439 & 0.9807 & 1.1157 & 1.0980 \\ 0.7439 & 0 & 0.7732 & 0.6231 & 0.5838 \\ 0.9807 & 0.7732 & 0 & 0.7556 & 0.8919 \\ 1.1157 & 0.6231 & 0.7556 & 0 & \mathbf{0.1797} \\ 1.0980 & 0.5838 & 0.7556 & \mathbf{0.1797} & 0 \end{bmatrix}$$

where Δc_{ij} is the Euclidean distance between centroids i and j. The Δc matrix indicates that fuzzy centroids 4 and 5 are much closer to each other than the other centroids, which implies that the corresponding membership functions overlap, and so they could be combined. Afterward, the neuro-fuzzy system should be retrained to compensate for the change in its structure.

4.4 Fine tuning using gradient information

The BBO algorithm that we used, like other Evolutionary Algorithms (EAs), does not depend on gradient information. Therein lies its strength relative to gradient-based optimization methods. Evolutionary Algorithms (EAs) can be used for global optimization since they do not rely on local gradient information. Since the neuro-fuzzy system shown in Figure 1 may have multiple optima, BBO training is less likely to get stuck in a local optima compared to gradient-based optimization.

However, additional performance improvement could be obtained in the neuro-fuzzy classifier by using gradient information in conjunction with EA-based optimization. Gradient-based methods can be combined with EAs in order to take advantage of the strengths of each method. First we can use BBO, as above, in order to find neuro-fuzzy parameters that are in the neighborhood of the global optimum. Then we can use a gradient-based method to fine tune the BBO result. The most commonly-used gradient-based method is gradient descent clustering (Chen, Linkens, 2001; Linkens, Chen, 1999). Gradient descent can be further improved by using an adaptive learning rate and momentum term (Nauck, Klawonn, Kruse, 1997).

Kalman filtering is a gradient-based method that can give better fuzzy system and neural network training results than gradient descent (Simon, 2002a, 2002b). Constrained Kalman filtering can further improve fuzzy system results by optimally constraining the network parameters (Simon, 2002c). H-infinity estimation is another gradient-based method that can be used for fuzzy system training to improve robustness to data errors (Simon, 2005).

4.5 Training criterion

The ultimate goal of the neuro-fuzzy network is to maximize correct classification percentage. If the neuro-fuzzy output is greater than 0, then the ECG is classified as cardiomyopathy;

otherwise, the ECG is classified as non-cardiomyopathy. The bottom plot in Figure 6 shows that while RMS training error is monotonically nondecreasing, the success rate for the training data is non-monotonic. We could more directly address the problem of ECG data classification by using classification success rate as our fitness function rather than trying to minimize the RMS error of Eq. (2). That is, in fact, one of the advantages of EA training relative to gradient-based methods – the fitness function does not have to be differentiable. However, if we use classification success rate as our fitness function, and then try to use a gradient-based method for fine-tuning, the cost functions of the two training methods would be inconsistent.

5. Conclusion

We have shown that clinical ECG data can be correctly classified as cardiomyopathy or non-cardiomyopathy using a neuro-fuzzy network training by biogeography-based optimization (BBO). Our results show a correct classification rate on test data of over 60%. Better results can undoubtedly be attained with further training, but the main goal of this initial research was to demonstrate feasibility and to establish a framework for further refinement.

Although our preliminary results are good, there are many enhancements that need to be made in order to improve performance and incorporate this work into a commercial product. For example, demographic information needs to be included with the ECG data. Some of the test ECGs were correctly classified 100% of the time, while others had a very low success rate. Figure 7 shows the classification success rate for the test data as a function of patient ID. Some patients generated ECG data that was successfully classified as cardiomyopathy / non-cardiomyopathy only 2% of the time, while others generated data that was successfully classified 100% of the time. This indicates that demographic data is important and that we should group patients into similar groups for testing and training. Some of these data include gender, race, medication usage, and age. This will become feasible as we perform more clinical studies and collect data from more patients.

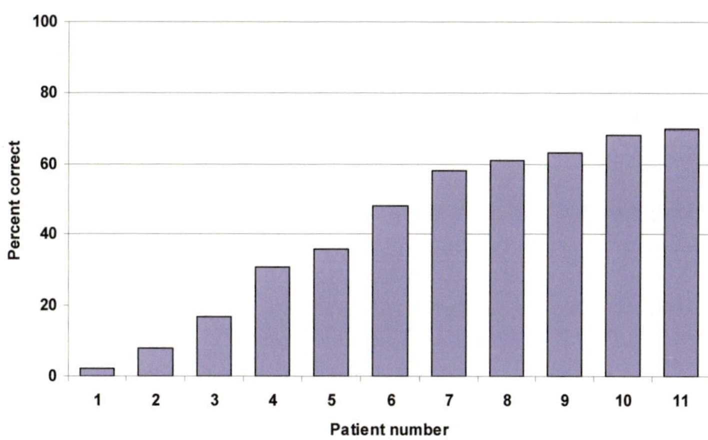

Fig. 7. ECG classification success rate for test patients.

We note that our results are based on snapshots of the data at single instants of time. We could presumably get better results by using a "majority rules" strategy for data collected over several minutes. For example, suppose that test accuracy is 60% for a given patient. We could use ECG data at three separate time instants and diagnose cardiomyopathy if the neuro-fuzzy network predicts cardiomyopathy for two or more of the data. This would boost test accuracy from 60% to 65%, assuming that the probability of correct classification is independent from one time instant to the next. We could then further improve accuracy by using more time instants.

A strong reason for investigating this cardiac anomaly is its association to Atrial Fibrillation occurrence. The availability of ECG registrations and efficiency in time and cost savings of such a different approach, especially in cardiovascular surgical patients would imply as a future work, the inclusion of this automated classification algorithm into a bed side monitor indicator that might be used in future classification and/or forecasting algorithms under investigation.

6. Acknowledgement

This work was partially supported by Grant 0826124 in the CMMI Division of the Engineering Directorate of the National Science Foundation and Grant NCRP 10CRP2600305 from American Heart Association.

7. References

Alvisi, S., Mascellani, G., Franchini, M., & Bardossy, A. (2006) - Water level forecasting through fuzzy logic and artificial neural network approaches, *Hydrology and Earth System Sciences*, 10 (1), pp. 1-17, 2006

American Heart Association, (2009). *Heart Disease and Stroke Statistics – 2009 Update*, www.americanheart.org/ presenter.jhtml?identifier=3018163

Bahl, O. (1972) - Electrocardiographic and vectorcardiographic pattern in cardiomyopathy, *Cardiovascular Clinics*, 4 (1), pp. 95-112, 1972

Bar-Cohen, Y., Silka, M. (2008) – Sudden cardiac death in pediatrics, *Current Opinion in Pediatrics*, 20 (5), pp. 517-521, 2008

Bashour, C., Visinescu, M., Gopakumaran, B., Wazni, O., Carragio, F., Yared, J., & Starr, N. (2004). Characterization of premature atrial contraction activity prior to the onset of postoperative atrial fibrillation in cardiac surgery patients, *Chest*, 126, 4 (2004), 831S.

Buckley, J. and Hayashi, Y. (1995) - Neural Nets for Fuzzy Systems, *Fuzzy Sets and Systems*, 71 (3), pp. 265-276, 1995

Chandy, J., Nakai, T., Lee, R., Bellows, W., Dzankic, S., & Leung, J. (2004) – Increases in P-wave Dispersion Predict Postoperative Atrial Fibrillation After Coronary Artery Bypass Graft Surgery, *Anesthesia & Analgesia*, 98, pp. 303-310, 2004

Chen, M. and Linkens, D. (2001). A systematic neuro-fuzzy modelling framework with application to material property prediction, *IEEE Transactions on Systems, Man, and Cybernetics – Part B: Cybernetics*, 31, 5 (2001), pp. 781-790.

Dische, M. R. (1972) - Observations on the morphological changes of the developing heart. *Cardiovascular Clinics*, 4 (3), pp. 175-191, 1972

Du, D., Simon, D., & Ergezer, M. (2009). Biogeography-based optimization combined with evolutionary strategy and immigration refusal. *In Proceedings of the IEEE Conference on Systems, Man, and Cybernetics (San Antonio, Texas, October 2009)*. pp. 1023–1028.

Ergezer, M., Simon D., & Du, D. (2009). Oppositional biogeography-based optimization. *In Proceedings of the IEEE Conference on Systems, Man, and Cybernetics (San Antonio, Texas, October 2009)*. pp. 1035–1040.

Feuring, T. and Lippe, W.-M. (1999) - The fuzzy neural network approximation lemma, *Fuzzy Sets and Systems*, 102 (2), pp. 227-236, 1999

Hancock, E.W., Mirvis, D.M., Okin, P., et al (2009) - AHA/ACCF/HRS recommendations for the standardization of interpretation of the electrocardiogram: part V: electrocardiogram changes associated with cardiac chamber hypertrophy: a scientific statement from the American Heart Association, Council on Clinical Cardiology; The American College of Cardiology Foundation, and the Heart Rhythm Society, *Journal of American College of Cardiology*, 53: pp. 992-1002, 2009

Heart Disease and Stroke Statistics, http://www.americanheart.org/presenter.jhtml?identifier=3018163, 2010

Ingles, J, Semsarian, C (2007) – Sudden cardiac death in the young: A clinical genetic approach, *Internal Medicine Journal*, 37 (1), pp. 32-37, 2007

Johnson, J. C., Horan, L. G., & Flowers, N. C. (1977) - Diagnostic accuracy of the electrocardiogram, *Cardiovascular Clinics*, 8 (3), pp. 25-40, 1977

Kennedy, J., Eberhart, R., & Shi, Y. (2001). *Swarm Intelligence*. Morgan Kaufmann,.

Kundra, H., Kaur, A., & Panchal, V. (2009). An integrated approach to biogeography based optimization with case based reasoning for retrieving groundwater possibility. In *Proceedings of the 8th Annual Asian Conference and Exhibition on Geospatial Information, Technology and Applications (Singapore, August 2009).*

Linkens, D. and Chen, M. (1999). Input selection and partition validation for fuzzy modelling using neural network. *Fuzzy Sets and Systems*, 107, 3 (1999), pp. 299–308.

Lomolino, M., Riddle, B., & Brown, J. (2009). *Biogeography*. Sinauer Associates.

Macfarlane, P. W. (2006) - Is electrocardiography still useful in the diagnosis of cardiac chamber hypertrophy and dilatation?, *Cardiology Clinics*, 24 (3), pp. 401-411, 2006

Magdic, K. S., Saul, L. M. (1997) - ECG Interpretation of chamber enlargement, *Critical Care Nurse*, 17 (1), 13, 16-25, 1997

Masson, J. M., Hancock, E. W., & Gettes, L. S. (2007) - AHA/ACC/HRS Scientific Statement, Recommendations for Standardization and Interpretation of the Electrocardiogram. Part II: Electrocardiography Diagnostic Statement List, A Scientific Statement From the American Heart Association Electrocardiography and Arrhythmias Committee, Council on Clinical Cardiology; The American College of Cardiology Foundation, and the Heart Rhythm Society, *Circulation*. 115: pp. 1325-1332, 2007

McKenna, W. J., Krikler, D. M., & Goodwin, J. F. (1982) - Arrhythmias in dilated and hypertrophic cardiomyopathy. *Medical Clinics of North America*, 68 (4), pp. 983-1000, 1984

Nauck, D., Klawonn, F., and Kruse, R. (1997). *Foundations of Neuro-Fuzzy Systems*. John Wiley & Sons.

Olson, E. N. (2004) - A decade of discoveries in cardiac biology, *Nature Medicine* 10, pp. 467-474, 2004

Ovreiu, M., Nair, B., Xu, M., Bakri, M., Li, L., Wazni, O., Fahmy, T., Petre, J., Sessler, D., Starr, N., & Bashour, A. (2008) Electrocardiographic Activity Before Onset of Postoperative Atrial Fibrillation in Cardiac Surgery Patients, *PACE*, November 2008, Vol. 31, issue 11, pp. 1371-1382 (with editorial comment of Lombardi, F. (2008) - "Atrial Fibrillation After cardiac Surgery: Prevention or Early Treatment of Patients at Risk", *PACE*, November 2008, Vol. 31, issue 11, pp. 1369-1370)

Panchal, V., Singh, P., Kaur, N., & Kundra, H. (2009). Biogeography based satellite image classification. *International Journal of Computer Science and Information Security*. 6, 2 (Nov. 2009), pp. 269–274.

Pereira, N., Barbosa, M., Ribeiro, A., Amorim, F., & Rocha, M. (2010) – Predictors of mortality in patients with dilated cardiomyopathy: Relevance of Chagas disease as an etiological factor, *Revista Espanola de Cardiologia*, 63 (7), pp. 788-797, 2010

Rahnamayan, S., Tizhoosh, H., & Salama, M. (2006). Opposition-based differential evolution for optimization of noisy problems, in *Proceedings of IEEE Congress on Evolutionary Computation (Vancounver, Canada, July 2006)*. pp. 1865–1872.

Rahnamayan, S., Tizhoosh, H., & Salama, M. (2007). Quasioppositional differential evolution, in *Proceedings of IEEE Congress on Evolutionary Computation (Singapore, September 2007)*. 2229–2236.

Rahnamayan, S., Tizhoosh, H., & Salama, M. (2008). Opposition-based differential evolution. *IEEE Transactions on Evolutionary Computation,* 12, 1 (2008), pp. 64–79.

Rarick, R., Simon, D., Villaseca, F. E., & Vyakaranam, B. (2009). Biogeography-based optimization and the solution of the power flow problem, In *Proceedings of the IEEE Conference on Systems, Man, and Cybernetics (San Antonio, Texas, October 2009)*. pp. 1029–1034.

Simon, D. (2002a). Training fuzzy systems with the extended Kalman filter. *Fuzzy Sets and Systems*, 132, 2 (December 2002), pp. 189–199.

Simon, D. (2002b). Training radial basis neural networks with the extended Kalman filter. *Neurocomputing*, 48, 1 (October 2002), pp. 455–475.

Simon, D. (2002c). Sum normal optimization of fuzzy membership functions. *International Journal of Uncertainty, Fuzziness, and Knowledge-Based Systems,* 10, 4 (August 2002), pp. 363–384.

Simon, D. (2005). H-infinity estimation for fuzzy membership function optimization, *International Journal of Approximate Reasoning*, 40, 3 (November 2005), pp. 224–242.

Simon, D. (2008). Biogeography-Based Optimization, *IEEE Transactions on Evolutionary Computation*, 12, 6 (December 2008), pp. 702–713.

Sox, H. C., Garber, A. M., & Littenberg, B. (1989). The resting Electrocardiogram as a Screening Test: A Clinical Analysis, *Annals of Internal Medicine*, 111, pp. 489-502, 1989

Tetko, I., Livingstone, D., & Luik, A. (1995). Neural network studies. 1. Comparison of overfitting and overtraining. *Journal of Chemical Information and Modeling,* 35, 5 (September 1995), pp. 826–833.

Tizhoosh, H. (2005). Opposition-based learning: A new scheme for machine intelligence, in *Proceedings of the International Conference on Computational Intelligence for Modelling, Control and Automation (Vienna, Austria, November 2005)*. pp. 695–701.

Visinescu, M., Bashour, A., Wazni, O., & Gopakumaran, B. (2004). Automatic detection of conducted premature atrial contractions to predict atrial fibrillation in patients after cardiac surgery, in *Proceedings of the 31st Annual International Conference on Computing in Cardiology (Chicago, Illinois, September 2004)*. pp. 429–432.

Visinescu, M. (2005). *Analysis of ECG to predict atrial fibrillation in post-operative cardiac surgical patients. Doctoral dissertation,* Cleveland State University, Cleveland, Ohio.

Visinescu, M., Bashour, A., Bakri, M., & Nair, B. (2006). Automatic detection of QRS complexes in ECG signals collected from patients after cardiac surgery, in *Proceedings of the 28th Annual International Conference of the IEEE Engineering in Medicine and Biology Society (New York, August 2006)*. pp. 3724–3727.

Ziegler, R. F. (1970). Electrocardiographic Clues in the diagnosis of congenital heart disease, *Cardiovascular Clinics*, 2 (1), pp. 97-114, 1970

Whittaker, R. (1998). *Island Biogeography*. Oxford University Press.

7

Prevention of Sudden Cardiac Death in Patients with Cardiomyopathy

M. Obadah Al Chekakie
University of Colorado, Cheyenne Regional Medical Center
United States

1. Introduction

Sudden cardiac death (SCD) is a major public health issue with an estimated annual incidence of 300,000 - 400,000 cases per year. The ACC/AHA/ESC 2006 guidelines define SCD as "death from an unexpected circulatory arrest, usually due to a cardiac arrhythmia occurring within an hour of the onset of symptoms"(Zipes et al. 2006). Most of the patients experiencing sudden cardiac arrest have an ejection fraction (LVEF) more than 50%, with the majority of these patients having a history of coronary artery disease (CAD). However, the risk of death in patients with LVEF of less than 35% is higher than patients with better preserved LVEF (Gorgels et al. 2003). Beta blocker therapy, Angiotensin enzymes inhibitors (ACE-I), angtiotensin receptor blockers as well as aldosteron antagonists have been shown to decrease the risk of sudden cardiac death especially in post myocardial infarction patients (Seidl et al. 1998; Domanski et al. 1999; Pitt et al. 2003; McMurray et al. 2005). In contrast antiarrhythmic drug therapy doesn't prevent sudden cardiac death in patients with cardiomyopathy. The focus of this chapter is to review the major implantable cardioverter defibrillator (ICD) and cardiac resynchronization therapy trials and their effects on sudden cardiac death prevention in patients with cardiomyopathy who are receiving optimal medical therapy.

2. Trials examining the benefits of ICD therapy in sudden cardiac death prevention

2.1 Secondary prevention trials of defibrillator therapy

The earlier trials examined the highest risk population of patients who had cardiac arrest due to ventricular fibrillation or sustained ventricular tachycardia (VT) and syncope. These trials helped establish the benefit of ICD therapy in prevention of sudden cardiac death as well as identify patients who are at high risk of dying suddenly and might benefit from ICD therapy as a primary prevention approach.
The first trial is the **Antiarrhythmic versus Implantable Defibrillators Trial (AVID)**. Patients were included if they were resuscitated from VT, had sustained VT with syncope or had sustained VT with LVEF < 40% and symptoms suggestive of hemodynamic compromise (angina or congestive heart failure or near syncope) (AVID 1997). Patients were excluded if the ventricular arrhythmia was due to a reversible cause, but those patients were followed in a registry. AVID enrolled 1016 patients and the primary end point was all cause mortality. Over

80% of the patients randomized to antiarrhythmic therapy (total of 509 patients) were on Amiodarone at end of follow up. AVID was terminated early when patients with ICD therapy (n=506) had a 38% reduction in all cause mortality compared to patients with antiarrhythmic drug therapy (HR 0.62, 95% CI of 0.47 to 0.81). Analysis of the AVID trial showed that patients with LVEF < 35% who received an ICD had significant reduction of sudden cardiac death while patients with LVEF > 35% who received an ICD did not see significant benefit compared to the antiarrhythmic drug therapy group (Domanski et al. 1999).

The patients with a reversible cause of ventricular arrhythmia who were not randomized were followed in a registry. These patients were in general younger, had a better mean LVEF and were more likely to have history of coronary artery disease and had underwent revascularization. Most of the reversible causes were due to ischemia or myocardial infarction (65%) or due to electrolytes imbalance (10%). Patients who were categorized as having VT/VF due to reversible causes had similar if not higher risk of sudden cardiac death compared to patients with no identifiable reversible cause(Wyse et al. 2001). Careful follow up and aggressive assessment for this patient group is advised.

The second study is the **Canadian Implantable Defibrillator Study (CIDS)**, which enrolled 659 patients who had VT, sustained VT with syncope or sustained VT with LVEF < 35%. Patients were excluded if they had recent myocardial infarction (MI) with in the past 72 hours or if they had electrolytes imbalance. Primary end point was all cause mortality. The patients were followed for an average of 36 months. There was a 20% relative risk reduction of death with ICD therapy compared to amiodarone (p=0.14)(Connolly et al. 2000). Analysis of CIDS showed that patients with low LVEF benefited from ICD therapy more than patient with better-preserved LVEF(O'Brien et al. 2001).

The third study is the **Cardiac Arrest Study Hamburg (CASH)**, which was a small trial randomizing 288 patients to ICD therapy with drug therapy. Inclusion criteria included patients successfully resuscitated from cardiac arrest due to documented sustained ventricular arrhythmia. Exclusion criteria included patients who had a cardiac arrest within 72 hours after MI or cardiac surgery or if they had a reversible cause due to electrolyte abnormality or proarrhythmic drug. There was a trend towards lower death with ICD therapy compared to drug therapy (23% relative risk reduction, p=0.16). Average follow up was 57 months. The lack of benefit in the CASH trial might be due to the fact that it had a small study population and better mean LVEF (45% ±18%) compared to the AVID trial(Kuck et al. 2000). Also, 44% of patient in CASH study had epicardial lead implantation as compared to only 4% in the AVID trial.

A pooled analysis of these trials demonstrated that all cause mortality was reduced by 27% (HR of ICD compared to Amiodarone of 0.73, 95% CI 0.60-0.87, p<0.001) (Connolly et al. 2000). Arrhythmic death was also reduced in the ICD group compared to the Amiodarone group (HR 0.49, 95% CI of 0.36 to 0.67, p<0.001). The metaanalysis also showed that patients with LVEF <35% had a significant benefit from ICD therapy compared to Amiodarone (HR 0.66, 95% CI of 0.53 to 0.83) while patients with LVEF >35% had no significant benefit from ICD therapy compared to Amiodarone therapy (HR of 1.2, 95% CI of 0.81 to 1.76). Furthermore, patients receiving epicardial lead systems had no benefit from ICD therapy compared to Amiodarone (HR 1.52, 95% CI of 0.92 to 2.50), while patients with transvenous lead had the most benefit (HR 0.69, 95% CI of 0.56 to 0.85). The three randomized trials examining the benefit of implantable cardioverter defibrillator (ICD) therapy in patients who survived cardiac arrest are summarized in Table 1.

Trial	N	Inclusion Criteria	Primary Endpoint	Age	Mean LVEF	HR (95% Confidence Interval)	P Value
Antiarrhythmics versus Implantable Defibrillators (AVID) (1016 patients)	1016	Resuscitated VF, sustained VT and syncope or sustained VT with LVEF < 40% and severe symptoms	All cause mortality	65	35%	0.62 (0.47-0.81)	0.02
Canadian Implatable Defibrillator Study (CIDS) (659 patients)	659	Resuscitated VF, sustained VT and syncope or sustained VT with LVEF < 35% or unmonitored syncope with subsequent inducible VT or sustained VT	All cause mortality	64	34%	0.82 (0.60 to 1.10)	0.14
Cardiac Arrest Study Hamburg (CASH)	288	cardiac arrest due to documented sustained ventricular arrhythmia	All cause mortality	58	45%		0.16

Table 1. Secondary prevention trials of ICD therapy. VT is for ventricular tachycardia, VF is for Ventricular Fibrillation, LVEF is for left Ventricular ejection Fraction. HR is for hazard Ratio, CI is confidence interval.

These trials established the benefits of ICD therapy in patients who survived cardiac arrest in the absence of reversible causes. Patients with reversible causes of the cardiac arrest remain high risk and should be followed closely. Even though the metaanalysis of these trials showed no benefits of ICD therapy in patients with LVEF >35%, this is not reflected in the guidelines due to the fact that LVEF was not an entry criterion in these trials. Furthermore, the mean time of cardiac arrest and measurement of LVEF was 3 days in the AVID trial, and the LVEF shortly after cardiac arrest might be depressed from myocardial injury and might improve over time. Table 2 lists current guidelines for ICD therapy.

Class I: (General agreement of benefit with ICD therapy)

1. ICD therapy is indicated in patients who are survivors of cardiac arrest due to VF or hemodynamically unstable sustained VT after evaluation to define the cause of the event and to exclude any completely reversible causes.
2. ICD therapy is indicated in patients with structural heart disease and spontaneous sustained VT, whether hemodynamically stable or unstable.
3. ICD therapy is indicated in patients with syncope of undetermined origin with clinically relevant, hemodynamically significant sustained VT or VF induced at electrophysiological study.
4. ICD therapy is indicated in patients with LVEF less than or equal to 35% due to prior

MI who are at least 40 days post-MI and are in NYHA functional Class II or III.

5. ICD therapy is indicated in patients with nonischemic dilated cardiomyopathy who have an LVEF less than or equal to 35% and who are in NYHA functional Class II or III.
6. ICD therapy is indicated in patients with LV dysfunction due to prior MI who are at least 40 days post-MI, have an LVEF less than or equal to 30%, and are in NYHA functional Class I.
7. ICD therapy is indicated in patients with nonsustained VT due to prior MI, LVEF less than or equal to 40%, and inducible VF or sustained VT at electrophysiological study.

Class IIa (Weight of evidence is in favor of usefulness of ICD therapy)

1. ICD implantation is reasonable for patients with unexplained syncope, significant LV dysfunction, and non-ischemic dilated cardiomyopathy.
2. ICD implantation is reasonable for patients with sustained VT and normal or near-normal ventricular function.
3. ICD implantation is reasonable for patients with hypertrophic cardiomyopathy (HCM) who have 1 or more major risk factors for SCD. [Major risk factors for SCD in patients with HCM are: prior cardiac arrest, spontaneous sustained VT, spontaneous non-sustained VT, Family history of SCD, LV thickness ≥ 30 mm and abnormal blood pressure response to exercise]
4. ICD implantation is reasonable for the prevention of SCD in patients with ARVD/C who have 1 or more risk factors for SCD. [Risk factors for SCD in patients with ARVD/C are: prior cardiac arrest, spontaneous sustained VT, spontaneous non-sustained VT, evidence of extensive RV disease, LV involvement, presentation with polymorphic VT and RV apical aneurysm and induction of VT during electrophysiologic testing]
5. ICD implantation is reasonable to reduce SCD in patients with long-QT syndrome who are experiencing syncope and/or VT while receiving beta blockers.
6. ICD implantation is reasonable for non hospitalized patients awaiting transplantation.
7. ICD implantation is reasonable for patients with Brugada syndrome who have had syncope.
8. ICD implantation is reasonable for patients with Brugada syndrome who have documented VT that has not resulted in cardiac arrest.
9. ICD implantation is reasonable for patients with catecholaminergic polymorphic VT who have syncope and/or documented sustained VT while receiving beta blockers.
10. ICD implantation is reasonable for patients with cardiac sarcoidosis, giant cell myocarditis, or Chagas disease.

Class IIb (Efficacy of the ICD therapy is less well established)

1. ICD therapy may be considered in patients with non-ischemic heart disease who have an LVEF of less than or equal to 35% and who are in NYHA functional Class I.
2. ICD therapy may be considered for patients with long-QT syndrome and risk factors for SCD.
3. ICD therapy may be considered in patients with syncope and advanced structural heart disease in whom thorough invasive and noninvasive investigations have failed

to define a cause.

4. ICD therapy may be considered in patients with a familial cardiomyopathy associated with sudden death.
5. ICD therapy may be considered in patients with LV noncompaction.

Class III (General agreement that an ICD is not effective and may be harmful)

1. ICD therapy is not indicated for patients who do not have a reasonable expectation of survival with an acceptable functional status for at least 1 year, even if they meet ICD implantation criteria specified in the Class I, IIa, and IIb recommendations above.
2. ICD therapy is not indicated for patients with incessant VT or VF.
3. ICD therapy is not indicated in patients with significant psychiatric illnesses that may be aggravated by device implantation or that may preclude systematic follow-up.
4. ICD therapy is not indicated for NYHA Class IV patients with drug-refractory congestive heart failure who are not candidates for cardiac transplantation or CRT-D.
5. ICD therapy is not indicated for syncope of undetermined cause in a patient without inducible ventricular tachyarrhythmias and without structural heart disease.
6. ICD therapy is not indicated when VF or VT is amenable to surgical or catheter ablation (e.g., atrial arrhythmias associated with the Wolff-Parkinson-White syndrome, RV or LV outflow tract VT, idiopathic VT, or fascicular VT in the absence of structural heart disease).
7. ICD therapy is not indicated for patients with ventricular tachyarrhythmias due to a completely reversible disorder in the absence of structural heart disease (e.g., electrolyte imbalance, drugs, or trauma).

Table 2. Recommendations for ICD therapy based on the ACC/AHA/HRS 2008 Guidelines for Device Based Therapy.

2.2 Primary prevention trials of defibrillator therapy

2.2.1 Primary prevention of SCD in patients with ischemic cardiomyopathy with and without prior myocardial infarction

The earlier primary prevention trials used electrophysiologic testing as well as a reduced LVEF as part of entry criterion. Electrophysiologic testing (EP study) was thought to be a reliable method of risk stratification of patients with coronary artery disease (CAD) who survived myocardial infarction.

The First of these trials is the **First Multicenter Automatic Defibrillator Implantation Trial (MADIT- I)** which compared ICD therapy to conventional care in 196 patients post MI, LVEF < 35%, non-sustained VT on ambulatory monitoring and inducible VT by programmed electrical stimulation and failure of intravenous procainamide to prevent inducibility (Moss et al. 1996). Patients were excluded if they had prior cardiac arrest or syncope due to ventricular tachycardia (VT) not related to myocardial infarction (MI). Patients were also excluded if they had suffered myocardial infarction within 3 weeks of randomization, had coronary artery bypass surgery within 2 months of randomization or if they had angioplasty within 3 months of randomization. MADIT I started enrolling patients in December 1990, with only transthoracic implantation of ICD was available at the time. Nonthoracotomy transvenous leads were implanted after being approved in August of 1993. Of the 196 patients enrolled, 95 patients were assigned to the ICD group and 101 patients were assigned to the conventional medical therapy group (which also included use of antiarrhythmic drugs). Primary endpoint was all cause mortality. After a mean follow up of 27 months, patients assigned to the ICD group had lower mortality than patients assigned to the conventional treatment group (Hazard Ratio (HR) of 0.46, 95% confidence interval (CI) 0.26 to 0.82, p=0.009). The interval from last MI was > 6 months in 75% of patients in each treatment group. The benefit of ICD was similar in patients with thoracotomy and non-thoracotomy ICD implantation (p=0.78). MADIT-I trail was the first trail to include patients who had purely low LVEF and inducible non-suppressible sustained ventricular arrhythmias during electrophysiologic testing.

The First Multicenter Unsustained Tachycardia Trial (MUSTT-I) trial was designed to determine whether inducibilty of VT identified risk of sudden cardiac death in patients with LVEF < 40%, prior myocardial infarction and non-sustained VT documented more than 4 days after MI. Patients were enrolled if they had a positive electrophysiology study (defined as an inducible monomorphic VT or inducible polymorphic VT with one or two extrastimuli). Those with negative EP study were followed in a registry. A total of 704 patients with positive EP study were randomized to electrophysiologic guided antiarrhythmic therapy (which included a drug or implantation of an ICD) versus best medial therapy (mainly beta blockers and angiotensin enzyme inhibitors but no antiarrhythmic drug therapy) (Buxton et al. 1999). Patients who failed suppression of inducibility of the ventricular arrhythmia after at least one antiarrhythmic drug trial could receive an ICD. The ICD implantation was not randomized in MUSTT-I. The primary endpoint was cardiac arrest or death from arrhythmia. Secondary endpoints included death from all causes, death from cardiac causes and spontaneous sustained VT. Over a follow up period of 39 months, patients assigned to electrophysiologic testing (n=351) had lower risk of arrhythmic death or cardiac arrest compared to patients receiving best medical therapy (n=353) (Relative risk 0.73, 95% CI 0.53 to 0.99, p =0.04). This is mostly attributable to lower risk of arrhythmic death or cardiac arrest in patients receiving an ICD compared to patients not receiving an ICD (relative risk 0.24, 95% CI of 0.13 to 0.45, p< 0.001). Patients who received an ICD had a lower risk of all cause mortality compared to patients with electrophysiology guided therapy who received antiarrhythmic drugs only (Relative risk 0.42, 95% CI of 0.29 to 0.61) This remained significant even after adjusting for all other clinical variables (Figure 1).

MUSTT-I showed that patients who had an inducible VT that was suppressed with antiarrhythmic drugs did not have any mortality benefit.

Patients who were screened for MUSTT-I but had a negative EP study were followed in a registry. Data was available for 1397 patients after 39 months of follow up. Total mortality was compared in this registry with the 353 patients in MUSTT-I with positive EP study that were assigned to best medical therapy. Only 35% of patients in the registry were on beta blockers compared to 51% of patients with inducible arrhythmias assigned to no antiarrhythmic therapy. The rate of used of ACE-I was similar (72% and 77% respectively). At 39 months, mortality was higher in patients with positive EP study assigned to best medical therapy (48%) compared to the patients with negative EP study in the registry (44%), (unadjusted p=0.09, adjusted p<0.001 for other clinical factors including use of beta blockers). Even though this difference was statistically significant, the absolute difference of 4% over 5 years is not clinically meaningful. Given these results as well as the consistency of LVEF <35% to predict a mortality benefit from ICD therapy, Electrophysiologic testing is not routinely performed in patients with coronary artery disease and LVEF < 35% as a risk stratifying tool. (Buxton et al. 2000).

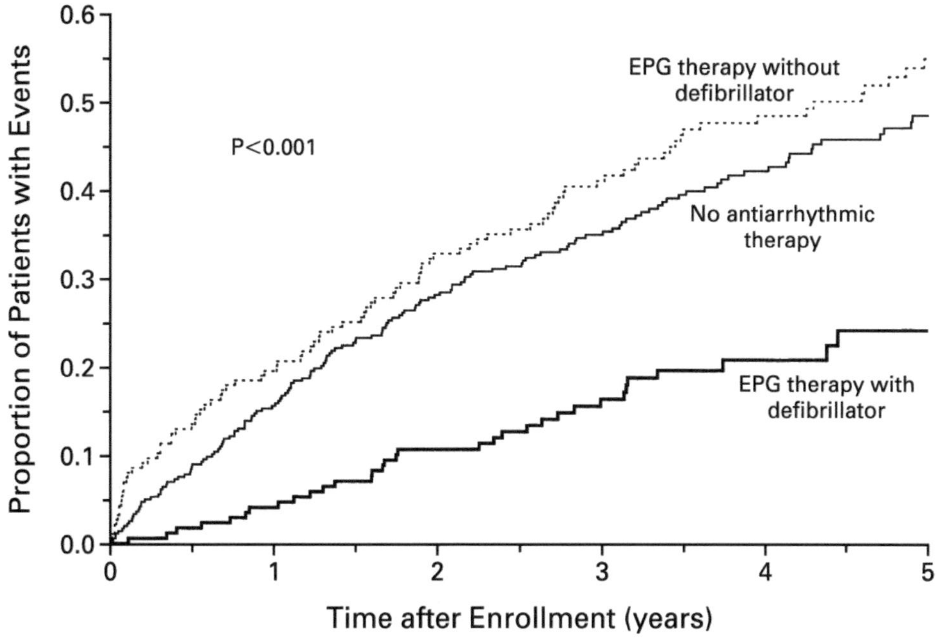

Fig. 1. Kaplan- Meier Estimates of the Rates of Death from All Causes. EPG denotes electrophysiologically guided. (From Buxton, A. E., Lee, K. L., Fisher, J. D., et al. (1999). "A randomized study of the prevention of sudden death in patients with coronary artery disease. Multicenter Unsustained Tachycardia Trial Investigators." New England Journal of Medicine, Vol. 341, No.25, (December, 1999): pp. 1882-1890, ISSN 0028-4793, with permission)

The Coronary Artery Bypass Graft Patch and The Second Multicenter Automatic Defibrillator Implantation Trial (MADIT- II) trials examined the benefits of ICD therapy in patients with reduced LVEF months after myocardial infarction and did not include electrophysiologic testing or arrhythmia suppression as part of entry criterion. **The Coronary Artery Bypass Graft-Patch Trial (CABG-Patch)** randomized 1055 patients undergoing coronary artery bypass surgery, LVEF <36% and positive signal-averaged electrocardiograms to receive ICD therapy (n=446) or conventional medical therapy (n=454) (Bigger 1997). Only 50% of the patients had prior myocardial infarction but all the patients received epicardial ICD systems. ICD therapy showed no survival benefit over conventional medical therapy (HR 1.06, 95% CI of 0.81 to 1.42, p=0.64). The lack of benefit of ICD therapy in this trial could be due to the methods used for patient selection, but most likely is due to the effects of complete revascularization on the risk of sudden cardiac death. In a subanalysis of **Studies of Left Ventricular Dysfunction (SOLVD)** trial, CABG was found to be associated with a 36% relative risk reduction of all cause mortality and a 46% reduction of sudden cardiac death regardless of the severity of heart failure or the decrease in the LVEF. This might have contributed to the lack of benefit from ICD early after coronary artery bypass surgery (Veenhuyzen et al. 2001).

The Second Multicenter Automatic Defibrillator Implantation Trial (MADIT- II) randomized 1232 patients in a 3:2 fashion with LVEF < 30% and prior MI to receive an ICD (n=742) compared to medical therapy (n=490). Patients were excluded if they had a recent MI

(<1 month), if they had revascularization in the past 3 months prior to randomization or if they were New York Heart Association (NYHA) class IV at enrollment. Mean follow up was for 30 months and primary end point was all cause mortality. ICD therapy was associated with a 31% reduction in relative risk of death at 20 months (HR 0.69, 95% confidence interval of 0.53 to 0.93, p = 0.02) (Moss et al. 2002). There was no difference in subgroup analysis based on age, gender, ejection fraction, QRS duration as well as NYHA class in terms of ICD benefit.

All ICD implantations were transvenous lead systems. No deaths were related to the implantation procedure and the complication of lead implantation was 1.8% and infection rate was 0.7%. Analysis of the mortality events showed that ICD therapy mainly prevented sudden cardiac death (HR 0.33, 95% CI of 0.2 to 0.53, p<0.001) but did not affect non-sudden cardiac death (p=0.32).

Even though MADIT-II did not require electrophysiologic testing as an entry criterion, the investigators sought to evaluate the predictive value of EP study to predict mortality and ICD efficacy as a pre-specified secondary endpoint. Patients assigned to the ICD group were encouraged to undergo an EP study and they received the ICD regardless of the results of the electrophysiologic testing. Of the 720 patients who received an ICD, only 593 patients underwent EP testing. A positive EP study was defined as sustained monomorphic or polymorphic VT induced with 3 or fewer extrastimuli or VF induced with 2 or fewer extrastimuli. A positive EP study according to this standard protocol did not predict the pre-specified primary endpoint of spontaneous VT or VF requiring treatment by the ICD (p=0.28). Patients with inducible VT were more likely to have VT during follow up (0.023) compared to patients with no inducible VT (Daubert et al. 2006). This confirms the findings of MUSTT-I trial in regards to the utility of EP testing in risk stratifying patients with coronary artery disease and LVEF < 35%.

Another subanalysis of MADIT-II trial showed that patients with ICD therapy who underwent coronary revascularization within 6 months of randomization had no survival benefit from ICD therapy compared to patients in the conventional treatment group (HR = 1.19; p = 0.76), while patients with ICD therapy who were randomized > 6 months after coronary revascularization had significant survival benefit from ICD therapy (HR =0.64, p = 0.01) after adjusting for other important clinical variables (Goldenberg et al. 2006). Furthermore, mortality risk in patients in MADIT II was shown to be time dependent, with benefit extending even for patients who had remote MI (>15 years) (Wilber et al. 2004). Two studies were conducted examine the benefits of ICD therapy early after myocardial infarction (MI). The first is **The Defibrillators in Acute Myocardial Infarction Trial (DINAMIT) which** was designed to evaluate the potential for ICD benefit early (6 to 40 days) after a MI in patients with LVEF <35%, and abnormal autonomic tone [high resting heart rate over 80 beats per minutes (bpm) or low heart rate variability]. Patients were excluded if they had three-vessel coronary intervention, if they already had an ICD or if they were planned to undergo coronary artery bypass graft surgery (CABG). A total of 647 patients were randomized to optimal medical therapy (n=342) or ICD therapy (n=332) (Hohnloser et al. 2004). The primary end point was all cause mortality and the secondary end point was arrhythmic death. After a mean follow up of 30 months, there was no overall survival benefit attributable to early implantation of an ICD compared to medical therapy [HR 1.08; 95% confidence interval (CI), 0.76 to 1.55; P=0.66]. The ICD group had less arrhythmic death compared to the medical therapy group (HR in the ICD group, 0.42; 95% CI, 0.22 to 0.83; P=0.009). There was an increase in non-sudden cardiac death in the ICD group compared to the medical therapy group (HR = 1.75; 95% CI, 1.11 to 2.76; P=0.02).

The second trial is **the Immediate Risk Stratification Improves Survival (IRIS) Trial**, which was a randomized, open label multicenter trial that studied the benefit of ICD therapy early after MI compared to optimal medical therapy. Patients were included if they had a history of myocardial infarction (5 to 31 days after MI), LVEF < 40% with either a baseline heart rate of > 90 bpm, non-sustained VT at >150 bpm on holter or both. A total of 898 patients were enrolled in the trial. Mean follow up was for 37 months, and almost 75% of the patients underwent revascularization. Most of the patients were on beta blockers (97% in the ICD group and 95% in the control group) and angiotensin receptor blockers (90% in ICD group and 91.1% in the control group). There was no difference in overall mortality between ICD group and the medical treatment group (HR 1.04, 95% CI of 0.81 to 1.35, p=0.78) (Steinbeck et al. 2009). Patients assigned to ICD therapy had lower incidence of sudden cardiac death (HR 0.55, 95% CI of 0.31 to 1.00, p = 0049) but higher incidence of non-sudden cardiac death (HR 1.92, 95% CI of 1.29 to 2.84).

The reasons for the lack of benefit of ICD therapy early after MI might never be known. Revascularization has a protective effect and leads to reverse remodeling especially if done in a timely fashion early after MI. Patients who died early in DINAMIT had pump failure. Other possibilities include side effects for ICD implantation early after MI or the negative effects of shocks or antitachycardia pacing on myocardial contractility.

In summary, the above trials support the use of ICD therapy for primary prevention of SCD in chronic ischemic cardiomyopathy. For patients who suffered a recent MI (<40 days), both IRIS and DINAMIT showed a decrease in arrhythmic death but no difference in all cause mortality. Currently, the guidelines support ICD therapy in patients with CAD who are > 40 days post MI and have LVEF < 35%.

Table 3 summarized the primary prevention trials in patients with coronary artery disease.

2.2.2 Primary prevention of SCD in patients with non-ischemic cardiomyopathy

The early trials examining the effects of ICD therapy compared to antiarrhythmic therapy in patients with non-ischemic cardiomyopathy (NICM) were small and not powered enough to show mortality benefit. The first trial is the **Amiodarone versus Implantable Cardioverter Defibrillator Trial (AMIOVERT)** which compared ICD therapy in 103 patients with NICM (with the diagnosis made > 6 months before enrollment) and non-sustained VT to amiodarone. The primary endpoint was all cause mortality. There was no difference in survival between the ICD group and the amiodarone group. The trial was terminated due to futility. The second trial is the **The Cardiomyopathy trial (CAT)** which was carried out in Germany and enrolled 104 patients with non-ischemic cardiomyopathy who were diagnosed within 9 months of enrollment. Mean follow up was 5.5 years and the primary end point was all cause mortality. Again there was no difference in survival between the ICD group and the control group. Both AMIOVERT and CAT trials were underpowered to detect a difference between groups, and in both of them the observed mortality was far lower than the predicted mortality used to design these trials.

Trial	N	Inclusion Criteria	Primary Endpoint	Age	Mean LVEF	NYHA Class	HR (95% CI)	P Value
First Multicenter Automatic Defibrillator Implantation Trial (MADIT-I)	196	NYHA I-III HF LVEF<35% MI > 4 weeks CABG > 3 months spontaneous NSVT and inducible VT	All cause mortality	63	26%	I, II and III	0.46 (0.26 to 0.82)	0.009
Multicenter Unsustained Tachycardia Trial (MUSTT)	704	NYHA I-III LVEF <40% MI>4 days spontaneous NSVT and inducible VT	Cardiac arrest or death from arrhythmia	65	28%	I, II and III	0.73 (0.53 -0.99)	0.04
The Coronary Artery Bypass Graft-Patch Trial (CABG-Patch)	1055	LVEF < 36%, Abnormal SAECG, undergoing CABG	All cause mortality	64	27%		1.06 (0.81 to 1.42)	0.64
Second Multicenter Automatic Defibrillator Implantation Trial (MADIT-II)	1232	NYHA I-III, LVEF < 30% MI > 1 month	All Cause mortality	64	23%	I, II and III	0.69 (0.53 to 0.93)	0.02
Defibrillators in Acute Myocardial Infarction Trial (DINAMIT)	674	NYHA I-III LVEF <35% recent MI (6-40 days) with depressed heart rate variability or elevated average Hear rate over 24 hrs	All Cause mortality	62	28%	I, II and III	1.08 (0.76 to 1.55)	0.66
the Immediate Risk Stratification Improves Survival (IRIS)	898	NYHA I-III LVEF <40% Recent MI (5 to 31 days after MI), with either a baseline heart rate of > 90 (bpm) or NSVT at >150 bpm on holter or both	All Cause mortality	62	30%	I, II and III	1.04 (0.81 to 1.35)	0.78

Table 3. Primary prevention trials of ICD therapy in patients with coronary artery disease. VT is for ventricular tachycardia, VF is for Ventricular Fibrillation, NSVT is for non sustained VT, LVEF is for left Ventricular ejection Fraction. HR is for hazard Ratio, CI is confidence interval.

The Defibrillators in Non-Ischemic Cardiomyopathy Treatment Evaluation Trial (DEFINITE) studied the efficacy of ICD therapy to prevent all cause mortality in patients with LVEF < 35% and non-sustained VT or frequent premature ventricular contractions (PVCs) on ambulatory monitoring (Kadish et al. 2004). A total of 488 patients (229 in the ICD group and 229 in the conventional treatment group) were enrolled and the primary end point was death from any cause and the secondary endpoint was sudden cardiac death. Most of the patients were receiving beta blocker (85%) and ACE-I (86%) There was a 35% relative risk reduction in mortality in the ICD group compared to the medical therapy group (HR, 0.65; 95% CI, 0.40 to

1.06; P=0.08) but it did not reach statistical significance. A significant reduction in SCD was observed (HR 0.20; 95% CI, 0.06 to 0.71; P=0.006). The DEFINITE trial didn't specify duration of heart failure as an entry criterion and it only required absence of a reversible cause of cardiomyopathy for enrollment. Patients in DEFINITE who had a recent diagnosis of non-ischemic cardiomyopathy (Using a 3 months cut point or a 9 months cut point) had similar benefit from ICD therapy when compared to patients who had a remote diagnosis of non-ischemic cardiomyopathy (p0.25) (Kadish et al. 2006)

The largest trial conducted to examine the effects of ICD therapy on sudden cardiac death prevention in patients with ischemic and non-ischemic cardiomyopathy is the **Sudden Cardiac Death-Heart Failure (SCD-HeFT) trial**. This trial enrolled 2521 patients with LVEF < 35%, NYHA II-III and it had similar proportion of patients with ischemic cardiomyopathy (52%) and non-ischemic cardiomyopathy (48%). Patients were randomized to receive a single chamber ICD (n=829), Amiodarone (n=845) or placebo (n=847) (Bardy et al. 2005). Patients with recent MI or revascularization (<1 month) were not eligible. Nearly 96% of patients were on ACE-I or angiotensin receptor blockers and 69% were receiving beta-blocker therapy. The primary endpoint was all cause mortality. The ICD group was programmed to shock therapy only. After mean follow up of 45.5 months, the ICD group had lower mortality compared to placebo (HR 0.77, 95% CI of 0.62-0.96, p=0.007) while amiodarone had no effect on mortality compared to placebo (HR 1.06, 95% CI 0.86 to 1.30, p=0.53) (Figure 2). Annual rate of appropriate ICD shocks occurred in 68% of patients with an average annual rate of 5.1%. The absolute reduction in mortality was similar in patients with ischemic (7.2%) and non-ischemic cardiomyopathy (6.5%).

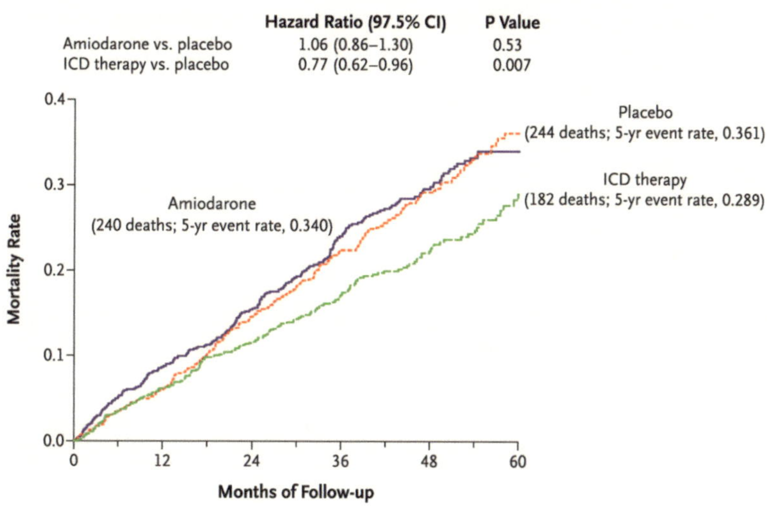

No. at Risk						
Amiodarone	845	772	715	484	280	97
Placebo	847	797	724	505	304	89
ICD therapy	829	778	733	501	304	103

Fig. 2. Kaplan-Meier Estimates of Death from Any Cause. CI denotes confidence interval. (From Bardy, G. H., Lee, K. L., Mark, D. B., et al. (2005). "Amiodarone or an implantable cardioverter-defibrillator for congestive heart failure." New England Journal of Medicine Vol. 352, No.3, (January, 2005): pp. 225-237, ISSN 1533-4406, with permission).

In a pooled analysis of 10 primary prevention trials (AMIOVERT, MADIT-I, MUSTT, MADIT-II, CABG PATCH, CAT, SCD-HeFT, COMPANION, DEFINITE and DINAMIT), ICD therapy was associated with 25% relative risk reduction of all cause mortality (RRR 9% to 37%, p=0.003) compared to the medical treatment group. The absolute risk reduction was 7.9%, which means 13 ICDs need to be implanted to save one life over about 3 years. This was not sensitive to removal of the any of the trials from the analysis. The benefit of ICD therapy in sudden cardiac death prevention is above and beyond the mortality benefit associated with use of beta blocker and ACE-I in patients with systolic heart failure (Nanthakumar et al. 2004). Table 4 summarized the primary prevention trials of ICD therapy in patients with non-ischemic cardiomyopathy.

Trial (N)	N	Inclusion Criteria	Primary Endpoint	Age	Mean LVEF	NYHA Class	HR (95% CI)	P Value
Amiodarone Versus Implantable Cardioverter Defibrillator Trial (AMIOVERT)	103	NYHA I-IV LVEF < 35% Dilated cardiomyopathy, NSVT	All cause mortality	52	23%	I, II ,III and IV		0.80
Cardiomyopathy Trial (CAT)	104	NYHA II-III, LVEF < 30%, Dilated cardiomyopathy, Recent onset heart failure < 9 months	All cause mortality	52	24%	II and III		0.54
The Defibrillators in Non-Ischemic Cardiomyopathy Treatment Evaluation Trial (DEFINITE)	488	NYHA I-III, LVEF < 35%, Dilated cardioyopathy, NSVT or frequent PVCs (>10 PVC /hr)	All cause mortality	58	21%	I, II and III	0.65 (0.40 to 1.06)	0.08
Sudden Cardiac Death-Heart Failure (SCD-HeFT) trial	2521	NYHA II-III, EF< 35%, non-recent MI or revascularization (>1 month), non-recent heart failure onset (> 3 months)	All Cause mortality	60	25%	II and III	0.77 (0.62-0.96)	0.007

Table 4. Primary prevention trials of ICD therapy in patients with non-ischemic cardiomyopathy. VT is for ventricular tachycardia, VF is for Ventricular Fibrillation, PVC is for premature ventricular contractions, LVEF is for left Ventricular ejection Fraction. HR is for hazard Ratio, CI is confidence interval.

2.2.3 Cost effectiveness of ICD therapy

ICD therapy adds to the costs of care of patients with cardiomyopathy. Analysis of cost effectiveness in the SCD-HeFT trial showed that ICD therapy is cost effective, with incremental cost of $38,400 (95% CI of $25,217 to $80,160). This was similar in patients with ischemic and non-ischemic cardiomyopathy (Mark et al. 2006). In a pooled analysis of eight primary prevention trials, ICD therapy was not found to be cost effective in CABG PATCH and in DINAMIT, which are the trials that showed no mortality benefit from ICD therapy compared to conventional medical therapy. When examining the primary prevention trials that showed mortality benefit (MADIT-I, MUSTT, MADIT-II, COMPANION, DEFINITE and SCD-HeFT), ICD therapy was found to be cost effective, adding between 1.01 and 2.99 quality-adjusted life years with costs ranging from $34,000 to $70,200. This analysis takes into account that the ICD generator will be replaced every 5 years and assumes that the mortality benefit persists throughout the patient's life time (Sanders et al. 2005). Careful patient selection with a focus on patients who best fit the trials and are likely to die from arrhythmia and not from other non cardiac causes is important to insure the best utilization of this important and life saving therapy.

3. Defibrillator therapy in less common types of cardiomyopathy

Some of the inherited cardiomyopathies carry an increased risk of sudden cardiac death. We will review in this section the data behind ICD therapy in patients with two inherited disorders, first is Hypertrophic cardiomyopathy (HCM) and the second is arrhythmogenic right ventricular dysplasia./ cardiomyopathy (ARVD/C).

3.1 Hypertrophic cardiomyopathy

Hypertrophic cardiomyopathy is an autosomal dominant disorder diagnosed by two-dimensional echocardiography and is characterized by hypertrophied and non-dilated LV in the absence of other causes of hypertrophy (no history of hypertension or aortic stenosis or any other cardiac or systemic disease causing hypertrophy) (Maron 2002; 2003). Histologically, there is myocardial disarray, abnormal microvascular circulation with mismatch between myocardial mass and blood supply as well as interstitial fibrosis (Maron et al. 1986; Varnava et al. 2001). All of these predispose to ventricular tachycardia and ventricular fibrillation putting the patients at risk of sudden cardiac death (Varnava et al. 2001). The disease can present at any age in life. Earlier registries from tertiary care centers overestimated the risk of sudden cardiac death due to selection bias (with the annual risk of death thought to be 3 to 6%). More recent population studies of unselected patients from community centers suggest a more benign prognosis (annual risk of death of 1%) (Maron et al. 1999; Kofflard et al. 2003). Despite all recent data, there is a subset of patients with HCM who are at high risk of sudden cardiac death. In fact HCM remains the most common etiology for SCD in patients younger than 40 years and it can be the first presentation in patients with HCM (Maron 2003). Patients who survived a cardiac arrest are particularly at high risk of dying suddenly. Data from registries suggest a number of markers that increase the risk of sudden cardiac death. These markers include one or more of the following: LV wall thickness > 30 mm (Maron et al. 1999), syncope (particularly exertional syncope) (Kofflard et al. 2003), family history of SCD, non-sustained VT on ambulatory holter of > 120 bpm and a blunted blood pressure response to exercise. High LV outflow gradient (> 30 mmHg) has also been considered as risk marker for sudden cardiac death (Maron et al. 2003).

There are no randomized trials examining the benefits of ICD therapy in this patient population, so the data supporting ICD therapy is derived from registry data in patients with HCM who received an ICD when found to be high risk by their treating cardiologist / Electrophysiologist (Maron et al. 2000). The last update from the registry included 506 patients with HCM with a mean age of 42 years. Patients received and ICD if they had survived a cardiac arrest due to ventricular tachycardia or ventricular fibrillation (secondary prevention cohort of 123 patients) or if they had one or more risk factors of sudden cardiac death: unexplained syncope, family history of sudden cardiac death in one or more first degree relatives, massive LV hypertrophy or non-sustained VT on holter monitoring (Primary prevention cohort of 383 patients) (Maron et al. 2007). Based on this registry, patients with HCM who survived cardiac arrest have a high appropriate ICD discharges (10.6% per year). This risk is lower in patients with HCM who had an ICD for primary prevention (3.6% per year). A third of these patients were 30 years or younger. Amiodarone was used based on the physicians judgment and it did not prevent arrhythmia occurrence (27% of patients who were on amiodarone had appropriate shocks). A third of the patients who received an ICD for primary prevention and had appropriate ICD discharges had one risk factor only for sudden cardiac death. There was no difference between the risk factors in the prediction of SCD. Since this is a young population of patients, they are at risk of inappropriate shocks, which occurred in 27% of the patients and were mainly due to sinus tachycardia, atrial fibrillation or lead malfunction. ICD implantation was shown to be safe with a rate of infection of 3.8% and the rate of lead fracture or dislodgement of 6.7%. Implantation of ICD has become an acceptable therapy in patients with HCM who survived cardiac arrest or who have two or more of the aforementioned risk factors of sudden cardiac death. For patients with only one risk factor of sudden cardiac death, the decision to implant an ICD is left to the physician's judgment and a careful discussion with the patient and his / her family in regards to the risks, benefits and alternatives of ICD therapy. In our experience, the presence of only one risk factor for SCD does not guarantee a recommendation for implanting an ICD. The clinical scenario is to be taken into account, as well as the patient's age and his / her wishes. The decision to implant is more favorable in a young patient with HCM with family history of sudden cardiac death or in a young patient with severe LV wall thickness (>30 mm) but still the discussion should take into account the young age of the patient and his / her wishes. On the other hand the discussion is more careful in an old patient with HCM in his / her 60s with history of non-exertional syncope that seems to be vasovagal in origin, the fact that the patient survived to that age without any major cardiac arrest indicates a more benign prognosis. Table 2 lists the current recommendations for ICD implantation for patients with hypertrophic cardiomyopathy.

3.2 Arrhythmogenic Right Ventricular Dysplasia / Cardiomyopathy (ARVD/C)

Arrhythmogenic right ventricular Dysplasia/ Cardiomyopathy (ARVD/C) is an inherited myopathy characterized by fibrofatty infiltration of the right ventricular (RV) wall, with left ventricular involvement over time in some patients (Gemayel et al. 2001; Sen-Chowdhry et al. 2004). The RV wall becomes thin, and the most areas affected are the RV inflow, apex and RV outflow, which form what is called the triangle of dysplasia. Ventricular tachycardia in general has left bundle branch morphology and is caused by macro-reentry and there is evidence that adrenergic stimulation acts as a trigger for these arrhythmias (Leclercq et al. 1996). ARVC/D accounts for 3 to 10% of death occurring in patients younger than 65 years (Tabib et al. 2003) and is one of the causes of sudden cardiac death in athletes (Maron 2003). The Most common presentation is with palpitations (due to frequent ventricular ectopy and ventricular tachycardia), chest pain, and syncope (mostly exertional). With time patients might develop RV dilatation, LV involvement and heart failure. Most of the data are obtained from registries in the United States and Europe (either single centers or multicenter registries). Diagnosis of

ARVD/C is based on the European Task Force criteria (McKenna et al. 1994). Risk factors of sudden cardiac death include prior cardiac arrest, hemodyamically unstable VT and prior syncope. Some studies suggested that LV involvement, development of heart failure and marked RV dilatation are risk factors for sudden cardiac death (Hulot et al. 2004). The role of electrophysiologic testing in risk stratification is less clear, with some studies showing a high positive predictive value and some showing low positive and low negative predictive values in predicting arrhythmias and appropriate ICD shocks (Corrado et al. 2003; Roguin et al. 2004). Beta blockers and sotalol were thought to be the best in suppressing these arrhythmias; however, this is challenged in more recent studies (Marcus et al. 2009). ICD therapy is clearly indicated in patients who survived cardiac arrest or have sustained VT and is a class IIa indication in patients with ARVD/C who have unexplained syncope. Some patients experience repetitive shocks requiring administration of antiarrhythmic drug therapy as well as VT ablation. Since this is a young population, they are also likely to experience inappropriate shocks due to sinus tachycardia or other supraventricular arrhythmias. In general ICD therapy is life saving and is well tolerated and has become accepted standard of care in patients with ARVD/C who experience cardiac arrest, sustained VT, unexplained syncope or marked RV dilatation or LV involvement (Epstein et al. 2008). Table 2 lists the current guidelines for ICD implantation in this patient population.

4. Cardiac Resynchronization Therapy (CRT) in patients with heart failure and its effects on mortality

Cardiac Resynchronization Therapy (CRT) aims at correcting mostly intraventricular dyssynchrony by stimulating the left ventricle (preferably basal stimulation) or by simultaneously stimulating the left and right ventricles after a sensed or paced atrial beat or during atrial fibrillation. CRT has been shown to improve the cardiac hemodynamics in patients with systolic heart failure, including improvements in the systolic blood pressure and decrease in the pulmonary capillary wedge pressure (by up to 20% in some patients) (Blanc et al. 1997). The early trials had endpoints related to heart failure functional status (including the 6 minute walk test, NYHA functional class), LV systolic function and improvement in the LV dimensions (including LVEF, LV end systolic volume and LV end systolic volume index as well as LV end diastolic dimension). Other studies relied on clinical composite score (which combines death from any cause, recent hospitalization for heart failure, NYHA class as well as the global assessment score) to define response to CRT (Chung et al. 2008). However, there is poor correlation between clinical and echocardiographic measurements of response and there is disagreement about the best way to measure response in patients with heart failure receiving CRT (Fornwalt et al.). So far QRS duration remains an important criterion for patient selection for CRT. Kass and colleagues demonstrated that baseline QRS duration correlated with enhancement in the isovolumetric dP/dt_{max} ($r = 0.6$, $p = 0.02$), while changes in the QRS duration with pacing did not predict hemodynamic response (Nelson et al. 2000). Most of the trials on CRT involved patients with systolic heart failure with LVEF < 35% and NYHA class III or IV as well as a QRS duration of > 120 msec. A trial studying patients with narrow QRS in patients with systolic heart failure failed to show any benefit. Later studies included patients with NYHA class I and class II heart failure with endpoints related to death or hospitalization. This section will focus mainly on the studies that included mortality as an endpoint.

4.1 Cardiac resynchronization therapy trials in patients with moderate to severe heart failure

The Multicenter InSync Randomized Clinical Evaluation (MIRACLE) trial involved implanting a CRT only device (with biventricular pacing only, no Defibrillator component). Patients were randomized if they had an LVEF < 35% and NYHA functional class III or IV heart failure despite optimal medical therapy and QRS duration of > 130 milliseconds (msec). a total of 453 patients were randomized after successful implantation of a CRT device to CRT ON (228 patients) and CRT OFF (225 patients) status for a period of 6 months (Abraham et al. 2002). The primary endpoint included the 6 minute walk test, quality of life score and NYHA class. A total of 453 patients were enrolled in the study. Patients assigned to CRT ON had 13% improvement in the 6-minute walk and in the quality of life score. The secondary endpoints also improved in the CRT ON arm including improvement in LVEF as well as peak oxygen consumption (VO2). The protocol specified safety variables that included an analysis of death or worsening heart failure. There was no difference in overall mortality (HR 0.73, 95% CI 0.34 to 1.54, p=0.40) but there was a decrease in hospitalization (HR 0.50, 95% CI 0.28 to 0.88, p= 0.02). The study did not specify mortality as a primary end point and was not powered enough to show differences in mortality.

The Multicenter Insync ICD randomized Clinical Evaluation (MIRACLE ICD) trial had a similar design to the MIRACLE study. Patients were included if they had LVEF < 35%, NYHA class III to IV despite optimal medical therapy and QRS duration of > 130 milliseconds and were at high risk of death from ventricular arrhythmias (Young et al. 2003). Almost two thirds of patients had an ischemic etiology and at least 60% were on beta blockers. All patients received a CRT-D device (total of 369 patients) of whom 182 had CRT OFF (controls) and 187 had CRT ON. At 6 months follow up, all patients with the CRT ON showed an improvement in the NYHA class (p=0.007) and the quality of life score (p=0.02). There was no difference in 6-minute walk distance (p=0.36) compared to the control group. Of the secondary endpoints, There was an improvement in the peak VO2 (p=0.04) and a trend towards reductions in the LV end systolic and end diastolic dimensions (p=0.06 for both) compared to the control group. The study did not show any difference in mortality (p=0.96) or hospitalization (p=0.69) between the two groups. Similar the to MIRACLE study, the MIRACLE ICD study had short follow up and was not powered enough to detect difference in mortality.

The CONTACT CD Biventricular Pacing study enrolled 490 patients with LVEF <35%, QRS > 120 msec and NYHA class II to IV despite optimal medical therapy and conventional indications for ICD implantation. Patients were assigned to CRT ON (245 patients) and CRT OFF (245 patients) for up to 6 months (Higgins et al. 2003). The primary endpoint was progression of heart failure, defined as all cause mortality, hospitalization for HF and ventricular tachycardia or ventricular fibrillation requiring device intervention. Secondary endpoints included peak oxygen consumption (VO2), 6-minute walk, NYHA class, quality of life as well as echocardiographic analysis. Patients with CRT ON had a 15% reduction in the composite HF progression but this was not statistically significant (p=0.35). However, patients with NYHA class III and IV had an improvement in the peak VO2 (p=0.003), 6-minute walk (p=0.03), NYHA class (p=0.0006) and QOL (0.02). Patients who had NYHA class I or II didn't show any improvement in any of the secondary parameters. One important finding in CONTACT CD trial is that patients with CRT ON had significant reductions in LV internal diameter in diastole (LVIDd) (p<0.001) LV internal diameter in systole (LVIDs) (p<0.001), and LVEF (p=0.02). Even patients with NYHA II had significant improvement in the LV dimensions with CRT ON. The study was not adequately powered to detect a statistical difference in the primary endpoint of composite HF progression. This was due to the fact that the observed event rates were half the expected while designing the trial.

The Comparison of Medical Therapy, Pacing and Defibrillation on Heart Failure Study (COMPANION) enrolled 1520 patients with LVEF< 35%, NYHA class III or IV heart failure despite optimal medical therapy and QRS duration of > 120 msec in a 1:2:2 fashion to medical therapy versus biventricular pacing alone (CRT only) versus biventricular pacing with defibrillation (CRT-D) (Bristow et al. 2004). Almost 59% of the patients had ischemic cardiomyopathy and 82% were NYHA class III. The primary endpoint was death or hospitalization for any cause while the secondary endpoints included death from any cause. As compared to the medical therapy group, patients with CRT only (Biventricular pacemaker only) decreased the risk of death or hospitalization from any cause (HR 0.81, p=0.014) as did CRT-D group (biventricular defibrillator group) (HR 0.80, p-0.01). CRT only decreased the risk of death by 24% (p=0.059) while CRT-D decreased the risk of death by 36% (p=0.003). COMPANION was the first trial to show that CRT improves the quality of life, symptoms as well as decrease the risk of death or hospitalization for heart failure.

The Cardiac Resynchronization-Heart Failure Study (CARE HF) randomized 813 patients with LVEF < 35%, NYHA class III to IV heart failure despite optimal medical therapy and QRS duration > 120 msec (patients with QRS between 120 to 149 msec had to have two of the three echocardiographic parameters of dys-synchrony: an aortic pre-ejection delay of > 140 msec, an interventricular mechanical delay of > 40 msec or delayed activation of the posterolateral wall of the LV (Cleland et al. 2005). Patients assigned to the CRT group received biventricular pacemaker (no defibrillators). The primary endpoint was the composite of death or unplanned hospitalization for a major cardiovascular event. Secondary endpoint was death from any cause. Other secondary endpoints included quality of life, improvement in NYHA class and echocardiographic parameters (mainly ventricular function, mitral regurgitation). After a mean follow up of 29.4 months, patients treated with CRT (total of 409 patients) had less death or hospitalization for cardiovascular event (HR 0.63, 95% CI 0.51 to 0.77, p< 0.001) compared to patients with medical therapy only (404 patients). CRT also improved survival (HR 0.64, 95% CI 0.48 to 0.85, p< 0.002) (Figure 3). Patients with CRT had improvement in NYHA class, better QOL, and showed smaller area of mitral regurgitation and an improvement in the LVEF at 3 and 18 months post CRT. CARE HF was the first CRT only trial to show that biventricular pacing alone can improve survival. The lack of mortality benefit from CRT only arm in COMPANION might be due to the fact that patients in COMPANION trial were sicker, with over 55% having ischemic cardiomyopathy with mean LVEF of 22% while patients in CARE HF had a mean LVEF of 25% and only a third of them had ischemic cardiomyopathy. The added benefits of CRT on survival will be examined later by the RAFT study.

The Cardiac Resynchronization Therapy in Patients with Heart Failure and Narrow QRS (RethinQ) study randomized 172 patients with history of NYHA class III heart failure, LVEF <35% despite optimal medical therapy and QRS duration of <130 msec with evidence of mechanical dys-synchrony on echocardiography (defined as septal to lateral or septal to inferior wall delay >65 msec as measured by tissue doppler or septal to posterior wall delay >130 msec as measured by M Mode echocardiography (Beshai et al. 2007). Primary outcome was the improvement of peak oxygen consumption of > 1 ml per kilogram of body weight

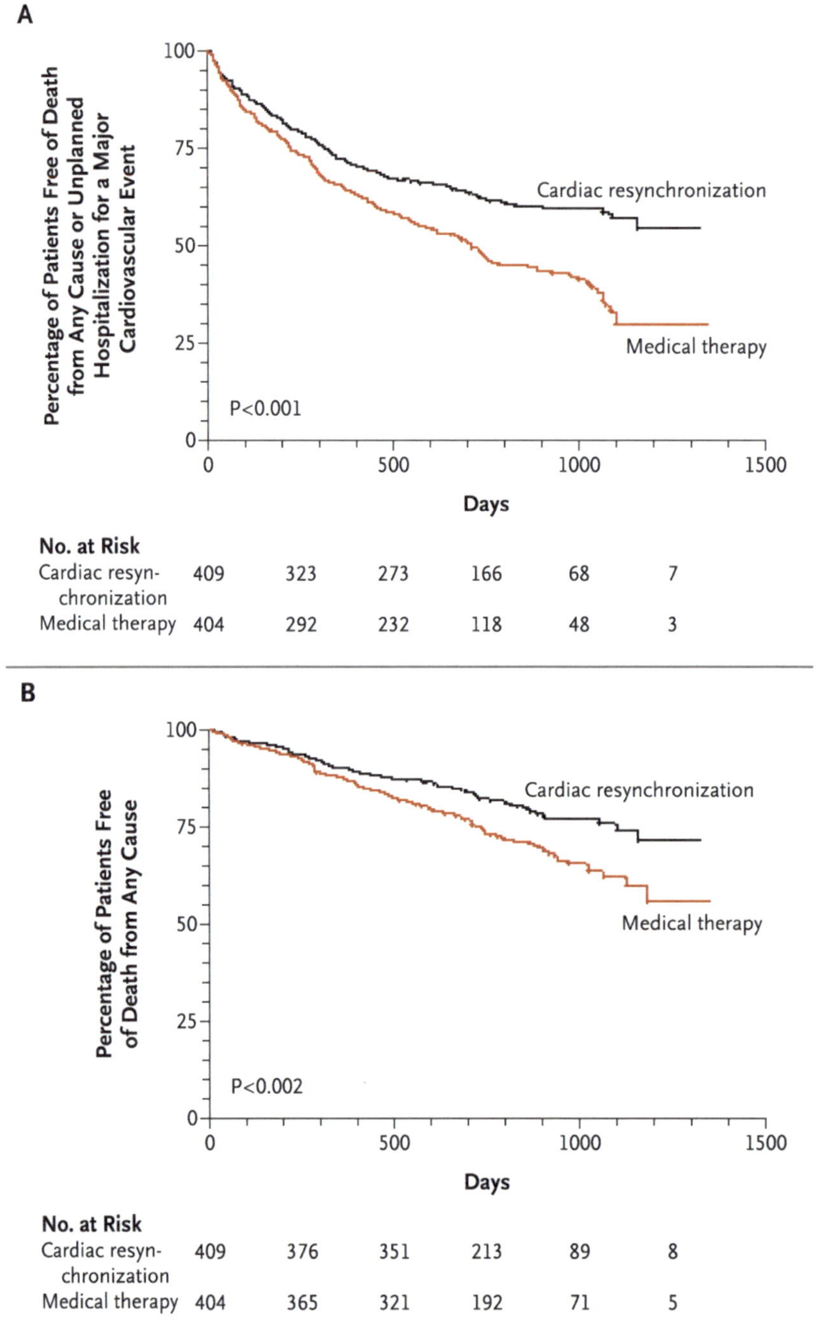

Fig. 3. Kaplan-Meier Estimates of the Time to the Primary End point of death or unplanned hospitalization for a major cardiovascular event (Panel A) and Death from any cause (Panel B). *(From Cleland, J. G., Daubert, J. C., Erdmann, E., et al. (2005). "The effect of cardiac resynchronization on morbidity and mortality in heart failure." New England Journal of Medicine, Vol. 352, No.15, (April, 2005): pp. 1539-1549, ISSN 1533-4406, with permission).*

per minute during cardiopulmonary exercise testing. The secondary outcomes were improvements in the 6 minute walk test, NYHA class and quality of life. All patients had a CRT device implantation and were assigned to CRT ON (n=76) or no CRT (n=80). After follow up of 6 months, there was no difference in the primary endpoint between patients with CRT and patients with no CRT (46% vs 44%, p=0.63). Patients in the CRT group with a QRS > 120 msec had significant improved in peak oxygen consumption at 6 months follow up (0.02) but patients in the CRT group with QRS <120 msec didn't have improvement in peak oxygen consumption at 6 months (p=0.45). There was no improvement in the quality of life measures (as measured by Minnesota living with Heart failure questionnaire) and in the 6-minute walk test in both groups of patients regardless of the QRS duration. Patients with CRT on had an improvement in the NYHA class at 6 months compared to patients with no CRT regardless of the QRS duration (p=0.006).

4.2 Cardiac resynchronization therapy trials in patients with mild heart failure

The Resynchronization Reverses Remodeling in Systolic Left Ventricular Dysfunction Study (REVERSE) trial was the first CRT trial to include patients with NYHA II and asymptomatic NYHA class I patients with LV dysfunction. A total of 610 patients underwent CRT device implantation and were randomized to CRT ON (419 patients) and CRT OFF (191 patients). Inclusion criteria included LVEF <40%, NYHA functional class I or II heart failure with a QRS 120 msec (Linde et al. 2008). Mean follow up was for 12 months. The primary end point was the heart failure (HF) clinical composite response (which included heart failure hospitalization, NYHA class and global assessment score). Secondary endpoints included LV end-systolic volume index and hospitalization for worsening HF. There was no difference between the two groups in the HF clinical composite score (which compared only the percent worsened) ($p = 0.10$). Patients assigned to CRT-ON experienced a greater improvement in LV end-systolic volume index (-18.4 ± 29.5 ml/m^2 vs. -1.3 ± 23.4 ml/m^2, $p < 0.0001$) and had a 53% relative risk reduction in time to first HF hospitalization (p=0.03). There was no difference between the two groups in the 6- minute walk test and in the quality of life scores. The improvement in LV end systolic volume index was similar in patients with NYHA I and NYHA II. The rate of LV lead implantation related complications was 10%. These complications were mostly due to LV lead dislodgement or diaphragmatic stimulation.

The Multicenter Automatic Defibrillator Implantation Trial with Cardiac Resynchronization therapy (MADIT-CRT) randomized 1820 patients with LVEF <30%, NYHA class I or II HF and QRS duration of > 130 msec in a 3:2 design to cardiac resynchronization therapy with defibrillation capacity (CRT-D) (1089 patients) and to ICD only group (731 patients). The primary endpoint was death from any cause or hospitalization for heart failure (Moss et al. 2009). Secondary endpoints included death from any cause and heart failure hospitalization alone. Follow up was for 4.5 years. Patients who received CRT-D had lower risk of death or hospitalization for heart failure (HR 0.66, 95% CI of 0.52 to 0.84, p=0.001) compared to the ICD only group. There was no difference in death from any cause between the two groups (HR 1.00, 95% CI of 0.69-1.44, p=0.99). The rate of hospitalization was significantly lower in the CRT-D group compared to the ICD only group (HR 0.59, 95% CI of 0.47 to 0.74, p<0.001). Patients with ischemic and non-ischemic cardiomyopathy benefited similarly from CRT. Subanalysis of MADIT CRT showed that female patients (n=453, 25%) were more likely to have non-ischemic cardiomyopathy and left bundle branch block (LBBB) compared to male patients. Female patients were more likely to have reverse remodeling by echocardiography and had a 69% relative risk reduction of death or heart failure (HR of 0.31, p<0.001) (Arshad et al.). Patients with QRS duration > 150 msec had greater benefit from CRT (HR 0.48, 95% CI 0.37 to 0.64) compared to patients with QRS duration < 150 msec (HR 1.06, 95% CI 0.74 to 1.52, p=0.001 for interaction). Patients assigned to the CRT-D arm had significant reduction in LV end diastolic volume index (-26.2 versus -7.4 mL/m^2), LV end systolic volume index (-28.7 versus -9.1 mL/m^2) as well as improvement in LVEF (11% versus 3%) compared to the ICD only group. After adjusting for baseline variables, for every 10% reduction in the LV end diastolic volume index, there was a 40% reduction in the risk of death or heart failure hospitalization (Solomon et al.). Furthermore MADIT CRT measured echocardiographic response as a decrease in LV end systolic volume > 25%. Using this definition, 529 patients assigned to the CRT-D arm responded to CRT and were less likely to have ventricular tachyarrhythmia (VT or VF) and inappropriate shocks. Analysis of the data showed that for every 10% reduction in LV end systolic volume, there is a 20% decrease in the risk of ventricular tachyarrhythmias (p<0.001) even after adjusting for other clinical risk factors including age, QRS duration, left bundle branch block, and blood urea nitrogen (BUN) (Barsheshet et al.).

The Resynchronization-Defibrillation for Ambulatory Heart Failure Trial (RAFT) randomized 1798 patients with LVEF <30%, NYHA II to III heart failure and QRS duration of >120 msec or a paced QRS duration of > 200 msec to either ICD alone or Biventricular defibrillator (CRT-D) (Tang et al.). Mean follow up was for 40 months and the primary endpoint was death or hospitalization for heart failure while secondary endpoints included death from any cause, death from cardiovascular cause and heart failure hospitalization. Most of the patient had NYHA class II (80%) and had ischemic etiology (64%). Patients with CRT-D had less death and heart failure hospitalization compared to the ICD group (HR 0.75, 95% CI of 0.64 to 0.87, p <0.001). CRT-D also improved survival compared to ICD alone (HR 0.75, 95% CI 0.62-0.91, p=0.003) (Figure 4). There was less heart failure hospitalizations with CRT-D group compared to ICD only group (HR 0.68, 95% CI of 0.56 to 0.83, p<0.001). There was no difference in the primary and secondary endpoints in patients with ischemic and non-ischemic cardiomyopathy. Patients with wider QRS (>150 milliseconds) had better survival than patients with QRS < 150 msec. However, patients with CRT-D had more 30 days adverse events compared to the ICD alone group (p<0.001), these were mostly device related complications.

These trails established CRT as an important therapy for patients with heart failure, LVEF < 35% and NYHA class III to IV. The only measure of dys-synchrony that stood the test of time is the QRS duration. Even though there is disagreement in the literature in the measurement of "response". At least two thirds of patients with CRT show clinical improvement in their functional status. CRT has been proven to improve survival independently as shown in the CARE HF trial, and it also improves survival above and beyond ICD therapy as shown in the RAFT trial. The guidelines for implantation for CRT in patients with systolic heart failure are listed in Table 5. These guidelines were written in 2008, and do not reflect the recent evidence of the benefits of CRT in milder forms of heart failure that was found in the REVERSE, MADIT CRT and RAFT trials.

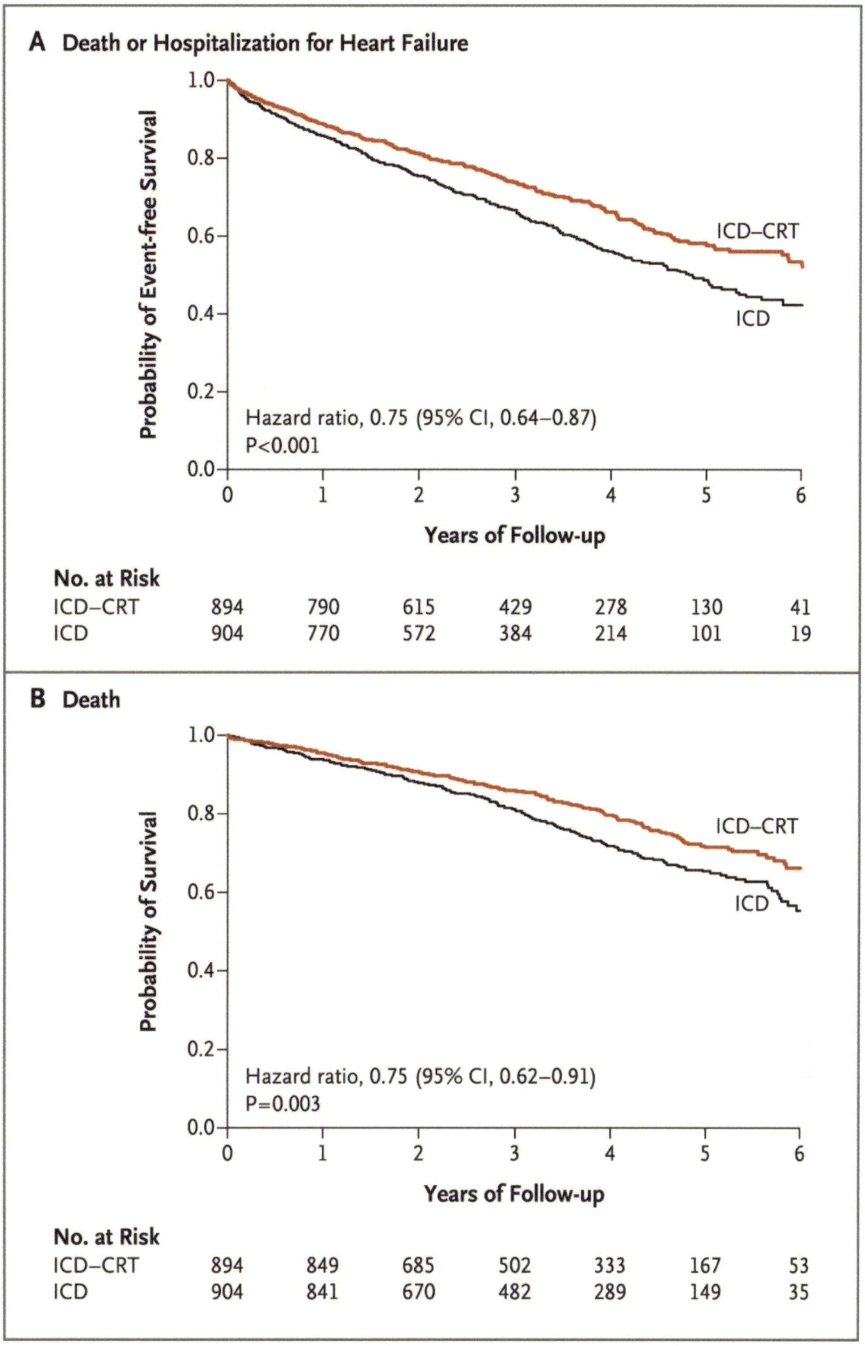

Fig. 4. Kaplan Meier Estimates of Death or Hospitalization for Heart Failure (Panel A) and Death from Any Cause (Panel B). (From Tang, A. S., Wells, G. A., Talajic, M., et al. "Cardiac-resynchronization therapy for mild-to-moderate heart failure." New England Journal of Medicine Vol. 363, No.25, (December, 2010): pp. 2385-2395, ISSN 1533-4406, with permission)

Class I (General agreement of benefit of CRT) 1. CRT with or without an ICD is indicated for the treatment of for patients are in sinus rhythm who have LVEF ≤ 35%, a QRS duration ≥ 120 milliseconds, NYHA functional Class III or ambulatory Class IV heart failure symptoms with optimal recommended medical therapy.
Class IIa (Weight of evidence is in favor of CRT) 1. CRT with or without an ICD is indicated for patients in sinus rhythm who have LVEF ≤ 35%, a QRS duration ≥ 120 msec, NYHA functional class III or ambulatory class IV heart failure symptoms with optimal recommended medical therapy. 2. CRT is reasonable for patients with LVEF ≤ 35%, QRS duration ≥120 milliseconds, NYHA functional Class III or ambulatory Class IV heart failure symptoms with optimal recommended medical therapy and who have frequent dependence on ventricular pacing.
Class IIb (Efficacy of CRT is less well established) 1. CRT may be considered for patients with LVEF ≤ 35% with NYHA functional Class I or II symptoms who are receiving optimal recommended medical therapy and who are undergoing implantation of a permanent pacemaker and/or ICD with anticipated frequent ventricular pacing.
Class III (General agreement that CRT is less effective and might be harmful) 1. CRT is not indicated for asymptomatic patients with reduced LVEF in the absence of other indications for pacing. 2. CRT is not indicated for patients whose functional status and life expectancy are limited predominantly by chronic non-cardiac conditions.

Table 5. Recommendations for cardiac resynchronization therapy based on the ACC/AHA/HRS 2008 Guidelines for Device Based Therapy. CRT: Cardiac Resynchronization Therapy. ICD: Implantable Cardioverter Defibrillator. NYHA: New York Heart Association

5. Defibrillator shocks, their impact on quality of life and prognosis

5.1 Impact of defibrillator shocks on quality of life

From all the studies presented earlier, it is clear that ICD therapy prevents sudden cardiac death. However, ICD shocks can be painful and have been shown to affect the quality of life in both primary and secondary prevention trials. Patients with ICD can receive inappropriate shocks due to atrial fibrillation (AF), supraventricular tachycardia (SVT) or inappropriate sensing from the device. The quality of life (QOL) was assessed in the AVID trial as a secondary endpoint using the Medical Outcomes Short Form 36 item questionnaire (SF-36). Of the 905 patients enrolled in QOL analysis, 800 survived for longer than 1 year. Both treatment groups (ICD group versus antiarrhythmic group) had significant impairment in both physical functioning and mental well-being(Schron et al. 2002). ICD shocks were independently associated with reduction in both physical functioning and mental well-being. The CIDS trial also measured QOL, in the 400 patients who survived for

> 1 year, patients assigned to the ICD group had an improvement in their quality of life scores compared to patients assigned to amiodarone. However, patients having frequent shocks (>5 shocks) had reduced QOL.
The SCD-HeFT trial also collected data on the quality of life using two different scales: The Duke Activity Scale Index (DASI) reflecting the overall physical functioning and the SF-36 Mental Health Inventory 5 which measures psychological well being (Mark et al. 2008). Data were collected at baseline, 3, 12 and 30 months of follow up. A total of 2479 patients (98%) enrolled in SCD-HeFT completed the quality of life portion of the study. Patients receiving ICD therapy and patients assigned to placebo had similar DASI scores and SF-36 MHI 5 scores at baseline. The psychological well being of patients receiving an ICD was significantly better at 3 months and 12 months compared to patients receiving placebo. There was no difference in the physical functioning at baseline or at 3, 12 or 30 months in the ICD group versus the placebo group. The quality of life of patients who received an ICD shock a month before the screening was significantly worse in multiple aspects (physical, psychological, social and self related health).

5.2 Impact of defibrillator shocks on prognosis

The SCD-HeFT Trial also evaluated the prognostic impact of ICD shocks in patients with ischemic and non-ischemic cardiomyopathy. Most of the patients received a single chamber ICD programmed to shock only therapy with no antitachycardia pacing involved. (Poole et al. 2008). Patients (n=811) were followed for 45.5 months and a third of patients (n=269) received ICD shocks. Patients who received appropriate ICD shock (n=128) were at increased risk of death (HR 5.68, 95% CI of 3.97 to 8.12, $p < 0.001$) compared to patients with no appropriate shocks. Patients who received inappropriate shocks were also at increased risk of death (HR 1.98, 95% CI of 1.29 to 3.05, p=0.002) compared to patients with no inappropriate shocks. Atrial fibrillation was the most common reason for inappropriate ICD shocks and the most common cause of death in patients receiving any shock was progressive heart failure.
Inappropriate shocks were examined in the MADIT-II trial. Of the 719 patients who received an ICD, inappropriate shocks occurred in 83 patients (11.5%). Inappropriate shocks represented a third (31.2%) of total shocks (Daubert et al. 2008). Independent predictors of inappropriate shocks included atrial fibrillation (HR = 2.9, $P<0.01$), smoking (HR 2.18, P=0.03), diastolic blood pressure of > 80 mmHg (HR = 1.61, P= 0.04) and antecedent appropriate shocks (HR = 2.25, P= 0.03). Again, inappropriate shocks were most likely due to AF (44%), SVT (36%) or abnormal sensing (20%). Implantation of a dual chamber ICD did not decrease the rate of inappropriate shocks compared to single chamber ICD implantation (38.6% versus 44% respectively, p=0.31). Any shock whether appropriate or inappropriate was associated with significant increase in mortality (HR 4.08, $p<0.01$). Inappropriate shocks were associated with a 2 fold increase in mortality (HR is 2.29, p=0.03) while appropriate shocks had a 3 fold increase in mortality (HR 3.36, $p<0.01$). Electrical instability in the form of VT or VF or atrial fibrillation could be markers of deteriorating heart function and pump failure(Obadah Al Chekakie 2009). It is unclear if the VT or VF that the patient experiences heralds progressive pump failure, or whether the fact that shocks my increase mortality due to their negative effect on contractility in this high risk population or if both assumptions are true.

5.3 Device programming studies: Safety, effectiveness and impact on quality of life

Since Shocks are associated with lower quality of life and increase mortality, attempts at reducing shocks (both appropriate and inappropriate) became the focus of several studies. Antitachycardia pacing (ATP) has been shown to terminate 78 to 94% of slow VTs (188 bpm) (Peinado et al. 1998). The PAINFREE RX II trial randomized 634 patients with ICDs to standardized ATP (n=313 patients) versus shocks (n=321 patients). The programming in the Standarized ATP arm included two main parameters: First programming ATP in the fast VT zone of 188 to 250 bpm, at 8 pulses and 88% of VT cycle length. Second is extending the detection to 18 of 24 beats to avoid shocking ventricular tachycardia that was going to terminate anyway. The primary objective was to demonstrate that ATP will not prolong treatment > 6 seconds compared to the shock arm. Secondary objectives included the QOL, ATP efficacy and acceleration and syncope (Sweeney et al. 2005). After mean follow up of 11+/- 3 months, 4230 ICD counters were retrieved, and electrograms were only available in 1827 episodes. A third of the shocks was deemed inappropriate and due to SVT and 0.2% were due to noise. Only 73% of total shocks were due to true ventricular arrhythmias. Of these, 431 (58%) were detected as VT, 32% as Fast VT and 10% as VF. ATP was successful as initial therapy in 81% of the episodes and failed in 54 episodes, of which 49 episodes were shocked while 5 were terminated by a second ATP therapy. ATP did not prolong therapy duration (median duration was 10 seconds in the ATP arm versus 9.7 seconds in the shock arm) and there was no significant difference in the acceleration of VT/VF between the two arms. Syncope was very rare in the two arms (2 in the ATP group and 1 in the shock arm) and the first shock success was identical between the two arms. There was no difference between the two groups at baseline in the QOL scores as assessed by the SF-36. Patients assigned to the shock arm had an improvement in the bodily pain scores at 12 months but no change in the other SF-36 subscales. While patients assigned to the ATP arm had significant improvement in 5 subscales (bodily pain, social functioning, role emotional, physical functioning and role physical). This trial established the safety and efficacy of ATP in the fast VT zone and the safety of extending the detection duration to 18 out of 24 beats, which led to a decrease in shocks (The patients assigned to the shock arm had 147 detected FVT episodes with only 99 episodes receiving therapy). This will be an important factor in the design and implementation of the PREPARE study.

The Primary Prevention Parameters Evaluation Study (PREPARE) study compared 700 patients who had received an ICD or Biventricular defibrillator for primary prevention within 6 months of enrollment (Wilkoff et al. 2008). The control group for the ICD patients was taken from the EMPIRIC trial while the control group for the Biventricular ICD (BiV ICD) arm was from the MIRACLE ICD trial. The cohort of the PREPARE study had the following programming parameters: Initial detection for VT at rate of >182 bpm, with ATP programmed to fast VT of 182 to 250 bpm, with detection prolonged to 30 of the 40 intervals to avoid shocking VT that was going to terminate anyway, programming SVT discriminators to arrhythmias < 200 bpm to prevent inappropriate shocks. The primary endpoint of the study was the morbidity index defined as 1) device related cardioversion or defibrillation whether appropriate or inappropriate, 2) syncope secondary to arrhythmia or presumed arrhythmia and 3) untreated sustained symptomatic VT/VF events. The PREPARE study patients were less likely to receive a shock for any cause in the first year as compared to the control cohort (8.5 % vs 16.9%, p<0.01) and were also less likely to receive inappropriate shocks even after correcting for differences in baseline variables including mean LVEF, hypertension, history of ischemic heart disease, syncope and baseline use of beta blockers. The morbidity index incidence density was significantly lower in the PREPARE cohort compared to the control cohorts (HR 0.26 versus 0.69, 95% CI of 0.2 to 0.72, p=0.003). Importantly, only 12 of the 40 syncope episodes were judged to be due to arrhythmia, and of those, only 11 were due to PREPARE programming. The PREPARE study established the efficacy of empirically programming the ICD detection and therapy to minimize both appropriate and inappropriate shocks. This is true for patients receiving ICD therapy for primary prevention only.

In summary: ICD therapy prevents sudden cardiac death but patients who receive an ICD shock have increased morbidity and mortality and poor quality of life. Programming the device can help minimize ICD shocks, whether appropriate or inappropriate. Patients with ICD therapy who receive a shock should be followed closely since they are at increased risk of pump failure.

6. Conclusion

Implantable cardioverter defibrillator therapy is important in sudden cardiac death prevention in patients with ischemic and non-ischemic cardiomyopathy as well as survivors of cardiac arrest. Cardiac resynchronization therapy with and without an ICD improves the quality of life and leads to reverse remodeling and independently prevents sudden cardiac death in patients with QRS > 120 msec and LVEF < 35% who are on optimal medical therapy. Defibrillator shocks are associated with adverse outcomes and pump failure. Careful patient selection and sophisticated programming can help prevent sudden cardiac death without compromising the quality of life of the patients.

7. References

Abraham, W. T., Fisher, W. G., Smith, A. L., et al. (2002). "Cardiac resynchronization in chronic heart failure." *New England Journal of Medicine* Vol. 346, No.24, (June, 2002): pp. 1845-1853, ISSN: 1533-4406

Arshad, A., Moss, A. J., Foster, E., et al. "Cardiac resynchronization therapy is more effective in women than in men: the MADIT-CRT (Multicenter Automatic Defibrillator Implantation Trial with Cardiac Resynchronization Therapy) trial." *Journal of The American College of Cardiology* Vol. 57, No.7, (February, 2011): pp. 813-820, ISSN 1558-3597

AVID Investigators (1997). "A comparison of antiarrhythmic-drug therapy with implantable defibrillators in patients resuscitated from near-fatal ventricular arrhythmias. The Antiarrhythmics versus Implantable Defibrillators (AVID) Investigators." *New England Journal of Medicine* Vol. 337, No.22, (November, 1997): pp. 1576-1583, ISSN 0028-4793

Bardy, G. H., Lee, K. L., Mark, D. B., et al. (2005). "Amiodarone or an implantable cardioverter-defibrillator for congestive heart failure." *New England Journal of Medicine* Vol. 352, No.3, (January, 2005): pp. 225-237, ISSN 1533-4406

Barsheshet, A., Wang, P. J., Moss, A. J., et al. "Reverse Remodeling and the Risk of Ventricular Tachyarrhythmias in the MADIT-CRT (Multicenter Automatic Defibrillator Implantation Trial-Cardiac Resynchronization Therapy)." *Journal of*

The American College of Cardiology Vol. 57, No.24, (June, 2011): pp. 2416-2423, ISSN 1558-3597

Beshai, J. F., Grimm, R. A., Nagueh, S. F., et al. (2007). "Cardiac-resynchronization therapy in heart failure with narrow QRS complexes." *New England Journal of Medicine* Vol. 357, No.24, (December, 2007): pp. 2461-2471, ISSN 1533-4406

Bigger, J. T., Jr. (1997). "Prophylactic use of implanted cardiac defibrillators in patients at high risk for ventricular arrhythmias after coronary-artery bypass graft surgery. Coronary Artery Bypass Graft (CABG) Patch Trial Investigators." *New England Journal of Medicine* Vol. 337, No.22, (November, 1997): pp. 1569-1575, ISSN 0028-4793

Blanc, J. J., Etienne, Y., Gilard, M., et al. (1997). "Evaluation of different ventricular pacing sites in patients with severe heart failure: results of an acute hemodynamic study." *Circulation* Vol. 96, No.10, (November, 1997): pp. 3273-3277, ISSN 0009-7322

Bristow, M. R., Saxon, L. A., Boehmer, J., et al. (2004). "Cardiac-resynchronization therapy with or without an implantable defibrillator in advanced chronic heart failure." *New England Journal of Medicine* Vol. 350, No.21, (May, 2004): pp. 2140-2150, ISSN 1533-4406

Buxton, A. E., Lee, K. L., DiCarlo, L., et al. (2000). "Electrophysiologic testing to identify patients with coronary artery disease who are at risk for sudden death. Multicenter Unsustained Tachycardia Trial Investigators." *New England Journal of Medicine* Vol. 342, No.26, (June, 2000): pp. 1937-1945, ISSN 0028-4793

Buxton, A. E., Lee, K. L., Fisher, J. D., et al. (1999). "A randomized study of the prevention of sudden death in patients with coronary artery disease. Multicenter Unsustained Tachycardia Trial Investigators." *New England Journal of Medicin* Vol. 341, No.25, (December, 1999): pp. 1882-1890, ISSN 0028-4793

Chung, E. S., Leon, A. R., Tavazzi, L., et al. (2008). "Results of the Predictors of Response to CRT (PROSPECT) trial." *Circulation* Vol. 117, No.20, (May, 2008): pp. 2608-2616, ISSN 1524-4539

Cleland, J. G., Daubert, J. C., Erdmann, E., et al. (2005). "The effect of cardiac resynchronization on morbidity and mortality in heart failure." *New England Journal of Medicine* Vol. 352, No.15, (April, 2005): pp. 1539-1549, ISSN 1533-4406

Connolly, S. J., Gent, M., Roberts, R. S., et al. (2000). "Canadian implantable defibrillator study (CIDS) : a randomized trial of the implantable cardioverter defibrillator against amiodarone." *Circulation* Vol. 101, No.11, (March, 2000): pp. 1297-1302, ISSN 1524-4539

Connolly, S. J., Hallstrom, A. P., Cappato, R., et al. (2000). "Meta-analysis of the implantable cardioverter defibrillator secondary prevention trials. AVID, CASH and CIDS studies. Antiarrhythmics vs Implantable Defibrillator study. Cardiac Arrest Study Hamburg . Canadian Implantable Defibrillator Study." *European Heart Journal* Vol. 21, No.24, (December, 2000): pp. 2071-2078, ISSN 0195-668X

Corrado, D., Leoni, L., Link, M. S., et al. (2003). "Implantable cardioverter-defibrillator therapy for prevention of sudden death in patients with arrhythmogenic right ventricular cardiomyopathy/dysplasia." *Circulation* Vol. 108, No.25, (December, 2003): pp. 3084-3091, ISSN 1524-4539

Daubert, J. P., Zareba, W., Cannom, D. S., et al. (2008). "Inappropriate implantable cardioverter-defibrillator shocks in MADIT II: frequency, mechanisms, predictors, and survival impact." *Journal of The American College of Cardiology* Vol. 51, No.14, (April, 2008): pp. 1357-1365, ISSN 1558-3597

Daubert, J. P., Zareba, W., Hall, W. J., et al. (2006). "Predictive value of ventricular arrhythmia inducibility for subsequent ventricular tachycardia or ventricular fibrillation in Multicenter Automatic Defibrillator Implantation Trial (MADIT) II patients." *Journal of The American College of Cardiology* Vol. 47, No.1, (January, 2006): pp. 98-107, ISSN 1558-3597

Domanski, M. J., Exner, D. V., Borkowf, C. B., et al. (1999). "Effect of angiotensin converting enzyme inhibition on sudden cardiac death in patients following acute myocardial infarction. A meta-analysis of randomized clinical trials." *Journal of The American College of Cardiology* Vol. 33, No.3, (March, 1999): pp. 598-604, ISSN 0735-1097

Domanski, M. J., Sakseena, S., Epstein, A. E., et al. (1999). "Relative effectiveness of the implantable cardioverter-defibrillator and antiarrhythmic drugs in patients with varying degrees of left ventricular dysfunction who have survived malignant ventricular arrhythmias. AVID Investigators. Antiarrhythmics Versus Implantable Defibrillators." *Journal of The American College of Cardiology* Vol. 34, No.4, (October, 1999): pp. 1090-1095, ISSN 0735-1097

Epstein, A. E., DiMarco, J. P., Ellenbogen, K. A., et al. (2008). "ACC/AHA/HRS 2008 Guidelines for Device-Based Therapy of Cardiac Rhythm Abnormalities: a report of the American College of Cardiology/American Heart Association Task Force on Practice Guidelines (Writing Committee to Revise the ACC/AHA/NASPE 2002 Guideline Update for Implantation of Cardiac Pacemakers and Antiarrhythmia Devices): developed in collaboration with the American Association for Thoracic Surgery and Society of Thoracic Surgeons." *Circulation* Vol. 117, No.21, (May, 2008): pp. e350-408, ISSN 1524-4539

Fornwalt, B. K., Sprague, W. W., BeDell, P., et al. "Agreement is poor among current criteria used to define response to cardiac resynchronization therapy." *Circulation* Vol. 121, No.18, (May, 2010): pp. 1985-1991, ISSN 1524-4539

Gemayel, C., Pelliccia, A. and Thompson, P. D. (2001). "Arrhythmogenic right ventricular cardiomyopathy." *Journal of The American College of Cardiology* Vol. 38, No.7, (December, 2001): pp. 1773-1781, ISSN 0735-1097

Goldenberg, I., Moss, A. J., McNitt, S., et al. (2006). "Time dependence of defibrillator benefit after coronary revascularization in the Multicenter Automatic Defibrillator Implantation Trial (MADIT)-II." *Journal of The American College of Cardiology* Vol. 47, No.9, (May, 2006): pp. 1811-1817, ISSN 1558-3597

Gorgels, A. P., Gijsbers, C., de Vreede-Swagemakers, J., et al. (2003). "Out-of-hospital cardiac arrest--the relevance of heart failure. The Maastricht Circulatory Arrest Registry." *European Heart Journal* Vol. 24, No.13, (July, 2003): pp. 1204-1209, ISSN 0195-668X

Higgins, S. L., Hummel, J. D., Niazi, I. K., et al. (2003). "Cardiac resynchronization therapy for the treatment of heart failure in patients with intraventricular conduction delay and malignant ventricular tachyarrhythmias." *Journal of The American College of Cardiology* Vol. 42, No.8, (October, 2003): pp. 1454-1459, ISSN 0735-1097

Hohnloser, S. H., Kuck, K. H., Dorian, P., et al. (2004). "Prophylactic use of an implantable cardioverter-defibrillator after acute myocardial infarction." *New England Journal of Medicine* Vol. 351, No.24, (December9, 2004): pp. 2481-2488, ISSN 1533-4406

Hulot, J. S., Jouven, X., Empana, J. P., et al. (2004). "Natural history and risk stratification of arrhythmogenic right ventricular dysplasia/cardiomyopathy." *Circulation* Vol. 110, No.14, (October, 2004): pp. 1879-1884, ISSN 1524-4539

Kadish, A., Dyer, A., Daubert, J. P., et al. (2004). "Prophylactic defibrillator implantation in patients with nonischemic dilated cardiomyopathy." *New England Journal of Medicine* Vol. 350, No.21, (May, 2004): pp. 2151-2158, ISSN 1533-4406

Kadish, A., Schaechter, A., Subacius, H., et al. (2006). "Patients with recently diagnosed nonischemic cardiomyopathy benefit from implantable cardioverter-defibrillators." *Journal of The American College of Cardiology* Vol. 47, No.12, (June, 2006): pp. 2477-2482, ISSN 1558-3597

Kofflard, M. J., Ten Cate, F. J., van der Lee, C., et al. (2003). "Hypertrophic cardiomyopathy in a large community-based population: clinical outcome and identification of risk factors for sudden cardiac death and clinical deterioration." *Journal of The American College of Cardiology* Vol. 41, No.6, (March, 2003): pp. 987-993, ISSN 0735-1097

Kuck, K. H., Cappato, R., Siebels, J., et al. (2000). "Randomized comparison of antiarrhythmic drug therapy with implantable defibrillators in patients resuscitated from cardiac arrest : the Cardiac Arrest Study Hamburg (CASH)." *Circulation* Vol. 102, No.7, (August, 2000): pp. 748-754, ISSN 1524-4539

Leclercq, J. F., Potenza, S., Maison-Blanche, P., et al. (1996). "Determinants of spontaneous occurrence of sustained monomorphic ventricular tachycardia in right ventricular dysplasia." *Journal of The American College of Cardiology* Vol. 28, No.3, (September, 1996): pp. 720-724, ISSN 0735-1097

Linde, C., Abraham, W. T., Gold, M. R., et al. (2008). "Randomized trial of cardiac resynchronization in mildly symptomatic heart failure patients and in asymptomatic patients with left ventricular dysfunction and previous heart failure symptoms." *Journal of The American College of Cardiology* Vol. 52, No.23, (December, 2008): pp. 1834-1843, ISSN 1558-3597

Marcus, G. M., Glidden, D. V., Polonsky, B., et al. (2009). "Efficacy of antiarrhythmic drugs in arrhythmogenic right ventricular cardiomyopathy: a report from the North American ARVC Registry." *Journal of The American College of Cardiology* Vol. 54, No.7, (August, 2009): pp. 609-615, ISSN 1558-3597

Mark, D. B., Anstrom, K. J., Sun, J. L., et al. (2008). "Quality of life with defibrillator therapy or amiodarone in heart failure." *New England Journal of Medicine* Vol. 359, No.10, (September, 2008): pp. 999-1008, ISSN 1533-4406

Mark, D. B., Nelson, C. L., Anstrom, K. J., et al. (2006). "Cost-effectiveness of defibrillator therapy or amiodarone in chronic stable heart failure: results from the Sudden Cardiac Death in Heart Failure Trial (SCD-HeFT)." *Circulation* Vol. 114, No.2, (July, 2006): pp. 135-142, ISSN 1524-4539

Maron, B. J. (2002). "Hypertrophic cardiomyopathy: a systematic review." *Journal of the American Medical Association* Vol. 287, No.10, (March, 2002): pp. 1308-1320, ISSN 0098-7484

Maron, B. J. (2003). "Sudden death in young athletes." *New England Journal of Medicine* Vol. 349, No.11, (September, 2003): pp. 1064-1075, ISSN 1533-4406

Maron, B. J., Casey, S. A., Poliac, L. C., et al. (1999). "Clinical course of hypertrophic cardiomyopathy in a regional United States cohort." *Journal of the American Medical Association* Vol. 281, No.7, (February, 1999): pp. 650-655, ISSN 0098-7484

Maron, B. J., McKenna, W. J., Danielson, G. K., et al. (2003). "American College of Cardiology/European Society of Cardiology clinical expert consensus document on hypertrophic cardiomyopathy. A report of the American College of Cardiology Foundation Task Force on Clinical Expert Consensus Documents and the European Society of Cardiology Committee for Practice Guidelines." *Journal of The American College of Cardiology* Vol. 42, No.9, (November, 2003): pp. 1687-1713, ISSN 0735-1097 (

Maron, B. J., Shen, W. K., Link, M. S., et al. (2000). "Efficacy of implantable cardioverter-defibrillators for the prevention of sudden death in patients with hypertrophic cardiomyopathy." *New England Journal of Medicine* Vol. 342, No.6, (February, 2000): pp. 365-373, ISSN 0028-4793

Maron, B. J., Spirito, P., Shen, W. K., et al. (2007). "Implantable cardioverter-defibrillators and prevention of sudden cardiac death in hypertrophic cardiomyopathy."*Journal of the American Medical Association* Vol. 298, No.4, (July, 2007): pp. 405-412, ISSN 1538-3598

Maron, B. J., Wolfson, J. K., Epstein, S. E., et al. (1986). "Intramural ("small vessel") coronary artery disease in hypertrophic cardiomyopathy." *Journal of The American College of Cardiology* Vol. 8, No.3, (September, 1986): pp. 545-557, ISSN 0735-1097

Maron, M. S., Olivotto, I., Betocchi, S., et al. (2003). "Effect of left ventricular outflow tract obstruction on clinical outcome in hypertrophic cardiomyopathy." *New England Journal of Medicine* Vol. 348, No.4, (January, 2003): pp. 295-303, ISSN 1533-4406

McKenna, W. J., Thiene, G., Nava, A., et al. (1994). "Diagnosis of arrhythmogenic right ventricular dysplasia/cardiomyopathy. Task Force of the Working Group Myocardial and Pericardial Disease of the European Society of Cardiology and of the Scientific Council on Cardiomyopathies of the International Society and Federation of Cardiology." *British Heart* Journal Vol. 71, No.3, (March, 1994): pp. 215-218, ISSN 0007-0769

McMurray, J., Kober, L., Robertson, M., et al. (2005). "Antiarrhythmic effect of carvedilol after acute myocardial infarction: results of the Carvedilol Post-Infarct Survival Control in Left Ventricular Dysfunction (CAPRICORN) trial." *Journal of The American College of Cardiology* Vol. 45, No.4, (Febrary, 2005): pp. 525-530, ISSN 0735-1097

Moss, A. J., Hall, W. J., Cannom, D. S., et al. (1996). "Improved survival with an implanted defibrillator in patients with coronary disease at high risk for ventricular arrhythmia. Multicenter Automatic Defibrillator Implantation Trial Investigators." *New England Journal of Medicine* Vol. 335, No.26, (December, 1996): pp. 1933-1940, ISSN 0028-4793

Moss, A. J., Hall, W. J., Cannom, D. S., et al. (2009). "Cardiac-resynchronization therapy for the prevention of heart-failure events." *New England Journal of Medicien* Vol. 361, No.14, (October, 2009): pp. 1329-1338, ISSN 1533-4406

Moss, A. J., Zareba, W., Hall, W. J., et al. (2002). "Prophylactic implantation of a defibrillator in patients with myocardial infarction and reduced ejection fraction." *New England Journal of Medicine* Vol. 346, No.12, (March, 2002): pp. 877-883, ISSN 1533-4406

Nanthakumar, K., Epstein, A. E., Kay, G. N., et al. (2004). "Prophylactic implantable cardioverter-defibrillator therapy in patients with left ventricular systolic dysfunction: a pooled analysis of 10 primary prevention trials." *Journal of The American College of Cardiology* Vol. 44, No.11, (December, 2004): pp. 2166-2172, ISSN 0735-1097

Nelson, G. S., Curry, C. W., Wyman, B. T., et al. (2000). "Predictors of systolic augmentation from left ventricular preexcitation in patients with dilated cardiomyopathy and intraventricular conduction delay." *Circulation* Vol. 101, No.23, (June, 2000): pp. 2703-2709, ISSN 1524-4539

O'Brien, B. J., Connolly, S. J., Goeree, R., et al. (2001). "Cost-effectiveness of the implantable cardioverter-defibrillator: results from the Canadian Implantable Defibrillator Study (CIDS)." *Circulation* Vol. 103, No.10, (March, 2001): pp. 1416-1421, ISSN 1524-4539

Al Chekakie, M. (2009). "Electrical instability heralding worsening heart failure in a patient with nonischemic dilated cardiomyopathy." *Congestive Heart Failure* Vol. 15, No.5, (September, 2009): pp. 249-251, ISSN 1751-7133

Peinado, R., Almendral, J., Rius, T., et al. (1998). "Randomized, prospective comparison of four burst pacing algorithms for spontaneous ventricular tachycardia." *American Journal of Cardiology* Vol. 82, No.11, (December, 1998): pp. 1422-1425, A1428-1429, ISSN 0002-9149

Pitt, B., Remme, W., Zannad, F., et al. (2003). "Eplerenone, a selective aldosterone blocker, in patients with left ventricular dysfunction after myocardial infarction." *New England Journal of Medicine* Vol. 348, No.14, (April, 2003): pp. 1309-1321, ISSN 1533-4406

Poole, J. E., Johnson, G. W., Hellkamp, A. S., et al. (2008). "Prognostic importance of defibrillator shocks in patients with heart failure." *New England Journal of Medicine* Vol. 359, No.10, (September, 2008): pp. 1009-1017, ISSN 1533-4406

Roguin, A., Bomma, C. S., Nasir, K., et al. (2004). "Implantable cardioverter-defibrillators in patients with arrhythmogenic right ventricular dysplasia/cardiomyopathy." *Journal of The American College of Cardiology* Vol. 43, No.10, (May, 2004): pp. 1843-1852, ISSN 0735-1097

Sanders, G. D., Hlatky, M. A. and Owens, D. K. (2005). "Cost-effectiveness of implantable cardioverter-defibrillators." *New England Journal of Medicine* Vol. 353, No.14, (October, 2005): pp. 1471-1480, ISSN 1533-4406

Schron, E. B., Exner, D. V., Yao, Q., et al. (2002). "Quality of life in the antiarrhythmics versus implantable defibrillators trial: impact of therapy and influence of adverse symptoms and defibrillator shocks." *Circulation* Vol. 105, No.5, (February, 2002): pp. 589-594, ISSN 1524-4539

Seidl, K., Hauer, B., Schwick, N. G., et al. (1998). "Comparison of metoprolol and sotalol in preventing ventricular tachyarrhythmias after the implantation of a cardioverter/defibrillator." *American Journal of Cardiology* Vol. 82, No.6, (September, 1998): pp. 744-748, ISSN 0002-9149

Sen-Chowdhry, S., Lowe, M. D., Sporton, S. C., et al. (2004). "Arrhythmogenic right ventricular cardiomyopathy: clinical presentation, diagnosis, and management." *American Journal of Medicine* Vol. 117, No.9, (November, 2004): pp. 685-695, ISSN 0002-9343

Solomon, S. D., Foster, E., Bourgoun, M., et al. "Effect of cardiac resynchronization therapy on reverse remodeling and relation to outcome: multicenter automatic defibrillator implantation trial: cardiac resynchronization therapy." *Circulation* Vol. 122, No.10, (September: pp. 985-992, ISSN 1524-4539

Steinbeck, G., Andresen, D., Seidl, K., et al. (2009). "Defibrillator implantation early after myocardial infarction." *New England Journal of Medicine* Vol. 361, No.15, (October, 2009): pp. 1427-1436, ISSN 1533-4406

Sweeney, M. O., Wathen, M. S., Volosin, K., et al. (2005). "Appropriate and inappropriate ventricular therapies, quality of life, and mortality among primary and secondary prevention implantable cardioverter defibrillator patients: results from the Pacing Fast VT REduces Shock ThErapies (PainFREE Rx II) trial." *Circulation* Vol. 111, No.22, (June 7, 2005): pp. 2898-2905, ISSN 1524-4539

Tabib, A., Loire, R., Chalabreysse, L., et al. (2003). "Circumstances of death and gross and microscopic observations in a series of 200 cases of sudden death associated with arrhythmogenic right ventricular cardiomyopathy and/or dysplasia." *Circulation* Vol. 108, No.24, (December, 2003): pp. 3000-3005, ISSN 1524-4539

Tang, A. S., Wells, G. A., Talajic, M., et al. "Cardiac-resynchronization therapy for mild-to-moderate heart failure." *New England Journal of Medicine* Vol. 363, No.25, (December, 2010: pp. 2385-2395, ISSN 1533-4406

Varnava, A. M., Elliott, P. M., Mahon, N., et al. (2001). "Relation between myocyte disarray and outcome in hypertrophic cardiomyopathy." *American Journal of Cardiology* Vol. 88, No.3, (August, 2001): pp. 275-279, ISSN 0002-9149

Veenhuyzen, G. D., Singh, S. N., McAreavey, D., et al. (2001). "Prior coronary artery bypass surgery and risk of death among patients with ischemic left ventricular dysfunction." *Circulation* Vol. 104, No.13, (September, 2001): pp. 1489-1493, ISSN 1524-4539

Wilber, D. J., Zareba, W., Hall, W. J., et al. (2004). "Time dependence of mortality risk and defibrillator benefit after myocardial infarction." *Circulation* Vol. 109, No.9, (March, 2004): pp. 1082-1084, ISSN 1524-4539

Wilkoff, B. L., Williamson, B. D., Stern, R. S., et al. (2008). "Strategic programming of detection and therapy parameters in implantable cardioverter-defibrillators reduces shocks in primary prevention patients: results from the PREPARE (Primary Prevention Parameters Evaluation) study." *Journal of The American College of Cardiology* Vol. 52, No.7, (August 12, 2008): pp. 541-550, ISSN 1558-3597

Wyse, D. G., Friedman, P. L., Brodsky, M. A., et al. (2001). "Life-threatening ventricular arrhythmias due to transient or correctable causes: high risk for death in follow-up." *Journal of The American College of Cardiology* Vol. 38, No.6, (November, 2001): pp. 1718-1724, ISSN 0735-1097

Young, J. B., Abraham, W. T., Smith, A. L., et al. (2003). "Combined cardiac resynchronization and implantable cardioversion defibrillation in advanced chronic heart failure: the MIRACLE ICD Trial." *JAMA* Vol. 289, No.20, (May, 2003): pp. 2685-2694, ISSN 0098-7484

Zipes, D. P., Camm, A. J., Borggrefe, M., et al. (2006). "ACC/AHA/ESC 2006 guidelines for management of patients with ventricular arrhythmias and the prevention of sudden cardiac death: a report of the American College of Cardiology/American Heart Association Task Force and the European Society of Cardiology Committee for Practice Guidelines (Writing Committee to Develop Guidelines for Management of Patients With Ventricular Arrhythmias and the Prevention of Sudden Cardiac Death)." *Journal of The American College of Cardiology* Vol. 48, No.5, (September, 2006): pp. e247-346, ISSN 1558-3597

8

Biomarker for Cardiomyopathy-B-Type Natriuretic Peptide

Mototsugu Nishii and Tohru Izumi
Kitasato University School of Medicine
Japan

1. Introduction

Cardiomyopathy is cardiac condition in which the normal muscular function of the myocardium has been altered by a variety of etiologies. Atherosclerotic coronary artery disease is the most common cause of cardiomyopathy in North America and Europe. Idiopathic cardiomyopathy is the second most common cause, although this may partially include undiagnosed etiologies such as viral infection, drug toxicity, and genetic factors. Other causes include endocrine diseases, collagen vascular diseases, metabolic disorders (hemochromatosis, amyloidosis, glycogen storage disease), neuromuscular disorders, and granulomatous diseases (sarcoidosis).

The cardiac malfunctions are variable, namely left ventricular (LV) systolic dysfunction, LV diastolic dysfunction, or both in accordance with etiologies and morphological findings (cardiac hypertrophy or dilatation). For example, hypertrophic cardiomyopathy initially has LV diastolic dysfunction, while amyloidosis that shows similar morphological change has LV systolic dysfunction. Ischemic or idiopathic cardiomyopathy with ventricular dilatation is represented by systolic dysfunction. Cardiac malfunctions are also altered on disease course. Initially, patients with cardiomyopathy may have asymptomatic LV systolic or diastolic dysfunction alone. However, adverse disease processes finally lead to both dysfunctions.

Imbalance between cardiac malfunctions and compensatory mechanisms worsens an outcome of cardiomyopathy. When abnormal LV filling pressure and volume is unable to be compensated by hemodynamic alterations such as the increases in heart rate and peripheral vascular tone by the accelerated vasoconstrictors including norepinephrine (NE), endothelin-1 (ET-1), and the renin-angiotensin-aldosterone (RAA), this imbalance precipitates decompensated heart failure (HF).

Early and simply identifying the decompensatory process is important therapeutic strategy in cardiomyopathy. Clinical utility of B-type natriuretic peptide (BNP) sensitively produced and secreted from heart in response to LV overload has been extended rapidly in patients with HF. At first, BNP emerged as a diagnostic marker for decompensated HF. Furthermore, BNP has been proved to predict a subsequent outcome in patients with HF. Recently, the efficiency of BNP-guided therapy in patients with HF has been demonstrated. In this chapter, we discuss about clinical utility of BNP assessments in patients with cardiomyopathy.

2. B-type natriuretic peptide (BNP)

BNP is predominantly secreted from the overloaded LV as a 76 aminoacid N-terminal fragment and a 32 aminoacid active hormone, and synthesis and release of BNP are adversely and rapidly accelerated in conjunction with the degree of LV wall stretch (1-2). In addition to this primary regulation, BNP synthesis can be also upregulated by tachycardia, glucocorticoids, thyroid hormones, vasoactive peptides such as ET-1, angiotensin II, and NE, and inflammatory cytokines. On the other hand, BNP is clearance via the binding to a natriuretic peptide receptor (NPR)-C of three NPRs (NPR-A, -B, -C). BNP is also inactivated by neutral endopeptidase, a zinc metallopeptidase which is expressed on the surface of endothelial cells, smooth-muscle cells, cardiac myocytes, renal epithelium, and fibroblasts.
BNP is included into compensatory mechanisms against HF. BNP promotes glomerular filtration and inhibits sodium reabsorption, resulting in natriuresis and diuresis. It reduces blood pressure through the relaxation of vascular smooth muscle and inhibits activations of not only central and peripheral sympathetic nerve systems but also cardiac sympathetic nervous system (3). Furthermore, it also inhibits the RAA system (4).

2.1 BNP as a diagnostic marker

2.1.1 BNP in heart failure

Plasma BNP levels have proven utility in the diagnostic evaluation of decompensated HF in patients with acute dyspnea (5-6). Particularly, BNP at a cutoff of 100 pg/ml could diagnose HF better than not only all other clinical parameters but also the clinical judgement by the emergency room physicians. However, BNP also has the diagostic limitation for HF. BNP is less accurate in detection of asymptomatic LV dysfunction than clinical parameters, because BNP has a close correlation with New York Heart Association (NYHA) functional class and patients with mild LV dysfunction often show normal range of BNP levels.

2.1.2 BNP in cardiomyopathy

BNP levels are raised in dilated, hypertrophic, and restrictive cardiomyopathies. Its increases seem to be different in accordance with cardiac malfunctions. BNP levels are generally higher in patients with systolic dysfunction than in those with isolated diastolic dysfunction, and highest in those with both dysfunctions (7). Furthermore, among patients with preserved LV systolic function, BNP correlates with the severity of diastolic dysfunction. BNP levels are raised in patients with impaired relaxation and especially highest in those with a restrictive filling pattern (8). BNP measurements may facilitate understanding the type and severity of cardiac malfunction on cardiomyopathy.
On the other hand, BNP measurement may be unavailable for distinguishing cardiomyopathies. Hypertrophic cardiomyopathy often shows extremely high levels of BNP, similarly to dilated cardiomyopathy (9). In addition, restrictive cardiomyopathy with systolic dysfunction also shows higher levels of BNP than that with diastolic dysfunction alone (8). However, several reports have demonstrated that BNP is able to distinguish constrictive pericarditis and restrictive cardiomyopathy, although these diseases overlap signs and symptoms of congestion (10). The level of BNP is elevated in patients with restriction, while level is nearly normal in those with constriction. The absence of cardiac stretch by constricting pericardium is thought to lead to lower BNP release.

2.2 BNP as a prognostic marker

Prognostic values of BNP have been identified in various heart diseases such as HF, cardiovascular diseases, and cardiomyopathy.

2.2.1 Heart failure

In patients with HF, higher levels of BNP have been implicated in increased risk of cardiovascular or all-cause mortality and readmission for decompensated HF. Furthermore, the cutoff points on the risk assessment curve are altered on time course after decompensated HF. In admitted patients for decompensated HF, the cutoff point of 800 pg/ml was associated with the increased risk of in-hospital mortality as shown by the ADHERE (Acute Decompensated Heart Failure National Registry) data (11). After the treatment, the predischarge cutoff point for the risk of readmission and mortality falls to about 500 pg/ml (12). The cutoff point further declined to abut 200 pg/ml in clinically stable outpatients after decompensated HF (13). These obsevations suggested that the therapeutic strategies for HF including a safe hospital discharge and the prevention of readmission or cardiac event may be guided by BNP measurement.

2.2.2 Cardiovascular diseases

In disorders other than HF, BNP also has prognostic value. BNP level is able to identify patients at the high risk group of adverse cardiac remodelling from patients with post-myocardial infarction, independent of age, history of HF, and LV ejection fraction (LVEF) (14). Even in patients with unstable angina alone, increased levels of BNP were associated with an increased risk of death (15). In right ventricular dysfunction resulting from pulmonary hypertension, BNP also provides similar prognostic information. These observations have extended the potential role of BNP measurement to risk stratification of cardiovascular events in patients with and without HF.

2.2.3 Cardiac inflammatory diseases; acute myocarditis

Acute myocarditis is able to be mainly divided into two disease conditions on a basis of clinicopathologic profiles, namely fulminant and non-fulminant myocarditis (16-17). Briefly, fulminant myocarditis is represented by the distinct onset of cardiac symptoms within 2 weeks following flu-like symptoms accompanied by histologically proven active myocarditis according to Dallas criteria and severe circulatory failure requiring high-dose intravenous catecholamines use (>5.0 γ) or mechanical circulatory assist devise, while non-fulminant myocarditis is by the indistinct onset of cardiac symptoms without those. Furthermore, these outcomes are distinguished by each unique clinical course (17). Non-fulminant myocarditis has been implicated in poorer long-term outcome than fulminant cases. A few patients with fulminant myocarditis lapsed into mortality from severely deteriorated circulatory collapse refractory to mechanical circulatory assist use or mechanical complications from its long-term use, including bleeding, infections, sepsis, and multiple organ failure. However, more than 80% of fulminant cases recover completely to an uncomplicated status, with cessation of myocardial inflammation and a generally favorable outcome, provided they are able to overcome poor cardiac condition successfully during acute phase (18). On the other hand, non-fulminant myocarditis without severe circulatory failure is likely to develop to chronic HF derived from dilated cardiomyopathy at chronic phase (16-17). Therefore, simple biomarkers to predict a requirement of mechanical assist devise use, outcome following its use, or the development to cardiomyopathy in patients with acute myocarditis have been sought.

Previously, we related various variables to short-term outcome in patients with fulminant myocarditis (19). In-hospital mortality was extremely higher in patients with fulminant myocarditis than in non-fulminant cases. Especially, extremely increased levels of interleukin-10, a major anti-inflammatory cytokine in serum on admission were associated with short-term outcome including mechanical assist use and in-hospital mortality in patients with acute myocarditis (Figure 1), which might be explained by its inhibitory effect on viral elimination from host. A major pathogenic factor of acute myocarditis and subsequent cardiomyopathy is viral infection, especially coxsackievirus B3 (Table 1).

		Patient positive (%)	
Virus	Type	Myocarditis	Dilated cardiomyopathy
Picornavirus	***Coxackie A, B***	***5-50%***	***5-15%***
	Echovirus	?	?
	Hepatitis A	?	?
	Hepatitis C	***0-15%***	***0-10%***
Orthomyxovirus	Influenza A, B	?	?
Paramyxovirus	RSV, Mumpus	?	<1%
Rubivirus/Toga virus	Rubella virus	?	<1%
Rhabdo virus	Rabies virus	?	?
Arbovirus/Tahyna	Dengue, yellow fever virus	?	?
Retrovirus/Lenti	HIV	Variable	?
Herpes virus	***Varicella-zoster***	***1-2%***	***1-2%***
	Cytomegalovirus	***1-15%***	***1-10%***
	Epstein-Barr virus	***1-3%***	***1-3%***
	Human herpes virus 6	***0-5%***	***0-5%***
	herpes simplex virus	0-3%	?
Mastadenovirus	***Adenovirus***	***5-20%***	***10-12%***
Parvovirus	***Parvo B 19 virus***	***10-30%***	***10-25%***

Table 1. Virus-induced myocarditis or cardiomyopathy

Hoffmann et al also reported that IL-10 expression in human peripheral monocytes was strongly and persistently induced by coxsackievirus B3 infection in spite of only slight production of other pro-inflammatory cytokines such as TNF-α, IL-1 and IL-6 (20). It has been reported that the inhibition of natural killer (NK) cells results in increased virus titers in the heart through delayed virus clearance (21). IL-10 inhibits the production of IFN-γ in NK cells, which has been demonstrated in association with susceptibility to Trypanosoma cruzi-induced myocarditis (22-23). In addition, it has been shown that IL-10 is transcribed in the myocardium parallel with viral replication in the acute and chronic stages of experimental Coxsackievirus B3 viral myocarditis (24-25). These findings imply that an extreme elevation of serum levels of IL-10, rather than TNF-α, on admission may reflect subsequent myocardial inflammation, which leads to the future deterioration of the disease, through delayed clearance of the virus.

On the other hand, high levels of IL-10 may reflect a favorable long-term outcome in patients with acute myocarditis. Studies using experimental models have demonstrated a protective role of IL-10 in the development of acute myocarditis (26-27). This mechanism was explained by its suppressive effect against excessive and persistent immune response to viral infection or a subsequent autoimmune response leading to chronic myocardial injury. Cases with high level of IL-10 during acute phase may be not likely to develop to chronic myocarditis or cardiomyopathy. So far, almost studies with human myocarditis have been limited to a small number of patients. Further large number prospective studies are required to prove our idea.

In our previous study, the association of BNP with outcome was examined, also. Its levels in plasma were significantly increased in fulminant cases than in non-fulminant cases. However, we could not confirm its prognostic utility. In such cases, BNP may simply reflect the existence of circulatory failure alone.

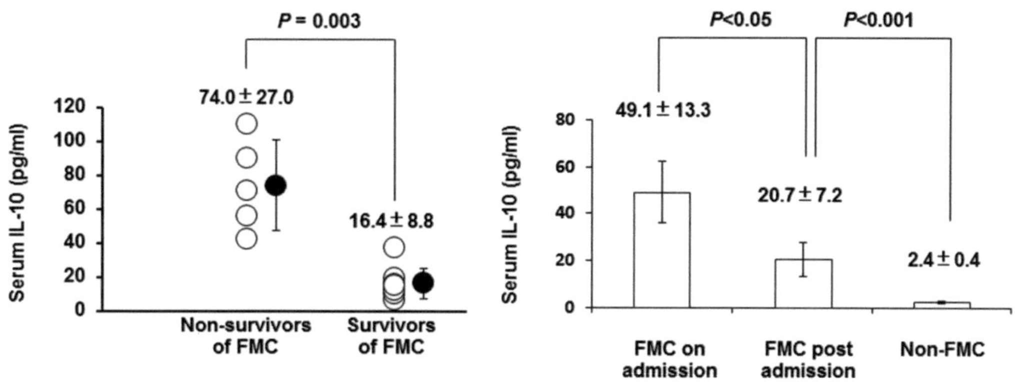

Serum levels of IL-10 were significantly increased in non-survivors than in survivors with fulminant myocarditis. IL-10 levels were significantly increased in not only patients with mechanical circulatory assist device on admission but also in those with it post admission, a few days after admission than in those without it throughout clinical course. IL: interleukin; FMC: fulminant myocarditis. (Nishii M, et al. J Am Coll Cardiol. 2004;44:1292-1297)

Fig. 1. Serum level of interleukin-10 in patients with acute myocarditis.

2.2.4 Cardiomyopathies

The HF is a major complication in cardiomyopathies such as dilated cardiomyopathy (DCM), hypertrophic cardiomyopathy (HCM), and restrictive cardiomyopathy (RCM). BNP must be a useful prognostic predictor for cardiomyopathies.

2.2.4.1 Dilated cardiomyopathy

Recently, we reported prognostic utility of BNP in clinically stable 83 outpatients with nonischemic DCM after decompensated HF (13). They were in a clinically stable status during at least 6 months after hospital discharge at relatively low BNP level, namely mean BNP level of about 200 pg/ml. This implied that pre-discharge BNP level may predict a post-discharge outcome in nonischemic DCM, as reported in general decompensated HF patients (12). Additionally, in this observation, the prognostic value of post-discharge BNP level was identified. Especially, among various predictors, levels at 6 months after hospital discharge showed the closest relation to the high risk of readmission for decompensated HF and mortality (Table 2). This association was explained by adverse cardiac remodeling. Persistently high levels of BNP during 6 months were related to poor improvement on cardiac remodeling (Figure 2).

Variable	Below vs. above median values			
	median level	HR	95% CI	*P* value
Univariate analysis				
Age	56	1.1895	0.7431-1.9246	0.47
Sex (Female)		1.0347	0.5886-2.0433	0.89
Hypertension		1.4902	0.8912-2.2819	0.18
Atrial fibrillation		1.2965	0.8885-2.0973	0.301
Ventricular tachycardia		1.2026	0.6132-2.1693	0.57
Beta-blocker use		1.6691	0.9056-2.5641	0.06
Diuretic use		1.3551	0.8086-2.1936	0.24
Echocardiographic parameters				
Left ventricular end-diastolic dimension at discharge	6.4 cm	0.8356	0.5189-1.3516	0.48
Left ventricular ejection fraction at discharge	30%	1.1629	0.7189-1.8729	0.54
Left atrial diastolic dimension at discharge	4.5 cm	1.3054	0.8106-2.1164	0.28
Left ventricular end-diastolic dimension at 6 months	6.0 cm	1.3866	0.8383-2.3598	0.22
Left ventricular ejection fraction at 6 months	36%	1.5019	0.9209-2.4641	0.11
Left atrial diastolic dimension at 6 months	4.25 cm	2.0003	1.2436-3.2233	0.0046
BNP measurements				
Plasma BNP level at discharge	180 pg/ml	1.2642	0.8051-1.9888	0.31
Plasma BNP level at 3 months	134 pg/ml	1.5097	0.9413-2.4212	0.09
Plasma BNP level at 6 months	174 pg/ml	2.2679	1.4336-3.5863	0.0005
Percentage change in BNP level between discharge and 3 months	-20.5%	1.4204	0.8863-2.2765	0.14
Percentage change in BNP level between discharge and 6 months	-11.5%	2.0127	1.2729-3.1757	0.0026
Multivariate analysis				
Plasma BNP level at 6 months	174 pg/ml	1.8427	1.1127-3.0426	0.0181
Percentage change in BNP level between discharge and 6 months	-11.5%	1.6538	0.9991-2.7214	0.051
Left atrial diastolic dimension at 6 months	4.25 cm	1.5678	0.9486-2.5904	0.0792

NYHA: New York Heart Association functional class; HR: hazard ratio; CI: confidence interval; BNP: B-type natriuretic peptide (Nishii M, et al. J Am Coll Cardiol. 2008;51:2329-2335)

Table 2. Univariate and multivariate Cox analyses of the incidence of death or readmission for heart failure.

2.2.4.2 Hypertrophic cardiomyopathy

Several reports have demonstrated that BNP levels reflect the severity of symptoms and HF in HCM (28-29). Additionally, high level of BNP has been related to cardiac events including silent myocardial ischemia (30), admission for HF, and mortality (31). On the other hand, our previous observation was unable to confirm these values, because even patients with high levels of BNP were in a clinically stable status. In HCM, BNP expression, however, is thought to occur as a response to not only hemodynamic changes resulting from diastolic dysfunction and obstruction but also histological changes such as myocardial fiber disarray, hypertrophy of myocytes, and fibrosis (32). Thus, even in clinically stable patients with HCM, extremely high levels may indicate a poor long-term outcome. Further studies are required to elucidate its prognostic value in HCM.

2.2.4.3 Restrictive cardiomyopathy

There is no report regarding prognostic value of BNP in RCM. However, when RCM had a further increase of LV end-diastolic pressure (LVEDP) or systolic dysfunction, BNP level would be more increased (7). BNP measurement may predict the occurrence of decompensated HF, although its value remains uncertain in RCM.

2.3 BNP-guided therapy

Efficiency of BNP-guided therapy on cardiomyopathies is not yet elucidated. However, BNP levels reflect therapeutic effect in patients with HF. Aggressive treatment with diuretics and vasodilators such as angiotensin-converting enzyme inhibitors (ACEIs) and angiotensin-II receptor antagonists reduce BNP level rapidly in conjunction with reduced intra-ventricular filling pressures. On the other hand, the effects of beta blockers on BNP concentrations are complex. Because adrenergic stimulation inhibits release of natriuretic peptides, beta blocking may initially increase BNP concentrations. By contrast, long-term use of beta blocker reduces BNP concentrations with the improvement in cardiac dysfunction. Thus, BNP measurement would help physicians to make clinical decisions to titrate pharmacological treatments.

BNP-guided therapy improves a treatment outcome in patients with HF. Two provocative pilot studies have prospectively assessed the utility of BNP to guide selection and intensity of pharmacotherapy. In one study, 69 symptomatic patients (NYHA class II to IV) with impaired systolic function defined as LVEF of <40% were randomly allocated to receive either standardised clinical assessment consist of symptoms and physical findings-guided therapy or N-terminal BNP-guided therapy (< 200 pmol/L) (33). During the follow up of at least 6 months, fewer patients had combined cardiovascular events (death, hospital admission, or heart failure decompensation) in the N-terminal BNP group than in the clinical group, which was associated with higher doses of ACEIs and diuretics. In a second multicenter randomised trial: The STARS-BNP Multicenter Study, 220 patients with symptomatic (NYHA class II to III) systolic HF defined as LVEF of <45% were randomized to medical treatments on either the basis of clinical findings from the physical examination and usual paraclinical and biological parameters or the basis of a decreasing BNP plasma levels of <100 pg/ml (34). After a mean follow-up of 15 months, significantly fewer patients had HF-related death in the BNP group than in the clinical group, which was in part associated with an increase in ACEIs and beta-blocker dosages.

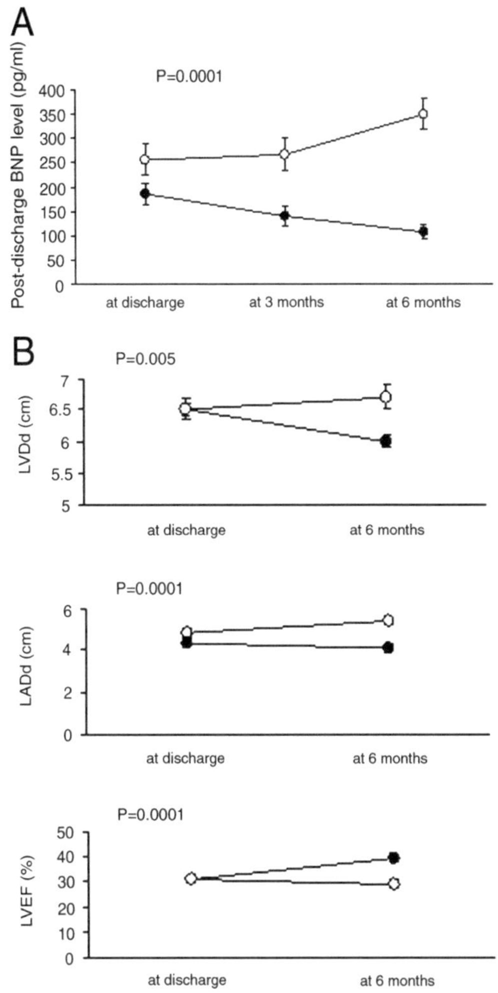

Fig. 2. Changes in B-type natriuretic peptide (BNP) levels and echocardiographic findings during a clinically compensated status in patients with dilated cardiomyopathy (Nishii M, et al. J Am Coll Cardiol. 2008;51:2329-2335)
Changes in BNP level at 3-month intervals after hospital discharge for decompensated heart failure (A) and in echocardiographic variables between discharge and 6 months (B). BNP levels were decreased during 6 months in event-free patients but not in readmitted patients, which was accompanied by the reduction of cardiac dimensions. Solid or open circles indicate BNP levels, echocardiographic dimensions (left ventricular end-diastolic dimension [LVDd]; left atrial diastolic dimension [LADd]), and left ventricular ejection fraction (LVEF) in event-free patients or patients readmitted for decompensated heart failure, respectively. Values are mean ± standard error of the mean. p values comparing changes in BNP and echocardiographic variables between readmitted patients and event-free patients are for repeated measures multivariate analysis of variance over 6 months.

On the other hand, it remained uncertain whether BNP guide is available for asymptomatic patients or not. We reported that in 83 outpatients with asymptomatic (NYHA class I to II) systolic HF defined as LVEF of <40%, BNP cutoff point of about 200 pg/ml at 6 months after the discharge for decompensated HF can identify patients at the high risk of readmission and sudden death (13) (Figure 3). Interestingly, Beta blocker use and its dosage were significantly lower in high risk patients [>200 vs. <200 pg/ml: 60 vs. 100%, P=0.001; 8 ± 5 vs. 16 ± 5 mg/day (carvedilol), P=0.0003; 64 ± 22 vs. 107 ± 40 mg/day (metoprolol), P=0.036; respectively]. The cutoff point might determine the requirement of initiation or titration of beta blockers. Even in asymptomatic HF setting, BNP-guided therapy may be also helpful.

2.4 The limitations on BNP-guided therapy

We have to consider the limitations on BNP-guided therapy, also. Recent multicenter trial (the randomized Trial of Intensified vs. Standard Medical Therapy in Elderly Patients with Congestive Heart Failure: TIME-CHF) could not identify the advantage of BNP-guided therapy over symptom-guided therapy in 499 elderly patients aged more than 60 years with symptomatic (NYHA class II or greater) systolic HF (LVEF of <45%) and prior hospitalization for decompensated HF (35). They were randomized to N-terminal BNP-guided HF therapy (levels of less than two times the upper limit of normal) and symptom-guided HF therapy (NYHA class of less than II). However, the improvements of outcomes including mortality, hospitalization, and quality of life were similar in both groups. Especially in patients aged more than 75 years, BNP-guided HF therapy did not improve outcome. In general, dosages of drugs such as ACEIs and beta-blockers are increased more in patients receiving BNP–guided therapy. Although persistence in intensifying medical therapy seems to be indispensable for better outcome in young and middle aged patients, it may be harmful to push dosages to the limits in elderly patients aged more than 75 years. Additionally, BNP-guided therapy may be disadvantageous in patients with low output syndrome resulting from severe systolic and diastolic dysfunctions. Because such cases require more ventricular load as a compensatory mechanism for congestive HF, rapid titration of ACEIs, beta blockers, and diuretics on the basis of BNP-guided HF therapy may lead to further deterioration of HF. Furthermore, edtablished cardiomyopathy with irreversible LV dilatation often shows persistently high level of BNP despite aggressive treatment for HF. A unified level of BNP-guided therapy would be unavailable for such cases. These emphasize the need of setting up individual BNP target level in accordance with cardiac conditions.

2.5 Individual target threshold of BNP

To set up individual target threshold of BNP for the risk reduction that were associated with cardiac dilatation and identify its prognostic utility, clinically stable 113 patients with systolic HF after decompensated HF represented by non-ischemic dilated cardiomyopathy were examined. Among these patients, 32 patients reached end-point composed of readmission for decompensated HF or death. Various variables were related to its combined event, including atrial fibrillation, low LVEF below the best cutoff value of 34%, cardiac dilatation (CD) indicated by left ventricular end-diastolic dimension×LAD/wall thickness/body surface area above the best cutoff value of 115 /m^2, high levels of BNP above the best cutoff value of 195 pg/ml. Furthermore, we found a significant positive correlation between BNP level and CD specific for event-free patients. The rage between 95% confidence interval on this specific linear regression line were closely associated with an incidence rate of readmission or death, also (Figure 4A, B). Thus, we defined this rage as individual target threshold of BNP.

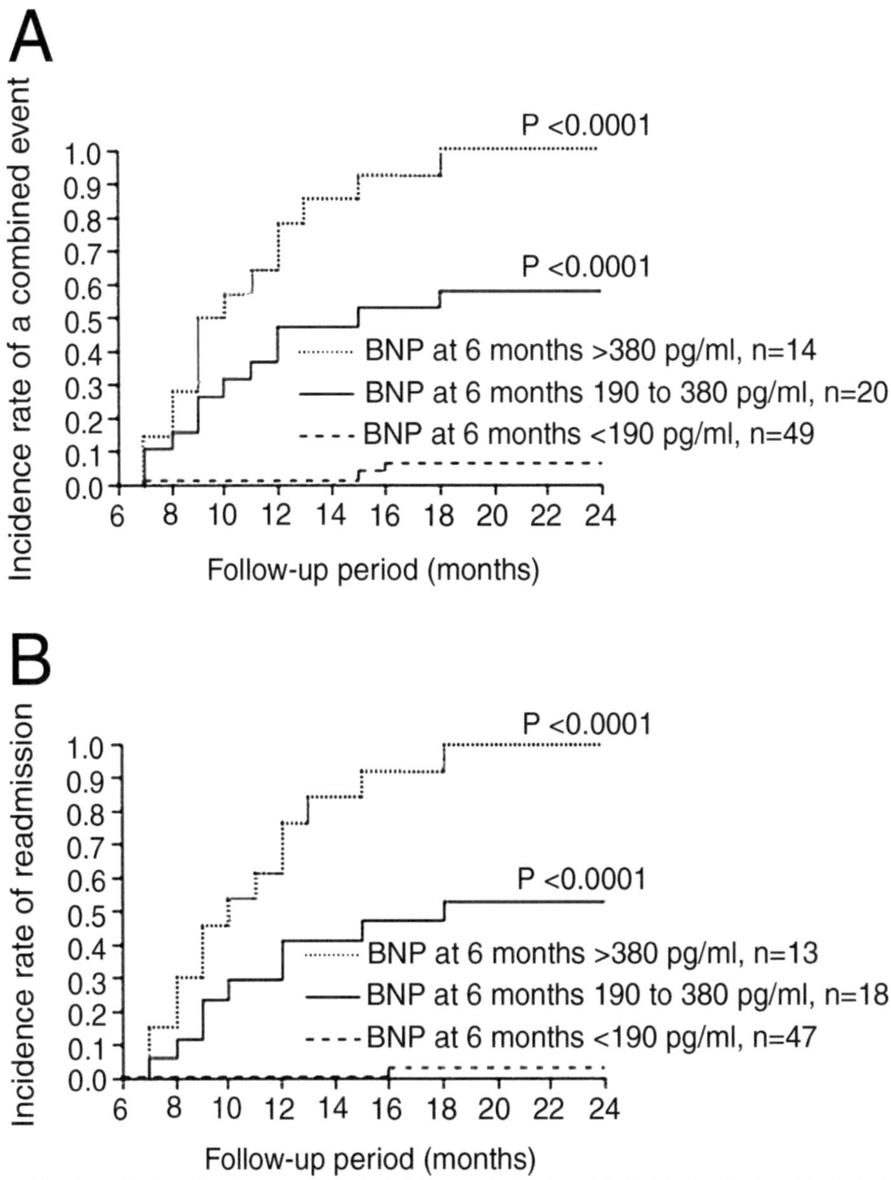

Fig. 3. Kaplan-Meier Analyses (Nishii M, et al. J Am Coll Cardiol. 2008;51:2329-2335) Kaplan-Meier curves showing the incidence rate of readmission for decompensated heart failure or sudden death (A) or of readmission alone (B) according to 6-month post-discharge B-type natriuretic peptide (BNP) ranges in outpatients with dilated cardiomyopathy. The risk of a combined event increased in a stepwise fashion across increasing ranges of 6-month post-discharge BNP, namely at <190 pg/ml, 190 to 380 pg/ml, and >380 pg/ml (Fig. 2A). Further, Kaplan-Meier curves for incidence of readmission alone (Fig. 2B) showed the same pattern. B-type natriuretic peptide ranges were <190 (the best cutoff level for predicting readmission or sudden death), 190 to 380, and >380 (its 2-fold level) pg/ml. p < 0.0001 (the log-rank test) versus a BNP range of <190 pg/ml.

Next, we examined its prognostic advantage over other variables. When adjusted to high-risk patients with advanced dilated cardiomyopathy, namely symptomatic non-ischemic systolic HF (LVEF below 34%) complicated by severe cardiac dilatation (CD above 115 /m^2), this individual target threshold alone was associated with the incidence rate (Figure 5). Based on Laplace Law (pressure x radius/2 wall thickness), this threshold may reflect individual optimal wall stretch for clinical stabilization. The left atrium (LA) acts as a reservoir during LV overload (36), and elevated LV filling pressure results in LA overload as well as LV diastolic dysfunction (37). Thus, LA dimension reflects intra-ventricular pressure, in part.

A combined assessment of BNP level and echocardiographic dimensions may facilitate individual disease management. Among overall patients, those with BNP levels over or under its target threshold required titration or withdrawal, respectively of pharmocological therapy including diuretics or vosadilators to keep a balance between ventricular load and cardiac function. Additionally, cases refractory to such pharmacological optimization may be considered application of mechanical circulatory assist device implantation or subsequent surgical intervention including heart transplantation.

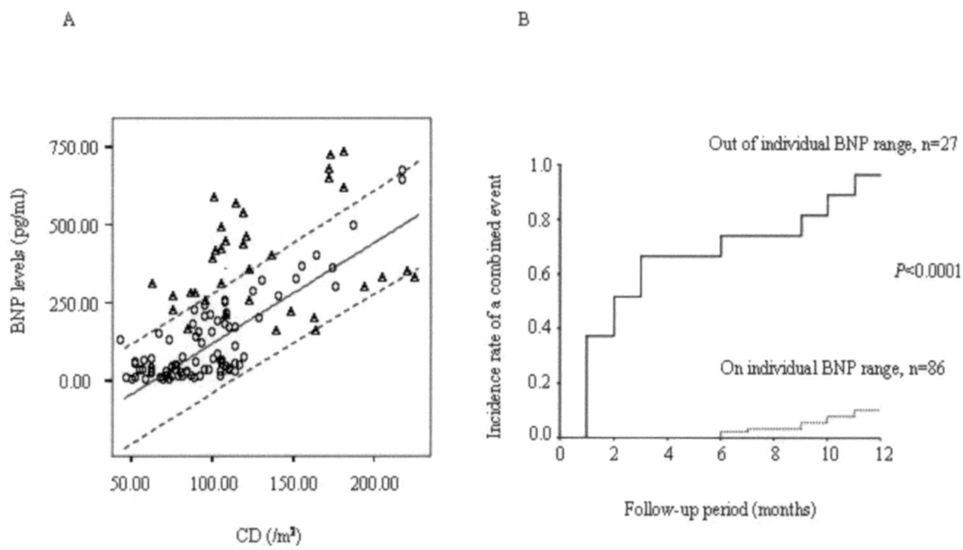

Fig. 4. Prognostic utility of individual target threshold of B-type natriuretic peptide (BNP) on readmission for decompensated heart failure or sudden death in patients with non-ischemic dilated cardiomyopathy

A: Individual target threshold of BNP. Event-free patients had a significantly positive correlation between BNP level and cardiac dilatation (CD) (r=0.88; *P*<0.0001), but event patients did not (r=0.26; *P*=0.421). BNP levels in event patients tended to be out of the range between dotted lines: 95% confidence interval (CI) on solid line: the linear regression line specific for event-free patients (BNP= -144.64 + 3.16×CD), namely individual target threshold of BNP. B: Kaplan-Meier curves showing the incidence rate of event according to individual target threshold of BNP. Out of this threshold was closely associated with an increase in event risk (the log-rank test: *P*<0.0001).

Open circles or triangles indicate even-free or event patients, respectively. CD was defined as left ventricular end-diastolic dimension×left atrial diastolic dimension/wall thickness/body surface area.

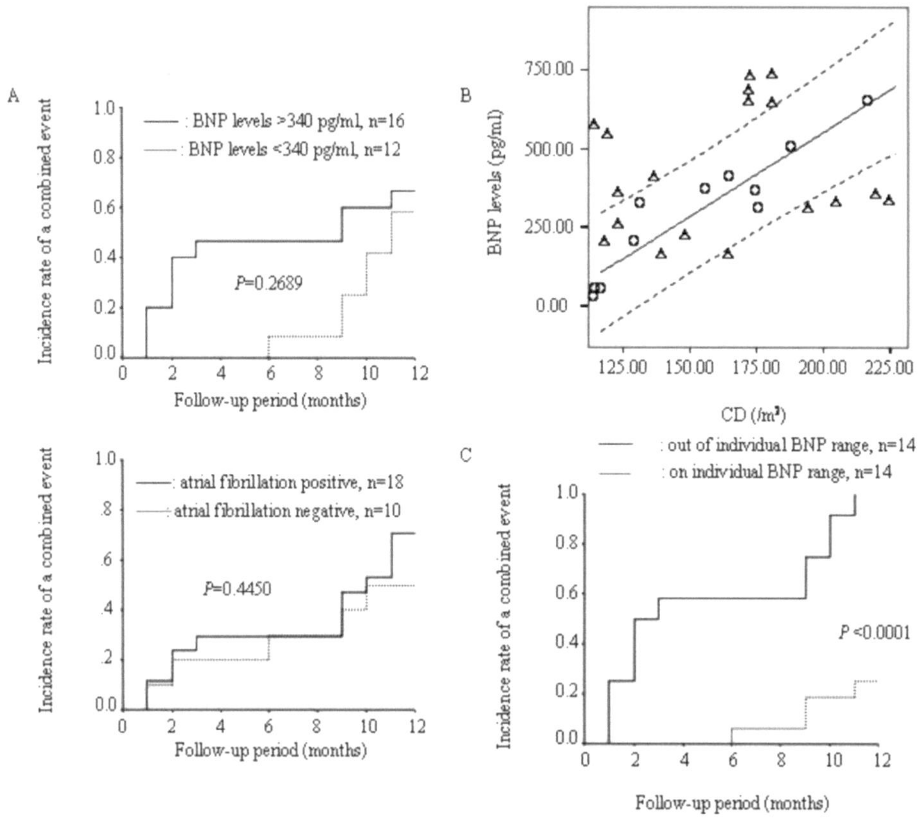

Fig. 5. Prognostic predictors on readmission for decompensated heart failure or death in patients with advanced dilated cardiomyopathy, namely symptomatic systolic heart failure (left ventricular ejection fraction below the best cutoff value of 34%) complicated by severe cardiac dilatation (CD) above the best cutoff value of 115 /m^2.
A: Kaplan-Meier curves showing the incidence rate of event according to levels of BNP above or below the best cutoff value of 340 pg/ml or atrial fibrillation. These variables had no significant association with an increase in event risk (the log-rank test; BNP levels: P=0.2689; atrial fibrillation: P=0.4450). B: Individual target threshold of BNP. Event-free patients had a significantly positive correlation between BNP level and CD (r=0.91; P<0.0001), independently of event patients (r=0.10; P=0.71). BNP levels in event patients tended to be out of individual target threshold of BNP between dotted lines: 95% confidence interval (CI) on solid line: the linear regression line specific for event-free patients C: Kaplan-Meier curves showing the incidence rate of event according to individual target threshold of BNP. Out of individual target threshold of BNP was significantly associated with an increase in event incidence (the log-rank test: P<0.0001).
Open circles or triangles indicate even-free or event patients. CD was defined as left ventricular end-diastolic dimension × left atrial diastolic dimension/wall thickness/body surface area.

The number of patients in our study is, however, relatively small, and our population was limited to only patients with non-ischemic dilated cardiomyopathy. Additional prospective multi-center studies including cases with ischemic heart disease would confirm our observation and extend it to various settings of systolic HF.

3. Conclusion

BNP measurement has facilitated the diagnosis of HF and decision of pharmacotherapy and improved outcome during the hospitalization and after the discharge for decompensated HF in cardiomyopathies, although BNP cutoff points for risk assessment are different on time course after decompensated HF and cardiac dysfunctions. On the other hand, availability of this BNP measurement was less especially in patients with advanced dilated cardiomyopathy as well as in elderly patients. However, individual target threshold of BNP for risk reduction related to cardiac dilatation exerted a strong prognostic power even in such advanced cases. This target threshold-guided therapy would facilitate individual disease management and thus contribute to further improvement of treatment outcome.

4. Acknowledgment

The authors thank Ms. Toshie Hashizume, Chiaki Notoya, and Kazumi Nakazato for their excellent technical assistance.

5. References

[1] Yoshimura, M.; Yasue, H.; Okumura, K.; Ogawa, H.; Jougasaki, M.; Mukoyama, M.; Nakao, K.; Imura, H. (1993). Different secretion pattern of atrial natriuretic peptide and brain natriuretic peptide in patients with congestive heart failure. *Circulation,* 87, 2, (Feb), pp. 464–469.

[2] Yasue, H.; Yoshimura, M and Sumida, H. (1994). Localization and mechanism of secretion of B-type natriuretic peptide in comparison with those of A-type natriuretic peptide in normal subjects and patients with heart failure. *Circulation,* 90, 1, (Jul), pp. 195–203.

[3] Brunner-La Rocca, HP.; Kaye, DM.; Woods, RL.; Hastings, J.; Esler, MD. (2001). Effects of intravenous brain natriuretic peptide on regional sympathetic activity in patients with chronic heart failure as compared with healthy control subjects. *J Am Coll Cardiol,* 37, 5, (Apr), pp. 1221–1227.

[4] Atarashi, K.; Mulrow, PJ.; Franco-Saenz, R. (1985). Effect of atrial peptides on aldosterone production. *J Clin Invest,* 76, 5, (Nov), pp. 1807–1811. .

[5] Maisel, AS.; Krishnaswamy, P.; Nowak, R.; McCord, J.; Hollander, JE.; Duc, P.; Omland, T.; Storrow, AB.; Abraham, WT.; Wu, AH.; Clopton, P.; Steg, PG.; Westheim, A.; Knudsen, CW.; Perez, A.; Kazanegra, R.; Herrmann, HC.; McCullough, PA. and Breathing Not Properly Multinational Study Investigators. (2002). Rapid measurement of B-type natriuretic peptide in the emergency diagnosis of heart failure. *N Engl J Med,* 347, 3, (Jul), pp. 161–167.

[6] Morrison LK, Harrison A, Krishnaswamy P, Kazanegra R, Clopton P, Maisel A. (2002). Utility of a rapid B-natriuretic peptide (BNP) assay in differentiating CHF from

lung disease in patients presenting with dyspnea. *J Am Coll Cardiol,* 39, 2, (Jan), pp. 202-209.

[7] Maisel, AS.; Koon, J.; Krishnaswamy, P.; Kazenegra, R.; Clopton, P.; Gardetto, N.; Morrisey, R.; Garcia, A.; Chiu, A.; De Maria, A. (2001). Utility of B-natriuretic peptide as a rapid, point-of-care test for screening patients undergoing echocardiography to determine left ventricular dysfunction. *Am Heart J,* 141, 3, (Mar), pp. 367-374.

[8] Yu CM, Sanderson JE, Shum IO, Chan S, Yeung LY, Hung YT, Cockram CS, Woo KS. (1996). Diastolic dysfunction and natriuretic peptides in systolic heart failure. Higher ANP and BNP levels are associated with the restrictive filling pattern. *Eur Heart J,* 17, 11, (Nov), pp. 1694-1702.

[9] Takeuchi, I.; Inomata, T.; Nishii, M.; Koitabashi, T.; Nakano, H.; Shinagawa, H.; Takehana, H.; Izumi, T. (2005). Clinical characteristics of heart disease patients with a good prognosis in spite of markedly increased plasma levels of type-B natriuretic peptide (BNP): anomalous behavior of plasma BNP in hypertrophic cardiomyopathy. Circ J, 69, 3, (Mar), pp. 277-282.

[10] Leya, FS.; Arab, D.; Joyal, D.; Shioura, KM.; Lewis, BE.; Steen, LH.; Cho, L. (2005). The efficacy of brain natriuretic peptide levels in differentiating constrictive pericarditis from restrictive cardiomyopathy. *J Am Coll Cardiol.* 45, 11, (Jun), pp. 1900-1902.

[11] Fonarow, GC.; Peacock, WF.; Phillips, CO.; Givertz, MM.; Lopatin, M.; ADHERE Scientific Advisory Committee and Investigators. (2007). Admission B-type natriuretic peptide levels and in-hospital mortality in acute decompensated heart failure. *J Am Coll Cardiol,* 49, 19, (May), pp. 1943-1950.

[12] Logeart, D.; Thabut, G.; Jourdain, P.; Chavelas, C.; Beyne, P.; Beauvais, F.; Bouvier, E.; Solal, AC. (2004). Predischarge B-type natriuretic peptide assay for identifying patients at high risk of re-admission after decompensated heart failure. *J Am Coll Cardiol,* 43, 4, (Feb), pp. 635-641.

[13] Nishii, M.; Inomata, T.; Takehana, H.; Naruke, T.; Yanagisawa, T.; Moriguchi, M.; Takeda, S.; Izumi, T. (2008). Prognostic utility of B-type natriuretic peptide assessment in stable low-risk outpatients with nonischemic cardiomyopathy after decompensated heart failure. *J Am Coll Cardiol,* 51, 24, (Jun), pp. 2329-2335.

[14] Richards, AM.; Nicholls, MG.; Yandle, TG.; Frampton, C.; Espiner, EA.; Turner, JG.; Buttimore, RC.; Lainchbury, JG.; Elliott, JM.; Ikram, H.; Crozier, IG.; Smyth, DW. (1998). Plasma N-terminal pro-brain natriuretic peptide and adrenomedullin: new neurohormonal predictors of left ventricular function and prognosis after myocardial infarction. *Circulation,* 97, 19, (May), pp. 1921-1929.

[15] de Lemos, JA.; Morrow, DA.; Bentley, JH.; Omland, T.; Sabatine, MS.; McCabe, CH.; Hall, C.; Cannon, CP.; Braunwald, E. (2001). The prognostic value of B-type natriuretic peptide in patients with acute coronary syndromes. *N Engl J Med,* 345, 14 (Oct), pp. 1014-1021.

[16] Lieberman, EB.; Hutchins, GM.; Herskowitz, A.; Rose, NR.; Baughman, KL. (1991). Clinicopathologic description of myocarditis. *J Am Coll Cardiol,* 18, 7, (Dec), pp. 1617-1626.

[17] McCarthy, RE 3 rd.; Boehmer, JP.; Hruban, RH.; Hutchins, GM.; Kasper, EK.; Hare, JM.; Baughman, KL. (2000). Long-term outcome of fulminant myocarditis as compared with acute (nonfulminant) myocarditis. *New Engl J Med*, 342, 10, (Mar), pp. 690-695.

[18] Woodruff, JF. Viral myocarditis: a review. (1980). Am J Pathol, 101, 2, (Nov), pp. 425-484.

[19] Nishii, M.; Inomata, T.; Takehana, H.; Takeuchi, I.; Nakano, H.; Koitabashi, T.; Nakahata, J.; Aoyama, N.; Izumi, T. (2004). Serum levels of interleukin-10 on admission as a prognostic predictor of human fulminant myocarditis. *Am J Coll Cardiol*, 44, 6, (Sep),pp. 1292-1297.

[20] Hofmann, P.; Schmidtke, M.; Stelzer, A.; Gemsa, D. (2001). Suppression of Proinflammatory cytokines and induction of IL-10 in human monocytes after coxsackievirus B3 infection. *J Med Virol*, 64, 4, (Aug), pp. 487-98.

[21] Godeny, EK.; Gauntt, CJ. (1987). Murine natural killer cells limit coxsackievirus B3 replication. *J Immunol*, 139, 3, (Aug), pp. 913-918.

[22] Reed, SG.; Brownell, CE.; Russo, DM.; Siva, JS.; Grabstein, KH.; Morrissey, PJ. (1994). IL-10 mediates susceptibility to Trypanosoma cruzi infection. *J Immunol*, 153, 7, (Oct), pp. 3135-3140.

[23] Silva, JS.; Aliberti, JC.; Martin, GA.; Souza, M.; Souto, JT.; Padua, MA. (1998). The role of IL-12 in experimental Trypanosoma cruzi infection. *Braz J Med Biol Res*, 31, 1, (Jan), pp. 111-115.

[24] Gluck, B.; Schmidtke, M.; Merkle, I.; Stelzner, A.; Gemsa, D. (2001). Persistent expression of cytokines in the chronic stage of CVB3-induced myocarditis in NMRI mice. *J Moll Cell Cardiol*, 33, 9, (Sep), pp. 1615-1626.

[25] Schmidtke, M.; Gluck, B.; Merkle, I.; Hoffmann, P.; Stelzner, A.; Gemsa, D. (2000). Cytokine profiles in heart, spleen, and thymus during the acute stage of experimental coxsackievirus B3-induced chronic myocarditis. *J Med Virol*, 61, 4, (Aug), pp. 518-526.

[26] Watanabe, K.; Nakazawa, M.; Fuse, K.; Hanawa, H.; Kodama, M.; Aizawa, Y.; Ohnuki, T.; Gejyo, F.; Maruyama, H.; Miyazaki, J. (2001). Protection against autoimmune myocarditis by gene transfer of interleukin-10 by electroporation. *Circulation*, 104, 10, (Sep), pp. 1098-1100.

[27] Nishio, R.; Matsumori, A.; Shioi, T.; Ishida, H.; Sasayama, S. (1999). Treatment of Experimental Viral Myocarditis With Interleukin-10. *Circulation*, 100, 10, (Sep), pp. 1102-1108.

[28] Maron, BJ.; Tholakanahalli, VN.; Zenovich, AG.; Casey, SA.; Duprez, D.; Aeppli, DM.; Cohn, JN. (2004). Usefulness of B-type natriuretic peptide assay in the assessment of symptomatic state in hypertrophic cardiomyopathy. *Circulation*, 109, 8, (Mar), pp. 984-989.

[29] Arteaga, E.; Araujo, AQ.; Buck, P.; Ianni, BM.; Rabello, R.; Mady, C. (2005). Plasma amino-terminal pro-B-type natriuretic peptide quantification in hypertrophic cardiomyopathy. *Am Heart J*, 150, 6, (Dec), pp. 1228-1232.

[30] Nakamura, T.; Sakamoto, K.; Yamano, T.; Kikkawa, M.; Zen, K.; Hikosaka, T.; Kubota, T.; Azuma, A.; Nishimura, T. (2002). Increased plasma brain natriuretic peptide level as a guide for silent myocardial ischemia in patients with non-obstructive hypertrophic cardiomyopathy. *J Am Coll Cardiol*, 39, 10, (May), pp. 1657-1663.

[31] Kubo, T.; Kitaoka, H.; Okawa, M.; Yamanaka, S.; Hirota, T.; Baba, Y.; Hayato, K.; Yamasaki, N.; Matsumura, Y.; Yasuda, N.; Sugiura, T.; Doi, YL. (2011). Combined measurements of cardiac troponin I and brain natriuretic Peptide are useful for predicting adverse outcomes in hypertrophic cardiomyopathy. *Circ J*, 75, 4, (Mar), pp. 919-926.

[32] Hasegawa, K.; Fujiwara, H.; Doyama, K.; Miyamae, M.; Fujiwara, T.; Suga, S.; Mukoyama, M.; Nakao, K.; Imura, H.; Sasayama, S. (1993). Ventricular expression of brain natriuretic peptide in hypertrophic cardiomyopathy. *Circulation*, 88, 2, (Aug), pp. 372-380.

[33] Troughton, RW.; Frampton, CM,; Yandle, TG.; Espiner, EA.; Nicholls, MG.; Richards, AM. (2000). Treatment of heart failure guided by plasma aminoterminal brain natriuretic peptide (N-BNP) concentrations. *Lancet*, 355, 9210, (Apr), pp. 1126–1130.

[34] Jourdain, P.; Jondeau, G.; Funck, F.; Gueffet, P.; Le Helloco, A.; Donal, E.; Aupetit, JF.; Aumont, MC.; Galinier, M.; Eicher, JC.; Cohen-Solal, A.; Juillière, Y. (2007). Plasma brain natriuretic peptide-guided therapy to improve outcome in heart failure: the STARS-BNP Multicenter Study. *J Am Coll Cardiol*, 49, 16, (Apr), pp. 1733-1739.

[35] Pfisterer, M.; Buser, P.; Rickli, H.; Gutmann, M.; Erne, P.; Rickenbacher, P.; Vuillomenet, A.; Jeker, U.; Dubach, P.; Beer, H.; Yoon, SI.; Suter, T.; Osterhues, HH.; Schieber, MM.; Hilti, P.; Schindler, R.; Brunner-La Rocca, HP.; TIME-CHF Investigators. (2009). BNP-guided vs. symptom-guided heart failure therapy: the Trial of Intensified vs. Standard Medical Therapy in Elderly Patients with Congestive Heart Failure (TIME-CHF) randomized trial. *JAMA*, 301, 4, (Jan), pp. 383–392.

[36] Hoit, BD.; Shao, Y.; Gabel, M.; Walsh, RA. (1994). In vivo assessment of left atrial contractile performance in normal and pathological conditions using a time-varying elastance model. *Circulation*, 89, 4, (Apr), pp. 1829-1838.

[37] Dernellis, JM.; Stefanadis, CI.; Zacharoulis, AA.; Toutouzas, PK. (1998). Left atrial mechanical adaptation to long-standing hemodynamic loads based on pressure-volume relations. *Am J Cardiol*, 81, 9, (May), pp. 1138-1143.

Part 2

Pathophysiology and Genetics of Cardiomyopathies

9

Heart Muscle and Apoptosis

Angelos Tsipis
1st Department of Pathology, Medical School, University of Athens
Greece

1. Introduction

Significant progress has been made in demonstrating the role of apoptosis in various heart diseases, and in elucidating the molecular mechanisms of cardiac apoptosis. Apoptosis has been attributed an essential role in cardiomyopathy. The progressive loss of cardiac myocytes is one of the most important pathogenic components of the heart failure. While initial studies reported unrealistically high levels of cell death, probably due to methodological problems, later work has consistently shown that approximately 80–250 heart muscle cells per 10^5 cardiac nuclei commit suicide at any given time in patients with late-stage dilated cardiomyopathy. In contrast, the base-line rate of apoptosis in healthy human hearts is only one to ten cardiac myocytes per 10^5 nuclei (Anversa & Kajstura, 1998; Yue et al., 1998). Even though the rate of apoptosis in heart failure is relatively low in absolute numbers, it is significantly higher than that in the normal heart, which has essentially negligible baseline apoptosis. Recently, animal models of heart failure incorporating transgenic technology have confirmed that myocyte apoptosis itself is sufficient to induce heart failure. Apoptosis has been implicated in a wide variety of physiological and pathological processes. The importance of apoptosis in cardiovascular system is also becoming increasingly clear, and the inhibition of apoptosis is emerging as a potential therapeutic tool for various forms of cardiovascular disease. In this chapter, we examine the evidence for apoptosis in cardiovascular disease and the molecular mechanisms of cardiac apoptosis.

2. Apoptosis

2.1 Concept and morphologic characteristics of apoptosis

There are two primary pathways by which cells die. The path for accidental cell death is called necrosis. Accidental cell death occurs when cells receive a structural or chemical insult from which they cannot recover. Examples of such insults include ischemia, extremes of temperature, and physical trauma. The hallmark of necrosis is that cells die because they are damaged. In contrast, cells that die by programmed cell death commit suicide actively as the results of activation of a dedicated intracellular program. For programmed cell death, the most commonly described pathway is apoptosis. Apoptosis begins with a signal that can come from within the cell (e.g., detection of radiation-induced DNA breaks) or from without (e.g., a decrease in the level of an essential growth factor or hormone). This pro-apoptotic signal induces the cell to make a decision to commit suicide. Initially, cells that are committed to undergo programmed cell death are in a latent phase of apoptosis. The latent phase can be subdivided into two stages: a condemned stage, during which the cell is proceeding on a pathway toward death but can still be rescued if it is exposed to anti-apoptotic activities, and a committed stage, beyond which rescue is impossible. Ultimately, the cells enter the execution phase of apoptosis, in which they undergo the dramatic morphologic and physiological changes (Pollard & Earnshaw, 2004). Apoptosis is characterized by a reproducible pattern of structural alterations of both the nucleus and cytoplasm. In order of appearance, these include: (1) Loss of microvilli and intercellular junctions. (2) Shrinkage of the cytoplasm. The cell is smaller in size. The cytoplasm is dense. The organelles, although relatively normal, are more tightly packed. (3) Dramatic changes in cytoplasmic motility with activation of a violent program of blebbing. (4) Loss of plasma membrane asymmetry, with the distribution of phosphatidyl serine being randomized so that it appears in the outer membrane leaflet. (5) Changes in the organization of the cell nucleus, typically involving the hypercondensation of the chromatin. This is the most characteristic feature of apoptosis. The chromatin aggregates peripherally, under the nuclear membrane, into dense masses of various shapes and sizes. The nucleus itself may break up, producing two or more fragments. (6) Formation of cytoplasmic blebs and apoptotic bodies. The apoptotic cell first shows extensive surface blebbing, then undergoes fragmentation into membrane-bound apoptotic bodies composed of cytoplasm and tightly packed organelles, with or without nuclear fragments. (7) Phagocytosis of apoptotic cells or cell bodies, usually by macrophages. The apoptotic bodies are rapidly degraded within lysosomes, and the adjacent healthy cells migrate or proliferate to replace the space occupied by the now deleted apoptotic cell. Because the vesicles remain membrane bound, the cellular contents are never released into the environment. As a result, apoptotic death does not lead to an inflammatory response. (Kumar et al., 2005; Pollard & Earnshaw, 2004).

2.2 Molecular mechanism and pathway description

The process of apoptosis may divided into an initiation phase, during which caspases become catalytically active, and an execution phase, during which these enzymes act to cause cell death. Initiation of apoptosis occurs principally by signals from two distinct but convergent pathways: the extrinsic, or receptor-initiated, pathway and the intrinsic or mitochondrial pathway. Both pathways converge to activate caspases and they may be interconnected at numerous steps.

2.2.1 The extrinsic (death receptors) pathway

This pathway is initiated by engagement of cell surface death receptors on a variety of cells. Death receptors are members of the tumor necrosis factor receptor family (Fas, TNFαR, DR3, DR4, DR5) that contain a cytoplasmic domain involved in protein-protein interactions that is called death domain because it is essential for delivering apoptotic signals.. Death receptor ligands characteristically initiate signaling via receptor oligomerization, which in turn results in the recruitment of specialized adaptor proteins and activation of caspase cascades. Binding of FasL induces Fas trimerization, which recruits initiator caspase-8 via the adaptor protein FADD. Caspase-8 then oligomerizes and is activated via autocatalysis. Activated caspase-8 stimulates apoptosis via two parallel cascades: it can directly cleave and activate caspase-3, or alternatively, it can cleave Bid, a pro-apoptotic Bcl-2 family protein. Truncated

Bid (tBid) translocates to mitochondria, inducing cytochrome c release, which sequentially activates caspase-9 and -3. TNF-α and DR-3L can deliver pro- or anti-apoptotic signals. TNFαR and DR3 promote apoptosis via the adaptor proteins TRADD/FADD and the activation of caspase-8. Interaction of TNF-α with TNFαR may activate the NF-κB pathway via NIK/IKK. The activation of NF-κB induces the expression of pro-survival genes including Bcl-2 and FLIP, the latter can directly inhibit the activation of caspase-8. Some viruses and normal cells produce FLIP, which binds to pro-caspase-8 but cannot cleave and activate the enzyme because it lacks enzymatic activity, and use this inhibitor to protect infected and normal cells from Fas-mediated apoptosis (Kumar et al., 2005). FasL and TNF-α may also activate JNK via ASK1/MKK7. Activation of JNK may lead to the inhibition of Bcl-2 by phosphorylation. In the absence of caspase activation, stimulation of death receptors can lead to the activation of an alternative programmed cell death pathway termed necroptosis by forming complex IIb. (Humphreys & Halpern, 2008; Logue & Martin, 2008; Yuan, 2010)

2.2.2 The intrinsic (mitochondrial) pathway

This pathway of apoptosis is the result of increased mitochondrial permeability and release of pro-apoptotic molecules into the cytoplasm, without a role for death receptors. Growth factors and other survival signals stimulate the production of anti-apoptotic members of the Bcl-2 family of proteins. The Bcl-2 family of proteins regulates apoptosis by controlling mitochondrial permeability. The anti-apoptotic proteins Bcl-2 and Bcl-xL reside in the outer mitochondrial wall and inhibit cytochrome c release. The proapoptotic Bcl-2 proteins Bad, Bid, Bax, and Bim may reside in the cytosol but translocate to mitochondria following death signaling, where they promote the release of cytochrome c. Bad translocates to mitochondria and forms a pro-apoptotic complex with Bcl-xL. This translocation is inhibited by survival factors that induce the phosphorylation of Bad, leading to its cytosolic sequestration. Cytosolic Bid is cleaved by caspase-8 following signaling through Fas; its active fragment (tBid) translocates to mitochondria. Bax and Bim translocate to mitochondria in response to death stimuli, including survival factor withdrawal. Activated following DNA damage, p53 induces the transcription of Bax, Noxa, and PUMA. Upon release from mitochondria, cytochrome c binds to Apaf-1 and forms an activation complex with caspase-9. Although the mechanism(s) regulating mitochondrial permeability and the release of cytochrome c during apoptosis are not fully understood, Bcl-xL, Bcl-2, and Bax may influence the voltage-dependent anion channel (VDAC), which may play a role in regulating cytochrome c release. Mule/ARF-BP1 is a DNA damage activated E3 ubiquitin ligase for p53, and Mcl-1, an anti-apoptotic member of Bcl-2 (Brenner & Mak, 2009; Chalah & Khosravi-Far, 2008; Yuan 2010). The essence of this intrinsic pathway is a balance between pro-apoptotic and protective molecules that regulate mitochondrial permeability and the release of death inducers that are normally sequestered within the mitochondria (Kumar et al., 2005).

2.2.3 The execution phase

The final phase of apoptosis is mediated by a proteolytic cascade, toward which the various initiating mechanisms converge. Caspases, a family of cysteine proteases, are the central regulators of apoptosis. They are mammalian homologues of the ced-3 in the nematode Caenorhabditis elegans. The caspase family, now including more than 10 members, can be divided functionally into two basic groups - initiator and executioner - depending on the order in which they are activated during apoptosis. Caspases exist as inactive pro-enzymes, or zymogens, and must undergo an activating cleavage for apoptosis to be initiated. Caspases have their own cleavage sites that can be hydrolyzed not only by other caspases but also autocatalytically. After an initiator caspase is cleaved to generate its active form, the enzymatic death program is set in motion by rapid and sequential activation of other caspases. Executioner caspases act on many cellular components. They cleave cytoskeletal and nuclear matrix proteins and thus disrupt the cytoskeleton and lead to breakdown of the nucleus. In the nucleus, the targets of caspase activation include proteins involved in transcription, DNA replication, and DNA repair (Haunstetter & Izumo, 1998; Kumar et al., 2005) (Table 1). Initiator caspases (including caspase-2, -8, -9, -10, -11, and -12) are closely coupled to pro-apoptotic signals. Once activated, these caspases cleave and activate downstream effector caspases (including caspase-3, -6, and -7), which in turn execute apoptosis by cleaving cellular proteins following specific Asp residues. Activation of Fas and TNFR by FasL and TNF, respectively, leads to the activation of caspase-8 and -10. DNA damage induces the expression of PIDD which binds to RAIDD and caspase-2 and leads to the activation of caspase-2. Cytochrome c released from damaged mitochondria is coupled to the activation of caspase-9. XIAP inhibits caspase-3, -7, and -9. Mitochondria release multiple pro-apoptotic molecules, such as Smac/ Diablo, AIF, HtrA2 and EndoG, in addition to cytochrome c. Smac/Diablo binds to XIAP which prevents it from inhibiting caspases. Caspase-11 is induced and activated by pathological proinflammatory and pro-apoptotic stimuli and leads to the activation of caspase-1 to promote inflammatory response and apoptosis by directly processing caspase-3. Caspase-12 and caspase-7 are activated under ER stress conditions. Anti-apoptotic ligands including growth factors and cytokines activate Akt and p90RSK. Akt inhibits Bad by direct phosphorylation and prevents the expression of Bim by phosphorylating and inhibiting the Forkhead family of transcription factors (Fox0). Fox0 promotes apoptosis by upregulating pro-apoptotic molecules such as FasL and Bim (Degterev & Yuan, 2008; Kurokawa & Kornbluth, 2009; Yuan 2010).

Nuclear proteins
Lamin, Rb protein, DNA-dependent protein kinase, 70-kDa subunit of U1 small nuclear ribonucleoprotein, Poly (ADP)-ribosylating protein (PARP), Mdm2
Regulatory proteins
MAPK/ERK kinase kinase 1 (MEKK1), Protein Kinase Cδ, G4-GDI GDP dissociation inhibitor, Sterol regulatory element binding protein, DNA fragmentation factor/inhibitor of caspase-activated DNAse
Cytoskeletal proteins
Fodrin, Gelsolin, Actin, Gas2

Table 1. Downstream targets of Caspases. (Haunstetter & Izumo, 1998)

2.3 Study of apoptosis

Light and electron microscopy are two of the classical techniques for the study of this process. Because of the lack of cellular synchronization in apoptosis and of the fact that the apoptotic cell is rapidly disposed of through phagocytosis, study methods based on morphologic criteria are adequate for the demonstration of the process, but are not useful for quantifying it. Further to these procedures, the study of DNA fragmentation in agarose gels has been considered to be identificative for apoptosis. A number of techniques take advantage of this DNA fragmentation for labelling the fragments and thus for quantifying the proportion of apoptotic cells. Each DNA fragment has a 3'OH terminal portion. This terminal fragment can be labelled in various ways (for instance, with the help of a modified terminal deoxynucleotidyl transferase), so that the labelling rate is proportional to the degree of DNA fragmentation. In TUNEL assay (terminal deoxyribonucleotidyl transferase [TdT]-mediated dUTP-digoxigeninnick end labeling), TdT transfers a fluorescent nucleotide to exposed breakpoints of DNA. Apoptotic cells that have incorporated the labeled nucleotide are then visualized by fluorescence microscopy or flow cytometry. Apoptotic cells that have extruded some of the DNA have less than their normal diploid content. Automated measurement of the amount of DNA in individual cells by flow cytometry thus produces a population distribution according to DNA content (cytofluorograph) (Rubin et al., 2005). At present, the most widely accepted and standardized technique takes advantage of the changes in the membrane phospholipids that occur early in apoptotic cells (Vermes et al., 1995). The negatively charged membrane phospholipids exposed to the external environment by the apoptotic cell are labeled with fluorochrome-conjugated molecules, and the percentage of fluorescent cells can be easily quantified (Chamond et al., 1999).

2.4 Apoptosis in developmental and physiological processes

Cell death is extremely important in embryonic development, maintenance of tissue homeostasis, establishment of immune self-tolerance, killing by immune effector cells, and regulation of cell viability by hormones and growth factors. Apoptosis is a normal phenomenon that serves to eliminate cells that are not longer needed and to maintain a steady number of various cell populations in tissues. It is important in the following physiologic situations. During molecular maturation of T-cell antigen receptors, immature T cells in the thymus rearrange the genes encoding the receptor α and β chains. Cells with receptors recognizing self-antigens are potentially harmful and are eliminated through programmed cell death. Cells with damaged DNA tend to accumulate mutations, and they are potentially harmful to the organism. DNA damage induces programmed cell death in many cell types. Furthermore one of the mechanisms to eliminate infected cells is through the action of cytotoxic T lymphocytes, which kill cells, by inducing them to undergo programmed cell death. T lymphocytes whose T-cell receptors cannot interact with the spectrum of MHC glycoproteins expressed in a given individual are ineffective in the immune response. Up to 95% of immature T cells die by apoptosis without leaving the thymus. Fetal development involves the sequential appearance and regression of many anatomical structures: some aortic arches do not persist, the mesonephros regresses in favor of the metanephros, interdigital tissues disappear to allow discrete fingers and toes, and excess neurons are pruned from the developing brain. Cells in these conditions serve no purpose in humans and are eliminated by programmed cell death. Excess neurons that do not make appropriate connections have no function and so are eliminated by apoptosis. Up to 80%of neurons in certain developing ganglia die this way (Rubin et al., 2005). Apoptosis also eliminates the constituent cells of mullerian ducts in males. Epithelial cells must die to allow fusion of palate and mammary and prostate cells die when deprived of hormones (Pollard & Earnshaw, 2004).

2.5 Apoptosis and disease

Death by apoptosis is also responsible for loss of cells in a variety of pathologic states. The diseases in which apoptosis has been involved can be divided into two groups: those in which there is an increase in cell survival (or diseases associated to inhibition of apoptosis), and those in which there is an increase in cell death (and hence hyperactive apoptosis) (Chamond et al., 1999). The group of diseases associated to apoptosis inhibition includes those diseases in which an excessive accumulation of cells occurs (neoplastic diseases, autoimmune diseases) (Table 2). It was classically believed that the excessive accumulation of cells in these diseases occurred because of an increased cell proliferation. In recent years, the study of apoptosis in these patients has led to a new and different approach, according to which this accumulation of cells would be due to defective apoptosis. Increased cell apoptosis has also been implicated in the aetiopathogenesis of a number of diseases.

A large group of neurodegenerative diseases, among them Alzheimer's disease, Parkinson's disease, amyotrophic lateral sclerosis and retinitis pigmentosa, are associated to selective apoptosis of the neurones. This neuronal death appears to be associated to increases susceptibility to apoptosis in these cells. Oxidative stress, mitochondrial defects and neurotoxic agents have been postulated as the inductors of neuronal death. The disease associated to infection by the Human Immunodeficiency Virus (HIV) has been defined as an imbalance between the number of CD4+ lymphocytes and the ability of the bone marrow to generate new mature cells. The CD4+ cells of the HIV(+) patients die through apoptosis when stimulated in vitro. Also, HIV infection of cells from healthy subjects induces apoptosis of CD4+ cells. However, further to this, not only the infected cells but also non-infected cells undergo apoptosis. Replicative exhaustion of the responding cell clones has been demonstrated in a number of diseases (among them AIDS, in which the responding clone is the CD4+ one); in these diseases the responding clone, after an initial phase of intense response to the stimulus, become exhausted and undergo apoptosis (Ameisen, 1995).

Through inhibition of apoptosis	Through excess apoptosis
Cancer	**AIDS**
Colorectal	T lymphocytes
Glioma	**Neurodegenerative diseases**
Hepatic	Alzheimer's disease
Neuroblastoma	Amyotrophic lateral sclerosis
Leukaemias and lymphomas	Parkinson's disease
Prostate	Retinitis pigmentosa
Autoimmune diseases	Epilepsy
Myastenia gravis	**Haematologic diseases**
Systemic lupus erythematosus	Aplastic anaemia
Inflammatory diseases	Myelodysplastic syndrome
Bronchial asthma	T CD4+ lymphocytopenia
Inflammatory intestinal disease	G6PD deficiency
Pulmonary inflammation	**Tissue damage**
Viral infections	Myocardial infarction
Adenovirus	Cerebrovascular accident
Baculovirus	Ischaemic renal damage
	Polycystic kidney

Table 2. Diseases associated to apoptosis

2.6 Apoptosis and cardiovascular disease

The myocardial cells allocate a limited faculty of proliferation and correspondingly, apoptosis is observed infrequently in adult hearts. On the contrary at the duration of organogenesis and in the formation of heart the apoptosis plays an important role, as an example in the formation of septa between the cardiac chambers and the valves. As consequence the defects in apoptosis can constitute basic causative factor of relatives of congenital heart disease. Apoptosis of myocardial cells is also observed afterwards the birth and concretely in the interventricular septum and right ventricular wall, at the duration of passage from the fetal circulation in the adult circulation. Moreover the phenomenon of apoptosis is also distinguished in the conducting system and can lead to congenital heart block, syndrome of long QT, and the existence of accessory pathways (Table 3) (Bennett, 2002). Until recently, the loss of myocytes was attributed to necrosis; however, it is now clear that apoptosis may play an important role in the pathogenesis of a variety of cardiovascular diseases. For instance, apoptosis has been detected in myocardial samples obtained from patients with end-stage congestive heart failure, arrhythmogenic right ventricular dysplasia and myocardial infraction. In addition, apoptosis has been detected in cardiac myocytes under hypoxia/reoxygenetion, mechanical stretch and in animal models of cardiac ischemia/reperfusion injury (Table 4) (Gustafsson & Gottlieb, 2003).

Myocyte
Idiopathic dilated cardiomyopathy Ischaemic cardiomyopathy Acute myocardial infarction Arrhythmogenic right ventricular dysplasia Myocarditis
Conducting tissues
Pre-excitations syndromes Congenital complete atrioventricular heart Long QT syndromes
Vascular
Atherosclerosis Restenosis after angioplasty / stenting Vascular graft rejection Arterial aneurysm formation

Table 3. Apoptosis and cardiovascular disease (Bennett, 2002; Haunstetter & Izumo, 1998)

Stimulus	Signaling pathway	Potential inhibitor
Ischaemia/reperfusion Pressure overload Neurohormonal factors Ischaemia Death receptor ligands	ERK/SARK ERK/SARK G protein coupling Lack of growth factor signaling Adapter molecules / caspases	Activation of ERK, inhibition of SARK signaling Activation of ERK, inhibition of SARK signaling β blockers Activation of Akt/ERK pathways Decoy receptors / receptor antagonists IAPs / caspase inhibitors
ERK, extracellular signal related kinase; IAP, inhibitor of apoptosis protein; SAPK, stress activated protein kinase		

Table 4. Potential inhibitors and signaling pathways of cardiomyocyte apoptosis (Bennett, 2002).

2.6.1 Apoptosis and atherosclerosis

Apoptosis constitutes basic characteristic of vessels remodeling that takes place in organogenesis and in pathological situations like injury and atherosclerosis. The significance of apoptosis in atherosclerosis depends on the stage of the plaque, localization and the cell types involved. Apoptosis of vascular smooth muscle cells (SMC), endothelial cells and macrophages may promote plaque growth and pro-coagulation and may induce rupture, the major consequence of atherosclerosis in humans. Apoptosis of macrophages is mainly present in regions showing signs of DNA synthesis/repair. SMC apoptosis is mainly present in less cellular regions and is not associated with DNA synthesis/repair. Even in the early stages of atherosclerosis SMC become susceptible to apoptosis since they increase different pro-apoptotic factors. Moreover, recent data indicate that SMC may be killed by activated macrophages. The loss of the SMC can be detrimental for plaque stability since most of the interstitial collagen fibres, which are important for the tensile strength of the fibrous cap, are produced by SMC. Rupture of atherosclerotic plaques is associated with a thinning of the SMC-rich fibrous cap overlying the core. Rupture occurs particularly at the plaque shoulders, which exhibit lack of SMCs and the presence of inflammatory cells. Apoptotic SMCs are evident in advanced human plaques including the shoulders regions, prompting the suggestion that SMC apoptosis may hasten plaque rupture. Indeed, increased SMC apoptosis occurs in unstable versus stable angina lesions. Apoptosis of macrophages could be beneficial for plaque stability if apoptotic bodies were removed. Apoptotic cells that are not scavenged in the plaque activate thrombin, which could further induce intraplaque thrombosis (Kockx & Knaapen, 2000). Most apoptotic cells in advanced lesions are macrophages next to the lipid core. Loss of macrophages from atherosclerotic lesions would be predicted to promote plaque stability rather than rupture, since macrophages can promote SMC apoptosis by both direct interactions and by release of cytokines (Bennett, 2002). It can be concluded that apoptosis in primary atherosclerosis is detrimental since it could lead to plaque rupture and thrombosis.

2.6.2 Apoptosis and ischaemia/infarction

Cardiac myocyte death during ischemic injury has been thought to occur exclusively by necrosis, but recently several studies have demonstrated that large numbers of myocytes undergo apoptosis in response to ischemic disorders (Saraste et al., 1997). In humans, apoptosis seems to occur primarily in the border zone of the ischemic region and, according to some studies, in the remote from ischemia regions. However, in vivo animal studies have demonstrated apoptosis both in the ischemic region and the ischemic border zone. Apoptosis of cardiomyocytes occurs in a temporally and spatially specific manner. The central, unperfused region also manifests apoptosis, particularly within the first six hours, although between 6-24 hours necrosis is more common (Bennett, 2002). In contrast, in some studies ischemia caused apoptosis in the ischemic region alone, whereas reperfusion caused a decrease in apoptotic cells in the ischemic region and an increase in apoptotic cells in the ischemic border zone and the remote from ischemia regions. These differences theoretically could be explained by the different methods of measuring apoptosis that were used (Krijnen et al., 2002). Apoptosis in the remote non-infarcted myocardium may be partly responsible for myocardial remodelling and dilatation after myocardial infarction, and may be amenable to treatment. Apoptosis is a highly regulated process in which several regulatory proteins play a significant part. P53 limits cellular proliferation by inducing cell cycle arrest and apoptosis in response to cellular stresses such as DNA damage, hypoxia, and oncogene activation. P53 mediates apoptosis through a linear pathway involving bax activation, cytochrome c release from mitochondria, and caspase activation (Shen & White, 2001). The Bcl-2 family of proteins constitutes a critical checkpoint in cell death. These proteins contain agonists and antagonists of apoptosis and alterations of their ratio determine the life or death of a cell (Anversa & Kajstura, 1998). Proapoptotic proteins include Bax, Bak, Bad, and Bcl-xs whereas Bcl-2 and Bcl-xL are antiapoptotic. Several studies have demonstrated that Bcl-2 protein is induced in salvaged myocytes surrounding infracted areas in the regions at risk in acute stage of infraction. Bcl-2 positive myocytes were not seen in the infracted myocytes in the heart with acute infraction. Bcl-2 positive immunoreactivity was not evident in salvaged myocytes of hearts with old infraction, in chronic ischemic disease or in normal hearts. P53 and Bax protein expression was rare in salvaged myocytes within the risk area at the acute stage of infraction. P53 and Bax positive immunoractivity was evident in the infracted myocytes. P53 protein is induced in salvaged myocytes at the old stage of infraction and in chronic ischemic disease. P53 positive immunoreactivity of normal control heart tissue was slight in most of myocytes. Myocytes exposed to various stress, such as chronic ischemia (salvaged myocytes at the old stage of infraction, myocytes at chronic ischemic disease) induced the overexpression of p53 protein (Tsipis et al., 2007). Consequently, the expression of bcl-2 or P53 protein in myocytes of human hearts with infarction may play an important role in the protection or the acceleration of cellular damage after infarction (Figure 1, Figure 2).

2.6.3 Apoptosis and heart failure

Congestive heart failure occurs as a late manifestation in diverse cardiovascular diseases characterized by volume or pressure overload and significant loss of contractile muscle mass. Cardiac output is initially maintained in these disorders by the development of compensatory myocardial hypertrophy and dilatation. However, the early mechanical adaptations to growth stimulus soon fall short of adequate compensation. The mechanism by which compensatory

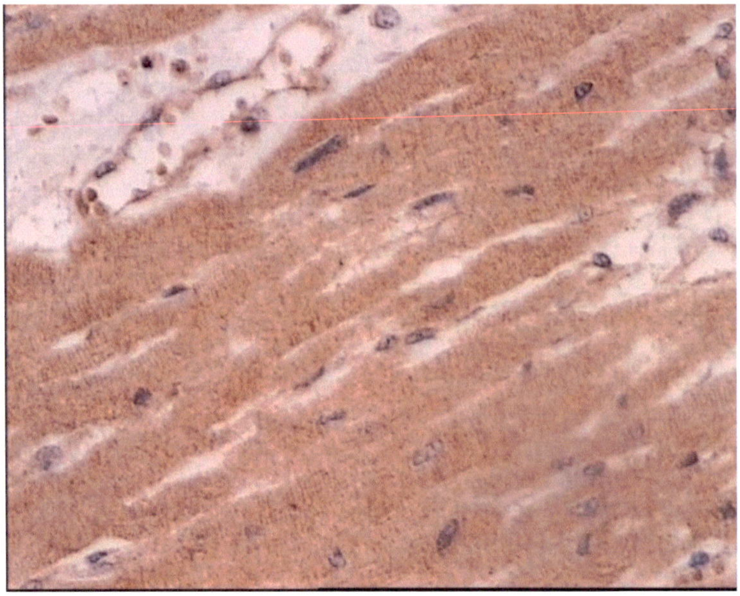

Fig. 1. Immunohistochemical staining for Bcl-2 in myocardial infarction (X400).

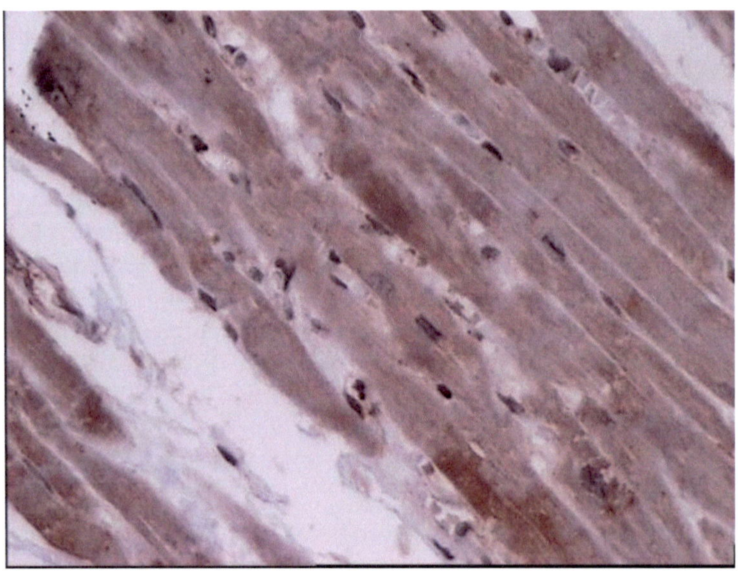

Fig. 2. Immunohistochemical staining for P53 in myocardial infarction (X400).

response triggered by myocardial failure culminates in myocardial dysfunction is not clear. In the past few years, several scientists have proposed apoptosis as the basis of the inexorable decline in ventricular systolic function (Narula et al., 2000). Although the initial studies reported unrealistically high levels of apoptosis in failed heart (as much as 35%), recent studies show an apoptosis rates of <1% (TUNEL-positive cells) during heart failure (Kang & Izumo, 2000). Because of the limitations with TUNEL staining and the difficulties in interpreting these findings, the use of TUNEL alone to detect the presence of apoptosis is not sufficient to define the role of apoptosis in heart failure. Later studies have consistently shown that approximately 80–250 heart muscle cells per 10^5 cardiac nuclei commit suicide at any given time in patients with late-stage dilated cardiomyopathy. In contrast, the base-line rate of apoptosis in healthy human hearts is only one to ten cardiac myocytes per 10^5 nuclei (Anversa & Kajstura, 1998; Yue et al., 1998). Even though the rate of apoptosis in heart failure is relatively low in absolute numbers, it is significantly higher than that in the normal heart, which has essentially negligible baseline apoptosis. Recently, animal models of heart failure incorporating transgenic technology have confirmed that very low levels of myocyte apoptosis, levels that are four- to tenfold lower than those seen in human heart failure, are sufficient to cause a lethal, dilated cardiomyopathy (Wencker et al., 2003).

It has been long believed that apoptosis does not occur in terminally differentiated cells such as adult cardiomyocytes. However, all mechanisms responsible for induction of apoptosis are operative in myocytes and are particularly activated during heart failure. Actually, the onset of myocardial failure leads to systemic and myocardial neurohumoral alterations and cytokine expression to maintain cardiac output. Upregulation of these adaptive responses also induces growth response and leads to compensatory myocardial hypertrophy and dilatation. Cardiac myocytes differentiate and withdraw from the cell cycle during the neonatal period, and persistent growth stimulus in the adult myocardium (such as that in heart failure) is perceived as a contradictory genetic demand, and programmed cell death occurs (Narula et al., 2000). P53 (tumor suppressor protein) is involved in the regulation of cell cycle progression in response to DNA damage. This p53 typically causes the cell to delay its entry into S phase until the damage has been repaired. P53 also is involved in triggering an apoptotic response in instances in which the damage is too severe to repair. P53 is a transcriptional regulator of the bcl-2 and bax genes. P53 mediates apoptosis through a linear pathway involving bax transactivation, Bax translocation from the cytosol to membranes, cytochrome c release from mitochondria, and caspase-9 activation, followed by the activation of caspase-3, -6, and -7 (Kim et al., 1994; Shen & White, 2001). P53 down-regulates the antiapoptotic gene product Bcl-2 and up-regulates the proapoptotic gene product Bax. Immunohistochemistry of p53 and antiapoptotic Bcl-2 protein demonstrated higher levels of both of these proteins in heart failure as compared with normal hearts (Figure 3, Figure 4). Tsipis et al. have observed that the percentage of p53- and bcl-2 positive samples in the end-stage dilated cardiomyopathy was 100% (20/20 diseased group samples). A 2- and 2.5-fold increase in p53 and bcl-2 positive samples was observed in the diseased group as compared with the control group. The diseased group had a larger number of samples with strong p53 staining as compared with the control group, which demonstrated weak p53 staining. Bcl-2 staining in the positive samples of the diseased group was generally weak as in the control group (Tsipis et al., 2010). Latif and colleagues, in a quantitation of the bcl-2 family of proteins after Western Immunoprobing, demonstrated a 2.9- and 5.35-fold increase in the levels of Bax and of Bcl-2, respectively,

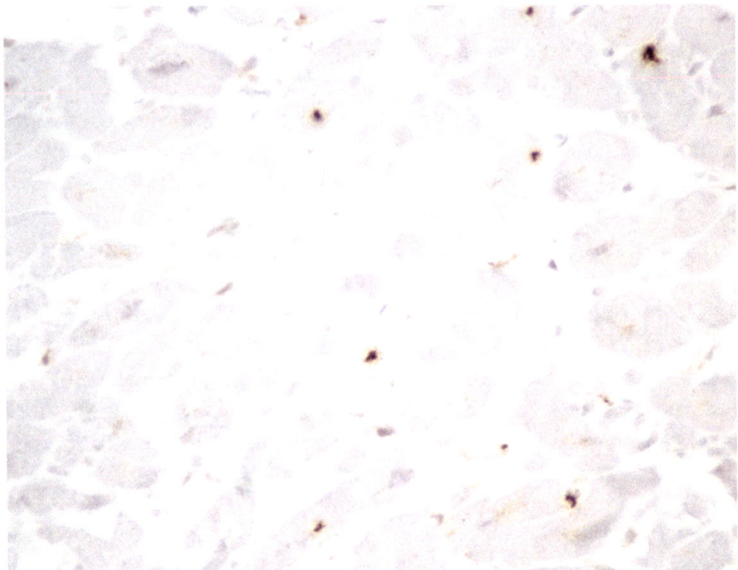

Fig. 3. Immunohistochemical staining for p53 protein in dilated cardiomyopathy (X400).

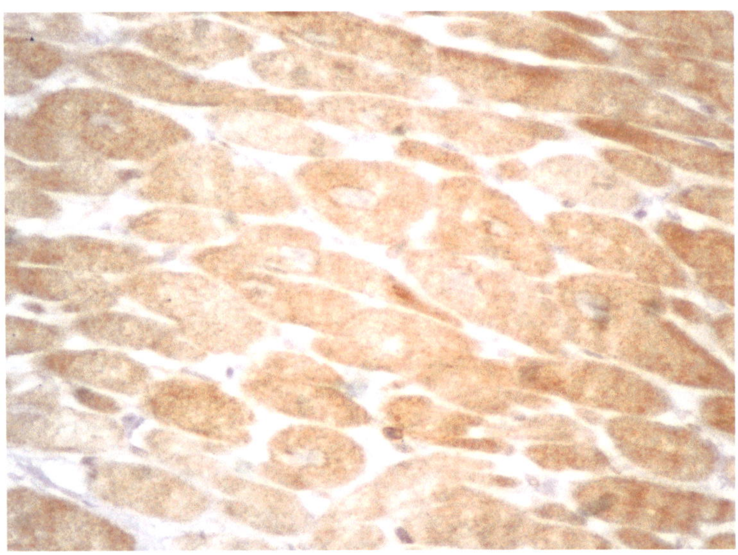

Fig. 4. Immunohistochemical staining for bcl-2 in dilated cardiomyopathy (X400).

in patients with dilated cardiomyopathy (Latif et al., 2000). Narula and colleagues demonstrated a release of cytochrome c from mitochondria in patients with heart failure (Narula et al., 2000). In the study of Tsipis et .al, increased expression of P53 protein was seen, but p53 up-regulates the proapoptotic gene product Bax (Tsipis et al., 2010). Elevated levels of Bax and Bak may mediate the release of cytochrome c, as it has been demonstrated that Bax and Bak accelerate the opening of the voltage-dependent anion channel (Latif et al., 2000; Shimizu et al., 1999). These results suggest that increased expression of p53 may be associated with apoptosis in heart failure of end-stage dilated cardiomyopathy. Moreover, various factors present in the failing myocardium have been shown to stimulate apoptosis in cardiac myocytes. Such factors include inflammatory cytokines, reactive oxygen species, nitric oxide, hypoxia, reperfusion, growth factors, and mechanical stretch (Foo et al., 2005). Ventricular decompensation and failure impose an elevated diastolic load on myocytes, resulting in stretching of sarcomeres and the stimulation of multiple second messenger systems which have been linked to the initiation of myocyte reactive hypertrophy in the pathologic heart. Abnormal levels of resting tension may lead to the local release of angiotensin II (Ang II) and the induction of programmed cell death in the myocardium. Sarcomere elongation in vitro results in Ang II release and activation of p53 and p53-dependent genes (Leri et al., 1998). Moreover, overstretching appears to be coupled with oxidant stress, expression of Fas, programmed cell death, architectural rearrangement of myocytes, and impairment in force development of the myocardium (Cheng et al., 1995). Using Western blotting, Olivetti et al. demonstrated a 2.4-fold increase in bcl-2 in patients with heart failure (Olivetti et al., 1997). However, the expression of Bax protein was not altered in the diseased group. This low expression of Bax protein may represent the prevalence of bcl-2 compensatory mechanism. The elevated presence of p53-positive cells, as demonstrated by immunohistochemistry, suggest that apoptosis may be significantly higher in dilated cardiomyopathy than that in the normal heart. On the other hand, increased expression of the antiapoptotic protein bcl-2 in human myocardium with dilated cardiomyopathy may be a compensation for the loss of myocytes and a possible compensatory antiapoptotic mechanism in the diseased group (Tsipis et al., 2010). In conclusion the etiology of heart failure in dilated cardiomyopathy involves multiple agents. The heart failure involves not only the contractile dysfunction, but also the progressive loss of myocytes by apoptosis. The elevated expression of proapoptotic is associated with progressive loss of myocytes in heart failure, and the increased expression of antiapoptotic proteins represent a possible compensatory mechanism. The prevalence of the apoptotic mechanism or this of compensatory antiapoptotic may influence the evolution of heart failure in cardiomyopathy.

3. Conclusions

Cells are poised between survival and apoptosis, and their fate rests on a balance of powerful intracellular and extracellular forces, whose signals constantly act upon and counteract each other. In many circumstances, apoptosis is a self-protective programmed mechanism that leads to the suicide of a cell when its survival is deemed detrimental to the organism. In other instances, apoptosis is a pathological process that contributes to many disorders. Thus, the pharmacological manipulation of apoptosis represents an active frontier of drug development. Recognition of the inducing mechanisms of apoptosis could open up ways to inhibit cell death in cardiovascular tissues and possibly help to define targets for future drug design. Furthermore, end-stage events of apoptosis, such as the activation of downstream caspases are essentially uniform in all cell types; although some regulatory mechanisms may be unique to cells in cardiovascular tissues. Elucidation of proapoptotic and antiapoptotic mechanisms in cardiomyocytes and vascular smooth muscle cells could delineate potential targets for intervention. In conclusion, various factors present in the diseased myocardium have been shown to stimulate apoptosis in cardiac myocytes. Changes in the induction of genes promoting or opposing apoptosis may modulate the total amount of myocyte damage. There is still a need to clarify the role played by different genetic and environmental factors implicated in cell death or survival.

4. References

Ameisen JC. From cell activation to cell depletion. The programmed cell death hypothesis of AIDS pathogenesis. Adv Exp Med Biol 1995; 374:139-163.

Anversa P & Kajstura J. Myocyte Cell Death in the Diseased Heart. Circulation Research. 1998;82:1231-1233.

Bennett Martin R. Apoptosis in the cardiovascular system, Heart 2002; 87: 480-487

Brenner D. & Mak TW. Mitochondrial cell death effectors. Curr. Opin. Cell Biol 2009; 21(6):871-7

Chalah & Khosravi-Far R. The mitochondrial death pathway. Adv. Exp. Med. Biol. 2008;615:25-45.

Chamond R.R, Añón J.C, Aguilary C.M. & Pasadas F.G. Apoptosis and disease. Alergol Inmunol Clin 1999; 14(6): 367-374

Cheng W, Li B, Kajstura J, Li P, Wolin MS, Sonnenblick EH, Hintze TH, Olivetti G & Anversa P. Stretch-induced programmed myocyte cell death. J Clin Invest. 1995;96:2247–2259.

Degterev A & Yuan J. Expansion and evolution of cell death programmes. Nat. Rev. Mol. Cell Biol. 2008;9(5), 378–90.

Foo RSY, Mani K. & Kitsis RN. Death begets failure in the heart. J Clin Invest. 2005;115: 565–571.

Gustafsson A.B. & Gottlieb R.A. Mechanisms of apoptosis in the heart. J Clin Immunol. 2003;23(6):447-59

Haunstetter A & Izumo S. Apoptosis: Basic mechanisms and implications for cardiovascular disease. Circulation Research. 1998;82:1111-1129.

Humphreys R.C. & Halpern W. Trail receptors: targets for cancer therapy. Adv. Exp. Med. Biol. 2008;615:127-58.

Kang P & Izumo S. Apoptosis and heart failure: A critical review of the literature. Circ Res. 2000;86 (11): 1107-13.

Kim KK, Soonpaa MH, Daud AI, Koh GY, Kim JS & Field LJ. Tumor suppressor gene expression during normal and pathologic myocardial growth. J Biol Chem. 1994; 269 (36): 22607-13.

Krijnen PA, Nijmeijer R, Meijer CJ, Visser CA, Hack CE & Niessen HW. Apoptosis in myocardial ischemia and infarction. J Clin Pathol. 2002;55(11):801-811.

Kockx M M & Knaapen MW. The role of apoptosis in vascular disease. J Pathol. 2000;190(3):267-80

Kumar V, Abbas Ak, Fausto N. Robbins and Cotran: Pathologic Basis Of Disease. 7th ed. Philadelphia: Elsevier Saunders;2005:26-32

Kurokawa M & Kornbluth S. Caspases and kinases in a death grip. Cell. 2009;138(5), 838–54.

Latif N, Khan MA, Birks E, O'Farrell A, Westbrook J, Dunn MJ & Yacoub MH. Upregulation of the Bcl-2 family of proteins in end stage heart failure. J Am Coll Cardiol. 2000;35 (7):1769-1777.

Leri A, Claudio PP, Li Q, Wang X, Reiss K, Wang S, Malhotra A, Kajstura J & Anversa P. Stretch-mediated release of Angiotensin II induces myocyte apoptosis by activating p53 that enhances the local renin-angiotensin system and decreases the bcl-2-to-bax Protein ratio in the cell. J Clin Invest. 1998;101(7): 1326-42.

Logue SE & Martin SJ. Caspase activation cascades in apoptosis. Biochem. Soc. Trans. 2008;36(1) :1-9

Narula J, kolodgie FD & Virmani R. Apoptosis And cardiomyopathy. Curr Opin in Cardiol 2000;15:183-88

Olivetti G, Abbi R, Quaini F, Kajstura J, Cheng W, Nitahara JA, Quaini E, Di Loreto C, Beltrami CA, Krajewski S, Reed JC & Anversa P. Apoptosis in the failing human heart. N Engl J Med. 1997;336(16): 1131-41.

Pollard T & Earnshaw W. Cell biology. Updated Edition 2004. Philadelphia: Saunders. An imprint of Elsevier, 2004; 772-776.

Rubin E, Gorstein F, Rubin R, Schwarting R, Strayer D. Rubin´s Pathology: Clinicopathologic Foundations of Medicine. 4th ed. Philadelphia: Lippincott Williams & Wilkins; 2005:566-70

Saraste A, Pulkki K, Kallajoki M, Hennksen K, Parvinen M & Voipio-Pulkki LM. Apoptosis in human acute myocardial infarction. Circulation 1997; 95(2):320–3.

Shen Y & White E. P53-dependent apoptosis pathways. Adv Cancer Res. 2001; 82:55-84.

Shimizu S, Narita M & Tsujimoto Y. Bcl-2 family proteins regulate the release of apoptogenic cytochrome c by the mitochondrial channel VDAC. Nature 1999;399:483-87

Tsipis A, Athanassiadou AM, Athanassiadou P, Kavantzas N, Agrogiannis G & Patsouris E. Apoptosis-related factors p53, Bcl-2 in acute and chronic ischemic cardiac disorders. Virchows Arch 2007;451(2):483-84

Tsipis A, Athanassiadou AM, Athanassiadou P, Kavantzas N, Agrogiannis G & Patsouris E. Apoptosis-related factors p53, Bcl-2 and the defects of force transmission in dilated cardiomyopathy. Pathol Res Pract 2010;206(9):625-30

Vermes I, Haanen C, Steffens-Nakken H & Reutelingsperger C. A novel assay for apoptosis. Flow cytometric detection of phosphatidilserine expression on early apoptotic cell using fluorescein labelled Annexin V. J Immunol Methods 1995; 184(1):39-51.

Wencker D, Chandra M, Nguyen K, Miao W, Garantziotis S, Factor SM, Shirani J, Armstrong RC & Kitsis RN. A mechanistic role for cardiac myocyte apoptosis in heart failure. J Clin Invest. 2003;111(10):1497–504

Yuan J. Apoptosis Pathway Description. Revised November 2010. www.Cellsignal.com

Yue TL, Ma XL, Wang X, Romanic AM, Liu GL, Louden C, Gu JL, Kumar S, Poste G , Ruffolo RR Jr & Feuerstein GZ. Possible involvement of stress-activated protein kinase signaling pathway and Fas receptor expression in prevention of ischemia/reperfusion-induced cardiomyocyte apoptosis by carvedilol. Circ Res. 1998;82(2): 166–74.

10

Cardiac Myocytes and Mechanosensation

Byambajav Buyandelger and Ralph Knöll
British Heart Foundation – Centre for Research Excellence, National Heart & Lung Institute, Imperial College, London, UK

1. Introduction

Mechanosensation is a fundamental process in biology and may have been developed by the early cells in response to hypo-osmotic stress [1]. With the evolution of different cell types and the appearance of multi-cellular organisms the mechanisms of mechanosensation and the corresponding transmission of signals became more complex and evolved in different cell types differently [2]. Particularly in cardiac myocytes different mechanosensory protein - complexes can be found: i) cell membrane associated ii) intracellular embedded iii) sarcomere related (figure 1). All these various signalosomes are sensitive to different types of mechanical signals. For example, a deformation of the cell membrane may be detected by cell membrane associated signalosomes, such as stretch activated channels (SAC), angiotensin receptors, the caveolae, and integrin mediated signalling. Depending on severity and duration, these events may also be sensed by intermediate filaments (IF) and or even by the sarcomere associated signalosomes. However it is important to differentiate between different types of stresses, such as the normal "stress" (σ) which is physically defined by:

$$\sigma = \frac{F}{A}$$

(where F is the applied force per unit area (A), dimension: N/m^2)
And "shear stress (τ)", where the applied force (F(S) = shear force) acts parallel to the area (A) (dimension: N/m^2):

$$\tau = \frac{F(S)}{A}$$

Other types of physical stresses such as compression and torsion may also occur and are equally important. Distinct from stress is "strain" (ε) which is physically defined by:

$$\varepsilon = \frac{\Delta L}{L}$$

(where L is the initial length and ΔL is the change in length, dimensionless)
Importantly different types of stress do cause strain or any type of deformation, or in other words, strain is the consequence of stress. Cells are able to detect strain via changes in conformation of proteins or macromolecular protein complexes, but the precise molecular mechanisms remains often unclear. In this regard two different models have been

developed to explain mechanosensory behaviour: i) the localized and ii) the decentralized model. The localized model proposes that changes at the cell membrane are sensed immediately and are transmitted from there to other parts of the cell. In contrast the decentralized model proposes that any force applied at the cell surface will cause deformations of elastic cytoskeletal components and as such can be sensed far away from the area of impact. The latter model is also called the "tensegrity" model (derived from: tensional integrity) based on Buckminster Fuller's geodesic dome.

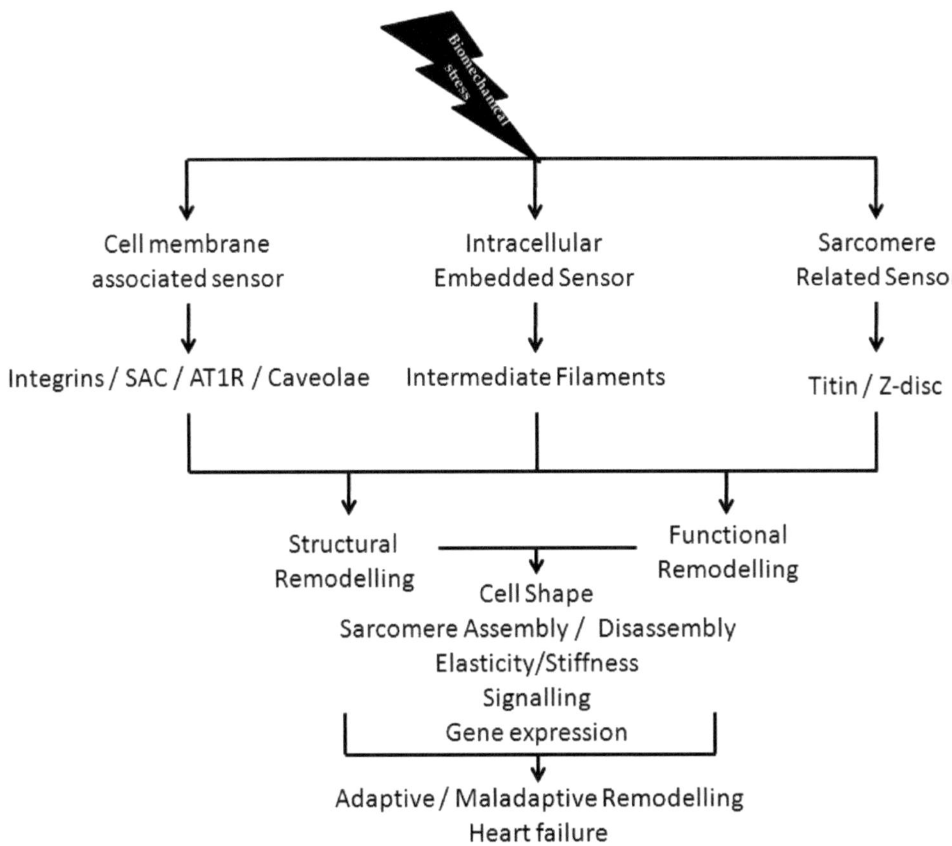

Legend to figure 1: The figure summarizes the most important stress and strain sensors present in cardiac myocytes. All sensors affect cell shape, sarcomere assembly and disassembly, elasticity and stiffness as well as gene expression which will finally decide whether adaptive or maladaptive remodelling will take place (abbreviations: SAC: stretch activated channels, AT1R: angiotensin II type 1 receptor).

Fig. 1. Summary of cardiac myocyte stress and strain sensors

Here we shall introduce the reader into different concepts of cardiac mechanosensation:

1. Receptor / cell membrane mediated mechanosensation (centralized models):
   i. Integrin mediated effects
   ii. Stretch activated channels
   iii. Angiotensin receptor mediated mechanosensation and other receptors
   iv. Caveolae
2. Intracellular stretch sensors:
   i. Intermediate filaments
3. Intrasarcomeric mechanosensors
   i. Z-disc associated mechanosensor complex
   ii. N2A and N2B - titin mechanosensor complex
   iii. Titin kinase mechanosensor complex

These different mechanosensory signalosomes integrate a variety of mechanical stimuli such as mechanical stress, shear stress, torsion and compression as well as the resulting strains into electrochemical and biochemical signals. They are translated into short term effects (i.e. changes in ion concentrations may lead to changes in action potential durations or changes in calcium concentration which may lead to changes in kinase and phosphatase activities) and long term effects via changes in gene expression.

1.1 Integrin mediated effects

Integrins are large heterodimeric transmembrane proteins, consisting of α and β subunits. They act as receptors and are enriched at focal adhesions or costameres, sites where the Z-discs become attached to the cell membrane. The extracellular part of the molecule interacts with fibronectin, laminin or collagen, whereas the intracellular domains interact with signalling proteins such as integrin linked kinase (ILK), focal adhesion kinase (FAK), or cytoskeletal components such as actin, talin and vinculin. As such, integrins link the extracellular matrix (ECM) to the cytoplasm and are able to respond to changes in the composition of the ECM as well as with regard to forces transmitted via the ECM and vice versa (inside out and outside in signalling). They are linked via Gα proteins to cAMP and protein kinase A (PKA) mediated effects, they activate via FAK and SH2 phospholipase C (PLC) as well as phosphatidyl inositol 3 kinase (PI3K) and Akt mediated survival pathways (figure 1, 2). Integrins activate as well Src kinase which phosphorylates particularly p130 CAS, which is an important mechanosensory element [3]. Indeed tyrosine kinase activation, such as Src activation, has been observed as early as one minute after stretch and as such is one of the earliest observable effects following mechanical stimuli [4]. It has been postulated, although not yet shown, that orphan tyrosine kinases such as Src might become activated via conformational changes upon membrane stretch. If verified, this could be another mechanism whereby stress is directly translated into enzyme activity (please see also titin kinase chapter). Integrins are also linked via Ras mediated signalling to mitogen activated protein kinases (MAPK) such as ERK and as such to serum response factor (SRF) mediated transcriptional events.

In this regard, it is no surprise that loss of integrins in genetically altered animals is associated with severe heart failure [5] and that human mutations in laminin alpha 4 (LAMA4) and ILK are associated with dilated cardiomyopathy (DCM) [6]. Although integrins are meanwhile well established mechanosensors, other transmembrane protein systems such as the dystrophin associated glycoprotein complex (DAG) are certainly as well important, but they are less well studied with regard to mechanosensation and mechanotransduction.

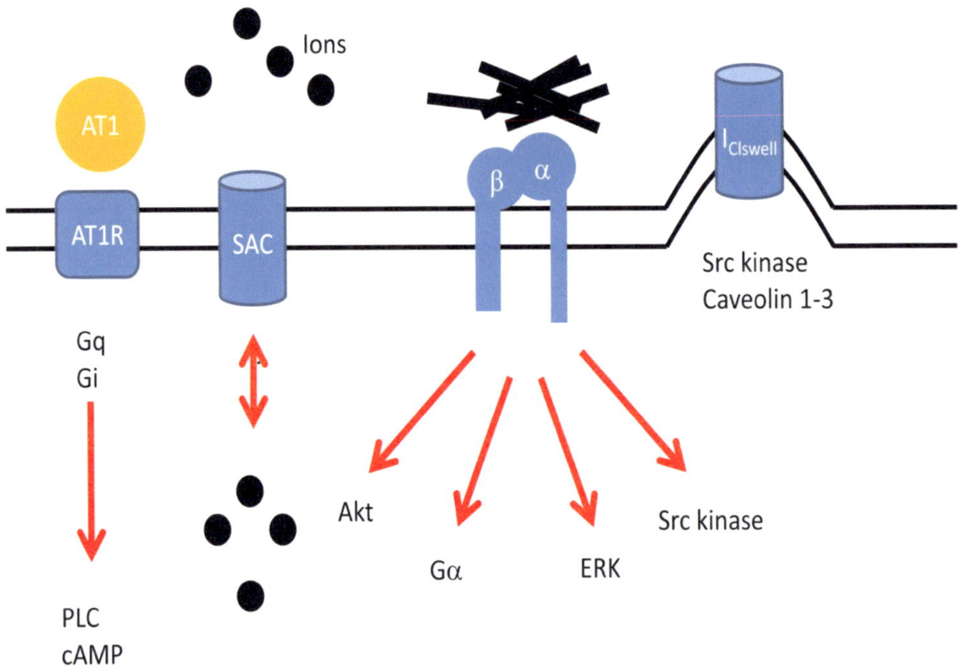

Legend to figure 2: The figure depicts four major membrane associated mechanosensory pathways, namely the angiotensin receptor (AT1R) mediated pathway, stretch activated channels (SAC), integrins and caveolae (abbreviations: Gq, Gi, Gα - Gq, Gi, and Gα mediated effects, PLC - phospholipase C, ERK - extracellular regulated kinase, Akt - Akt kinase, black dots indicate ions such as K^+, Na^+, Ca^{++}, Cl^-, etc.).

Fig. 2. Membrane associated mechanosensory pathways

1.2 Stretch activated channels (SAC)

Stretch activated or stretch gated ion channels respond to strain by opening or closing their pores. They were first found in skeletal muscle [7] and since then have been identified in every living cell of every kingdom, including Archaea, Bacteria, Plant, Fungi and Eukaryote (figure 1, 2). These channels open, or even close, upon membrane stretch and allow ions such as chloride, calcium, potassium, and sodium which are permeable to this channel, to follow the electrochemical gradient and to change the membrane potential. However mechanosensitivity is not restricted to a small subset of ion channels, in fact many proteins and voltage gated channels are mechanosensitive. The difficulty is to identify whether or not the mechanosensitivity of a single protein or channel is biologically relevant [8].

At least two different mechanisms can be made responsible for the opening mechanism:

i. stretch from the plasma membrane is transferred directly to the channel resulting in a conformational change (lipid bilayer tension or stretch model) and
ii. a spring like tether, connecting ECM, channel and intracellular space, responds to changes by opening the channel (spring like tether model).

Mechanosensitive channels such as the L-type calcium channel are particularly important in cardiac myocytes where they have been made at least partially responsible for post-ischemic arrhythmias. Other effects include their ability to respond to a stretch early in the action potential and to produce a repolarizing tendency whereas if stretched late, the channel causes depolarization, an effect called: "reversal potential" [9-10]. Although it is a general principle in biology to amplify a signal via changes in ion concentrations, which supports a role for SAC in mechanosensation, inhibition of SAC by using Gadolinium is unable to inhibit major stretch induced features such as immediate early gene expression or the increase in protein synthesis [11]. Therefore additional effects must be at play.

1.3 Angiotensin receptor mediated mechanosensation and other receptors

While mechanical activation affects directly transmembrane proteins and causes via direct or indirect effects conformational changes which elicit profound intracellular signaltransduction cascades, another mechanism proposes that mechanical stimulation leads to autocrine angiotensin II release which activates the angiotensin II type 1 (AT1) receptor [12]. As such $G_{q/11}$ and G_i mediated effects, which lead to phospholipase C activation and increased intracellular calcium concentrations and/or a decrease in cAMP via adenylyl cyclase inhibition, may cause long term effects such as cardiac myocyte hypertrophy.
However an even more important mechanism has been discovered only recently when it was demonstrated that the AT1 receptor, even without binding to its ligand, can be activated by mechanical stimulation [13]. In addition, beta receptors have also been implicated in mechanosensation, although evidence for their role here is available, but they are less well studied with regard to mechanosensation (please see for a brief overview [14]). Angiotensin converting enzyme (ACE) inhibitors, angiotensin receptor blockers and beta blockers belong to the most powerful therapeutic tools in cardiovascular medicine. Based on the direct involvement of the AT1 receptor in mechanosensation, their actions might at least be partially attributable to their effects here.

1.4 Caveolae

Caveolae are small (50 - 100 nm) invaginations of the plasma membrane found in a variety of different cell types, including cardiac myocytes. They may represent a cellular compartment where ion channels such as the mechanosensitive $I_{Clswell}$, signal transduction components such as Src kinase and caveolins 1-3, among others, can be found enriched (figure 2). $I_{Clswell}$ channels are important for intracellular homeostasis, particularly during hypo-osmotic conditions. Only recently it was shown that caveolae provide significant membrane reserve [15] and that caveolae are important for proper activation of $I_{Clswell}$ channel and as such can be seen as a mechanosensitive structure [16].

2. Intracellular stretch sensors

2.1 Intermediate filaments

Intermediate filaments (IF) are a group of related proteins that share common structural and sequence features, such as amino and carboxy-terminus globular parts which surround the alpha helical rod domain. They were initially named after their diameter which is with ~ 10 nm in the between of actin filaments and myosins and were subdivided into types I - VI. Most types of IFs are cytoplasmic, except for the lamins which are present in the nucleus or in the nuclear membrane. At least 91 different diseases are associated with mutations in these genes and as such a comprehensive discussion of all of them within the context of this chapter is impossible. However desmin is a major IF and present in almost every cell type. In cardiac myocytes desmin connects desmosomes with other organelles such as the Z-disc or the nucleus. Mutations in this gene result in a variety of different cardiac diseases such as desmin related myopathy [17-18], limb girdle muscular dystrophy [19], dilated cardiomyopathy (DCM) [20], arrhythmogenic right ventricular cardiomyopathy (ARVC) [21], cardiomyopathy with advanced AV block and arrhythmia [22], familial restrictive cardiomyopathy [23] and DCM with conduction system defects [24]. IFs interact with a variety of different proteins and because of their elasticity they are able to sense any deformation of cellular structure. As such, IFs have been linked to mechanosensation and might well have a function via "tensegration", i. e. their elasticity may enable them to change their conformation in response to any type of mechanical stimulation. As such, lamin A/C knockout animals develop severe heart failure most probably due to defects in mechanosensation. In this regard, lamin A/C mutations are one of the major causes of DCM and associated arrhythmia and it is interesting to note, that treatment of animals carrying human LMN A/C mutations with carvedilol an agent with alpha and beta receptor blocking properties improves heart failure significantly [25].

3. Intrasarcomeric mechanosensors

3.1 Z-disc associated mechanosensor complex (MLP/Telethonin)

While all other so far discussed mechanosensors are associated with cell structures found in almost every other cell types, the intrasarcomeric mechanosensors are skeletal and cardiac myocyte specific (figure 3). Any pharmacological intervention at this level might offer the possibility of targeting cross striated myocytes specifically.

Moreover, all other mechanosensors are probably able to sense primarily "external stimuli", whereas the sarcomere associated signalosomes are able to sense force, stress and strain produced primarily within the cell. In addition, all sarcomere associated sensors are directly or indirectly associated with titin, the giant molecular ruler which spans half the sarcomere from the Z-disc to the M-band.

In this regard, the sarcomeric Z-disc which is probably one of the most complex macromolecular structures in biology contains at its periphery a variety of small molecules, namely muscle LIM protein (MLP, CSRP3) and telethonin (TCAP), which interact with the very aminoterminus of titin [26]. Interestingly MLP deficient papillary muscles develop a defect in passive elasticity and isolated cardiac myocytes have a defect in their BNP response following stretch whereas other signal transduction pathways, such as G_q mediated effects are still able to induce this gene. A human mutation in the MLP gene (W4R-MLP), significantly associated with DCM, was also identified and shown to lead to a significant loss of affinity between MLP and telethonin (TCAP). In comparison to the MLP knockout animals, W4R-MLP knock in mice develop a similar phenotype, for example they develop myocardial hypertrophy followed by heart failure, their papillary muscles develop less stiffness when stretched and isolated cardiac myocytes exhibit a similar defect in BNP response [27-28], albeit the effects are smaller and are gene dosage and age dependent. In this regard, MLP was also shown to shuttle into the nucleus and to be necessary for myocardial hypertrophy [29,28].

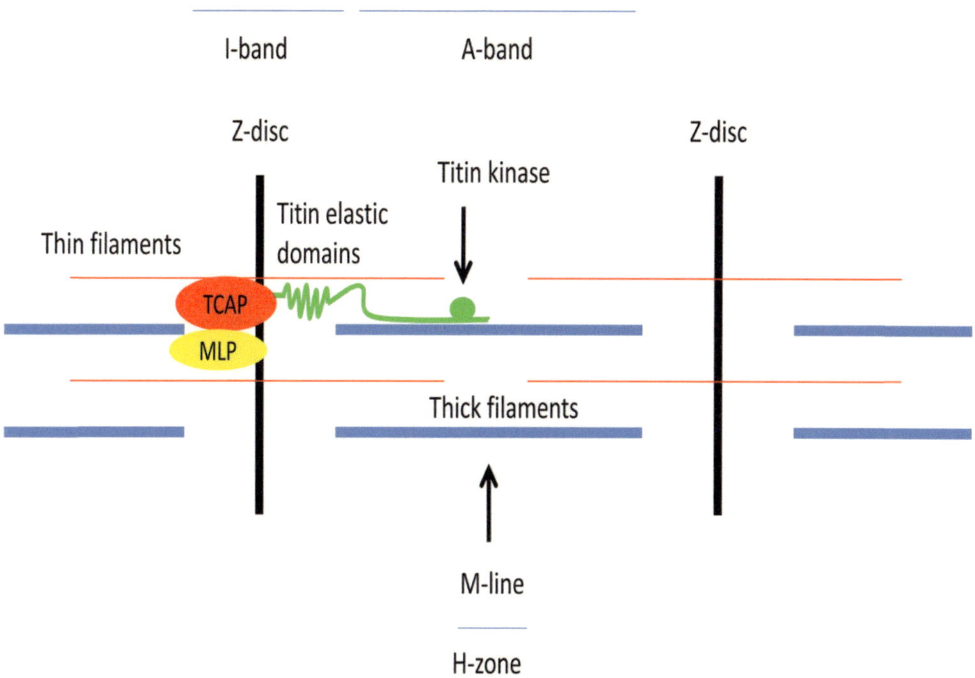

Legend to figure 3: The figure shows a schematic diagram of a sarcomere and depicts major structural elements. Please note the green titin molecule, spanning from the Z-disc to the M-line. At the aminoterminus TCAP (Telethonin) and MLP (muscle LIM protein) are localized. Titin's elastic domains are localized within the I-band and the kinase domain is localized close to the M-line.

Fig. 3. Sarcomere associated mechanosensors

Moreover, it was also shown that MLP interacts with and is necessary for the activation of the serine threonine phosphatase calcineurin (PP2A), which is an important link to myocardial hypertrophy via transcription factors such as nuclear factor of activated T-cells (NFAT) [30].
In addition, MLP interacts with the integrin linked kinase (ILK) and as such provides a molecular link between the sarcomeric Z-disc and integrin mediated signalling (please see also chapter integrins) [6]. However, in addition to MLP mutations, telethonin mutations have also been shown to be associated with types of muscular dystrophy as well as with hypertrophic cardiomyopathy (HCM) and DCM [31-32,27,33-34].
In summary, MLP and telethonin are likely to be involved in Z-disc mediated stress sensation, and mutations in these genes are involved in the pathogenesis of various diseases, but the precise molecular mechanism remains to be defined [35].

3.2 N2A and N2B – Titin mechanosensor complexes (FHL1/MARP)

With a molecular mass of up to 4.2 MDa, titin is the largest molecule in biology and well known for its multiple functions such as serving as a molecular ruler, its importance during embryonic development, and for its role in providing mechanical stability - just to name a few. However the molecule contains at its I-band region several elastic domains, such as the distal and proximal Immunoglobulin (Ig) domains, the N2B and N2BA domains, the N2A domain, which is embedded within the N2BA domain, as well as the PEVK domain. All of

these domains unfold upon stretch and release and/or store energy during every cycle of contraction and relaxation (i. e. entropic springs [36]). Differential splicing particularly of the N2B and the more compliant N2BA domains add an additional level of complexity, which is of course species specific, depends on the developmental stage, the environment as well as on different states of disease, where DCM and hypothyroidism lead to increased stiffness [37]. Moreover, PKA and PKG mediated phosphorylation causes the elastic domains to "soften" whereas PKC mediated effects causes them to "stiffen" (figure 3).
The N2B domain binds specifically to four and a half LIM protein 1 (FHL1), which in turn is the core of a signalosome consisting of RAF, MEK1/2, and ERK2, thus connecting growth factor mediated Gq signalling to titin extensibility and finally to changes in gene expression. Interestingly, loss of FHL1 blunts pathologic hypertrophy and as such inhibition of this pathway might be beneficial [38].
Another important pathway is linked to the N2A elastic titin domain, were the muscle ankyrin repeat proteins (MARP) including cardiac ankyrin repeat protein (CARP), ankrd2/Arpp and DARP interact to constitute a signalosome which responds to passive stretch *in vitro* [39].

3.3 Titin kinase mechanosensor complex

While titin's elastic I-band domains may be able to sense strain, titin's amino-terminus, which is anchored within the Z-disc and its carboxy-terminus, anchored within the M-line, may well be able or may at least be involved in the sensation of stress. Interestingly titin's M-line (or better H-band) domain contains a mechanically modulated kinase able to bind and to phosphorylate nbr1 and p62 (SQSTM1) *in vitro*. MURF1 and 2 (and probably MURF3 which has not been analyzed yet) also bind to this complex and will translocate into the nucleus upon mechanical inactivity, where they downregulate and or induce the nuclear export of SRF and as such aggravate the transcriptional atrophy programme [40]. This is supported by the R279W-Titin kinase mutation which is associated with hereditary myopathy with early respiratory failure (HMERF) and which leads to a dramatic loss of affinity to nbr1 [41]. Additional evidence for this model is supported by in vitro experiments whereby stretching of the kinase domain leads to activation of the kinase, thus effectively linking mechanosensation to kinase activity ("mechanozymatics") [42]. Moreover titin's kinase domain is linked via nbr1 and p62 to autophagy, a process of regulated protein and or organelle turnover [43].

4. Summary

Every cell is capable of mechanical stress sensation either via local or decentralized molecular mechanisms and to transform these signals into electrochemical and biochemical mediators. Because of their force generating ability cardiac myocytes developed additional sarcomere titin I-band related strain and Z-disc as well as M-line related stress sensors. It is a general principle in biology to amplify a signal via an increase in local ion concentrations as such SAC play certainly a major role in nerve and muscle cells. Mechanical stimulation also might lead via conformational changes to the direct activation of tyrosine kinases and or the titin kinase - an effect which might be called "mechanozymatics". Direct activation of AT1 receptors via mechanical stimuli has been shown and in this context it might well be possible that other receptors, such as β-receptors, play a role in mechanosensation as well.

Mutations in components of any of the above mentioned systems have been found to cause muscle and or heart failure phenotypes (figure 1, 2) [44-45].

5. Abbreviations

Cardiovascular disease: CVD
Dilated cardiomyopathy: DCM
Extracellular matrix: ECM
Focal adhesion kinase: FAK
Hypertrophic cardiomyopathy: HCM
Immunoglobulin: Ig
Integrin linked kinase: ILK
Muscle Ankyrin Repeat Proteins: MARP
Muscle LIM protein: MLP, CSRP3
Nuclear factor of activated T-cells: NFAT
Protein kinase A, C, G: PKA/C/G
Sarcomere length: SL
Serum response factor: SRF
Telethonin: TCAP

6. References

[1] Kung C (2005) A possible unifying principle for mechanosensation. Nature 436 (7051):647-654. doi:nature03896 [pii] 10.1038/nature03896
[2] Knöll R, Hoshijima M, Chien K (2003) Cardiac mechanotransduction and implications for heart disease. J Mol Med Dec;81(12):750-756.
[3] Sawada Y, Tamada M, Dubin-Thaler BJ, Cherniavskaya O, Sakai R, Tanaka S, Sheetz MP (2006) Force sensing by mechanical extension of the Src family kinase substrate p130Cas. Cell 127 (5):1015-1026. doi:S0092-8674(06)01405-X [pii] 10.1016/j.cell.2006.09.044
[4] Sadoshima J, Izumo S (1997) The cellular and molecular response of cardiac myocytes to mechanical stress. Annu Rev Physiol 59:551-571.
[5] Shai SY, Harpf AE, Babbitt CJ, Jordan MC, Fishbein MC, Chen J, Omura M, Leil TA, Becker KD, Jiang M, Smith DJ, Cherry SR, Loftus JC, Ross RS (2002) Cardiac myocyte-specific excision of the beta1 integrin gene results in myocardial fibrosis and cardiac failure. Circulation research 90 (4):458-464.
[6] Knöll R, Postel R, Wang J, Kratzner R, Hennecke G, Vacaru AM, Vakeel P, Schubert C, Murthy K, Rana BK, Kube D, Knoll G, Schafer K, Hayashi T, Holm T, Kimura A, Schork N, Toliat MR, Nurnberg P, Schultheiss HP, Schaper W, Schaper J, Bos E, Den Hertog J, van Eeden FJ, Peters PJ, Hasenfuss G, Chien KR, Bakkers J (2007) Laminin-alpha4 and integrin-linked kinase mutations cause human cardiomyopathy via simultaneous defects in cardiomyocytes and endothelial cells. Circulation 116 (5):515-525
[7] Guharay F, Sachs F (1984) Stretch-activated single ion channel currents in tissue-cultured embryonic chick skeletal muscle. J Physiol 352:685-701
[8] Sachs F (2010) Stretch-activated ion channels: what are they? Physiology (Bethesda) 25 (1):50-56. doi:25/1/50 [pii] 10.1152/physiol.00042.2009

[9] Lab MJ (1978) Mechanically dependent changes in action potentials recorded from the intact frog ventricle. Circulation research 42 (4):519-528
[10] Zabel M, Koller BS, Sachs F, Franz MR (1996) Stretch-induced voltage changes in the isolated beating heart: importance of the timing of stretch and implications for stretch-activated ion channels. Cardiovasc Res 32 (1):120-130. doi:0008636396000892 [pii]
[11] Sadoshima J, Takahashi T, Jahn L, Izumo S (1992) Roles of mechano-sensitive ion channels, cytoskeleton, and contractile activity in stretch-induced immediate-early gene expression and hypertrophy of cardiac myocytes. Proc Natl Acad Sci U S A 89 (20):9905-9909
[12] Sadoshima J, Xu Y, Slayter HS, Izumo S (1993) Autocrine release of angiotensin II mediates stretch-induced hypertrophy of cardiac myocytes in vitro. Cell 75 (5):977-984
[13] Yasuda N, Akazawa H, Qin Y, Zou Y, Komuro I (2008) A novel mechanism of mechanical stress-induced angiotensin II type 1-receptor activation without the involvement of angiotensin II. Naunyn Schmiedebergs Arch Pharmacol 377 (4-6):393-399. doi:10.1007/s00210-007-0215-1
[14] Lab MJ (2006) Mechanosensitive-mediated interaction, integration, and cardiac control. Ann N Y Acad Sci 1080:282-300. doi:1080/1/282 [pii] 10.1196/annals.1380.022
[15] Kohl P, Cooper PJ, Holloway H (2003) Effects of acute ventricular volume manipulation on in situ cardiomyocyte cell membrane configuration. Prog Biophys Mol Biol 82 (1-3):221-227. doi:S0079610703000245 [pii]
[16] Kozera L, White E, Calaghan S (2009) Caveolae act as membrane reserves which limit mechanosensitive I(Cl,swell) channel activation during swelling in the rat ventricular myocyte. PLoS One 4 (12):e8312. doi:10.1371/journal.pone.0008312
[17] Dalakas MC, Dagvadorj A, Goudeau B, Park KY, Takeda K, Simon-Casteras M, Vasconcelos O, Sambuughin N, Shatunov A, Nagle JW, Sivakumar K, Vicart P, Goldfarb LG (2003) Progressive skeletal myopathy, a phenotypic variant of desmin myopathy associated with desmin mutations. Neuromuscul Disord 13 (3):252-258. doi:S0960896602002717 [pii]
[18] Dalakas MC, Park KY, Semino-Mora C, Lee HS, Sivakumar K, Goldfarb LG (2000) Desmin myopathy, a skeletal myopathy with cardiomyopathy caused by mutations in the desmin gene. N Engl J Med 342 (11):770-780. doi:10.1056/NEJM200003163421104
[19] Walter MC, Reilich P, Huebner A, Fischer D, Schroder R, Vorgerd M, Kress W, Born C, Schoser BG, Krause KH, Klutzny U, Bulst S, Frey JR, Lochmuller H (2007) Scapuloperoneal syndrome type Kaeser and a wide phenotypic spectrum of adult-onset, dominant myopathies are associated with the desmin mutation R350P. Brain 130 (Pt 6):1485-1496. doi:awm039 [pii] 10.1093/brain/awm039
[20] Li D, Tapscoft T, Gonzalez O, Burch P, Quinones M, Zoghbi W, Hill R, Bachinski L, Mann D, Roberts R (1999) Desmin mutation responsible for idiopathic dilated cardiomyopathy. Circulation 100 (5):461-464
[21] Klauke B, Kossmann S, Gaertner A, Brand K, Stork I, Brodehl A, Dieding M, Walhorn V, Anselmetti D, Gerdes D, Bohms B, Schulz U, Zu Knyphausen E, Vorgerd M, Gummert J, Milting H (2010) De novo desmin-mutation N116S is associated with arrhythmogenic right ventricular cardiomyopathy. Hum Mol Genet 19 (23):4595-4607. doi:ddq387 [pii] 10.1093/hmg/ddq387
[22] Otten E, Asimaki A, Maass A, van Langen IM, van der Wal A, de Jonge N, van den Berg MP, Saffitz JE, Wilde AA, Jongbloed JD, van Tintelen JP (2010) Desmin

mutations as a cause of right ventricular heart failure affect the intercalated disks. Heart Rhythm 7 (8):1058-1064. doi:S1547-5271(10)00398-X [pii] 10.1016/j.hrthm.2010.04.023

[23] Pruszczyk P, Kostera-Pruszczyk A, Shatunov A, Goudeau B, Draminska A, Takeda K, Sambuughin N, Vicart P, Strelkov SV, Goldfarb LG, Kaminska A (2007) Restrictive cardiomyopathy with atrioventricular conduction block resulting from a desmin mutation. Int J Cardiol 117 (2):244-253. doi:S0167-5273(06)00565-1 [pii] 10.1016/j.ijcard.2006.05.019

[24] Taylor MR, Slavov D, Ku L, Di Lenarda A, Sinagra G, Carniel E, Haubold K, Boucek MM, Ferguson D, Graw SL, Zhu X, Cavanaugh J, Sucharov CC, Long CS, Bristow MR, Lavori P, Mestroni L (2007) Prevalence of desmin mutations in dilated cardiomyopathy. Circulation 115 (10):1244-1251. doi:CIRCULATIONAHA.106.646778 [pii] 10.1161/CIRCULATIONAHA.106.646778

[25] Chandar S, Yeo LS, Leimena C, Tan JC, Xiao XH, Nikolova-Krstevski V, Yasuoka Y, Gardiner-Garden M, Wu J, Kesteven S, Karlsdotter L, Natarajan S, Carlton A, Rainer S, Feneley MP, Fatkin D (2010) Effects of mechanical stress and carvedilol in lamin A/C-deficient dilated cardiomyopathy. Circulation research 106 (3):573-582. doi:CIRCRESAHA.109.204388 [pii] 10.1161/CIRCRESAHA.109.204388

[26] Zou P, Pinotsis N, Lange S, Song YH, Popov A, Mavridis I, Mayans OM, Gautel M, Wilmanns M (2006) Palindromic assembly of the giant muscle protein titin in the sarcomeric Z-disk. Nature 439 (7073):229-233

[27] Knöll R, Hoshijima M, Hoffman HM, Person V, Lorenzen-Schmidt I, Bang ML, Hayashi T, Shiga N, Yasukawa H, Schaper W, McKenna W, Yokoyama M, Schork NJ, Omens JH, McCulloch AD, Kimura A, Gregorio CC, Poller W, Schaper J, Schultheiss HP, Chien KR (2002) The cardiac mechanical stretch sensor machinery involves a Z disc complex that is defective in a subset of human dilated cardiomyopathy. Cell 111 (7):943-955.

[28] Knöll R, Kostin S, Klede S, Savvatis K, Klinge L, Stehle I, Gunkel S, Kotter S, Babicz K, Sohns M, Miocic S, Didie M, Knoll G, Zimmermann WH, Thelen P, Bickeboller H, Maier LS, Schaper W, Schaper J, Kraft T, Tschope C, Linke WA, Chien KR (2010) A common MLP (muscle LIM protein) variant is associated with cardiomyopathy. Circulation research 106 (4):695-704. doi:CIRCRESAHA.109.206243 [pii] 10.1161/CIRCRESAHA.109.206243

[29] Boateng SY, Senyo SE, Qi L, Goldspink PH, Russell B (2009) Myocyte remodeling in response to hypertrophic stimuli requires nucleocytoplasmic shuttling of muscle LIM protein. J Mol Cell Cardiol 47 (4):426-435. doi:S0022-2828(09)00154-0 [pii] 10.1016/j.yjmcc.2009.04.006

[30] Heineke J, Ruetten H, Willenbockel C, Gross SC, Naguib M, Schaefer A, Kempf T, Hilfiker-Kleiner D, Caroni P, Kraft T, Kaiser RA, Molkentin JD, Drexler H, Wollert KC (2005) Attenuation of cardiac remodeling after myocardial infarction by muscle LIM protein-calcineurin signaling at the sarcomeric Z-disc. Proc Natl Acad Sci U S A 102 (5):1655-1660

[31] Bos JM, Poley RN, Ny M, Tester DJ, Xu X, Vatta M, Towbin JA, Gersh BJ, Ommen SR, Ackerman MJ (2006) Genotype-phenotype relationships involving hypertrophic cardiomyopathy-associated mutations in titin, muscle LIM protein, and telethonin. Mol Genet Metab 88 (1):78-85. doi:S1096-7192(05)00342-2 [pii] 10.1016/j.ymgme.2005.10.008

[32] Hayashi T, Arimura T, Itoh-Satoh M, Ueda K, Hohda S, Inagaki N, Takahashi M, Hori H, Yasunami M, Nishi H, Koga Y, Nakamura H, Matsuzaki M, Choi BY, Bae SW,

You CW, Han KH, Park JE, Knoll R, Hoshijima M, Chien KR, Kimura A (2004) Tcap gene mutations in hypertrophic cardiomyopathy and dilated cardiomyopathy. J Am Coll Cardiol 44 (11):2192-2201. doi:S0735-1097(04)01749-8 [pii] 10.1016/j.jacc.2004.08.058

[33] Moreira ES, Wiltshire TJ, Faulkner G, Nilforoushan A, Vainzof M, Suzuki OT, Valle G, Reeves R, Zatz M, Passos-Bueno MR, Jenne DE (2000) Limb-girdle muscular dystrophy type 2G is caused by mutations in the gene encoding the sarcomeric protein telethonin. Nat Genet 24 (2):163-166

[34] Olive M, Shatunov A, Gonzalez L, Carmona O, Moreno D, Quereda LG, Martinez-Matos JA, Goldfarb LG, Ferrer I (2008) Transcription-terminating mutation in telethonin causing autosomal recessive muscular dystrophy type 2G in a European patient. Neuromuscul Disord 18 (12):929-933. doi:S0960-8966(08)00607-X [pii] 10.1016/j.nmd.2008.07.009

[35] Buyandelger B, Ng KE, Miocic S, Piotrowska I, Gunkel S, Ku CH, Knoll R (2011) MLP (muscle LIM protein) as a stress sensor in the heart. Pflugers Arch. doi:10.1007/s00424-011-0961-2

[36] Linke WA, Grutzner A (2008) Pulling single molecules of titin by AFM--recent advances and physiological implications. Pflugers Arch 456 (1):101-115. doi:10.1007/s00424-007-0389-x

[37] LeWinter MM, Granzier H (2010) Cardiac titin: a multifunctional giant. Circulation 121 (19):2137-2145. doi:121/19/2137 [pii] 10.1161/CIRCULATIONAHA.109.860171

[38] Sheikh F, Raskin A, Chu PH, Lange S, Domenighetti AA, Zheng M, Liang X, Zhang T, Yajima T, Gu Y, Dalton ND, Mahata SK, Dorn GW, 2nd, Heller-Brown J, Peterson KL, Omens JH, McCulloch AD, Chen J (2008) An FHL1-containing complex within the cardiomyocyte sarcomere mediates hypertrophic biomechanical stress responses in mice. J Clin Invest 118 (12):3870-3880

[39] Miller MK, Bang ML, Witt CC, Labeit D, Trombitas C, Watanabe K, Granzier H, McElhinny AS, Gregorio CC, Labeit S (2003) The muscle ankyrin repeat proteins: CARP, ankrd2/Arpp and DARP as a family of titin filament-based stress response molecules. J Mol Biol 333 (5):951-964. doi:S0022283603011380 [pii]

[40] Braun T, Gautel M (2011) Transcriptional mechanisms regulating skeletal muscle differentiation, growth and homeostasis. Nat Rev Mol Cell Biol 12 (6):349-361. doi:nrm3118 [pii] 10.1038/nrm3118

[41] Lange S, Xiang F, Yakovenko A, Vihola A, Hackman P, Rostkova E, Kristensen J, Brandmeier B, Franzen G, Hedberg B, Gunnarsson LG, Hughes SM, Marchand S, Sejersen T, Richard I, Edstrom L, Ehler E, Udd B, Gautel M (2005) The Kinase Domain of Titin Controls Muscle Gene Expression and Protein Turnover. Science

[42] Puchner EM, Alexandrovich A, Kho AL, Hensen U, Schafer LV, Brandmeier B, Grater F, Grubmuller H, Gaub HE, Gautel M (2008) Mechanoenzymatics of titin kinase. Proc Natl Acad Sci U S A 105 (36):13385-13390. doi:0805034105 [pii] 10.1073/pnas.0805034105

[43] Gautel M (2011) Cytoskeletal protein kinases: titin and its relations in mechanosensing. Pflugers Arch. doi:10.1007/s00424-011-0946-1

[44] Buyandelger B, Ng KE, Miocic S, Gunkel S, Piotrowska I, Ku CH, Knoll R (2011) Genetics of Mechanosensation in the Heart. J Cardiovasc Transl Res. doi:10.1007/s12265-011-9262-6

[45] Kimura A (2010) Molecular basis of hereditary cardiomyopathy: abnormalities in calcium sensitivity, stretch response, stress response and beyond. J Hum Genet 55 (2):81-90. doi:jhg2009138 [pii] 10.1038/jhg.2009.138

11

Dobutamine-Induced Mechanical Alternans

Akihiro Hirashiki and Toyoaki Murohara
Nagoya Graduate School of Medicine
Japan

1. Introduction

We investigated the relationship between the occurrence of dobutamine-induced mechanical alternans (MA) and prognosis in ambulatory patients with idiopathic dilated cardiomyopathy (IDCM).

Recent American College of Cardiology and American Heart Association guidelines for the management of heart failure have emphasized the need for earlier identification and therapy for patients at high risk of systolic dysfunction, as well as for those with symptomatic heart failure.

MA, a condition characterized by beat-to-beat oscillation in the strength of cardiac muscle contraction at a constant heart rate, has been observed in patients with severe heart failure and in animal models of this condition.

Although MA is rare under resting conditions in individuals with controlled heart failure, at higher heart rates it is more prevalent and likely to be sustained, as exemplified by pacing-induced MA or dobutamine-induced MA. However, few studies have addressed the clinical implications of dobutamine-induced MA in patients with heart failure. We therefore prospectively examined the prognostic value of dobutamine- and pacing- induced MA in ambulatory patients with IDCM in sinus rhythm.(1)

2. Methods

2.1 Patient population

We studied 90 patients with IDCM (mean age, 50 years; range, 20 to 76 years) and an New York Heart Association (NYHA) functional class of I or II. Thirty-eight of the patients had previously been admitted to hospital because of heart failure with dyspnea on exertion, palpitations, or peripheral edema, whereas the remaining 52 were asymptomatic and were identified on the basis of electrocardiogram abnormalities detected at annual health checkups. All patients had normal sinus rhythms. IDCM was defined by the presence of both a reduced left ventricular (LV) ejection fraction (<50%, as determined by contrast left ventriculography) and a dilated LV cavity.

2.2 Cardiac catheterization

All patients initially underwent routine diagnostic left and right heart catheterization. A 6F fluid-filled pigtail catheter with a high-fidelity micromanometer was advanced into the left ventricle through the right radial artery to measure LV pressure. Right atrial pacing was initiated at 80 beats per minute (bpm) and was increased in increments of 10 bpm. We selected steady-state LV pressure data for at least 2 min at the baseline and at each pacing rate for analysis.(2) We calculated the maximum first derivative of LV pressure (LV dP/dt_{max}) as an index of contractility. To evaluate LV isovolumic relaxation, we computed the pressure half-time ($T_{1/2}$) directly, as previously described.(3) The peak pacing rate was defined as the heart rate at which second-degree atrioventricular block occurred. After the hemodynamic values had returned to baseline, dobutamine was infused intravenously at incremental doses of 5, 10, and 15 μg kg^{-1} b.w. min^{-1} and hemodynamic measurements were performed at the end of each 5-min infusion period. MA was diagnosed if the pressure difference between the strong and weak beats was ≥4 mm Hg continuously in the analyzed LV pressure data, as previously described.(4)

2.3 Quantitative RT-PCR analysis

Quantitative reverse transcription (RT) and polymerase chain reaction (PCR) analysis of the mRNAs for sarcoplasmic reticulum Ca^{2+}-ATPase (SERCA2a), ryanodine receptor 2, phospholamban, calsequestrin, and the Na^{+}-Ca^{2+} exchanger was performed as previously described.(5) The amount of each mRNA was normalized against the corresponding amount of glyceraldehyde-3-phosphate dehydrogenase (GAPDH) mRNA.

2.4 Follow-up

We prospectively followed up all patients for the occurrence of primary events, which were defined as cardiac death (death from worsening heart failure or sudden death), unscheduled hospital readmission for worsening heart failure, or receipt of an implantable cardioverter defibrillator (ICD) because of life-threatening arrhythmia.

3.Results

3.1 Classification of IDCM patients on the basis of MA

To identify on the basis of the classification by hemodynamic response to pacing or dobutamine stress testing, patients were classified into three groups: those who exhibited neither pacing- nor dobutamine-induced MA (n = 60, group N), those who manifested only pacing-induced MA (n = 20, group P), and those who developed both pacing- and dobutamine-induced MA (n = 10, group D). All patients who did not develop pacing-induced MA also did not exhibit dobutamine-induced MA. LV pressure waveforms during atrial pacing at 120 bpm or after dobutamine infusion at 10 μg kg^{-1} min^{-1} are shown for representative patients from each group (Fig. 1).

3.2 Baseline clinical data

There were no significant differences in age and sex among the three groups of patients (Table 1). All patients were classified as NYHA functional class I or II at the time of cardiac catheterization. The LV ejection fraction (LVEF) in groups P and D was significantly lower than that in group N. There were also no significant differences in plasma brain natriuretic peptide (BNP) or norepinephrine levels among the three groups.

3.3 Abundance of Ca^{2+}-handling protein mRNAs in endomyocardial biopsy specimens

The amounts of Ca^{2+}-handling protein mRNAs in endomyocardial biopsy specimens were determined by using quantitative RT-PCR and were normalized against that of GAPDH mRNA (Table 2). The abundance of phospholamban mRNA was significantly lower in group D than in group P. The SERCA2a/phospholamban mRNA ratio was significantly higher in group D than in groups N and P.

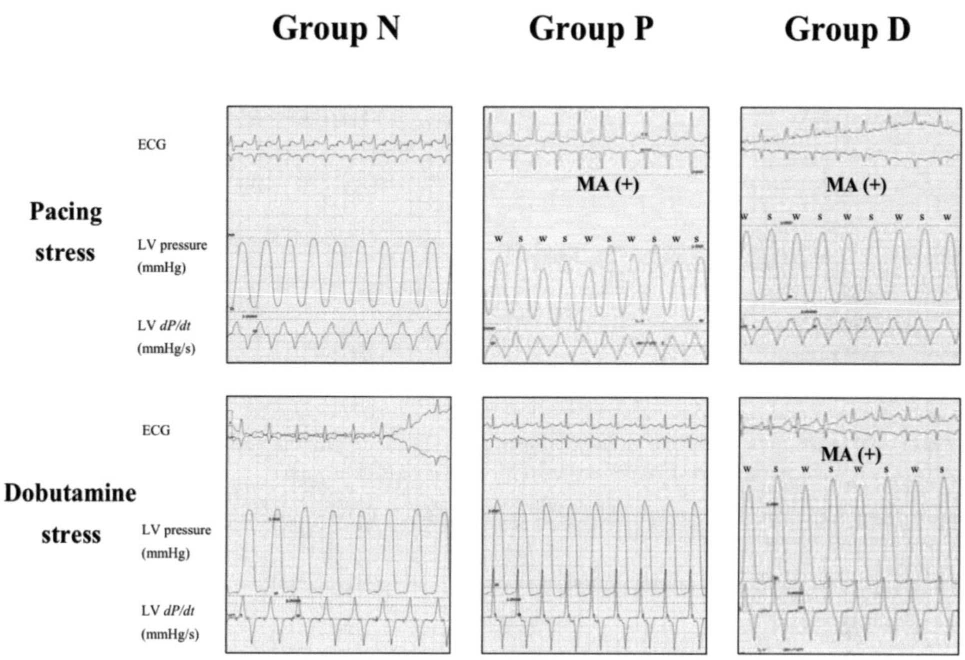

Fig. 1. LV pressure waveforms during atrial pacing at 120 bpm and after infusion of dobutamine at a dose of 10 μg kg^{-1} min^{-1} in representative patients of three study groups. The traces represent the lead II electrocardiogram (ECG), LV pressure, and LV dP/dt. Both LV dP/dt_{max} and LV dP/dt_{min} showed alternating changes with LV pressure. Strong and weak beats are indicated by s and w, respectively.

Characteristic	Group N (n = 60)	Group P (n = 20)	Group D (n = 10)
Age (years)	51 ± 12	50 ± 13	45 ± 11
Sex (M/F)	44 / 16	16 / 4	6 / 4
NYHA functional class I	32 (53%)	9 (45%)	5 (50%)
class II	28 (47%)	11 (55%)	5 (50%)
Medication			
Diuretics	30 (50%)	17* (85%)	9* (90%)
ACE inhibitors or ARBs	42 (70%)	19 (95%)	7 (70%)
Beta blockers	22 (37%)	10 (50%)	5 (50%)
PAWP (mmHg)	10.7 ± 4.7	14.6 ± 6.2*	13.9 ± 7.2
Cardiac index (L min^{-1} m^{-2})	3.07 ± 0.55	2.83 ± 0.58	3.26 ± 0.66
LVEF (%)	38.9 ± 8.1	32.9 ± 9.6*	30.3 ± 9.0*
Plasma BNP (pg/mL)	100 ± 173	179 ± 186	249 ± 262
Plasma norepinephrine (pg/mL)	440 ± 221	689 ± 764	664 ± 324

*P < 0.05 versus group N. Abbreviations not defined in text: ACE, angiotensin-converting enzyme; ARB, angiotensin-II receptor blocker; PAWP, pulmonary artery wedge pressure.

Table 1. Baseline clinical characteristics of patients in the three study groups

mRNA ratio	Group N	Group P	Group D
SERCA2a/GAPDH	0.42 ± 0.15	0.41 ± 0.13	0.43 ± 0.13
Phospholamban/GAPDH	0.82 ± 0.45	1.01 ± 0.13	0.42 ± 0.24*
Ryanodine receptor 2/GAPDH	0.50 ± 0.19	0.53 ± 0.21	0.75 ± 0.17
SERCA2a/phospholamban	0.63 ± 0.31	0.59 ± 0.40	1.32 ± 0.95*†
SERCA2a/Na^+-Ca^{2+} exchanger	0.57 ± 0.79	0.50 ± 0.56	0.27 ± 0.14

*P < 0.05 versus group P, †P < 0.05 versus group N.

Table 2. Quantitative RT-PCR analysis of the abundance of Ca^{2+}-handling protein mRNAs in endomyocardial biopsy specimens.

3.4 Follow-up evaluation and event-free survival

Of the 90 patients who were followed up, 4 individuals (4%) experienced cardiac death, 10 (11%) manifested worsening heart failure, and 4 (4%) received ICDs. The probability of event-free survival in group D was significantly lower than that in groups N or P (P = 0.002) (Fig. 2).

3.5 Univariate and multivariate analysis of cardiac events

Univariate analysis revealed that dobutamine-induced MA, pacing-induced MA, NYHA functional class, plasma BNP levels, mitral regurgitation, pulmonary artery wedge pressure, LV end-diastolic volume index, LV end-systolic volume index, LVEF, LV end-diastolic pressure and T½ were significant predictors of cardiac events (Table 3). Then, stepwise multivariate analysis identified dobutamine-induced MA (odds ratio, 4.05; 95% confidence interval, 1.35 to 12.2) as a significant independent predictor of cardiac events (Table 4). Both $T_{1/2}$ (odds ratio, 1.079; 95% confidence interval, 1.003 to 1.161) and plasma BNP level (odds ratio, 1.002; 95% confidence interval, 1.0004 to 1.0038) were also significant independent predictors of cardiac events, but with smaller odds ratios than that of dobutamine-induced MA.

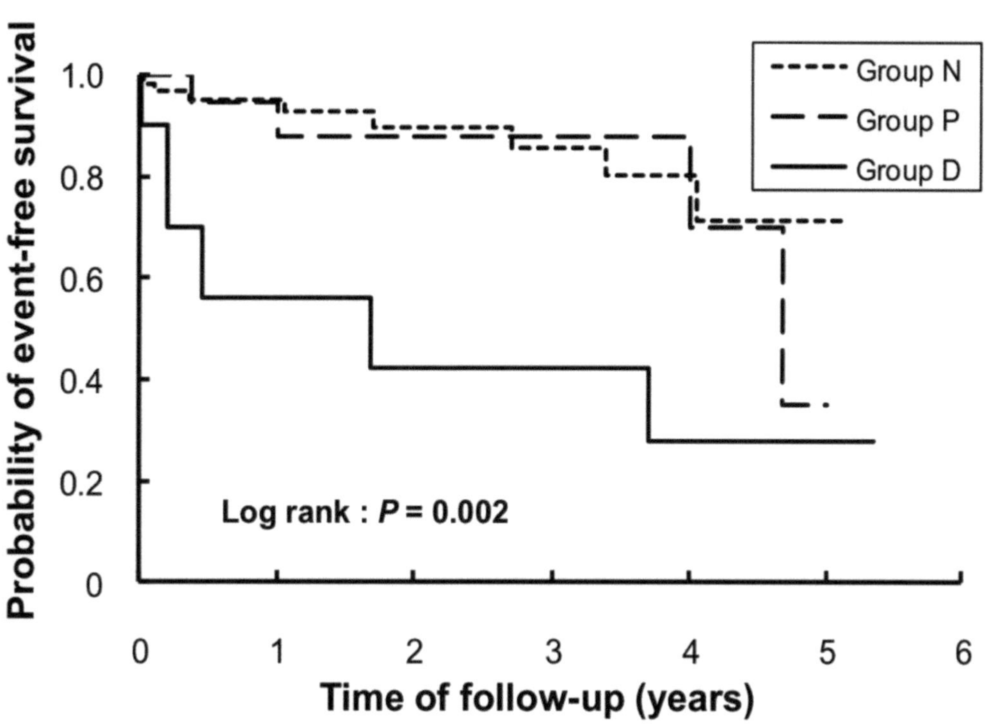

Fig. 2. Kaplan-Meier analysis of the cumulative probability of event-free survival of the 90 IDCM study patients. The probability of event-free survival in group D was significantly lower than that in groups P and N by the log-rank test (P = 0.002).

Parameter	Univariate analysis		
	Event-free group (n = 72)	Cardiac-event group (n = 18)	P
Dobutamine-induced MA (group D/groups P and N)	4 / 68	6 / 12	0.0019
Pacing-induced MA (groups D and P/group N)	20 / 52	10 / 8	0.04
Age (years)	50 ± 12	53 ± 14	0.34
Sex (M/F)	53 / 19	13 / 5	0.86
Body mass index (kg/m^2)	24.4 ± 4.9	22.5 ± 2.6	0.15
NYHA functional class	1.3 ± 0.5	1.6 ± 0.4	0.011
QRS duration (ms)	113 ± 27	112 ± 22	0.88
Beta blockers	55 (76%)	10 (56%)	0.58
Diuretics	52 (72%)	16 (89%)	0.88
Plasma BNP (pg/mL)	123 ± 238	228 ± 162	0.0013
eGFR (mL min^{-1} 1.73 m^{-2})	74 ± 17	68 ± 18	0.089
Plasma norepinephrine (pg/mL)	521 ± 452	524 ± 292	0.32
Mitral regurgitation	0.56 ± 0.64	0.94 ± 0.94	0.022
E/E'	15.6 ± 8.6	24.2 ± 8.4	0.227
PAWP (mmHg)	11.5 ± 5.3	13.7 ± 6.6	0.044
Cardiac index (L min^{-1} m^{-2})	3.02 ± 0.57	3.13 ± 0.64	0.85
LVEDVI (mL m^{-2})	73 ± 52	115 ± 79	0.02
LVESVI (mL m^{-2})	43 ± 36	84 ± 62	0.018
LVEF (%)	38.2 ± 8.7	32.8 ± 6.8	0.003
Heart rate (bpm)	76 ± 17	75 ± 14	0.34
LVEDP (mmHg)	12 ± 8	15 ± 9	0.019
LVSP (mmHg)	119 ± 19	116 ± 23	0.62
LV dP/dt_{max} (mmHg/s)	1114 ± 263	1160 ± 263	0.73
$T_{1/2}$ (ms)	39 ± 7	44 ± 4.7	0.0086

Table 3. Univariate of predictors of cardiac events.

Parameter	Multivariate analysis			
	β	OR	(95% CI)	*P*
Dobutamine-induced MA (group D/groups P and N)	1.4	4.05	(1.35–12.2)	0.0126
Plasma BNP (pg/mL)	0.0021	1.002	(1.0004–1.0038)	0.014
$T_{1/2}$ (ms)	0.076	1.079	(1.0033–1.161)	0.041

Table 4. Multivariate analysis of predictors of cardiac events.

4. Discussion

We found that the occurrence of dobutamine-induced MA was a clinical predictor of poor prognosis in ambulatory patients with IDCM in sinus rhythm. Although there was no significant difference in LVEF between patients who manifested only pacing-induced MA and those who developed both pacing- and dobutamine-induced MA, the probability of event-free survival in the latter group was significantly lower than that in the former. Multivariate analysis also revealed that the occurrence of dobutamine-induced MA was a significant independent predictor of cardiac events.

Our study included a group of 90 ambulatory patients with IDCM (mean LVEF of 36.5% and plasma BNP concentration of 132 pg/mL). We sought to investigate whether the hemodynamic response to dobutamine stress testing was associated with prognosis in such patients and could thereby serve as a physiological phenomenon on which risk stratification could be based. Three general mechanisms have been proposed to account for the development of MA: alteration of action potential duration, impaired ventricular relaxation, and abnormal intracellular Ca^{2+} handling.(6) The low relative ratio of phospholamban to SERCA reduces the inhibition of SERCA and increases Ca^{2+} -uptake; this enhances relaxation and contraction in the human atrium. However, humans lacking phospholamban develop lethal IDCM.(7) SERCA2a and ryanodine receptor 2 mRNA levels were similar in all three of our groups, whereas the relative ratio of SERCA to phospholamban was significantly higher in patients with pacing- and dobutamine-induced MA than in those with only pacing-induced MA or with no MA. Our results suggest that an imbalance between phospholamban and SERCA mRNA levels in the abundant Ca^{2+}-handling proteins is associated with dobutamine-induced MA. We also recently found that the amounts of mRNAs for the β_1-adrenergic receptor and SERCA2a in the myocardium were smaller in asymptomatic or mildly symptomatic IDCM patients with reduced adrenergic myocardial contractile reserve than in those with preserved adrenergic contractile reserves.(8) The occurrence of dobutamine-induced MA in our patients in the present study might also reflect abnormal β_1-adrenergic receptor signaling in the myocardium. However, steady-state mRNA levels do not necessarily reflect the corresponding protein levels, in particular because both mRNA and protein synthesis or degradation may be altered in the failing heart.(9, 10) Further studies are needed to elucidate these issues.

In patients with heart failure, dobutamine-induced MA is highly prevalent(4) and mechanical and visible T-wave alternans is detectable under tachycardia or catecholamine exposure.(2, 11) Dobutamine-induced MA may be attributed various factors, including an increase in the heart rate as a result of dobutamine infusion, impaired LV contraction, the influence of preload, and abnormal Ca^{2+} under pathophysiological conditions. Dobutamine is a β-stimulator that increases both heart rate (HR) and LV contraction. The increase in HR, but not that in LV contraction, is likely to be a trigger for the occurrence of dobutamine-induced MA. Therefore, the increased occurrence of dopamine-induced MA in heart failure patients might be related to their poor myocardial contractile reserve

We reported previously that the occurrence of pacing-induced MA is a potentially useful indicator of poor prognosis in patients with mild-to-moderate IDCM in sinus rhythm.(2) Here, we found that, among our ambulatory IDCM patients, those with both pacing- and dobutamine-induced MA had the least favorable clinical course, whereas those with only pacing-induced MA had a moderate clinical course, even though the mean value of baseline LVEF did not differ significantly between these two groups.

Our results show that the occurrence of dobutamine-induced MA is a potentially useful clinical predictor of cardiac events in ambulatory patients with IDCM in sinus rhythm. Recent guidelines for the management of heart failure emphasize the need for earlier identification of and therapy for patients who are at high risk of developing heart failure or who have asymptomatic LV systolic dysfunction.(12) We showed here that the prevalence of cardiac events or cardiac death was higher in patients with dobutamine- and pacing-induced MA than in those without it. Assessment of dobutamine-induced MA in addition to routine clinical evaluation in patients with IDCM may thus contribute to stratification of individuals into low- or high-risk groups.

Our study had several limitations. First, it included only a small number of patients. Second, the identification of pacing- or dobutamine-induced MA requires an invasive examination and time-consuming hemodynamic stress assessment. The current trend in clinical medicine is to find a non-invasive test with prognostic consequences. However, these results of the present study suggested that the hemodynamic phenomenon by dobutamine stress testing might be also potentially useful marker for predicting the occurrence of cardiac events. The fact that such examinations are not amenable to being repeated over time is a potential limitation of their prognostic utility. Whether our findings will also hold for patients with more severe heart failure requires further investigation.

In conclusion, the occurrence of dobutamine-induced MA is a potentially useful clinical predictor of poor prognosis in ambulatory patients with IDCM in sinus rhythm.

5. References

[1] Hirashiki A, Izawa H, Cheng XW, Unno K, Ohshima S, Murohara T. Dobutamine-induced mechanical alternans is a marker of poor prognosis in idiopathic dilated cardiomyopathy. *Clin Exp Pharmacol Physiol* 2010; 37(10):1004–1009.

[2] Hirashiki A, Izawa H, Somura F, Obata K, Kato T, Nishizawa T, Yamada A, Asano H, Ohshima S, Noda A, Iino S, Nagata K, Okumura K, Murohara T, Yokota M. Prognostic value of pacing-induced mechanical alternans in patients with mild-to-moderate idiopathic dilated cardiomyopathy in sinus rhythm. *J Am Coll Cardiol* 2006; 47(7):1382–1389.

[3] Mirsky I. Assessment of diastolic function: suggested methods and future considerations. *Circulation* 1984; 69(4):836–841.

[4] Kodama M, Kato K, Hirono S, Okura Y, Hanawa H, Ito M, Fuse K, Shiono T, Watanabe K, Aizawa Y. Mechanical alternans in patients with chronic heart failure. *J Card Fail* 2001; 7(2):138–145.

[5] Somura F, Izawa H, Iwase M, Takeichi Y, Ishiki R, Nishizawa T, Noda A, Nagata K, Yamada Y, Yokota M. Reduced myocardial sarcoplasmic reticulum Ca(2+)-ATPase mRNA expression and biphasic force-frequency relations in patients with hypertrophic cardiomyopathy. *Circulation* 2001; 104(6):658–663.

[6] Lab MJ, Lee JA. Changes in intracellular calcium during mechanical alternans in isolated ferret ventricular muscle. *Circ Res* 1990; 66(3):585–595.

[7] Haghighi K, Kolokathis F, Pater L, Lynch RA, Asahi M, Gramolini AO, Fan GC, Tsiapras D, Hahn HS, Adamopoulos S, Liggett SB, Dorn GW II, MacLennan DH, Kremastinos DT, Kranias EG. Human phospholamban null results in lethal dilated cardiomyopathy revealing a critical difference between mouse and human. *J Clin Invest* 2003; 111(6):869–876.

[8] Kobayashi M IH, Cheng XW Asano H, Hirashiki A, Unno K, Ohshima S,Yamada T, Murase Y, Kato ST, Obata K, Noda A, Nishizawa T, Isobe S, Nagata K, Matsubara T, Murohara T, Yokota M. Dobutamine stress testing as a diagnostic tool for evaluation of myocardial contractile reserve in asymptomatic or mildly symptomatic patients with dilated cardiomyopathy. *J Am Coll Cardiol Imaging* 2008; (6):718–726.

[9] Linck B, Boknik P, Eschenhagen T, Muller FU, Neumann J, Nose M, Jones LR, Schmitz W, Scholz H. Messenger RNA expression and immunological quantification of phospholamban and SR-Ca(2+)-ATPase in failing and nonfailing human hearts. *Cardiovasc Res* 1996; 31(4):625–632.

[10] Hasenfuss G. Alterations of calcium-regulatory proteins in heart failure. *Cardiovasc Res* 1998; 37(2):279–289.

[11] Kodama M, Kato K, Hirono S, Okura Y, Hanawa H, Yoshida T, Hayashi M, Tachikawa H, Kashimura T, Watanabe K, Aizawa Y. Linkage between mechanical and electrical alternans in patients with chronic heart failure. *J Cardiovasc Electrophysiol* 2004; 15(3):295–299.

[12] Radford MJ, Arnold JM, Bennett SJ, Cinquegrani MP, Cleland JG, Havranek EP, Heidenreich PA, Rutherford JD, Spertus JA, Stevenson LW, Goff DC, Grover FL, Malenka DJ, Peterson ED, Redberg RF. ACC/AHA key data elements and definitions for measuring the clinical management and outcomes of patients with chronic heart failure: a report of the American College of Cardiology/American Heart Association Task Force on Clinical Data Standards

(Writing Committee to Develop Heart Failure Clinical Data Standards): developed in collaboration with the American College of Chest Physicians and the International Society for Heart and Lung Transplantation: endorsed by the Heart Failure Society of America. *Circulation* 2005; 112(12):1888-1916.

12

MicroRNAs Telltale Effects on Signaling Networks in Cardiomyopathy

Manveen K. Gupta[2], Zhong-Hui Duan[1],
Sadashiva S. Karnik[2] and Sathyamangla V. Naga Prasad[2]
[1]*Department of Computer Sciences, University of Akron, Akron, OH,*
[2]*Department of Molecular Cardiology, Lerner Research Institute,*
Cleveland Clinic, Cleveland, OH,
USA

1. Introduction

MicroRNAs (miRNAs) are single-stranded, highly conserved, short non-coding RNAs (~ 22 nucleotides) regulating target gene expression by base pairing with specific sequences of target mRNAs (Ambros, 2004). miRNAs negatively regulate gene expression post-transcriptionally by suppressing translation and/or inducing mRNA degradation. Bioinfomatically, it is estimated that human genome may contain approximately 1000 miRNAs (Bartel, 2004; Berezikov et al., 2005; Griffiths-Jones et al., 2008) and consistently, additional miRNAs are continually being identified (Griffiths-Jones et al., 2006). miRNAs modulate the expression of target proteins in a non-canonical manner by binding to specific sequences regulating functional networks. Consequentially, a single miRNA might target hundreds of distinct genes or alternatively expression of a single coding gene can be regulated by many different miRNAs (Lewis et al., 2005; Miranda et al., 2006). Recent studies show the important role of miRNAs in the regulation of a variety of physiological functions ranging from stem cell differentiation to cardiac muscle development and stress (Krichevsky et al. 2006; Chen et al., 2006; Zhao et al., 2005; Pedersen et al., 2007; Kloosterman et al., 2007; Felli et al., 2005; Tay et al., 2008). Furthermore, aberrant expression of miRNAs has been found in various diseases including cancer, diabetes and cardiac hypertrophy/failure.

The binding specificity of miRNAs depend on complementary base pairing of ~ 7 nucleotide seed sequence region at the 5′ end of the miRNA with the corresponding mRNA target. Another caveat that needs to be considered in the miRNA regulation is the miRNA sequences outside the 7 nucleotide seed region which pairs with the mRNA that may also play a role in determining the strength/efficacy of regulating the target mRNA. The binding of miRNAs to their cognate target mRNAs commonly results in decreased expression of target genes through translational repression or mRNA degradation (Fig. 1). Conversely, decreased expression of miRNAs will lead to increased target gene expression (Gregory et al., 2008).

This realm of knowledge has allowed for studies on miRNAs on their tissue specificity and disease specificity but critically little information is available with regards to temporal or spatial expression profiles of miRNAs in the heart. By and large studies have used micro-array analysis to identify altered miRNAs to define signature of altered miRNAs in a specific cardiac phenotype. As miRNAs target multiple proteins, these signatures have been used to predict the array of molecules altered. Over time sophisticated computational approaches have been developed that has lead to identification of previously unrecognized targets within disease pathways of interest (Ivanovska and Cleary, 2008; Gusev et al., 2007). Among the computational tools the most commonly used target prediction algorithms include DIANA-microT (Kiriakidou et al., 2004), miRanda (Griffiths-Jones et al., 2006), TargetScan (Lewis et al., 2003), TargetScanS (Lewis et al., 2005), PicTar (Krek et al., 2005) and PITA (Kertesz et al., 2007). These algorithms rely on criteria like conservation among species, seed complementarity, thermo-stability of miRNA-mRNA hybrids, delta G of target mRNA binding site, and multiple miRNA binding sites in the 3'UTR (cooperativity) to predict targets (Bartel, 2009; Cacchiarelli et al., 2008; Ivanovska and Cleary, 2008; Gusev et al., 2007). Thus, use of these algorithms provide hundreds of targets indicating that miRNA alteration in expression could have wide ranging effects on molecules belonging to multiple signaling pathways. It is important to note that target prediction with these algorithms remains challenging but these are the tools currently available in field to provide a window into understanding the role of miRNAs. These predicted targets can then be used as a platform for identifying signaling pathways and networks that are altered manifesting in the phenotype. Critically these bioinformatic tools are evolving with the field and are pivotal to understanding the global role of miRNAs in cardiomyopathy. Although miRNA regulation adds another layer of complexity to the already complex etiology, understanding the regulation could provide novel therapeutic strategies due to miRNAs ability to target multiple molecules. In this regard, the focus of our article is to provide an overview of altered miRNAs in cardiac stress and the available tools that could be used to understand their global implications.

2. miRNA generation

2.1 Genome distribution, miRNA processing and nuclear export

miRNAs are encoded by their own genes which are an integral part of cell's genetic make up and are evolutionarily conserved (Ambros, 2004; Bartel, 2004). miRNAs can be transcribed as polycistronic primary transcripts or as individual transcripts from intergenic regions, exon sequences of non-coding strand or intronic sequences (Kim and Nam, 2006; Altuvia, et al., 2005) (Fig. 1). Intronic miRNAs are generally transcribed coincidentally with the gene and excised by the splicing machinery from the larger gene transcript in which they are embedded (Rodriguez et al., 2004). Indeed, intronic miRNAs may represent a simple way for a protein-coding gene to regulate other protein-coding genes in a non-canonical manner. miRNAs are transcribed by the RNA polymerase II as a primary transcript several kilobases long characterized by stem-loop hairpin structures called pri-miRNAs that are 5' capped and a poly (A) to stabilize these pre-miRNAs similar to that of the traditional mRNAs (Lee et al., 2004). The generated pre-miRNA is processed in the nucleus and exported out through a regulated process. The stem-loop structures of pre-miRNAs are recognized by Drosha (a double-stranded specific RNase III) and its partner DGCR8 (a double stranded RNA binding protein) that cleave at the hair-pin base to release ~ 70-90 nucleotide stem-loop pri-miRNA precursor (Lee et al., 2003, 2004). In addition to this classical pathway, recent studies have identified alternate pathway wherein intronic pre-miRNA precursors "mirtrons" uses the cellular splicing machinery to bypass Drosha mediated processing (Ruby et al., 2007; Okamura et al., 2007) . The cleaved stem-loop pre-miRNA hairpins are exported into the cytoplasm by the exportin-5 (a Ran-GTP-dependent nuclear transport receptor) (Yi et al., 2003). The interaction of exportin-5 with the pre-miRNA 'minihelix motif' (~14 nucleotide stem and a short 30 nucleotide overhang) is thought to stabilize the pre-miRNAs (Yi et al., 2003; Filipowicz, 2005) manifesting in efficient transport.

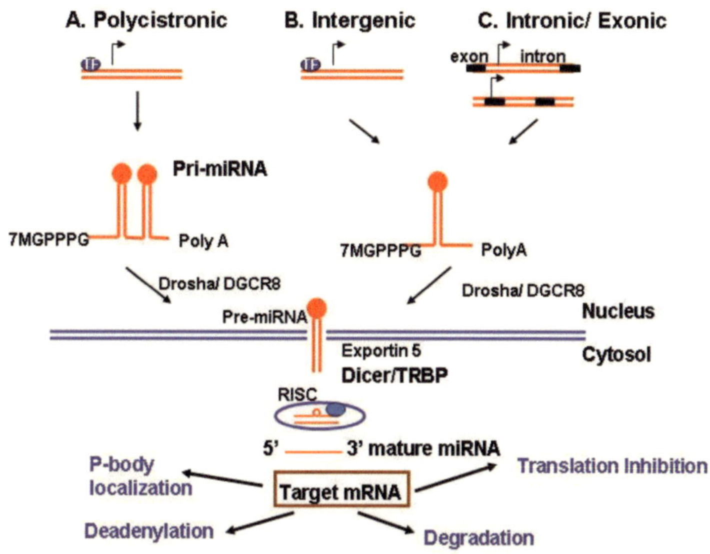

Fig. 1. MicroRNA (miRNA) genomic organization, biogenesis and function
Genomic distribution of miRNA genes. TF: transcription factor. (A) Clusters throughout the genome transcribed as polycistronic primary transcripts and subsequently cleaved into multiple miRNAs; (B) intergenic regions transcribed as independent transcriptional units; (C) intronic sequences of protein-coding or -non-coding transcription units or exonic sequences (black cylinders) of non-coding genes. Primary miRNAs(pri-miRNAs) transiently have a 7- methylguanosine (7mGpppG) cap and a poly(A) tail. The pri-miRNA is processed into a precursor miRNA (pre-miRNA) stem-loop of 60 nucleotides (nt) in length by the nuclear RNase III enzyme Drosha and its partner DiGeorge syndrome critical region gene 8 (DGCR8). Exportin-5 actively transports pre-miRNA into the cytosol, where it is processed by the Dicer RNaseIII enzyme, together with its partner TAR (HIV) RNA binding protein (TRBP), into mature, 22 nt-long double strand miRNAs. The RNA strand (in red) is recruited as a single-stranded molecule into the RNA-induced silencing (RISC) effector complex and assembled through processes that are dependent on Dicer and other double strand RNA binding domain proteins, as well as on members of the Argonaute family. Mature miRNAs then guide the RISC complex to the 3′ untranslated regions (3′-UTR) of the complementary messenger RNA (mRNA) targets and repress their expression by several mechanisms: repression of mRNA translation, destabilization of mRNA transcripts through cleavage, de-adenylation, and localization in the processing body (P-body), where the miRNA-targeted mRNA can be sequestered from the translational machinery and degraded or stored for subsequent use. Nuclear localization of mature miRNAs has also been described and is a novel mechanism of action for miRNAs.

2.2 Generation of mature miRNA, activation and target recognition

The pre-miRNA is processed into a mature miRNA of ~22 nucleotides long by another double stranded RNase III called the Dicer (Hutvagner et al., 2001). Single stranded RNA is assembled into a RNA-inducing silencing complex (RISC) with the help of Dicer, TAR (HIV) RNA binding protein (TRBP), and dsRNA-binding proteins of the argonaute (AGO) family (Chapman and Carrington, 2007; Filipowicz, 2005; Schwarz et al., 2003; MacRae et al., 2008; Okamura et al., 2004). Additional factors have also been isolated and implicated (Chapman and Carrington, 2007; Filipowicz, 2005; Schwarz et al., 2003; MacRae et al., 2008; Okamura et al., 2004) to be a part of RISC complex bringing about miRNA-mediated silencing of gene expression that could be either a translational repression or degradation of mRNA. miRNAs recognize their target mRNAs through specific interaction of the 5′ end 'seed' region (2–8 nt from the 5′ end) and the complementary sequences of conserved target mRNAs (Bartel, 2004). Since only a few miRNAs have perfect complementarity to the target mRNAs leading to degradation, majority of the miRNAs have imperfect match resulting in translational repression (Nilsen, 2007). Another caveat in the miRNA silencing dynamics is the ability of multiple miRNAs to bind to the same mRNA initiating translational repression with different potencies. Repressed mRNAs are sequestered from translational machinery, degraded or stored for subsequent use in large macroscopic cytoplasmic foci, named processing bodies (P-bodies) upon silencing by miRNAs. The P-bodies contain a wide range of enzymes involved in RNA turnover, including de-capping enzymes, de-adenylases and exonucleases (Eulalio et al., 2007). In addition to their cytoplasmic role, miRNAs with nuclear localization sequence have been identified demonstrating their role in transcriptional control of gene expression (Chapman and Carrington, 2007; Volpe et al., 2002; Zilberman, et al., 2003; Aravin et al., 2007; Yu et al., 2008; Hwang et al., 2007; Calin et al., 2007).

3. miRNAs and cardiac development

3.1 miRNA expression in cardiac development

Studies have shown that miRNA mediated fine tuning leads to critical cell lineage commitment and embryonic tissue development (Latronico, et al., 2007; Farh et al., 2005; Ivey et al., 2008). Consistent with the role of miRNA in development, deletion of Dicer leads to embryonic lethality resulting from defects in cardiogenesis due to deficiencies in miRNAs biogenesis (Giraldez et al., 2006; Ebert et al., 2007). In tune with complex process of cardiogenesis many miRNAs are shown to be involved and the selection of miRNAs enriched during the differentiation of mouse embryonic stem cells to cardiomyocytes are detailed in Table 1 (Lakshmipathy et al., 2007; Thum et al., 2007). Significant increase in miRNA expression with development shows that miRNAs play an important role in early embryonic patterning and orchestrating organogenesis (Ivey et al., 2008). Expression pattern of miRNA-1 and -133 show that these two miRNAs play a key role in skeletal muscle proliferation and differentiation (Chen et al., 2006). Specifically, miRNA-1 promotes myogenesis by targeting histone deacetylase (HDAC4), a transcriptional repressor while miRNA-133 enhances myoblast proliferation by repressing serum response factor (SRF) (Zhao et al., 2005, 2007; Kwon et al., 2005; Niu et al., 2007). In this context, loss of function of miRNA-1 in Drosophila results in embryonic/larval lethality due to altered sarcomeric gene expression and increased number of undifferentiated muscle progenitors (Kwon et al., 2005). Where as miRNA-1 gain of function results in embryonic lethality due to insufficient numbers of cardioblasts indicating that cardiogenesis and differentiation is a spatio-temporal process tightly regulated by miRNA-1 mediated by cardiac transcription factor Hand2 (Zhao et al., 2005; Srivastava et al., 1997). Another important component of miRNA expression is the Dicer mediated generation of miRNA during development. Dicer expression during development determines miRNA expression and its regulation. Indeed, Dicer-deficient animals fail to synthesize new miRNAs resulting in embryonic lethality in zebrafish (Giraldez et al., 2005) and mice (Bernstein et al., 2003). More importantly cardiac specific deletion of Dicer results in aberrant cardiac contractile protein expression and severe sarcomere disarray, leading to progressive dilated cardiomyopathy (DCM), failure and postnatal lethality (Chen et al., 2008).

Downregulated miRs		Upregulated miRs		Species
Development	Disease	Development	Disease	
	1, 7d*, 10a/b, 26a/b, 29a/b/c, 30a-3p/a-5p/b/ c/d/e/e*, 30e, 93, 126-5p, 133a/b, 139, 149, 150, 151, 155, 181b, 185, 187, 194, 218, 292-5p, 373, 378, 451, 466, 486	1, 18, 20, 23b, 24, 26a, 30c, 133, 43, 182, 183, 200a/b, 292-3p, 293, 295, 335	10b, 15b, 17-5p, 18b, 19a/b, 20b, 21, 23a/b, 24, 25, 27a/b, 29a, 31, 103, 106a, 107, 125b, 126, 127, 140/*, 142-3p, 146, 153, 154, 195, 199a/a*/b, 200a, 208, 210, 211, 214, 217, 218, 221, 222, 330, 341, 351, let-7b/c, 424	Mouse
	16, 17-5p, 19b, 22, 23b, 24, 27a, 30a-5p/b/c/e-5p, 107, 126, 130b, 135a, 136, 148a, 150, 182, 186, 192, 199a*, 218, 299-5p, 302b*, 302c*, 325, 339, 342, 452/ *, 494, 495, 497, 499, 507, 512-5p, 515-5p, 520d*/h, 520, 523, 526b/b*, 378,7	1, 20, 21, 26a, 92, 127, 129, 130a, 199b, 200a, 335, 424	1, 7a/b/c/d/e/f, 10b, 17-3p, 21, 23, 24, 26a, 28, 29a/b/c, 32, 34b, 98, 106b, 125a/b, 126*, 129/-3p, 130a, 132, 195, 196a, 199a/b, 200c, 204, 205, 208, 210, 211, 212, 213, 214, 215, 292-3p, 294, 295, 296, 297, 300, 302a, 320, 322, 330, 331, 333, 340, 341, 343, 365, 367, 372, 373, 377, 381, 382, 423, 424, 429, 432, 500, 520c, 525*,	Human

Upregulated (enriched) miRNA during mouse cardiac development as shown by Srivastava and colleagues. Data about altered miRNAs in heart failure and animal models of heart disease originate from different results published earlier. Note that in some cases results were not consistent between the different laboratories.

Table 1. Summary of regulated microRNAs (miRNAs) in cardiac development and disease.

3.2 Regulation of miRNA transcription

Understanding transcriptional regulation of miRNAs is critical as expression of miRNAs is a major determinant of miRNA dependent regulatory mechanisms. As miRNAs are transcribed like other genes, they are regulated by transcription factors and expression of transcription factors determines the miRNA expression. SRF is a cardiac enriched transcription factor that regulates sarcomere organization in the heart and SRF expression follows a restrictive pattern during development (Olson and Schneider, 2003; Niu et al., 2007; Barron et al., 2005). SRF expression is very important as multiple SRF binding sites have been identified in promoters of genes regulating contractility, cell movement, and growth signaling (Sun et al., 2006; Zhang et al., 2005). Consistent with the role of SRF in cardiac development, several miRNAs have been identified to contain SRF binding sites in their promoter including miRNA-1-1, -1-2, -21, -206, -214, -133 and others (Niu et al., 2007). In addition, studies have unequivocally have shown that miRNA-1-1, -1-2 and -133 are regulated by SRF transcription factor alone or in conjunction with co-factors like GATA5, MyoD, Nkx 2.5 or MEF2 (Fig. 2) (Zhao et al., 2005; Chen et al., 2006; Niu et al., 2007; Rao et al., 2006; Xiao et al., 2007). It is important to note that the outlined co-factors of SRF by themselves can act as transcriptional regulators in their own right increasing complexity of regulation. For example, MEF2 along with MyoD is known to regulate miRNA-1-2/133a-1 in myotomes during embryogenesis and all skeletal fibers in adulthood (Liu et al., 2007).

3.3 miRNA expression patterns

miRNA expression is greatly enriched in a tissue/cell-specific manner indicating unique signature patterns for each type. This enrichment and signature pattern suggests that miRNAs play a critical role in regulating and maintaining the specific cellular phenotype which is of essence in an organ with diverse cell/tissue types contributing to effective functioning. In this regard, heart as an organ contains many "non-cardiomyocyte" cell types like endothelial cells, smooth muscle cells and fibroblasts and each of which have distinct function in the heart. Consistently, differential enrichment of miRNAs are observed in cardiomyocyte versus cardiac fibroblasts indicating important role in cellular specificity (Landgraf et al., 2007; Kuehbacher et al., 2007; Harris et al., 2008). Although specific miRNA enrichments are being found in different cell types (Kuehbacher et al., 2007; Harris et al., 2008), lot more work needs to be done to determine contribution of miRNAs towards regulation of global networking pathways that defines specific fingerprints for each cell type. The current studies have all been focused on one or two miRNAs (Chen et al., 2006; Gregory et al., 2008; Harris et al., 2008) which by themselves may not be sufficient to determine a cellular phenotype indicating requirement of more comprehensive studies on specific miRNAs signature for cellular phenotype.

4. miRNAs and cardiac disease

The heart is responsive to physiological stimuli or pathological stress and accordingly undergoes remodeling to meet the demand (Catalucci et al., 2008). Following stress, the heart undergoes extensive remodeling in the form of physiological or pathological hypertrophy defined as an augmentation of ventricular mass due to increased cardiomyocyte size. Cardiac hypertrophy is characterized by initial compensatory mechanisms that adapt the heart towards sustaining the cardiac output. However, this process is only an initial 'adaptive' response and chronic exposure to stress eventually leads to impaired function that, in many cases, progresses to failure. This maladaptive change is accompanied by alterations in the underlying molecular map including a switch in the gene expression program leading to reexpression of fetal genes (Catalucci et al., 2008; Thum et al., 2007). The involvement of miRNAs in this pathological process has been recognized and is thought to be integral 'switch' in the gene expression program. Intense efforts have been put into identifying miRNAs altered in pathology and evolving signature of deregulated miRNAs identified cardiac disease is detailed in Table 2.

4.1 Myocardial hypertrophy, remodeling, and heart failure

Cardiac remodeling is characterized by structural alterations of myocardial tissue, modification of the extracellular matrix, and reshaping of left ventricle geometry and performance (Catalucci et al., 2008; Dash et al., 2001). The presence of chronic stress results in deleterious remodeling.

microRNA	Experiment	Phenotype
miRNA-1-2	Mouse knockout	Cardiac septal defects, hyperplasia and delay between atrial an ventricular repolarizations (PR interval) was shortened (Zhao et al.,2007)
miRNA-1	Neonatal cardiomyocyte	Inhibits FBS/endothelin/isoproterenol overexpression mediated hypertrophy (Ikeda et al., 2009)
miRNA-21	TAC and isoproterenol induced hypertrophy	Upregulated in compensatory hypertrophy and reduced in decompensation (Sayed et al., 2008)
	Neonatal cardiomyocyte overexpression	Outgrowths in the cardiomyocytes accompanied by connections via gap junctions (Sayed et al., 2008)
	Transgenic cardiomyocyte-specific expression	No specific phenotype indicating minimal role for miRNA21 in cardiomyocytes (Thum et al., 2008)
	Cardiac fibroblast overexpression	Anti-apoptotic (Thum et al., 2008)
miRNA-23a	Antagomir infusion using minipumps	Isoproterenol-induced cardiac hypertrophy is attenuated with miRNA23a antagomirs (Lin et al., 2009)
	Neonatal cardiomyocyte overexpression	Induces hypertrophy (van Rooij et al., 2006;, Lin et al., 200955)
miRNA-23b	Neonatal cardiomyocyte overexpression	Induces hypertrophy (van Rooij et al., 2006)
miRNA-24	Antagomir infusion using minipumps	Isoproterenol-induced cardiac hypertrophy is not altered (Lin et al., 2009)
	Neonatal cardiomyocyte overexpression	Induces hypertrophy (van Rooij et al., 2006)
miRNA-27	Antagomir infusion using minipumps	Isoproterenol-induced cardiac hypertrophy is not attenuated (Lin et al., 2009)
miRNA-92	miRNA inhibitor treatment of neonatal cardiomyocytes	Minimal effect on fetal gene expression (Sucharov et al., 2008)
miRNA-100	miRNA mimic treatment of neonatal cardiomyocytes	Results in re-expression of fetal genes (Sucharov et al., 2008)
miRNA-129	Neonatal cardiomyocyte transfection	Induces hypertrophy (Thum et al., 2007)
miRNA-133	Neonatal cardiomyocyte transfection	Inhibited hypertrophy (Care et al., 2007)
	Antagomir infusion using minipumps	Induces cardiac hypertrophy (Care et al., 2007)
	Double knockout of miRNA-133-a/b	Embryonic myocyte proliferation, septal defects, and surviving adults have severe dilated cardiomyopathy (Liu et al., 2008)
	Transgenic cardiomyocyte specific expression	Inhibitor of cardiomyocyte proliferation (Liu et al., 2008)
	Transgenic cardiomyocyte-specific expression subjected to TAC	Cardiac hypertrophy is not inhibited, but decreases myocardial fibrosis and cardiomyocyte apoptosis (Matkovich et al., 2010)
miRNA-195	Neonatal cardiomyocyte overexpression	Induces hypertrophy (van Rooij et al., 2006)
	Transgenic cardiomyocyte specific expression	Induces cardiac hypertrophy and dilated cardiomyopathy (van Rooij et al., 2006)
miRNA-199a	Neonatal cardiomyocyte overexpression	Cardiomyocyte enlargement (van Rooij et al., 2006)]
miRNA-208	Knockout mice subjected to TAC or bred to mouse model of hypertrophy	No hypertrophic response in both the cases [van Rooij et al., 2007)
miRNA-214	Neonatal cardiomyocyte overexpression	Cardiomyocyte hypertrophy (van Rooij et al., 2006)
	Transgenic cardiomyocyte specific expression	No phenotype (van Rooij et al., 2006)

Table 2. miRNAs experimentally determined to play a role in cardiac hypertrophy/ cardiomyopathy

Multiple studies have been carried out to reveal important roles of miRNAs in cardiac hypertrophy and heart failure. Studies have found that a unique set of miRNAs are upregulated, downregulated or unaltered during the adaptive response of the heart to stress stimuli (Latronico et al., 2007). Furthermore, unique subset of miRNAs are known to be altered within the various etiologies of heart failure indicating significant role of miRNAs in these disease states (Sucharo et al., 2008). Consistent with the reexpression of fetal gene program, a high degree of similarity has been found between the miRNA expression pattern occurring in failing human hearts and those observed in the 12- 14 week-old hearts (Thum et al., 2007). Approximately, 80% of the analyzed miRNAs are similarly altered in failing adult and fetal human hearts compared to non-failing hearts. Multiple miRNAs have been implicated in cardiomyocyte hypertrophy and studies have consistently found upregulation of miRNA-21, -23a, -23b, -24, -195, -199a and miR-214 and downregulation of miRNA-1, -7, -133 and 378 (Naga Prasad and Karnik, 2010). Many of these miRNAs have been tested for hypertrophic response in neonatal cardiomyocytes. Concordant data from human and mice samples indicate that miRNAs may be involved in common pathway mediating hypertrophic response (Thum et al., 2007; van Rooij et al., 2006; Chen et al., 2008; Ikeda et al., 2007; Tatsuguchi et al., 2007; Sayed et al., 2007; Cheng et al., 2007) .

Among the miRNAs altered in various cardiac etiologies, some of them have been studied indepth and these include miRNA-1, -21, -133 and -208. It is well known that miRNA-1 is downregulated with a week of transverse aortic banding and its expression is inversely correlated with cardiac hypertrophy (Table 2) (Sayed et al., 2007; Catalucci et al., 2008; Ikeda et al., 2009, Naga Prasad et al., 2009 after al., 2009)). Similarly, Care et al., observed impaired expression of both miR-1 and miR-133 in patients with hypertrophic cardiomyopathy and atrial dilatation as well as in 3 different murine models of cardiac hypertrophy (Catalucci et al., 2008). In vitro cellular overexpression of miRNA-133 resulted in suppression of protein synthesis and block in hypertrophic response. Contrastingly, utilization of a decoy for miRNA-133 resulted in cellular hypertrophy and in vivo administration resulted in significant myocardial hypertrophy associated with reexpression of the fetal gene program (Catalucci et al., 2008). Some of targets of miRNA-133 have been validated and many are still being validated to provide evidence of miRNA-133 targeting multiple molecules to bring about hypertrophic response. miRNA-133 is encoded by 133a-1 and –2 and deletion of individual miRNA have no obvious cardiac abnormalities but combined deletion results in severe cardiac malformations with embryonic and post-natal lethality (Care et al., 2007). In contrast, overexpression of miRNA-133a results in embryonic lethality (E 15.5) caused by ventricular septal defected and impaired cardiomyocyte proliferation resulting in thinning of ventricular walls unable to meet hemodynamic needs (Care et al., 2007). These studies reveal that miRNA-133 plays a key role in myocardial development, hypertrophy and function. miRNA-208 is unique as it is a cardiac-specific miRNA encoded within the intron of α-myosin heavy chain (α-MHC) gene. miR-208 knockout mice are viable and do not show any obvious cardiac phenotype, but they fail to undergo stress-induced cardiac remodeling, hypertrophic growth, and α-MHC upregulation following transverse aortic constriction (Table 2) (van Rooij et al., 2007). It is believed that miRNA-208 regulation of this process involves α-MHC alterations balancing α-MHC.

While miRNA-208 mediates cardiac function by cardiomyocyte specific expression, miRNA-21 regulates cardiac function by its expression in both myocytes as well as cardiac fibroblasts. Recent studies (Thum et al., 2008) have shown progressive upregulation of miR-21 during late stages of heart failure, with an expression profile restricted exclusively to cardiac fibroblasts (Table 2). Upregulation of miR-21 was shown to be responsible for increased extracellular signal-regulated kinase (ERK) signaling through inhibition of its target, spry1 (sprouty 1), an inhibitor of the ERK/extracellular signal-regulated kinase pathway. These studies suggest that miRNA-21 expression results in increased fibroblast survival and reduced interstitial fibrosis independent of cardiomyocyte loss that may provide protective effects (Thum et al., 2008). Likewise, it has been (van Rooij et al., 2008) recently demonstrated that downregulation of the fibroblast-enriched miRNA-29 family in fibrotic areas surrounding a cardiac infarct is responsible for the regulation of mRNAs that encode a multitude of proteins involved in fibrosis such as collagens, fibrillins, and elastins. In addition to these miRNAs, we have recently shown that 8 miRNAs are differentially expressed in human dilated cardiomyopathy (DCM) (Naga Prasad et al., 2009). The miRNA-1, -29b, -7, and -378 were significantly down-regulated in the DCM samples compared with non-failing controls. In contrast, miRNA-214, -342, -125b and -181b were significantly upregulated in DCM compared with non-failing controls. These studies identified miRNA-7 and -378 as novel miRNAs which are significantly downregulated during end stage cardiac dysfunction whose role in cardiac pathology remains to be determined.

4.2 Arrhythmia

One of the well known contributing factors for heart failure are the changes in ion channel function and expression leading to electrophysiological remodeling in both atria and ventricles. Although the role of miRNAs with regard to arrhythmia is not yet well established, recent evidence supports their role in the induction of arrhythmia. Expression of miRNA-1 by viral transduction following myocardial infarction in rat resulted in significant enlargement of the QRS complex, prolongation of the QT interval, and an increased incidence of arrhythmias (Yang et al., 2007). Conversely, a low incidence of fatal arrhythmias was obtained when antisense for miRNA-1 was used. These studies further identified that miRNA-1 targets GJA1 (connexin 43) and KCNJ2 a critical K^+ channel subunit both of which are required for maintenance of membrane potential. Consistently, miRNA-1 and -2 double knockout mice that survived until birth had high incidence of electrophysiological abnormalities resulting in sudden death (Zhao et al., 2007). In addition to miRNA-1, miRNA-133 has been implicated in contributing towards cardiac disease by altering electrophysiological remodeling. In particular, downregulation of miRNA-133 in hypertrophic hearts has been associated with an increase in ion channels HCN2/HCN4 which when upregulated, enhance automaticity and the development of arrhythmia (Luo et al., 2008). Moreover, in a model of diabetic cardiomyopathy, overexpression of miR-133 has been shown to downregulate the ERG (ether a-go-go-related gene) with consequent QT prolongation responsible for arrhythmias (Xiao et al., 2007). Although only two miRNAs have been extensively studied with regards to arrhythmia, it is only matter of time that more miRNAs will be found to play a critical contributing role in complex electrophysiological remodeling that may cause heart failure and sudden death.

5. Cardiac microRNA targets

5.1 Identification of microRNA targets

To comprehensively understand the miRNA function and potential therapeutic use in heart disease, identification and validation of miRNA targets is of fundamental importance. A large number of bioinformatic methods have been developed to predict miRNA targets based on the assumption that the 5′-nucleotides of miRNAs are most critical for target recognition (Lai, 2002; Lewis et al., 2003). Such methods easily result in the prediction of hundreds of potential miRNA targets which are difficult to validate using conventional means. Target accessibility is an important factor for miRNA target repression as nearly all the miRNA binding sites reside in the 3′-UTRs of target mRNA that is located in the unstable regions of mRNA structure calculated on the basis of free energy predictions and RNA structure (Zhao et al., 2005; Lee et al., 2002). Although various target prediction algorithms use the sequence complimentarity as a major determinant, newer tools are being developed as our understanding of the miRNA biology improves. In addition to the previous tools a novel miRNA target identification algorithms are being developed that also include target accessibility by evaluation of energy states of sequences flanking the miRNA target (Lewis et al., 2003; Lai, 2002). Such a tool has become a necessity as previous prediction algorithms seem to have higher levels of false positives. In this context, however it remains to be determined whether this stringent approach may identify less false-positive targets without missing others (Bruneau, 2005). A potential relationship between altered miRNA expression and changes in messenger RNA expression profiles in failing human left ventricles has recently been explored (Thum et al., 2007). Computational prediction identified multiple potential target genes with at least one binding site for highly upregulated miRNAs during heart failure. In contrast, transcriptome analysis conducted in parallel showed that theoretically predicted target genes were upregulated, demonstrating no obvious preponderance of gene repression (Thum et al., 2007). This obvious disconnect could be because the analysis was carried out at transcriptome level and not at a proteome level. It is potentially possible that the target proteins are significantly altered in response to miRNA alterations. The observed increase in miRNA transcripts could be due to feed back mechanism of reduced protein levels of the respective target proteins. These observations bring to focus our incomplete understanding of mRNA targeting by miRNA and we still have lot more to learn with regards to determining the underlying mechanisms regulating these processes. However, simultaneous use of current prediction algorithms and proteomic analysis should be able to provide a realistic idea on the target proteins. An important caveat that needs consideration is the sensitivity of proteome analysis which may still miss out on proteins altered at lower potency by miRNAs.

5.2 MicroRNA targets in cardiac disease

Despite the shortcomings of the tools available to accurately predict the targets, various studies have used traditional and non-traditional tools to verify and validate the targets of miRNAs. In many cases the targets have been identified in the knock-out or overexpression system which provides validity to the targets and it is further strengthened by the function of the target protein. We quote some of the examples below that provide a view point the way studies are currently being carried to unequivocally show that a specific protein is a miRNA target. Targeted deletion of miR-1-2 in mice causes 50% lethality mainly because of ventricular wall defects (Zhao et al., 2007) along with arrhythmias leading to sudden death. This has been linked to upregulation of Irx5, which is a target of miR-1 (Zhao et al., 2007). Conversely, it is also known that miRNA-1 expression resulted in repression of target KCNJ2 and GJA1 channels that code for the main potassium channel subunit Kir2.1 and connexin (Yang et al., 2007). This to a certain degree explains higher degree of arrhythmias found in patients with coronary artery disease where miRNA-1 expression is elevated and similar elevation is observed in mice following myocardial infarction. In contrast to these findings our studies in end-stage dilated cardiomyopathy and studies by others on aortic stenosis have found reduction in miRNA-1 expression (Naga Prasad et al., 2009). A preview of these studies show varied expression pattern of miRNA-1 based on the variations of diseases, biopsy locations, technical differences, or altered cellular composition of the biopsies. This indicates a need for appreciation of the differences so that in future a much more representative pattern develops for each of the altered miRNAs. In this context, miRNA-1 targets have been very well summarized that includes Ras GTPase-activating protein (RasGAP), cyclin-dependent kinase 9 (Cdk9), Ras homolog enriched in brain (Rheb), and fibronectin (Latronico et al., 2007).

On a similar note, miRNA-133 targets have also been well studied and they have been identified using in vitro and in vivo techniques (Care et al., 2007). They include Cdc42 (implicated in cytoskeletal modifications during cardiac remodelling), Rho-A (a GTP-GDP-binding molecule, also critical for hypertrophy), and NELF-A/WHSC2 (a nuclear factor involved in heart genesis). While Rho-A and Cdc42 have already been established as fundamental factors for cell growth, cytoskeletal reorganization, and regulation of contractility in cardiomyocytes, (Brown et al., 2006; Ke et al., 2004) the role of NELF-A/WHSC2 in cardiac hypertrophy is yet to be defined. Transduction of cardiomyocytes both in vitro and in vivo with an adenoviral vector containing a Whsc2 transgene resulted in protein synthesis inhibition, but induced the fetal gene program and upregulation of Rho-A, (Care et al., 2007) supporting the postulation that WHSC2 could play a selective role in hypertrophy. In addition to targeting molecules modulating cardiac hypertrophy, miRNA-133 also targets molecules regulating cardiac conductance. In the diabetic heart, upregulation of miR-133 expression results in downregulation of protein expression of the ether-a-go-go-related gene (ERG), encoding the rapid delayed rectifier potassium channel (Xiao et al., 2007) .

The studies on miRNA-133 targets are interesting suggesting a lot needs to be understood in terms of alteration of these miRNAs in stress results in a unique pathological phenotype. Such a view is further supported by studies on miRNA-208 which is expressed specifically in the cardiomyocytes (van Rooij et al., 2007). A major target of miRNA-208 is thrap1 [thyroid hormone receptor (THR)-associated protein 1] and reduction in the expression of miRNA-208 results in loss of negative regulation on THRAP-1 (van Rooij et al., 2007). The resulting increase in THRAP 1 protein affects the THR-regulated expression of α-MHC and β-MHC, which are inversely regulated through a positive and negative thyroid hormone response element on their promoters. This shift in expression is thought to be the underlying factor for the blunted response to pressure overload in miR-208 knockout mice. In this context, our studies have shown that miRNA-7 is significantly down-regulated in end-stage human heart failure and upon TAC in mice and consistently its targets ERBB2 (epidermal growth factor receptor 2) and COL1A (Collagen 1) are upregulated (Naga Prasad et al., 2009). The above discussed studies are only a representative window on plethora of studies identifying targets for various miRNAs altered in conditions of cardiac stress. These studies have been discussed with an aim to provides a bird eye view of the complexity in regulation of target protein expression by miRNAs and to appreciate the diverse effects miRNA alteration can have in a pathology accounting for the phenotype.

6. Specific molecules and network pathways altered in cardiac disease

In this section we will specifically discuss the study initiated by our group to uncover the specific set of molecules and pathways altered during end stage human heart failure. Our published study comprehensively showed alterations in eight miRNAs which are significantly altered in heart failure out of which two new miRNAs that are yet to be implicated in cardiac pathophysiology. We have built signaling pathway networks using predicted targets for the miRNAs and identified nodal molecules that control these networks. Genome-wide profiling of miRNAs was performed using custom-designed miRNA microarray followed by validation on an independent set of samples. To gain an unbiased global perspective on regulation by altered miRNAs, predicted targets of eight miRNAs were analyzed using the Ingenuity Pathways Analysis network algorithm to build signaling networks and identify nodal molecules. The majority of nodal molecules identified in our analysis were targets of altered miRNAs and well known regulators of cardiovascular signaling. A heart failure gene expression data base was used to analyze changes in the expression patterns for these target nodal molecules (Naga Prasad et al., 2009). Indeed, expression of nodal molecules was altered in heart failure and inversely correlated to miRNA changes validating our analysis. Importantly, using network analysis we were successful in identification of a limited number of key functional targets that may regulate expression of the myriad proteins in heart failure and could be potential therapeutic targets. Furthermore, we have been able to independently see these 2 new miRNAs mir-7 and -378 in TAC mice hearts (Naga Prasad et al., 2009). We have shown miRNA-7 and -378 to be downregulated in the end stage human heart failure and targets of miRNA-7, ERBB2 and Col1A to be upregulated. miRNA-7-1 is encoded by the intron-1 of the HNRNPk gene. Similarly, we found miRNA-378 target SLC2A to be upregulated. Out of 1785 predicated targets, 1716 could be mapped to signaling networks in the IPATM, and 995 predicated targets were found to be network-eligible. The 995 network-eligible candidates mapped to 43 networks that are predicted to be involved in the cross-talk with the peripheral molecules bridging different networks. A representative network with NFkB, a known mediator in cardiac dysfunction (Naga Prasad et al., 2009) as a central node, is shown in Fig. 2 wherein the members that network with NFkB are targets for the miRNAs 1, 29b, 125b, 181b 214, 342, and 378. As individual miRNA acts on each target, the net effect on the node would be the collective influence of all the members connected to the central node, NFkB (Fig. 2) Based on this consideration, we predicted that the complete NFkB regulatory signaling network (Fig. 2) would be significantly down-regulated in DCM since molecules in this network are predicted targets for up-regulated miRNAs 125b, 181b, 214, and 243.

To directly evaluate whether nodal molecules are potential targets for altered miRNAs, immunoblotting studies in the end-stage human heart failure samples revealed an inverse co-relation with the level of respective miRNAs (Fig. 3). Immunoblotting showed ERBB2, HDAC4, COL1, MMP2, and TIMP2 were significantly up-regulated in human DCM (Fig. 3) and were inversely correlated to the down-regulation of their respective miRNAs. In contrast, STAT3 and E2F3 are down-regulated, consistent with the observation of up-regulation of their respective miRNAs suggesting that expression of these molecules may be regulated by miRNAs. Interestingly, we did not observe changes in expression levels of RB1 or EZH2 (Fig. 4) despite being predicted targets for miRNAs consistent with our data.

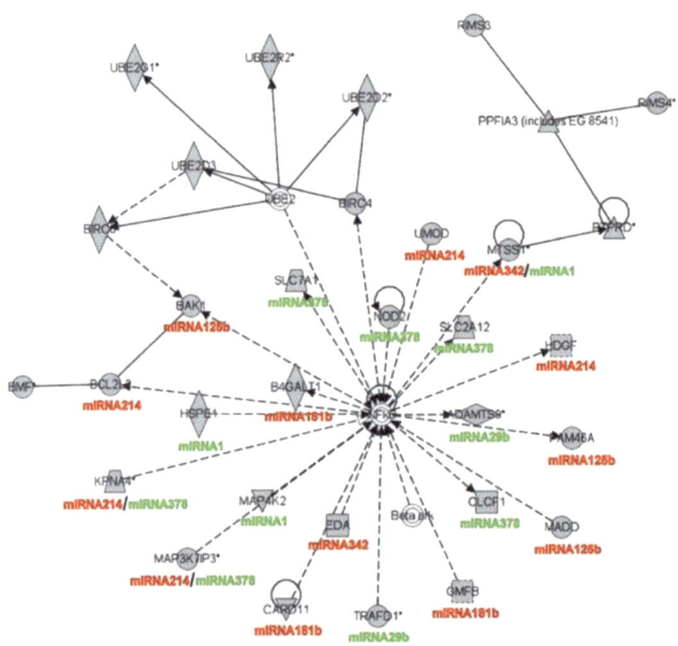

Fig. 2. A representative network showing NF-κB as high connectivity node: The hub is the center of the web of signaling connections and NF-κB is connected to nearly all the molecules in the network. Altered miRNAs in end-stage heart failure are overlaid with their respective predicted targets. miRNA represented in green are downregulated and in red are upregulated in end-stage human dilated cardiomyopathy. Importantly, NF-κB is not a predicted target to any of the altered miRNAs in DCM, yet it could be regulated by alterations in miRNA targets.

7. miRNA databases and computational tools

In recent years, many miRNA database systems have been developed and each of the databases has unique capabilities as they distinguish themselves by the types of data collected, the organization principles, and sources of the data contents. Therefore, it is important for researchers to use all of them to make an informed decision regarding execution of their experimental plan. These databases provide valuable resources to the research community towards understanding the functions of miRNAs in gene regulation. Critically, these databases contain miRNA sequences, annotations and nomenclature, miRNA targets and their relationships, as well as in some cases miRNA expression profiles in different cell types and tissues.

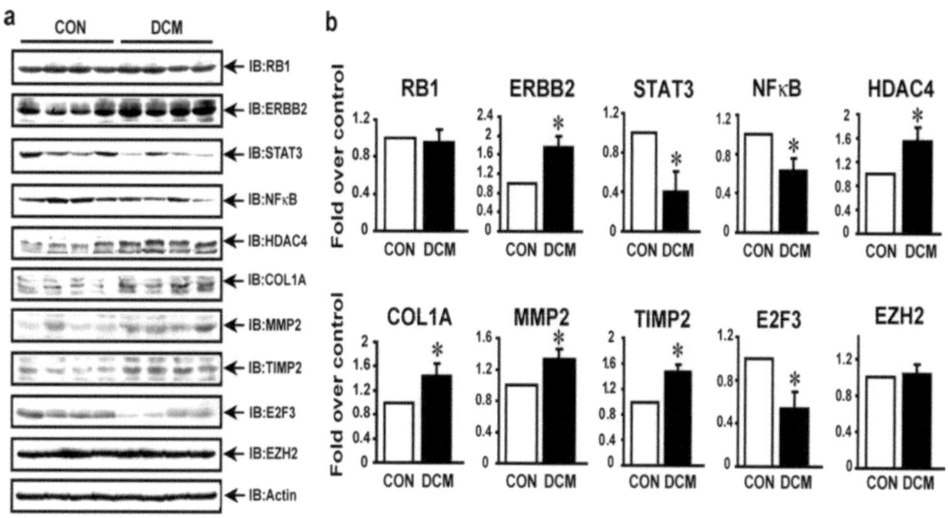

Fig. 3. Immunoblotting in end stage human heart failure *a,* Western immunoblotting analysis was carried out on nonfailinghuman hearts (*CON,* controls; *n*=8), and hearts from patients diagnosed with DCM (*n*=8). 170 microgram of myocardial lysate was resolved with SDS-polyacrylamide gel and immunoblotted (*IB*) with respective antibodies. The blots were stripped and re-probed multiple times with various antibodies, including beta-actin antibody that was used to ensure equal loading. *b,* densitometric analysis in the DCM samples is represented as fold over nonfailing controls.*, $p < 0.001$ control *versus* DCM.

miRBase (Griffiths-Jones et al., 2008) and Rfam (Gardner et al.,) are two major databases containing miRNA sequences and their annotations. miRBase database is an online repository for miRNA sequences and annotations that provides naming service for new miRNA genes isolated by researchers prior to publication. As of April 2011, miRBase contains 16772 mRNA entries from 153 species. Each entry represents a predicted hairpin portion of a miRNA transcript with information on the location and sequence of the mature miRNA as well as functional information/references. In this regard, Rfam database contains information about non-coding RNA families and annotations for family of RNA genes. As of June 2011, Rfam contains 1973 RNA families annotating over 2,756,313 regions in 1,723 unique species. Each family in Rfam is represented by multiple sequence alignments, its consensus secondary structures, and the associated probabilistic covariance models. In addition, Rfam coordinates a community annotation system providing access through Wikipedia allowing researchers to update entries and create families in the database.

An essential aspect of the functional analysis of miRNAs is the annotation of their targets. Increasing number of miRNA target genes are being identified and confirmed experimentally and simultaneously numerous target prediction algorithms are being developed to enhance the certainty of prediction. miRNA target prediction data base TargetScan (Lewis et al., 2003) predicts miRNA targets in mammals by searching for the presence of conserved 8-mer and 7-mer sites that match the seed region of the miRNA. The criteria for prediction and ranking include stringent seed sequence base pairing, untranslated region (UTR) context, the degree of target sequence conservation across the range of species and finally the thermodynamic stability of the predicted pairings. In addition to TargetScan, there are also several other miRNA target prediction algorithms like PicTar (Lall et al., 2006), MiRanda (John et al., 2004) , EMBL (Stark et al., 2005). They all adopt similar criteria (of rigorous seed pairing, site number, site type and context, likelihood of preferential conservation, and predicted site accessibility) for the target prediction. Historically, during the early phases of target prediction algorithm development, the predicted targets would vary remarkably with many non-overlapping predictions. But with time, utilization of similar criteria has significantly reduced the discrepancies with many overlaps of predicted targets. Such cross-references across the data bases for the miRNA targets is provided by miRecords. This computational tool provides an integrated view of experimentally validated miRNA targets and displays predicted targets generated by 11 established miRNA target prediction programs.

Since targets for many miRNAs are being identified, there is an ongoing simultaneous effort to develop databases that exclusively provides information on validated miRNA targets like TarBase (Sethupathy et al., 2006) and miRTarBase. TarBase database collects manually curated and experimentally supported miRNA targets in animal species, plants and viruses. It includes more than 1300 targets and each target is described by the miRNA it binds, the experiments that tested this relationship and the link to citation. Database miRTarBase (Hsu et al.,) curates 3576 experimentally validated microRNA-target interactions between 657 microRNAs and 2297 target genes among 17 species. In order to provide a disease perspective on the role of miRNA and their targets in pathology, a unique database miR2Disease [miR2Disease] has been generated. miR2Disease (Jiang et al., 2009) documents 1939 curated miRNA-disease relationships between 299 human miRNAs and 94 human diseases. Each entry in the database contains information on the miRNA ID, the disease name, validated targets, expression patterns of the miRNA, a brief description of the miRNA-disease relationship and citation.

Another important issue the readers need to appreciate is that despite the knowledge that there may be 1000 potential miRNA genes in the human genome, all of them have not yet been experimentally validated. These miRNA encoding gene predictions come from the sequence based curation of the genome to determine whether a specific DNA sequence characteristically fits the requirement for encoding a miRNA. RepTar (Elefant et al.,) is one such database that curates genome-wide predicted miRNAs of human and mouse. Furthermore, it can also predict cellular targets of human and mouse viral miRNAs. In addition to the miRNA sequence and target databases, a growing number of entries have been recorded at gene expression databases such as Gene Expression Omnibus (GEO) (Barrett et al.,) at NCBI and ArrayExpress (Brazma et al., 2006) Archive at EBI.

Although we are a long way away from validating all the predicted targets of altered miRNAs in heart failure, the predicted targets provide us a window to assess the global signaling pathways that could potentially be altered by the miRNAs in the heart failure. We have used this idea to build signaling networks of predicted targets of miRNAs altered in human heart failure which involves the role of miRNA target interaction with the biological pathways which ultimately generate the phenotype. A well known web-based tool is the Ingenuity Pathway Analysis (IPA) which is commonly used to model, analyze, and understand biological data derived from mRNA/miRNA gene expression arrays, SNP microarrays, proteomics, as well as small scale experiments. The core of IPA is its knowledge database on genes, proteins, chemicals, and molecular relationships. The database contains highly structured information about molecular interactions and functional annotations as well as contextual details of the biological interactions. IPA provides modules that can be used to integrate data at multiple levels to obtain insight into the molecular interactions, cellular phenotypes and disease processes of the biological system like heart failure. The main analysis modules include 1) IPA Core Analysis for identifying signaling and metabolic pathways, molecular networks, and biological processes that are related to the biological data; 2) IPA-Metabolomics for extracting biological insight into cell physiology and metabolism; 3) IPA-Tox for analyzing toxicity of candidate compounds; and 4) IPA-Biomarker for identifying the most promising and relevant biomarker candidates within experimental datasets. In addition, IPA's Path Designer provides researchers with help for transforming customized networks/pathways into pathway graphics for easy representation. It is well known historically that as the field evolves, so also the tools and miRNA target filter in the IPA analysis is one such evolution. miRNA Target Filter was introduced in the recent version of IPA (IPA 9.0) that allows researcher to examine both predicted and experimentally confirmed miRNA targets. Furthermore, it prioritizes targets based on related biological context and allows visualization of molecular interactions between miRNAs, their targets and other related molecules. IPA uses TargetScan database for predicted targets and TarBase for experimentally confirmed targets.

8. miRNAs as therapeutic targets

The current evidence from multiple studies show that miRNAs are altered with cardiac stress and genetic manipulation shows that miRNAs may actively contribute towards the deleterious cardiac phenotype. The regulation of cardiac phenotype by miRNAs, indicates that miRNAs can be used in therapeutic strategies to ameliorate deleterious outcomes. Since miRNAs are RNAs, they can be manipulated using the existing antisense and gene therapy approaches in vivo. Modified antisense oligonucleotides targeting the mature miRNA sequence, antimiRs, can reduce the levels of pathogenic or aberrantly expressed miRNAs (Krutzfeldt et al., 2005). Conversely, miRNA mimics can elevate the levels of miRNAs with beneficial outcomes (Xiao et al., 2007). Since miRNAs typically act as inhibitors of gene expression, the effect of adding specific miRNA mimics to a system is to decrease the expression of the mRNAs controlled by the miRNA. Conversely, the effect of inhibitors of specific miRNAs is to relieve the inhibition of the genes normally targeted by the miRNA. Thus, the primary effect of a miRNA inhibitor is activation of gene expression and a miRNA mimic is suppression of gene expression.

8.1 Antisense miRNA oligonucleotides and miRNA mimics

Disease condition is contributed by upregulation or downregulation of miRNAs. In conditions of upregulation specific reduction of the miRNA would be therapeutically desirable. One of the efficient ways to inhibit miRNAs would be the use of chemically modified single-stranded reverse complement oligonucleotides. The synthetic reverse complement oligonucleotide approach affects miRNA levels by (1) binding the mature miRNA within the RISC and acting as a competitive inhibitor; (2) binding to the pre-miRNA and preventing its processing or entry into the RISC; (3) interfering with the processing or export of the pre- or pri-miRNA from the nucleus. In any case, the net result is a reduction in the concentration of a specific miRNA-programmed RISC. This approach is similar in concept to traditional antisense targeting of mRNAs, except the number of targeting sites for a miRNA is very limited. Although conceptually comparable, only a handful of modifications have been achieved for inhibition of miRNAs. Such a technique has been effectively used to knock down let-7 in Drosophila (Hutvagner, Simard et al. 2004) while miRNA-122 was the first mammalian miRNA to be targeted for liver (Krutzfeldt et al., 2005). In this context, miRNA-133 (Altuvia et al., 2005) and miRNA-29 (van Rooij et al., 2008) have been effectively used to alter cardiac phenotype suggesting that this specific technique would be a viable option for therapeutic strategy. More recently, the technique of modifying the oligonucleotides with 2'O-methoxyethyl phosphorothioate is being extensively used as it seems to provide long term stability for the administered oligos thus extending the beneficial effects in vivo.

Anti-sense oligos can be used in conditions of targeting upregulated miRNAs and in conditions where reduction in miRNA level causes a disease state, beneficial therapeutic approach would be to increase its concentration. Instead of delivering the single-stranded oligonucleotide equivalent of the mature miRNA, an increase in the effective concentration of a reduced miRNA can be achieved through the use of synthetic RNA duplexes in which 1 strand is identical to the native miRNA. In this case, short double stranded oligonucleotides are designed in which 1 strand is the mature miRNA sequence (guide strand) and a complimentary or partially complementary stand is complexed with the mature miRNA sequence (passenger strand). The double stranded structure is required for recognition and loading into the RISC (Martinez et al., 2002). The only caveat in this kind of the design is to make sure that the passenger strand is eliminated and does not act as a new miRNA that may complicate the interpretation. Alternatively, approaches similar to that undertaken with siRNA using bioinformatic and chemical modification can be used and provides attractive means to elevate miRNA levels.

8.2 Therapeutic targeting of miRNA and challenges

Despite the ability to manipulate miRNAs in vivo to provide unique opportunities therapeutically, miRNA-based therapeutics pose challenges that are different from those associated with classic drugs. One of the major stumbling blocks for miRNA targeting is the issue of specificity. While specificity for a single cellular target is vital in classic drugs, miRNAs have numerous molecular targets raising the possibility that targeting of a miRNA may perturb multiple cellular functions both deleterious as well as beneficial. Since miRNAs are new set of molecules that are being targeted, better understanding of pharmacokinetics, biodistribution, and cell penetration is required to develop these as therapeutics. It is known that native nucleic acids are rapidly degraded by a variety of nucleases and phosphodiesterases in blood. Furthermore, biological environments and requirement of chemical modifications on the synthetic nucleotide derivatives may alter miRNA biophysical properties reducing the efficiency of therapeutic function. In this regards, several modifications that increase the stability of the oligonucleotides, including phosphorothioate, 2′-O-methyl, and 2′-fluoro substitutions can be effectively put to use in developing therapeutic strategies (Soutschek et al., 2004).

8.3 Methods of Delivery

In addition to efforts on developing miRNAs that are stable by modification, intense efforts are also ongoing to identify agents capable of targeted delivery of nucleic acids to tissues and cells. Delivery approaches can be broadly divided into 2 categories, conjugation and formulation. Conjugation strategies include direct attachment of targeting and cell-penetrating peptides, antibodies, and other bioactive molecules to the oligonucleotide. Formulation approaches vary broadly and include complex lipid emulsions from natural sources, synthetic liposomes, polyplexes, polymers and nanoparticles. To enter mammalian cells, the reverse-complement oligonucleotide needs to cross the lipid bilayer of the cell membrane and can be achieved by packaging the oligonucleotide into liposomes or nanoparticles that facilitates endocytosis. Alternatively, the oligonucleotide can be linked to a lipophilic moiety or receptor ligand, such as cholesterol that seems to greatly enhance cellular uptake (Soutschek et al., 2004). Despite significant advances in systemic delivery technology, most nucleic acid delivery agents developed to date have demonstrated efficacy in delivery to the liver. Therefore, effective delivery approaches especially to the heart would be a great stepping stone in the direction towards use of synthetic nucleic acids as therapeutics for cardiovascular disease. Interestingly, heart failure affords a unique opportunity to expand the potential for local delivery through the use of catheters providing additional level of sophistication.

9. Conclusions

It is remarkable to consider that miRNAs were first shown to function in mammals less than a decade ago, and the concept of miRNA manipulation in vivo to regulate disease-related processes is already becoming a feasible future therapeutic approach. Moreover, the rapidly expanding number of miRNAs makes it likely that the relatively few miRNAs studied to date represent only a subset of the miRNAs of interest in human disease. Given the established involvement of miRNAs in many facets of heart disease, it becomes pertinent to understand the underlying basis for its contributing role before taking on miRNA based human trials. Understanding the role of miRNAs in regulating various targets is the weakest link in this chain of fast moving area of miRNA that needs effort and resources. We believe the efforts are needed simultaneously in the direction of indepth contemporary proteomics along with assessment of miRNAs providing platform for linking miRNA to target protein expression which are the ultimate determinants of the phenotype. Therefore, identifying and validating miRNA targets are of paramount importance and establishment of the miRNA targets will provide a sound foundation for development of global signaling networks. Understanding the global regulation of networks by a miRNA rather than a specific target would be a more feasible approach to understand the overall function of miRNAs in development and disease conditions as a single miRNA could target both synergistic as well as antagonistic pathways. Appreciation of this unique regulation by miRNAs in physiology as well as pathology is the incentive to develop tools and technology to better understand the role of miRNAs in effecting global change rather than specific molecules in a given pathway.

10. Acknowledgement

This work was supported in part by Department of Molecular Cardiology Startup Funds, LRI, Cleveland Clinic Foundation NIH RO1 HL089473 (S.V.NP), RO1 HL083243 (S.S.K) and AHA 10POST3610049 (M.K.G).

11. References

Altuvia, Y., P. Landgraf, et al. (2005). "Clustering and conservation patterns of human microRNAs." *Nucleic Acids Res* 33(8): 2697-706.

Ambros, V. (2004). "The functions of animal microRNAs." *Nature* 431(7006): 350-5.

Aravin, A. A., G. J. Hannon, et al. (2007). "The Piwi-piRNA pathway provides an adaptive defense in the transposon arms race." *Science* 318(5851): 761-4.

Barrett, T., D. B. Troup, et al. "NCBI GEO: archive for functional genomics data sets--10 years on." *Nucleic Acids Res* 39(Database issue): D1005-10.

Barron, M. R., N. S. Belaguli, et al. (2005). "Serum response factor, an enriched cardiac mesoderm obligatory factor, is a downstream gene target for Tbx genes." *J Biol Chem* 280(12): 11816-28.

Bartel, D. P. (2004). "MicroRNAs: genomics, biogenesis, mechanism, and function." *Cell* 116(2): 281-97.

Bartel, D. P. (2009). "MicroRNAs: target recognition and regulatory functions." *Cell* 136(2): 215-33.

Berezikov, E., V. Guryev, et al. (2005). "Phylogenetic shadowing and computational identification of human microRNA genes." *Cell* 120(1): 21-4.

Bernstein, E., S. Y. Kim, et al. (2003). "Dicer is essential for mouse development." *Nat Genet* 35(3): 215-7.

Brazma, A., M. Kapushesky, et al. (2006). "Data storage and analysis in ArrayExpress." *Methods Enzymol* 411: 370-86.

Brown, J. H., D. P. Del Re, et al. (2006). "The Rac and Rho hall of fame: a decade of hypertrophic signaling hits." *Circ Res* 98(6): 730-42.

Bruneau, B. G. (2005). "Developmental biology: tiny brakes for a growing heart." *Nature* 436(7048): 181-2.

Cacchiarelli, D., D. Santoni, et al. (2008). "MicroRNAs as prime players in a combinatorial view of evolution." *RNA Biol* 5(3): 120-122.

Calin, G. A., C. G. Liu, et al. (2007). "Ultraconserved regions encoding ncRNAs are altered in human leukemias and carcinomas." *Cancer Cell* 12(3): 215-29.

Care, A., D. Catalucci, et al. (2007). "MicroRNA-133 controls cardiac hypertrophy." *Nat Med* 13(5): 613-8.

Catalucci, D., M. V. Latronico, et al. (2008). "Physiological myocardial hypertrophy: how and why?" *Front Biosci* 13: 312-24.

Chapman, E. J. and J. C. Carrington (2007). "Specialization and evolution of endogenous small RNA pathways." *Nat Rev Genet* 8(11): 884-96.

Chen, J. F., E. M. Mandel, et al. (2006). "The role of microRNA-1 and microRNA-133 in skeletal muscle proliferation and differentiation." *Nat Genet* 38(2): 228-33.

Chen, J. F., E. P. Murchison, et al. (2008). "Targeted deletion of Dicer in the heart leads to dilated cardiomyopathy and heart failure." *Proc Natl Acad Sci U S A* 105(6): 2111-6.

Cheng, Y., R. Ji, et al. (2007). "MicroRNAs are aberrantly expressed in hypertrophic heart: do they play a role in cardiac hypertrophy?" *Am J Pathol* 170(6): 1831-40.

Dash, R., V. Kadambi, et al. (2001). "Interactions between phospholamban and beta-adrenergic drive may lead to cardiomyopathy and early mortality." *Circulation* 103(6): 889-96.

Ebert, M. S., J. R. Neilson, et al. (2007). "MicroRNA sponges: competitive inhibitors of small RNAs in mammalian cells." *Nat Methods* 4(9): 721-6.

Elefant, N., A. Berger, et al. "RepTar: a database of predicted cellular targets of host and viral miRNAs." *Nucleic Acids Res* 39(Database issue): D188-94.

Eulalio, A., I. Behm-Ansmant, et al. (2007). "P-body formation is a consequence, not the cause, of RNA-mediated gene silencing." *Mol Cell Biol* 27(11): 3970-81.

Farh, K. K., A. Grimson, et al. (2005). "The widespread impact of mammalian MicroRNAs on mRNA repression and evolution." *Science* 310(5755): 1817-21.

Felli, N., L. Fontana, et al. (2005). "MicroRNAs 221 and 222 inhibit normal erythropoiesis and erythroleukemic cell growth via kit receptor down-modulation." *Proc Natl Acad Sci U S A* 102(50): 18081-6.

Filipowicz, W. (2005). "RNAi: the nuts and bolts of the RISC machine." *Cell* 122(1): 17-20.

Gardner, P. P., J. Daub, et al. "Rfam: Wikipedia, clans and the "decimal" release." *Nucleic Acids Res* 39(Database issue): D141-5.

Giraldez, A. J., R. M. Cinalli, et al. (2005). "MicroRNAs regulate brain morphogenesis in zebrafish." *Science* 308(5723): 833-8.

Giraldez, A. J., Y. Mishima, et al. (2006). "Zebrafish MiR-430 promotes deadenylation and clearance of maternal mRNAs." *Science* 312(5770): 75-9.

Gregory, P. A., A. G. Bert, et al. (2008). "The miR-200 family and miR-205 regulate epithelial to mesenchymal transition by targeting ZEB1 and SIP1." *Nat Cell Biol* 10(5): 593-601.

Griffiths-Jones, S., R. J. Grocock, et al. (2006). "miRBase: microRNA sequences, targets and gene nomenclature." *Nucleic Acids Res* 34(Database issue): D140-4.

Griffiths-Jones, S., H. K. Saini, et al. (2008). "miRBase: tools for microRNA genomics." *Nucleic Acids Res* 36(Database issue): D154-8.

Gusev, Y., T. D. Schmittgen, et al. (2007). "Computational analysis of biological functions and pathways collectively targeted by co-expressed microRNAs in cancer." *BMC Bioinformatics* 8 Suppl 7: S16.

Harris, T. A., M. Yamakuchi, et al. (2008). "MicroRNA-126 regulates endothelial expression of vascular cell adhesion molecule 1." *Proc Natl Acad Sci U S A* 105(5): 1516-21.

Hsu, S. D., F. M. Lin, et al. "miRTarBase: a database curates experimentally validated microRNA-target interactions." *Nucleic Acids Res* 39(Database issue): D163-9.

Hutvagner, G., J. McLachlan, et al. (2001). "A cellular function for the RNA-interference enzyme Dicer in the maturation of the let-7 small temporal RNA." *Science* 293(5531): 834-8.

Hutvagner, G., M. J. Simard, et al. (2004). "Sequence-specific inhibition of small RNA function." *PLoS Biol* 2(4): E98.

Hwang, H. W., E. A. Wentzel, et al. (2007). "A hexanucleotide element directs microRNA nuclear import." *Science* 315(5808): 97-100.

Ikeda, S., A. He, et al. (2009). "MicroRNA-1 negatively regulates expression of the hypertrophy-associated calmodulin and Mef2a genes." *Mol Cell Biol* 29(8): 2193-204.

Ikeda, S., S. W. Kong, et al. (2007). "Altered microRNA expression in human heart disease." *Physiol Genomics* 31(3): 367-73.

Ivanovska, I. and M. A. Cleary (2008). "Combinatorial microRNAs: working together to make a difference." *Cell Cycle* 7(20): 3137-42.

Ivey, K. N., A. Muth, et al. (2008). "MicroRNA regulation of cell lineages in mouse and human embryonic stem cells." *Cell Stem Cell* 2(3): 219-29.

Jiang, Q., Y. Wang, et al. (2009). "miR2Disease: a manually curated database for microRNA deregulation in human disease." *Nucleic Acids Res* 37(Database issue): D98-104.

John, B., A. J. Enright, et al. (2004). "Human MicroRNA targets." *PLoS Biol* 2(11): e363.

Ke, Y., L. Wang, et al. (2004). "Intracellular localization and functional effects of P21-activated kinase-1 (Pak1) in cardiac myocytes." *Circ Res* 94(2): 194-200.

Kertesz, M., N. Iovino, et al. (2007). "The role of site accessibility in microRNA target recognition." *Nat Genet* 39(10): 1278-84.

Kim, V. N. and J. W. Nam (2006). "Genomics of microRNA." *Trends Genet* 22(3): 165-73.

Kiriakidou, M., P. T. Nelson, et al. (2004). "A combined computational-experimental approach predicts human microRNA targets." *Genes Dev* 18(10): 1165-78.

Kloosterman, W. P., A. K. Lagendijk, et al. (2007). "Targeted inhibition of miRNA maturation with morpholinos reveals a role for miR-375 in pancreatic islet development." *PLoS Biol* 5(8): e203.

Krek, A., D. Grun, et al. (2005). "Combinatorial microRNA target predictions." *Nat Genet* 37(5): 495-500.

Krichevsky, A. M., K. C. Sonntag, et al. (2006). "Specific microRNAs modulate embryonic stem cell-derived neurogenesis." *Stem Cells* 24(4): 857-64.

Krutzfeldt, J., N. Rajewsky, et al. (2005). "Silencing of microRNAs in vivo with 'antagomirs'." *Nature* 438(7068): 685-9.

Kuehbacher, A., C. Urbich, et al. (2007). "Role of Dicer and Drosha for endothelial microRNA expression and angiogenesis." *Circ Res* 101(1): 59-68.

Kwon, C., Z. Han, et al. (2005). "MicroRNA1 influences cardiac differentiation in Drosophila and regulates Notch signaling." *Proc Natl Acad Sci U S A* 102(52): 18986-91.

Lai, E. C. (2002). "Micro RNAs are complementary to 3' UTR sequence motifs that mediate negative post-transcriptional regulation." *Nat Genet* 30(4): 363-4.

Lakshmipathy, U., B. Love, et al. (2007). "MicroRNA expression pattern of undifferentiated and differentiated human embryonic stem cells." *Stem Cells Dev* 16(6): 1003-16.

Lall, S., D. Grun, et al. (2006). "A genome-wide map of conserved microRNA targets in C. elegans." *Curr Biol* 16(5): 460-71.

Landgraf, P., M. Rusu, et al. (2007). "A mammalian microRNA expression atlas based on small RNA library sequencing." *Cell* 129(7): 1401-14.

Latronico, M. V., D. Catalucci, et al. (2007). "Emerging role of microRNAs in cardiovascular biology." *Circ Res* 101(12): 1225-36.

Lee, N. S., T. Dohjima, et al. (2002). "Expression of small interfering RNAs targeted against HIV-1 rev transcripts in human cells." *Nat Biotechnol* 20(5): 500-5.

Lee, Y., C. Ahn, et al. (2003). "The nuclear RNase III Drosha initiates microRNA processing." *Nature* 425(6956): 415-9.

Lee, Y., M. Kim, et al. (2004). "MicroRNA genes are transcribed by RNA polymerase II." *EMBO J* 23(20): 4051-60.

Lewis, B. P., C. B. Burge, et al. (2005). "Conserved seed pairing, often flanked by adenosines, indicates that thousands of human genes are microRNA targets." *Cell* 120(1): 15-20.

Lewis, B. P., I. H. Shih, et al. (2003). "Prediction of mammalian microRNA targets." *Cell* 115(7): 787-98.

Liu, N., A. H. Williams, et al. (2007). "An intragenic MEF2-dependent enhancer directs muscle-specific expression of microRNAs 1 and 133." *Proc Natl Acad Sci U S A* 104(52): 20844-9.

Luo, X., H. Lin, et al. (2008). "Down-regulation of miR-1/miR-133 contributes to re-expression of pacemaker channel genes HCN2 and HCN4 in hypertrophic heart." *J Biol Chem* 283(29): 20045-52.

MacRae, I. J., E. Ma, et al. (2008). "In vitro reconstitution of the human RISC-loading complex." *Proc Natl Acad Sci U S A* 105(2): 512-7.

Martinez, J., A. Patkaniowska, et al. (2002). "Single-stranded antisense siRNAs guide target RNA cleavage in RNAi." *Cell* 110(5): 563-74.

Miranda, K. C., T. Huynh, et al. (2006). "A pattern-based method for the identification of MicroRNA binding sites and their corresponding heteroduplexes." *Cell* 126(6): 1203-17.

Naga Prasad, S. V., Z. H. Duan, et al. (2009). "Unique microRNA profile in end-stage heart failure indicates alterations in specific cardiovascular signaling networks." *J Biol Chem* 284(40): 27487-99.

Naga Prasad and Karnik SS (2010). ''MicroRNAs--regulators of signaling networks in dilated cardiomyopathy.''*J Cardiovasc Transl Res.* 3(3):225-34.

Nilsen, T. W. (2007). "Mechanisms of microRNA-mediated gene regulation in animal cells." *Trends Genet* 23(5): 243-9.

Niu, Z., A. Li, et al. (2007). "Serum response factor micromanaging cardiogenesis." *Curr Opin Cell Biol* 19(6): 618-27.

Okamura, K., J. W. Hagen, et al. (2007). "The mirtron pathway generates microRNA-class regulatory RNAs in Drosophila." *Cell* 130(1): 89-100.

Okamura, K., A. Ishizuka, et al. (2004). "Distinct roles for Argonaute proteins in small RNA-directed RNA cleavage pathways." *Genes Dev* 18(14): 1655-66.

Olson, E. N. and M. D. Schneider (2003). "Sizing up the heart: development redux in disease." *Genes Dev* 17(16): 1937-56.

Pedersen, I. M., G. Cheng, et al. (2007). "Interferon modulation of cellular microRNAs as an antiviral mechanism." *Nature* 449(7164): 919-22.

Rao, P. K., R. M. Kumar, et al. (2006). "Myogenic factors that regulate expression of muscle-specific microRNAs." *Proc Natl Acad Sci U S A* 103(23): 8721-6.

Rodriguez, A., S. Griffiths-Jones, et al. (2004). "Identification of mammalian microRNA host genes and transcription units." *Genome Res* 14(10A): 1902-10.

Ruby, J. G., C. H. Jan, et al. (2007). "Intronic microRNA precursors that bypass Drosha processing." *Nature* 448(7149): 83-6.

Sayed, D., C. Hong, et al. (2007). "MicroRNAs play an essential role in the development of cardiac hypertrophy." *Circ Res* 100(3): 416-24.

Schwarz, D. S., G. Hutvagner, et al. (2003). "Asymmetry in the assembly of the RNAi enzyme complex." *Cell* 115(2): 199-208.

Sethupathy, P., B. Corda, et al. (2006). "TarBase: A comprehensive database of experimentally supported animal microRNA targets." *RNA* 12(2): 192-7.

Soutschek, J., A. Akinc, et al. (2004). "Therapeutic silencing of an endogenous gene by systemic administration of modified siRNAs." *Nature* 432(7014): 173-8.

Srivastava, D., T. Thomas, et al. (1997). "Regulation of cardiac mesodermal and neural crest development by the bHLH transcription factor, dHAND." *Nat Genet* 16(2): 154-60.

Stark, A., J. Brennecke, et al. (2005). "Animal MicroRNAs confer robustness to gene expression and have a significant impact on 3'UTR evolution." *Cell* 123(6): 1133-46.

Sucharov, C., M. R. Bristow, et al. (2008). "miRNA expression in the failing human heart: functional correlates." *J Mol Cell Cardiol* 45(2): 185-92.

Sun, Q., G. Chen, et al. (2006). "Defining the mammalian CArGome." *Genome Res* 16(2): 197-207.

Tatsuguchi, M., H. Y. Seok, et al. (2007). "Expression of microRNAs is dynamically regulated during cardiomyocyte hypertrophy." *J Mol Cell Cardiol* 42(6): 1137-41.

Tay, Y. M., W. L. Tam, et al. (2008). "MicroRNA-134 modulates the differentiation of mouse embryonic stem cells, where it causes post-transcriptional attenuation of Nanog and LRH1." *Stem Cells* 26(1): 17-29.

Thum, T., P. Galuppo, et al. (2007). "MicroRNAs in the human heart: a clue to fetal gene reprogramming in heart failure." *Circulation* 116(3): 258-67.

Thum, T., C. Gross, et al. (2008). "MicroRNA-21 contributes to myocardial disease by stimulating MAP kinase signalling in fibroblasts." *Nature* 456(7224): 980-4.

van Rooij, E., L. B. Sutherland, et al. (2006). "A signature pattern of stress-responsive microRNAs that can evoke cardiac hypertrophy and heart failure." *Proc Natl Acad Sci U S A* 103(48): 18255-60.

van Rooij, E., L. B. Sutherland, et al. (2007). "Control of stress-dependent cardiac growth and gene expression by a microRNA." *Science* 316(5824): 575-9.

van Rooij, E., L. B. Sutherland, et al. (2008). "Dysregulation of microRNAs after myocardial infarction reveals a role of miR-29 in cardiac fibrosis." *Proc Natl Acad Sci U S A* 105(35): 13027-32.

Volpe, T. A., C. Kidner, et al. (2002). "Regulation of heterochromatic silencing and histone H3 lysine-9 methylation by RNAi." *Science* 297(5588): 1833-7.

Xiao, J., X. Luo, et al. (2007). "MicroRNA miR-133 represses HERG K+ channel expression contributing to QT prolongation in diabetic hearts." *J Biol Chem* 282(17): 12363-7.

Yang, B., H. Lin, et al. (2007). "The muscle-specific microRNA miR-1 regulates cardiac arrhythmogenic potential by targeting GJA1 and KCNJ2." *Nat Med* 13(4): 486-91.

Yi, R., Y. Qin, et al. (2003). "Exportin-5 mediates the nuclear export of pre-microRNAs and short hairpin RNAs." *Genes Dev* 17(24): 3011-6.

Yu, W., D. Gius, et al. (2008). "Epigenetic silencing of tumour suppressor gene p15 by its antisense RNA." *Nature* 451(7175): 202-6.

Zhang, S. X., E. Garcia-Gras, et al. (2005). "Identification of direct serum-response factor gene targets during Me2SO-induced P19 cardiac cell differentiation." *J Biol Chem* 280(19): 19115-26.

Zhao, Y., J. F. Ransom, et al. (2007). "Dysregulation of cardiogenesis, cardiac conduction, and cell cycle in mice lacking miRNA-1-2." *Cell* 129(2): 303-17.

Zhao, Y., E. Samal, et al. (2005). "Serum response factor regulates a muscle-specific microRNA that targets Hand2 during cardiogenesis." *Nature* 436(7048): 214-20.

Zilberman, D., X. Cao, et al. (2003). "ARGONAUTE4 control of locus-specific siRNA accumulation and DNA and histone methylation." *Science* 299(5607): 716-9.

13

Intercellular Connections in the Heart: The Intercalated Disc

Maegen A. Ackermann, Li-Yen R. Hu and
Aikaterini Kontrogianni-Konstantopoulos
Department of Biochemistry and Molecular Biology, University of Maryland, School of Medicine, Baltimore, MD, USA

1. Introduction

Proper cardiac function requires the synchronous mechanical and electrical activity of individual cardiomyocytes to ensure the coordinated excitation and contractile performance of the heart, as an organ. The intercalated disc (ID), a unique membrane structure forming at the edges of mammalian cardiomyocytes (Li and Radice, 2010), fulfills this role by allowing the transmission of mechanical and electrical activity between neighboring cells; (reviewed in Delmar and McKenna, 2010; Noorman et al., 2009).

1.1 A brief history of the ID

The ID was first depicted in 1866 by Karl Josef Ebhert *et al.* as "verdichtungsstreifen", which literally translates to "compression strips", but was later referred to as a homogeneous "cementing material" found at the ends of cardiac myocytes (Saphir and Karsner, 1924). A decade later, Engelman described the heart as a continuous syncytium, while a century later Weidmann suggested the presence of "membrane areas of synchronicity", characterized by low resistance that allows the transmission of electrical potential (Engelmann, 1875; Weidmann, 1952).

The idea of a continuous region connecting two cells was challenged in the mid 1950's by several groups who used electron microscopy to show that cardiac cells are separated from one another by a specialized extension of the sarcoplasm oriented transversely with respect to the cell's boundaries (Sjostrand and Andersson, 1954; Van Breemen, 1953). Since the middle of the 20th century, we have significantly advanced our understanding of the structure and composition of the ID. Accordingly, the ID was found to be a highly organized structure composed of three main junctional complexes; the gap junctions, which enable the propagation of electrical stimuli throughout heart cells, the adherens junctions, and the desmosomes, which provide mechanical coupling and stability to cardiomyocytes, respectively. The advent of electron microscopy in the 1950's to 1970's further provided detailed visualizations of the regions connecting two cardiomyocytes (Fawcett and McNutt, 1969; McNutt et al., 1970; Muir, 1957; Rayns et al., 1969; Sjostrand and Andersson, 1954; Van Breemen, 1953). Recently, novel cellular isolation techniques combined with scanning or transmission electron microscopy (SEM and TEM, respectively) have yielded three-dimensional images of the ID (Hoyt et al., 1989; Shimada et al., 2004; Tandler et al., 2006), showing that in the mammalian ventricular heart, IDs are arranged both transversely and longitudinally in a stairwell like fashion with steps and risers. Transverse or plicate segments, resembling the steps, run in a zigzag arrangement with finger-like micro-projections, and contain mainly adherens junctions and desmosomes with smaller regions of gap junction plaques. Longitudinal or interplicate segments resemble the risers and contain mainly desmosomes and larger areas of gap junction plaques. The many folds and projections found within this region, increase the surface area of the ID, providing the cardiac cells with superior intercellular communication.

1.2 Spatiotemporal distribution of ID components

During cardiomyocyte development and maturation, major changes occur in structures associated with the ID. Studies using human myocardium showed that during embryonic development adherens junction and desmosomal organization follows that of gap junctions (Pieperhoff and Franke, 2007). However, during postnatal development proteins of the adherens and gap junctions appear to orient themselves at IDs simultaneously (Peters et al., 1994). Moreover, *in vivo* studies of lower mammals (including rodent, bovine and canine) have shown that at embryonic stages and postnatal day 1, components of gap junctions, desmosomes and adherens junctions are uniformly distributed throughout the sarcolemma, mutually exclusive from one another (Angst et al., 1997; Hirschy et al., 2006). However, at later postnatal stages (days 6-20), proteins of the adherens junctions and desmosomes begin to concentrate towards the termini of cardiomyocytes, leaving proteins of gap junctions uniformly distributed at the plasma membrane. By postnatal day 90, all components of the three junctions are segregated and organized at IDs. These findings were also supported by *in vitro* studies using primary cultures of rat and mouse cardiomyocytes (Geisler et al., 2010; Kostin et al., 1999). Interestingly, the latter further demonstrated that when individual cardiocytes are allowed to make contact in culture, proteins of the adherens junctions are the first to assemble and "mark" the location of the developing ID, closely followed by desmosomal proteins and finally proteins of gap junctions (Geisler et al., 2010; Kostin et al., 1999). Supporting this, the organization of adherens junctions and desmosomes is independent of gap junctions; however, gap junction organization requires that of adherens junctions and desmosomes (Gutstein et al., 2003; Wei et al., 2005). Taken together, these observations suggest that proteins necessary for mechanical coupling, i.e. components of adherens junctions and desmosomes, create the appropriate environment for proteins mediating electro-chemical coupling, i.e. those associated with gap junctions.

1.3 Organization of the ID

Gap junctions mediate the direct communication between neighboring cells by forming a low resistance pathway for the transmission of signals and electrical current (Rohr, 2004). A gap junction is composed of twelve connexin proteins, with connexin-43 being the most prominent in mammalian cardiomyocytes, along with low amounts of connexin-45 and 40 (Beyer et al., 1987; Vozzi et al., 1999). Each cardiomyocyte contributes six connexin molecules to form a hemi-channel, or a connexon; two connexons join to form a pore or gap junction channel, which is isolated from the extracellular space and connects the cytosol of two neighboring cells (Sohl and Willecke, 2004). These channels are responsible for the occurrence of synchronous contractions throughout the heart (Sohl and Willecke, 2004).

Consequently, in the absence of connexin-43 channels, normal propagation of contraction is disrupted, and lethal arrhythmias develop (Gutstein et al., 2001a; Gutstein et al., 2001b).

Adherens junctions facilitate the transmission of contractile force from one cell to the next and are crucial in maintaining mechanical strength uniformly across the heart (Tepass et al., 2000). They are mainly composed of transmembrane cadherins and cytosolic catenins (Niessen, 2007). N-cadherin, the main cardiac isoform, is a transmembrane protein, with extracellular and intracellular components (Niessen, 2007). Its extracellular portion forms homodimers bringing together the membranes of two opposing cells, while its intracellular segment forms a complex with various members of the catenin family (α-, β-, γ- and p120) present in the cytosol, which in turn are linked to the actin cytoskeleton (Bass-Zubek et al., 2009). Consequently, adherens junctions serve as anchors between the extracellular space and the actin cytoskeleton (Noorman et al., 2009).

Desmosomes provide structural support to cardiomyocytes, which are subjected to strong contractile stress (Delmar, 2004). Desmosomes, similar to adherens junctions, are composed of intercellular and intracellular components (Rayns et al., 1969). The intercellular component consists of desmosomal cadherins, desmocollin and desmoglein, which form a hetero-complex within the extracellular space joining together two bordering cells (Green and Simpson, 2007), while the intracellular component consists of proteins of the armadillo/catenin (plakoglobin and plakophilin) and plakin (desmoplakin) families (Bass-Zubek et al., 2009). Desmoplakin directly interacts with intermediate filaments to stabilize the desmosomal structure. Importantly, a high incidence of mutations within genes encoding desmosomal proteins has been linked to the development of arrhythmogenic right ventricular cardiomyopathy (ARVC).

Although, the ID has been traditionally described to contain three distinct structures (i.e. gap junctions, adherens junctions and desmosomes), recent technological advancements indicate that they are more interwined than originally proposed (Delmar and McKenna, 2010). Consistent with this, adherens junctions and desmosomes are intimately associated in the "*area composita*" where proteins from both structures are present (Borrmann et al., 2006; Franke et al., 2006). Similarly, proteins of the adherens and gap junctions have been shown to interact directly (Delmar, 2004). Taken together, these observations suggest that the ID is actually a single functional unit where macromolecular complexes interact to maintain structural integrity and synchronous contraction throughout the heart.

Bridging the gap between the ID and the sarcomeric cytoskeleton is a newly defined region termed the transitional junction. This area is rich in structural proteins, including spectrin, ankyrin-G, α-actinin and the NH_2-terminal region of titin, which typically localizes to the Z-disc (Bennett et al., 2006). The transitional junction is suggested to connect the ID with the contractile apparatus, mediating the transmission of force between adjacent cardiocytes.

The high degree of complexity and organization of junctions at the ID suggests a tight interplay between mechanical and electrical activities. Disruption of either mechanical or electrical coupling leads to irregular conduction of electrical impulses and deterioration of cardiac function, subsequently resulting in the development of cardiac arrhythmias. Various mutations in genes encoding for ID proteins have been causatively linked to these complex disorders, many of which manifest themselves as ARVC; (recently reviewed in Protonotarios et al., 2011).

There are ~200 known proteins that are associated with the ID (Dowling et al., 2008; Estigoy et al., 2009; Geisler et al., 2007; Lin et al.; Kargacin et al., 2006; Satomi-Kobayashi et al., 2009;

Schroen et al., 2007; Seeger et al., 2010). Herein, we provide a summation of the current knowledge on the junctional structures present in the ID, focusing on their most prominent and influential components, and how these relate to each other and the sarcomeric cytoskeleton in normal and disease states.

2. Gap junctions

Gap junctions were first described by Revel and Karnovsky in 1967, as "hexagonal arrays" that localize to the ID and mediate the electrical and metabolic coupling of adjacent cardiomyocytes by allowing the diffusion of small molecules (<1000 Da) (Elfgang et al., 1995; Ravel and Karnovsky, 1967). At gap junctions, the distance between opposing membranes is ~3 nm (Fig. 1; Perkins et al., 1997). Gap junction plaques can contain from a few up to 200,000 connexon channels (Evans et al., 2006).

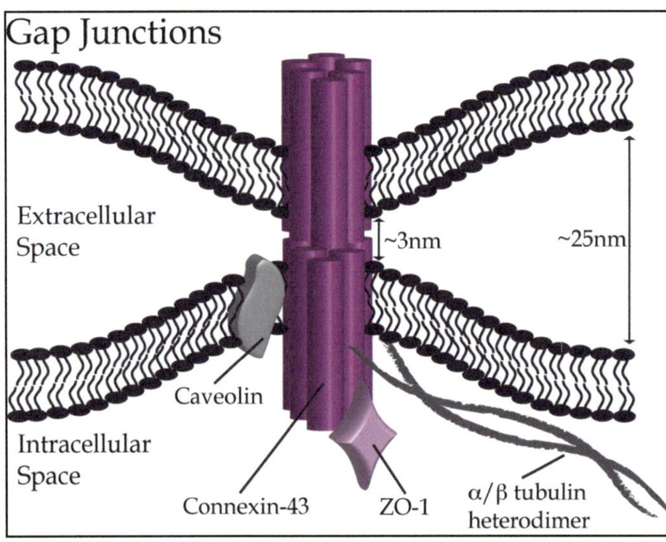

Fig. 1. Gap junctions in ventricular cardiomyocytes are composed of two homo-hexameric hemi-channels. forming a channel or a connexon. Each hemi-channel consists of six connexin-43 monomers (shown in dark purple), allowing the transmission of electrical current and small signalling molecules from adjoining cardiomyocytes. Zona Occludens-1 (ZO-1) (depicted in light purple) interacts directly with connexin-43. In addition, the connexin-43 complex interacts with members of the caveolin family (shown in light grey) that target gap junctions to lipid rafts, and cytosolic α/β tubulin heterodimers (shown in dark grey) that link gap junctions to the microtubular network.

2.1 Structural organization of connexons: Connexin-43

Connexin-43: The human connexin super-family is composed of at least twenty-one members. Connexin-43 is the predominant form expressed in the human heart, while connexins 40 and 45 are present in lower amounts (reviewed in Sohl and Willecke, 2004). Connexin-43 is a four-pass transmembrane protein that contains a cytoplasmic loop and two extracellular loops (Fig. 2A). Notably, both its NH_2- and COOH- termini are located in the cytosol (reviewed in Sohl and Willecke, 2004). Three conserved cysteine residues, located in the extracellular loops, have been implicated in disulfide bond formation between neighboring connexins of adjacent cells, and contribute to the development of a tight seal that prevents the exchange of materials with the extracellular matrix (Unger et al., 1999). Consistent with this, a constitutive connexin-43 null murine model is embryonic lethal (Reaume et al., 1995), while a cardiac-specific knock-out model exhibits sudden cardiac death by 2 months of age (Gutstein et al., 2001a; Gutstein et al., 2001b).

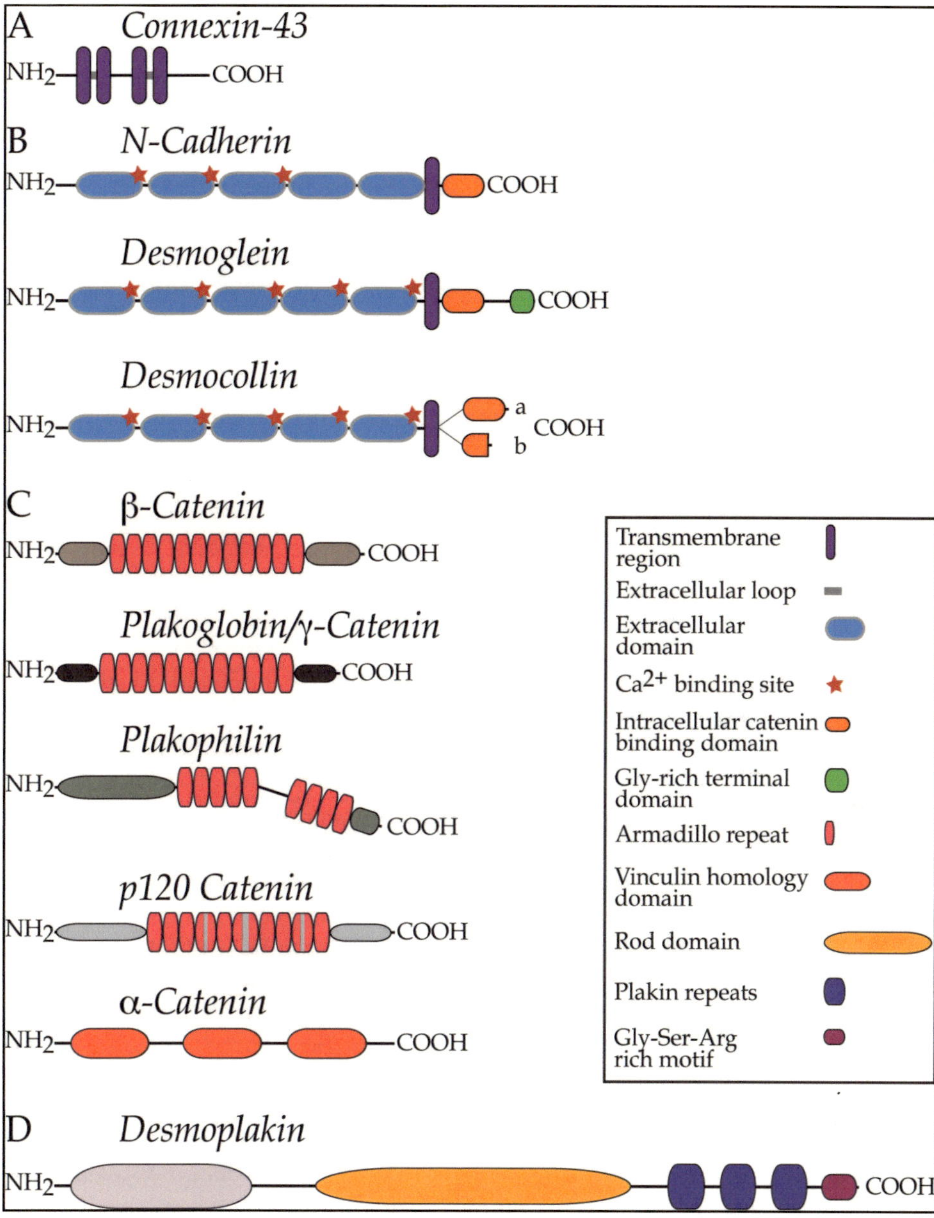

Fig. 2. Schematic representation of the domain structure of major ID proteins. Grey ovals denote protein specific domains.

NMR studies have demonstrated the presence of short, flexible α-helical segments in the cytoplasmic loop and the COOH-terminus of connexin-43, which provide binding sites for several proteins and mediate gating of the connexon (Duffy et al., 2002; reviewed in Gonzalez et al., 2007). Consequently, connexons can exist in a closed or open conformation; at high Ca^{2+} concentrations (i.e. 1.8 mM), they tend to adapt a closed conformation, however, in the absence of Ca^{2+} they exist in an open state (Thimm et al., 2005). Importantly, the gating of connexons is regulated by additional factors, including pH, levels of Mg^{2+}, voltage as well as the phosphorylation status of connexins (please see below; Bukauskas and Verselis, 2004; Delmar, 2004; Ek et al., 1994; Ek-Vitorin et al., 1996; Gonzalez et al., 2007; Matsuda et al., 2010).

2.2 Propagation of electrical stimulation throughout the heart

The propagation of electrical stimulation is the driving force for heart contraction. It originates at the sinoatrial (SA) node, traverses through the atria, crosses the atrioventricular (AV) node and propagates through the bundle of His and the Purkinje fibers before it activates the ventricles. The coordinated contraction of the atria and ventricles is achieved by conduction of the electrical impulse at variable speeds, mediated by the different forms of connexins, which confer to gap junction plaques distinct electrophysiological properties. As such, connexin-45 is preferentially expressed in the SA and AV nodes, but co-expressed with connexin-43 in the bundle of His and the Purkinje fibers. Conversely, connexin-43 is primarily present in the ventricles, but also co-expressed with connexin-40 in the atria; (reviewed in Severs et al., 2008).

Conferring low conductance in a single homotypic channel, connexin-45 is distributed at SA node in a sparse and scattered pattern that ensures poor coupling between adjacent cardiocytes. Similarly at the AV node, connexin-45 contributes to the sequential activation of the atria and ventricles reducing the occurrence of arrhythmias; (reviewed in Severs et al., 2008). On the contrary, the rapid propagation of electrical signals through the Purkinje fibers is mediated by gap junctions mainly consisting of connexins 43 and 40, which confer relatively large conductance, and to a lesser extent connexin-45, thus maintaining the regular contractions of the heart (Gonzalez et al., 2007; Kirchhoff et al., 1998).

2.3 Phosphorylation regulates the permeability of connexons

Several kinases modulate the function of connexons. Although a complete listing of all identified kinases is beyond the scope of this chapter, we will refer to major ones, highlighting their roles during normalcy and stress. Connexin-43 is a substrate of Src tyrosine kinase, which phosphorylates Tyr-265 to disrupt its interaction with ZO-1 (discussed below, Toyfuku et al., 2001), and suppress gap junction communication in the failing heart (Giepmans et al., 2001a; Toyofuku et al., 2001). Similarly, mitogen-activated protein kinase (MAPK) phosphorylates connexin-43 at Ser-255, Ser-279 and Ser-282 to repress gap junction communication (Warn-Cramer et al., 1998; Warn-Cramer et al., 1996). Conversely, phosphorylation of Ser-365 by protein kinase A (PKA) promotes gap junction assembly and communication (Burghardt et al., 1995; Solan et al., 2007; TenBroek et al., 2001). Although several isozymes of protein kinase C (PKC) phosphorylate connexin-43 in diverse cell types and tissues, PKCε is the only isoform that phosphorylates it at the ID (Bowling et al., 2001; Doble et al., 2000; Lampe et al., 2000; Lin et al., 2003; Saez et al., 1997). Consistent with this, PKCε suppresses gap junction communication in the ischemic heart through phosphorylation of connexin-43 at Ser-368 (Ek-Vitorin et al., 2006; Hund et al., 2007; Hund et al., 2008).

Several phosphorylation sites (i.e. Ser-306 and Ser-325/Ser-328/Ser-330) on connexin-43 are non- or de-phosphorylated in ischemic and hypertrophic hearts (Lampe et al., 2006; Procida et al., 2009). The absence of phosphorylation at these sites has been suggested to correlate with reduced cardiac conductance (Lampe et al., 2006; Procida et al., 2009). In agreement with this, transgenic mice in which Ser-325/Ser-328/Ser-300 were substituted by glutamic acid (phosphomimetic residue) were less susceptible to arrhythmia. Yet, the kinase(s) that is responsible for these phosphorylation events remain(s) to be identified. Importantly, Ser-325/Ser-328/Ser-330 are substrates of casein kinase 1 (CK1) in normal rat kidney cells (Cooper and Lampe, 2002), however, its role in cardiac muscle remains to be defined. Moreover, Ca^{2+}/Calmodulin-dependent protein kinase II (CaMKII) is capable of phosphorylating many Ser residues on connexin-43 *in vitro*, including Ser-306, Ser-325, Ser-328 and Ser-330 (Huang et al., 2011), however the physiological significance of these results requires further investigation.

The phosphatases acting upon and regulating the activities of connexin-43 have been also long sought after. Receptor protein tyrosine phosphatase μ (RPTPμ) has been suggested to dephosphorylate Tyr residues present in connexin-43 in lung cells (Giepmans et al., 2003), however, its physiological relevance in the myocardium remains to be established. Moreover, serine/threonine phosphatase type 1 and type 2A (PP1 and PP2A, respectively) have been implicated in the dephosphorylation of connexin-43 (Ai and Pogwizd, 2005; Duthe et al., 2001; Jeyaraman et al., 2003). For instance, PP1, but not PP2A, modulates the phosphorylation status of Ser-368 (Jeyaraman et al., 2003). Conversely, PP2A exists in a complex with connexin-43 in homogenates prepared from patients suffering from dilated cardiomyopathy (DCM) or idiopathic dilated cardiomyopathy (IDCM), as well as from a non-ischemic heart failure rabbit model (Ai and Pogwizd, 2005; Ai et al., 2011). Consistent with this, application of specific PP2A inhibitors prevented uncoupling of cardiocytes in the rabbit failing heart (Ai and Pogwizd, 2005).

2.4 Connexin-43 interacts with ZO-1, caveolins and microtubules at the ID

Zona occludens-1: Zona occludens-1 (ZO-1) interacts with connexin-43 in cardiac myocytes via its PDZ2 domain that directly binds to the last five residues present in the COOH-terminus of connexin-43 (Giepmans and Moolenaar, 1998; Giepmans et al., 2001a; Toyofuku et al., 1998). Interestingly though, their interaction is not abolished in a transgenic murine model that expresses a truncated form of connexin-43 that is missing the last 124 amino acid residues (Maass et al., 2007), suggesting that additional domains contribute to binding.

The interaction of ZO-1 and connexin-43 mainly takes place at the periphery of the gap junctional plaque (Hunter et al., 2005; Zhu et al., 2005). Notably, their binding is suppressed in the presence of Src (Sorgen et al., 2004; Toyofuku et al., 2001). A number of early studies suggested that ZO-1 targets or retains connexin-43 to the ID, while others proposed that it regulates the size of gap junctions or the internalization of connexin-43 (Barker et al., 2002; Hunter et al., 2005; Rhett et al., 2011; Toyofuku et al., 1998). Intriguingly, recent studies from failing human hearts have provided conflicting results. Bruce *et al.* reported that in hearts of DCM and IDCM patients, ZO-1 interacts more extensively with connexin-43 compared to healthy ones (Bruce et al., 2008), whereas Laing *et al.* and Kostin, described diminished colocalization of connexin-43 and ZO-1 in hearts from patients with DCM, ischaemic cardiomyopathy and end-stage heart failure (Kostin, 2007; Laing et al., 2007). In support of this, transgenic mice lacking ZO-1 are embryonic lethal, exhibiting cardiac developmental challanges (Katsuno et al., 2008; Xu et al., 2008). Recently, Rhett *et al.* proposed a model, whereby ZO-1 interacts with connexin-43 to inhibit the incorporation of additional connexons into gap junctional plaques (Rhett et al., 2011).

Caveolin-1: Caveolins are the main scaffolding components of caveolae in lipid rafts, and have been found to interact with connexin-43 in different cell types (Langlois et al., 2008; Liu et al., 2010; Schubert et al., 2002). While the caveolin scaffolding domain along with the COOH-terminus of caveolin-1 are sufficient to support binding to connexin-43, the respective interacting region of the latter has yet to be defined (Schubert et al., 2002). Contrary to epithelial cells, the interaction between caveolins and connexin-43 in the myocardium is less understood. Along these lines, caveolin-3, which is specifically expressed in heart and skeletal muscle (Tang et al., 1996), has been shown to interact with connexin-43 in a yeast-two-hybrid study and confirmed by co-immunoprecipitation assays using heart homogenates (Liu et al., 2010). As caveolin-3 is present at the sarcolemma, but not the ID, the physiological relevance of this interaction remains to be examined (Abi-Char et al., 2007; Yarbrough et al., 2002). Moreover, a murine model lacking caveolin develop DCM at early stages (Zhao, 2002).

Microtubules: First characterized as binding partners of connexin-43 in RAT-1 cells and other fibroblast and epithelial cell lines, α/β-tubulins have been shown to specifically interact with the tubulin-binding motif present in the COOH-terminus of connexin-43 (Giepmans et al., 2001a; Giepmans et al., 2001b). Immunofluorescence studies and live-cell imaging further demonstrated that connexin-43 co-localizes with tubulins along microtubule tracks, as it traverses from the Golgi apparatus to other membranes (Giepmans et al., 2001b; Lauf et al., 2002; Shaw et al., 2007). To date, only a handful of studies have described the interaction between tubulins and connexin-43 in the heart. Accordingly, a recent study by Smyth *et al.* proposed that EB1, a microtubule plus-end tracking protein, is required to deliver connexin-43 to the ID (Smyth et al., 2010). Consistent with this, disruption of the interaction between EB1 and microtubules (e.g. during ischemia) significantly decreases the surface expression of connexin-43 at the ID (Smyth et al., 2010).

3. Adherens junctions

Adherens junctions are specialized structures necessary for cell-cell adhesion that provide uniform mechanical strength to the heart. Unlike gap junctions where membranes remain relatively close, opposing membranes at adherens junctions are separated by ~20 nm (Niessen, 2007). Adherens junctions frequently alternate with gap junctions along the sarcolemma at the ID, and are typically oriented perpendicular to the long axis of cardiomyocytes, optimizing the transmission of mechanical force (Hoyt et al., 1989). In addition, they can be found with desmosomes at the *area composita.* Functional adherens junctions require two main anchor points, one within the extracellular space where cadherins from adjacent cells tightly interact in a homophillic manner, and the other within the cytoplasmic region linking the adherens junction complex to the actin cytoskeleton through direct interactions with members of the catenin family (Fig. 3; reviewed in Niessen, 2007; Noorman et al., 2009).

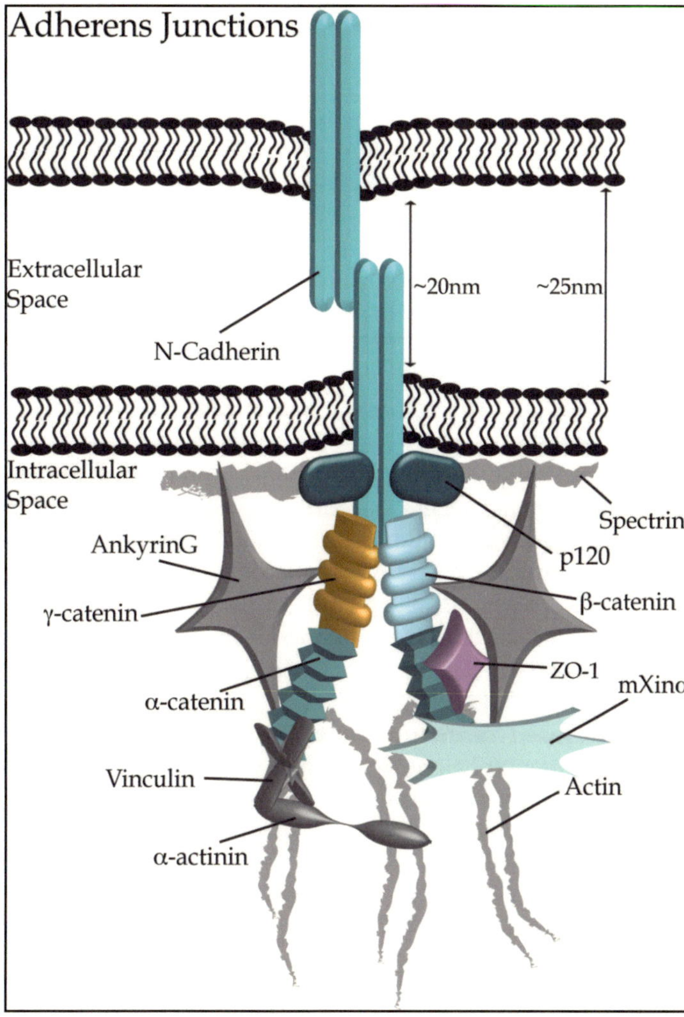

Fig. 3. Adherens Junctions connect neighbouring cardiomyocytes through homophilic dimers of N-cadherin. Connections within the intracellular space link N-cadherin to the actin cytoskeleton (depicted in grey), via additional adherens junction proteins (shown in hues of teal), ie. p120 catenin, β-catenin, α-catenin and mXinα. Proteins not traditionally considered as components of adherens junctions, but localizing to the ID are shown in grey. Proteins of other ID structures, ZO-1 (gap junctions) and γ-catenin (desmosomes), are depicted in light purple and gold, respectively.

3.1 N-cadherin

N-Cadherin: Cadherins are a super-family of transmembrane glycoproteins that mediate Ca^{2+}-dependent adhesion between neighbouring cells. In the early 1980s, N-cadherin was identified as a major component of the myocardium, that localizes to the ID (Volk and Geiger, 1984). Five extracellular domains are present in N-cadherin, with the first three possessing Ca^{2+} binding sites; each domain is composed of up to ~110 amino acids (Fig. 2B). The extreme NH_2-terminus of N-cadherin contains a highly conserved ligand recognition site composed of repeating motifs of His-Ala-Val residues, necessary for homophilic dimer formation (Nose et al., 1990). Two cadherin monomers, one from each adjacent myocyte, form a Ca^{2+}-dependent, zipper-like homodimer (Takeichi, 1994). Although Ca^{2+} is necessary for maintaining cadherin homodimers, it does not mediate their initial interaction (Nagaraj et al., 1996). Following the extensive extracellular domain, N-cadherin contains a single-pass transmembrane region and a short cytoplasmic segment that associates with the actin cytoskeleton via proteins of the catenin family (Ozawa et al., 1990).

The importance of N-cadherin in the stability of IDs is evidenced in various animal models. A murine systemic knock-out model of N-cadherin resulted in embryonic lethality due to improper development of the heart tube among other abnormalities, despite the development of primitive myocardial tissue (Radice et al., 1997). Interestingly, isolated murine myocytes from the same model were able to weakly contract and aggregate in culture (Radice et al., 1997). Taken together, these results suggested that N-cadherin is critical for embryonic development of the heart and other tissues, however it is not required for electrical coupling and cell adhesion at this stage. Moreover, in a murine conditional cardiac-specific knock-out model where N-cadherin was deleted in 6-10 week old mice, sudden death occurred after ~2 months (Li et al., 2005). A significant decrease in the expression levels of gap junction proteins was also observed in this model, which was accompanied by the development of dilated cardiomyopathy and impaired left ventricular function (Li et al., 2005). In addition, the amounts of other proteins at ID were reduced, including plakoglobin and α-, β-, and p120 catenins, resulting in dissolution of the ID structure (Kostetskii et al., 2005; Li et al., 2005). Similarly, mice overexpressing N-cadherin developed early onset dilated cardiomyopathy (Ferreira-Cornwell et al., 2002), and N-cadherin/connexin-43 compound heterozygous mice were prone to cardiac arrhythmias (Li et al., 2008). Collectively, these studies suggested that N-cadherin is necessary for the maintenance and stabilization of the ID, while its absence may lead to the development of heart failure and ultimately death.

3.2 Proteins of the catenin family

Within adherens junctions, N-cadherin associates with the actin cytoskeletal network through direct interactions mediated by members of the catenin/armadillo family; these include β-, α-, p120 and γ-catenin (also called plakoglobin). β- and p120 catenin bind directly to the cytoplsmic domain of N-cadherin, whereas α-catenin links the actin cytoskeleton to N-cadherin, via its direct interactions with both components (reviewed in Aho et al., 1999; Butz and Larue, 1995; Niessen, 2007).

β-Catenin: β-Catenin, like other members of the catenin/armadillo family, is characterized by a series of central domains, referred to as armadillo (arm) repeats, each composed of 42 amino acids, that form an elongated superhelix when repeated in tandem (Huber et al., 1997). β-Catenin contains twelve arm repeats (Fig. 2C; Peifer et al., 1994); deletion mutagenesis has mapped the binding site for N-cadherin to the central repeat region of β-catenin (Hulsken et al., 1994). Flanking the arm repeats are small, ~100 amino acids long, NH_2- and COOH- termini that mediate the regulatory functions of β-catenin.

p120 Catenin: p120 Catenin shares a similar organization with β-catenin, and a ~22% identity within the arm repeats region (Peifer et al., 1994; Reynolds et al., 1992). Alternative splicing gives rise to four similar p120 catenin isoforms (Keirsebilck et al., 1998). Each isoform is composed of ten arm repeats that are responsible for their direct interaction with the COOH-terminus of cadherins (Fig. 2C; Daniel and Reynolds, 1995; Finnemann et al., 1997; Reynolds et al., 1992; Shibamoto et al., 1995; Staddon et al., 1995; Thoreson et al., 2000). p120 catenin does not interact with α-catenin or the actin cytoskeleton (Daniel and Reynolds, 1995), suggesting a novel, yet unidentified, function within adherens junctions.

α-Catenin: α-Catenin is a subfamily of proteins that differs significantly in both primary sequence and structural organization from the other members of the traditional catenin/armadillo family (reviewed in Kobielak and Fuchs, 2004). Instead of arm repeats, α-catenin contains three vinculin homology (VH) domains, therefore sharing considerable homology with vinculin (Fig. 2C; Rudiger, 1998). Of the main α-catenin isoforms, αT-catenin is the most prominent in the mammalian heart and localizes to the ID (Janssens et al., 2001). Through its most NH_2-terminal VH domain, α-catenin dimerizes and interacts directly with β- and γ-catenin (Koslov et al., 1997; Pokutta and Weis, 2000), while through its middle VH domain supports binding to vinculin and α-actinin, both of which are present within the transitional junction of the ICD (McGregor et al., 1994; Weiss et al., 1998). Similar to vinculin, α-catenin associates with filamentous actin through its last VH domain and its COOH-terminus (Rimm et al., 1995). In addition, its COOH-terminus interacts with ZO-1, which is also complexed with connexin-43 at gap junctions (Imamura et al., 1999; Talhouk et al., 2008). Taken together, these observations indicate that α-catenin functions as an intracellular adhesion protein.

It is well established that β- and p120 catenins play essential roles in diverse signaling pathways, including modulation of cell-cell adhesion; (reviewed in Anastasiadis and Reynolds, 2000; Niessen, 2007). Recently, α-catenin was also implicated in the regulation of cell adhesion and proliferation (reviewed in Kobielak and Fuchs, 2004). Although many of their suggested signaling roles originate from studies in non-cardiac cells, it is presumed that catenins may have similar regulatory activities at the ID of cardiomyocytes. In support of this, transgenic mice lacking either β- or α-catenin result in detrimental effects on the longevity of the animals, with phenotypes ranging from embryonic lethality to the development of early onset DCM (Haegel et al., 1995; Piven et al., 2011; Sheikh et al., 2006). Future studies are necessary to continue addressing this question.

4. Desmosomes

Similar to adherens junctions, desmosomes are also symmetrical protein complexes with intercellular elements connecting adjacent cells, and intracellular components associating with intermediate filaments. First identified as adhesive structures of epithelial cells by Giulio Bizzozero in the late 19th century, the term desmosomes was initially coined in 1920 by Josef Schaffer from the Greek words "desmo" and "soma" meaning bond or fastening and body, respectively; (reviewed in Delva et al., 2009). In the middle of the 20th century, desmosomes were identified as a major component of the cardiac ID (Fawcett and McNutt, 1969; Grimley and Edwards, 1960; Muir, 1957; Sjostrand and Andersson, 1954), where its main function is to provide structural support to neighboring cardiomyocytes (reviewed in Delmar and McKenna, 2010; Delva et al., 2009; Thomason et al., 2010). Desmosomes bring apposing cells within 20-35 nm of each other (Noorman et al., 2009), and are typically found in close proximity to gap junctions, although recent studies indicate that they are also present next to adherens junctions within the *area composita*. They consist of proteins from three families: the desmosomal cadherins, the catenin/armadillo family and the plakins (Fig. 4).

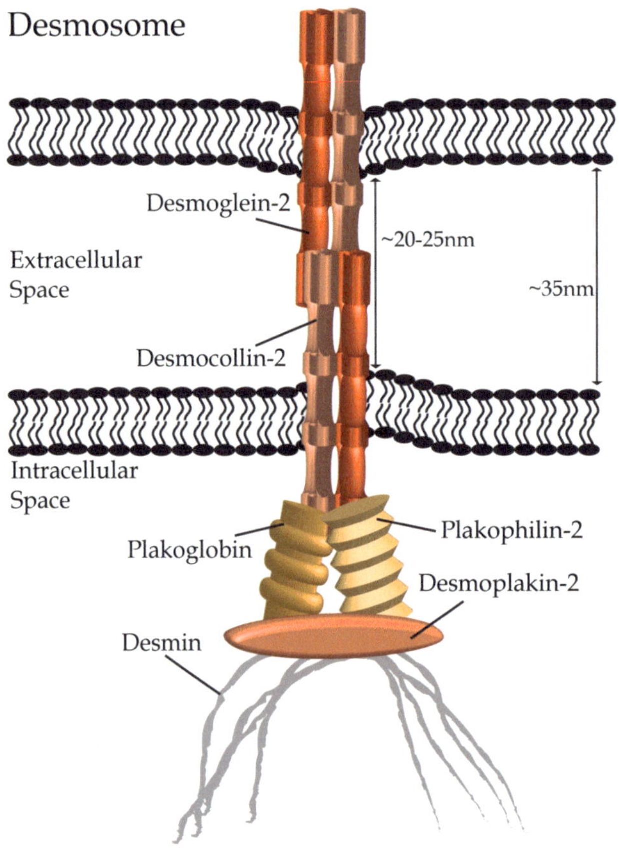

Fig. 4. Desmosomes connect neighbouring cardiomyocytes through heterophilic dimers of desmocollin-2 and desmoglein-2 (shown in hues of orange) forming within the extracellular space. Interactions with plakophilin-2, plakoglobin (a.k.a. γ-catenin) and desmoplakin-1 (depicted in hues of gold and orange) link the desmosomal complex to the intermediate filament protein desmin (shown in gray) in cardiomyocytes.

4.1 Desmosomal cadherins

Desmosomal cadherins are a superfamily of Ca^{2+}-dependent adhesion molecules, which form dimers to make up the core of desmosomal junctions (Dusek et al., 2007). Desmogleins and desmocollins, the two main types of desmosomal cadherins, possess several isoforms (4 and 3 respectively in humans, Green and Simpson, 2007; Lorimer et al., 1994; Schmelz et al., 1986) with desmoglein-2 and desmocollin-2 being the main isoforms expressed in mammalian cardiomyocytes (Garrod and Chidgey, 2008).

Desmoglein and Desmocollin: These classical cadherins are highly homologous; desmogleins and desmocollins share ~30% identity with each other and with other members of the cadherin family (Garrod et al., 2002). Much of their homology is found within their extracellular domains. They possess five extracellular domains or cadherin repeats of ~110 amino acids and are separated by Ca^{2+} binding motifs, which are necessary for dimerization (Fig 2B; Pokutta and Weis, 2007). A single-pass transmembrane domain and an intracellular anchoring segment follow the extracellular domains (Green and Simpson, 2007; Kowalczyk et al., 1999). Within their intracellular regions, desmogleins and desmocollins possess a cadherin-like sequence capable of binding catenins, or in the case of desmosomal cadherins, plakoglobin (Mathur et al., 1994).

Desmoglein and desmocollin differ significantly within their COOH-termini, however. In particular, the COOH-terminal region of desmoglein contains a proline-rich linker region, a series of short (~29 amino acids long) repeats and a glycine-rich terminal domain (Garrod and Chidgey, 2008; Holthofer et al., 2007), which likely mediates weak interactions with other desmosomal proteins (Kami et al., 2009). Conversely, alternative splicing within the COOH-terminus of desmocollin gives rise to two forms (Collins et al., 1991; Parker et al., 1991); the "b" or shorter form does not contain the traditional catenin-binding domain, however, the longer "a" form possesses a normal catenin-binding domain and has been shown to bind plakoglobin with high affinity (Troyanovsky et al., 1993).

Many studies suggest that both desmoglein and desmocollin are necessary for desmosomal formation (Getsios et al., 2004; Marcozzi et al., 1998; Tselepis et al., 1998). However, it is unclear if homophilic or heterophilic interactions maintain desmosomal adhesion. Although heterophilic complexes between desmoglein-2 and desmocollin-2 have been reported, it has been suggested that homophilic interactions between desmogleins mediate complex formation (Heupel et al., 2008; Syed et al., 2002; Waschke et al., 2005). Nonetheless, the importance of both desmoglein and desmocollin in cardiac function is further evidenced by the numerous mutations identified in their respective genes that lead to cardiomyopathies, mainly manifested as ARVC. Consistent with this, mice harbouring a mutation resulting in a truncated form of desmoglein-2 develop ARVC (Krusche et al., 2011), while a systemic knockout mouse model of desmoglein-2 is embryonic lethal (Eshkind et al., 2002).

4.2 Proteins of the catenin/armadillo family

Desmosomal cadherins form cytoplasmic connections with intermediate filaments in part through proteins of the armadillo family. Armadillo proteins include plakoglobin (also called γ-catenin) and plakophilin, which are found at desmosomal structures (Cowin et al., 1986; Hatzfeld, 2005; Hatzfeld, 2007; Mertens et al., 1996; Mertens et al., 1999; Peifer et al., 1992), in addition to β-catenin, α–catenin and p120 catenin, which are mainly associated with adherens junctions (Hatzfeld, 2005; Hatzfeld, 2007). In addition to facilitating the anchoring of desmosomes to intermediate filaments, desmosomal armadillo proteins function in diverse signal transduction pathways.

Plakoglobin: Plakoglobin contains 12 arm repeats, which share 65% identity with the ones present in β-catenin, and are flanked by Pro-Lys-Gly rich NH_2- and COOH-terminal domains (Fig. 2C; Garrod and Chidgey, 2008; Huber et al., 1997; Peifer et al., 1992). Mutation analysis suggested that plakoglobin interacts with desmosomal cadherins through its NH_2-terminal domain as well as the arm repeats near its COOH-terminus (Chitaev et al., 1996; Wahl et al., 1996). Although the Pro-Lys-Gly motif interacts with both desmosomal and adherens junction cadherins, it has a higher affinity for desmoglein supporting plakoglobin's mainly desmosomal localization (Chitaev et al., 1996; Choi et al., 2009). Moreover, through its central arm repeats plakoglobin interacts with desmoplakin, which in turn binds to intermediate filaments.

Plakophilin: Plakophilins undergo alternative splicing giving rise to four products, referred to as plakophilin 1-4; (reviewed in Bass-Zubek et al., 2009), with plakophilin-2 being the most prominent form in mammalian cardiomyocytes (Mertens et al., 1996). Plakophilins contain 9 arm repeats flanked by an NH_2-terminal head and a short COOH-terminal region (Fig. 2C; Bass-Zubek et al., 2009). In addition, plakophilins 1-3 possess a flexible insertion between repeats 5 and 6, which introduces a major bend to their overall structure (Choi and Weis, 2005). Plakophilins bind to several desmosomal proteins through their NH_2-terminal regions, including desmocollin, desmoplakin and plakoglobin as well as actin and the intermediate filament proteins keratin and desmin (Hofmann et al., 2000). Notably, plakophilin-2 also interacts with ankyrin-G at the ID, a sodium channel anchoring protein and with connexin-43 (Sato et al., 2011). Consequently, loss of plakophilin-2 leads to a decrease in the level of the α-subunit of the sodium channel ($Na_V1.5$) at the membrane, which results in slow propagation of the action potential in cardiocytes (Sato et al., 2009). In addition to ankyrin-G, plakophilin-2 interacts with PKCα, which is necessary for phosphorylation and recruitment of desmoplakin to newly forming desmosomes in the developing heart and during repair of myocardial injury (reviewed in Garrod and Chidgey, 2008). Thus, through its multiple interactions, plakophilin-2 may serve as a scaffold to contribute to adhesion and signalling at the ID by facilitating the lateral interaction between desmosomes and adherens junctions (Kowalczyk et al., 1999).

The critical roles of both plakoglobin and plakophilin-2 in desmosomal assembly and maintenance is evidenced by the severe phenotypes that relevant transgenic mice models exhibit and the different forms of heart disease associated with mutations in their respective genes (please see Tables 1 and 2). Consistent with this, both plakoglobin and plakophilin-2 null mice show premature death during embryogenesis because of myocardial fragility (Bierkamp et al., 1996; Grossmann et al., 2004; Ruiz et al., 1996). Similarly, cardiac-specific knockout of plakoglobin results in progressive development of cardiac dysfunction (Li et al., 2011).

4.3 Plakins

Desmoplakin: Plakins are large multi-domain proteins that mediate the interaction of intermediate filaments (desmin in heart) with desmosomes. Desmoplakin, the main plakin protein expressed in heart, is characterized by a central α-helical coiled-coil rod domain, which is flanked by globular NH_2- and COOH-termini (Fig. 2D; Franke et al., 1982). Through its coiled-coil region, desmoplakin has been suggested to form homodimers (Kowalczyk et al., 1994), while its NH_2-terminal region binds to plakoglobins and plakophilins, targeting them to desmosomes (Bornslaeger et al., 1996; Bornslaeger et al., 2001; Holthofer et al., 2007; Kowalczyk et al., 1999). Its COOH-terminal tail is composed of three plakin-repeat domains and a Gly-Ser-Arg rich motif; both shown to mediate binding to desmin (Choi et al., 2002; Getsios et al., 2004). Interestingly, mice lacking desmoplakin exhibit embryonic lethality characterized by reduced number of desmosomes with residual structures separated from intermediate filaments (Gallicano et al., 1998). These results, along with the various desmoplakin mutations associated with human genetic disorders (please see below) support a strong role for desmoplakin in the assembly and interlinking of desmosomes to desmin intermediate filaments in cardiomyocytes.

	Major Proteins	References	Animal Models	Phenotype	References
Gap Junctions	Connexin-43	Beyer et al., 1987	Systemic KO	Embryonic lethal	Reaume et al., 1995
			Cardiac Specific KO	Sudden cardiac death ~2 months	Gutstein et al., 2001b
	ZO-1	Giepmans et al., 1998; Toyofuku et al., 1998	Systemic KO	Embryonic lethal	Xu et al., 2008; Katsuno et al., 2008
	Caveolin	Schubert et al., 2002	Systemic KO	Development of DCM	Zhao et al., 2002
	Microtubule	Shaw et al., 2007	N/A	N/A	N/A
Adherens Junctions	N-Cadherin	Volk et al., 1984	Systemic KO	Embryonic lethal	Radice et al., 1997
			Cardiac specific KO	Sudden cardiac death ~2 months	Li et al., 2005; Kostetskii et al., 2005
			Dual heterozygote with connexin-43	Develop arythmias	Li et al., 2008
	β-catenin	Butz et al., 1995	Systemic KO	Embryonic lethal	Haegel et al., 1995
			Cardiac specific KO	Low survival rate	Piven et al., 2011
	α-catenin	Butz et al., 1995	Cardiac specific KO	Development of DCM	Piven et al., 2011; Sheikh et al., 2006
	P120 catenin	Aho et al., 1999	N/A	N/A	N/A
Desmosomes	Desmocollin-2	Lorimer et al., 1994	N/A	N/A	N/A
	Desmoglein-2	Schmelz et al., 1986	Transgenic lacking extracellular domains	Develop ARVC	Krusche et al., 2011
			Systemic KO	Embryonic lethal	Eshkind et al., 2002
	Plakoglobin	Peifer et al., 1992; Cowin et al., 1986	Systemic KO	Embryonic lethal	Bierkamp et al., 1996; Ruiz et al., 1996
			Cardiac Specific KO	Premature death due to cardiac dysfunction	Li et al., 2011
	Plakophilin-2	Mertens et al., 1996; Mertens et al., 1999	Systemic KO	Embryonic lethal	Grossmann et al., 2004
	Desmoplakin	Franke et al., 1982	Systemic KO	Embryonic lethal	Gallicano et al., 1998; Uzumcu et al., 2006
			Tetraploid rescue of systemic KO	Embryonic lethal	Gallicano et al., 2001
			Val30Met & Gln90Arg cardiac specific mutations	Embryonic lethal	Yang et al., 2006

Table 1. Listing of major proteins found at the ID and associated animal models with appropriate references; DCM: Dilated Cardiomyopathy, N/A: not applicable, and KO: knock-out.

Gene Product	Mutations	Disease	References
Plakophilin-2	Arg79Stop Arg735Stop IVSAS10, G-C, -1 (nt 2146) IVS12, G-A, +1 (nt 2489)	ARVC	Gerull et al., 2004
Desmocollin-2	1bp deletion, 1430C 1bp deletion, 1841G 2bp deletion, 2687GA IVS5AS, A-G, -2 (nt 631)	ARVC	Syrris et al, 2006 Simpson et al. , 2009
Desmoglein-2	Arg45Gln Arg48His Val56Met Asn266Ser Glu331Lys Trp305Stop Cys506Tyr Gly811Cys IVS12AS, A-G, -2 (nt 1881)	ARVC	Awad et al., 2006 Pilichou et al., 2006 Syrris et al., 2007 Posch et al., 2008
Plakoglobin	3bp deletion, 118GCA Ser39Lys40insSer	ARVC	McKoy et al., 2000
	2bp deletion, 2157TG	Naxos disease	Asimaki et al., 2007
Desmoplakin	Val30Met Ser299Arg Lys959Met Arg1255Lys Arg1267X Arg1775Ile Arg2834His Gly2375Arg 2034insA Arg1934Stop 1bp deletion, 7901G IVS, G-A, +1 (nt 423)	ARVC/ Carvajal syndrome	Norgett et al., 2000 Rampazzo et al., 2002 Norman et al., 2005 Yang et al., 2006 Uzumcu et al., 2006 Bolling et al., 2010 Bauce et al., 2010

Table 2. Listing of mutations found in desmosomal genes that have been causally linked to the development of ARVC or variations of it; bp: base pair, IVS or AVSAS: denotes a splice site mutation, IVS: intervening sequence, AS: acceptor splice site, nt: nucleotide, ins: insertion.

5. ID proteins in human heart disease

Arrhythmogenic Right Ventricular Cardiomyopathy (ARVC) is a progressive disease characterized by loss of the right ventricular myocardium, and at advanced stages of the left ventricular myocardium as well, accompanied by fibro-fatty tissue infiltration and replacement. Its clinical manifestations include ventricular arrhythmias, syncope, heart failure and sudden cardiac death (Delmar and McKenna, 2010; Estigoy et al., 2009; Lombardi and Marian, 2011). ARVC has an estimated prevalence of 1 in 5,000 (Sen-Chowdhry et al., 2010), although in some regions (e.g. northern Italy) it reaches 1 in 2,000 (Thiene et al., 2007). Genetic studies have indicated that ~50% of the diagnosed ARVC cases are familial, with an autosomal dominant inheritance (Marcus et al., 1982). Accordingly, a number of mutations have been identified in the genes that encode cardiac desmosomal proteins, and thus ARVC is also referred to as "a disease of the desmosome" (Li and Radice, 2010). These mutations not only affect the number, structural integrity and proper localization of desmosomes, but also of gap junctions, resulting in impaired intercellular conductance and thus development of arrhythmias. To date, five desmosomal genes have been identified that carry inherited mutations causing different variations of ARVC, including: plakophilin-2, desmocollin-2, desmoglein-2, plakoglobin and desmoplakin. Table 2 includes a comprehensive list of mutations identified to date in these five desmosomal genes; for updated listing please refer to: http://www.ncbi.nlm.nih.gov/omim.

More than 70% of the identified desmosomal mutations associated with the development of familial ARVC are present in the gene encoding plakophilin-2 (Gerull et al., 2004; Sen-Chowdhry et al., 2010; van Tintelen et al., 2007). These account for ~20% of diagnosed ARVC cases, while mutations in the genes encoding desmocollin-2 (Simpson et al., 2009; Syrris et al., 2006) and desmoglein-2 (Awad et al., 2006; Posch et al., 2008; Syrris et al., 2006) account for ~10-15% of cases each (Lombardi and Marian, 2011; Pilichou et al., 2006).

Plakoglobin was the first desmosomal protein to be causally associated with a cardiocutaneous subtype of ARVC, known as Naxos disease, which was first characterized by Protonotarios *et al.* (Protonotarios et al., 1986). Genetic studies of patients from the Greek island Naxos, where the syndrome took its name from, revealed a homozygous two-base-pairs deletion (2157-2158delGT) in the gene encoding plakoglobin that was inherited in an autosomal recessive manner (McKoy et al., 2000). In addition to developing ARVC, these individuals also suffered from palmoplantar keratoderma and woolly hair. Recently though, a variation of the Naxos syndrome was diagnosed in a German family that carried a dominantly inherited mutation in the plakoglobin gene (Ser39Lys40insSer) that caused ARVC without the accompanying cutaneous abnormalities (Asimaki et al., 2007). Importantly, the reduced expression or complete absence of plakoglobin from the ID of ARVC patients is a consistent feature, making it a valuable marker for its diagnosis, which still remains problematic with many cases being un- or misdiagnosed.

Mutations in the gene encoding desmoplakin have been identified as the underlying cause of a variation of Naxos disease, referred to as Carvajal syndrome that is also characterized by woolly hair, palmoplantar keratoderma and cardiac disease (Kaplan et al., 2004a; Kaplan et al., 2004b; Norman et al., 2005; Rampazzo et al., 2002; Saffitz, 2009; Yang et al., 2006; Bauce et al., 2010; Bolling et al., 2010; Norgett et al., 2000; Uzumcu et al., 2006). Notably, cardiac disease is presented as a generalized hypertrophy and dilation, involving both the right and left ventricles, and accompanied by focal ventricular aneurysms without any apparent fibro-fatty tissue replacement (Kaplan et al., 2004a; Yang et al., 2006). A major feature of the

Carvajal syndrome is the virtual absence of desmoplakin in the affected hearts, indicating that the missense or nonsense mutations identified result in truncated and/or unstable forms of the protein (Norman et al., 2005; Rampazzo et al., 2002).
Alterations in the amounts, localization and functional properties of desmosomal proteins not only affect intercellular adhesion, but also promote remodelling of gap junctions by leading to abnormal expression and distribution of gap junctional proteins, and primarily connexin-43, which in turn induces defects in the electrochemical coupling of neighbouring cardiocytes and leads to the development of severe arrhythmias (Kaplan et al., 2004a; Pieperhoff et al., 2008; Saffitz, 2009). On the contrary, changes in gap junctions do not affect the structural integrity or proper function of desmosomes and adherens junctions, and thus mechanical coupling of adjacent cardiocytes is not disrupted (Delmar and McKenna, 2010; Li and Radice, 2010; Noorman et al., 2009).
A number of mutations have also been identified in the gene encoding connexin-43, which are associated with the development of oculodentodigital dysplasia (ODDD) that is frequently accompanied by hair and skin defects, too (Kelly et al., 2006). Some of these mutations have been further linked to the development of cardiac disturbances. In such patients, the expression levels of connexin-43, and thus the number of gap junctions, are moderately decreased (Manias et al., 2008); however, cardiac conduction is not affected. Thus, sole mutations in the gene encoding connexin-43 cannot be the primary inducers of electrical or mechanical defects underlying arrhythmogenesis. Interestingly, neither loss- nor gain-of-function mutations have been identified in proteins of adherens junctions that are causally associated with the development of cardiac disease. A plausible explanation is that dysfunctional adherens junctions may be detrimental to the developing myocardium and thus may result in embryonic lethality. Consistent with this, a constitutive null model of N-cadherin was embryonic lethal, while a developmental and cardiac tissue specific model developed dilated cardiomyopathy and died 2 months following excision of the gene, due to mechanical and electrical abnormalities (Li et al., 2005; Radice et al., 1997); for review of available animal models of N-cadherin and their phenotypic characterization, please refer to (Li et al., 2006).

6. Concluding remarks: The intercalated disc is a single functional unit

Although traditionally depicted as a composition of three separate units, data from the last decade suggest that the ID of cardiomyocytes is in fact a single functional unit. Several studies have begun to describe *area composita* as a hybrid between proteins of adherens junctions and desmosomes that form a single anchoring unit (Delmar, 2004; Franke et al., 2006; Pieperhoff and Franke, 2007; Saffitz, 2005). Consistent with this, plakophilin-2 and desmoglein, which typically localize to desmosomes, interact with β- or α-catenin and p120 catenin, respectively, present in adherens junctions (Chen et al., 2002; Goossens et al., 2007). Similarly, molecular linkages between desmosomes and gap junctions have also been identified (Rohr, 2007; Saffitz, 2005). As such, desmocollin-2 directly interacts with connexin-43 (Gehmlich et al., 2011). Taken together, these studies clearly suggest that there is a three-way exchange and cross-talk of junctional proteins, supporting the idea of the ID being a single functional unit.
During the last decade, there have been significant advancements concerning the structural composition of the ID. A plethora of new proteins has been identified as integral or peripheral components of the ID that directly or indirectly contributes to the mechanical and

electrical coupling of neighbouring cardiocytes. The challenge of the future lies in the characterization of the precise roles that these proteins play to ensure the synchronous contraction of the myocardium. A combination of sophisticated molecular, genetic and cellular approaches will be needed to address this unequivocally important question.

7. Acknowledgments

Our research has been supported by grants to A.K.K. through the National Institutes of Health (R21 HL106197) and the American Heart Association (GRNT 3780035), to M.A.A from the National Institutes of Health (F32 AR058079) and to L.-Y.R.H. from the National Institutes of Health (Training Grant 2T32AR7592-16).

8. References

Abi-Char J., Maguy A., Coulombe A., Balse E., Ratajczak P., Samuel J.L., Nattel S., Hatem S.N. (2007) Membrane cholesterol modulates Kv1.5 potassium channel distribution and function in rat cardiomyocytes. J Physiol 582:1205-17.

Aho S., Rothenberger K., Uitto J. (1999) Human p120ctn catenin: tissue-specific expression of isoforms and molecular interactions with BP180/type XVII collagen. J Cell Biochem 73:390-9.

Ai X., Pogwizd S.M. (2005) Connexin 43 downregulation and dephosphorylation in nonischemic heart failure is associated with enhanced colocalized protein phosphatase type 2A. Circ Res 96:54-63.

Ai X., Jiang A., Ke Y., Solaro R.J., Pogwizd S.M. (2011) Enhanced activation of p21-activated kinase 1 in heart failure contributes to dephosphorylation of connexin 43. Cardiovasc Res, In Press.

Anastasiadis P.Z., Reynolds A.B. (2000) The p120 catenin family: complex roles in adhesion, signaling and cancer. J Cell Sci 113 (Pt 8):1319-1334.

Angst B.D., Khan L.U., Severs N.J., Whitely K., Rothery S., Thompson R.P., Magee A.I., Gourdie R.G. (1997) Dissociated spatial patterning of gap junctions and cell adhesion junctions during postnatal differentiation of ventricular myocardium. Circ Res 80:88-94.

Asimaki A., Syrris P., Wichter T., Matthias P., Saffitz J.E., McKenna W.J. (2007) A novel dominant mutation in plakoglobin causes arrhythmogenic right ventricular cardiomyopathy. Am J Hum Genet 81:964-73.

Awad M.M., Dalal D., Cho E., Amat-Alarcon N., James C., Tichnell C., Tucker A., Russell S.D., Bluemke D.A., Dietz H.C., Calkins H., Judge D.P. (2006) DSG2 mutations contribute to arrhythmogenic right ventricular dysplasia/cardiomyopathy. Am J Hum Genet 79:136-42.

Barker R.J., Price R.L., Gourdie R.G. (2002) Increased association of ZO-1 with connexin43 during remodeling of cardiac gap junctions. Circ Res 90:317-24.

Bass-Zubek A.E., Godsel L.M., Delmar M., Green K.J. (2009) Plakophilins: multifunctional scaffolds for adhesion and signaling. Curr Opin Cell Biol 21:708-716.

Bauce B., Nava A., Beffagna G., Basso C., Lorenzon A., Smaniotto G., De Bortoli M., Rigato I., Mazzotti E., Steriotis A., Marra M.P., Towbin J.A., Thiene G., Danieli G.A., Rampazzo A. (2010) Multiple mutations in desmosomal proteins encoding genes in arrhythmogenic right ventricular cardiomyopathy/dysplasia. Heart Rhythm 7:22-9.

Bennett P.M., Maggs A.M., Baines A.J., Pinder J.C. (2006) The transitional junction: a new functional subcellular domain at the intercalated disc. Mol Biol Cell 17:2091-2100.

Beyer E.C., Paul D.L., Goodenough D.A. (1987) Connexin43: a protein from rat heart homologous to a gap junction protein from liver. J Cell Biol 105:2621-9.

Bierkamp C., McLaughlin K.J., Schwarz H., Huber O., Kemler R. (1996) Embryonic heart and skin defects in mice lacking plakoglobin. Dev Biol 180:780-5.

Bolling M.C., Veenstra M.J., Jonkman M.F., Diercks G.F., Curry C.J., Fisher J., Pas H.H., Bruckner A.L. (2010) Lethal acantholytic epidermolysis bullosa due to a novel homozygous deletion in DSP: expanding the phenotype and implications for desmoplakin function in skin and heart. Br J Dermatol 162:1388-94.

Bornslaeger E.A., Corcoran C.M., Stappenbeck T.S., Green K.J. (1996) Breaking the connection: displacement of the desmosomal plaque protein desmoplakin from cell-cell interfaces disrupts anchorage of intermediate filament bundles and alters intercellular junction assembly. J Cell Biol 134:985-1001.

Bornslaeger E.A., Godsel L.M., Corcoran C.M., Park J.K., Hatzfeld M., Kowalczyk A.P., Green K.J. (2001) Plakophilin 1 interferes with plakoglobin binding to desmoplakin, yet together with plakoglobin promotes clustering of desmosomal plaque complexes at cell-cell borders. J Cell Sci 114:727-38.

Borrmann C.M., Grund C., Kuhn C., Hofmann I., Pieperhoff S., Franke W.W. (2006) The area composita of adhering junctions connecting heart muscle cells of vertebrates. II. Colocalizations of desmosomal and fascia adhaerens molecules in the intercalated disk. Eur J Cell Biol 85:469-85.

Bowling N., Huang X., Sandusky G.E., Fouts R.L., Mintze K., Esterman M., Allen P.D., Maddi R., McCall E., Vlahos C.J. (2001) Protein kinase C-alpha and -epsilon modulate connexin-43 phosphorylation in human heart. J Mol Cell Cardiol 33:789-98.

Bruce A.F., Rothery S., Dupont E., Severs N.J. (2008) Gap junction remodelling in human heart failure is associated with increased interaction of connexin43 with ZO-1. Cardiovasc Res 77:757-65.

Bukauskas F.F., Verselis V.K. (2004) Gap junction channel gating. Biochim Biophys Acta 1662:42-60.

Burghardt R.C., Barhoumi R., Sewall T.C., Bowen J.A. (1995) Cyclic AMP induces rapid increases in gap junction permeability and changes in the cellular distribution of connexin43. J Membr Biol 148:243-53.

Butz S., Larue L. (1995) Expression of catenins during mouse embryonic development and in adult tissues. Cell Adhes Commun 3:337-52.

Chen X., Bonne S., Hatzfeld M., van Roy F., Green K.J. (2002) Protein binding and functional characterization of plakophilin 2. Evidence for its diverse roles in desmosomes and beta -catenin signaling. J Biol Chem 277:10512-22.

Chitaev N.A., Leube R.E., Troyanovsky R.B., Eshkind L.G., Franke W.W., Troyanovsky S.M. (1996) The binding of plakoglobin to desmosomal cadherins: patterns of binding sites and topogenic potential. J Cell Biol 133:359-69.

Choi H.J., Weis W.I. (2005) Structure of the armadillo repeat domain of plakophilin 1. J Mol Biol 346:367-76.

Choi H.J., Gross J.C., Pokutta S., Weis W.I. (2009) Interactions of plakoglobin and beta-catenin with desmosomal cadherins: basis of selective exclusion of alpha- and beta-catenin from desmosomes. J Biol Chem 284:31776-88.

Choi H.J., Park-Snyder S., Pascoe L.T., Green K.J., Weis W.I. (2002) Structures of two intermediate filament-binding fragments of desmoplakin reveal a unique repeat motif structure. Nat Struct Biol 9:612-20.
Collins J.E., Legan P.K., Kenny T.P., MacGarvie J., Holton J.L., Garrod D.R. (1991) Cloning and sequence analysis of desmosomal glycoproteins 2 and 3 (desmocollins): cadherin-like desmosomal adhesion molecules with heterogeneous cytoplasmic domains. J Cell Biol 113:381-91.
Cooper C.D., Lampe P.D. (2002) Casein kinase 1 regulates connexin-43 gap junction assembly. J Biol Chem 277:44962-8.
Cowin P., Kapprell H.P., Franke W.W., Tamkun J., Hynes R.O. (1986) Plakoglobin: a protein common to different kinds of intercellular adhering junctions. Cell 46:1063-73.
Daniel J.M., Reynolds A.B. (1995) The tyrosine kinase substrate p120cas binds directly to E-cadherin but not to the adenomatous polyposis coli protein or alpha-catenin. Mol Cell Biol 15:4819-24.
Delmar M. (2004) The intercalated disk as a single functional unit. HRTHM 1:12-13.
Delmar M., McKenna W.J. (2010) The cardiac desmosome and arrhythmogenic cardiomyopathies: from gene to disease. Circ Res 107:700-714.
Delva E., Tucker D.K., Kowalczyk A.P. (2009) The desmosome. Cold Spring Harbor perspectives in biology 1:a002543.
Doble B.W., Ping P., Kardami E. (2000) The epsilon subtype of protein kinase C is required for cardiomyocyte connexin-43 phosphorylation. Circ Res 86:293-301.
Dowling J.J., Gibbs E., Russell M., Goldman D., Minarcik J., Golden J.A., Feldman E.L. (2008) Kindlin-2 is an essential component of intercalated discs and is required for vertebrate cardiac structure and function. Circ Res 102:423-431.
Duffy H.S., Sorgen P.L., Girvin M.E., O'Donnell P., Coombs W., Taffet S.M., Delmar M., Spray D.C. (2002) pH-dependent intramolecular binding and structure involving Cx43 cytoplasmic domains. J Biol Chem 277:36706-14.
Dusek R.L., Godsel L.M., Green K.J. (2007) Discriminating roles of desmosomal cadherins: beyond desmosomal adhesion. J Derm Sci 45:7-21.
Duthe F., Plaisance I., Sarrouilhe D., Herve J.C. (2001) Endogenous protein phosphatase 1 runs down gap junctional communication of rat ventricular myocytes. Am J Physiol Cell Physiol 281:C1648-56.
Ek J.F., Delmar M., Perzova R., Taffet S.M. (1994) Role of histidine 95 on pH gating of the cardiac gap junction protein connexin43. Circ Res 74:1058-64.
Ek-Vitorin J.F., King T.J., Heyman N.S., Lampe P.D., Burt J.M. (2006) Selectivity of connexin 43 channels is regulated through protein kinase C-dependent phosphorylation. Circ Res 98:1498-505.
Ek-Vitorin J.F., Calero G., Morley G.E., Coombs W., Taffet S.M., Delmar M. (1996) PH regulation of connexin43: molecular analysis of the gating particle. Biophys J 71:1273-84.
Elfgang C., Eckert R., Lichtenberg-Frate H., Butterweck A., Traub O., Klein R.A., Hulser D.F., Willecke K. (1995) Specific permeability and selective formation of gap junction channels in connexin-transfected HeLa cells. J Cell Biol 129:805-17.
Engelmann T. (1875) Uber die Leitung der Erregung im Herzmuskel. Pfugers Arch Physiol 11.
Eshkind L., Tian Q., Schmidt A., Franke W.W., Windoffer R., Leube R.E. (2002) Loss of desmoglein 2 suggests essential functions for early embryonic development and proliferation of embryonal stem cells. Eur J Cell Biol 81:592-8.

Estigoy C.B., Pontén F., Odeberg J., Herbert B., Guilhaus M., Charleston M., Ho J.W.K., Cameron D., dos Remedios C.G. (2009) Intercalated discs: multiple proteins perform multiple functions in non-failing and failing human hearts. Biophys Rev 1:43-49.

Evans W.H., De Vuyst E., Leybaert L. (2006) The gap junction cellular internet: connexin hemichannels enter the signalling limelight. Biochem J 397:1-14.

Fawcett D.W., McNutt N.S. (1969) The ultrastructure of the cat myocardium. I. Ventricular papillary muscle. J Cell Biol 42:1-45.

Ferreira-Cornwell M.C., Luo Y., Narula N., Lenox J.M., Lieberman M., Radice G.L. (2002) Remodeling the intercalated disc leads to cardiomyopathy in mice misexpressing cadherins in the heart. J Cell Sci 115:1623-1634.

Finnemann S., Mitrik I., Hess M., Otto G., Wedlich D. (1997) Uncoupling of XB/U-cadherin-catenin complex formation from its function in cell-cell adhesion. J Biol Chem 272:11856-62.

Franke W.W., Borrmann C.M., Grund C., Pieperhoff S. (2006) The area composita of adhering junctions connecting heart muscle cells of vertebrates. I. Molecular definition in intercalated disks of cardiomyocytes by immunoelectron microscopy of desmosomal proteins. Eur J Cell Biol 85:69-82.

Franke W.W., Moll R., Schiller D.L., Schmid E., Kartenbeck J., Mueller H. (1982) Desmoplakins of epithelial and myocardial desmosomes are immunologically and biochemically related. Differentiation 23:115-27.

Gallicano G.I., Kouklis P., Bauer C., Yin M., Vasioukhin V., Degenstein L., Fuchs E. (1998) Desmoplakin is required early in development for assembly of desmosomes and cytoskeletal linkage. J Cell Biol 143:2009-22.

Garrod D., Chidgey M. (2008) Desmosome structure, composition and function. Biochim Biophys Acta 1778:572-87.

Garrod D.R., Merritt A.J., Nie Z. (2002) Desmosomal adhesion: structural basis, molecular mechanism and regulation. Mol Membr Biol 19:81-94.

Gehmlich K., Lambiase P.D., Asimaki A., Ciaccio E.J., Ehler E., Syrris P., Saffitz J.E., McKenna W.J. (2011) A novel desmocollin-2 mutation reveals insights into the molecular link between desmosomes and gap junctions. Heart Rhythm 8:711-718.

Geisler S.B., Robinson D., Hauringa M., Raeker M.O., Borisov A.B., Westfall M.V., Russell M.W. (2007) Obscurin-like 1, OBSL1, is a novel cytoskeletal protein related to obscurin. Genomics 89:521-531.

Geisler S.B., Green K.J., Isom L.L., Meshinchi S., Martens J.R., Delmar M., Russell M.W. (2010) Ordered assembly of the adhesive and electrochemical connections within newly formed intercalated disks in primary cultures of adult rat cardiomyocytes. J Biomed Biotechnol 2010:624719.

Gerull B., Heuser A., Wichter T., Paul M., Basson C.T., McDermott D.A., Lerman B.B., Markowitz S.M., Ellinor P.T., MacRae C.A., Peters S., Grossmann K.S., Drenckhahn J., Michely B., Sasse-Klaassen S., Birchmeier W., Dietz R., Breithardt G., Schulze-Bahr E., Thierfelder L. (2004) Mutations in the desmosomal protein plakophilin-2 are common in arrhythmogenic right ventricular cardiomyopathy. Nat Genet 36:1162-4.

Getsios S., Amargo E.V., Dusek R.L., Ishii K., Sheu L., Godsel L.M., Green K.J. (2004) Coordinated expression of desmoglein 1 and desmocollin 1 regulates intercellular adhesion. Differentiation 72:419-33.

Giepmans B.N., Moolenaar W.H. (1998) The gap junction protein connexin43 interacts with the second PDZ domain of the zona occludens-1 protein. Curr Biol 8:931-934.

Giepmans B.N., Verlaan I., Moolenaar W.H. (2001a) Connexin-43 interactions with ZO-1 and alpha- and beta-tubulin. Cell Commun Adhes 8:219-223.

Giepmans B.N., Feiken E., Gebbink M.F., Moolenaar W.H. (2003) Association of connexin43 with a receptor protein tyrosine phosphatase. Cell Commun Adhes 10:201-5.

Giepmans B.N., Verlaan I., Hengeveld T., Janssen H., Calafat J., Falk M.M., Moolenaar W.H. (2001b) Gap junction protein connexin-43 interacts directly with microtubules. Curr Biol 11:1364-1368.

Gonzalez D., Gomez-Hernandez J.M., Barrio L.C. (2007) Molecular basis of voltage dependence of connexin channels: an integrative appraisal. Prog Biophys Mol Biol 94:66-106.

Goossens S., Janssens B., Bonné S., De Rycke R., Braet F., van Hengel J., van Roy F. (2007) A unique and specific interaction between alphaT-catenin and plakophilin-2 in the area composita, the mixed-type junctional structure of cardiac intercalated discs. J Cell Sci 120:2126-2136.

Green K.J., Simpson C.L. (2007) Desmosomes: new perspectives on a classic. J Invest Dermatol 127:2499-515.

Grimley P.M., Edwards G.A. (1960) The ultrastructure of cardiac desnosomes in the toad and their relationship to the intercalated disc. J Biophys Biochem Cytol 8:305-318.

Grossmann K.S., Grund C., Huelsken J., Behrend M., Erdmann B., Franke W.W., Birchmeier W. (2004) Requirement of plakophilin 2 for heart morphogenesis and cardiac junction formation. J Cell Biol 167:149-60.

Gutstein D.E., Liu F.-Y., Meyers M.B., Choo A., Fishman G.I. (2003) The organization of adherens junctions and desmosomes at the cardiac intercalated disc is independent of gap junctions. J Cell Sci 116:875-885.

Gutstein D.E., Morley G.E., Vaidya D., Liu F., Chen F.L., Stuhlmann H., Fishman G.I. (2001a) Heterogeneous expression of Gap junction channels in the heart leads to conduction defects and ventricular dysfunction. Circ 104:1194-9.

Gutstein D.E., Morley G.E., Tamaddon H., Vaidya D., Schneider M.D., Chen J., Chien K.R., Stuhlmann H., Fishman G.I. (2001b) Conduction slowing and sudden arrhythmic death in mice with cardiac-restricted inactivation of connexin43. Circ Res 88:333-9.

Haegel H., Larue L., Ohsugi M., Fedorov L., Herrenknecht K., Kemler R. (1995) Lack of beta-catenin affects mouse development at gastrulation. Development 121:3529-37.

Hatzfeld M. (2005) The p120 family of cell adhesion molecules. Eur J Cell Biol 84:205-14.

Hatzfeld M. (2007) Plakophilins: Multifunctional proteins or just regulators of desmosomal adhesion? Biochim Biophys Acta 1773:69-77.

Heupel W.M., Baumgartner W., Laymann B., Drenckhahn D., Golenhofen N. (2008) Different Ca2+ affinities and functional implications of the two synaptic adhesion molecules cadherin-11 and N-cadherin. Mol Cell Neurosci 37:548-58.

Hirschy A., Schatzmann F., Ehler E., Perriard J.-C. (2006) Establishment of cardiac cytoarchitecture in the developing mouse heart. Dev Biol 289:430-441.

Hofmann I., Mertens C., Brettel M., Nimmrich V., Schnolzer M., Herrmann H. (2000) Interaction of plakophilins with desmoplakin and intermediate filament proteins: an in vitro analysis. J Cell Sci 113 (Pt 13):2471-83.

Holthofer B., Windoffer R., Troyanovsky S., Leube R.E. (2007) Structure and function of desmosomes. Int Rev Cytol 264:65-163.

Hoyt R.H., Cohen M.L., Saffitz J.E. (1989) Distribution and three-dimensional structure of intercellular junctions in canine myocardium. Circ Res 64:563-574.

Huang R.Y.C., Laing J.G., Kanter E.M., Berthoud V.M., Bao M., Rohrs H.W., Townsend R.R., Yamada K.A. (2011) Identification of CaMKII Phosphorylation Sites in Connexin43 by High-Resolution Mass Spectrometry. J Proteome Res 10:1098-1109.

Huber A.H., Nelson W.J., Weis W.I. (1997) Three-dimensional structure of the armadillo repeat region of beta-catenin. Cell 90:871-882.

Hulsken J., Birchmeier W., Behrens J. (1994) E-cadherin and APC compete for the interaction with beta-catenin and the cytoskeleton. J Cell Biol 127:2061-9.

Hund T.J., Lerner D.L., Yamada K.A., Schuessler R.B., Saffitz J.E. (2007) Protein kinase Cepsilon mediates salutary effects on electrical coupling induced by ischemic preconditioning. Heart Rhythm 4:1183-93.

Hund T.J., Decker K.F., Kanter E., Mohler P.J., Boyden P.A., Schuessler R.B., Yamada K.A., Rudy Y. (2008) Role of activated CaMKII in abnormal calcium homeostasis and I(Na) remodeling after myocardial infarction: insights from mathematical modeling. J Mol Cell Cardiol 45:420-8.

Hunter A.W., Barker R.J., Zhu C., Gourdie R.G. (2005) Zonula occludens-1 alters connexin43 gap junction size and organization by influencing channel accretion. Mol Biol Cell 16:5686-98.

Imamura Y., Itoh M., Maeno Y., Tsukita S., Nagafuchi A. (1999) Functional domains of alpha-catenin required for the strong state of cadherin-based cell adhesion. J Cell Biol 144:1311-22.

Janssens B., Goossens S., Staes K., Gilbert B., van Hengel J., Colpaert C., Bruyneel E., Mareel M., van Roy F. (2001) alphaT-catenin: a novel tissue-specific beta-catenin-binding protein mediating strong cell-cell adhesion. J Cell Sci 114:3177-88.

Jeyaraman M., Tanguy S., Fandrich R.R., Lukas A., Kardami E. (2003) Ischemia-induced dephosphorylation of cardiomyocyte connexin-43 is reduced by okadaic acid and calyculin A but not fostriecin. Mol Cell Biochem 242:129-34.

Jung-Ching Lin J., Gustafson-Wagner E.A., Sinn H.W., Choi S., Jaacks S.M., Wang D.-Z., Evans S., Li-Chun Lin J. (2005) Structure, Expression, and Function of a Novel Intercalated Disc Protein, Xin. J Med Sci 25:215-222.

Kami K., Chidgey M., Dafforn T., Overduin M. (2009) The desmoglein-specific cytoplasmic region is intrinsically disordered in solution and interacts with multiple desmosomal protein partners. J Mol Biol 386:531-43.

Kaplan S.R., Gard J.J., Carvajal-Huerta L., Ruiz-Cabezas J.C., Thiene G., Saffitz J.E. (2004a) Structural and molecular pathology of the heart in Carvajal syndrome. Cardiovasc Pathol 13:26-32.

Kaplan S.R., Gard J.J., Protonotarios N., Tsatsopoulou A., Spiliopoulou C., Anastasakis A., Squarcioni C.P., McKenna W.J., Thiene G., Basso C., Brousse N., Fontaine G., Saffitz J.E. (2004b) Remodeling of myocyte gap junctions in arrhythmogenic right ventricular cardiomyopathy due to a deletion in plakoglobin (Naxos disease). Heart Rhythm 1:3-11.

Kargacin G.J., Hunt D., Emmett T., Rokolya A., McMartin G.A., Wirch E., Walsh M.P., Ikebe M., Kargacin M.E. (2006) Localization of telokin at the intercalated discs of cardiac myocytes. Arch Biochem Biophys 456:151-160.

Katsuno T., Umeda K., Matsui T., Hata M., Tamura A., Itoh M., Takeuchi K., Fujimori T., Nabeshima Y., Noda T., Tsukita S. (2008) Deficiency of zonula occludens-1 causes embryonic lethal phenotype associated with defected yolk sac angiogenesis and apoptosis of embryonic cells. Mol Biol Cell 19:2465-75.

Keirsebilck A., Bonne S., Staes K., van Hengel J., Nollet F., Reynolds A., van Roy F. (1998) Molecular cloning of the human p120ctn catenin gene (CTNND1): expression of multiple alternatively spliced isoforms. Genomics 50:129-46.

Kelly S.C., Ratajczak P., Keller M., Purcell S.M., Griffin T., Richard G. (2006) A novel GJA 1 mutation in oculo-dento-digital dysplasia with curly hair and hyperkeratosis. Eur J Dermatol 16:241-5.

Kirchhoff S., Nelles E., Hagendorff A., Kruger O., Traub O., Willecke K. (1998) Reduced cardiac conduction velocity and predisposition to arrhythmias in connexin40-deficient mice. Curr Biol 8:299-302.

Kobielak A., Fuchs E. (2004) Alpha-catenin: at the junction of intercellular adhesion and actin dynamics. Nature Rev 5:614-625.

Koslov E.R., Maupin P., Pradhan D., Morrow J.S., Rimm D.L. (1997) Alpha-catenin can form asymmetric homodimeric complexes and/or heterodimeric complexes with beta-catenin. J Biol Chem 272:27301-6.

Kostetskii I., Li J., Xiong Y., Zhou R., Ferrari V.A., Patel V.V., Molkentin J.D., Radice G.L. (2005) Induced deletion of the N-cadherin gene in the heart leads to dissolution of the intercalated disc structure. Circ Res 96:346-354.

Kostin S. (2007) Zonula occludens-1 and connexin 43 expression in the failing human heart. J Cell Mol Med 11:892-5.

Kostin S., Hein S., Bauer E.P., Schaper J. (1999) Spatiotemporal development and distribution of intercellular junctions in adult rat cardiomyocytes in culture. Circ Res 85:154-167.

Kowalczyk A.P., Stappenbeck T.S., Parry D.A., Palka H.L., Virata M.L., Bornslaeger E.A., Nilles L.A., Green K.J. (1994) Structure and function of desmosomal transmembrane core and plaque molecules. Biophys Chem 50:97-112.

Kowalczyk A.P., Hatzfeld M., Bornslaeger E.A., Kopp D.S., Borgwardt J.E., Corcoran C.M., Settler A., Green K.J. (1999) The head domain of plakophilin-1 binds to desmoplakin and enhances its recruitment to desmosomes. Implications for cutaneous disease. J Biol Chem 274:18145-8.

Krusche C.A., Holthöfer B., Hofe V., van de Sandt A.M., Eshkind L., Bockamp E., Merx M.W., Kant S., Windoffer R., Leube R.E. (2011) Desmoglein 2 mutant mice develop cardiac fibrosis and dilation. Bas Res Cardiol 106:617-633.

Laing J.G., Saffitz J.E., Steinberg T.H., Yamada K.A. (2007) Diminished zonula occludens-1 expression in the failing human heart. Cardiovasc Pathol 16:159-64.

Lampe P.D., Cooper C.D., King T.J., Burt J.M. (2006) Analysis of Connexin43 phosphorylated at S325, S328 and S330 in normoxic and ischemic heart. J Cell Sci 119:3435-42.

Lampe P.D., TenBroek E.M., Burt J.M., Kurata W.E., Johnson R.G., Lau A.F. (2000) Phosphorylation of connexin43 on serine368 by protein kinase C regulates gap junctional communication. J Cell Biol 149:1503-12.

Langlois S., Cowan K.N., Shao Q., Cowan B.J., Laird D.W. (2008) Caveolin-1 and -2 interact with connexin43 and regulate gap junctional intercellular communication in keratinocytes. Mol Biol Cell 19:912-28.

Lauf U., Giepmans B.N., Lopez P., Braconnot S., Chen S.C., Falk M.M. (2002) Dynamic trafficking and delivery of connexons to the plasma membrane and accretion to gap junctions in living cells. Proc Natl Acad Sci U S A 99:10446-51.

Li J., Radice G.L. (2010) A New Perspective on Intercalated Disc Organization: Implications for Heart Disease. Dermatol Res Pract 2010:1-5.
Li J., Patel V.V., Radice G.L. (2006) Dysregulation of cell adhesion proteins and cardiac arrhythmogenesis. Clin Med Res 4:42-52.
Li J., Levin M.D., Xiong Y., Petrenko N., Patel V.V., Radice G.L. (2008) N-cadherin haploinsufficiency affects cardiac gap junctions and arrhythmic susceptibility. J Mol Cell Cardiol 44:597-606.
Li J., Swope D., Raess N., Cheng L., Muller E.J., Radice G.L. (2011) Cardiac tissue-restricted deletion of plakoglobin results in progressive cardiomyopathy and activation of {beta}-catenin signaling. Mol Cell Biol 31:1134-1144.
Li J., Patel V.V., Kostetskii I., Xiong Y., Chu A.F., Jacobson J.T., Yu C., Morley G.E., Molkentin J.D., Radice G.L. (2005) Cardiac-specific loss of N-cadherin leads to alteration in connexins with conduction slowing and arrhythmogenesis. Circ Res 97:474-481.
Lin D., Zhou J., Zelenka P.S., Takemoto D.J. (2003) Protein kinase Cgamma regulation of gap junction activity through caveolin-1-containing lipid rafts. Invest Ophthalmol Vis Sci 44:5259-68.
Liu L., Li Y., Lin J., Liang Q., Sheng X., Wu J., Huang R., Liu S., Li Y. (2010) Connexin43 interacts with Caveolin-3 in the heart. Mol Biol Reports 37:1685-1691.
Lombardi R., Marian A.J. (2011) Molecular genetics and pathogenesis of arrhythmogenic right ventricular cardiomyopathy: a disease of cardiac stem cells. Pediatr Cardiol 32:360-5.
Lorimer J.E., Hall L.S., Clarke J.P., Collins J.E., Fleming T.P., Garrod D.R. (1994) Cloning, sequence analysis and expression pattern of mouse desmocollin 2 (DSC2), a cadherin-like adhesion molecule. Mol Membr Biol 11:229-36.
Maass K., Shibayama J., Chase S.E., Willecke K., Delmar M. (2007) C-terminal truncation of connexin43 changes number, size, and localization of cardiac gap junction plaques. Circ Res 101:1283-91.
Manias J.L., Plante I., Gong X.Q., Shao Q., Churko J., Bai D., Laird D.W. (2008) Fate of connexin43 in cardiac tissue harbouring a disease-linked connexin43 mutant. Cardiovasc Res 80:385-95.
Marcozzi C., Burdett I.D., Buxton R.S., Magee A.I. (1998) Coexpression of both types of desmosomal cadherin and plakoglobin confers strong intercellular adhesion. J Cell Sci 111 (Pt 4):495-509.
Marcus F.I., Fontaine G.H., Guiraudon G., Frank R., Laurenceau J.L., Malergue C., Grosgogeat Y. (1982) Right ventricular dysplasia: a report of 24 adult cases. Circ 65:384-98.
Mathur M., Goodwin L., Cowin P. (1994) Interactions of the cytoplasmic domain of the desmosomal cadherin Dsg1 with plakoglobin. J Biol Chem 269:14075-80.
Matsuda H., Kurata Y., Oka C., Matsuoka S., Noma A. (2010) Magnesium gating of cardiac gap junction channels. Prog Biophys Mol Biol 103:102-10.
McGregor A., Blanchard A.D., Rowe A.J., Critchley D.R. (1994) Identification of the vinculin-binding site in the cytoskeletal protein alpha-actinin. Biochem J 301 (Pt 1):225-33.
McKoy G., Protonotarios N., Crosby A., Tsatsopoulou A., Anastasakis A., Coonar A., Norman M., Baboonian C., Jeffery S., McKenna W.J. (2000) Identification of a deletion in plakoglobin in arrhythmogenic right ventricular cardiomyopathy with palmoplantar keratoderma and woolly hair (Naxos disease). Lancet 355:2119-24.

McNutt D.P., Feldman P.D., Houck J.R., Harwit M. (1970) Far-infrared observations of the night sky: different data. Science 167:1277.

Mertens C., Kuhn C., Franke W.W. (1996) Plakophilins 2a and 2b: constitutive proteins of dual location in the karyoplasm and the desmosomal plaque. J Cell Biol 135:1009-25.

Mertens C., Kuhn C., Moll R., Schwetlick I., Franke W.W. (1999) Desmosomal plakophilin 2 as a differentiation marker in normal and malignant tissues. Differentiation 64:277-90.

Muir A.R. (1957) An electron microscope study of the embryology of the intercalated disc in the heart of the rabbit. J Biophys Biochem Cytol 3:193-202.

Nagaraj R.H., Shipanova I.N., Faust F.M. (1996) Protein cross-linking by the Maillard reaction. Isolation, characterization, and in vivo detection of a lysine-lysine cross-link derived from methylglyoxal. J Biol Chem 271:19338-45.

Niessen C.M. (2007) Tight junctions/adherens junctions: basic structure and function. J Invest Dermatol 127:2525-2532.

Noorman M., van der Heyden M.A.G., van Veen T.A.B., Cox M.G.P.J., Hauer R.N.W., de Bakker J.M.T., van Rijen H.V.M. (2009) Cardiac cell-cell junctions in health and disease: Electrical versus mechanical coupling. J Mol Cell Cardiol 47:23-31.

Norgett E.E., Hatsell S.J., Carvajal-Huerta L., Cabezas J.C., Common J., Purkis P.E., Whittock N., Leigh I.M., Stevens H.P., Kelsell D.P. (2000) Recessive mutation in desmoplakin disrupts desmoplakin-intermediate filament interactions and causes dilated cardiomyopathy, woolly hair and keratoderma. Hum Mol Genet 9:2761-6.

Norman M., Simpson M., Mogensen J., Shaw A., Hughes S., Syrris P., Sen-Chowdhry S., Rowland E., Crosby A., McKenna W.J. (2005) Novel mutation in desmoplakin causes arrhythmogenic left ventricular cardiomyopathy. Circ 112:636-42.

Nose A., Tsuji K., Takeichi M. (1990) Localization of specificity determining sites in cadherin cell adhesion molecules. Cell 61:147-55.

Ozawa M., Ringwald M., Kemler R. (1990) Uvomorulin-catenin complex formation is regulated by a specific domain in the cytoplasmic region of the cell adhesion molecule. Proc Natl Acad Sci U S A 87:4246-50.

Parker A.E., Wheeler G.N., Arnemann J., Pidsley S.C., Ataliotis P., Thomas C.L., Rees D.A., Magee A.I., Buxton R.S. (1991) Desmosomal glycoproteins II and III. Cadherin-like junctional molecules generated by alternative splicing. J Biol Chem 266:10438-45.

Peifer M., Berg S., Reynolds A.B. (1994) A repeating amino acid motif shared by proteins with diverse cellular roles. Cell 76:789-91.

Peifer M., McCrea P.D., Green K.J., Wieschaus E., Gumbiner B.M. (1992) The vertebrate adhesive junction proteins beta-catenin and plakoglobin and the Drosophila segment polarity gene armadillo form a multigene family with similar properties. J Cell Biol 118:681-91.

Perkins G., Goodenough D., Sosinsky G. (1997) Three-dimensional structure of the gap junction connexon. Biophys J 72:533-44.

Peters N.S., Severs N.J., Rothery S.M., Lincoln C., Yacoub M.H., Green C.R. (1994) Spatiotemporal relation between gap junctions and fascia adherens junctions during postnatal development of human ventricular myocardium. Circ 90:713-725.

Pieperhoff S., Franke W.W. (2007) The area composita of adhering junctions connecting heart muscle cells of vertebrates - IV: coalescence and amalgamation of desmosomal and adhaerens junction components - late processes in mammalian heart development. Eur J Cell Biol 86:377-391.

Pieperhoff S., Schumacher H., Franke W.W. (2008) The area composita of adhering junctions connecting heart muscle cells of vertebrates. V. The importance of plakophilin-2 demonstrated by small interference RNA-mediated knockdown in cultured rat cardiomyocytes. Eur J Cell Biol 87:399-411.

Pilichou K., Nava A., Basso C., Beffagna G., Bauce B., Lorenzon A., Frigo G., Vettori A., Valente M., Towbin J., Thiene G., Danieli G.A., Rampazzo A. (2006) Mutations in desmoglein-2 gene are associated with arrhythmogenic right ventricular cardiomyopathy. Circ 113:1171-1179.

Piven O.O., Kostetskii I.E., Macewicz L.L., Kolomiets Y.M., Radice G.L., Lukash L.L. (2011) Requirement for N-cadherin-catenin complex in heart development. Exp Biol Med 236:816-22.

Pokutta S., Weis W.I. (2000) Structure of the dimerization and beta-catenin-binding region of alpha-catenin. Mol Cell 5:533-43.

Pokutta S., Weis W.I. (2007) Structure and mechanism of cadherins and catenins in cell-cell contacts. Annu Rev Cell Dev Biol 23:237-61.

Posch M.G., Posch M.J., Geier C., Erdmann B., Mueller W., Richter A., Ruppert V., Pankuweit S., Maisch B., Perrot A., Buttgereit J., Dietz R., Haverkamp W., Ozcelik C. (2008) A missense variant in desmoglein-2 predisposes to dilated cardiomyopathy. Mol Genet Metab 95:74-80.

Procida K., Jorgensen L., Schmitt N., Delmar M., Taffet S.M., Holstein-Rathlou N.H., Nielsen M.S., Braunstein T.H. (2009) Phosphorylation of connexin43 on serine 306 regulates electrical coupling. Heart Rhythm 6:1632-8.

Protonotarios N., Tsatsopoulou A., Patsourakos P., Alexopoulos D., Gezerlis P., Simitsis S., Scampardonis G. (1986) Cardiac abnormalities in familial palmoplantar keratosis. Br Heart J 56:321-6.

Protonotarios N., Anastasakis A., Antoniades L., Chlouverakis G., Syrris P., Basso C., Asimaki A., Theopistou A., Stefanadis C., Thiene G., McKenna W.J., Tsatsopoulou A. (2011) Arrhythmogenic right ventricular cardiomyopathy/dysplasia on the basis of the revised diagnostic criteria in affected families with desmosomal mutations. Eur Heart J 32(9):1097-104.

Radice G.L., Rayburn H., Matsunami H., Knudsen K.A., Takeichi M., Hynes R.O. (1997) Developmental defects in mouse embryos lacking N-cadherin. Dev Biol 181:64-78.

Rampazzo A., Nava A., Malacrida S., Beffagna G., Bauce B., Rossi V., Zimbello R., Simionati B., Basso C., Thiene G., Towbin J.A., Danieli G.A. (2002) Mutation in human desmoplakin domain binding to plakoglobin causes a dominant form of arrhythmogenic right ventricular cardiomyopathy. Am J Hum Genet 71:1200-6.

Ravel J., Karnovsky M. (1967) Hexagonal array of subunits in intercellular junctions of the mouse heart and liver. J Cell Biol 22:1516-1528.

Rayns D.G., Simpson F.O., Ledingham J.M. (1969) Ultrastructure of desmosomes in mammalian intercalated disc; appearances after lanthanum treatment. J Cell Biol 42:322-326.

Reaume A.G., de Sousa P.A., Kulkarni S., Langille B.L., Zhu D., Davies T.C., Juneja S.C., Kidder G.M., Rossant J. (1995) Cardiac malformation in neonatal mice lacking connexin43. Science 267:1831-4.

Reynolds A.B., Herbert L., Cleveland J.L., Berg S.T., Gaut J.R. (1992) p120, a novel substrate of protein tyrosine kinase receptors and of p60v-src, is related to cadherin-binding factors beta-catenin, plakoglobin and armadillo. Oncogene 7:2439-45.

Rhett J.M., Jourdan J., Gourdie R.G. (2011) Connexin 43 connexon to gap junction transition is regulated by zonula occludens-1. Mol Biol Cell 22:1516-28.

Rimm D.L., Koslov E.R., Kebriaei P., Cianci C.D., Morrow J.S. (1995) Alpha 1(E)-catenin is an actin-binding and -bundling protein mediating the attachment of F-actin to the membrane adhesion complex. Proc Natl Acad Sci U S A 92:8813-7.

Rohr S. (2004) Role of gap junctions in the propagation of the cardiac action potential. Cardiov Res 62:309-322.

Rohr S. (2007) Molecular crosstalk between mechanical and electrical junctions at the intercalated disc. Circulation research 101:637-639.

Rudiger M. (1998) Vinculin and alpha-catenin: shared and unique functions in adherens junctions. Bioessays 20:733-40.

Ruiz P., Brinkmann V., Ledermann B., Behrend M., Grund C., Thalhammer C., Vogel F., Birchmeier C., Gunthert U., Franke W.W., Birchmeier W. (1996) Targeted mutation of plakoglobin in mice reveals essential functions of desmosomes in the embryonic heart. J Cell Biol 135:215-25.

Saez J.C., Nairn A.C., Czernik A.J., Fishman G.I., Spray D.C., Hertzberg E.L. (1997) Phosphorylation of connexin43 and the regulation of neonatal rat cardiac myocyte gap junctions. J Mol Cell Cardiol 29:2131-45.

Saffitz J.E. (2005) Dependence of Electrical Coupling on Mechanical Coupling in Cardiac Myocytes: Insights Gained from Cardiomyopathies Caused by Defects in Cell-Cell Connections. Ann New York Acad Sci 1047:336-344.

Saffitz J.E. (2009) Arrhythmogenic cardiomyopathy and abnormalities of cell-to-cell coupling. Heart Rhythm 6:S62-5.

Saphir O., Karsner H.T. (1924) An Anatomical and Experimental Study of Segmentation of the Myocardium and its Relation to the Intercalated Discs. J Med Res 44:539-556.5.

Sato P.Y., Musa H., Coombs W., Guerrero-Serna G., Patiño G.A., Taffet S.M., Isom L.L., Delmar M. (2009) Loss of plakophilin-2 expression leads to decreased sodium current and slower conduction velocity in cultured cardiac myocytes. Circ Res 105:523-526.

Sato P.Y., Coombs W., Lin X., Nekrasova O., Green K.J., Isom L.L., Taffet S.M., Delmar M. (2011) Interactions between ankyrin-g, plakophilin-2, and connexin43 at the cardiac intercalated disc. Circ Res 109:193-201.

Satomi-Kobayashi S., Ueyama T., Mueller S., Toh R., Masano T., Sakoda T., Rikitake Y., Miyoshi J., Matsubara H., Oh H., Kawashima S., Hirata K.-i., Takai Y. (2009) Deficiency of nectin-2 leads to cardiac fibrosis and dysfunction under chronic pressure overload. Hypertension 54:825-831.

Schmelz M., Duden R., Cowin P., Franke W.W. (1986) A constitutive transmembrane glycoprotein of Mr 165,000 (desmoglein) in epidermal and non-epidermal desmosomes. I. Biochemical identification of the polypeptide. Eur J Cell Biol 42:177-83.

Schroen B., Leenders J.J., van Erk A., Bertrand A.T., van Loon M., van Leeuwen R.E., Kubben N., Duisters R.F., Schellings M.W., Janssen B.J., Debets J.J., Schwake M., Høydal M.A., Heymans S., Saftig P., Pinto Y.M. (2007) Lysosomal integral membrane protein 2 is a novel component of the cardiac intercalated disc and vital for load-induced cardiac myocyte hypertrophy. J Exper Med 204:1227-1235.

Schubert A.-L., Schubert W., Spray D.C., Lisanti M.P. (2002) Connexin family members target to lipid raft domains and interact with caveolin-1. Biochemistry 41:5754-5764.

Seeger T.S., Frank D., Rohr C., Will R., Just S., Grund C., Lyon R., Luedde M., Koegl M., Sheikh F., Rottbauer W., Franke W.W., Katus H.A., Olson E.N., Frey N. (2010) Myozap, a Novel Intercalated Disc Protein, Activates Serum Response Factor-Dependent Signaling and Is Required to Maintain Cardiac Function In Vivo. Circ Res 106:880-890.

Sen-Chowdhry S., Morgan R.D., Chambers J.C., McKenna W.J. (2010) Arrhythmogenic cardiomyopathy: etiology, diagnosis, and treatment. Annu Rev Med 61:233-53.

Severs N.J., Bruce A.F., Dupont E., Rothery S. (2008) Remodelling of gap junctions and connexin expression in diseased myocardium. Cardiovasc Res 80:9-19.

Shaw R.M., Fay A.J., Puthenveedu M.A., von Zastrow M., Jan Y.N., Jan L.Y. (2007) Microtubule plus-end-tracking proteins target gap junctions directly from the cell interior to adherens junctions. Cell 128:547-60.

Sheikh F., Chen Y., Chen Y., Liang X., Hirschy A., Stenbit A.E., Gu Y., Dalton N.D., Yajima T., Lu Y., Knowlton K.U., Peterson K.L., Perriard J.-C., Chen J. (2006) alpha-E-catenin inactivation disrupts the cardiomyocyte adherens junction, resulting in cardiomyopathy and susceptibility to wall rupture. Circ 114:1046-1055.

Shibamoto S., Hayakawa M., Takeuchi K., Hori T., Miyazawa K., Kitamura N., Johnson K.R., Wheelock M.J., Matsuyoshi N., Takeichi M., et al. (1995) Association of p120, a tyrosine kinase substrate, with E-cadherin/catenin complexes. J Cell Biol 128:949-57.

Shimada T., Kawazato H., Yasuda A., Ono N., Sueda K. (2004) Cytoarchitecture and intercalated disks of the working myocardium and the conduction system in the mammalian heart. Anatom Rec 280:940-951.

Simpson M.A., Mansour S., Ahnood D., Kalidas K., Patton M.A., McKenna W.J., Behr E.R., Crosby A.H. (2009) Homozygous mutation of desmocollin-2 in arrhythmogenic right ventricular cardiomyopathy with mild palmoplantar keratoderma and woolly hair. Cardiology 113:28-34.

Sjostrand F.S., Andersson E. (1954) Electron microscopy of the intercalated discs of cardiac muscle tissue. Experientia 10:369-70.

Smyth J.W., Hong T.T., Gao D., Vogan J.M., Jensen B.C., Fong T.S., Simpson P.C., Stainier D.Y., Chi N.C., Shaw R.M. (2010) Limited forward trafficking of connexin 43 reduces cell-cell coupling in stressed human and mouse myocardium. J Clin Invest 120:266-79.

Sohl G., Willecke K. (2004) Gap junctions and the connexin protein family. Cardiovasc Res 62:228-32.

Solan J.L., Marquez-Rosado L., Sorgen P.L., Thornton P.J., Gafken P.R., Lampe P.D. (2007) Phosphorylation at S365 is a gatekeeper event that changes the structure of Cx43 and prevents down-regulation by PKC. J Cell Biol 179:1301-9.

Sorgen P.L., Duffy H.S., Sahoo P., Coombs W., Delmar M., Spray D.C. (2004) Structural changes in the carboxyl terminus of the gap junction protein connexin43 indicates signaling between binding domains for c-Src and zonula occludens-1. J Biol Chem 279:54695-701.

Staddon J.M., Smales C., Schulze C., Esch F.S., Rubin L.L. (1995) p120, a p120-related protein (p100), and the cadherin/catenin complex. J Cell Biol 130:369-81.

Syed S.E., Trinnaman B., Martin S., Major S., Hutchinson J., Magee A.I. (2002) Molecular interactions between desmosomal cadherins. Biochem J 362:317-27.

Syrris P., Ward D., Evans A., Asimaki A., Gandjbakhch E., Sen-Chowdhry S., McKenna W.J. (2006) Arrhythmogenic right ventricular dysplasia/cardiomyopathy associated with mutations in the desmosomal gene desmocollin-2. Am J Hum Genet 79:978-84.

Takeichi M. (1994) The cadherin cell adhesion receptor family: roles in multicellular organization and neurogenesis. Progr Clin Biol Res 390:145-153.

Talhouk R.S., Mroue R., Mokalled M., Abi-Mosleh L., Nehme R., Ismail A., Khalil A., Zaatari M., El-Sabban M.E. (2008) Heterocellular interaction enhances recruitment of alpha and beta-catenins and ZO-2 into functional gap-junction complexes and induces gap junction-dependant differentiation of mammary epithelial cells. Exper Cell Res 314:3275-3291.

Tandler B., Riva L., Loy F., Conti G., Isola R. (2006) High resolution scanning electron microscopy of the intracellular surface of intercalated disks in human heart. Tissue Cell 38:417-420.

Tang Z., Scherer P.E., Okamoto T., Song K., Chu C., Kohtz D.S., Nishimoto I., Lodish H.F., Lisanti M.P. (1996) Molecular cloning of caveolin-3, a novel member of the caveolin gene family expressed predominantly in muscle. J Biol Chem 271:2255-61.

TenBroek E.M., Lampe P.D., Solan J.L., Reynhout J.K., Johnson R.G. (2001) Ser364 of connexin43 and the upregulation of gap junction assembly by cAMP. J Cell Biol 155:1307-18.

Tepass U., Truong K., Godt D., Ikura M., Peifer M. (2000) Cadherins in embryonic and neural morphogenesis. Nat Rev Mol Cell Biol 1:91-100.

Thiene G., Corrado D., Basso C. (2007) Arrhythmogenic right ventricular cardiomyopathy/dysplasia. Orphanet J Rare Dis 2:45.

Thimm J., Mechler A., Lin H., Rhee S., Lal R. (2005) Calcium-dependent open/closed conformations and interfacial energy maps of reconstituted hemichannels. J Biol Chem 280:10646-54.

Thomason H.A., Scothern A., McHarg S., Garrod D.R. (2010) Desmosomes: adhesive strength and signalling in health and disease. Biochem J 429:419-433.

Thoreson M.A., Anastasiadis P.Z., Daniel J.M., Ireton R.C., Wheelock M.J., Johnson K.R., Hummingbird D.K., Reynolds A.B. (2000) Selective uncoupling of p120(ctn) from E-cadherin disrupts strong adhesion. J Cell Biol 148:189-202.

Toyofuku T., Yabuki M., Otsu K., Kuzuya T., Hori M., Tada M. (1998) Direct association of the gap junction protein connexin-43 with ZO-1 in cardiac myocytes. J Biol Chem 273:12725-31.

Toyofuku T., Akamatsu Y., Zhang H., Kuzuya T., Tada M., Hori M. (2001) c-Src regulates the interaction between connexin-43 and ZO-1 in cardiac myocytes. J Biol Chem 276:1780-8.

Troyanovsky S.M., Eshkind L.G., Troyanovsky R.B., Leube R.E., Franke W.W. (1993) Contributions of cytoplasmic domains of desmosomal cadherins to desmosome assembly and intermediate filament anchorage. Cell 72:561-74.

Tselepis C., Chidgey M., North A., Garrod D. (1998) Desmosomal adhesion inhibits invasive behavior. Proc Natl Acad Sci U S A 95:8064-9.

Unger V.M., Kumar N.M., Gilula N.B., Yeager M. (1999) Three-dimensional structure of a recombinant gap junction membrane channel. Science 283:1176-80.

Uzumcu A., Norgett E.E., Dindar A., Uyguner O., Nisli K., Kayserili H., Sahin S.E., Dupont E., Severs N.J., Leigh I.M., Yuksel-Apak M., Kelsell D.P., Wollnik B. (2006) Loss of desmoplakin isoform I causes early onset cardiomyopathy and heart failure in a Naxos-like syndrome. J Med Genet 43:e5.

Van Breemen V. (1953) Intercalated discs in heart muscle studied with the electron microscope. Anatom Rec 117:49-63.

van Tintelen J.P., Hofstra R.M., Wiesfeld A.C., van den Berg M.P., Hauer R.N., Jongbloed J.D. (2007) Molecular genetics of arrhythmogenic right ventricular cardiomyopathy: emerging horizon? Curr Opin Cardiol 22:185-192.

Volk T., Geiger B. (1984) A 135-kd membrane protein of intercellular adherens junctions. EMBO J 3:2249-2260.

Vozzi C., Dupont E., Coppen S.R., Yeh H.I., Severs N.J. (1999) Chamber-related differences in connexin expression in the human heart. J Mol Cell Cardiol 31:991-1003.

Wahl J.K., Sacco P.A., McGranahan-Sadler T.M., Sauppe L.M., Wheelock M.J., Johnson K.R. (1996) Plakoglobin domains that define its association with the desmosomal cadherins and the classical cadherins: identification of unique and shared domains. J Cell Sci 109 (Pt 5):1143-54.

Warn-Cramer B.J., Cottrell G.T., Burt J.M., Lau A.F. (1998) Regulation of connexin-43 gap junctional intercellular communication by mitogen-activated protein kinase. J Biol Chem 273:9188-96.

Warn-Cramer B.J., Lampe P.D., Kurata W.E., Kanemitsu M.Y., Loo L.W., Eckhart W., Lau A.F. (1996) Characterization of the mitogen-activated protein kinase phosphorylation sites on the connexin-43 gap junction protein. J Biol Chem 271:3779-86.

Waschke J., Bruggeman P., Baumgartner W., Zillikens D., Drenckhahn D. (2005) Pemphigus foliaceus IgG causes dissociation of desmoglein 1-containing junctions without blocking desmoglein 1 transinteraction. J Clin Invest 115:3157-65.

Wei C.-J., Francis R., Xu X., Lo C.W. (2005) Connexin43 associated with an N-cadherin-containing multiprotein complex is required for gap junction formation in NIH3T3 cells. J Biol Chem 280:19925-19936.

Weidmann S. (1952) The electrical constants of Purkinje fibres. J Physiol 118:348-60.

Weiss E.E., Kroemker M., Rudiger A.H., Jockusch B.M., Rudiger M. (1998) Vinculin is part of the cadherin-catenin junctional complex: complex formation between alpha-catenin and vinculin. J Cell Biol 141:755-64.

Xu J., Kausalya P.J., Phua D.C., Ali S.M., Hossain Z., Hunziker W. (2008) Early embryonic lethality of mice lacking ZO-2, but Not ZO-3, reveals critical and nonredundant roles for individual zonula occludens proteins in mammalian development. Mol Cell Biol 28:1669-78.

Yang Z., Bowles N.E., Scherer S.E., Taylor M.D., Kearney D.L., Ge S., Nadvoretskiy V.V., DeFreitas G., Carabello B., Brandon L.I., Godsel L.M., Green K.J., Saffitz J.E., Li H., Danieli G.A., Calkins H., Marcus F., Towbin J.A. (2006) Desmosomal dysfunction due to mutations in desmoplakin causes arrhythmogenic right ventricular dysplasia/cardiomyopathy. Circ Res 99:646-55.

Yarbrough T.L., Lu T., Lee H.C., Shibata E.F. (2002) Localization of cardiac sodium channels in caveolin-rich membrane domains: regulation of sodium current amplitude. Circ Res 90:443-9.

Zhao Y.Y., Liu Y., Stan R. V., Fan L., Gu Y., Dalton N., Chu P.H., Peterson K., Ross J., Chien K.R. (2002) Defects in *caveolin-1* cause dilated cardiomyopathy and pulmonary hypertension in knockout mice. Proc Natl Acad Sci USA 99:11375-80.

Zhu C., Barker R.J., Hunter A.W., Zhang Y., Jourdan J., Gourdie R.G. (2005) Quantitative analysis of ZO-1 colocalization with Cx43 gap junction plaques in cultures of rat neonatal cardiomyocytes. Microsc Microanal 11:244-8.

14

Familial Hypertrophic Cardiomyopathy-Related Troponin Mutations and Sudden Cardiac Death

Laura Dewar, Bo Liang, Yueh Li, Shubhayan Sanatani and Glen F. Tibbits
Simon Fraser University
Canada

1. Introduction

Hypertrophic cardiomyopathy (HCM) is a common structural anomaly of the myocardium that is unexplained by an underlying condition such as hypertension. The main findings in HCM are varying degrees of ventricular and/or septal hypertrophy, myocyte disarray and increased myocardial fibrosis (Maron et al., 1995). There is significant variation in the clinical manifestation among patients, from asymptomatic, to mild dyspnea upon exertion, to substantive heart failure. While many individuals will present with clinical symptoms, including a cardiac murmur related to outflow tract obstruction, in some families, diagnosis is not established until the sudden death of, or incidental finding of hypertrophy within, a family member. Transthoracic echocardiography has traditionally been the clinician's primary tool for determination of asymmetric hypertrophy of the left interventricular septum, with or without left ventricular outflow tract obstruction. Given the heterogeneity in severity of disease and penetrance within HCM-affected families, it is important to rule out other secondary causes of hypertrophy, such as hypertension or aortic stenosis. Diagnosis can be difficult, especially in elite athletes who may present with physiological left ventricular hypertrophy (Maron, 2009). Clinically identifiable HCM has a prevalence of 1:500 in young adults in the general population, making it the most common genetic cardiovascular disease in many countries (Maron et al., 1995).

Although familial hypertrophic cardiomyopathy (FHC) was first described clinically more than half a century ago (Teare, 1958), it was only about 20 years ago that the underlying molecular causes of FHC began to be established, with the finding of a mutation in the beta-myosin heavy chain (*MYH7*) gene (Geisterfer-Lowrance et al., 1990). Since this seminal discovery, there have been more than 900 different mutations identified in over 20 FHC candidate genes (Tester & Ackerman, 2009). Historically, attempts to establish the link between genotype and phenotype were based on studying FHC cohorts with severe, well established disease with cardiac remodelling and in some patients, progression to end-stage cardiac dilatation and failure. It is increasingly apparent that focussing on the end phenotype as a link to genotype is problematic; families are highly heterogeneous in their disease presentation with, in many cases, low penetrance (at least on echocardiography diagnoses) and with novel mutations not seen in other families. There are few large FHC-affected families, leading to linkage analysis difficulties. When a pathogenic FHC mutation is uncovered in the proband, genetic testing of all first degree relatives is highly recommended. When other family members are genotyped, mutation-positive relatives can be closely monitored for disease progression (Colombo et al., 2008).

Up to 60% of patients with a high index of suspicion for FHC are found to have a genetic mutation in one of the FHC-susceptibility genes. A subset of FHC patients do not have identifiable mutations, perhaps because of reduced screening sensitivity that does not incorporate deep intronic sequencing, identify large insertions or deletions in the known candidate genes or include non-hot spot encoding regions. In addition, some patients may have mutations in as-yet unrecognized candidate genes (Rodriguez et al., 2009). The majority of documented FHC mutations occur as single nucleotide substitutions or "missense" mutations, although nucleotide deletions and insertions have also been identified. Insertions and deletions can potentially truncate the gene product by causing a shift in the reading frame leading to a premature stop codon. Mutations that occur at exon/intron boundaries can cause splice anomalies, leading to abnormal and potentially dysfunctional protein products (Wheeler et al., 2009).

Two prominent hypotheses have been developed to explain how sarcomere protein mutations cause the FHC phenotype: first is the "poison polypeptide" hypothesis, in which a single mutant protein disrupts the function of the entire sarcomere unit in a dominant negative manner (Thierfelder et al., 1994). The mutant protein is translated and incorporated into the sarcomere, where it can impair contraction. The second hypothesis is that sarcomeric protein mutations can lead to haploinsufficiency, in which mutations disrupt one copy of the gene, leaving the wild-type gene copy to produce the protein product in inadequate quantities for a balanced sarcomere unit (Thierfelder et al., 1994). In this situation, there is a 50% reduction in peptide concentration due to disruption in translation or trafficking of the mutant. Inadequate levels of incorporated wild-type protein create an imbalance in thin filament stoichiometry.

2. Sudden cardiac death in FHC

FHC is the most common cause of sudden cardiac death (SCD) in young people, affecting approximately 1-2% of children and adolescents, and up to 1% of young adults in HCM community cohorts (Elliott et al., 2000; Maron, 2002). Although SCD is considered rare in competitive athletes (1 in 200,000), HCM is associated with nearly one third of such occurrences (Maron, 2003). Children have the highest SCD rates of FHC patients suggesting that early onset can result from a more severe phenotype that includes lethal arrhythmias (Maron et al., 1999; Ostman-Smith et al., 2008). The highest mortality rates are seen in children aged 9 to 14 years, averaging 7.2%. The SCD risk peaks in girls at 10 to 11 years of age and occurs in boys at 15 to 16 years of age, leading to some researchers to propose that the surge in androgens that occurs prior to puberty may be associated with rapid disease progression and increased SCD risk (Ostman-Smith et al., 2008). There is a male preponderance for FHC-related SCD, especially among athletes (Maron et al., 1996). FHC patients with 2 or more mutations (Hershberger, 2010; Van Driest et al., 2004), and homozygous mutation patients, have more severe disease phenotypes with higher penetrance and greater incidence of SCD over single mutation patients (Ho et al., 2000; Ingles et al., 2005). Modifier gene polymorphisms such as angiotensin I converting enzyme (ACE) D allele, (Marian et al., 1993) and lifestyle/environmental factors such as diet, exercise, body mass and hypertension may also affect the FHC phenotype. With such complexities in disease manifestation, SCD risk assessment has been problematic. Younger age at onset, history of syncope with exertion, history of SCD within close relatives, severity of symptoms and degree of ventricular and septal wall thickness have been used in risk stratification algorithms; however, many risk factor studies involved non-genotyped patients with sometimes conflicting or confusing results and frequently with no single risk factor being identified. Prognosis for genotyped patients varies with the gene and in many cases, specific mutations within a gene; however, the mechanisms by which such mutations have an increased propensity for sudden death in some individuals, while in others appear to be relatively benign, are not well understood. The primary prevention risk factors for SCD in FHC include family history of SCD, unexplained recent syncope, runs of non-sustained ventricular tachycardia on ambulatory 24 hour Holter monitor, hypotensive response to exercise and severe left ventricular wall thickness (over 30 mm) (Maron, 2010). With respect to the latter, mild ventricular hypertrophy, however, does not correlate with low SCD risk, especially with thin filament mutations, as discussed later.

3. The role of the troponin complex in cardiac dynamics

The focus of this chapter is on three genes that encode the troponin complex found within the sarcomere; *TNNT2*, encoding cardiac troponin T, *TNNI3*, encoding cardiac troponin I and *TNNC1*, encoding troponin C. These genes encode the cardiac troponin genes that are unique from their skeletal counterparts and have evolved to help regulate excitation-contraction coupling in the heart. The troponin (Tn) proteins are part of a thin filament regulatory unit of the sarcomere. Cardiac troponin C (cTnC) is the Ca^{2+}-binding subunit that acts as a cytosolic Ca^{2+} sensor, cardiac troponin I (cTnI) is the inhibitory subunit that inhibits contraction when intracellular Ca^{2+} levels are below activation levels and cardiac troponin T (cTnT) is the subunit responsible for attaching the troponin complex to the thin filament via binding with tropomyosin (Tm) and believed responsible for movement of Tm on the thin filament modulating binding of the myosin head to actin. The subunits are arranged in a 1:1:1 stoichiometric ratio along the thin filament with one Tn:Tm complex bound to every seven actin monomers. Actin monomers are arranged in a double helix oriented in parallel to myosin-containing thick filaments. These protein-protein configurations allow for thin filament activation (Figure 1), which in turn facilitates cross-bridge cycling through the action of myosin binding to actin and the production of force (Gordon et al., 2000).

Takeda and collaborators (Takeda et al., 2003) successfully crystallized the globular core of the Tn complex, which revealed that the complex is highly flexible, an inherent feature crucial to its role in heart muscle contraction. The structure consists of two domains: the regulatory head composed of the N-terminus of TnC (residues 3 – 84) and two α-helices of TnI (denoted as H3 and H4, residues 150 - 188), and the highly conserved IT arm composed of the C-terminus of TnC (residues 93-161), two α-helices of TnI (H1 and H2, residues 42-136) and two α-helices of TnT (H3 and H4, residues 203-271). Although crystallography allowed most of the Tn complex structure to be observed, some regions remain unresolved, including the inhibitory region of TnI, and both the N- and C-terminal regions of TnT. These regions are likely highly flexible, allowing them to bind to other thin filament proteins (i.e. actin) to modulate thin filament activation. The primary role of the regulatory domain is as the "Ca^{2+} sensor", while the rigid IT domain appears to be sensitive to myosin binding during contraction (Sun, Bradmeier & Irving, 2006, as cited in Willott et al., 2010).

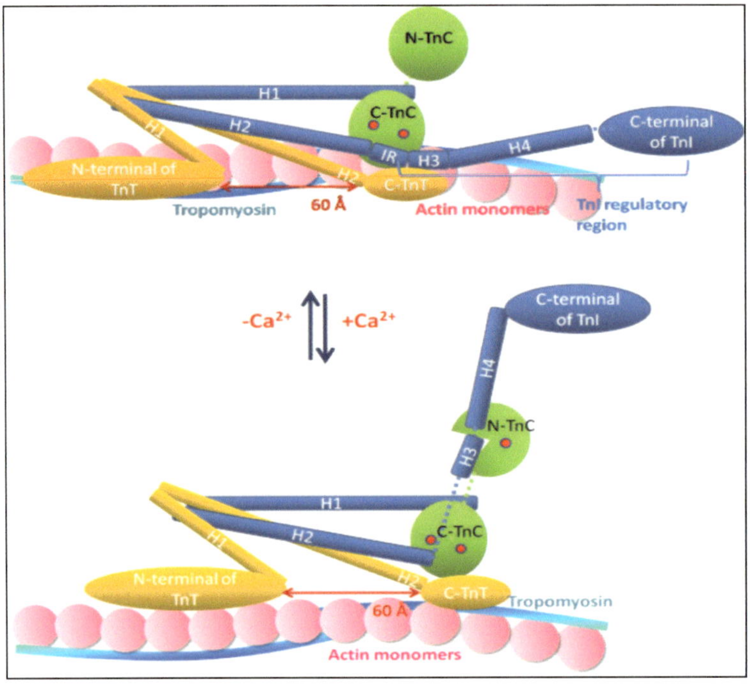

Fig. 1. A schematic representation of cardiac troponin in relation to the thin filament in the absence and presence of Ca^{2+}. The inhibitory region of TnI (IR), and the N-terminal and C-terminal domains of TnT are not clearly observed in the crystal structure, likely due to their inherent flexibility (see text). The red dots represent Ca^{2+} ions. The figure is adapted from Takeda, 2003 (Li, 2009).

Most researchers believe that a "3 state model" exists to explain myofilament contraction. Interestingly, it was the study of how various mutations disrupt these interactions that lead to further development and confirmation of the 3 state model (Gordon et al., 2000). During diastole, the ventricles fill with blood to their end-diastolic volumes. The sarcomeres are stretched to longer lengths but without developing significant diastolic pressures. Cross-bridge cycling is physically blocked by the Tm:Tn complex at this stage and is referred to as the "blocked" or "B" state. Recently it has been postulated that perhaps only 50% of the cross-bridges are sterically blocked. The rest may be in a weakly-bound non-force generating state that facilitates the transition of cross-bridge cycling into the systolic state. There are two actin-binding regions on cTnI that play an essential role in diastole. There is an inhibitory region (residues 137-148) and a downstream helix (H3, residues 150-159) that tightly binds to actin, which along with cTnT, anchor Tm into the blocking position (see review by Parmacek & Solaro, 2004).

Calcium initially enters the cell mainly through L-type Ca^{2+} channels and initiates Ca^{2+}-induced Ca^{2+} release from the sarcoplasmic reticulum. As cytosolic Ca^{2+} levels rise, the sarcomeres develop tension that increases ventricular isovolumic pressure until the aortic and pulmonary valves open. Blood is expelled from the ventricles by sarcomeres shortening to their end-systolic lengths. At the subcellular level, myofilament activation begins with Ca^{2+} binding to cTnC site II, exposing a hydrophobic region at the N lobe of cTnC and creating a new binding site for cTnI. Cardiac TnI then dissociates from actin and binds tightly to the hydrophobic region of cTnC, causing a cascade of protein-protein interactions that allows Tm to move closer into the thin filament groove. This stage is referred to as the "closed" or "C" state. This movement exposes myosin binding sites on actin and also appears to alter thin filament structure, allowing more cross-bridges to occur and moving Tm further into the thin filament groove (thus shifting into the "open" or "M" state). Positive feedback may arise from bound cross-bridges causing an increased affinity for Ca^{2+} by cTnC (Pan & Solaro, 1987 as cited in Solaro & Kobayashi, 2011). At basal states of contractility, only 25% of available cTnC regulatory (site II) Ca^{2+} binding sites are occupied due to low cytosolic Ca^{2+} levels, resulting in a substantial cardiac reserve for recruitment of blocked cross-bridges when required.

After the valves close, the sarcomeres are quiescent as the ventricles prepare for refilling. This relaxation phase is highly dependent upon the rate of cytosolic Ca^{2+} removal, the off-loading of Ca^{2+} from cTnC, and the cross-bridges returning to the weakly bound or blocked state. Phosphorylation of the thin filament proteins, in particular the N-terminus of cTnI, plays a crucial role in drawing upon cardiac reserve, cross-bridge cycling rate and hence, relaxation, in a signaling cascade initiated by β-adrenergic stimulation (see review by Tardiff, 2011). These mechanisms are critically important when increased heart rate is required during exercise. Considering that SCD in young FHC patients frequently occurs during exercise (Cha et al., 2007), thin filament mutations may have an inhibitory effect on phosphorylation signalling and cardiac reserve as well as other cross-bridge cycling effects.

4. Mechanisms of Sudden Cardiac Death in FHC troponin mutations

Various mechanisms for SCD due to FHC have been suggested including arrhythmias arising from sinus nodal and atrioventricular nodal conduction abnormalities, and tachycardia due to re-entrant depolarization pathways from myocardial disarray and fibrosis, abnormal Ca^{2+} homeostasis, ventricular diastolic dysfunction or left ventricular outflow tract obstruction (Fatkin & Graham, 2002). With several underlying mechanisms leading to SCD, research is only beginning to define the link between the underlying molecular pathology and arrhythmogenesis in FHC-associated troponin mutations.

One emerging issue is that studying patients with well established disease for the purpose of linking phenotype to genotype has proven extremely difficult. Like all monogenic disorders, there are myriad disease modifiers including genetic, environmental and lifestyle factors that influence disease progression and severity in a manner that is poorly understood. What is also becoming apparent is that ventricular hypertrophy, fibrosis and obstructive disease are likely compensatory FHC features and based on complex signalling cascades arising from pathologies within the sarcomere, as discussed later in this chapter. Perhaps longitudinal studies of patients prior to the onset of structural disease may uncover mutation-specific disease progression that parallels the molecular and biophysical effects observed in *in vitro* experiments, animal models and *in silico* predictions (Tardiff, 2011). There is likely a less complex phenotype in FHC patients in the early disease stages allowing a more discernable link between genotype and phenotype. A study of preclinical FHC patients provides evidence for this hypothesis (Ho et al., 2002). In their study, most FHC cohorts presented with one common phenotype, namely prolonged diastolic relaxation on echocardiography, despite patients having different mutations within different genes. This approach may also benefit treatment outcomes for preclinical FHC cohorts with targeted mutation-specific treatment to attenuate disease progression. It makes sense to treat pre-symptomatic FHC patients long before gross phenotype becomes established. Diltiazem, a calcium channel blocker, normalized Ca^{2+} regulation and attenuated ventricular hypertrophy in a mouse model (Semsarian et al., 2002) and formed the basis of an ongoing clinical trial, in which preclinical FHC patients receive diltiazem therapy while being monitored for disease progression (http://clinicaltrials.gov/ct2/show/NCT00319982).

Recent approaches to identifying the pathophysiology of FHC mutations includes investigation of the dynamic properties of cross-bridge cycling at the molecular level and how Tn mutations disrupt precise molecular movements. Such high resolution investigations commonly incorporate computational approaches to examine protein flexibility and to predict changes in protein mobility caused by mutations, using molecular dynamics simulation programs such as GROMACS (Van Der Spoel et al., 2005) and CHARMM (Brooks et al., 2009). Another approach is Nuclear Magnetic Resonance (NMR) imaging, allowing investigators to compare recombinant wild-type and mutated Tn complexes in different metal-binding states to measure conformational changes (Lassalle, 2010).

4.1 Troponin T mutations

Since the identification of *cTNNT2* in 1993 as the first Tn-based gene associated with FHC (Thierfelder et al., 1993), cTnT mutations have been extensively studied and account for up to 15% of all FHC mutations (Watkins et al., 1995). To date, there are at least 68 cTnT mutations identified associated with FHC (Willott et al., 2010), with a subset that present with a high frequency of SCD and/or ventricular arrhythmia in humans (Table 1). Alternative splicing of exons 4 and 5 of the *cTNNT2* gene in the human heart results in four temporally regulated isoforms: one adult isoform (TnT3) and 3 fetal isoforms (TnT1,TnT2 and TnT4). The variable cTnT N-domain contributes to the Ca^{2+} sensitivity of force development and the presence of fetal isoforms in adult myofilaments has been associated with increased myofilament Ca^{2+} sensitivity and diastolic dysfunction (Gomes et al., 2002 as cited in Gomes et al., 2004). Tn complexes with fetal isoforms TnT1 and TnT2 (containing exon 5) have a reduced inhibition of actomyosin ATPase activity compared with the adult TnT3 isoform which suggests that the TnT isoforms have varying ability to modulate cross-bridge cycling and hence, cardiac contraction (Gomes et al., 2002). These findings are noteworthy in that increased myofilament Ca^{2+} sensitivity and diastolic dysfunction occur with many FHC causing Tn mutations; however, studies investigating the expression of cTnT isoforms in diseased hearts and a possible contributory role in altered contractile performance remain unresolved with no as-yet obvious correlation between fetal isoform TnT4 expression and Ca^{2+} sensitivity in diseased hearts (see review by Parmacek & Solaro, 2004).

The majority of cTnT mutations occur within the two structurally poorly resolved regions with a clustering of mutations within residues 69 to 110. There are three "hot spots" occurring at residues 92, 94 and 110, of which R92L and F110I have been associated with high rates of SCD and/or ventricular arrhythmia (Table 1). Another mutational "hotspot" occurs at residues 160 to 163, which is found within a highly charged and a highly conserved sequence from 157 to 166. This region is believed to be a flexible linker between H1 and H2 and whose structure has so far eluded resolution. Closer to the C terminus is a scattering of mutations associated with dilated cardiomyopathy (DCM) as well as several FHC mutations. It is believed that residues in this particular region affect Ca^{2+} sensitivity via allosteric interactions with the cTnC C domain, although actual evidence is lacking (Tardiff, 2011).

Troponin subunit	Mutation(s)	SCD or Ventricular Arrhythmia	References
cTnT	I79N, F87L, R92L, R92W, R94L, A104V, ΔE160*, S179F, Intron 16G1→AŦ	SCD	(Gimeno et al., 2009; Knollmann & Potter, 2001; Moolman et al., 1997; Thierfelder et al., 1993; Thierfelder et al., 1994)
	F110I	Ventricular arrhythmia	(Watkins et al., 1995)
cTnI	R145G, A157V, R162Q, ΔK183*, R186Q, S199N	SCD	(Ashrafian et al., 2003; Niimura et al., 2002; Van Driest et al., 2003)
	R141Q, G203R	Ventricular arrhythmia	(Alcalai et al., 2008; Ashrafian et al., 2003)
cTnC	Q122AfsX30¥	SCD	(Chung et al., 2011)

Table 1. Troponin mutations associated with SCD and ventricular arrhythmia. *Δ denotes deletion of the noted residue causing an in-frame mutation; Ŧ denotes a splice donor site mutation that removes 28 residues at the C terminus and replaces them with 7 nonsense codons resulting in a truncated cTnT mutant; ¥ denotes a nucleotide duplication (G) at position 363, causing a frame-shift substitution on residue 122 (Q122A) and a premature stop codon (X) at residue 30 resulting in a truncated cTnC mutant.

4.1.1 *In vitro* and *in vivo* approaches, animal models and *in silico* predictions

Cardiac TnT mutations are predicted to affect the regulatory role of the Tn-Tm complex on sarcomere activation given that TnT functions to attach the Tn complex to Tm and actin (Tobacman, 1996). *In vitro* studies with different FHC mutations (including cTnT mutants) show faster contraction kinetics and increased Ca^{2+} sensitivity of force generation. Some studies show increased sarcomeric activation at lower Ca^{2+} levels, resulting in myofilament activation and contraction at shorter sarcomere lengths against an increased passive force (Haim et al., 2007; Tardiff et al., 1999). The shorter baseline sarcomere length may be an important factor in why cTnT R92Q transgenic mutant mice have smaller myocytes and negligent or minimal ventricular hypertrophy (Tardiff et al., 1999).

Abnormal Ca^{2+} homeostasis may result from a variety of factors including altered Ca^{2+} availability and altered myofibrillar Ca^{2+} sensitivity. *In vitro* studies of skinned myocardial fibres reconstituted with mutant cTnT mutations (I79N, R92Q, F110I, ΔE160) show increased myofilament Ca^{2+} sensitivity, which researchers postulate is an important mechanism for the high incidence of SCD even with mild or absent hypertrophy and fibrosis (Gomes & Potter, 2004a; Gomes & Potter, 2004b; Knollmann & Potter, 2001). *In silico* studies based on results from *in vivo* transgenic I79N cTnT mouse fibres predict a higher basal contractility, increased rate of force development, delayed relaxation and increased resting tension compared with wild-type fibres (Miller et al., 2001).

In intact transgenic mouse hearts and in isolated voltage-clamped cardiomyocytes, Knollmann et al. produced compelling evidence that ventricular arrhythmias may arise from action potential remodelling related to altered Ca^{2+} regulation in mice carrying the human cTnT I79N mutation (Knollmann et al., 2003). A more recent study elegantly demonstrated that the degree of myofilament sensitivity may be correlated positively with the risk of developing ventricular tachycardia (Baudenbacher et al., 2008). Given that the transgenic mice had no evidence of hypertrophy, fibrosis or myocyte disarray, this study provided further evidence that altered myofilament function is the underlying pathophysiological mechanism of FHC and may be the causal link of FHC to SCD. Many of the most "deleterious" cTnT mutations are located within the H1 domain of the N-terminus. Previous studies have demonstrated that the N-terminus plays an important role in the inhibition of myofilament activation (reviewed in Tardiff, 2011). It stands to reason that disruption of this inhibitory N-terminal function by mutations in this region may allow Tm movement (and hence, cross-bridge cycling) under conditions of low Ca^{2+}, exhibiting an apparent increased Ca^{2+} sensitivity of myofilament activation (Tardiff, 2011).

4.1.2 Human cardiac TnT mutation studies

FHC patients harbouring the I79N cTnT mutation commonly present with minimal or absent hypertrophy on echocardiography and are frequently asymptomatic (i.e. no syncope, dyspnea or chest pain at rest or with exertion), yet have the highest incidence of SCD among young cTnT mutation carriers (Watkins et al., 1995) and is one of the most investigated of all FHC mutations (see review by Gomes et al., 2004). The F87L mutation also presents with mild hypertrophy (less than 16 mm ventricular wall thickness) but with a high incidence of SCD, including sub-adult patients, in a study of one multigenerational family (Gimeno et al., 2009). Of great significance, the youngest mutation carriers were completely asymptomatic. The R94L was also studied within a single family and found to have marked myocyte disarray and frequent SCD in the absence of ventricular hypertrophy (Varnava et al., 1999 as cited in Gomes et al., 2004). FHC patients with the A104V cTnT mutation also have a high incidence of SCD with only moderate left ventricular hypertrophy (Szczesna et al., 2000 as cited in Gomes & Potter, 2004; Gomes et al., 2004). A longitudinal study involving R92W cTnT FHC patients revealed that clinically identifiable hypertrophy did not occur in this cohort until after 35 years of age and yet the highest occurrence of SCD was prior to cardiac remodelling, particularly in young males (Revera et al., 2007, as cited in Revera et al., 2008). Another study by the same group (Revera et al., 2008) reported that phenotype-negative R92W patients had higher basal contractility and delayed relaxation compared to their genotype-negative relatives. Given the mild phenotype of many cTnT mutation patients, there is likely a reporting and referral bias in these patients and are therefore likely under-recognized in FHC clinics where the majority of patients have substantial hypertrophy and outflow obstruction that are relatively easy to diagnose non-invasively by echocardiography (Tardiff, 2011).

A study comparing FHC cTnT mutation patients with other FHC patients who died suddenly revealed that the cTnT mutation patients were younger, had less hypertrophy and fibrosis, but more myocardial disarray than other patients (Varnava, Elliott, Baboonian et al., 2001). Such findings suggest that the pathological mechanism is essentially myocellular as opposed to being related to the sequelae of ventricular hypertrophy and that ventricular wall thickness may not be an appropriate risk factor for SCD in cTnT patients.

4.2 Troponin I mutations

The first report of FHC-causing mutations in the *TNNI3* gene was in 1997 (Kimura et al., 1997), in which 5 missense mutations were discovered that co-segregated with FHC. Since then, approximately 35 mutations have been reported linked to FHC, of which several missense and deletion mutations are associated with SCD and/or ventricular arrhythmia (Table 1). There are 3 genes encoding 3 TnI protein isoforms, of which two are expressed in the human heart on a temporal basis. The slow skeletal TnI (ssTnI from the *TNNI1* gene) is the predominant isoform expressed within the fetal heart. This isoform declines rapidly after birth and is generally replaced by the cardiac isoform (cTnI from the *TNNI3* gene) by approximately 9 months of age in humans (Bhavsar et al., 1991, Hunkeler, Kullman and Murphy, 1991 and Sasse et al., 1993 in Parmacek & Solaro, 2004). The 31 residue N-terminus in cTnI is entirely absent in ssTnI and contains two serine residues at positions 23 and 24, that are substrates for phosphorylation by protein kinase A (PKA). Given that PKA phosphorylation of these serine residues reduces myofilament Ca^{2+} sensitivity and accelerates cross-bridge cycling during high heart rates (see below), it is not surprising that fetal myofilaments have an increased Ca^{2+} sensitivity and reduced length dependence of Ca^{2+} activation (Arteaga et al., 2000, Fentzke et al., 1999 and Wolksa et al., 2001 as cited in Parmacek & Solaro, 2004). However, increased ssTnI expression is not observed in hearts with severe FHC phenotype (Sasse et al., 1993 as cited in Parmacek & Solaro, 2004), suggesting that other factors, such as myocellular modifications due to FHC mutations, are at play.

The clustering of FHC mutations within the highly flexible inhibitory domain and the mobile region of cTnI with its actin-Tm binding site are of extreme interest to researchers. Perhaps this clustering represents a "tolerance" to alterations of the highly mobile regions of the thin filament, providing evidence that Tn mutations frequently modulate, but do not obliterate, thin filament movements. Some researchers have proposed that under sub-maximal cardiac loads, many of the discussed mutations are relatively benign. However, increased cardiac loads can create the arrhythmogenic substrate leading to SCD in a subset of FHC patients, which is in keeping with the observed high frequency of SCD occurring during or following physical activity (Maron, 2003).

PKA phosphorylation of cTnI affects the cross-bridge cycling rate in response to β-adrenergic activation and represents a post-translational mechanism through which mutations can cause adverse effects to cardiac output and response to increased cardiac demands. Phosphorylation of cTnI at S23 and S24 causes a decrease in Ca^{2+} sensitivity of force generation, increase in off-rates of Ca^{2+} from TnC site II, increase in cross-bridge cycling rate and increase in relaxation rate (Metzger & Westfall, 2004 in Tardiff, 2011). Functional studies with the FHC cTnI R145G mutation provide evidence of an interaction between the N-terminus and the inhibitory domain of cTnI, as the expected desensitization after PKA-mediated phosphorylation was not observed with this mutant. Perhaps the loss of a basic residue (arginine to glycine) depresses inhibition in the inhibitory domain and alters electrostatic interactions with the N-terminal of cTnI (Deng, Y. et al., 2001 as cited in Tardiff, 2011).

4.2.1 *In vitro* and *in vivo* approaches

Similar to other FHC mutations, cTnI mutations demonstrate increased myofilament Ca^{2+} sensitivity which is believed to contribute to pathological hypertrophy and SCD (Parmacek

& Solaro, 2004). Elliot et al. (2000) reported that R145G and R162G mutations demonstrated significantly increased Ca^{2+} sensitivity of ATPase regulation (i.e. force generation) and reduced inhibition of actomyosin ATPase activity *in vitro*. Skinned reconstituted rabbit fibres incorporating R145G, R162G and ΔK183 mutants provide further evidence with increased Ca^{2+} sensitivity consistent with myofilament activation at lower Ca^{2+} levels and predicting an impairment in cardiac relaxation (Takahashi-Yanaga et al., 2001). An *in vivo* study with a cTnI R145G transgenic mouse model also confirmed these results (James et al., 2000). Other animal models recapitulate human FHC findings of myocellular dysfunction preceding structural phenotype; young transgenic cTnI G203S mice display abnormal Ca^{2+} cycling with prolonged decay rates of Ca^{2+} transients long before phenotypic expression of hypertrophy, fibrosis and myocyte disarray (Tsoutsman et al., 2006). Transgenic rabbits expressing low protein levels of R145G cTnI displayed apical myocyte disarray, interstitial fibrosis, but with only mild ventricular hypertrophy at later ages (1.5 to 2 years of age) (Sanbe et al., 2005). Rabbit models more closely resemble human cardiac physiology in that myocellular Ca^{2+} handling and alterations in Ca^{2+} flux during heart failure is much more similar to humans than mouse models (Bers, 2002, as cited in Sanbe et al., 2005). Another limitation for mouse models is their heart rate is roughly 10 times faster than humans, which in turn influences the refractory period associated with arrhythmia incidence (Boyett and Jewell, 1978 as cited in Sanbe et al., 2005).

4.2.2 Human cardiac TnI mutation studies

As with cTnT mutations, studies into patients with cTnI mutations are confounded by small family sizes and referral biases. Nonetheless, characterization of the ΔK183 mutation in several families lead to striking discoveries of high penetrance, age-independent SCD and highly variable ventricular remodeling with some patients, particularly in patients over 40 years, progressing to left ventricular dilatation (referred to as "burned out" hypertrophic cardiomyopathy) within single, multigenerational families (Kokado et al., 2000). A landmark study (Mogensen et al., 2004) reported the phenotype with 748 families ranging from severe restrictive cardiomyopathy, biventricular hypertrophy, or apical hypertrophy in some relatives to no disease features in others, complicating treatment options and risk stratification within families and suggesting that other genetic and/or environmental factors play a role in disease manifestation (Parmacek & Solaro, 2004). Unlike cTnT mutations, however, there have been no reported cases of SCD with mild disease presentation (Mogensen et al., 2004). Interestingly, most of the 13 cTnI mutations within this large cohort are found with the relatively narrow range of exons 7 and 8 encompassing the inhibitory and mobile domains of the C terminal domain.

4.3 Troponin C mutations

Cardiac TnC has only recently joined the list of FHC-causing genes and so far, 6 mutations have been identified (Chung et al., 2011; Chung et al., 2011; Hoffmann et al., 2001; Landstrom et al., 2008; Willott et al., 2010). Cardiac TnC is a highly conserved protein found in all striated muscle among vertebrate species. In mammals, there are two paralogs of TnC: the fast skeletal TnC (sTnC) and the cardiac/slow skeletal TnC (cTnC), consisting of N- and C-terminal domains connected by a long central α-helix. Each domain contains a pair of EF-hand (helix-loop-helix) motifs that bind Ca^{2+} (Kretsinger & Nockolds, 1973, as cited in Li, 2009) and are numbered I to IV (Potter & Gergely, 1975; Zot & Potter, 1982 as cited in Li,

2009). Site III and site IV in the C-terminal domain have high Ca^{2+} binding affinity and are generally occupied by Mg^{2+} and Ca^{2+} ions under physiological conditions. Thus, the C-terminal domain almost always adopts a more open conformation, making it a "structural" domain that maintains the integrity of the Tn complex (Potter & Gergely, 1975; Zot & Potter, 1982 as cited in Li, 2009). The N-terminal domain exhibits a lower Ca^{2+} binding affinity of 10^6 M^{-1} (more than one order of magnitude lower affinity than sites III and IV) and is therefore sensitive to changes in cytosolic Ca^{2+} concentration, making it the "regulatory domain" (Potter & Gergely, 1975; Zot & Potter, 1982 as cited in Li, 2009). It was proposed that the N-terminal domain changes from a "closed" state to an "open" state upon Ca^{2+} binding. A reorientation of helices exposes the hydrophobic residues of the central helix, where the inhibitory domain of TnI binds and triggers the overall conformational change of the Tn complex. As cTnC does not have a functional Ca^{2+} binding site I, it tends to have a more closed conformation compared to sTnC even when site II is coordinating Ca^{2+} (Herzberg, Moult & James, 1986 in Li, 2009).

4.3.1 *In vitro* analyses and human cardiac TnC mutation studies

What makes cTnC mutations unique is that they are dispersed relatively evenly throughout the gene. As with other Tn mutations, investigations into cTnC mutations are confounded by small family sizes and in some cases, are limited to a single patient. Commercial and research laboratories have only recently added cTnC to their molecular genetic testing platforms (and some continue to omit cTnC from their screenings), leading one to propose perhaps some purportedly genotype-negative FHC patients could potentially harbour cTnC mutations.

The first observed FHC related cTnC mutation, L29Q, was discovered in a 59 year old man who presented with dyspnea upon exertion (Hoffmann et al., 2001). An ECG revealed an abnormal QRS complex suggestive of ventricular hypertrophy and confirmed by echocardiography. There has yet to be any follow-up study with this patient who would now be approximately 70 years of age, which limits knowledge of disease progression with this mutation.

Leucine 29 of cTnC is located in the dysfunctional Ca^{2+} binding site I of the N-domain. Although it is not Ca^{2+} binding, it is important in maintaining the structural integrity of the first helix of cTnC (Sia et al., as cited in Li, 2009). It is located at the cTnI binding site (Schmidtmann et al., 2005). Replacement of a non-polar leucine with a polar glutamine is predicted to have an impact on overall function of the Tn complex with Tm. However, several studies show that in the absence of phosphorylated cTnI, the L29Q mutation can decrease, increase, or have no affect on Ca^{2+} sensitivity (Baryshnikova et al., 2008; Liang et al., 2008; Schmidtmann et al., 2005) leading to scepticism of its status as a pathogenic FHC mutation. For example, *in vitro* assays conducted on L29Q show that the Ca^{2+} sensitivity of ATPase in reconstituted thin filaments is not affected by PKA-dependent phosphorylation of cTnI (Schmidtmann et al., 2005). This finding implies that L29Q may decrease the Ca^{2+} sensitivity and disrupt the signal from the phosphorylated cTnI to cTnC. However, this finding contradicts other reports of FHC mutations generally having higher myofilament Ca^{2+} sensitivities (Chang et al., 2005; Gomes & Potter, 2004; Karibe et al., 2001). Recent NMR and ultraviolet/visual spectrum titration studies showed that L29Q essentially has the same Ca^{2+} affinity as that of wild-type cTnC (Baryshnikova et al., 2008) although this technique presents challenges for measuring Ca^{2+} affinity (see below).

Conversely, our research group demonstrated that L29Q significantly increases the Ca^{2+} sensitivity of force generation using single skinned cardiac myocytes, but in a manner that was extremely sarcomere length dependent (Liang et al., 2008). Cardiac TnC F27W was used as a fluorescence reporter to monitor the *in vitro* Ca^{2+} binding and exchange with binding site II of cTnC. Our results showed that L29Q has a significantly increased Ca^{2+} binding affinity compared to the wild-type, and its response to sarcomere length change was significantly reduced. The increased Ca^{2+} sensitivity suggests that L29Q mutants bind Ca^{2+} more tightly and cause Ca^{2+} to dissociate more slowly from cTnC site II. Reduced length dependence of myofilament Ca^{2+} sensitivity likely influences the heart's ability to regulate ventricular output in response to changes in ventricular filling (Liang et al., 2008). Overall, the heart is maintained in systole longer, resulting in diastolic dysfunction (Wen et al., 2008 in Pinto et al., 2009). Changes in Ca^{2+} affinity is hypothesized to disrupt myocellular homeostasis, triggering Ca^{2+}-regulated pathways leading to SCD (Baudenbacher et al., 2008) and/or hypertrophy (Heineke & Molkentin, 2006) as discussed later in this chapter.

Choice of experimental techniques may account for the conflicting results. Compared to studies using single cardiac myocytes, ATPase and *in* vitro motility assays are excellent techniques for defining molecular interactions, but lack the geometric and mechanical constraints from other proteins within the sarcomere (Liang et al., 2008). Additionally, NMR techniques are limited in terms of accurate Ca^{2+} measurement as Ca^{2+} chelators, such as EGTA, cannot be utilized in NMR studies (Liang et al., 2008). The reduced length dependence of Ca^{2+} sensitivity is likely why other researchers, who had no or only marginal sarcomeric length control in their experimental techniques, have observed such variable results. Our experimental technique using single cardiac myocytes held at a constant sarcomere length may be more precise and closer to physiological conditions. Further to this, our work on cTnC and the L29Q mutation precedes the discovery of a human L29Q cTnC FHC patient. Salmonid cTnC has a greater than two-fold Ca^{2+} affinity over mammalian cTnC (Gillis et al., 2003) with four sequence differences between the mammalian and salmonid homologues responsible for the high Ca^{2+} affinity: D2N, V28I, L29Q, and G30D (NIQD). When the mammalian residues were mutated to the salmonid-equivalent, including L29 to Q29, the Ca^{2+}-binding affinities of the mammalian cTnC mutants increased to the level of the salmonid cTnC (Gillis et al., 2005).

Seven years after the initial FHC cTnC report, a large study cohort of 1025 unrelated patients was screened for FHC mutations and four novel cTnC mutations were reported: A8V, C84Y, E134D and D145E (Landstrom et al., 2008). All four patients were symptomatic for FHC, with findings of syncope upon exertion (C84Y) and dyspnea and chest pain in the other three patients. They were all positive for varying degrees of ventricular hypertrophy. All were young or relatively young (17, 22, 37 and 58 years old) when diagnosed, but SCD was not reported in any patients or relatives. Functional analysis of the four variants using skinned porcine papillary fibres revealed increased Ca^{2+} sensitivity of force development for A8V, C84Y and D145E mutations, and A8V and D145E also showed increases in maximal force consistent with other *in vitro* studies of FHC-associated mutants (Landstrom et al., 2008). Actomyosin ATPase activity in reconstituted thin filaments and spectroscopic properties of the four mutants confirmed increased myofilament Ca^{2+} sensitivity, except for E134D which was not significantly different from wild-type (Pinto et al., 2009). Isolated cTnC, Tn complex and thin filament assays, however, did not recapitulate the Ca^{2+} sensitivity findings observed in the reconstituted fibre assays, suggesting that the entire reconstituted myofilament (that included the S1 myosin head) is required to recreate the increased Ca^{2+} sensitivity changes observed in skinned fibre assays.

This research group also proposed that the D145E mutation influences regulation of contraction by disrupting Ca^{2+} binding to site IV of cTnC and demonstrated that this mutation reduced the cTnC α helicity in the metal-bound state as determined by circular dichroism (Pinto et al., 2009). Another report investigated the effects of IAANS-labeled cTnC mutants on Ca^{2+} off-rate kinetics and concluded that both A8V and D145E mutations had significantly slower off-rate kinetics over the wild-type, suggesting that both mutations alter muscle relaxation properties by reducing ventricular filling time which correlates with the diastolic dysfunction seen in FHC patients (Pinto et al., 2011).

Only one cTnC mutation so far has been directly linked to the SCD of a previously undiagnosed and asymptomatic 19 year old man who had a witnessed collapse while working at his computer (Chung et al., 2011). Autopsy revealed ventricular hypertrophy. Genetic testing of his family revealed a novel cTnC duplication at nucleotide 363, leading to a frameshift mutation at Q122A and causing a premature stop codon at position 30 in the new reading frame (Q122AfsX30) in 4 out of 7 relatives. The primary concern was for his 16 year old genotype-positive, phenotype-negative sister, who can be monitored for disease manifestation (Chung et al., 2011). To date, no functional analysis has been done on this mutation finding. The premature stop codon created by this frameshift mutation is close to the C terminus, leading to speculation that the mutant protein is successfully translated, incorporated into the thin filament and creates adverse effects on Ca^{2+} sensitivity of force production similar to other cTnC mutations. One could also propose that the protein undergoes nonsense-mediated decay, leading to haploinsufficiency of cTnC within the cardiac myocytes. Future investigations will hopefully provide further insight to the pathogenic mechanisms of this newest cTnC mutation finding.

5. Arrhythmogenic mechanisms in FHC

Many studies comparing FHC phenotype with suspected underlying mechanisms are plagued by the lack of genotyping of cardiomyopathy patients, perhaps related to the high cost and time-consuming work of genetic testing. To address this issue, Colombo et al. (Colombo et al., 2008) argue that some genotype-phenotype correlations can provide important information to target DNA analyses in specific FHC candidate genes. Genetic testing may also clarify diagnosis and assist with optimal treatment strategies for more malignant phenotypes. In addition, genetic screening of first-degree relatives can assist in early identification and diagnosis of individuals at greatest risk for developing cardiomyopathy, allowing physicians to focus clinical resources on high-risk family members. Determining the underlying mechanism of SCD resulting from FHC remains elusive, though recent studies have begun to focus on the three cardinal manifestations of FHC separately (i.e. cardiac hypertrophy, myocyte disarray and fibrosis), as researchers are postulating that they may arise from distinct and independent mechanisms (Varnava, Elliott, Baboonian et al., 2001; Varnava, Elliott, Mahon et al., 2001; Wolf et al., 2005). Myocyte hypertrophy is postulated by some to increase arrhythmia vulnerability through intrinsic automaticity changes, as some studies demonstrate that hypertrophied myocytes exhibit pacemaker current up-regulation (re-expression) and action potential prolongation by down-regulation of the potassium transient outward I_{to} current (Sanguinetti, 2002 as cited in Wolf et al., 2005).

Triggered arrhythmias can occur as delayed after-depolarizations (DADs), early after-depolarizations (EADs) or increased automaticity in non-ischemic FHC and are likely related to myocellular Ca^{2+} signalling and transport (Bers, 2008). DADs are commonly believed to be caused by spontaneous Ca^{2+} release from the SR that occurs as a consequence of high SR Ca^{2+} levels. This SR Ca^{2+} release causes a transient inward current (I_{ti}) that can cause a threshold depolarization leading to an action potential. Several studies suggest that the Na^+/ Ca^{2+} exchanger current (I_{NCX}) is responsible for I_{ti} in human ventricular myocytes (Pogwizd et al., 2001). Further to this, Ter Keurs' research group has been investigating myofilament arrhythmogenic Ca^{2+} release to determine if non-uniform excitation-contraction coupling plays a role in the initiation of extra-systoles that create arrhythmias ((Ter Keurs et al., 2006). Ter Keurs developed a model of non-uniform excitation-contraction using rat trabeculae and exposed a small muscle segment to BDM, a cross-bridge inhibitor (Backx et al., 1995 as cited in Ter Keurs et al., 2006), to recapitulate non-contracting myocardium as found in diseased hearts. Triggered propagating contractions were observed in the border zone of myocardium between non-contractile and contractile tissue when the trabeculae were stimulated to contract. The triggered contractions may be due to a quick release-induced Ca^{2+} dissociation from cTnC site II, leading to a local Ca^{2+} surge that is above the threshold for inducing Ca^{2+}-induced Ca^{2+} release. This mechanism, referred to as "reverse excitation contraction coupling" (RECC), occurs when Ca^{2+} reuptake mechanisms have sufficiently recovered from the previous contraction during diastole (Boyden & ter Keurs, 2001). In FHC, the myocardium may have focal regions of non-uniformity due to structural anomalies, such as fibrosis or myocardial disarray, or perhaps due to electrical remodelling or gene dosage effects from Tn mutations. Increased Ca^{2+} binding to cTnC leading to a high Ca^{2+} buffering capacity may cause a large Ca^{2+} surge during rapid myofilament shortening during RECC. Hence, RECC may be an underlying pathological mechanism of arrhythmogenesis seen in FHC patients and warrants further investigation.

Electrical alternans, in which there is alternating long and short action potential duration (APD), increases the risk of ventricular tachycardia that can degrade to ventricular fibrillation and SCD. The underlying mechanism may to be related to Ca^{2+} transient amplitude alternans. At high pacing frequencies, slow ryanodine receptor and/or Ca^{2+} current recovery may result in alternating SR Ca^{2+} release, due to alternating availability of ryanodine receptors (RyR). Prolonged Ca^{2+} transient decay rates, as seen in some transgenic FHC animal models may play a role here (see below). Spatially discordant alternans is thought to be a prerequisite to dangerous arrhythmias, as there is a non-synchronous electrical substrate within the heart (Bers, 2008). Animal models support this hypothesis; increased myofilament Ca^{2+} sensitivity was associated with an arrhythmogenic substrate in transgenic cTnT mice, despite the absence of structural heart disease (Baudenbacher et al., 2008). Addition of a myofilament Ca^{2+} sensitizing agent, EMD, resulted in repolarization alternans at high pacing rates, beat to beat variation in APD, shorter effective refractory periods and increased spatial conduction velocity dispersion in wild-type cat and mouse hearts, paralleling the findings as observed in mutant cTnT I79N transgenic mice. Several mechanisms were proposed for the induction of ventricular tachyarrhythmias: increased Ca^{2+} binding to cTnC resulting in reduced Ca^{2+} transients with slower decay rates responsible for the shorter APD seen in transgenic I79N cTnT mice, and dysfunctional myocardial relaxation as seen in transgenic mice and in human patients also causing APD shortening. However, transgenic mice have differing ion channel and Ca^{2+}-handling protein expression from human hearts (Wetzel & Klitzner, 1996). The high heart rates of mice, roughly 10 times faster than humans, can influence the refractory period associated with the incidence of arrhythmias, as mentioned previously. Additionally, studies of human HCM patients suggested that T-wave alternans (surface ECG recording associated with action potential alternans) may not be a useful SCD prediction tool (Fuchs & Torjman, 2009).

5.1 Clinical findings in FHC patients

It has proven difficult to elucidate the exact mechanisms linking FHC pathology and arrhythmogenicity in humans with limited access to fresh cardiac tissue from FHC patients. Studies currently utilize tissue from myectomy samples and explanted hearts in which there is profound disease phenotype. Thus, explorations of disease progression in pre-clinical patients are normally limited to non-invasive imaging techniques and electrophysiology. In addition, there is inherent patient referral bias for research studies as most FHC patients seen in surgical referral centres already have profound disease manifestation (Tardiff, 2011).

Stored electrograms from implantable cardiac defibrillators indicate that SCD largely results from sustained ventricular tachycardia and/or ventricular fibrillation (B.J. Maron, 2010). One suggested trigger for SCD is sympathetic excitation, given that the initiating rhythm in many cases is sinus tachycardia, which may underlie the high SCD rate in athletes and sub-adult FHC populations (Cha et al., 2007). Several studies of HCM patients wearing Holter monitors identified a higher rate of SCD for younger patients (age 30 and under) with non-sustained ventricular tachycardia (NSVT) detected at least once during the 48 hour monitoring period. While NSVT is usually asymptomatic and frequently occurs during periods of increased parasympathetic (vagal) tone, it is associated with an increased SCD risk, especially in children and young adults (Elliott et al., 2000; Monserrat et al., 2003). However, most SCDs occur in patients without ambulatory ECG episodes of NSVT; clearly other contributory factors leading to risk of SCD are at play. A more recent study identified an increased SCD risk with ventricular arrhythmias triggered by exercise (Gimeno, Tome-Esteban et al., 2009), which is more in keeping findings of triggered arrhythmias during sinus tachycardia, implicating sympathetic excitation during physical activity (Cha et al., 2007). This is also in keeping with the *in vitro* experimental evidence of a blunted response to β-adrenergic stimulation through phosphorylation of cTnI (i.e. reduced inhibitory response of phosphorylated cTnI on Ca^{2+} sensitivity for cTnC) and the resultant diastolic dysfunction as discussed previously.

Cardiac magnetic resonance (CMR) imaging has allowed clinicians to precisely determine myocyte fibrosis and scarring in non-ischemic FHC, including phenotype-negative FHC patients who have experienced life-threatening arrhythmias (Makhoul et al., 2011; Strijack et al., 2008). Detection of fibrosis by late gadolinium enhancement in CMR is associated with increased propensity for VT on ambulatory ECG monitoring (Adabag et al., 2008) and is being considered as a clinical SCD risk marker (Maron, 2010). Fibrosis and scarring may promote localized zones of slowed conduction resulting in re-entrant arrhythmias (Cha et al., 2007). NMR imaging can detect focal or diffuse regions of fibrosis and hypertrophy morphologies that are missed by traditional echocardiography (M. S. Maron, 2009) and will likely continue to improve in resolution leading to improved risk stratification for FHC patients.

Myocyte disarray is another common feature in FHC patients and a recent study of myectomy samples from a small pediatric HCM cohort suggests that myocyte disarray has a significantly higher correlation with diastolic dysfunction than either hypertrophy or fibrosis (Menon et al., 2009). Extensive myocyte disarray has been linked to SCD in younger FHC patients (Varnava, Elliott, Mahon et al., 2001), especially those with cTnT mutations (Varnava, Elliott, Baboonian et al., 2001) in the absence of, or with minimal hypertrophy.

6. Future considerations

Of interest to investigators is the potential role of Ca^{2+} dysregulation in ER stress pathways. The SR in myocardial cells has long been thought to be the cardiac equivalent to ER with its main role as the intracellular regulator of Ca^{2+} fluxes and hence, excitation-contraction coupling in the heart. Some researchers propose that the SR contains a functional ER "compartment" with physiological roles such as protein synthesis, translocation and integration into membranes, folding and post-translational modifications including glycosylation and Ca^{2+} homeostasis (Mesaeli et al., 2001), although studies are lacking. ER stress occurs in response to environmental or genetic factors causing ER metabolic disturbances, accumulation of misfolded proteins, oxidative stress and/or depletion of ER Ca^{2+} stores. The "unfolded protein response" (UPR) is one mechanism by which the ER attempts to reestablish homeostasis by reducing protein expression, by increasing production of chaperones to handle accumulation of misfolded protein, promoting ER-associated degradation to remove misfolded proteins (Schroder & Kaufman, 2005). This initial response of protein synthesis, suppression and upregulation of ER resident chaperones is designed to resolve the ER stress and enhance survival, but if the ER stress is severe or prolonged, the UPR may stimulate apoptosis (cell death). Do FHC mutations play a role in ER stress pathways, such as through Ca^{2+} dysregulation? Activation of the "fetal gene program" is a response to elevated Ca^{2+} to increase cardiac efficiency in the stressed heart. This response, unfortunately, also commonly results in detrimental cardiac hypertrophy (Eizirik et al., 2008; Wang et al., 2000). Elevated Ca^{2+} activates calcineurin A that dephosphorylates the transcription factor NFAT which translocates to the nucleus to stimulate cardiac remodelling and hypertrophy associated with the fetal gene program (Heineke & Molkentin, 2006). Other factors, such as MEF2, GATA and CamKII are also activated which initiate transcription programs associated with hypertrophy, remodelling and heart failure with increased risk of cardiac death (Molkentin et al., 1998). GATA-4 may play a significant role in FHC pathogenesis due to its ability to stimulate transcription of the cardiac-specific Tn genes (Liang et al., 2001; Molkentin & Olson, 1997; Molkentin et al., 1998). Therefore, ER stress may turn on the fetal gene program in response to pathological insult. MicroRNAs (miRs) likely play a role in these regulatory processes with miRNA coding sequences often located within the newly transcribed genes (Eizirik et al., 2008; Wang et al., 2000). The hypothesis of elevated Ca^{2+} causing transcriptional activation of hypertrophy and perhaps pathological arrhythmia substrates (see below) is provocative and will likely continue to be an area of active investigation.

Research into miRs that play a role in regulation of cardiac function and the recent findings that miR expression is deranged in cardiac disease may help to uncover the pathways to FHC disease progression and arrhythmogenesis. MiRs are short, non-coding RNA sequences that regulate expression of genes involved in orchestrating growth, development, function and stress responses in a spatio-temporal manner. MiRs target specific mRNA sequences generally to inhibit protein expression, either by degradation of the bound mRNA target or by directly inhibiting translation of the mRNA sequence (Bartel, 2004). To date, there are at least 4 miRs shown to be involved in cardiac development, apoptosis and hypertrophy, namely: miR-1, miR-133, miR-208 and miR-499 (van Rooij et al., 2006). Several important target genes for miRs related to cardiac electrophysiology have been identified, including connexin 43 and inwardly-rectifying potassium channel Kir2.1 (Zhao et al., 2007) and miR-1 expression changes have been associated with arrhythmogenesis due to up-regulation or down-regulation of these gene products (Girmatsion et al., 2009; Yang et al., 2007). Recent studies are beginning to elucidate the link between miRs and SCD due to arrhythmias by identifying the effects of altered expression levels of miRs in the heart on cardiac conduction and excitability (Callis et al., 2009; Matkovich et al., 2010; Zhao et al., 2007). A database has been developed online (http://www.mir2disease.org/) for miRs involved in human disease, including FHC.

Sudden Infant Death Syndrome (SIDS) refers to the sudden death of an infant under 1 year of age which remains unexplained after a thorough medicolegal investigation (Willinger et al., 1991). Researchers are now considering inherited cardiac arrhythmia syndromes in its etiology. Recent research has revealed that up to 20% of SIDS cases may be associated with inheritable arrhythmia syndromes, such as long QT syndrome (Klaver et al., 2011). Given that FHC is the most common cause of SCD in young individuals, it stands to reason that some infants may die from SCD attributed to FHC. Further to this, as discussed earlier, some Tn mutants, particularly the cTnT mutants, have negligible or mild hypertrophy that may not be observed grossly during the post mortem exam. To date, only one study has screened SIDS cases for FHC mutations (Brion et al., 2009). Their findings of 14 cases with 7 genetic variants from 4 different FHC genes, including cTnT and cTnI, from 140 SIDS tissues suggests that some SIDS cases may be associated with FHC-causing mutations. The relatively recent emergence of FHC-associated Tn (in particular, cTnC) gene mutations make these candidate genes previously unrecognized and perhaps under-represented factors to be considered in future SIDS investigations. Besides SIDS cases, how many FHC mutation positive cases have gone unrecognized in post mortem investigations following the sudden, unexpected death of children and young adults?

7. Conclusions

Sudden cardiac death affects approximately 1-2% of children and adolescents, and up to 1% of young adults in FHC-affected populations. *In vitro* analysis of single molecule mechanics and reconstituted skinned myocytes have identified intracellular Ca^{2+} dysregulation, altered myofibrillar Ca^{2+} sensitivity and altered energy metabolism as potential mechanisms at the sarcomere and cellular level. Animal models incorporating specific FHC mutations have broadened our understanding of the pathogenesis of FHC, including structural and electrophysiological remodelling associated with the arrhythmogenic substrate. There are, however, caveats to using in vitro and animal model analyses, given that some may not necessarily recapitulate the physiological substrate in human FHC patients. Most models, however, share a consistent molecular phenotype, namely increased myofilament Ca^{2+} sensitivity and increased energetic cost of force development, that underlies the complex and heterogeneous phenotype that exists at the human patient level. Other genetic, environmental and biological factors such as age, lifestyle and other health issues are also likely disease-modifying factors. Research into molecular approaches and post-translational mechanisms associated with FHC, including effects of phosphorylation and a potential role in ER stress mechanisms, will likely continue to elucidate the link between genotype and phenotype.

8. Acknowledgements

GFT is a Canada Research Chair and the authors acknowledge the generous support of the Heart and Stroke Foundation of BC and Yukon.

9. References

Adabag, A. S., Maron, B. J., Appelbaum, E., Harrigan, C. J., Buros, J. L., Gibson, C. M., Maron, M. S. (2008). Occurrence and frequency of arrhythmias in hypertrophic cardiomyopathy in relation to delayed enhancement on cardiovascular magnetic resonance. *Journal of the American College of Cardiology, 51*(14), 1369-1374. doi:10.1016/j.jacc.2007.11.071

Alcalai, R., Seidman, J. G., & Seidman, C. E. (2008). Genetic basis of hypertrophic cardiomyopathy: From bench to the clinics. *Journal of Cardiovascular Electrophysiology, 19*(1), 104-110. doi:10.1111/j.1540-8167.2007.00965.x

Ashrafian, H., Redwood, C., Blair, E., & Watkins, H. (2003). Hypertrophic cardiomyopathy:A paradigm for myocardial energy depletion. *Trends in Genetics : TIG, 19*(5), 263-268.

Bartel, D. P. (2004). MicroRNAs: Genomics, biogenesis, mechanism, and function. *Cell, 116*(2), 281-297.

Baryshnikova, O. K., Li, M. X., & Sykes, B. D. (2008). Modulation of cardiac troponin C function by the cardiac-specific N-terminus of troponin I: Influence of PKA phosphorylation and involvement in cardiomyopathies. *Journal of Molecular Biology, 375*(3), 735-751. doi:10.1016/j.jmb.2007.10.062

Baudenbacher, F., Schober, T., Pinto, J. R., Sidorov, V. Y., Hilliard, F., Solaro, R. J., Knollmann, B. C. (2008). Myofilament Ca2+ sensitization causes susceptibility to cardiac arrhythmia in mice. *The Journal of Clinical Investigation, 118*(12), 3893-3903. doi:10.1172/JCI36642

Bers, D. M. (2008). Calcium cycling and signaling in cardiac myocytes. *Annual Review of Physiology, 70*, 23-49. doi:10.1146/annurev.physiol.70.113006.100455

Boyden, P. A., & ter Keurs, H. E. (2001). Reverse excitation-contraction coupling: Ca2+ ions as initiators of arrhythmias. *Journal of Cardiovascular Electrophysiology, 12*(3), 382-385.

Brion, M., Allegue, C., Gil, R., Torres, M., Santori, M., Poster, S., .. Carracedo, A. (2009). Involvement of hypertrophic cardiomyopathy genes in sudden infant death syndrome (SIDS). *Forensic Science International: Genetics Supplement Series, 2*(1), 495-496. doi:DOI: 10.1016/j.fsigss.2009.09.040

Brooks, B. R., Brooks, C. L.,3rd, Mackerell, A. D.,Jr, Nilsson, L., Petrella, R. J., Roux, B., Karplus, M. (2009). CHARMM: The biomolecular simulation program. *Journal of Computational Chemistry, 30*(10), 1545-1614. doi:10.1002/jcc.21287

Callis, T. E., Pandya, K., Seok, H. Y., Tang, R. H., Tatsuguchi, M., Huang, Z. P., .. Wang, D. Z. (2009). MicroRNA-208a is a regulator of cardiac hypertrophy and conduction in mice. *The Journal of Clinical Investigation, 119*(9), 2772-2786. doi:10.1172/JCI36154; 10.1172/JCI36154

Cha, Y. M., Gersh, B. J., Maron, B. J., Boriani, G., Spirito, P., Hodge, D. O., .. Shen, W. K. (2007). Electrophysiologic manifestations of ventricular tachyarrhythmias provoking appropriate defibrillator interventions in high-risk patients with hypertrophic cardiomyopathy. *Journal of Cardiovascular Electrophysiology, 18*(5), 483-487. doi:10.1111/j.1540-8167.2007.00780.x

Chang, A. N., Harada, K., Ackerman, M. J., & Potter, J. D. (2005). Functional consequences of hypertrophic and dilated cardiomyopathy-causing mutations in alpha-tropomyosin. *The Journal of Biological Chemistry, 280*(40), 34343-34349. doi:10.1074/jbc.M505014200

Chung, W. K., Kitner, C., & Maron, (2011). Novel frameshift mutation in troponin C (TNNC1) associated with hypertrophic cardiomyopathy and sudden death. *Cardiology in the Young*, , 1-4. doi:10.1017/S1047951110001927

Colombo, M. G., Botto, N., Vittorini, S., Paradossi, U., & Andreassi, M. G. (2008). Clinical utility of genetic tests for inherited hypertrophic and dilated cardiomyopathies. *Cardiovascular Ultrasound, 6*, 62. doi:10.1186/1476-7120-6-62

Elliott, P. M., Poloniecki, J., Dickie, S., Sharma, S., Monserrat, L., Varnava, A., .. McKenna, W. J. (2000). Sudden death in hypertrophic cardiomyopathy: Identification of high risk patients. *Journal of the American College of Cardiology, 36*(7), 2212-2218.

Eizirik, D. L., Cardozo, A. K., & Cnop, M. (2008). The role for endoplasmic reticulum stress in diabetes mellitus. *Endocrine Reviews, 29*(1), 42-61. doi:10.1210/er.2007-0015

Fatkin, D., & Graham, R. M. (2002). Molecular mechanisms of inherited cardiomyopathies. *Physiological Reviews, 82*(4), 945-980. doi:10.1152/physrev.00012.2002

Fuchs, T., & Torjman, A. (2009). The usefulness of microvolt T-wave alternans in the risk stratification of patients with hypertrophic cardiomyopathy. *The Israel Medical Association Journal : IMAJ, 11*(10), 606-610.

Geisterfer-Lowrance, A. A., Kass, S., Tanigawa, G., Vosberg, H. P., McKenna, W., Seidman, C. E., & Seidman, J. G. (1990). A molecular basis for familial hypertrophic cardiomyopathy: A beta cardiac myosin heavy chain gene missense mutation. *Cell, 62*(5), 999-1006.

Gillis, T. E., Liang, B., Chung, F., & Tibbits, G. F. (2005). Increasing mammalian cardiomyocyte contractility with residues identified in trout troponin C. *Physiological Genomics, 22*(1), 1-7. doi:10.1152/physiolgenomics.00007.2005

Gillis, T. E., Moyes, C. D., & Tibbits, G. F. (2003). Sequence mutations in teleost cardiac troponin C that are permissive of high Ca2+ affinity of site II. *American Journal of Physiology.Cell Physiology, 284*(5), C1176-84. doi:10.1152/ajpcell.00339.2002

Gimeno, J. R., Monserrat, L., Perez-Sanchez, I., Marin, F., Caballero, L., Hermida-Prieto, M., Valdes, M. (2009). Hypertrophic cardiomyopathy. A study of the troponin-T gene in 127 spanish families. *Revista Espanola De Cardiologia, 62*(12), 1473-1477.

Gimeno, J. R., Tome-Esteban, M., Lofiego, C., Hurtado, J., Pantazis, A., Mist, B., .. Elliott, P. M. (2009). Exercise-induced ventricular arrhythmias and risk of sudden cardiac death in patients with hypertrophic cardiomyopathy. *European Heart Journal, 30*(21), 2599-2605. doi:10.1093/eurheartj/ehp327

Girmatsion, Z., Biliczki, P., Bonauer, A., Wimmer-Greinecker, G., Scherer, M., Moritz, A., Ehrlich, J. R. (2009). Changes in microRNA-1 expression and IK1 up-regulation in human atrial fibrillation. *Heart Rhythm : The Official Journal of the Heart Rhythm Society, 6*(12), 1802-1809. doi:10.1016/j.hrthm.2009.08.035

Gomes, A. V., Guzman, G., Zhao, J., & Potter, J. D. (2002). Cardiac troponin T isoforms affect the Ca2+ sensitivity and inhibition of force development. insights into the role of troponin T isoforms in the heart. *The Journal of Biological Chemistry, 277*(38), 35341-35349. doi:10.1074/jbc.M204118200

Gomes, A. V., Barnes, J. A., Harada, K., & Potter, J. D. (2004). Role of troponin T in disease. *Molecular and Cellular Biochemistry, 263*(1-2), 115-129.

Gomes, A. V., & Potter, J. D. (2004). Molecular and cellular aspects of troponin cardiomyopathies. *Annals of the New York Academy of Sciences, 1015*, 214-224. doi:10.1196/annals.1302.018

Gordon, A. M., Homsher, E., & Regnier, M. (2000). Regulation of contraction in striated muscle. *Physiological Reviews, 80*(2), 853-924.

Haim, T. E., Dowell, C., Diamanti, T., Scheuer, J., & Tardiff, J. C. (2007). Independent FHC-related cardiac troponin T mutations exhibit specific alterations in myocellular contractility and calcium kinetics. *Journal of Molecular and Cellular Cardiology, 42*(6), 1098-1110. doi:10.1016/j.yjmcc.2007.03.906

Heineke, J., & Molkentin, J. D. (2006). Regulation of cardiac hypertrophy by intracellular signalling pathways. *Nature Reviews.Molecular Cell Biology, 7*(8), 589-600. doi:10.1038/nrm1983

Hershberger, R. E. (2010). A glimpse into multigene rare variant genetics: Triple mutations in hypertrophic cardiomyopathy. *Journal of the American College of Cardiology, 55*(14), 1454-1455. doi:10.1016/j.jacc.2009.12.025

Ho, C. Y., Lever, H. M., DeSanctis, R., Farver, C. F., Seidman, J. G., & Seidman, C. E. (2000). Homozygous mutation in cardiac troponin T: Implications for hypertrophic cardiomyopathy. *Circulation, 102*(16), 1950-1955.

Ho, C. Y., Sweitzer, N. K., McDonough, B., Maron, B. J., Casey, S. A., Seidman, J. G., .. Solomon, S. D. (2002). Assessment of diastolic function with doppler tissue imaging to predict genotype in preclinical hypertrophic cardiomyopathy. *Circulation, 105*(25), 2992-2997.

Hoffmann, B., Schmidt-Traub, H., Perrot, A., Osterziel, K. J., & Gessner, R. (2001). First mutation in cardiac troponin C, L29Q, in a patient with hypertrophic cardiomyopathy. *Human Mutation, 17*(6), 524. doi:10.1002/humu.1143

Ingles, J., Doolan, A., Chiu, C., Seidman, J., Seidman, C., & Semsarian, C. (2005). Compound and double mutations in patients with hypertrophic cardiomyopathy: Implications for genetic testing and counselling. *Journal of Medical Genetics, 42*(10), e59. doi:10.1136/jmg.2005.033886

James, J., Zhang, Y., Osinska, H., Sanbe, A., Klevitsky, R., Hewett, T. E., & Robbins, J. (2000). Transgenic modeling of a cardiac troponin I mutation linked to familial hypertrophic cardiomyopathy. *Circulation Research, 87*(9), 805-811.

Karibe, A., Tobacman, L. S., Strand, J., Butters, C., Back, N., Bachinski, L. L., .. Fananapazir, L. (2001). Hypertrophic cardiomyopathy caused by a novel alpha-tropomyosin mutation (V95A) is associated with mild cardiac phenotype, abnormal calcium binding to troponin, abnormal myosin cycling, and poor prognosis. *Circulation, 103*(1), 65-71.

Kimura, A., Harada, H., Park, J. E., Nishi, H., Satoh, M., Takahashi, M., .. Sasazuki, T. (1997). Mutations in the cardiac troponin I gene associated with hypertrophic cardiomyopathy. *Nature Genetics, 16*(4), 379-382. doi:10.1038/ng0897-379

Klaver, E. C., Versluijs, G. M., & Wilders, R. (2011). Cardiac ion channel mutations in the sudden infant death syndrome. *International Journal of Cardiology*, doi:10.1016/j.ijcard.2010.12.051

Knollmann, B. C., Kirchhof, P., Sirenko, S. G., Degen, H., Greene, A. E., Schober, T., .. Morad, M. (2003). Familial hypertrophic cardiomyopathy-linked mutant troponin T causes stress-induced ventricular tachycardia and Ca2+-dependent action potential remodeling. *Circulation Research*, *92*(4), 428-436. doi:10.1161/01.RES.0000059562.91384.1A

Knollmann, B. C., & Potter, J. D. (2001). Altered regulation of cardiac muscle contraction by troponin T mutations that cause familial hypertrophic cardiomyopathy. *Trends in Cardiovascular Medicine*, *11*(5), 206-212.

Kokado, H., Shimizu, M., Yoshio, H., Ino, H., Okeie, K., Emoto, Y., .. Mabuchi, H. (2000). Clinical features of hypertrophic cardiomyopathy caused by a Lys183 deletion mutation in the cardiac troponin I gene. *Circulation*, *102*(6), 663-669.

Landstrom, A. P., Parvatiyar, M. S., Pinto, J. R., Marquardt, M. L., Bos, J. M., Tester, D. J., .. Ackerman, M. J. (2008). Molecular and functional characterization of novel hypertrophic cardiomyopathy susceptibility mutations in TNNC1-encoded troponin C. *Journal of Molecular and Cellular Cardiology*, *45*(2), 281-288. doi:DOI: 10.1016/j.yjmcc.2008.05.003

Lassalle, M. W. (2010). Defective dynamic properties of human cardiac troponin mutations. *Bioscience, Biotechnology, and Biochemistry*, *74*(1), 82-91.

Li, Y. A. (2009). *Crystallographic analysis of the regulatory domain of human cardiac troponin C.* (Master of Science, Simon Fraser University).

Liang, B., Chung, F., Qu, Y., Pavlov, D., Gillis, T. E., Tikunova, S. B., .. Tibbits, G. F. (2008). Familial hypertrophic cardiomyopathy-related cardiac troponin C mutation L29Q affects Ca2+ binding and myofilament contractility. *Physiological Genomics*, *33*(2), 257-266. doi:10.1152/physiolgenomics.00154.2007

Liang, Q., De Windt, L. J., Witt, S. A., Kimball, T. R., Markham, B. E., & Molkentin, J. D. (2001). The transcription factors GATA4 and GATA6 regulate cardiomyocyte hypertrophy in vitro and in vivo. *The Journal of Biological Chemistry*, *276*(32), 30245-30253. doi:10.1074/jbc.M102174200

Makhoul, M., Ackerman, M. J., Atkins, D. L., & Law, I. H. (2011). Clinical spectrum in a family with tropomyosin-mediated hypertrophic cardiomyopathy and sudden death in childhood. *Pediatric Cardiology*, *32*(2), 215-220. doi:10.1007/s00246-010-9843-1

Marian, A. J., Yu, Q. T., Workman, R., Greve, G., & Roberts, R. (1993). Angiotensin-converting enzyme polymorphism in hypertrophic cardiomyopathy and sudden cardiac death. *Lancet*, *342*(8879), 1085-1086.

Maron, (2002). Hypertrophic cardiomyopathy: A systematic review. *JAMA : The Journal of the American Medical Association*, *287*(10), 1308-1320.

Maron, (2003). Sudden death in young athletes. *The New England Journal of Medicine*, *349*(11), 1064-1075. doi:10.1056/NEJMra022783

Maron, (2009). Distinguishing hypertrophic cardiomyopathy from athlete's heart physiological remodelling: Clinical significance, diagnostic strategies and implications for preparticipation screening. *British Journal of Sports Medicine*, *43*(9), 649-656. doi:10.1136/bjsm.2008.054726

Maron, (2010). Contemporary insights and strategies for risk stratification and prevention of sudden death in hypertrophic cardiomyopathy. *Circulation, 121*(3), 445-456. doi:10.1161/CIRCULATIONAHA.109.878579

Maron, B. J., Casey, S. A., Poliac, L. C., Gohman, T. E., Almquist, A. K., & Aeppli, D. M. (1999). Clinical course of hypertrophic cardiomyopathy in a regional united states cohort. *JAMA : The Journal of the American Medical Association, 281*(7), 650-655.

Maron, B. J., Gardin, J. M., Flack, J. M., Gidding, S. S., Kurosaki, T. T., & Bild, D. E. (1995). Prevalence of hypertrophic cardiomyopathy in a general population of young adults. echocardiographic analysis of 4111 subjects in the CARDIA study. coronary artery risk development in (young) adults. *Circulation, 92*(4), 785-789.

Maron, B. J., Shirani, J., Poliac, L. C., Mathenge, R., Roberts, W. C., & Mueller, F. O. (1996). Sudden death in young competitive athletes. clinical, demographic, and pathological profiles. *JAMA : The Journal of the American Medical Association, 276*(3), 199-204.

Maron, M. S. (2009). The current and emerging role of cardiovascular magnetic resonance imaging in hypertrophic cardiomyopathy. *Journal of Cardiovascular Translational Research, 2*(4), 415-425. doi:10.1007/s12265-009-9136-3

Matkovich, S. J., Wang, W., Tu, Y., Eschenbacher, W. H., Dorn, L. E., Condorelli, G., .. Dorn, G. W.,2nd. (2010). MicroRNA-133a protects against myocardial fibrosis and modulates electrical repolarization without affecting hypertrophy in pressure-overloaded adult hearts. *Circulation Research, 106*(1), 166-175. doi:10.1161/CIRCRESAHA.109.202176

Menon, S. C., Eidem, B. W., Dearani, J. A., Ommen, S. R., Ackerman, M. J., & Miller, D. (2009). Diastolic dysfunction and its histopathological correlation in obstructive hypertrophic cardiomyopathy in children and adolescents. *Journal of the American Society of Echocardiography : Official Publication of the American Society of Echocardiography, 22*(12), 1327-1334. doi:10.1016/j.echo.2009.08.014

Mesaeli, N., Nakamura, K., Opas, M., & Michalak, M. (2001). Endoplasmic reticulum in the heart, a forgotten organelle? *Molecular and Cellular Biochemistry, 225*(1-), 1-6.

Miller, T., Szczesna, D., Housmans, P. R., Zhao, J., de Freitas, F., Gomes, A. V., .. Potter, J. D. (2001). Abnormal contractile function in transgenic mice expressing a familial hypertrophic cardiomyopathy-linked troponin T (I79N) mutation. *The Journal of Biological Chemistry, 276*(6), 3743-3755. doi:10.1074/jbc.M006746200

Mogensen, J., Murphy, R. T., Kubo, T., Bahl, A., Moon, J. C., Klausen, I. C., .. McKenna, W. J. (2004). Frequency and clinical expression of cardiac troponin I mutations in 748 consecutive families with hypertrophic cardiomyopathy. *Journal of the American College of Cardiology, 44*(12), 2315-2325. doi:10.1016/j.jacc.2004.05.088

Molkentin, J. D., Lu, J. R., Antos, C. L., Markham, B., Richardson, J., Robbins, J., .. Olson, E. N. (1998). A calcineurin-dependent transcriptional pathway for cardiac hypertrophy. *Cell, 93*(2), 215-228.

Molkentin, J. D., & Olson, E. N. (1997). GATA4: A novel transcriptional regulator of cardiac hypertrophy? *Circulation, 96*(11), 3833-3835.

Monserrat, L., Elliott, P. M., Gimeno, J. R., Sharma, S., Penas-Lado, M., & McKenna, W. J. (2003). Non-sustained ventricular tachycardia in hypertrophic cardiomyopathy: An independent marker of sudden death risk in young patients. *Journal of the American College of Cardiology, 42*(5), 873-879.

Moolman, J. C., Corfield, V. A., Posen, B., Ngumbela, K., Seidman, C., Brink, P. A., & Watkins, H. (1997). Sudden death due to troponin T mutations. *Journal of the American College of Cardiology, 29*(3), 549-555.

Niimura, H., Patton, K. K., McKenna, W. J., Soults, J., Maron, B. J., Seidman, J. G., & Seidman, C. E. (2002). Sarcomere protein gene mutations in hypertrophic cardiomyopathy of the elderly. *Circulation, 105*(4), 446-451.

Ostman-Smith, I., Wettrell, G., Keeton, B., Holmgren, D., Ergander, U., Gould, S., .. Verdicchio, M. (2008). Age- and gender-specific mortality rates in childhood hypertrophic cardiomyopathy. *European Heart Journal, 29*(9), 1160-1167. doi:10.1093/eurheartj/ehn122

Parmacek, M. S., & Solaro, R. J. (2004). Biology of the troponin complex in cardiac myocytes. *Progress in Cardiovascular Diseases, 47*(3), 159-176.

Pinto, J. R., Parvatiyar, M. S., Jones, M. A., Liang, J., Ackerman, M. J., & Potter, J. D. (2009). A functional and structural study of troponin C mutations related to hypertrophic cardiomyopathy. *The Journal of Biological Chemistry, 284*(28), 19090-19100. doi:10.1074/jbc.M109.007021

Pinto, J. R., Reynaldo, D. P., Parvatiyar, M. S., Dweck, D., Liang, J., Jones, M. A., .. Potter, J. D. (2011). Strong cross-bridges potentiate the ca(2+) affinity changes produced by hypertrophic cardiomyopathy cardiac troponin C mutants in myofilaments: A fast kinetic approach. *The Journal of Biological Chemistry, 286*(2), 1005-1013. doi:10.1074/jbc.M110.168583

Pogwizd, S. M., Schlotthauer, K., Li, L., Yuan, W., & Bers, D. M. (2001). Arrhythmogenesis and contractile dysfunction in heart failure: Roles of sodium-calcium exchange, inward rectifier potassium current, and residual beta-adrenergic responsiveness. *Circulation Research, 88*(11), 1159-1167.

Revera, M., van der Merwe, L., Heradien, M., Goosen, A., Corfield, V. A., Brink, P. A., & Moolman-Smook, J. C. (2008). Troponin T and beta-myosin mutations have distinct cardiac functional effects in hypertrophic cardiomyopathy patients without hypertrophy. *Cardiovascular Research, 77*(4), 687-694. doi:10.1093/cvr/cvm075

Rodriguez, J. E., McCudden, C. R., & Willis, M. S. (2009). Familial hypertrophic cardiomyopathy: Basic concepts and future molecular diagnostics. *Clinical Biochemistry,* doi:10.1016/j.clinbiochem.2009.01.020

Sanbe, A., James, J., Tuzcu, V., Nas, S., Martin, L., Gulick, J., .. Robbins, J. (2005). Transgenic rabbit model for human troponin I-based hypertrophic cardiomyopathy. *Circulation, 111*(18), 2330-2338. doi:10.1161/01.CIR.0000164234.24957.75

Schmidtmann, A., Lindow, C., Villard, S., Heuser, A., Mugge, A., Gessner, R., .. Jaquet, K. (2005). Cardiac troponin C-L29Q, related to hypertrophic cardiomyopathy, hinders the transduction of the protein kinase A dependent phosphorylation signal from cardiac troponin I to C. *The FEBS Journal, 272*(23), 6087-6097. doi:10.1111/j.1742-4658.2005.05001.x

Schroder, M., & Kaufman, R. J. (2005). The mammalian unfolded protein response. *Annual Review of Biochemistry, 74*, 739-789. doi:10.1146/annurev.biochem.73.011303.074134

Semsarian, C., Ahmad, I., Giewat, M., Georgakopoulos, D., Schmitt, J. P., McConnell, B. K., .. Seidman, J. G. (2002). The L-type calcium channel inhibitor diltiazem prevents cardiomyopathy in a mouse model. *The Journal of Clinical Investigation, 109*(8), 1013-1020. doi:10.1172/JCI14677

Solaro, R. J., & Kobayashi, T. (2011). Protein phosphorylation and signal transduction in cardiac thin filaments. *The Journal of Biological Chemistry,* doi:10.1074/jbc.R110.197731

Strijack, B., Ariyarajah, V., Soni, R., Jassal, D. S., Greenberg, C. R., McGregor, R., & Morris, A. (2008). Late gadolinium enhancement cardiovascular magnetic resonance in genotyped hypertrophic cardiomyopathy with normal phenotype. *Journal of Cardiovascular Magnetic Resonance : Official Journal of the Society for Cardiovascular Magnetic Resonance, 10,* 58. doi:10.1186/1532-429X-10-58

Takahashi-Yanaga, F., Morimoto, S., Harada, K., Minakami, R., Shiraishi, F., Ohta, M., .. Ohtsuki, I. (2001). Functional consequences of the mutations in human cardiac troponin I gene found in familial hypertrophic cardiomyopathy. *Journal of Molecular and Cellular Cardiology, 33*(12), 2095-2107. doi:10.1006/jmcc.2001.1473

Takeda, S., Yamashita, A., Maeda, K., & Maeda, Y. (2003). Structure of the core domain of human cardiac troponin in the ca(2+)-saturated form. *Nature, 424*(6944), 35-41. doi:10.1038/nature01780

Tardiff, J. C. (2011). Thin filament mutations: Developing an integrative approach to a complex disorder. *Circulation Research, 108*(6), 765-782. doi:10.1161/CIRCRESAHA.110.224170

Tardiff, J. C., Hewett, T. E., Palmer, B. M., Olsson, C., Factor, S. M., Moore, R. L., .. Leinwand, L. A. (1999). Cardiac troponin T mutations result in allele-specific phenotypes in a mouse model for hypertrophic cardiomyopathy. *The Journal of Clinical Investigation, 104*(4), 469-481. doi:10.1172/JCI6067

Teare, D. (1958). Asymmetrical hypertrophy of the heart in young adults. *British Heart Journal, 20*(1), 1-8.

Ter Keurs, H. E., Wakayama, Y., Miura, M., Shinozaki, T., Stuyvers, B. D., Boyden, P. A., & Landesberg, A. (2006). Arrhythmogenic ca(2+) release from cardiac myofilaments. *Progress in Biophysics and Molecular Biology, 90*(1-3), 151-171. doi:10.1016/j.pbiomolbio.2005.07.002

Tester, D. J., & Ackerman, M. (2009). Cardiomyopathic and channelopathic causes of sudden, unexpected death in infants and children. *Annual Review of Medicine,* doi:10.1146/annurev.med.60.052907.103838

Thierfelder, L., MacRae, C., Watkins, H., Tomfohrde, J., Williams, M., McKenna, W., .. Bowcock, A. (1993). A familial hypertrophic cardiomyopathy locus maps to chromosome 15q2. *Proceedings of the National Academy of Sciences of the United States of America, 90*(13), 6270-6274.

Thierfelder, L., Watkins, H., MacRae, C., Lamas, R., McKenna, W., Vosberg, H. P., .. Seidman, C. E. (1994). Alpha-tropomyosin and cardiac troponin T mutations cause familial hypertrophic cardiomyopathy: A disease of the sarcomere. *Cell, 77*(5), 701-712.

Tobacman, L. S. (1996). Thin filament-mediated regulation of cardiac contraction. *Annual Review of Physiology, 58,* 447-481. doi:10.1146/annurev.ph.58.030196.002311

Tsoutsman, T., Chung, J., Doolan, A., Nguyen, L., Williams, I. A., Tu, E., .. Semsarian, C. (2006). Molecular insights from a novel cardiac troponin I mouse model of familial hypertrophic cardiomyopathy. *Journal of Molecular and Cellular Cardiology, 41*(4), 623-632. doi:10.1016/j.yjmcc.2006.07.016

Van Der Spoel, D., Lindahl, E., Hess, B., Groenhof, G., Mark, A. E., & Berendsen, H. J. (2005). GROMACS: Fast, flexible, and free. *Journal of Computational Chemistry, 26*(16), 1701-1718. doi:10.1002/jcc.20291

Van Driest, S. L., Ellsworth, E. G., Ommen, S. R., Tajik, A. J., Gersh, B. J., & Ackerman, M. J. (2003). Prevalence and spectrum of thin filament mutations in an outpatient referral population with hypertrophic cardiomyopathy. *Circulation, 108*(4), 445-451. doi:10.1161/01.CIR.0000080896.52003.DF

Van Driest, S. L., Vasile, V. C., Ommen, S. R., Will, M. L., Tajik, A. J., Gersh, B. J., & Ackerman, M. J. (2004). Myosin binding protein C mutations and compound heterozygosity in hypertrophic cardiomyopathy. *Journal of the American College of Cardiology, 44*(9), 1903-1910. doi:10.1016/j.jacc.2004.07.045

van Rooij, E., Sutherland, L. B., Liu, N., Williams, A. H., McAnally, J., Gerard, R. D., .Olson, E. N. (2006). A signature pattern of stress-responsive microRNAs that can evoke cardiac hypertrophy and heart failure. *Proceedings of the National Academy of Sciences of the United States of America, 103*(48), 18255-18260. doi:10.1073/pnas. 0608791103

Varnava, A. M., Elliott, P. M., Baboonian, C., Davison, F., Davies, M. J., & McKenna, W. J. (2001). Hypertrophic cardiomyopathy: Histopathological features of sudden death in cardiac troponin T disease. *Circulation, 104*(12), 1380-1384.

Varnava, A. M., Elliott, P. M., Mahon, N., Davies, M. J., & McKenna, W. J. (2001). Relation between myocyte disarray and outcome in hypertrophic cardiomyopathy. *The American Journal of Cardiology, 88*(3), 275-279.

Wang, Y., Shen, J., Arenzana, N., Tirasophon, W., Kaufman, R. J., & Prywes, R. (2000). Activation of ATF6 and an ATF6 DNA binding site by the endoplasmic reticulum stress response. *The Journal of Biological Chemistry, 275*(35), 27013-27020. doi:10.1074/jbc.M003322200

Watkins, H., McKenna, W. J., Thierfelder, L., Suk, H. J., Anan, R., O'Donoghue, A., Seidman, J. G. (1995). Mutations in the genes for cardiac troponin T and alpha-tropomyosin in hypertrophic cardiomyopathy. *The New England Journal of Medicine, 332*(16), 1058-1064. doi:10.1056/NEJM199504203321603

Wetzel, G. T., & Klitzner, T. S. (1996). Developmental cardiac electrophysiology recent advances in cellular physiology. *Cardiovascular Research, 31 Spec No*, E52-60.

Wheeler, M., Pavlovic, A., DeGoma, E., Salisbury, H., Brown, C., & Ashley, E. A. (2009). A new era in clinical genetic testing for hypertrophic cardiomyopathy. *Journal of Cardiovascular Translational Research, 2*(4), 381-391. doi:10.1007/s12265-009-9139-0

Willinger, M., James, L. S., & Catz, C. (1991). Defining the sudden infant death syndrome (SIDS): Deliberations of an expert panel convened by the national institute of child health and human development. *Pediatric Pathology / Affiliated with the International Paediatric Pathology Association, 11*(5), 677-684. doi:10.3109/15513819109065465

Willott, R. H., Gomes, A. V., Chang, A. N., Parvatiyar, M. S., Pinto, J. R., & Potter, J. D. (2010). Mutations in troponin that cause HCM, DCM AND RCM: What can we learn about thin filament function? *Journal of Molecular and Cellular Cardiology, 48*(5), 882-892. doi:10.1016/j.yjmcc.2009.10.031

Wolf, C. M., Moskowitz, I. P., Arno, S., Branco, D. M., Semsarian, C., Bernstein, S. A., Seidman, J. G. (2005). Somatic events modify hypertrophic cardiomyopathy pathology and link hypertrophy to arrhythmia. *Proceedings of the National Academy of Sciences of the United States of America, 102*(50), 18123-18128. doi:10.1073/pnas.0509145102

Yang, B., Lin, H., Xiao, J., Lu, Y., Luo, X., Li, B., Wang, Z. (2007). The muscle-specific microRNA miR-1 regulates cardiac arrhythmogenic potential by targeting GJA1 and KCNJ2. *Nature Medicine, 13*(4), 486-491. doi:10.1038/nm1569

Zhao, Y., Ransom, J. F., Li, A., Vedpantham, V., von Drehle, M., Muth, A. N., Srivastava, D. (2007). Dysregulation of cardiogenesis, cardiac conduction, and cell cycle in mice lacking miRNA-1-2. *Cell, 129*(2), 303-317. doi:10.1016/j.cell.2007.03.030

15

Consequences of Mutations in Genes Encoding Cardiac Troponin C, T and I – Molecular Insights

Kornelia Jaquet and Andreas Mügge
Molecular Cardiology & Clinic of Cardiology, St. Josef-Hospital & Bergmannsheil, University Hospitals of the Ruhr-University of Bochum, Germany

1. Introduction

Cardiac troponin is the main regulatory protein of the thin filament and mediates the Ca^{2+}-sensitivity of the actin-myosin interaction. Troponin forms a heterotrimeric complex composed of the tropomyosin binding subunit (cTnT), the inhibitory subunit (cTnI) and the Ca^{2+}-binding subunit (cTnC). A complex interplay between the cardiac troponin subunits and other thin filament proteins, as tropomyosin (Tm) and actin, is essential to regulate muscle contraction, which can be described by cross bridge cycling on the molecular level. Troponin is located on both sides of the thin filament with a stagger of about 27 Angstroms between two adjacent troponin molecules (Ebashi, 1972; Paul et al., 2009). In the thin filament each troponin binds to one tropomyosin, which covers 7 actin monomers. It is no surprise that mutations in genes encoding proteins, which participate in crossbridge cycling and its regulation, derange interactions and lead to contractile dysfunction and disease. In all three cardiac troponin subunits, changes in amino acid sequence have been identified in families with hypertrophic (HCM), restrictive (RCM) and dilated cardiomyopathy (DCM). Therefore knowledge of structure, function and interactions of the proteins is a prerequisite to understand dysfunction in disease.

1.1 Cardiac troponin T (cTnT)

One of the main tasks of cardiac troponin T (30-35kDa) is to fix the troponin complex to the thin filament. Furthermore cTnT participates in conferring calcium sensitivity to actin/myosin (Tobacman, 1988). Tobacman also showed that the N-terminal half of cTnT, TnT1 (amino acids 1-158, skeletal muscle numbering), was able to keep the thin filament in the blocked state without TnI. In the blocked state of the thin filament no interaction between actin and myosin is possible, i.e. no force production occurs. Thus cTnT plays an active role in inhibition of actin/myosin interaction in the resting state. It further promotes tropomyosin polymerization and binding of tropomyosin to actin.
Structural information on cTnT is poor. According to EM analysis of thin filaments and low resolution co-crystallization of Tm in complex with cTnT, cTnT is highly asymmetric. It is a 180-202 nm long comma –shaped molecule, with the N-terminal rod like part arranged along the thin filament and a C-terminal more globular domain (Ohtsuki, 1979, Flicker et al., 1982, White et al., 1987). The high resolution crystal structure available for the core troponin complex contains only the less flexible C-terminal part of cTnT, which binds the other two

troponin subunits, cTnI and cTnC (Takeda et al., 2003). There is strong evidence from latest single particle reconstruction studies of the thin filament by Paul et al., (2009), that the N-terminal tail of cTnT points to the M-band of the sarcomere, whereas the core domain of the troponin complex is oriented versus the Z-band.

The N-terminal tail fraction of cTnT contains a hypervariable N-terminal part and a highly conserved region, which is located in the central region of the cTnT molecule (Fig. 1). This conserved region contains the main interaction site for tropomyosin (Biesiadecki et al., 2007, Perry, 1998) comprising 39 amino acids (residues 98-136 (human cardiac sequence)) (Jin & Chong, 2010). The Tm interaction site forms a helix according to Murakami et al., (2008) and binds to the overlapping region of two tropomyosin molecules (Jin & Chong, 2010). Crystal structure of the tropomyosin overlap region and the Tm binding helix reveals the formation of a four helix bundle between tropomyosin ends and cTnT (Murakami et al., 2008). The hypervariable region of the cTnT tail fraction does not bind to tropomyosin and can be truncated without losing binding ability of the rest of the molecule (Zhang et al., 2006). Phylogenetically the hypervariable region might be added to the conserved core region of cTnT (Conserved tail region and C-terminal domain) (Jin & Samanez, 2001; Biesiadecki et al., 2007). Its function is not completely elucidated, but the hypervariable region may play a role as modulator of the core molecule thus subtly affecting binding affinities of Tm and cTnT (Biesiadecki et al, 2007; Feng et al., 2008).

A second interaction site for tropomyosin is located at the beginning of the C-terminal half of cTnT and has lately been analysed by Jin & Chong (2010) using antibodies. They showed that highly conserved amino acid sequences are involved comprising amino acid residues 197-236 (human sequence). This interaction site binds to the middle part of tropomyosin near Cys190. Earlier studies (Pearlstone et al., 1983; Morris & Lehrer, 1984) propose the second interaction with tropomyosin at the very C-terminus of cTnT involving residues 272-288. Whichever amino acids are included in the cTnT/Tm interactions, in the presence of cTnC binding of the TnT-C-Terminus to tropomyosin near Cys190 is Ca^{2+} dependent (Chong & Hodges, 1982). Ca^{2+} weakens its binding to tropomyosin though the molecular mechanism, i.e. conformational changes which lead to alteration in Tm/TnT -binding, is not known yet. The TnT-C-Terminus also contains the binding site for the other two troponin subunits, TnI and TnC. According to the 3 D structure of the core cardiac troponin complex, the helix in the C-terminal region of cTnT (residues 226-271), which is highly conserved (Jin et al., 2008) forms a rigid coiled coil with a cTnI-helix (residues 90-136) and is part of a rigid structure within the troponin complex, called the IT-arm (Takeda et al., 2003). At the C-terminal end of the coiled coil the interaction site for cTnC is located and comprises amino acid residues 256- 270. The organisation of cTnT is summarized in Fig.1.

In cardiac muscle the mammalian cTnT- gene (TNNT2) is composed of 17 exons. Exon 5 is absent in adult cTnT (Cooper & Ordahl, 1985). Exon 5 encodes a 10 amino acid long region within the hypervariable N-terminus of cTnT. This sequence contains several acidic residues and contributes to a more negatively charged cTnT. Such a charge difference may modulate function. Indeed fetal cTnT, which contains exon 5, exhibits a higher Ca^{2+}-sensitivity compared to adult cTnT and shows a higher tolerance towards acidic pH (Gomes et al., 2002). Mainly 4 variants of human cTnT ($cTnT_{1-4}$) have been described due to alternative splicing of exons 4 and 5, whereby TnT_1 and TnT_3 are the major isoforms present in fetal and in the adult human cardiac muscle, respectively (Townsend et al., 1995; Anderson et al., 1991). The expression pattern of cTnT isoforms seems to be altered in heart failure and correlates with changes in Ca^{2+}- sensitivity. The modification in Ca^{2+}- sensitivity however, seems not to be caused by an alteration in the isoform expression pattern. Differences in the phosphorylation status of sarcomeric proteins, especially of myosin light chain 2 (MLC-2) may be decisive (van der Velden et al., 2003). Also cTnT itself is a phospho protein (Fig. 1) which is constitutively phosphorylated at Ser1 in several species inclusive men due to the action of casein kinase- 2 (Gusev et al., 1980; Risnik & Gusev, 1984, Swiderek et al., 1990). The function of this phosphorylation is not known up to date. It might prevent degradation and/or interaction of the hypervariable region. At least one further reversible phosphorylation site for PKC is located in the C-terminal region of cTnT near the second Ca^{2+}- dependent interaction site for Tm and thus may affect Ca^{2+}- sensitivity of the actin/myosin interaction. Indeed, according to Sumandea et al., reversible phosphorylation of Thr206 (mouse sequence) is critical for function (Sumandea et al., 2003). *In vitro* experiments showed that phosphorylation by PKCα decreases maximal tension, myofilament Ca^{2+} -sensitivity, actomyosin ATPase activity and cooperativity (Sumandea et al., 2003). Other protein kinases than PKC, as for example ROCKII (Vahebi et al., 2005), phosphorylate cTnT *in vitro*. The physiological role of cTnT phosphorylation by different protein kinases is not yet clarified. cTnT, however, is not a target of cAMP dependent protein kinase (PKA), which is activated upon ß-adrenergic stimulation. But as recently described by Sumandea et al., (2011) cTnT forms an AKAP for PKA with either regulatory subunit I or II (PKA-RI, PKA-RII) and thus provides a platform for sarcomeric protein phosphorylation upon ß-adrenergic stimulation. Binding of PKA might occur within the amino acid region 202-226 which forms an amphiphilic helix needed for the docking of PKA RI and—II (Feliciello et al., 2001). The interaction site for PKA-R would then be located just near the second interaction site with tropomyosin described by (Jin & Chong, 2010) and the PKC phosphorylation site. This implies that PKA-R binding might be affected by PKC phosphorylation and vice versa.

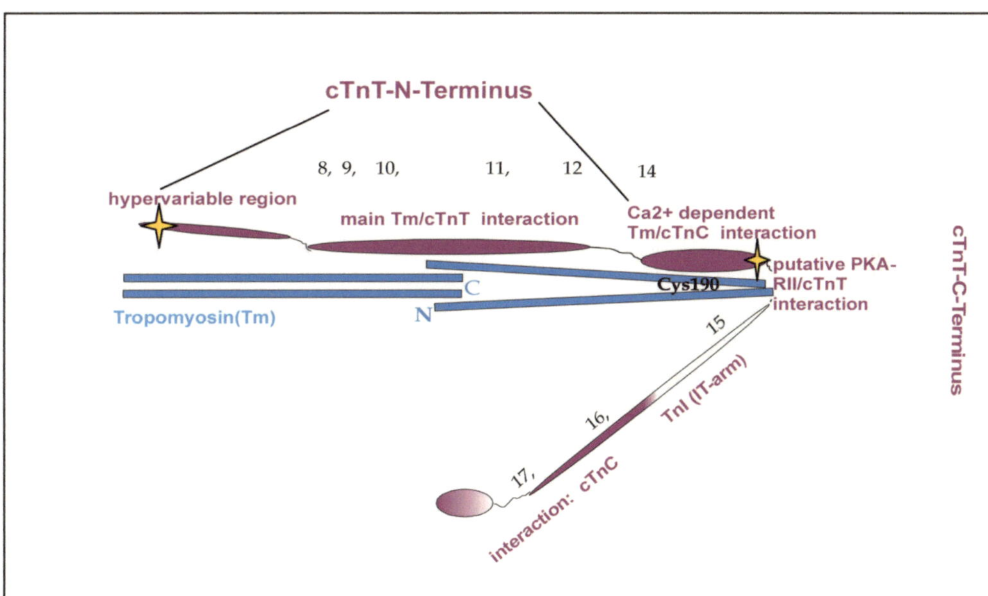

Fig. 1. Organisation , interaction and phosphorylation sites of cardiac troponin T. Exons known to contain cardiomyopathy mutations are indicated by numbers

1.2 Cardiac troponin C (cTnC)

cTnC is the calcium binding subunit of the cardiac troponin complex. Structurally the protein belongs to the EF-hand calcium binding protein super family together with parvalbumin, the first described protein of this family, Calmodulin, skeletal muscle troponin C etc. cTnC is composed of two lobes connected by a flexible linker (Sia et al., 1997) (Fig.2).

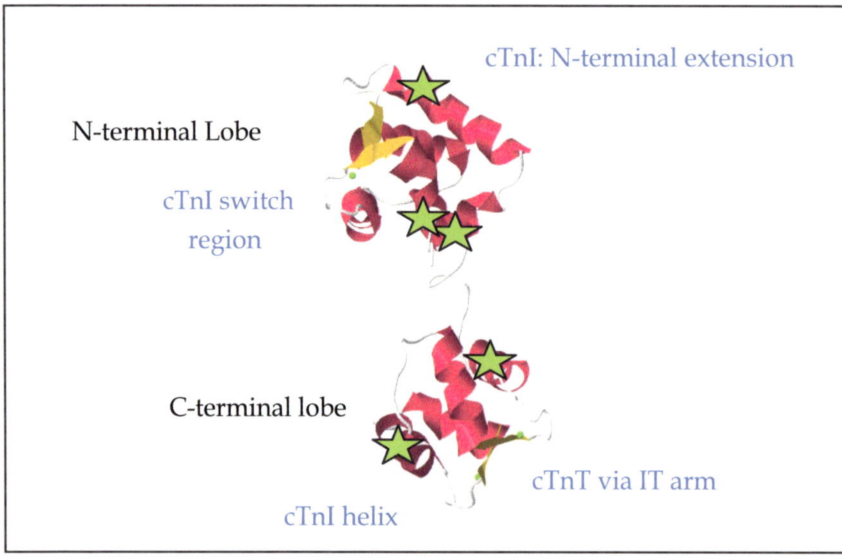

Fig. 2. Interaction sites and cardiomyopathy inducing single amino acid exchanges in cTnC

The structure was taken from PDP 1AJ4 based on the work of (Sia et al., 1997). The 3 D structure of cTnC in calcium (green points) saturated from is shown. Helices are given as magenta ribbons. The position of cardiomyopathy mutations is indicated by stars. Interacting proteins are given in blue.

Each lobe contains two parallel EF hands, each of which forms the helix-loop-helix divalent metal binding domain. Helices in a protein have been labeled by capital letters, with A assigned to the most N-terminally located helix. Thus E and F are the loop flanking helices in parvalbumin forming the metal binding motif. The name EF-hand for the helix loop helix metal binding motif is based on this nomenclature. The short helices of about 10-12 residues are arranged perpendicular. The loop is composed of 12 residues essential for calcium coordination in a pentagonal bipyramidal configuration. The residues 1, 3, 5, 7, 9 and 12 (X, Y, Z, -Y, -X, -Z) are involved in Ca^{2+}-coordination. In position 12 there is a conserved glutamate or aspartate residue providing two oxygens for calcium binding (Structure Reference: PDB: 2PMY). The calcium binding residues preferentially have an acidic side chain, but also the protein backbone is involved. In cTnC the two EF hands (III, IV) in the C-terminal lobe are the high affinity Ca^{2+}-, Mg^{2+}-binding sites, which contain metal ions also at low (relaxing) intracellular Ca^{2+}-concentration. This C-terminal domain of cTnC provides the platform for binding of cTnI and of cTnT and therefore is pivotal for the integrity of the troponin complex. Helices of the metal bound C-terminal domain exhibit a hydrophobic pocket, where cTnI is bound (Gasmi-Seabrook et al., 1999). cTnT binds to Calcium sites III and IV at the end of the rigid coiled coil. Besides the structural role of the C-terminal lobe, there is now strong evidence that it plays an active part in thin filament activation (Fuchs &

Grabarek, 2011). Alteration in Ca^{2+}-/Mg^{2+}-binding to sites III and IV might alter the interaction with cTnT and the coiled coil structure. Also the identification of cardiomyopathy causing alterations in this part of cTnC points to the involvement in regulation.
The N-terminal EF-hand I is not able to bind Ca^{2+} due to an insertion of Val and the replacement of two Asp residues involved in Ca^{2+}-coordination by Ala and Leu residues. Therefore there is only one functional active Ca^{2+}-binding site (site II) in the N-terminal domain of cTnC, which is a high affinity Ca^{2+}-specific binding site. Binding and release kinetics of Ca^{2+} to cTnC within the thin filament are such that Ca^{2+}-binding and release occurs within one contraction cycle (Davis & Tikunova, 2008). Saturation of cTnC with Ca^{2+} is obtained upon increase in intracellular Ca^{2+}-concentration after influx from sarcoplasmatic Ca^{2+}-store upon membrane depolarization. Therefore site II is named the regulatory Ca^{2+}-binding site. Due to the non functional site I there is no conformational switch from closed to open solely upon Ca^{2+} -binding as is observed for skeletal muscle TnC and the C-terminal lobe of cTnC (Sia et al., 1997). For the stabilization of the open conformation of the N-terminal lobe cTnI binding is required (Dong et al., 1999; Li et al., 1999). There exist multiple interaction sites for cTnI throughout the complete cTnC molecule. The amphiphilic part of helix 1 in cTnI (residues 43-65) binds via several polar and van der Waals interaction to the C-terminal cTnC lobe and around residue 10 of the N-terminal helix of cTnC. Furthermore residues 93-161 in the C-terminal lobe of cTnC interact with the IT-arm (Takeda et al., 2003), The N-terminal lobe of cTnC forms the Ca^{2+}-dependent binding site for the cTnI switch region (Takeda et al., 2003) and a phosphorylation dependent binding site near the nonfunctional Ca^{2+}-binding loop with the flexible heart specific N-terminal cTnI extension (see below) (Schmidtmann et al., 2005).

1.3 Cardiac troponin I (cTnI)

cTnI, the inhibitory subunit of the troponin complex is a very flexible molecule consisting of helices and random coils. In solution cTnI exhibits no tertiary structure. A specific spatial orientation is only obtained within the ternary troponin complex. cTnI is build up in a modular fashion (Fig. 3).

1.3.1 The N-terminal extension

The N-terminal extension of about 31 amino acids (length is dependent on species) is heart specific and resembles the hypervaraible region of cTnT. It contains conserved amino acid stretches; thus at the very N-terminus there is a acidic region (Sadayappan et al., 2008) followed by a proline rich sequence, which forms a polyprolin helix and functions as a rigid spacer to keep the N-terminus extended (Howarth et al., 2007). Then the phosphorylation region follows, which contains two adjacent located serine residues at position 22 and 23 (numbered without starter methionine). Both residues are substrates for PKA (Swiderek et al., 1990; Mittmann et al., 1990). In its dephosphorylated state the N-terminal cTnI arm interacts between residues 10-30 with cTnC around amino acid residue 29 (Fig. 2) (Finley et al., 1999; Gaponenko et al., 1999; Abbott et al., 2000; Ward et al.,2003, 2004; Schmidtmann et al., 2002, 2005). This interaction also seems to stabilize the open conformation of the cTnC-N-terminal lobe (Abbott et al., 2000, 2001; Ward et al., 2004). Bisphosphorylation of the two serine residues 22 and 23 by PKA upon ß- adrenergic stimulation releases the interaction with cTnC. According to Howarth et al, (2007) the bisphosphorylated arm contains a helix comprising amino acids 21-30 being stabilized by salt bridges between phosphate and preceeding arginine residues (Jaquet et al. 1998). The release of the extension from cTnC takes place due to the insertion of negative charges followed by conformational changes. This allows a different interaction, which is directed by the acidic part of the N-terminal cTnI arm and therefore needs a positively charged partner (Sadayappan et al., 2008). Clusters of basic amino acid residues are provided by the regulatory C-terminal domain of cTnI itself, but also an additional interaction with actin cannot be excluded. The release of the N-terminal arm from cTnC leads to a reduction of the Ca^{2+} -affinity of cTnC, in myofilament Ca^{2+}-sensitivity (Zhang et al 1995; Reiffert et al., 1996) and to enhanced cross bridge cycling (Kentish et al.,2001; Turnbull et al., 2002). There is evidence that the main action occurs via interaction with cTnI, which stabilizes cTnI binding to the thin filament (Sakthivel et al., 2005).

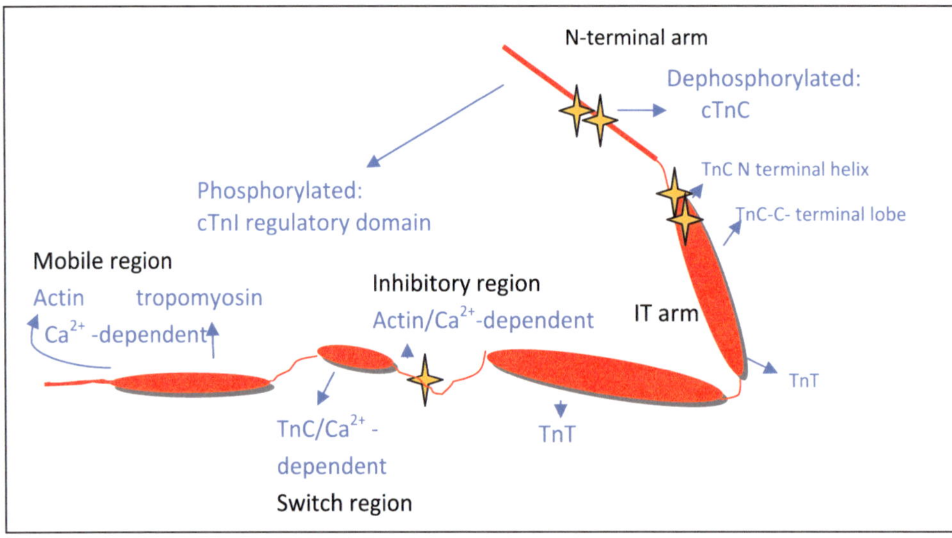

Fig. 3. Organization of cTnI, its interactions (blue) and phosphorylation sites (indicated by ✧)

1.3.2 Constitutive cTnC and cTnT binding sites

The cTnC binding site is located subsequent to the N-terminal extension. It forms a helix (helix 1 according to the nomenclature of Takeda et al., 2003) which contacts the N-terminal cTnC helix and reaches to the C-terminal lobe of cTnC. It strongly binds to the hydrophobic pocket of the C-terminal cTnC lobe. The C-terminal part of helix 1 also interacts with cTnT via several hydrogen bonds and hydrophobic interactions. This helix is followed by another helical binding site for cTnT (helix 2). Helix 2 forms a coiled coil with a helix located in the C-terminal half of cTnT. The two helices are part of the IT arm (Takeda et al., 2003). Both these binding sites in cTnI are independent on reversible Ca^{2+} -binding to the regulatory Ca^{2+} binding loop in cTnC. In helix 1 there are two serine residues (Ser43/45) which are phosphorylated by PKC upon alpha adrenergic stimulation. Ser43/45 are positioned near residue 10 of the N-terminal helix in cTnC-N-terminal lobe as well as near the C-terminal lobe. Thus, phosphorylation might alter these interactions. In mice phosphorylation of these sites by PKC upon α-adrenergic stimulation is responsible for the negative inotropic effect and might be influenced by the cTnT phosphorylation state. The physiological effect of PKA dependent phosphorylation at Ser22/23 seems not to be impaired by Ser43/45 phosphorylation (Montgomery et al., 2002).

1.3.3 Regulatory C-terminal region

The C-terminal region of cTnI can functionally be subdivided into the inhibitory region comprising amino acids 137-148, the helical switch region (amino acids 150-159) and the C-terminal mobile region. The inhibitory region binds to actin/tropomyosin in the relaxed state, i.e. when the regulatory Ca^{2+} binding loop of cTnC contains no Ca^{2+}. Within this region there is another heart specific PKC phosphorylation site at Thr 144. The physiological role of this phosphorylation site is not quite clear (Solaro & Kobayashi, 2011), though investigations by Tachampa et al., (2007) imply that Thr144 is involved in length dependent activation of tension development in thin filament bundles. Phosphorylation might modulate this function probably by loosening the interaction of cTnI inhibitory region with actin.
Upon Ca^{2+}- saturation of cTnC the inhibitory region is released from actin and the switch region binds to the cTnC-N-terminal lobe inducing the formation of the hydrophic pocket. Strength of interaction is sensible to small conformational changes in the cTnC-N-lobe also affecting Ca^{2+}-binding affinity. The C-terminal mobile region following the switch region is a very important cTnI region for regulation of muscle contraction, though not much is known about this region. It provides a second actin binding site and a tropomyosin binding site. Under relaxing conditions, this mobile region is fixed to tropomyosin (Pirani et al., 2005; Galinska et al., et al., 2008) and actin, and is released from actin/tropomyosin upon Ca^{2+}-saturation of cTnC. Thus the C-Terminus stabilizes the blocked state of the thin filament (Galinska et al., 2010). Probably this effect is intensified by the interaction of cTnT binding to tropomyosin actin. Thus cTnT- N-terminus and cTnI-C-terminus both support the inhibitory region of cTnI in keeping tropomyosin in the blocking position. Hereby troponin complexes on opposite sites cooperate, one complex providing cTnT/tropomyosin interaction the other cTnI/tropomyosin/actin interaction (Paul et al., 2009; Solaro & Kobayashi, 2011). But cardiac TnI is not only involved in regulation of inhibition, but also of activation. Evidence came from investigations of Galinska et al., (2010) using truncated cTnI and normal length cTnI. They showed that the C-terminus is also involved in stabilization of tropomyosin in the active state (Ca^{2+} - saturated cTnC). Truncation may occur *in vivo* due to proteolysis in myocardial stunning (reversible ischemia/reperfusion injury) (Foster et al., 2003) and due to cardiomyopathy mutations.

2. Cardiomyopathy inducing troponin mutations

A large number of mutations have been detected in genes encoding for the three cTn subunits in patients suffering of cardiomyopathies (tables 1-6). Resulting phenotypes are highly variable, even within a family carrying the same mutation (see below), indicating that modifiers, environment or polymorphisms are involved in disease development. Wang et al., (2005) was the first group who detected a polymorphism in the MYBPC3 (cardiac myosin binding protein C gene) that might be able to modify the expression of hypertrophy. Also combinations of more than one mutation determine the disease development. Therefore it is still impossible to correlate phenotype and genotype, though an immense progress has been made in the understanding of molecular pathogenesis. The goal to understand phenotype development remains. Since the disease is primarily caused by mutations, it is crucial to improve knowledge on the dysfunctions on molecular level in detail of as many mutants as possible. Thus one might be able to detect common features and mechanisms which might allow detection of a link to phenotype development. Though the molecular effects of only a couple of mutations have been thoroughly investigated a first common rule, namely an enhancement in Ca^{2+}- sensitivity of the myofilament for HCM/RCM-mutants and a decrease in Ca^{2+}- sensitivity for DCM mutants has been stated by Robinson et al., (2007). However it seems to be too simple and does not explain the development of HCM or RCM or the often very low degree of hypertrophy despite large Ca2+ sensitivity changes and susceptibility to malignant arrhythmia. Furthermore, the rule does not apply to all mutations investigated. One problem is that analysis of Ca^{2+} - sensitivity resulted in many opposing statements. Thus for example Nakaura et al., 1999 did not observe enhanced Ca^{2+} -sensitivity of force in skinned fibres with cTnT-F110I, whereas Hernandez et al., 2005 described enhanced Ca^{2+} -sensitivity of force development as well as of actomyosin ATPase activity. One main reason lies in the complexity of the systems used, as reconstituted proteins, skinned fibers, myofibrils, isolated cardiomyocytes (adult or neonatal), transgenic animals. In general results obtained with higher organised system sseem to be more reliable. But additionally species differences might account for differing results. For example according to Rust et al., (1999) overexpression of cTnT-I79N in rat cardiomyocytes resulted in suppressed contractile performance, whereas others using mice myofibrils suggested hypercontractility.

2.1 Mutations in TNNT2, the gene encoding cTnT

Most mutations in TNNT2 detected in patients lead to familial hypertrophic cardiomyopathy (HCM), only a few to restricted cardiomyopathy (RCM) or dilated hypertrophic cardiomyopathy (DCM) (Table 1). Families with DCM mutations in TNNT2 mostly exhibit a severe disease progression with poor prognosis.

2.1.1 HCM inducing mutations

HCM-mutations in TNNT2 are found in about 10% of the HCM cases, and thus TNNT2 belongs to the more abundant troponin disease genes. There is no known HCM mutation which is located within the hypervariable N-terminal region of cTnT. All mutations identified in patients suffering from HCM are located either near or within the N-terminal main interaction site for tropomyosin (amino acids 79-182) or within the C-terminal half (amino acids 203-288) which contains multiple interaction and putative phosphorylation sites (Table 1; Fig. 1). This distribution of mutations implies that they affect the interaction either with tropomyosin (Tm) and/ or the other troponin subunits and might influence phosphorylation dependent effects. The majority of gene loci, where mutations have been identified in patients encode the N-terminal region of cTnT interacting with the overlap of Tm (Table 1; Fig. 1). Mutations in the Tm binding region of cTnT (amino acids 92-183) destabilize Tm binding to actin filaments (Palm et al., 2001). Mutations within the main Tm binding site further weaken the end-to-end Tm interaction, which is responsible for the cooperativity (Palm et al., 2001). Also a lowered affinity of troponin to actin/Tm could be expected. Indeed cTnT-F110I, located at the C-terminal end of the main Tm binding region, impairs binding of troponin to actin/Tm by altering the dynamic properties of the tail region (Hinkle & Tobacman, 2002). It reduces its flexibility. Flexibility of the cTnT-tail is an important feature for its interaction with Tm overlap region (Hinkle & Tobacman, 2002).

Mutation	Disease	Exon/Intron	Reference
Phe70Leu (F70L)	HCM	8	Richard et al., (2003) Circ. 107: 2227-32
Pro77Leu (P77L)	HCM	8	Varnava et al., (2001) Circ. 104: 1380-4
Ile79Asn (I79N)	HCM , RCM, DCM	8	Thierfelder et al., (1994) Cell 77:701-12; Watkins et al., (1995) NEJM. 332: 1058-64; Rust et al., (1999) JCI. 104: 1459-67; Yanaga et al., JBC. (1999) 74:8806-12; Varnava et al., (2001) Circ. 104: 1380-4 ; Palm et al., (2001) Biophys J. 81: 827-37 ; Westermann et al., (2006) Eur J Heart Fail. 8:115-21 ; Menon et al., (2008) Clin Genet, 74(5): 445-54 ; Baudenbacher et al.,(2008) JCI. 118 :3893-903 ; Midde et al., (2011) JMCC [Epub ahead of print]
Glu83Lys (E83K)	HCM	8	Mogensen et al., (2003) J Med Genet 40: e59
Val85Leu (V85L)	HCM	8	Konno et al., (2005) J Intern Med. 258: 216-24.
Asp86Ala (D86A)	HCM	8	Van Driest et al., (2003) Circ. 108: 445-51
Arg92Trp (R92W)	HCM	9	Moolman et al., (1997) JACC. 29: 549-55; Moolman-Smook et al., (1999) Am J Hum Genet. 65:1308-20; Fujino et al., (2001) Clin Cardiol. 24: 397-402; Varnava et al., (2001) Circ. 104:1380-4; Palm et al., (2001) Biophys J. 81:2827-37; Waldmuller et al., Hum Mutat (2002) 19:560-9; Ackerman et al., (2002) JACC. 39: 2042-8; Van Driest et al., (2003) Circ. 108: 445-51; Shimizu et al., (2003) Clin Cardiol 26: 536-9; Konno et al., (2005) J Intern Med. 258:216-24
Arg92Leu (R92L)	HCM	9	Forissier et al., (1996) Circ. 94: 3069-73 ; Varnava et al., (2001) Circ. 104: 1380-4 ; Palm et al., (2001) Biophys J. 81:2827-37 ; Richard et al., (2003) Circ. 107: 2227-32
Arg92Gln (R92Q)	HCM	9	Thierfelder et al., (1994) Cell 77:701-12; Watkins et al., (1995) NEJM. 332:1058-64; Yanaga et al., (1999) JBC. 274: 8806-12; Palm et al., (2001) Biophys J. 81:2827-37 ; Cuda et al., (2002) Hum Mutat 19:309-10; Robinson et al., (2002) JBC. 277: 40710-6; Hinkle & Tobacman (2003)JBC. 278: 506-13; Javadpour et al., (2003) JCI. 112: 768-75; Torricelli et al., (2003) Am J Cardiol 92:1358-62; Van Driest et al., (2004) JACC. 44: 1903-10
Arg94Leu (R94L)	HCM	9	Varnava et al., (1999) Heart 82: 621-4; Varnava et al., (2001) Circ. 104:1380-4 ; Palm et al., (2001) Biophys J. 81:2827-37
Arg94Cys (R94C)	HCM	9	Mogensen et al., (2003) J Med Genet. 40: e59
Lys97Asn (K97N)	HCM	9	Barr, Seidman et al., (2001) originally posted on URL: http://www.cardiogenomics.org
Ala104Val (A104V)	HCM	9	Nakajima-Taniguchi et al., (1997) JMCC. 29: 839-43; Palm et al., (2001) Biophys J. 81: 2827-37 ; Hinkle & Tobacman (2003) JBC. 278: 506-13.

Mutation	Disease	Exon/Intron	Reference
Phe110Ile (F110I)	HCM	9	Watkins et al., (1995) NEJM. 332: 1058-64; Anan et al., (1998) Circ. 98: 391-7; Yanaga et al., (1999) JBC. 274: 8806-12; Lin et al., (2000) Cardiol. 93:155-62 ; Palm et al., (2001) Biophys J. 81: 2827-37 ; Hinkle & Tobacman (2003) JBC. 278: 506-13; Konno et al., (2005) J Intern Med. 258: 216-24; Hernandez et al., (2005) JBC. 280: 37183-94
Phe110Leu (F110L)	HCM	9	Torricelli et al., (2003) Am J Cardiol. 92: 1358-62
Phe110Val (F110V)	HCM	9	Richard et al., (2003) Circ. 107: 2227-32 ; Torricelli F et al., (2003) Am J Cardiol. 92: 1358-62
Lys124Asn (K124N)	HCM	9	An et al., (2004) Zhonghua Xue Za Zhi 84:1 340-3
Arg130Cys (R130C)	HCM	10	Torricelli et al., (2003) Am J Cardiol. 92: 1358-62 ; Song et al., (2005) Clin Chim Acta 351: 209-16
Glu163Lys (E163K)	HCM	11	Watkins et al., (1995) NEJM. 332: 1058-64; Palm et al., (2001) Biophys J. 81: 2827-37
Glu160del (ΔE160)	HCM	11	Watkins et al., (1995) NEJM. 332: 1058-64; Palm et al., (2001)Biophys J. 81: 2827-37 ; Richard et al., (2003) Circ. 107: 2227-32 ; Mogensen et al., (2003) J Med Genet. 40:e59; Torricelli et al., (2003) Am J Cardiol. 92:1358-62; Capek & Skvor (2006) Meth Inf Med. 45: 169-72
Ser179Phe (S179F)	HCM	11	Ho et al., (2000) Circ. 102:1950-5
Glu244Asp (E244D)	HCM	14	Watkins et al., (1995) NEJM. 332: 1058-64; Yanaga et al., (1999) JBC. 274: 8806-12; Moore, Seidman et al., (2004) URL: http://www.cardiogenomics.org
Lys247Arg (K247R)	HCM	14	Garcia-Castro et al., (2003) Clin Chem. 49: 1279-85
Asn271Ile (N271I)	HCM	15	Richard (2003) Circ. 107:2227-32
Lys273Glu (K273E)	HCM	15	Fujino et al., (2002) Am J Cardiol. 89:29-33; Venkatraman et al., (2003) JBC 278: 41670-6; Konno et al., (2005) J Intern Med. 258: 216-24
IVS15+1G>A	HCM	15	Thierfelder et al., (1994) Cell 77: 701-12; Watkins et al., (1995) NEJM. 332: 1058-64; Watkins et al., (1996) JCI. 98: 2456-61. ; Mukherjea et al., (1999) Biochem. 38: 13296-301; Redwood et al., (2000) Circ Res. 86: 1146-52; Varnava et al., (2001) Circ. 104: 1380-4

Mutation	Disease	Exon/Intron	Reference
Arg278Cys (R278C)	HCM	16	Watkins et al., (1995) NEJM. 332:1058-64; Yanaga et al., (1999) JBC. 274:806-12; Elliott et al., (1999) NEJM. 341: 1855-6; Barr, Seidman et al., 2002 and Moore, Seidman et al., (2003, 2004) URL:http://www. cardiogenomics.org; Van Driest et al., (2003) Circ. 108: 445-51; Garcia-Castro et al., (2003) Clin Chem 49: 1279-85; Garcia-Castro et al., (2003) Rev Esp Cardiol. 56: 1022-5; Torricelli (2003) Am J Cardiol 92: 1358-62; Theopistou et al., (2004) Am J Cardiol 94: 246-9; Miliou et al., (2005) Heart 91: 966-7; Hernandez et al., (2005) JBC. 280:371 83-94; Ingles et al., . (2005) J Med Genet. 42:e59, Sirenko et al., (2006) J Physiol. 5755.1: 201-13
Arg278Pro (R278P)	HCM	16	Erdmann et al., 1998. (on-line); Van Driest et al., (2003) Circ. 108: 445-51; Miliou et al., (2005) Heart 91: 966-7
Arg286Cys (R286C)	HCM	16	Richard et al., (2003) Circ. 107: 2227-32 ; Miliou et al., (2005) Heart 91: 966-7
Arg286His (R286H)	HCM	16	Van Driest et al., (2003) Circ. 108: 445-51 ; Van Driest et al., (2004) JACC. 44: 1903-10
Trp287ter (W287ter)	HCM	16	Richard et al., (2003) Circ. 107: 2227-32.
Arg113Trp (R113W)	DCM	9	Mogensen et al., (2004) JACC. 44: 2033-40 ; Mirza et al., (2005) JBC. 280 :28498-506
Arg141Trp (R141W)	DCM	10	Li et al., (2001) Circ. 104:2188-93 ; Venkatraman et al., (2003) JBC. 278: 41670-6 ; Villard et al., (2005) EHJ. 26: 794-803 ; Mirza et al., (2005) JBC. 280 :28498-506
Ala172Ser (A172S)	DCM	11	Stefanelli et al., (2004) Mol Genet Metab. 83: 188-96
Arg205Leu (R205L)	DCM	13	Mogensen et al., (2004) JACC 44: 2033-40; Mirza et al., (2005) JBC. 280 :28498-506
Lys210del (ΔK210)	DCM	13	Kamisago et al., (2000) NEJM. 343: 1688-96; Hanson et al., (2002) J Card Fail. 8 : 28-32 ; Venkatraman et al., (2003) JBC 278: 41670-6 ; Mogensen et al., (2004) JACC 44: 2033-40.
Asp270Asn (D270N)	DCM	15	Mirza et al., (2005) JBC. 280 :28498-506
Glu96del (ΔE96)	RCM	9	Peddy et al., (2006) Pediatrics 117:1830-3; Pinto et al., (2008) JBC. 283:2156-66
Asn100del/Glu101 Del (ΔN100/ΔE101)	RCM	9	Pinto et al., (2011)JBC 286:20901-12 (double mutation)
Glu136Lys (E136K)	RCM	10	Kaski et al., (2008) Heart 94:1478-84

Updated from: Genomics of Cardiovascular Development, Adaptation, and Remodeling. NHLBI Program for Genomic Applications, Harvard Medical School. [*june, 2011 accessed*] and OMIM database. ter designates termination of sequence resulting in a truncated protein, del and Δ are synonyms for a deleted amino acid. The one letter code is given in brackets.

Table 1. Mutations in TNNT2

Since the cTnT- N-terminus contributes to the inhibition of the actin/myosin interaction (Tobacman, 1988), one might assume that also inhibition is affected by mutations. Indeed inhibition of is reduced due to cTnT-F110I (Knollmann & Potter, 2001; Gomes et al., 2004). A similar decrease in inhibition has been described for I79N (Yanaga et al., 1999), though this amino acid exchange is positioned N-terminally of the main Tm interaction site. Nevertheless I79N and F110I exhibit several similarities. Thus, Midde et al., 2011 showed that rigor crossbridges in I79N or F110I containing filaments were disordered, indicating that disruption in thin filament structure may lead to severe contractile dysfunction. I79N, as most investigated HCM mutants, enhances the Ca^{2+}- sensitivity of force development and actomyosin ATPase activity, which might contribute to enhanced contractility and higher energy consumption (Lin et al., 1996; Sweeney et al., 1998; Chandra et al., 2005). Furthermore, mouse hearts with I79N or R92Q could not increase cardiac performance upon ß-adrenergic stimulation (Knollmann et al., 2001; Javadpour et al., 2003), performance of I79N transgenic even worsened upon isoproterenol treatment (Sirenko et al., 2006). Such an effect as well as Ca^{2+} –sensitivity increase has not been observed with a R278C, a mutation located in the cTnT-C-terminus. These findings suggest that the region around amino acids 79 and 92 is important for Ca^{2+} -signal transmission and affects Ca^{2+}-regulation. Furthermore dysfunction is especially prominent under ß-adrenergic stimulation, which might explain the high risc for cardiac sudden death of these mutations. Causality between enhanced Ca^{2+}-sensitivity and the potential for the development of malignant arrhythmias has been shown by Baudenbacher et al., (2008) for I79N. They described altered action potential duration due to the mutation.

Mutations in TNNT2 gene encoding the C-terminal half of cTnT might affect the interaction with tropomyosin at the second Ca^{2+} -dependent binding site, as well as binding to cTnI and cTnC. Most mutations in this part lead either to single amino acid exchanges, deletions of single amino acids or to C-terminally truncated cTnT molecules due to splice site mutations. IVS15+1G>A is a splicing donor mutant which might result in two truncated proteins. In one mutant exon 16 is skipped encoding the C-terminal 14 amino acids, in the other mutants seven amino acids replace the C-terminal 28 amino acids encoded by exon 15 and 16 (Thierfelder et al., 1994). Both mutants are able to form a heterotrimeric troponin complex, however their affinity towards cTnI is drastically reduced (Mukherjea et al., 1999). The impaired interaction with cTnI may be the cause for reduced inhibitory capacity of troponin at low Ca^{2+}-concentrations described by Redwood et al., (2000) and accelerated cross bridge kinetics (Stelzer et al., 2004). Furthermore a reduced binding of troponin to the thin filament has been reported dependent on its regulatory states (Knollmann & Potter, 2001; Burhop et al., 2001), indicating that the C-terminal part of cTnT stabilizes binding of cTn to the thin filament and affects Ca^{2+} -regulation. Increased Ca^{2+}-sensitivity and cooperativity (Nakaura et al., 1999)) and impaired switching off myosin cycling at low Ca^{2+}-concentrations is observed (Burhop et al., 2001). Up to date nearly nothing is known on how cardiomyopathy inducing mutations in TNNT2 influence phosphorylation dependent effects of PKC dependent cTnT or PKA dependent cTnI phosphorylation. According to a study of Nakaura et al., (1999) effects of truncated cTnT were independent on PKA dependent cTnI phosphorylation.

2.1.2 RCM inducing mutations

There are only few RCM mutations detected in TNNT2 (Table 1). Most RCM mutations in genes encoding for cardiac troponin subunits are found in TNNI3 (see below). However, interestingly I79N, originally listed as HCM mutation, might also cause RCM or DCM even in members of the same family. This indicates that other factors besides the mutation, as for example polymorphisms etc. (see below) are determinant for the development of the specific disease. Also in mice RCM might be evolved by I79N (Table 1). The other two RCM mutations (Table 1), a deletion of an acidic residue (E96del) and replacement of a glutamic acid residue by a basic lysine (E136K) have been detected in children developing RCM with very poor prognosis. E96del poorly inhibited actomyosin activity at low Ca^{2+} -concentrations (Pinto et al., 2008) confirming that the cTnT N-terminus is important for the inhibitory capacity of the cardiac troponin complex. A first double deletion (Table 1) leads to the deletion of two amino acids, located adjacently within the main Tm binding site. In filaments with adult, not fetal cTnT an increase in Ca^{2+}-sensitivity and decrease in cooperativity has been observed so far (Pinto et al., 2011).

2.1.3 DCM inducing mutations

Patients with DCM mutations in cTNNT2 exhibit a malignant prognosis as do also most of the FHC mutations in cTNNT2. Investigations on molecular level are largely missing to date. All patients showed decreased cardiac function (Kamisago et al., 2000) in contrast to enhanced contractility often observed in patients and transgenic animals carrying HCM mutations. In accordance *in vitro* analysis of DCM-mutations revealed a decreased Ca^{2+}-sensitivity (Mirza et al., 2005). Venkatraman et al., 2005 showed that ΔK210, the most prominent example for DCM causing cTnT-variation, decreases Ca^{2+}-sensitivity of force and actomyosin ATPase activity as well as maximal force and ATPase activity not only with adult, but also with fetal cTnT. The deletion of K210 occurs in the second Ca^{2+} -sensitive tropomyosin binding region near the PKC phosphorylation site and possibly near the binding site for PKA regulatory subunit II. This implies that Ca^{2+} -regulation as well as PKC dependent phosphorylation of cTnT and/or PKA dependent phosphorylation of other sarcomeric proteins might be affected. Detailed information is missing.

2.2 Mutations in TNNC1, the gene encoding cTnC

Mutations in the TNNC1 gene occur seldom. Far less than 1% of the genetic disorders leading to familial cardiomyopathies in patients are due to mutations in TNNC1. Up to date only six HCM and one DCM inducing mutations, all single amino acid exchanges, have been identified (Fig.2; Table 2). A8V, L29Q and C84Y are located in the N-terminal and N122fs, E134D, D145E and G159D in the C-terminal domain of cTnC (Fig. 2). L29Q was the first mutation detected in the cTnC gene (Hoffmann et al., 2001). Since there was only one family showing this mutation, it is not clear if this mutation causes HCM. However, according to Schmidtmann et al., 2005 and Liang et al., 2008 this amino acid replacement has the potential to cause a cardiomyopathy. Replacement of leucine by glutamine destabilizes the interaction of the N-terminal cTnI arm with cTnC (Schmidtmann et al., 2005; Baryshnikova et al., 2008). The release of the N-terminal cTnI arm occurs also upon bisphosphorylation of cTnI after ß-adrenergic stimulation and contributes to a reduction in Ca^{2+}-sensitivity of the actomyosin ATPase activity (see below). Consistent with this effect for L29Q a small reduction of Ca^{2+}- sensitivity has been described (Schmidtmann et al., 2005). However, in the phosphorylated state of cTnI, an enhanced Ca^{2+}-sensitivity of the actomyosin ATPase activity was observed, indicating an altered ß-adrenergic responsiveness. Divergent results might be obtained in systems differing in complexity

mutation	disease	exon	reference
Leu29Gln (L29Q)	HCM	3	Hoffmann et al., (2001). Hum. Mutat. 17: 524; Dweck et al., (2008). J Biol Chem. 283: 33119-28; Liang et al., (2008). Physiol. Gen. 33:257-66; Schmidtmann et al., (2005). *FEBS J.* 272(23):6087-97.
Ala8Val (A8V)	HCM	1	Landstrom et al., (2008). JMCC 45: 281-288 ; Pinto et al., (2009) JBC. 284(28):19090-100; Pinto et al., (2011).JBC. 286(2):1005-13.
Cys84Tyr (C84Y)	HCM	4	Landstrom et al., (2008). JMCC 45: 281-288. Pinto et al., (2009) JBC. 284(28):19090-100
Gln122Alafsx30 (Q122fs)	HCM	4	Chung et al., (2011) Cardiol. Young [Ehead of print]
Glu134Asp (E134D)	HCM		Pinto et al., (2009) JBC. 284(28):19090-100
Asp145Glu (D145E)	HCM	5	Landstrom et al., (2008). JMCC 45: 281-288. Pinto et al., (2009) JBC. 284(28):19090-100; Pinto et al., (2011).JBC. 286(2):1005-13.
Gly159Asp (G159D)	DCM	6	Mogensen et al., (2004). JACC 44: 2033-2040; Mirza et al., (2005). JBC 280: 28498- 506.

Modified from: OMIM database (http://omim.org); the one letter code is given in brackets; fs designates frameshift.

Table 2. Mutations in TNNC1

(Dweck et al., 2008). Thus, in a higher organized system, namely mouse cardiomyocytes, Liang et al. (2008) described an enhanced Ca^{2+}-sensitivity of force generation dependent on sarcomere length. They showed that also Ca^{2+}- binding affinity to site II was higher in cTnC-L29Q than in cTnC wild type, whereas Ca^{2+}-dissociation rate was not affected. This is in agreement with former findings of Gillis et al., 2005, that residues 2, 28-30 affect Ca^{2+}-binding properties of the regulatory Ca^{2+}-binding site. Replacement of these residues might increase cardiomyocyte contractility. Also the other FHC mutation in TNNC1, leading to A8V, C84Y and D145E replacements in cTnC, enhance Ca^{2+} -sensitivity of force development (Landstrom et al., 2008). For E134D no influence on Ca^{2+}-sensitivity could be observed. It remains unclear how this mutation leads to contractile dysfunction. Since E134 is located near contact sites of cTnI around Ser43/45 effects of PKC dependent phosphorylation might be influenced. Also A8V in the N-terminal helix of cTnC- N-lobe is located near a contact site with cTnI- Ser43 in H1 of cTnI (Li et al., 2004, Takeda et al., 2003). No data on the impact of these mutations on PKC phosphorylation are available up to date.

The proximity of A8 and E134 to the same cTnI region underlines findings of Smth et al. (1999) that the cTnC-N-terminal helix is spatially near the C-lobe. Latest kinetical investigations by Pinto et al, (2011a) showed that Ca^{2+} off rates are delayed for A8V and D145E, both stabilizing cross bridges. Thus structural disturbances at the cTnC-N-terminus not only alter structure of the N- but also of the C-terminal lobe and vice versa and may impair cTnC-cTnI interaction. C84Y is located at the end of the EF hand helix flanking regulatory Ca^{2+}- binding loop at the transition to the central linker region. This residue probably is involved in forming the binding platform for the cTnI switch region and thus might destabilize binding of cTnI in Ca^{2+} -saturated state of cTnC (Fig. 2). D145E is located in Ca^{2+} -binding loop IV, in +Z position (see above) indicating that divalent cation binding might be affected (Pinto et al., 2009). Another amino acid exchange in the C-terminal lobe, G159D, is linked to DCM. Consistent with all other investigated DCM causing mutations G159D reduces Ca^{2+}-sensitivity of the actin-myosin interaction and decreases contractility (Mirza et al., 2005). The hydrophobic residues at position 156,157 and 160 make contact to cTnI (Gasmi-Seabrook et al., 1999). Thus the G156D exchange may considerably disturb the hydrophobic interaction with cTnI and also might affect interaction with cTnT. In the troponin complex G159D reduced the opening (Ca2+ binding) and closing rates (Ca2+ dissociation) of the N-terminal domain of cTnC. Alteration in opening rate was also observed for L29Q, indicating that both mutants alter structural transition kinetics (Dong et al., 2008). PKA dependent phosphorylation of cTnI also affects kinetics in that it enhances the closing rate. This effect was abolished by L29Q and G159D implying that phosphorylation signal transduction is impaired as was earlier proposed for L29Q by Schmidtmann et al. (2005).

2.3 Mutations in TNNI3, the gene encoding cTnI

Most mutations in the gene encoding cTnI, are located in exon 7 and 8, which encode the regulatory C-terminal region of cTnI a few are located in the N-terminal heart specific extension. In patients they mostly induce either HCM or RCM. There are only three mutations identified up to date in TNNI3, which are linked to DCM.

2.3.1 Mutations in TNNI3 linked to HCM

Only one mutation has been identified in exon 3 encoding part of the heart specific N-terminal cTnI arm (Table 3). This mutation results in an R20C (numbering without starter methionine) amino acid exchange, which is located within the consensus sequence for PKA (Fig. 3). The consensus sequence is present in cTnI in a dublicated form (Mittmann et al., 1992) enabling phosphorylation of two adjacent located serine residues (Ser22, 23) by PKA (Fig. 4). The exchange of the middle arginine in a series of three arginine residues (position 20 or 21 dependent on the inclusion of the starter methionine) impairs phosphorylation of the two serine residues and reduces the phosphorylation effect *in vitro* as shown by Gomes et al. (2005). Since both phosphorylation sites are affected, susceptibility towards proteolysis is enhanced. Phosphorylation protects to a certain extent towards proteolysis (Barta et al., 2003). But also the amino acid exchange itself might enhance susceptibility towards protein degradationas proposed by Gomes et al. (2005). Thus probably impairment of PKA dependent phosphorylation as well as enhanced protein digestion might be the main effect of this mutant protein for disease development.

...RRRSSNY.....
▲
20 * *

*Designates phosphorylation sites, arg 20 is indicated

Fig. 4. Consensus sequence in cTnI for PKA.

The first 6 mutations in TNNI3 causing HCM were described by Kimura et al. (1997) (Table 3). R145G, for example, is located within the inhibitor region of cTnI, which binds to actin/tropomyosin at low intracellular Ca^{2+} -concentrations (relaxed state) and blocks actin/myosin interaction (Fig. 3). Mutations located in the inhibitory region most probably affect inhibitory capacity of cTnI by altering actin/cTnI interaction in the relaxed state. Indeed R145G in fibers resulting from transgenic mice reduce inhibition (James et al., 2000; Wen et al., 2008) and binding affinity towards actin. Ca^{2+} -sensitivity of force development in skinned papillary muscles from these mice was enhanced with maximal force being decreased (Krüger et al., 2005; Wen et al ., 2008). These findings are in accordance with enhanced Ca^{2+}-sensitivity and reduced maximal actomyosin ATPase activity described by Deng et al. (2001). Also energy consumption in transgenic mice was increased as shown by Wen et al., 2008, indicating hypercontractility. In isolated rat cardiomyocytes as in myofibrils from transgenic mice contractile parameters were reduced (James et al., 2000; Kruger et al., 2005; Reis et al., 2008) and Ca^{2+} -regulation and ß -adrenergic response was impaired (Lang et al., 2002; Reis et al., 2008). The dynamic properties of contraction were severely suppressed upon ß- adrenergic stimulation (Reis et al., 2008). This again supports the idea that impairment of ß- adrenergic signaling might be important for disease development. Furthermore, R145G might also affect PKC dependent phosphorylation at Thr144, which has not been investigated thoroughly yet. Kobayashi et al. (2004) showed that effects of exchange of all PKC sites Thr144/ Ser43/45 by a glutamic acid residue, which is thought to mimic phosphorylation, are reduced due to the mutation. Pseudophosphorylated PKC sites reduce the Ca^{2+} -dependent opening of the N-terminal lobe of cTnC (Kobayashi et al., 2004). However, a more differentiated analysis is needed.

Mutations in the switch region (Table 3, Fig. 3), which binds to the N-terminal lobe of cTnC upon Ca^{2+}-saturation, are thought to impair binding to N-terminal lobe of cTnC under Ca^{2+}-saturating conditions. Thus, they probably affect Ca^{2+}- dissociation from cTnC and the conformational switch of cardiac troponin I needed for transmission of the Ca^{2+}- signal. An example for such a mutation is Ala157Val.

Mutations located in the mobile C terminal cTnI region may alter cTnI Tm/actin interaction. This may affect inhibition as well as activation. The mobile C-terminus together with N-terminal part of cTnT of the opposing troponin complex stabilizes the tropomyosin position in the blocked state. Indeed for C-terminally truncated cTnI impaired relaxation kinetics, enhanced Ca^{2+} sensitivity and disturbed cooperativity has been observed (Narolska et al., 2006, Tachampa et al., 2009). A small decrease in inhibitory capacity has been described for R162W and K185del (Redwood et al., 1998). Mutations located at the very C-terminus of cTnI as G203S or K206Q do not exhibit an effect on inhibition (Deng et al., 2003, Köhler et al, 2003). Again there are conflicting results concerning Ca^{2+}-sensitivity alterations. Transgenic mice with cTnI-G203S exhibit altered Ca^{2+} -regulation and show prominent altered expression of cytosketetal, contractile proteins and of proteins involved in energy production (Tsoutsman et al., 2006; Lam et al., 2007). Not much is known about other mutations at the same position, G203R (replacement of glycin by the positively charged larger and less flexible amino acid arginine) and a frameshift (fs) mutation (table 3). One would expect that dysfunction due to these sequence alterations are more prominent than for G203S. Also K206Q is not well characterized. It enhances maximal actomyosin ATPase activity and alters dynamics of the actin myosin interaction (Deng et al., 2003). According to our own latest investigations (abstract, Saes et al., DGK, Mannheim April 2011) this part of cTnI interacts with actin; the replacement of lysine in position 206 by glutamine abolishes cTnI-C-terminus/actin interaction indicating a stabilization of the activated state. Furthermore, K206Q as well as G203S impair transduction of the PKA dependent phosphorylation signal *in vitro* (Deng et al., 2003). This implies that PKA dependent phosphorylation at the cTnI-N-terminus modulates not onlyfunction of inhibitory and switch region, but also of the mobile domain.

2.3.2 Mutations in TNNI3 linked to RCM

Mutations linked to RCM occur mostly in the regulatory domain as do HCM inducing mutations and may share even the same locus (Table 3). Thus for example R145G induces FHC and R145W, RCM. Indeed RCM and HCM have some clinical as well as molecular characteristics in common. Both diseases show diastolic dysfunction and all RCM mutations investigated lead to enhanced Ca^{2+}- sensitivity as do most of the HCM inducing mutations. Many of them reduce maximal tension a well as maximal actomyosin ATPase activity and impair inhibition (Gomes et al., 2005; Davis et al., 2008; Kobayashi & Solaro, 2006; for review see Parvatayar et al., 2010). Thus it is unclear how the RCM phenotype develops. But it indicates that the type of exchange (for example R145G HCM and R145W RCM) might be important for the disease development. A glycine exhibits a much smaller van der Waals volume, higher flexibility and higher hydrophilicity than a tryptophan at the same position and thus may alter interactions and dynamic properties very differently. Ca^{2+}-regulation is accompanied by allosteric transitions which are dependent on dynamic properties of the proteins involved. Thus alteration in dynamic properties affects Ca^{2+} regulation and might determine the type of dysfunction (Lassalle, 2010).

2.3.3 Mutations in TNNI3 linked to DCM

The first mutation identified (autosomal recessive) is located at the very N-terminal end of the heart specific N-terminal arm of cTnI and leads to a conservative replacement of the amino acid alanine by valine, which both are hydrophobic (Table 3). However, in contrast to alanine, valine is branched, takes double of the van der Waals volume and has a higher hydropathy index. These altered physicochemical properties might produce local structure disturbances and therefore modify interactions. According to Murphy et al., 2004 this amino acid exchange affects cTnI/cTnT interaction, though no direct interaction of the N-terminal arm with cTnT has been described so far. There are several contacts of the non phosphorylated N-terminus with cTnC- N-terminal lobe and of the phosphorylated N-terminus with the regulatory C-terminal region of cTnI. The mechanism how this mutation may alter cTnI/cTnI interaction is not clear. Further investigations are needed. Lately Carballo et al. (2009) described two new DCM mutations in cTNNI3 with an autosomal dominant trait leading to a severe onset of the disease. K36Q is located near constitutive cTnC interaction site and in the putative hinge region important for phosphorylation dependent movement of the cTnI-N-terminal arm. Therefor this mutation possibly might affect structural integrity of the troponin complex and ß-adrenergic responsiveness. N185K is located within the mobile cTnI C-terminal region. *In vitro* both amino acid replacements reduce Ca^{2+} -sensitivity of the actomyosin ATPase and decreased maximal ATPase activity (Carballo et al., 2009) considered as typical for DCM.

mutation	disease	exon	reference
Arg21Cys (R21C / R20C)	HCM	3	Barr, Seidman et al. (2001) first posted on URL: http: //www. cardiogenomics.org; Arad et al., (2005) Circ. 112:2805-1 ; Gomes et al.,(2005) JMCC 39 :754-65
Arg141Gln (R141Q)	HCM	7	Richard et al., (2003) Circ. 107:2227-32 ; Van Driest et al., (2003) Circ. 108 : 445-51
Leu144Pro (L144P)	HCM	7	Merk, Seidman et al., (2005) first posted on URL:http://www. cardiogenomics.org
Arg145Gly (R145G/R146G)	HCM	7	Kimura et al., (1997) Nat Genet. 16:379-82. Takahashi-Yanaga, et al., (2000) J Biochem (Tokyo) 127:355-7, Elliott et al. (2000) JBC 275:22069-74 ; Deng et al., (2001) Biochem. 40:14593-602; Takahashi-Yanaga et al., (2001)JMCC 33:2095-107 ; Lang et al., (2002) JBC 277(4):11670-8 ; Burton et al., (2002) Biochem J 362:443-51 ; Lindhout et al., (2002) Biochem 41:7267-74 and (2005) Biochem 44:14750-9; Kruger et al., (2005) J Physiol 564: 347-57, Wen et al.,(2008) JBC 283: 20484-94; Reis et al., (2008) *Pflugers Arch.* 457:17-24
Arg145Gln (R145Q)	HCM	7	Kimura et al., (1997) Nat Genet 16:379-82 ; Taka-hashi-Yanaga et al., (2001) JMCC 33: 2095-107; Mogensen et al., (2004) JACC 44: 2315-25.
Ala157Val (A157V)	HCM	7	Richard et al., (2003) Circ. 107: 2227-32 ; Mogensen et al., (2004) JACC 44:2315-25; Brito & Madeira (2005)Rev Port Cardiol. 24:1137-46 ; Meder et al., (2009) J Cardiol 15: 274-8
Arg162Trp (R162W)	HCM	7	Kimura et al., (1997) Nat Genet 16: 379-82; Elliott et al., (2000) JBC 275: 22069-74; Takahashi-Yanaga et al., (2001) JMCC 33: 2095-107
Arg162Gln (R162Q)	HCM	7	Van Driest et al., (2003) Circ.108: 445-51; Mogensen et al., (2004) JACC 44: 2315-25 ; Doolan et al., (2005) JMCC 2005 38: 387-93; Cheng et al., (2005) JACC 46:180-1; Ingles et al., (2005) J Med Genet. 42 :e59.
Arg162Pro (R162P)	HCM	7	Richard et al., (2003)Circ. 2003 107: 2227-32; Doolan et al., (2005) JMCC 38: 387-93; Ingles et al., (2005) J Med Genet. 42: e59
Ser166Phe (S166F)	HCM	7	Van Driest et al., (2003) Circ. 108: 445-51; Van Driest et al., (2004) JACC 44: 1903-10; Mogensen et al., (2004) JACC 44: 2315-25
Lys178del (ΔK178)	HCM	7	Richard et al., (2003) Circ. 107: 2227-32
Lys183Glu (K183E)	HCM	7	Mogensen et al., (2004) JACC 44: 2315-25

mutation	disease	exon	reference
Lys183del (ΔK183)	HCM	7	Kimura et al., (1997) Nat Genet. 16: 379-82; Kokado et al., (2000) Circ. 102: 663-9; Takahashi-Yanaga et al., (2001) JMCC 33: 2095-107; Kohler et al., (2003) Physiol Gen. 14: 117-28 ; Konno et al., (2005) J Int Med. 258: 216-24.
Arg186Gln (R186Q)	HCM	8	Richard et al., (2003) Circ. 107:2227-32; Mogensen et al., (2004) JACC 44: 2315-25
Ile195Met (I195M)	HCM	8	Barr, Seidman et al., (2001) first posted on URL: http://www. cardiogenomics.org
Asp196Asn (D196N)	HCM	8	Richard et al., (2003) Circ. 107: 2227-32; Mogensen et al., (2004) JACC 44: 2315-25; Nimura et al., (2002) Circ. 105 : 446-51
Leu198Val (L198V)	HCM	8	Merk, Seidman et al., (2005) first posted on URL:http://www. cardiogenomics.org
Leu198Pro (L198P)	HCM	8	Doolan et al., (2005) JMCC 38: 387-93
Ser199Gly (S199G)	HCM	8	Mogensen et al., (2004) JACC 44: 2315-25
Ser199Asn (S199N)	HCM	8	Mogensen et al., (2004) JACC 44: 2315-25; Brito & Madeira (2005) Rev Port Cardiol. 24: 1137-46
Glu202Gly (E202G)	HCM	8	Mogensen et al., (2004) JACC 44: 2315-25
Gly203Arg (G203R)	HCM	8	Mogensen et al., (2004) JACC 44: 2315-25
Gly203Ser (G203S)	HCM/ Wolff Parkinson syndrom	8	Kimura et al., (1997) Nat Genet. 16:379-82; Kokado et al., (2000) Circ. 102: 663-9 ; Takahashi-Yanaga et al., (2001) JMCC 33: 2095-107 ; Burton D et al., (2002) Biochem J 362: 443-51; Kohler et al., (2003) Physiol Gen. 14: 117-28, Deng et al., (2003) JMCC 35: 1365-74; Tsoutsman et al., (2006) JMCC 41: 623-32; Nguyen et al., (2007) Int J Cardiol. 119: 245-8; Lam et al., (2010) JMCC 48: 1014-22
Gly203fs (G203fs)	HCM	8	Morner et al., (2000) JMCC 32: 521-5 and (2003) 35: 841-9; Richard et al., (2003) Circ. 107: 2227-32
Arg204Cys (R204C)	HCM	8	Barr, Seidman et al., (2002) first posted on URL: http://www. cardiogenomics.org
Arg204His (R204H)	HCM	8	Doolan et al., (2005) JMCC 38: 387-93; Ingles et al., (2005) J Med Genet. 42: e59
Lys206Gln (K206Q)	HCM	8	Kimura et al., (1997) Nat Genet. 16:379-82; Taka-hashi-Yanaga et al., (2001) JMCC 33: 2095-107; Kohler et al., (2003) Physiol Gen. 14: 117-28; Deng et al., (2003) JMCC 35: 1365-74
Ala2Val (A2V)	DCM, recessive	1	Murphy et al., (2004) Lancet 363: 371-2
Lys36Gln (K36Q)	DCM, dominant	3	Carballo et al., (2009) Circ. 105 : 375-82
Asn135Lys (N135K)	DCM dominant	7	Carballo et al., (2009) Circ. 105 : 375-82
Leu144Gln (L144Q)	RCM	7	Mogensen et al., (2003) JCI 111:209-16; Gomes et al., (2005) JBC 280: 30909-15
Arg145Trp (R145W)	RCM	7	Mogensen et al., (2003) JCI 111: 209-16; Mogensen et al., (2004) JACC 44: 2315-25; Gomes et al., (2005) JBC 280: 30909-15; Cheng (2005) J Am Coll Cardiol 46: 180-1

mutation	disease	exon	reference
Ala171Thr (A171T)	R CM	7	Mogensen et al., (2003) JCI 111: 209-16; Gomes et al., (2005) JBC 280: 30909-15
Lys178Glu (K178E)	RCM	7	Mogensen et al., (2003) JCI 111: 209-16; Gomes et al., (2005) JBC 280: 30909-15
Asp190His (R190H)	RCM	8	Mogensen et al., (2003) JCI 111: 209-16; Gomes et al., (2005) JBC 280: 30909-15
Asp190Gly (D190G)	RCM	8	Davis et al., (2008) JMCC 44: 891-904
Arg192His (R192H)	RCM	8	Mogensen et al., (2003) JCI 111: 209-16; Gomes et al., (2005) JBC 280: 30909-15

In brackets the one letter code and positions due to species specifities are given; fs designates frameshift.

Table 3. Mutations in TNNI3

In summary, there seem to be three major factors on the molecular level which help to understand phenotype development and might be directive for future investigations. 1) Mutations might severely affect affinity to other thin filament proteins and/or enhance susceptibility to proteolysis. In both cases structural integrity of the thin filament would be disturbed, which would in turn affect contractile function. It might even affect sarcomeric structure. 2) Mutations alter dynamical properties of the protein. Changes in dynamics might affect inter- and intramolecular interactions, Ca^{2+}-regulation, ß -adrenergic responsiveness and PKC mediated phosphorylation and thereby may induce contractile dysfunction in various degrees. 3) Combinations of mutations might lead to additive or compensatory effects.

3. Clinical presentation

3.1 Diagnosis of HCM

In 1989 (Jarcho et al., 1989) and 1990 (Geisterfer-Lowrance et al., 1990), the first "disease genes" have been identified in family members with inherited hypertrophic cardiomyopathy (HCM). This identification of disease genes has raised many expectations, among others in the better understanding of the molecular mechanisms of disease development, in a more reliable identification of patients at risk, and in new concepts of treatment (Keren et al.; 2008, Lippi et al., 2009; Marian, 2010; Ho, 2010a; Watkins et al, 1995; 2011). The following paragraphs will focus on the clinical presentation of patients with mutations in the genes encoding troponin C, T and I (TNNC1, TNNT2, and TNNI3) in the context of HCM. For clinical presentation of HCM patients in general the reader is referred to an excellent book chapter from Fatkin et al., (2007).

HCM is clinically suggested in patients by the presence of unexplained left ventricular hypertrophy (LVH, usually defined as ventricular wall thickness ≥ 15 mm or ≥ 13 mm in relatives of a HCM patient; Elliott et al., 2008) and a non-dilated left ventricle with preserved or even enhanced global systolic function (Fig.5). Diagnosis relies on the electrographic and echocardiographic demonstration of hypertrophy. LVH may be diffuse or more segmentally distributed (proximal and/or midportion of the interventricular septum, apex, anterior or lateral wall), but no single morphologic expression appears to be specific (Klues et al., 1995). In fact, differentiation of LVH secondary to HCM may be difficult from other diseases affecting the ventricles, e.g. hypertrophy secondary to infiltrative diseases (e.g. amyloidosis),

Fabry's disease (Monserrat et al., 2007), glycogen storage disorders (Arad et al., 2005a), or systemic arterial hypertension. These diagnostic difficulties may rise with advanced age.

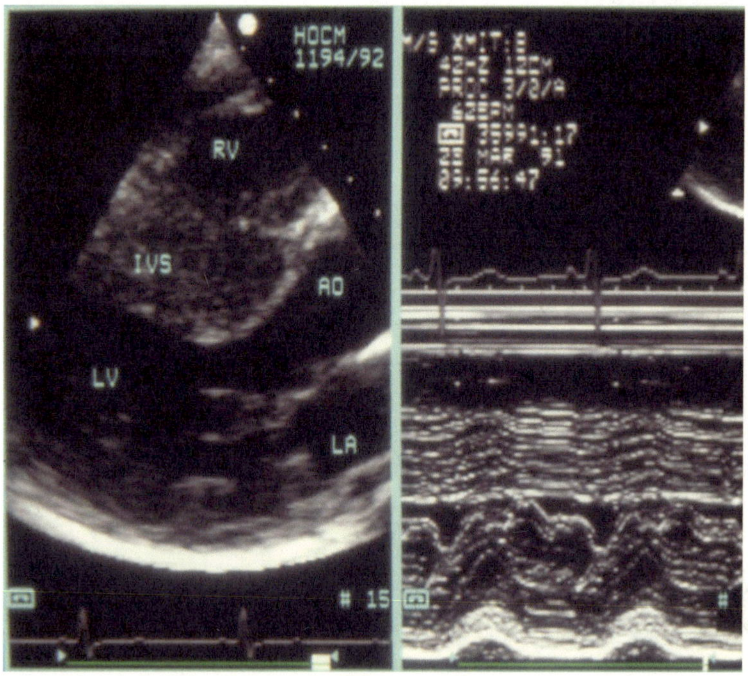

(IVS=septum, LV/RV=left/right ventricles, Ao=aorta ascendens, LA=left atrium)

Fig. 5. 2D and M-mode echocardiogram demonstrating severe hypertrophy (> 25 mm) of the septum

Besides LVH, left ventricular outflow obstruction is one of the most suspicious features of this disease. Braunwald & Ebert (1962) noted first the dynamic component of this obstruction. Later on the systolic anterior motion ("SAM") of the anterior leaflet of the mitral valve was recognized as the major contributor of left ventricular outflow obstruction and the more or less significant accompanying mitral regurgitation (Marian 2010). In a series of 320 consecutive HCM patients, this obstructive pathology at resting conditions (defined as a gradient ≥ 50 mmHg at rest) was found in 37% of patients (Maron et al., 2006). In the remaining patients, 52% developed dynamic outflow gradients during exercise or maneuvers which decrease afterload or increase contractility. These high numbers, however, should be cautiously extrapolated for the general HCM population because of referral bias and patients selection criteria.

Abnormal diastolic function (prolonged LV relaxation and increased LV chamber stiffness) is an almost universal feature of HCM. It appears that diastolic dysfunction is a very early manifestation of HCM, even before morphological evidence of hypertrophy occurs (Nagueh et al., 2001; Ho et al., 2009). Today, diastolic dysfunction is suggested if the ratio between early diastolic peak filling velocity (the E wave in transmitral Doppler) and early diastolic peak velocity of the mitral annulus (the E′ derived from tissue Doppler) exceeds the value 15 in the presence of normal systolic function (Fig. 6; Ommen et al., 2000; Paulus et al., 2007).

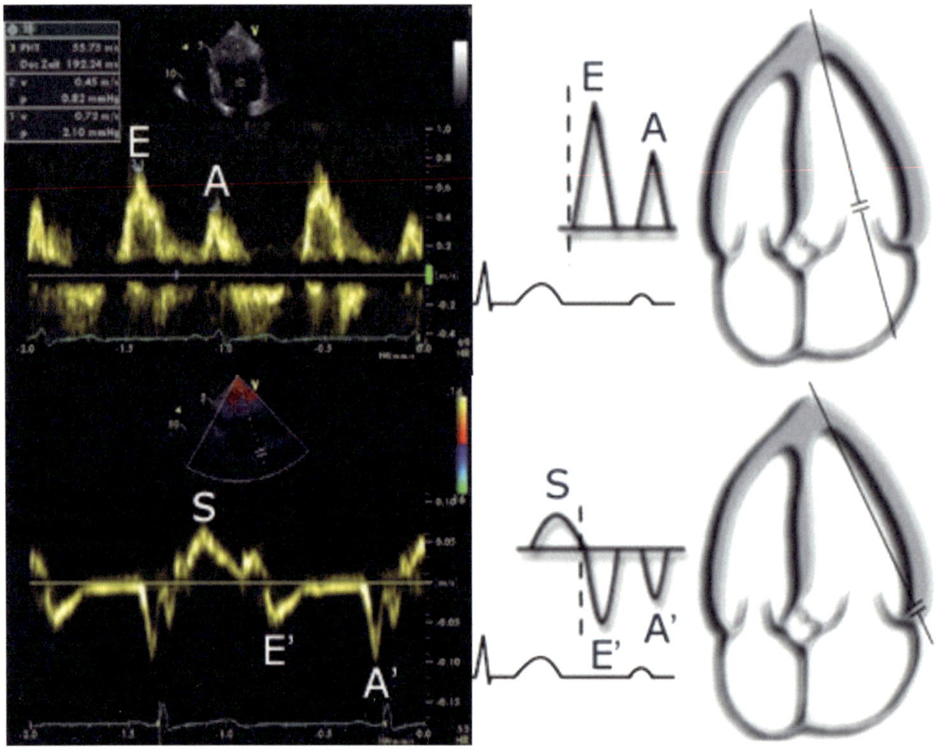

Fig. 6. Transmitral Doppler (top) and tissue Doppler (bottom) allowing quantification of the early diastolic peak filling velocity (E) and early diastolic peak velocity of the mitral annulus (E′). The ratio E/E′ is used to determine diastolic dysfunction.

The clinical presentation of HCM patients shows a remarkable diversity: some individuals experience none or minor symptoms, others may develop dyspnoe at exercise or at rest, angina pectoris, palpitations, atrial fibrillation, dizziness, presyncope and syncope, fatigue or finally end stage heart failure requiring cardiac transplantation (Ho, 2010a).

The changes on ECG are very variable and include left axis deviation, occurrence of Q waves, a positive Sokolow index for hypertrophy, conduction abnormalities, ST-T depression or other abnormalities, negative T waves and giant T waves (particularly observed in Japanese patients with apical type of HCM (Sakamoto et al., 1976). The ECG abnormalities may not parallel hypertrophy in all cases. In fact, ECG abnormalities are more frequently found in HCM patients as echocardiographic abnormalities. Konno et al. (2005) observed ECG abnormalities (in particular ST-T abnormalities) in about 54% of genetically affected, but nonhypertrophic patients at echocardiography. However, almost all of ECG abnormalities (perhaps except giant T waves) are unspecific, and do also occur in patients with advanced age for various other reasons.

The underlying histopathology is characterized by gross cardiac hypertrophy, myocyte hypertrophy, disarray of cardiac cells, interstitial fibrosis, hyperplasia of the media of coronary arteries. The cardiac myocyte disarray (Fig. 7) appears to be a hallmark of HCM, not infrequently involving up to 20% of the ventricles (Maron & Roberts, 1979; Elliot & McKenna, 2004).

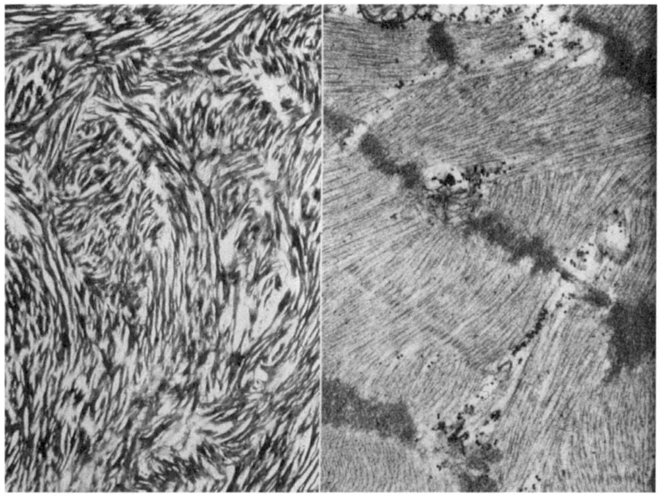

Fig. 7. Histology of the heart of a patient with HCM demonstrating typical disarray of the myocytes and myofibrils.

3.2 Complications and general prognosis in HCM

A major concern in the management of patients with HCM is prognosis. Sudden cardiac death (which may account for 50% of the disease-related death), atrial fibrillation with the risk of stroke, and congestive heart failure (CHF) are the leading contributors to the morbidity and mortality associated with HCM (Keren et al., 2008; Marian 2010). Overall, HCM is a "benign" disease with an annual mortality rate of 0.5-1% in unselected HCM-affected subjects (Cannan et al. 1995). However, sudden death may the first clinical manifestation of this disease, particularly in young otherwise healthy appearing subjects (Maron et al., 1996). In a meta-analysis by Liberthson (1996), HCM was the most frequent single cause of sudden death in children and young adults. This was supported by a large series of Maron (2003) who analyzed 387 young athletes who died suddenly, and found that HCM was the cause in 26.4%. The overall risk of sudden death appears to be similar in males and females (Olivotto et al., 2005), by contrast, 90% of 134 athletes with sudden cardiac death were males (Maron et al., 1996).

The risk for sudden cardiac death can be effectively reduced by the prophylactic implantation of an internal automated defibrillator (ICD), the main problem is, however, to identify those who will profit from this device. So far, no single risk factor (except surviving cardiac arrest) has been identified which may clearly justify prophylactic ICD implantation. Nowadays, a more comprehensive approach is used combining informations/findings (family history of sudden death, severe cardiac hypertrophy, history of presynope or syncope, non-sustained or sustained ventricular tachycardia) (Kofflard et al., 2003; Marian 2003; Frenneaux 2004; Marian 2010). It is a new challenge to integrate genotype testing in this risk assessment algorithm, although the power of genetic testing appears to be up to now more the identification of non-carriers in HCM families obviating the need for clinical screening and follow-up examinations (Keren et al., 2008; Pinto et al., 2011). The ethical, legal and societal implications of genetic testing for cardiac diseases in clinical practice has been discussed elsewhere (Tester & Ackerman, 2011). Furthermore, the pro and contra of genotyping in predicting prognosis in HCM has been recently discussed in Circulation (Ho, 2010b; Landstrom & Ackerman, 2010).

The true penetrance of all clinical presentations is not known and may be underestimated because the clinical diagnosis of HCM is not robust. Furthermore, clinical findings may either vary over time or the disease-related abnormalities may have a variable onset during life. For example, progressive increase in LV wall thickness has been observed in adolescents and young adults with HCM, whereas wall thickness remains to be more stable in the elderly (Maron et al., 1986; Semsarian et al., 1997). This may, however, not be true for all mutations. Revera et al. (2007) re-evaluated 22 carriers with an Arg92Trp (TNNT2 gene) mutation after an average of 11 years. With age, left ventricular hypertrophy increased (≥ 5 mm wall thickness, as assessed by echocardiography) in 50% of individuals. These later points are of particular importance since most clinical studies have a cross-sectional design, and prospective longitudinal studies are scarce.

All groups are in agreement that the phenotypic heterogeneity in HCM patients/families cannot be explained by the genetic defect alone. Other factors must be involved including sex, additional disease such as arterial hypertension, and environmental factors. This heterogeneity is particularly striking in families with one genetic defect, but demonstrating phenotypes of different cardiomyopathies. For example, Menon et al. (2008) identified a large family with a mutation in the TNNT2 gene (Ile79Asn). This mutation affected 9 family members. Mutation carries showed clinically a restrictive cardiomyopathy in 2, a non-obstructive HCM in 3, dilated cardiomyopathy in 2, a mixed cardiomyopathy in 1, and mild concentric hypertrophy in 1 family member. Genetic factors others than the causal sarcomere mutation may affect the penetrance and severity of cardiac abnormalities, referred as the modifier genes. In this regard, variants of the angiotensin-1 converting enzyme (ACE-1) gene are discussed as potential modifiers, increasing the risk for sudden cardiac death (Marian et al., 1993) and the severity of LVH (Lechin et al., 1995). Beside modifier genes, others factors must also determine the phenotype, as pressure or volume load, since manifestations of HCM are predominantly restricted to the LV, although the mutant sarcomeric protein is expressed in both ventricles. Finally, homozygous mutations (as it has been described for a child with a Ser179Phe mutation in the TNNT2 gene who died suddenly at the age of 17 (Ho et al., 2000)), or multiple mutations within the sarcomere protein encoding genes may cause a more severe type of HCM. For example, Girolami et al. (2010) identified in a cohort of 488 unrelated index HCM patients 4 patients (0.8%) who harbored triple mutations of the sarcomere proteins. The triple sarcomere defects were associated with an adverse outcome.

Mutations in the troponin genes (TNNC1, TNNT2, TNNI3) are accounting for less than 10% of patients with HCM. In a large series of 197 index patients living in France, Richard et al. (2003) detected disease-casing mutations in 63%, whereby mutations within the TNNT2 and TNNI3 gene accounted for 4% each.

3.3 TNNT2

In MEDLINE, reports on approx. 194 HCM patients from various living areas with a mutation of the TNNT2 gene have been published so far (Thierfelder et al., 1994; Watkins et al., 1995; Forissier et al., 1996; Moolman et al., 1997; Anan et al., 1998; Elliott et al., 1999; Ho et al., 2000; Varnava et al., 2001; Richard et al., 2003; Van Driest et al, 2003; Garcia-Castro et al., 2003; Torricelli et al., 2003; An et al., 2004; Theopistou et al., 2004; Miliou et al., 2005; Konno et al., 2005; Capek & Skvor, 2006; Menon et al., 2008; Xu et al., 2008; Gimeno et al., 2009). Table 4 summarizes those reports (86 families, 188 genetically affected subjects) which provided at least prognostic informations and/or some data on the phenotype. The median age (at the time of examination) is 40 years, 56.1% are females. Maximal left ventricular wall thickness was less than 15 mm in 49.5% of genetically affected subjects, only in 9.7% of patients, the wall thickness exceeded 25 mm. The ECG was abnormal in the majority of affected subjects (78.8%). Congestive heart failure (CHF, NYHA class ≥ II) was present in 42.9% of subjects. Prognostic data were available for 30 affected families, 19 lamented sudden cardiac death within their families. In additional 31 index patients, sudden cardiac death, heart transplantation or an ICD implantation was reported on 11 patients. Watkins et al. (1995) overlooked a series of 67 subjects over the age of 16 years who had TnT mutations. He noted that 24% of these individuals did not fulfill the clinical diagnostic criteria of HCM. The risk for disease-related death, however, was high (sudden cardiac death, death related to CHF). Varnava et al. (2001) investigated histologically 75 hearts with HCM. Blood samples from relatives and/or affected patients (before death) were available in 50 cases, allowing genotyping. Mutations in the TNNT2 gene were found in 9/50 patients, 8 of the 9 patients died suddenly. The heart weight was less, but the degree of disarray was significantly more in those patients with a mutation of the TNNT2 gene as compared to mutations of other genes. Other authors confirmed this constellation "minor LVH and high risk for sudden cardiac death" particularly for the following mutations: Phe87Leu (Gimeno et al., 2009), Arg92Trp (Moolman et al., 1997), Ala104Val (Nakajima-Taniguchiet et al., 1997), and Lys273Glu (Fujino et al., 2002).

3.4 TNNI3

Reports on approx. 99 patients have been published so far (Kimura et al., 1997; Kokado et al., 2000; Mörner et al., 2000; Niimura et al., 2002; Richard et al., 2003; Van Driest et al., 2003; Mogensen et al., 2004; Arad et al., 2005b; Brito & Madeira, 2005; Doolan et al., 2005; Sheng et al., 2008). Table 5 summarizes the reports (41 families, 87 genetically affected subjects) which provided prognostic informations or some data on phenotype. The median age (at the time of examination) is 46 years, 55.1% are females. Maximal left ventricular wall thickness was less than 15 mm in 53.2% of genetically affected subjects, in none the wall thickness exceeded 25 mm. An abnormal ECG was observed in 90.5% of genetically affected patients. Congestive heart failure was present in 36.4% subjects. In 24 of 37 families, sudden cardiac death or cardiac arrest occurred.

3.5 TNNC1

Only six cases with mutations of the TNNC1 gene have been published so far (Hoffmann et al., 2001; Landstrom et al., 2008; Chung et al., 2011) (Table 6). The first missense mutation within the TNNC1 gene (Leu29Gln) was described by Hoffmann et al. (2001) in a 60 year-old man with a moderate LV hypertrophy, ECG abnormalities and heart failure. The number of cases is too low to characterize a typical phenotype. Three of the 6 cases underwent myectomie, in a 19 year-old man, sudden cardiac death occurred.

3.6 Prognosis in patients with mutations of the genes encoding cTnT and cTnI

Overall, patients with mutations within the gene encoding cardiac troponin T and I are characterized by minor/moderate left ventricular hypertrophy, the maximal wall thickness of the LV does exceed 25 mm in a small percentage only. Despite the presence of minor/moderate LV hypertrophy, the rate of abnormal ECGs is high (> 75%). Furthermore,

congestive heart failure is not an infrequent complication (35-40% of the genetically affected patients). The rate of sudden cardiac death/arrest appears to be very high (> 30% of index patients or in related family members). Whereas some mutations are associated with sudden cardiac death at any age (e.g. the Lys183 deletion mutation in he TNNI3 gene; Kokado et al., 2000), others are associated with disease-related death predominantly in older carriers (e.g. the Phe87Leu mutation within the TNNT2 gene; Gimeno et al., 2009), or at younger age (e.g. the Arg92Trp mutation within troponin T; Moolman et al., 1997). Of note, the degree of disarray of the myocytes may not parallel the magnitude of hypertrophy: Gambrin et al. (2008) described a 22 year old women who underwent cardiac transplantation for restrictive filling pattern and CHF. Histology revealed severe disarray in the absence of hypertrophy. Genetic analysis disclosed an Arg204His mutation in the TNNI3 gene.
The mechanism of sudden cardiac death in patients with HCM is still under debate (Ho, 2010 a,b). For many years, the ischemia hypothesis has been proposed, that is increased oxygen demand due to increased LV mass and wall stress, combined with reduced oxygen supply due to reduced capillary density and abnormal narrowed intramural coronary arteries. This balance may further deteriorate if myocardial bridging with systolic compression of epicardial coronary artery is present (Yetman et al., 1998). The ischemia hypothesis is supported by a study of Spirito et al. (2000). These authors investigated the relation between the magnitude of hypertrophy and mortality in 480 consecutive patients with HCM. Over a follow-up period of 6.5 years, 65 patients died (23 sudden death, 15 CHF-related, 27 noncardiac cause or stroke). The risk of sudden death increased progressively with the wall thickness (0 per 1000 person-years for a wall thickness ≤ 15 mm, up to 18.2 per 1000 person-years for those with a wall thickness ≥ 30 mm).

3.7 What we can learn from patients with troponin mutations

What can we learn from the patients with troponin mutations? One important message to the clinicians is that the risk of sudden cardiac death does not go along with the severity of left ventricular hypertrophy/wall thickness. Furthermore, sudden cardiac death may occur in all age groups with troponin mutations. These observations imply that other mechanisms than ischemia-triggered rhythm disturbances may account for the excessive risk of sudden cardiac death in this subgroup (and other subgroups?) of patients with HCM. In transgenic mice expressing the TnT-I79N (Ile79Asn) mutation, no ventricular hypertrophy or fibrosis was detected, but ventricular ectopy and the rate of stress-induced ventricular tachycardia were significantly increased (Knollmann et al, 2003). Baudenbacher et al. (2008) showed in this mouse model that the risk of developing ventricular tachycardia appears to be directly proportional to the degree of Ca^{2+} sensitization caused by different troponin T mutations (TnT-I79N, TnT-F110I, and TnT-R278C). They gave first evidence that reduction of Ca^{2+} -sensitivity (by blebbistatin) in myofilaments acts "antiarrhythmic". This work by Baudenbacher and coworkers clearly demonstrates that changes in the intracellular Ca^{2+} -sensor cardiac troponin are associated with arrhythmias, and histological/anatomical changes which do often later develop in the course of hypertrophic cardiomyopathy, are not a prerequisite for these life-threatening arrhythmias. In our laboratory, we studied the effects of the cTnI-R145G mutation on adrenergic signalling in isolated rat ventricular cardiomyocytes (Reis et al., 2008). This mutation hinders the transduction of the phosphorylation signal from troponin to the thin filament. Upon adrenergic stimulation of the cardiomyocytes, rates of shortening and relengthening were significantly suppressed.

This suppression was evident in response to ß2- but not ß1-adrenergic stimulation. These data demonstrate that adrenoceptor-mediated signalling may be altered by troponin mutations. Since sudden cardiac death in patients with HCM often occurs during exercise or physical activity, thus conditions with increased sympathetic activity, altered adrenergic signalling may be a potential player in the pathogenesis of life-threatening arrhythmias.
Many other mechanism are currently under investigation, including the role of the myocyte enhancer factor 2, transforming growth factor, connective tissue factor, and periostin in the development of hypertrophy, diastolic dysfunction, and myocardial scarring (Seidman & Seidman, 2011); also altered intracellular calcium handling and abnormalities in myocardial energetics are under discussion to participate in this complex phenotype (Ho, 2010a,b). Despite obvious progress, the precise link between the molecular defect and the complex phenotype HCM is still not understood.

Patients/ Family	Clinical Presentation							References
	Age/Sex	Septum (mm)	Wall (mm)	LVH type+	ECG	CHF	Prognosis	
Ser69Phe								
n=1 (9 unrelated SCD) Area: U.K.	29 M	n.a.	n.a.	n.a.	n.a.	n.a.	SCD	Varnava et al., 2001
Pro77Leu								
n=1 (9 unrelated SCD) Area: U.K.	37 M	n.a.	n.a.	n.a.	n.a.	n.a.	SCD	Varnava et al., 2001
Ile79Asn								
n=9 (1 family + unrelated p.) Area: multi-ethnic/racial	n.a.	13.4±4 (n=4)	n.a.	n.a.	n.a.	n.a.	4 SCD in family	Watkins et al., 1995
n=1 (9 unrelated SCD) Area: U.K.	16 M	n.a.	n.a.	n.a.	n.a.	n.a.	SCD	Varnava et al., 2001
n=9 (1 family) Area: U.S.A.	50 F[1]	n.a.	n.a.	n.a.	n.a.	+	DCM, death at age 64	Menon et al., 2008
	68 F	10	9	normal	+	+	DCM, death at age 73	
	66 F[1]	18	10	n.a.	+	+	-	
	46 M[1]	16	12	n.a.	+	+	mixed DCM/HCM	
	58 M[1]	12	10	normal	+	+	RCM type	
	53 F[1]	14	11	n.a.	+	+	RCM type	
	49 F[1]	16	9	n.a.	+	+	-	
	40 F[1]	24	8	n.a.	+	+	-	
	48 F	14	10	n.a.	-	-	-	

Patients/ Family	Clinical Presentation							References
	Age/Sex	Septum (mm)	Wall (mm)	LVH type+	ECG	CHF	Prognosis	
Asp86Ala								
n=1(389 unrelated p.) Area: U.S.A.	39 M	n.a.	30	n.a.	n.a.	+	-	Van Driest et al., 2003
Phe87Leu								
n=7 (1 family) Area: Spain	52 F	14	n.a.	n.a.	+	+	SCD in family	Gimeno et al., 2009
	39 M	13	n.a.	n.a.	+	+	"	
	40 F	14	n.a.	n.a.	+	+	", ICD	
	30 F	18	n.a.	n.a.	+	+	", ICD	
	30 M	27	n.a.	n.a.	+	-	"	
	29 F	25	n.a.	n.a.	+	+	"	
	9 M	12	n.a.	n.a.	+	-	"	
Arg92Gln								
n=1 (150 unrelated p.) Area: Toscana	23 M	29	n.a.	III	+	-	-	Thierfelder et al., 1994; Torricelli et al., 2003
n=32 (3 families + unrelated p.) Area : multi-ethnic/racial	n.a.	n.a.	15.0±6 (n=21)	n.a.	n.a.	n.a.	SCD in 11 p	Watkins et al., 1995
Arg92Trp								
n=18 (2 families) Area: South Africa	56 F	14	12	n.a.	+	n.a.	SCD in family	Moolman et al., 1997
	57 F	13	12	n.a.	+	n.a.	"	
	41 F	12	13	n.a.	+	n.a.	"	
	28 F	24	11	n.a.	+	n.a.	"	
	35 F	13.8	7.5	n.a.	-	n.a.	"	
	23 F	6	6	-	+	n.a.	"	
	21 M	normal	normal	-	+	n.a.	"	
	38 M	9	9	-	+	n.a.	"	
	35 F	8	8	-	+	n.a.	"	
	28 M	7	8	-	+	n.a.	"	
	47 F	7	7	-	-	n.a.	"	
	27 F	6	6	-	-	n.a.	"	
	9 F	4	4	-	-	n.a.	"	
	28 M	8.5	8.5	-	-	n.a.	"	
	15 F	5	5	-	-	n.a.	"	
	11 F	7	7	-	-	n.a.	"	
	34 F	18-20	11	n.a.	+	n.a.	"	
	56 F	8	7	-	+	n.a.	"	
n=1 (389 unrelated p.) Area : U.S.A.	27 F	n.a.	32	n.a.	n.a.	-	-	Van Driest et al., 2003
n=2(9 unrelated SCD) Area.U.K.	22 M	n.a.	n.a..	n.a.	n.a.	n.a.	SCD	Varnava et al., 2001
	6 F	n.a.	n.a.	n.a.	n.a.	+	transplant	

Patients/ Family	Age/Sex	Clinical Presentation Septum (mm)	Wall (mm)	LVH type+	ECG	CHF	Prognosis	References
Arg92Leu								
n=1 (9 unrelated SCD) Area: U.K.	26 M	n.a.	n.a.	n.a.	n.a.	n.a.	SCD	Varnava et al., 2001
n=4 (1 family) Area: France	43 F	n.a.	19	n.a.	-	+	CHF at 44 y	Forissier et al., 1996
	23 M	n.a.	35	n.a.	+	+	n.a	
	20 F	n.a.	n.a.	apical	+	+	n.a.	
	45 F	n.a.	10	n.a.	+	-	n.a.	
Arg94Leu								
n=2 (9 unrelated SCD) Area: U.K.	17 M	n.a.	n.a.	n.a.	n.a.	n.a.	SCD	Varnava et al., 2001
	21 F	n.a.	n.a.	n.a.	n.a.	n.a.	SCD	
Ala104Val								
n=4 (1 family) Area: Japan	50 F	15	8	n.a.	+	+	SCD at age 50	Nakajima-Taniguchi et al., 1997
	36 F	17	6	n.a.	+	+	SCD at age 36	
	54 F	17	8	n.a.	+	+	ventricular tachycardia	
	33 F	20	12	n.a.	+	-	-	
Phe110Ile								
n=2 (1 family) Area : multi-ethnic/racial	n.a.	n.a.	17 (n=2)	n.a.	n.a.	n.a.	-	Watkins et al., 1995
n=16 (6 families) Area : Japan	38 F	27	17	III	+	-	-	Anan et al., 1998
	69 F	22	14	III	+	-	SCD in family	
	47 F	20	13	III	+	-	SCD in family	
	87 F	9	9	IV	+	-	-	
	48 M	10	10	IV	+	-	-	
	42 F	11	11	normal	-	-	-	
	64 M	23	10	II	+	-	-	
	70 M	20	11	II	+	-	-	
	47 F	13	13	III	+	-	-	
	45 M	12	10	normal	+	-	-	
	39 F	13	13	III	+	-	-	
	24 F	11	11	IV	+	-	-	
	56 F	19	11	II	+	-	SCD in family	
	53 M	15	13	III	+	-	"	
	31 F	21	12	II	+	-	"	
	28 F	10	10	normal	+	-	"	
Phe110Val								
n=3 (150 unrelated p.) Area: Italy	28 F	32	n.a.	III	+	-	-	Torricelli et al., 2003
	48 F	21	n.a.	III	+	n.a.	-	
	82 M	15	n.a.	II	+	n.a.	-	

Patients/ Family	Clinical Presentation							References
	Age/Sex	Septum (mm)	Wall (mm)	LVH type+	ECG	CHF	Prognosis	
Lys124Asn n=1 (71 unrelated p.) Area : China	41 F	n.a.	n.a.	LVH	n.a.	n.a.	-	An et al., 2004
Arg130Cys n=2 (150 unrelated p.) Area: Italy	55 M	23	n.a.	III	+	-	-	Torricelli et al., 2003
	58 F	13	n.a.	n.a.	+	-	-	
Glu160 n=32 (2 families +unrelated p.) Area : multi-ethnic/racial	n.a.	n.a.	17.5±5 (n=14)	n.a.	n.a.	n.a.	SCD in 14	Watkins et al., 1995
n=2 (150 unrelated p.) Area: Italy	50 F	20	n.a.	III	+	-	-	Torricelli et al., 2203
	55 M	22	n.a.	III	+	+	-	
Glu163Lys n=5(1 family + unrelated p.) Area. multi-ethnic/racial	n.a.	n.a.	19.8±8 (n=5)	n.a.	n.a.	n.a.	SCD in 0	Watkins et al., 1995
Ser179Phe n=1 (1 family) Area: Kuwait	17 M	25	11	n.a	+	-	SCD	Ho et al., 2000
Glu244Asp n=1 (1 family) Area: multi-ethnic/racial	n.a.	n.a.	n.a.	n.a.	n.a.	n.a.	SCD in 0	Watkins et al., 1995
Lys247Arg n=1 (30 unrelated p.) Area: Spain	60 F	23	n.a.	n.a.	n.a.	n.a.	-	Garcia-Castro et al., 2003
Intron 15 G1→A n=28 (1 family +unrelated p.) Area: multi-ethnic/racial	n.a.	n.a.	17.5±5 (n=17)	n.a.	n.a.	n.a.	SCD in 9	Watkins et al., 1995
n=1 (9 unrelated SCD) Area. U.K.	15 M	n.a.	n.a.	n.a.	n.a.	n.a.	SCD	Varnava et al., 2001
Asn271Ile 3 (1 family) Area: Spain	62 M	22	n.a.	n.a.	+	-	-	Gimeno et al., 2009
	36 M	14	n.a.	n.a.	+	-	-	
	31 F	9	n.a.	n.a.	-	-	-	

Patients/ Family	Clinical Presentation							References
	Age/Sex	Septum (mm)	Wall (mm)	LVH type+	ECG	CHF	Prognosis	
Lys273Glu								
n=8 (2 families) Area: Japan	58 F	7	8	n.a.	n.a.	n.a.	DCM features	Fujino et al., 2002
	32 F	23	7	asym.	n.a.	n.a	-	
	29 F	23	10	asym.	n.a.	n.a.	-	
	75 F	15	13	n.a.	n.a.	n.a.	SCD in family	
	78 F	15	11	asym.	n.a.	n.a.	"	
	75 F	16	9	asym.	n.a.	n.a.	"	
	49 F	20	9	asym	n.a.	n.a.	"	
	46 M	21	10	asym	n.a.	n.a.	"	
Arg278Cys								
n=3 (1 family + unrelated p.) Area: multi-ethnic/racial	n.a.	n.a.	16.3±6 (n=3)	n.a.	n.a.	n.a.	SCD in 1	Watkins et al., 1995
n=3(389 unrelated p.) Area: U.S.A.	57 M	n.a.	20	n.a.	n.a.	-	-	Van Driest et al.,, 2003
	66 M	n.a.	15	n.a.	n.a.	+	pacemaker	
	74 M	n.a.	23	n.a.	n.a.	+	TASH	
n=1 Area: U.K.	57 M	12	n.a.	n.a.	+	+	late onset HCM	Elliott et al., 1999
n=1 (30 unrelated p.) Area: Spain	60 F	22	n.a.	n.a.	n.a.	n.a.	-	Garcia-Castro et al., 2003
n=8 (2 families) Area: Spain	55 F	22	n.a.	n.a.	+	+	-	Gimeno et al., 2009
	59 M	22	n.a.	n.a.	+	+	-	
	27 M	12	n.a.	n.a.	-	-	-	
	30 M	10	n.a.	n.a.	-	-	-	
	29 M	10	n.a.	n.a.	-	-	-	
	21 M	40	n.a.	n.a.	+	+	ICD-Impl.	
	64 M	26	n.a.	n.a.	+	-	-	
	33 M	11	n.a.	n.a.	+	-	-	
n=6 (2 families) Area: Greek	40 M	20	11	asym	+	+	SCD in family	Theopistou et al., 2004
	71 F	13	12	conc.	+	+	"	
	41 M	10	8	normal	-	n.a.	"	
	38 M	10	10	normal	-	n.a.	"	
	14 F	7	8	normal	-	n.a.	"	
	13 M	22	11	asym.	+	-	SCD age 15	
n=1 (150 unrelated p.) Area: Italy	66 M	24	n.a.	III	+	+	-	Torricelli et al., 2003

Patients/ Family	Age/Sex	Clinical Presentation Septum (mm)	Wall (mm)	LVH type+	ECG	CHF	Prognosis	References
Arg278Pro								
n=1 (389 unrelated p.) Area: U.S.A.	47 M	n.a.	19	n.a.	n.a.	+	ICD	Van Driest et al., 2003
n=1 (143 unrelated p.) Area : Greek	18 M	n.a.	n.a.	LVH	n.a.	n.a.	-	Miliou et al., 2005
Arg286Cys								
n=1 (143 unrelated p.) Area : Greek	26 F	n.a.	n.a.	LVH	n.a.	n.a.	-	Miliou et al., 2005
Arg286His								
n=2 (389 unrelated p.) Area: U.S.A.	49 M	n.a.	20	n.a.	n.a.	-	-	Van Driest et al., 2003
	39 M	n.a.	25	n.a.	n.a.	+	myectomy	

Table 4. Mutations in the TNNT2 Gene Associated with HCM

Number of affected patients is given (out of a group of unrelated HCM patients or families with HCM). Age=age at investigation if not otherwise noted; [1]age at diagnosis; n.a.=data not available; SCD=sudden cardiac death; DCM=dilated cardiomyopathy like-type; RCM=restrictive cardiomyopathy like-type; CHF=congestive heart failure; TASH=transcoronary septal ablation; ICD=internal automated defibrillator; area=living area of study patients. +Left ventricular hypertrophy (LVH) is classified according to according to Maron et al. (1981) type I=confined to the anterior segment of the ventricular septum, type II=involved anterior and posterior septum, type III=involvement of both the septum and the free wall of the left ventricle, and type IV=regions other than the basal and anterior septum (e.g. apical area).

Patients/Family	Age/Sex	Clinical Presentation Septum (mm)	Wall (mm)	LVH type+	ECG	CHF	Prognosis	Reference
Arg21Cys								
n=1 (15 unrelated p.) Area: Europa	40 F	n.a.	n.a.	apical	n.a.	n.a.	SCD in family	Arad et al., 2005
Pro82Ser								
1 pt. with late-onset HCM Area: n.a.	> 40	n.a.	n.a.	LVH	+	+	n.a.	Niimura et al., 2002
Arg141Gln								
n=1 (389 unrelated p.) Area: U.S.A	41 M	n.a.	25	n.a.	n.a.	-	-	Van Driest et al., 2003
Arg145Gln								
n=1 (1 family) Area : U.K.	n.a.	21	n.a	apical	+	n.a.	n.a	Mogensen et al., 2004

Patients/Family	Clinical Presentation							Reference
	Age/Sex	Septum (mm)	Wall (mm)	LVH type+	ECG	CHF	Prognosis	
Ala157Val								
n=5 (3 families) Area : U.K.	n.a.	n.a.	n.a.	n.a.	+	n.a.	SCD in family	Mogensen et al., 2004
n=1 (1 family) Area: Portugal	24 M	n.a.	n.a.	LVH	*	*	SCD at age 44	Brito & Madeira, 2005
Arg162Gln								
n=7 (3 families) Area: U.K.	n.a.	n.a.	n.a.	n.a.	n.a.	n.a	SCD in family	Mogensen et al., 2004
n=2 (389 unrelated p.) Area: U.S.A.	76 F	n.a.	17	n.a.	n.a.	+	myectomy	Van Driest et al., 2003
	33 M	n.a.	19	n.a.	n.a.	+	SCD in family	
n=3 (1 family) Area: Australia	70 M	n.a.	n.a.	n.a.	n.a.	n.a.	n.a.	Doolan et al., 2005
	44 M	n.a.	10	normal	-	-	-	
	40 M	n.a.	10	normal	-	-	-	
Arg162Pro								
n=2 (1 family) Area: Australia	52 F	n.a.	9	normal.	-	-	-	Doolan et al., 2005
	25 F	n.a.	14	n.a.	+	-	cardiac arrest at age 21	
Ser166Phe								
n=3 (389 unrelated p.) Area: U.S.A.	48 F	n.a.	22	n.a.	n.a.	+	myectomy	Van Driest et al., 2003
	79 F	n.a.	14	n.a.	n.a.	+	myectomy	
	21 F	n.a.	17	n.a.	n.a.	+	myectomy	
n=1 (1 family) Area: U.K.	n.a.	19	n.a.	n.a.	+	n.a	-	Mogensen et al., 2004
Lys183Glu								
n=3 (1 family) Area: U.K.	n.a.	n.a.	n.a.	n.a.	+	n.a	-	Mogensen et al., 2004
Lys183del								
n=25 (7 families) Area: Japan	65 F	13	7	I/II	+	n.a.	SCD in family	Kokado et al., 2000
	61 F	17	12	I/II	+	n.a.	"	
	51 F	9	10	normal	+	n.a.	"	
	46 F	20	10	I/II	+	n.a.	"	
	36 F	16	8	I/II	+	n.a.	"	
	48 F	7	7	normal	+	n.a.	"	
	36 M	18	13	III	+	n.a.	"	
	33 F	21	9	I/II	+	n.a.	"	
	47 F	10	8	normal	+	n.a.	"	
	27 F	13	9	III	+	n.a.	"	
	8 M	5	5	normal	-	n.a.	"	
	85 M	14	10	I/II	+	n.a.	"	
	56 F	23	11	IV	+	n.a.	"	
	48 F	13	14	IV	+	n.a.	"	
	71 F	11	10	normal	+	n.a.	"	

Patients/Family	Clinical Presentation							Reference
	Age/Sex	Septum (mm)	Wall (mm)	LVH type+	ECG	CHF	Prognosis	
	49 M	5	9	normal	+	n.a.	"	
	24 F	20	11	I/II	+	n.a.	"	
	23 F	9	8	normal	+	n.a.	"	
	66 F	11	11	normal	+	n.a.	"	
	62 M	13	12	normal	+	n.a.	"	
	35 M	12	11	normal	-	n.a.	"	
	48 M	10	13	LVH	+	n.a.	"	
	24 M	13	10	LVH	+	n.a.	"	
	68 F	19	11	I/II	+	n.a.	"	
	78 F	22	13	I/II	+	n.a.	"	
Arg186Gln n=5 (2 families) Area: U.K.	n.a.	n.a.	n.a.	n.a.	n.a.	n.a	SCD in family	Mogensen et al., 2004
Asp196Asn n=4 (2 families) Area: U.K.	n.a.	n.a.	n.a.	n.a.	+	n.a	-	Mogensen et al., 2004
n=1 with late-onset HCM Area: n.a.	>40	n.a.	LVH	+	+	n.a.	n.a.	Niimura et al., 2002
Leu198Pro n=1 (1 family) Area: Australia	15 M	n.a.	22	n.a.	+	-	SCD at age 15	Doolan et al., 2005
Ser199Gly n=1 (1 family) Area: U.K.	n.a.	n.a.	n.a.	apical	+	n.a.	-	Mogensen et al., 2004
Ser199Asn n=8 (2 families) Area: U.K.	n.a.	n.a.	n.a.	n.a.	+	n.a.	SCD in family	Mogensen et al., 2004
n=1 (1 family) Area: Portugal	52 M	n.a.	n.a.	LVH	+	-	cardiac arrest at age 61	Brito & Madeira, 2005
Glu202Gly n=1 (1 family) Area: U.K.	n.a.	19	n.a.	n.a.	+	n.a.	-	Mogensen et al., 2004
Gly203Arg n=2 (1 family) Area: U.K.	n.a.	n.a.	n.a.	n.a.	+	n.a.	-	Mogensen et al., 2004
Gly203 frameshift n=4 (1 family) Area: Sweden	71 F	9	9	normal	+	+	-	Mörner et al., 2000
	61 M	15	8	LVH	+	-	-	
	64 M	16	14	LVH	+	-	-	
	27 F	8	7	normal	-	-	-	
Arg204His n=3 (1 family) Area: Australia	37 M	n.a.	17	n.a.	+	-	cardiac arrest at age 17	Doolan et al., 2005
	9 M	n.a.	7	normal	+	-	-	
	5 M	n.a.	5	normal	+	-	-	

Table 5. Mutations in the TNNI3 Gene Associated with HCM

Patients/ Family	Age/Sex	Clinical Presentation					Prognosis	Reference
		Septum (mm)	Wall (mm)	LVH type+	ECG	CHF		
Ala8Val n=1 (1025 unrelated p.) Area: U.S.A./ Caucasian	37M	18	n..a	n.a.	n.a.	+	myectomy	Landstrom et al., 2008
Leu29Gln n=1 Area: Germany	60 M	15	15	n.a.	+	+	n.a.	Hoffmann et al. ,2001
Cys84Tyr n=1 (1025 unrelated p.) Area: U.S.A./ Caucasian	17 M	19	n.a.	n.a.	n.a.	-	n.a.	Landstrom et al., 2008
Glu134Asp n=1 (1015 unrelated p.) Area: U.S.A./ Caucasian	22 F	26	n.a.	n.a.	n.a.	+	myectomy	Landstrom et al., 2008
Asp145Glu n=1 (1025 unrelated p.) Area: U.S.A./ Caucasian	58 M	22	n..a	n.a.	n.a.	+	myectomy	Landstrom et al., 2008
c.363dupG frameshift n=1(1 family) Area: U.S.A.	19 M	n.a.	n.a.	n.a.	n.a.	n.a.	SCD	Chung et al., 2011

Table 6. Mutations in the TNNC1 Gene Associated with HCM

4. References

Abbott, M. B., Gaponenko, V., Abusamhadneh, E., Finley, N., Li, G., Dvoretsky, A., Rance, M., Solaro, R. J. & Rosevear, P. R. (2000). Regulatory domain conformational exchange and linker region flexibility in cardiac troponin C bound to cardiac troponin I. *J. Biol. Chem.*, 275, pp. 20610-7

Abbott, M. B., Dong, W. J., Dvoretsky, A., DaGue, B., Caprioli, R. M., Cheung, H. C. & Rosevear, P. R. (2001). Modulation of cardiac troponin C-cardiac troponin I regulatory interactions by the amino-terminus of cardiac troponin I. *Biochemistry*, 40, pp. 5992-6001

An, F. S., Zhang, Y., Li, D. Q., Yang, X. S., Li L, Zhang, C, Yan, M.L., Wang, Y. & An, G. P. (2004). A novel missense mutation, K124N, in the troponin T gene of Chinese populations with hypertrophic cardiomyopathy. *Zhonghua Yi Xue Za Zhi.* 84(16), pp. 1340-3

Anan, R., Shono, H., Kisanuki, A., Arima, S., Nakao, S. &Tanaka, H. (1998). Patients with familial hypertrophic cardiomyopathy caused by a Phe110Ile missense mutation in the cardiac troponin T gene have variable cardiac morphologies and a favorable prognosis. *Circulation*, 98, pp. 391-7-3

Anderson, P. A., Malouf, N. N., Oakeley, A.E., Pagani, E. D. & Allen, P. D. (1991). Troponin T isoform expression in humans. A comparison among normal and failing adult heart, fetal heart, and adult and fetal skeletal muscle. *Circ. Res.*, 69(5), pp. 1226-33

Arad, M., Maron, B. J., Gorham, J. M., Johnson, W. H., Saul, J. P., Perez-Atayde, A. R., Spirito, P., Wright, G. B., Kanter, R.J., Seidman, C. E., Seidman, J. G. (2005a). Glycogen storage diseases presenting as hypertrophic cardiomyopathy. *N Engl J Med.*, 352(4), pp. 362-72

Arad, M., Penas-Lado, M., Monserrat, L., Maron, B. J., Sherrid, M., Ho, C. Y., Barr, S., Karim, A., Olson, T. M., Kamisago, M., Seidman, J. G. &, Seidman C. E. (2005b). Gene mutation in apical hypertrophic cardiomyopathy. *Circulation*, 112, pp. 2805-2811

Baudenbacher, F., Schober, T., Pinto, J.R., Sidorov, V.Y., Hilliard, F., Solaro, R. J., Potter, J. D. & Knollmann, B. C. (2008). Myofilament Ca2+ sensitization causes susceptibility to cardiac arrhythmia in mice. *J. Clin. Invest.*, 118(12), pp. 3893-903

Barta, J., Tóth, A., Jaquet, K., Redlich, A., Edes, I. & Papp, Z. (2003). Calpain-1-dependent degradation of troponin I mutants found in familial hypertrophic cardiomyopathy. *Mol Cell Biochem,*. 251(1-2), pp. 83-8

Baryshnikova, O. K., Li, M. X. & Sykes, B. D. (2008). Modulation of Cardiac Troponin C Function by the Cardiac-Specific N-Terminus of Troponin I: Influence of PKA Phosphorylation and Involvement in Cardiomyopathies. *J. Mol. Biol.*, 375(3), pp. 735-51

Biesiadecki, B. J., Chong, S. M., Nosek, T. M. & Jin, J. P. (2007). Troponin T core structure and the regulatory NH2-terminal variable region. *Biochemistry*, 46(5), pp. 1368-79

Braunwald, E. & Ebert, P. A. (1962). Hemodynamic alterations in idiopathic hypertrophic subaortic stenosis induced by sympathomimetic drugs. *Am. J. Cardiol.*, 10, pp. 489-95

Brito, D. & Madeira, H. (2005). Malignant mutations in hypertrophic cardiomyopathy: fact or fancy? *Rev. Port. Cardiol.*, 24(9), pp. 1137-46

Burhop, J., Rosol, M., Craig, R., Tobacman, L. S. & Lehman W. (2001). Effects of a cardiomyopathy-causing troponin t mutation on thin filament function and structure. *J. Biol. Chem.*, 276(23), pp. 20788-94

Cannan, C. R., Reeder, G. S., Bailey, K. R., Melton, L. J. & Gersh, B. J. (1995). Natural history of hypertrophic cardiomyo-pathy. A population-based study, 1976 through 1990. *Circulation*, 92, pp. 2488-95

Capek, P. & Skvor, J. (2006). Hypertrophic cardiomyoptahy. Molecular genetic analysis of exons 9 and 11 of the TNNT2 gene in Czech patients. *Methods Inf. Med.*, 45, pp. 169-72

Carballo, S., Robinson, P., Otway, R., Fatkin, D., Jongbloed, J. D., de Jonge, N., Blair, E., van Tintelen, J. P., Redwood, C. & Watkins, H. (2009). Identification and functional characterization of cardiac troponin I as a novel disease gene in autosomal dominant dilated cardiomyopathy. *Circ. Res.*, 105(4), pp. 375-82

Chandra, M., Tschirgi, M. L. & Tardiff, J. C. (2005). Increase in tension dependent ATP consumption induced by cardiac troponin T mutation. *AJP Heart*, 289(5), pp. H2112-9

Chong, P. C. & Hodges, R. S. (1982). Photochemical cross-linking between rabbit skeletal troponin and alpha-tropomyosin. Attachment of the photoaffinity probe N-(4-

azidobenzoyl-[2-3H]glycyl)-S-(2-thiopyridyl)-cysteine to cysteine 190 of alpha-tropomyosin. *J. Biol. Chem.*, 257(15), pp. 9152-60

Chung, W. K., Kitner, C. & Maron, B. J. (2011). Novel frameshift mutation in troponin C (TNNC1) associated with hypertrophic cardiomyopathy and sudden death. *Cardiol. Young*, Jan 25, epub ahead of print

Cooper, T. A. & Ordahl, C. P. (1985). A single cardiac troponin T gene generates embryonic and adult isoforms via developmentally regulated alternate splicing. *J. Biol. Chem.*, 260(20), pp. 11140-8

Davis, J. P. & Tikunova, S. B. (2008). Ca(2+) exchange with troponin C and cardiac muscle dynamics. *Cardiovasc. Res.*, 77(4), pp. 619-26. Review.

Davis, J. & Metzger, J. M. (2010). Combinatorial effects of double cardiomyopathy mutant alleles in rodent myocytes: a predictive cellular model of myofilament dysregulation in disease. *PLoS One*, 5(2), pp e9140

Deng, Y., Schmidtmann, A., Redlich, A., Westerdorf, B., Jaquet, K. & Thieleczek, R. (2001). Effects of phosphorylation and mutation R145G on human cardiac troponin I function. *Biochemistry*, 40(48), pp. 14593-602

Deng, Y., Schmidtmann, A., Kruse, S., Filatov, V., Heilmeyer, L. M. Jr., Jaquet, K. & Thieleczek, R. (2003). Phospho-rylation of human cardiac troponin I G203S and K206Q linked to familial hypertrophic cardiomyopathy affects actomyosin interaction in different ways. *J Mol Cell Cardiol.*, 35(11), pp. 1365-74

Doolan, A., Tebo, M., Ingles, J., Nguyen, L., Tsoutsman, T., Lam, L., Chiu, C., Chung, J., Weintraub, R. G., Semsarian, C. (2005). Cardiac troponin I mutations in Australian families with hypertrophic cardiomyopathy: clinical, genetic and functional consequences. *J Mol Cell Cardiol.*, 38(2), pp. 387-393

Dong, W. J., Xing, J., Villain, M., Hellinger, M., Robinson, J. M., Chandra, M., Solaro, R. J., Umeda, P. K. & Cheung, H. C. (1999). Conformation of the regulatory domain of cardiac muscle troponin C in its complex with cardiac troponin I. *J Biol Chem.*, 274(44), pp. 31382-90

Dong, W. J., Xing, J., Ouyang, Y., An, J. & Cheung, H. C. (2008). Structural kinetics of cardiac troponin C mutants linked to familial hypertrophic and dilated cardiomyopathy in troponin complexes. *J Biol Chem.*, 283(6), pp. 3424-32

Dweck, D., Hus, N. & Potter, J. D. (2008). Challeging current paradigm related to cardiomyopathies. *J Biol Chem.*, 283, pp. 33119-28

Ebashi, S. (1972). Calcium ions and muscle contraction. *Nature*, 240, pp. 217-8

Elliott, P. M, D'Cruz, L. & McKenna, W. J. (1999). Late-onset hypertrophic cardiomyopathy caused by a mutation in the cardiac troponin T gene. *N Engl J Med.*, 341, pp. 1855 (letter)

Elliott, P. M., Andersson, B., Arbustini, E., Bilinska, Z., Cecchi, F., Charron, P., Dubourg, O., Kühl, U., Maisch, B., McKenna, W. J., Monserrat, L., Pankuweit, S., Rapezzi, C., Seferovic, P., Tavazzi, L. & Keren, A. (2008). Classification of the cardiomyopathies: a position statement from the European Society Of Cardiology Working Group on myocardial and pericardial diseases. *Eur Heart J.*, 29, pp. 270–6

Elliott, P. M., McKenna, W. J. (2004). Hypertrophic cardiomyopathy. *Lancet*, 363, pp. 1881-91

Fatkin, D., Seidman, J. G. & Seidman, C. E. Hypertrophic cardiomyopathy. In: Willersen, J. T., Cohn, J. N., Wellens, H. J. J. & Holmes, D. R. (eds.) Cardiovascular Medicine, 3rd edition, 2007, pp. 1261-84

Feliciello, A., Gottesman, M. E. & Avvedimento, E. V. (2001). The biological functions of A-kinase anchor proteins. *J Mol Biol.,* 308(2), pp. 99-114

Feng, H. Z., Biesiadecki, B. J., Yu, Z. B., Hossain, M. M. & Jin, J. P. (2008). Restricted N-terminal truncation of cardiac troponin T: a novel mechanism for functional adaptation to energetic crisis. *J Physiol.,* 586(14), pp. 3537-50

Finley, N., Abbott, M. B., Abusamhadneh, E., Gaponenko, V., Dong, W., Gasmi-Seabrook, G., Howarth, J. W., Rance, M., Solaro, R. J., Cheung, H. C., Rosevear, P. R. (1999). NMR analysis of cardiac troponin C-troponin I complexes: effects of phosphorylation. *FEBS Lett.* 453,107-112.

Flicker, P. F., Phillips, G. N., Jr. & Cohen, C. (1982). Troponin and its interactions with tropomyosin. An electron microscope study. *J Mol Biol.,* 162(2), pp. 495-501

Forissier, J. F., Carrier, L., Farza, H., Bonne, G., Bercovici, J., Richard, P., Hainque, B., Townsend, P. J., Yacoub, M. H., Faure, S., Dubourg, O., Millaire, A., Hagege, A. A., Desnos, M., Komajda, M. & Schwartz, K. (1996). Codon 102 of the cardiac troponin T gene is a putative hot spot for mutations in familial hypertrophic cardiomyopathy. *Circulation,* 94, pp. 3069-3073

Foster, D. B., Noguchi, T., VanBuren, P., Murphy, A. M. & Van Eyk, J. E. (2003). C-terminal truncation of cardiac troponin I causes divergent effects on ATPase and force: implications for the pathophysiology of myocardial stunning. *Circ Res.,* 93, pp. 917–24

Frenneaux, M. P. (2004). Assessing the risk of sudden cardiac death in a patient with hypertrophic cardiomyopathy. *Heart,* 90, pp. 570-5

Fuchs, F. & Grabarek, Z. (2011). The Ca2+/Mg2+ sites of troponin C modulate crossbridge-mediated thin filament activation in cardiac myofibrils. *Biochem Biophys Res Commun.* 408(4), pp. 697-700

Fujino, N., Shimizu, M., Ino, H., Okeie, K., Yamaguchi, M., Yasuda, T., Kokado, H. & Mabuchi, H. (2001). Cardiac troponin T Arg92Trp mutation and progression from hypertrophic to dilated cardiomyopathy. *Clin Cardiol.,* 24(5), pp. 397-402

Fujino, N., Shiizu, M., Ino, H., Yamaguchi, M., Yasuda, T., Nagata, M., Konno, T. & Mabuchi, H. (2002). A novel mutation Lys273Glu in the cardiac troponin T gene shows high degree of penetrance and transition from hypertrophic to dilated cardiomyopathy. *Am J Cardiol.,* 89, 29-33

Galinska-Rakoczy, A., Engel, P., Xu, C., Jung, H., Craig, R., Tobacman, L. S. & Lehman, W. (2008). Structural basis for the regulation of muscle contraction by troponin and tropomyosin. *J Mol Biol.* , 379, pp. 929–35

Galińska, A., Hatch, V., Craig, R., Murphy, A. M., Van Eyk, J. E., Wang, C. L., Lehman, W. & Foster, D. B. (2010). The C terminus of cardiac troponin I stabilizes the Ca2+-activated state of tropomyosin on actin filaments. *Circ Res.,* 106(4), pp. 705-11

Gambarin, F. I., Tagliani, M. & Arbustini, E. (2008). Pure restrictive cardiomyopathy associated with cardiac troponin I gene mutation: mismatch between the lack of hypertrophy and the presence of disarray. *Heart,* 94(10), pp. 1257

Gaponenko, V., Abusamhadneh, E., Abbott, M. B., Finley, N., Gasmi-Seabrook, G., Solaro, R. J., Rance, M. & Rosevear, P. R. (1999) Effects of troponin I phosphorylation on conformational exchange in the regulatory domain of cardiac troponin C. *J. Biol. Chem.,* 274, pp. 16681-4

Garcia-Castro, M., Ruguero, J. R., Batalla, A., Diaz-Molina, B., Gonzalez, P., Alvarez, V., Cortina, A., Cubero, G. I. & Coto, E. (2003). Hypertrophic cardiomyopathy: low frequency of mutations in the ß-myosin heavy chain (MYH7) and cardiac troponin T (TNNT2) genes among Spanish patients. *Clin Chem.*, 49(8), pp. 1279-85

Gasmi-Seabrook, G. M., Howarth, J. W., Finley, N., Abusamhadneh, E., Gaponenko, V., Brito, R. M., Solaro, R. J. & Rosevear, P. R. (1999). Solution structures of the C-terminal domain of cardiac troponin C free and bound to the N-terminal domain of cardiac troponin I. *Biochemistry*, 38(26), pp. 8313-22. Erratum in: *Biochemistry*. (1999) 38(43), pp. 14432

Geisterfer-Lowrance, A. A, Kass, S., Tanigawa, G., Vosberg, H. P., McKenna, W., Seidman, C. E. & Seidman, J. G. (1990). A molecular basis for familial hypertrophic cardiomyopathy: a beta cardiac myoson heavy chain gene missense mutation. *Cell*, 62 (5), pp. 999-1006

Gimeno, J. R., Monserrat, L., Perez-Sanchez, I., Marin, F., Caballero, L., Hermida-Prieto, M., Castro, A. & Valdes, M. (2009). Hypertrophic cardiomyopathy: a study of the troponin-T gene in 127 Spanish families. *Rev Esp Cardiol.*, 62(12), pp. 1473-7

Gillis, T. E., Liang, B., Chung, F. & Tibbits, G. F. (2005). Increasing cardiomyocyte contractility with residues identified in trout troponin C. *Physiol Gen.*, 22, pp. 1-7

Girolami, F., Ho, C. Y., Semsarian, C., Baldi, M., Will, M. L., Baldini, K., Torricelli, F., Yeates, L., Cecchi, F., Ackerman, M. J. & Olivotto, I. (2010). Clinical features and outcome of hypertrophic cardiomyopathy associated with triple sarcomere protein gene mutations. *J Am Coll Cardiol.*, 55(14), pp. 1444-53

Gomes, A. V., Guzman, G., Zhao, J. & Potter, J. D. (2002). Cardiac troponin T isoforms affect the Ca^{2+} sensitivity and inhibition of force development. Insights into the role of troponin T isoforms in the heart. *J Biol Chem.*, 277, pp. 35341–49

Gomes, A. V., Barnes, J. A., Harada, K. & Potter, J. D. (2004). Role of troponin T in disease. *Mol Cell Biochem.* ,263(1-2), pp. 115-29. Review.

Gomes, A. V. & Potter, J. D. (2004). Cellular and molecular aspects of familial hypertrophic cardiomyopathy caused by mutations in the cardiac troponin I gene. *Mol Cell Biochem.*, 263(1-2), pp. 99-114. Review.

Gomes, A. V. & Potter, J. D. (2004). Molecular and cellular aspects of troponin cardiomyopathies. *Ann N Y Acad Sci.* 1015, pp. 214-24. Review.

Gomes, A. V., Harada, K. & Potter, J. D. (2005). A mutation in the N-terminus of troponin I that is associated with hypertrophic cardiomyopathy affects the Ca2+-sensitivity, phosphorylation kinetics and proteolytic susceptibility of troponin. *J Mol Cell Cardiol.*, 39, pp. 754-5

Gomes, A. V., Venkatraman, G., Davis, J. P., Tikunova, S. B., Engel, P., Solaro, R. J. & Potter, J. D. (2004). Cardiac troponin T isoforms affect the Ca(2+) sensitivity of force development in the presence of slow skeletal troponin I: insights into the role of troponin T isoforms in the fetal heart. *J Biol Chem.*, 279(48), pp. 49579-87

Gusev, N. B, Dobrovolskii, A. B & Severin, S. E. (1980). Isolation and some properties of troponin T kinase from rabbit skeletal muscle. *Biochem J.*, 189(2), pp. 219-26

Hernandez, O. M., Szczesna-Cordary, D., Knollmann, B. C., Miller, T., Bell, M., Zhao, J., Sirenko, S. G., Diaz, Z., Guzman, G., Xu, Y., Wang, Y., Kerrick, W. G. & Potter, J. D. (2005). F110I and R278C troponin T mutations that cause familial hypertrophic cardiomyopathy affect muscle contraction in transgenic mice and reconstituted human cardiac fibers. *J Biol Chem.*, 280(44):, pp. 37183-94

Hinkle, A. & Tobacman, L. S. (2003). Folding and function of the troponin tail domain. Effects of cardiomyopathic troponin T mutations. *J Biol Chem.* , 278(1), pp. 506-13

Ho, C. Y. (2010a). Hypertrophic cardiomyopathy: for Heart Failure Clinics. Genetics of cardiomyopathy and heart failure. *Heart Fail Clin.*, 6(2), pp. 141-59

Ho, C. Y.(2010b). Is genotype clinically useful in predicting prognosis in hypertrophic cardiomyopathy? Genetics and clinical destiny: improving care in hypertrophic cardiomyopathy. *Circulation.*122, pp. 2430-40

Ho, C. Y., Lever, H. M., DeSanctis, R., Farver, C. F., Seidman, J. G. & Seidman, C. E. (2000). Homozygous mutation in cardiac troponin T: implications for hypertrophic cardiomyopthyy. *Circulation.* 102, pp. 1950-5

Ho, C. Y., Carlsen, C., Thune, J. J., Havndrup, O., Bundgaard, H., Farrohi, F., Rivero, J., Cirino, A. L, Andersen, P. S., Christiansen, M., Maron, B. J., Orav, E. J. & Kober, L. (2009). Echocardiographic strain imaging to assess early and late consequences of sarcomere mutations in hypertrophic cardiomyopathy. *Circ Cardiovasc Genet.* 2, pp. 314-21

Hoffmann, B., Schmidt-Traub, H., Perrot, A., Osterziel, K. J. & Gessner, R. (2001). First mutation in cardiac troponin C, L29Q, in a patient with hypertrophic cardiomyopathy. Hum. Mutat. , 17, pp. 524 only

Howarth, J. W., Meller, J., Solaro, R. J., Trewhella, J. & Rosevear, P. R. (2007). Phosphorylation-dependent conformational transition of the cardiac specific N-extension of troponin I in cardiac troponin. *J. Mol. Biol.*, 373, pp. 706-22

James, J., Zhang, Y., Osinska, H., Sanbe, A., Klevitsky, R., Hewett, T. E. & Robbins, J. (2000). Transgenic modeling of a cardiac troponin I mutation linked to familial hypertrophic cardiomyopathy. *Circ Res.*, 87(9), pp. 805-11

Jaquet, K., Lohmann, K., Czisch, M., Holak, T., Gulati, J. & Jaquet, R. (1998). A model for the function of the bisphos-phorylated heart-specific troponin-I N-terminus. *J Muscle Res Cell Motil.* , 19(6), pp. 647-59

Jarcho, J. A., McKenna, W., Pare, J. A., Solomon, S. D, Holcombe, R. F, Dickie, S., Levi, T., Donis-Keller, H., Seidman, J. G. & Seidman, C. E.(1989). Mapping a gene for familial hypertrophic cardiomyopathy to chromosome 14q1. *N Engl J Med.*, 321 (20), pp. 1372-8

Javadpour, M. M, Tardiff, J. C, Pinz, I. & Ingwall, J. S. (2003). Decreased energetics in murine hearts bearing the R92Q mutation in cardiac troponin T. *J Clin Invest.*, 112(5), pp. 768-75

Jin, J. P. & Chong, S. M. (2010). Localization of the two tropomyosin-binding sites of troponin T. *Arch Biochem Biophys.*, 500(2), pp. 144-50

Jin, J. P & Samanez, R. A. (2001). Evolution of a metal-binding cluster in the NH(2)-terminal variable region of avian fast skeletal muscle troponin T: functional divergence on the basis of tolerance to structural drifting. *J Mol Evol.* , 52(2), pp. 103-16

Jin, J. P., Zhang, Z. & Bautista, J. A. (2008). Isoform diversity, regulation, and functional adaptation of troponin and calponin. *Crit Rev Eukaryot Gene Expr.*, 18(2), pp. 93-124. Review.

Kamisago, M., Sharma, S. D., DePalma, S. R., Solomon, S., Sharma, P., McDonough, B., Smoot, L., Mullen, M. P., Woolf, P. K., Wigle, E. D., Seidman, J. G. & Seidman, C. E.

(2000). Mutations in sarcomeric protein genes as a cause of dilated cardiomyopathy. *N. Engl. J. Med.*, 343(23), pp. 1888-96

Kentish, J. C., McCloskey, D. T., Layland, J., Palmer, S., Leiden, J. M., Martin, A. F. & Solaro, R. J. (2001). Phosphorylation of troponin I by protein kinase A accelerates relaxation and crossbridge cycle kinetics in mouse ventricular muscle. *Circ. Res.* 88, pp. 1059-65

Keren, A., Syrris, P. & McKenna, W. J. (2008). Hypertrophic cardiomyopathy: the genetic determinants of clinical disease expression. *Nature Clin Pract.*, 5(3), pp. 158-68

Kimura, A., Harada, H., Park, J-E., Nishi, H., Satoh, M., Takahashi, M,, Hiroi, S., Sasaoka, T., Ohbuchi, N., Nakamura, T., Koyanagi, T., Hwang, T-H., Choo, J., Chung, K-S., Hasegawa, A., Nagai, R., Okazaki, O., Nakamura, H., Matsuzaki, M., Sakamoto, T., Toshima, H., Koga, Y., Imaizumi, T. & Sasazuki, T. (1997). Mutations in the cardiac troponin I gene associated with hypertrophic cardiomyopathy. Nature Genet., 16, pp. 379-82

Knollmann, B. C. & Potter, J. D. (2001). Altered regulation of cardiac muscle contraction by troponin T mutations that cause familial hypertrophic cardiomyopathy. *Trends Cardiovasc Med.*, 11(5), pp. 206-12

Knollmann, B. C., Blatt, S. A., Horton, K., de Freitas, F., Miller, T., Bell, M., Housmans, P. R., Weissman, N. J, Morad, M. &, Potter, J. D. (2001). Inotropic stimulation induces cardiac dysfunction in transgenic mice expressing a troponin T (I79N) mutation linked to familial hypertrophic cardiomyopathy. *J Biol Chem.*, 276(13), pp. 10039-48

Knollmann, B. C., Kirchhof, P., Sirenko, S. G., Degen, H., Greene, A. E., Schober, T., Mackow, J. C., Fabritz, L., Potter, J. D. & Morad, M. (2003). Familial hypertrophic cardiomyopathy-linked mutant troponin T causes stress-induced ventricular tachycardia and Ca2+-dependent action potential remodeling. *Circ Res.*, 92(4), pp. 428-36

Klues, H. G, Schiffers, A. & Maron, B. J. (1995). Phenotypic spectrum and patterns of left ventricular hypertrophy in hypertrophic cardiomyopathy: morphologic observations and significance as assessed by two-dimensional echocardiography in 600 patients. *J Am Coll Cardiol.*, 26(7), pp. 1699-1708

Kobayashi, T., Dong, W. J., Burkart, E. M., Cheung, H. C. & Solaro, R. J. (2004). Effects of protein kinase C dependent phosphorylation and a familial hypertrophic cardiomyopathy-related mutation of cardiac troponin I on structural transition of troponin C and myofilament activation. *Biochemistry*, 43 (20), pp. 5996-6004

Kobayashi, T. & Solaro, R. J. (2006). Increased Ca2+ affinity of cardiac thin filaments reconstituted with cardiomyopathy-related mutant cardiac troponin I. *J Biol Chem.*, 281(19), pp. 13471-7

Köhler, J., Chen, Y., Brenner, B., Gordon, A. M., Kraft, T., Martyn, D. A., Regnier, M., Rivera, A. J., Wang, C. K. & Chase, P. B. (2003). Familial hypertrophic cardiomyopathy mutations in troponin I (K183D, G203S, K206Q) enhance filament sliding. *Physiol Genomics*,. 14(2), pp. 117-28

Kofflard, M. J. M., ten Cate, F. J., van der Lee, C. & van Domburg, R. T. (2003). Hypertrophic cardiomyopathy in a large community-based population: clinical outcome and identification of risk factors for sudden death and clinical deterioration. *J Am Coll Cardiol.*, 41, pp. 987-93

Kokado, H., Shimizu, M., Yoshio, H., Ino, H., Okeie, K., Emoto, Y., Matsuyama, T., Yamaguchi, M., Ysuda, T., Fujino, N., Ito, H., Mabuchi, H. (2000). Clinical features of hypertrophic cardiomyopathy caused by a Lys183 deletion mutation in the cardiac troponin I gene. *Circulation*, 102, pp. 663-9

Konno, T., Shimizu, M., Ino, H., Fujino, N., Hayashi, K., Uchiyama, K., Kaneda, T., Inoue, M., Masuda, E., Mabuchi, H. (2005). Phenotypic differences between electrocardiographic and echocardiographic determination of hypertrophic cardiomyopathy in genetically affected subjects. *J Intern Med.*, 258, pp. 216-24

Kruger, M., Zittrich, S., Redwood, C., Blaudeck, N., James, J., Robbins, J., Pfitzer, G. & Stehle, R. (2005). Effects of the mutation R145G in human cardiac troponin I on the kinetics of the contraction-relaxation cycle in isolated cardiac myofibrils. *J Physiol.*, 564(Pt 2), pp. 347-57

Lam, L., Tsoutsman, T., Arthur, J. & Semsarian, C. (2010). Differential protein expression profiling of myocardial tissue in a mouse model of hypertrophic cardiomyopathy. *J Mol Cell Cardiol.*, 48(5), pp. 1014-22

Landstrom, A. P. & Ackerman, M. J. (2010). Is genotype clinically useful in predicting prognosis in hypertrophic cardiomyopathy? Mutation type is not clinically useful in predicting prognosis in hypertrophic cardiomyopathy. *Circulation*, 122, pp. 2441-50

Landstrom, A. P., Parvatiyar, M. S., Pinto, J. R., Marquardt, M. L., Bos, J. M., Tester, D. J., Ommen, S. R., Potter, J. D. & Ackerman, M. J. (2008). Molecular and functional characterization of novel hypertrophic cardiomyopathy susceptibility mutations in TNNC1-encoded troponin C. *J Mol Cell Cardiol.* , 45, pp. 281-288

Lang, R., Gomes, A. V., Zhao, J., Housmans, P. R., Miller, T. & Potter, J. D. (2002). Functional analysis of a troponin I (R145G) mutation associated with familial hypertrophic cardiomyopathy. *J Biol Chem.*, 277(14), pp. 11670-8

Lassalle, M. W. (2010). Defective dynamic properties of human cardiac troponin mutations. *Biosci Biotechnol Biochem.*, 74(1), pp. 82-91

Lechin, M., Quinones, M. A., Omran, A., Yu, Q. T., Rakowski, H., Wigle, D., Liew, C. C., Sole, M., Roberts, R. & Marian, A. J. (1995). Angiotensin-I conversing enzyme genotypes and left ventricular hypertrophy in patients with hypertrophic cardiomyopathy. *Circulation*, 92, pp. 1808-12

Li, M. X., Spyracopoulos, L. & Sykes, B. D. (1999). Binding of cardiac troponin-I147-163 induces a structural opening in human cardiac troponin-C. *Biochemistry*, 38(26), pp. 8289-98

Liang, B., Chung, F., Qu, Y., Pavlov, D., Gillis, T. E., Tikunova, S. B., Davis, J. P. & Tibbits, G. F. (2008). Familial hypertrophic cardiomyopathy- related cardiac troponin C mutation L29Q affects Ca2+ binding and myofilament contractility. *Physiol. Gen.*, 33, pp. 257-66

Liberthson, R. R.(1996). Sudden death from cardiac causes in children and young adults. *N Engl J Med.*, 334, pp. 1039-44

Lin, D., Bobkova, A., Homsher, E. & Tobacman, L. S. (1996). Altered cardiac troponin T in vitro function in the presence of a mutation implicated in familial hypertrophic cardiomyopathy. *J Clin Invest.* 97(12), pp. 2842-8

Lindhout, D. A., Li, M. X., Schieve, D. & Sykes, B. D. (2002). Effects of T142 phosphorylation and mutation R145G on the interaction of the inhibitory region of human cardiac troponin I with the C-domain of human cardiac troponin C. *Biochemistry*, 41(23), pp. 7267-74. Erratum in: *Biochemistry* (2003), 42(1), pp. 238

Lindhout DA, Boyko RF, Corson DC, Li MX & Sykes BD. (2005).The role of electrostatics in the interaction of the inhibitory region of troponin I with troponin C. *Biochemistry*, 44(45): 14750-9.

Lippi, G., Targher, G., Franchini, M. & Plebani, M. (2009). Genetic and biochemical heterogeneity of cardiac troponins: clinical and laboratory implications. *Clin Chem Lab Med.*, 47(10), pp. 1183-94

Marian, A. J. (2003). On predictors of sudden cardiac death in hypertrophic cardiomyopathy. *J Am Coll Cardiol.*, 41, pp. 994-6

Marian, A. J. (2010). Hypertrophic cardiomyopathy: from genetics to treatment. *Eur J Clin Invest.* 40(4), pp. 360-9

Marian, A. J., Yu, Q. T., Workman, R., Greve, G. & Roberts, R. (1993). Angiotensin-converting enzyme polymorphism in hypertrophic cardiomyopathy and sudden cardiac death. *Lancet*, 342, pp. 1085-6

Maron, B. J., Shirani, J., Poliac, L. C., Mathenge, R., Roberts, W. C. & Mueller, F. O. (1996). Sudden death in young competitive atheletes : clinical, demographic, and pathological profiles. *JAMA*, 276(3), pp. 199-204

Maron, B. J. (2003). Sudden death in young athletes. *N Engl J Med.*, 349,pp. 1064-75

Maron, B. J. & Roberts, W. C. (1979). Quantitative analysis of cardiac muscle cell disorganization in the ventricular septum of patients with hypertrophic cardiomyopathy. *Circulation*, 59, pp. 689-706

Maron, B. J., Gottdiener, J. S. & Epstein, S. E. (1981). Patterns and significance if distribution of left ventricular hypertrophy in hypertrophic cardiomyopathy. A wide angle, two dimensional echocardiographic study of 125 patients. *Am J Cardiol.*, 48(3), pp. 418-28

Maron, M. S., Olivotto, I., Zenovich, A. G., Link, M. S., Pandian, N. G., Kuvin, J. T., Nistri, S., Cecchi, F., Udelson, J. E. & Maron, B. J. (2006). Hypertrophic cardiomyoptahy is predominantly a disease of the left ventricular outflow tract obstruction. *Circulation*, 114, pp. 2232-9

Maron, B. J., Spirito, P., Wesley, Y. & Arce, J. (1986). Development and progression of left ventricular hypertrophy in children with hypertrophic cardiomyopathy. *N Engl J Med.*, 315(10), pp. 610-4

Menon, S. C., Michels, V. V., Pellikka, P. A., Ballew, J. D., Karst, M. L., Herron, K. J., Nelson, S. M., Rodeheffer, R. J. & Olson, T. M. (2008). Cardiac troponin T mutation in familial cardiomyopathy with variable remodeling and restrictive physiology. *Clin Genet.*, 74(5), pp. 445-54

Midde, K., Dumka, V., Pinto, J. R., Muthu, P., Marandos, P., Gryczynski, I., Gryczynski, Z., Potter J. D. & Borejdo, J. (2011). Myosin cross-bridges do not form precise rigor bonds in hypertrophic heart muscle carrying Troponin T mutations. *J Mol Cell Cardiol.*, Jun 12 [Epub ahead of print]

Miller, T., Szczesna, D., Housmans, P. R., Zhao, J., de Freitas, F., Gomes, A. V., Culbreath, L., McCue, J., Wang, Y., Xu, Y., Kerrick, W. G. & Potter, J. D. (2001). Abnormal contractile function in transgenic mice expressing a familial hypertrophic cardiomyopathy-linked troponin T (I79N) mutation. *J Biol Chem.*, 276(6), pp. 3743-55

Miliou, A., Anastasakis, A., D'Cruz, L. G., Theopistou, A., Rigopoulos, A., Rizos, I., Stamatelpoulos, S., Toutouzas, P., Stefanadis, C. (2005). Low prevalence of cardiac troponin T mutations in a Greek hypertrophic cardiomyopathy cohort. *Heart,* 91, pp. 966-7

Mittmann, K., Jaquet, K. & Heilmeyer, L. M., Jr. (1990). A common motif of two adjacent phosphoserines in bovine, rabbit and human cardiac troponin I. *FEBS Lett.*, 273(1-2), pp. 41-5

Mittmann, K., Jaquet, K. & Heilmeyer, L. M., Jr. (1992). Ordered phosphorylation of a duplicated minimal recognition motif for cAMP-dependent protein kinase present in cardiac troponin I. *FEBS Lett.*, 302(2), pp. 133-7

Mirza, M., Marston, S., Willott, R., Ashley, C., Mogensen, J., McKenna, W., Robinson, P., Redwood, C. & Watkins, H. (2005). Dilated cardiomyopathy mutations in three thin filament regulatory proteins result in a common functional phenotype. *J. Biol. Chem.*, 280, pp. 28498- 506

Mörner, S., Richard, P., Kazzam, E., Hainque, B., Schwartz, K., Waldenström, A. (2000). Deletion in he cardiac troponin I gene in a family from northern Sweden with hypertrophic cardiomyopathy. *J Mol Cell Cardiol.*, 32(3), pp. 521-5

Mogensen, J., Murphy, R. T., Kubo, T., Bahl, A., Moon, J. C., Klausen, I. C., Elliot, P. M., McKenna, W. J. (2004). Frequency and clinical expression of cardiac troponin I mutations in 748 consecutive falilies with hypertrophic cardiomyopathy. *J Am Coll Cardiol.*, 44, pp. 2315-25

Mogensen, J., Murphy, R. T., Shaw, T., Bahl, A., Redwood, C., Watkins, H., Burke, M., Elliott, P. M. & McKenna, W. J. (2004). Severe disease expression of cardiac troponin C and T mutations in patients with idiopathic dilated cardiomyopathy. J. Am. Coll. Cardiol., 44, pp. 2033-40

Monserrat, L., Gimeno-Blanes, J. R., Marin, F., Hermida-Prieto, M., Garcia-Honrubia, A., Perez, I., Fernandez, I., de Nicolas, R., de la Morena, G., Paya, E., Yague, J. & Egido, J.(2007).Prevalence of Fabry disease in a cohort of 508 unrelated patients with hypertrophic cardiomyopathy. *J Am Coll Cardiol.*, 50(25), 2399-403

Montgomery, D. E., Wolska, B. M., Pyle, W. G., Roman, B. B., Dowell, J. C., Buttrick, P. M., Koretsky, A. P., Del Nido, P. & Solaro, R. J. (2002). alpha-Adrenergic response and myofilament activity in mouse hearts lacking PKC phosphorylation sites on cardiac TnI. *Am J Physiol Heart Circ Physiol.*, 282(6), pp. H2397-405

Moolman, J. C., Corfield, V. A., Posen, B., Ngumbela, K., Seidman, C., Brink, P. A., & Watkins, H. (1997). Sudden death due to troponin T mutations. *J Am Coll Cardiol.*, 29, pp. 549-55.

Morris, E. P. & Lehrer, S. S. Troponin-tropomyosin interactions. Fluorescence studies of the binding of troponin, troponin T, and chymotryptic troponin T fragments to specifically labeled tropomyosin. *Biochemistry* 23, 2214-20.

Mukherjea, P., Tong, L., Seidman, J. G., Seidman, C. E. & Hitchcock-DeGregory, S. E. (1999). Altered regulatory function of two familial hypertrophic cardiomyopathy troponin T mutants. *Biochemistry,* 38(49), pp. 13296-301

Murakami, K., Stewart, M., Nozawa, K,, Tomii, K., Kudou, N., Igarashi, N., Shirakihara, Y., Wakatsuki, S., Yasunaga, T. & Wakabayashi, T. (2008). Structural basis for tropomyosin overlap in thin (actin) filaments and the generation of a molecular swivel by troponin-T. *Proc Natl Acad Sci U.S.A.* 105(20), pp. 7200-5

Murphy, R. T., Mogensen, J., Shaw, A., Kubo, T., Hughes, S. & McKenna, W, J. (2009). Novel mutation in cardiac troponin I in recessive idiopathic dilated cardiomyopathy. *Circ Res.*, 105(4), pp. 375-82

Nagueh, S. F., Bachinski, L. L., Meyer, D., Hill, R., Zoghbi, W. A., Tam, J. W., Quinones, M. A., Roberts, R., Marian, A. J. (2001). Tissue Doppler imaging consistently detects myocardial abnormalities in patients with hypertrophic cardiomyopathy and provides a novel means for an early diagnosis before and independently of hypertrophy. *Circulation*, 104(2), pp. 128-30

Nakajima-Taniguchi, C., Matsui, H., Fujio, Y, Nagata, S, Kishimoto T, Yamauchi-Takihara, K. (1997). Novel missense mutation in cardiac troponin T gene found in Japanese patient with hypertrophic cardiomyopathy. *J Mol Cell Cardiol.*, 29, 839-43

Nakaura, H., Yanaga, F., Ohtsuki, I. & Morimoto, S. (1999). Effects of missense mutations Phe110Ile and Glu244Asp in human cardiac troponin T on force generation in skinned cardiac muscle fibers. *J Biochem.*, 126(3), pp. 457-60

Narolska, N. A., Piroddi, N., Belus, A., Boontje, N. M., Scellini, B., Deppermann, S., Zaremba, R., Musters, R. J., dos Remedios, C., Jaquet, K., Foster, D. B., Murphy, A. M., van Eyk, J. E., Tesi, C., Poggesi, C., van der Velden, J. & Stienen, G. J. (2006). Impaired diastolic function after exchange of endogenous troponin I with C-terminal truncated troponin I in human cardiac muscle. *Circ Res.*, 99(9), pp. 1012-20

Niimura, C., Patton, K. K., McKenna, W. J., Soults, J., Maron, B. J., Seidman, J. G. & Seidman, C. E. (2002). Sarcomere protein gene mutations in hypertrophic cardiomyopathy of the elderly. *Circulation*, 105, 446-51

Nguyen, L., Chung, J., Lam, L., Tsoutsman, T. & Semsarian, C. (2006). Abnormal cardiac response to exercise in a murine model of familial hypertrophic cardiomyopathy. *J Mol Cell Cardiol.*, 41(4), pp. 623-32

Ohtsuki, I. (1979). Molecular Arrangement of Troponin-T in the Thin Filament. *J. Biochem.*, 86(2), pp. 491-7

Olivotto, I., Maron, B. S., Adabag, A. S., Casey, S. A., Vargiu, D., Link, M. S., Udelson, S. E, Cecchi, F. & Maron, B. J. (2005). Gender- related differences in the clinical presentation and outcome of hypertrophic cardiomyopathy. *J. Am Coll Cardiol.*, 46(3), pp. 480-7

Ommen, S. R., Nishimura, R. A., Appelton, C. P., Miller, F. A., Oh, J. K., Redfield, M. M. & Tajik, A. J. (2000). Clinical utility of Doppler echocardiography and tissue Doppler imaging in the estimation of left ventricular filling pressures: a comparative simultaneous Doppler-catheterization study.*Circulation*, 102, pp. 1788-94

Palm, T., Graboski, S., Hitchcock-DeGregori, S. E., Greenfield, N. J. (2001). Disease-causing mutations in cardiac troponin T: identification of a critical tropomyosin-binding region. *Biophys J.*, 81(5), 2827-37. Erratum in *Biophys. J.* (2002) 82(5), pp. 2826

Paul, D. M., Morris, E. P., Kensler, R. W. & Squire, J. M. (2009). Structure and orientation of troponin in the thin filament. *J Biol Chem.*, 284(22), pp. 15007-15.

Paulus, W. J., Tschöpe, C., Anderson, J. E., Rusconi, C., Flachskampf, F. A., Rademakers, F. E., Marino, P., Smiseth, O. A., De Keulenaer, G., Leite-Moreira, A. F., Borbely, A., Edes, I., Handoko, M. L., Heymans, S., Pezzali, N., Pieske, B., Dickstein, K., Fraser, A. G. & Brutsaert, D. L. (2007). How to diagnose diastolic heart failure: a consensus statement on the diagnosis of heart failure with normal left ventricular ejection fraction by the Heart Failure and Echocardiography Associations of the European Society of Cardiology. *Eur Heart J.*, 28, pp. 2539-50

Parvatiyar, M. S., Pinto, J. R., Dweck, D. & Potter, J. D. (2010). Cardiac troponin mutations and restrictive cardiomyopathy. *J Biomed Biotechnol.*, 2010, 350706. Review.

Pearlstone, J. R. & Smillie, L. B. (1983) Effects of troponin-I plus-C on the binding of troponin-T and its fragments to alpha-tropomyosin. Ca^{2+} sensitivity and cooperativity. *J. Biol. Chem.*, 258, pp. 2534-42

Perry, S. V. (1998). Troponin T: genetics, properties and function. *J Muscle Res Cell Motil.*, 19, pp. 575–602

Pinto, J. R., Parvatiyar, M. S., Jones, M. A., Liang, J. & Potter, J. D. (2008). A troponin T mutation that causes infantile restrictive cardiomyopathy increases Ca2+ sensitivity of force development and impairs the inhibitory properties of troponin. *J. Biol. Chem.*, 283(4), pp. 2156-66

Pinto, J. R., Parvatiyar, M. S., Jones, M. A., Liang, J., Ackerman, M. J. & Potter, J. D. (2009). A functional and structural study of troponin C mutations related to hypertrophic cardiomyopathy. *J Biol Chem.*, 284(28), pp. 19090-100

Pinto, J. R., Reynaldo, D.P., Parvatiyar, M. S., Dweck, D., Liang, J., Jones, M. A., Sorenson, M. M. & Potter, J. D. (2011a). Strong cross-bridges potentiate the Ca(2+) affinity changes produced by hypertrophic cardiomyopathy cardiac troponin C mutants in myofilaments: a fast kinetic approach. *J Biol Chem.*, 286(2), pp. 1005-13

Pinto, J. R., Yang, S.W., Hitz, M.P., Parvatiyar, M.S., Jones, M.A., Liang,J., Kokta, V., Talajic, M., Tremblay, N., Jaeggi, M., Andelfinger, G. & Potter, J. D. (2011). Fetal cardiac troponin isoforms rescue the increased Ca2+ sensitivity produced by a novel double deletion in cardiac troponin T linked to restrictive cardiomyopathy: a clinical, genetic, and functional approach. *J Biol Chem.*, 286(23), pp. 20901-12

Pinto, Y. M., Wilde, A. M., van Rijsingen, I. A. W., Christaans, I., Lekanne, Deprez, R. H. & Elliot, P. M. (2011). Clinical utility gene card for: hypertrophic cardiomyopathy (type 1-4). *Eur J Hum Genet.*, epub ahead of print.

Pirani, A., Xu, C., Hatch, V., Craig, R., Tobacman, L. S. & Lehman, W. (2005). Single particle analysis of relaxed and activated muscle thin filaments. *J Mol Biol., 346,* pp. *761*–72

Redwood, C., Lohmann, K., Bing, W., Esposito, G. M., Elliott, K., Abdulrazzak, H., Knott, A., Purcell, I., Marston, S. & Watkins, H. (2000). Investigation of a truncated cardiac troponin T that causes familial hypertrophic cardiomyopathy. Ca(2+) regulatory properties of reconstituted thin filaments depend on the ratio of mutant to wild-type protein. *Circ Res.*, 86(11), pp. 1148-52

Reiffert, S. U., Jaquet, K., Heilmeyer, L. M., Jr., Ritchie, M. D., Geeves, M. A. (1996). Bisphosphorylation of cardiac troponin I modulates the Ca(2+)-dependent binding of myosin subfragment S1 to reconstituted thin filaments. *FEBS Lett.*, 384(1), 43-7

Reis, S., Littwitz, C., Preilowski, S., Mügge, A., Stienen, G. J., Pott, L. & Jaquet, K. (2008). Expression of cTnI-R145G affects shortening properties of adult rat cardiomyocytes. *Pflugers Arch.*, 457(1), pp. 17-24

Revera, M., Van der Merwe, L., Heradien, M., Goosen, A., Corfield, V. A., Brink, P. A. & Moolman-Smook, J. C. (2007). Long-term follow-up of R403WMYH7 and R92WTNNT2 HCM families: mutations determine left ventricular dimensions but not wall thickness during disease progression. *Cardiovasc J Afr.*, 18(3), pp. 146-53

Richard, P., Charron, P., Carrier, L., Ledeuil, C., Cheav, T., Picherau, C., Benaiche, A., Isnard, R., Dubourg, O., Burban, M., Gueffet, J. P., Millaire, A., Desnos, M., Schwartz, K., Hainque, B. & Komajda, M. for the EUROGENE Heart Failure Project: Hypertrophic cardiomyopathy. (2003). Distribution of disease genes, spectrum of mutations, and implications for a molecular diagnosis strategy. *Circulation.*, 107, pp. 2227-32

Risnik, V. V. & Gusev, N. B. (1984). Some properties of the nucleotide-binding site of troponin T kinase-casein kinase type II from skeletal muscle. *Biochim Biophys Acta.*, 790(2), pp. 108-16

Robinson, P., Griffiths, P. J., Watkins, H. & Redwood, C. S. (2007). Dilated and hypertrophic cardiomyopathy mutations in troponin and alpha-tropomyosin have opposing effects on the calcium affinity of cardiac thin filaments. *Circ Res.*, 101(12), 1266-73

Rust, E. M., Albayya, F. P. & Metzger, J. M. (1999). Identification of a contractile deficit in adult cardiac myocytes expressing hypertrophic cardiomyopathy-associated mutant troponin T proteins. *J Clin Invest.*, 103(10), 1459-67

Sadayappan, S., Finley, N., Howarth, J. W., Osinska, H., Klevitsky, R., Lorenz, J. N., Rosevear, P. R. & Robbins, J. (2008). Role of the acidic N' region of cardiac troponin I in regulating myocardial function. *FASEB J.*, 22(4), pp. 1246-57

Sakthivel, S., Finley, N. L., Rosevear, P. R., Lorenz, J. N., Gulick, J., Kim, S., VanBuren, P., Martin, L. A. & Robbins, J. (2005). In vivo and in vitro analysis of cardiac troponin I phosphorylation. *J. Biol. Chem.* 280, pp. 703-14

Sakamoto, T., Tei, C., Murayama, M., Ischiyasu, H. & Hada, Y. (1976). Giant negative T-wave inversion as a manifestation of asymmetric apical hypertrophy of the left ventricle: echocardiographic and ultrasonocardiotomography. *Jpn Heart J.*, 17(5), pp. 611-29

Schmidtmann, A., Lohmann, K. & Jaquet, K. (2002). The interaction of the bisphosphorylated N-terminal arm of cardiac troponin I-A 31P-NMR study. *FEBS Lett.*, 513(2-3), pp. 289-93

Schmidtmann, A., Lindow, C., Villard, S., Heuser, A., Mügge, A., Gessner, R., Granier, C. & Jaquet, K. (2005). Cardiac troponin C-L29Q, related to hypertrophic cardiomyopathy, hinders the transduction of the protein kinase A dependent phosphorylation signal from cardiac troponin I to C. *FEBS J.*, 272(23), 6087-97

Sia, S. K., Li, M. X., Spyracopoulos, L., Gagné, S. M., Liu, W., Putkey, J. A. & Sykes, B. D. (1997). Structure of cardiac muscle troponin C unexpectedly reveals a closed regulatory domain. *J Biol Chem.*, 272(29), pp. 18216-21

Sirenko, S. G., Potter, J. D. & Knollmann, B. C. (2006). Differential effect of troponin T mutations on the inotropic responsiveness of mouse hearts--role of myofilament $Ca2+$ sensitivity increase. *J Physiol.* 575(Pt 1), pp. 201-13

Seidman, C. E. & Seidman, J. G. (2011). Identifying sarcomere gene mutations in hypertrophic cardiomyopathy. A personal history. *Circ Res.* 108, pp. 743-50

Semsarian, C., French, J., Trent, R. J., Richmond, D. R. & Jeremy, R. W. (1997). The natural history of left ventricular wall thickening in hypertrophic cardiomyopathy. *Aust NZ J Med.*, 27(1), 51-58

Sheng, H. Z., Shan, Q. J., Wu, X. & Cao, K. J. (2008). Cardiac troponin I gene mutation (Asp127Tyr) in a Chinese patient with hypertrophic cardiomyopathy). *Zhonghua Xin Xue Guan Bing Za Zhi.* 36(12): 1063-5

Spirito, P., Bellone, P., Harris, K. M., Bernabo, P., Bruzzi, P. & Maron, B. J. (2000). Magnitude of left ventricular hypertrophy and risk of sudden death in hypertrophic cardiomyopathy. *N Engl J Med.*, 342(24), pp. 1778-85

Smith, L., Greenfield, N. J. & Hitchcock-DeGregori, S. E. (1999). Mutations in the N- and D-helices of the N-domain of troponin C affect the C-domain and regulatory function. *Biophys J.*, 76(1 Pt 1), pp. 400-8

Solaro, R. J. & Kobayashi, T. (2011). Protein Phosphorylation and signal transduction in cardiac filaments. *J. Biol. Chem.*, 286(12), pp. 9935-40

Stelzer, J. E., Patel, J. R., Olsson, M. C., Fitzsimons, D. P., Leinwand, L. A. & Moss, R. L. (2004). Expression of cardiac troponin T with COOH-terminal truncation accelerates cross-bridge interaction kinetics in mouse myocardium. *AJP Heart*, 287(4), pp. H1756-61

Sumandea, M. P., Pyle, W. G., Kobayashi, T., de Tombe, P. P. & Solaro, R. J. (2003). Identification of a functionally critical protein kinase C phosphorylation residue of cardiac troponin T. *J Biol Chem.*, 278(37), pp. 35135-44. Review.

Sumandea, C. A., Garcia-Cazarin, M. L., Bozio, C. H., Sievert, G. A., Balke, C. W. & Sumandea, M. P. (2011). Cardiac troponin T, a sarcomeric AKAP, tethers protein kinase A at the myofilaments. *J Biol Chem*. 286(1), pp. 530-41

Sweeney, H. L., Feng, H. S., Yang, Z. & Watkins, H. (1998). Functional analyses of troponin T mutations that cause hypertrophic cardiomyopathy: insights into disease pathogenesis and troponin function. *Proc Natl Acad Sci U S A.*, 95(24), 14406-10

Swiderek, K., Jaquet, K., Meyer, H. E., Schächtele, C., Hofmann, F. & Heilmeyer, L. M., Jr. (1990). Sites phosphorylated in bovine cardiac troponin T and I. Characterization by 31P-NMR spectroscopy and phosphorylation by protein kinases. *Eur J Biochem.*, 190(3), 575-82

Szczesna, D., Zhang, R., Zhao, J., Jones, M., Guzman, G., Potter, J. D. (2000). Altered regulation of cardiac muscle contraction by troponin T mutations that cause familial hypertrophic cardiomyopathy. *J Biol Chem.*, 275(1), pp. 624-30

Tachampa, K., Wang, H., Farman, G. P. & de Tombe, P. P. (2007). Cardiac troponin I threonine 144: role in myofilament length dependent activation. *Circ Res.*, 101(11), pp. 1081-3

Takeda, S., Yamashita, A., Maeda, K. & Maéda, Y. (2003). Structure of the core domain of human cardiac troponin in the Ca(2+)-saturated form. *Nature*, 424(6944), pp. 35-41

Tester, D. J., Ackeman, M. J. (2011). Genetic testing for potentially lethal, highly treatable inherited cardiomyopathies/channelopathies in clinical practice. *Circulation*, 123, 1021-37

Theopistou, A., Anastasakis, A., Miliou, A., Rigopoulos, A., Toutouzas, P. & Stefanadis, C. (2004). Clinical features of hypertrophic cardiomyopathy caused by an Arg278Cys missense mutation in the cardiac troponin T gene. *Am J Cardiol.*, 94, 246-9

Thierfelder, L., Watkins, H., MacRae, C., Lamas, R., Mc Kenna, W., Vosberg, H. P., Seidman, J. G. & Seidman, C. E. (1994). Alpha-tropomyosin and cardiac troponin T mutations cause familial hypertrophic cardiomyopathy: a disease of the sarcomere. *Cell*, 77(5), 701-12

Tobacman, L. S. (1988). Structure-function studies of the amino-terminal region of bovine cardiac troponin T. *J Biol Chem.*, 263(6), 2668-72

Torricellli, F., Girolami, F., Olivotto, I., Passerini, I., Frusconi, S., Vardiu, D., Richard, P. & Cecchi, F. (2003). Prevalence and clinical profile of troponin T mutations among patients with hypertrophic cardiomyopathy in Tuscany. *Am J Cardiol.*, 92, pp. 1358-62

Townsend, P. J., Barton, P. J., Yacoub, M. H. & Farza, H. (1995). Molecular cloning of human cardiac troponin T isoforms: expression in developing and failing heart. *J Mol Cell Cardiol.*, 27(10), pp. 2223-36

Turnbull, L., Hoh, J. F., Ludowyke, R. I. & Rossmanith, G. H. (2002). Troponin I phosphorylation enhances crossbridge kinetics during beta-adrenergic stimulation in rat cardiac tissue. *J. Physiol.*, 542, pp. 911-20

Tsoutsman, T., Chung, J., Doolan, A., Nguyen, L., Williams, I.A., Tu, E., Lam, L., Bailey, C. G., Rasko, J. E., Allen, D. G. & Semsarian, C. (2006). Molecular insights from a novel cardiac troponin I mouse model of familial hypertrophic cardiomyopathy. *J Mol Cell Cardiol.*, 41(4), pp. 623-32

Tsoutsman, T., Bagnall, R. D. & Semsarian, C. (2008). Impact of multiple gene mutations in determining the severity of cardiomyopathy and heart failure. *Clin Exp Pharmacol Physiol.*, 35(11), pp. 1349-57. Review.

Tsoutsman, T., Kelly, M., Ng, D. C., Tan, J. E., Tu, E., Lam, L., Bogoyevitch, M. A., Seidman, C. E., Seidman, J. G. & Semsarian, C. (2008). Severe heart failure and early mortality in a double-mutation mouse model of familial hypertrophic cardiomyopathy. *Circulation*, 117(14), pp. 1820-31

Vahebi, S., Kobayashi, T., Warren, C. M., de Tombe, P. P. & Solaro, R. J. (2005). Functional effects of rho-kinase-dependent phosphorylation of specific sites on cardiac troponin. *Circ Res.*, 96(7), pp. 740-7

van der Velden, J., Papp, Z., Zaremba, R., Boontje, N. M., de Jong, J. W., Owen, V. J., Burton, P. B., Goldmann, P., Jaquet, K. & Stienen, G. J. (2003) Increased Ca2+-sensitivity of the contractile apparatus in end-stage human heart failure results from altered phosphorylation of contractile proteins. *Cardiovasc Res.*, 57(1), pp. 37-47

Van Driest, S. L., Ellsworth, E. G., Ommen, S. R., Tajik, J., Gersh, B. J. & Ackerman, M. J. (2003). Prevalence and spectrum of thin filament mutations in an outpatient referral population with hypertrophic cardiomyopathy. *Circulation*, 108, pp. 445-51

Varnava, A. M., Elliot, P. M., Baboonian, C., Davison, F., Davies, M. J. & McKenna, W. J. (2001). Hypertrophic cardiomyopathy. Histological features of sudden death in cardiac troponin T disease. *Circulation*, 104, pp. 1380-4

Venkatraman, G., Gomes, A. V., Kerrick, W. G. & Potter J. D. (2005). Characterization of troponin T dilated cardiomyopathy mutations in the fetal troponin isoform. *J Biol. Chem.*, 280(18), pp. 17584-92

Wang, P., Zou, Y., Fu, C. Y., Zhou, X. & Hui, R. (2005). MYBPC3 polymorphism is a modifier for expression of cardiac hypertrophy in patients with hypertrophic cardiomyopathy. *Biochem Biophys Res Comm.*, 329(2), pp. 796-9

Ward, D. G., Brewer, S. M., Cornes, M. P. & Trayer, I. P. (2003) .A cross-linking study of the N-terminal extension of human cardiac troponin I. *Biochemistry*, 42, pp. 10324-32

Ward, D. G., Brewer, S. M., Gallon, C. E., Gao, Y., Levine, B. A., Trayer & I. P. (2004). NMR and mutagenesis studies on the phosphorylation region of human cardiac troponin I. *Biochemistry*, 43, pp. 5772-81

Ward, D. G., Brewer, S. M., Calvert, M. J., Gallon, C. E., Gao, Y. & Trayer, I. P. (2004). Characterization of the interaction between the N-terminal extension of human cardiac troponin I and troponin C. *Biochemistry*, 43, pp. 4020-7

Watkins, H., McKenna, W. J, Thierfelder, L., Suk, H. J., Anan, R., O'Donoghue, A., Spirito, P., Matsumori, A., Moravec, C. S., Seidman, J. G. & Seidman, C. E. (1995). Mutations in the genes for cardiac troponin T and α-tropomyosin in hypertrophic cardiomyopathy. *N Engl J Med.*, 332, pp. 1058-64

Watkins, H., Ashrafian, H. & Redwood, C. (2011). Inherited cardiomyopathies. *N Engl J Med.*, 364, pp. 1643-56

Wen, Y., Pinto, J. R., Gomes, A. V., Xu, Y., Wang, Y., Wang, Y., Potter, J. D. & Kerrick, W. G. (2008). Functional consequences of the human cardiac troponin I hypertrophic cardiomyopathy mutation R145G in transgenic mice. *J Biol Chem.*, 283(29), pp. 20484-94

Westermann, D., Knollmann, B. C., Steendijk, P., Rutschow, S., Riad, A., Pauschinger, M., Potter, J. D., Schultheiss, H. P. & Tschöpe, C. (2006). Diltiazem treatment prevents diastolic heart failure in mice with familial hypertrophic cardiomyopathy. *Eur J Heart Fail.*, 8(2), pp. 115-21

White, S. P., Cohen, C. & Phillips, G. N., Jr. (1987). Structure of co-crystals of tropomyosin and troponin. *Nature*, 325(6107), pp. 826-8

Xu, C., Wie, M., Su, B., Hua, X. W., Zhang, G. W., Xue, X. P., Pan, C. M., Liu, R., Sheng, Y., Lu, Z. G., Jin, L. R. & Song, H. D. (2008). Ile90Met, a novel mutation in the cardiac troponin T gene for familial hypertrophic cardiomyopathy in a Chinese pedigree. *Genet Res.*, 90(5), pp. 445-50

Yanaga, F., Morimoto, S. & Ohtsuki, I. (1999). Ca2+ sensitization and potentiation of the maximum level of myofibrillar ATPase activity caused by mutations of troponin T found in familial hypertrophic cardiomyopathy. *J Biol Chem.* , 274(13), pp. 8806-12

Yetman, A. T., McCrindle, B. W., MacDonald, C., Freedom, R. M. & Gow, R.(1998). Myocardial bridging in children with hypertrophic cardiomyopathy - a risk factor for sudden death. *N Engl J Med.*, 339, pp. 1201-9

Zhang R, Zhao J & Potter JD. (1995). Phosphorylation of both serine residues in cardiac troponin I is required to decrease the Ca2+ affinity of cardiac troponin C. *J Biol Chem,*. 270(51), pp. 30773-80

Zhang, Z., Biesiadecki, B. J. & Jin, J. P. (2006). Selective deletion of the NH_2-terminal variable region of cardiac troponin T in ischemia reperfusion by myofibril-associated mu-calpain cleavage. *Biochemistry*, 45, pp. 11681–94

16

Cardiomyopathies Associated with Myofibrillar Myopathies

Lilienbaum Alain[1] and Vernengo Luis[2]
[1]*Univ. Paris Diderot-Paris 7, Unit of Functional and Adaptive Biology (BFA) affiliated with CNRS (EAC4413), Laboratory of Stress and Pathologies of the Cytoskeleton, Paris*
[2]*Clinical Unit, Department of Genetics, Faculty of Medicine, University of the Republic, Montevideo*
[1]*France*
[2]*Uruguay*

1. Introduction

The aim of this chapter is to describe cardiomyopathies associated with myofibrillar myopathies (MFM, OMIM 601419). Myofibrillar myopathies are a group of heterogeneous neuromuscular disorders usually characterized by a severe myopathy, and generally associated with cardiomyopathy in 15% to 30% of the affected individuals. These familial or sporadic muscle disorders are characterized morphologically by focal disintegration of the myofibrils and abnormal ectopic accumulation of multiple proteins due to their degradation. The six genes that are held responsible so far for this clinically heterogenous, genetically heterogenous and morphologically homogeneous disorders are desmin, αB-crystallin, myotilin, LDB3 (ZASP), FLNC and BAG3. In the first part of the chapter the normal function in skeletal and cardiac muscles of the six genes will be discussed as well as physiopathological consequences of their mutations. The second part will describe how proteins encoded by these genes, together with main contractile proteins such as actin, tropomyosin, myosin, troponin, integrate into functional sarcomeric structures, which in turn determine the main cardiac functions : force generation, force transmission, nervous influx conduction, energy metabolism. Special emphasis will be put on a dynamic point of view, including protein turnover, protein quality control, with the involvement of ubiquitin-proteasome and autophagic systems. The third part gives a view of the latest insight of the clinical and therapeutic perspectives.

2. Clinical manifestations of myofibrillar myopathies

Myofibrillar myopathies represent a group of muscular dystrophies, generally associated with cardiomyopathy. They present specific but not always identical morphologic features. Because aggregates present desmin with other proteins, it has been called desmin-related myopathy.

2.1 Clinical and histopathological features of DRMs

Diagnosis is based on clinical observations of patients and histologic studies using histochemistry and electron microscopy. Common symptoms of the disease are weakness and atrophy of the distal muscles of the lower limbs which progress to the hands and arms, then the trunk, neck and face. Wasting, muscle stiffness, cramps can also be found. The myopathy may progress to facial, cervical, velopharyngeal, truncal and respiratory muscles. The vast majority of MFM patients have an adult onset of their progressive muscle symptoms (Goldfarb et al., 2004). Cardiomyopathy is associated in 15 to 30 % of the affected individuals. However, in some patients, the cardiomyopathy may precede the muscle weakness. Therefore, distal muscle involvement, cardiomyopathy and peripheral neuropathy are important clinical clues, although they are not present in all patients (Bar et al., 2004; Finsterer & Stollberger, 2008; Schroder et al., 2007).

2.1.1 Skeletal

The abnormal size of muscular fibers, with few atrophic fibers, are the characteristics of the disorder. These fibers present amorphous, granular or hyaline deposits that vary in shape and size. As abnormal fibers can be focally distributed, the symptomatic changes may be missed in small samples. Many abnormal fibers show alteration in oxidative enzymes activity, which are diminished or absent. Reduced oxidative activity is often associated with the presence of hyaline structures, and conversely, enhanced activity around the larger inclusions. Some muscular fibers harbor small to large vacuoles containing membranous materials. Many hyaline structures are stained blue or blue-red with Trichome or intensively stained with Congo red, which is an important diagnostic feature of MFM biopsies (Schroder & Schoser, 2009).

Immunohistochemical studies reveal accumulations of desmin, myotilin, dystrophin, sarcoglycans, actin, plectin, gelsolin, filamin C, syncoilin, Bag3, synemin, αB-crystallin, Hsp27 and DNAJB2. Additional pathologic markers may be observed, including phosphorylated tau proteins, β amyloids, ubiquitin, glycoxidation and lipoxidation can be found, more specifically in desmin- and myotilin-opathies (Selcen, 2011).

Electron microscopy shows a marked disorganization of the myofibrils ultrastructure, beginning at the Z-disc. Accumulation of dense materials is found in the close proximity of the Z-disc. In patients with desmin, αB-crystallin or Bag3 mutations, small pleiomorphic dense structures or granulofilamentous materials are found between the myofibrils. At later stages, Z-disc are disintegrated and sarcomeres disorganized, a prelude to myofibrils dislocation (Goldfarb & Dalakas, 2009). Electromyogram (EMO) studies of affected muscles reveal myopathic motor units potentials and abnormal electrical irritability, often with myotonic discharges (Schroder & Schoser, 2009).

2.1.2 Cardiac

All the genes cited in paragraph 2.3 cause cardiomyopathy. In 15 to 30 % of patients, the disorder presents with cardiomyopathy. There are also cases with only cardiomyopathic signs without skeletal muscle involvement. In advanced stages of the disease, cardiomyopathies develop in up to 60 % of the patients. MFM-associated atrioventricular conduction blocks can be associated with dilated (17 %), restricted (12 %), or hypertrophic (6 %) cardiomyopathy (van Spaendonck-Zwarts et al., 2010). When the cardiac muscle is involved, impaired conduction, arrhythmia, cardiac hypertrophy or dilation, secondary valvular insufficiency, intracardial formation of thrombi and heart failure can be observed. The least severe cases are caused by myotilin mutations. Atrioventricular conduction abnormalities may occur, and require urgent implantation of permanent pacemaker. This feature of MFMs can be attributed to the fact that the conduction system is rich in desmin (Finsterer & Stollberger, 2008; Goldfarb & Dalakas, 2009).

2.1.3 Respiratory

As the diaphragm is the main muscle involved in the respiratory cycle, progressive respiratory muscle impairment can occur, sometimes at early stages. Respiratory insufficiency can therefore be a major cause of disability and death with hypoventilation and ultimately respiratory failure, caused for example by mutations A357P, L370P in the desmin gene, or P209L in the BAG3 gene. Respiratory muscle weakness leads to a restrictive ventilatory failure when there is a mutation on the genes causing any of the myopathies except on ZASPopathy in which respiratory muscle involvement has not yet been described (Goldfarb & Dalakas, 2009).

2.2 Inheritance

The majority of cases follow an autosomal dominant mode of inheritance, and very few an autosomal recessive pattern. However, a significant number of MFMs shows sporadic disease manifestation.

2.2.1 Autosomal dominant mode

80 % of families with MFMs present an autosomal dominant pattern of inheritance, mostly with full penetrance (Goldfarb & Dalakas, 2009). Depending on the mutation, however, these facts can be modulated: for example, in families with the I451M mutation in the desmin gene, incomplete penetrance was demonstrated for the first time (Li et al., 1999). It is not possible, however, to link a specific mutation of the affected genes to clinical signs, although certain mutations are more frequently associated with specific signs. For example, the desmin A350P mutation predisposes male patients to higher risks of sudden cardiac death (Walter et al., 2007), as it is also the case for men and women in mutations p.E114del and N116S of the segment 1A of the desmin gene (Klauke et al., 2010; Vernengo et al., 2010).

2.2.2 Autosomal recessive mode

In a restricted number of families (6%), mutations are autosomal recessive (Goldfarb & Dalakas, 2009). The disease generally develops in childhood with severe clinical symptoms (Goldfarb et al., 2004). This is the case, for example, of the deletion A173_G179del of 21 nucleotides in the 1B helical segment of desmin (Muñoz-Marmol et al., 1998). Another intriguing report indicate two mutations A360P and N393I in the desmin protein, which are not pathogenic in heterozygous state, but give rise to a highly aggressive cardioskeletal myopathy when combined in the same child (Goldfarb et al., 1998). There is also a case reported for αB-crystallin (mutation S21AfsX24) (Selcen, 2011).

2.2.3 Modifying genes

Lamin A/C mutations have been involved in muscular dystrophies but can also lead to completely different pathologies, depending on the mutations involved. A patient with a combination of Lamin A/C A644C and desmin V469M mutations developed severe muscle weakness and complete heart block, requiring heart transplantation (Muntoni et al., 2006). Lamin A/C and desmin networks are supposed to be indirectly connected (Costa et al., 2004), and therefore may interact in the development of the disease. As individuals from the same family are diversely affected by the disease, one can suspect their individual history (practice of sport) or differential genetic background. The question of the identity of modifying genes remains, however, largely unresolved.

2.3 Molecular genetics

So far, six genes have been formally identified and are held responsible for MFMs associated with cardiomyopathy, but for around 80 % of the patients, the disease still awaits a molecular diagnosis (Selcen, 2011). Schröder et al. include FHL1 and plectin in MFM-causing genes (Schröder, 2009). The knowledge of the structure and function of the already identified genes is, therefore, a prerequisite for the understanding of human MFMs.

2.3.1 Desmin

The human *DES* gene (NM_001927.3), on chromosome 2q35, comprises nine exons within an 8.4 kb region that encodes a 470 amino acids (53 kDa) muscle-specific protein (Li et al., 1989). Desmin belongs to the family of type III intermediate filaments (IF) proteins, which polymerize into 10 nm filaments, a size intermediate between thick (15 nm) and thin (5-6 nm) filaments. Desmin is synthetized only in cardiac, skeletal and smooth muscles (Lazarides & Hubbard, 1976 ; Paulin & Li, 2004). It is organized into three domains, a highly conserved α helical core of 303 amino acids residues flanked by globular N- and C- terminal structures. The helical structure, called the rod domain, is interrupted by three short polypeptide linkers (L1, L12, L2), which determine four consecutive helical segments (1A, 1B, 2A, 2B). Desmin is more abundant in heart muscle (2% of total proteins) of mammals than in their skeletal muscle (0.35%) (Paulin et al., 2004). It forms a three-dimensional scaffold around the myofibrillar Z-disc, and interconnects the entire contractile apparatus with the subsarcolemmal cytoskeleton and the nuclei (Lazarides & Hubbard, 1976). Desmin also forms longitudinal connections between the peripheries of successive Z-discs and along the plasma membrane. In addition, desmin IFs bind and participate to the location of mitochondria. In the heart, desmin is particularly abundant in Purkinje conduction fibers, and at intercalated discs, where it forms a double-banded structure (Thornell & Eriksson, 1981). Since the first description of desminopathy by Goldfarb et al. (Goldfarb et al., 1998) and Muñoz-Marmol et al. (Muñoz-Marmol et al., 1998), more than 50 mutations (45 missenses, 4 in frame deletions, 1 exon skipping, 2 single nucleotide insertion with premature termination) have been described (Klauke et al., 2011; Selcen, 2011; van Spaendonck-Zwarts et al., 2010).

Studies of DES-knockout mice have shown that defects develop in skeletal, smooth and cardiac muscle after birth, principally characterized by a loss of lateral alignment and anchorage of myofibrils, swollen mitochondria and loss of nuclear shape. The hearts develop a myopathy with impaired force generation, increased diastolic pressure with thicker ventricle walls (Li et al., 1996; Milner et al., 1996). Few transgenic mice have been described. With the Arg173_Glu179del desmin mutant transgene, aggregates containing desmin and other cytoskeletal proteins have been found in the heart (Wang et al., 2001a). A clear explanation of the molecular pathogenesis remains to be found.

Misfolded desmin molecules escape regular degradation mechanisms and accumulate with other proteins as aggregates. Cellular transfection studies have demonstrated that aggregates inhibit the proteasome system (Liu et al., 2006). In general, aggregates may accumulate through an active transport mechanism into perinuclear bodies called aggresomes (Johnston et al., 1998). Aggregates and proteasome impairement trigger autophagy (macroautophagy) as a mechanism of cellular cleaning (Tannous et al., 2008a), but recent studies have shown that this process is stalled at least with the desmin S13F mutant used in these studies (Wong et al., 2008).

2.3.2 αB-crystallin

AlphaB-crystallin is a small heat shock protein (sHSP) of 20 kDa that assembles into 500 - 800 kDa homo and heterodimers with other sHSPs. It is encoded by the CRYAB gene (NM_001885.1), a three-exon gene on chromosome 11 (11q21-23) in human beings. αB-crystallin proteins contain a conserved α crystallin domain (residues 67 to 149), surrounded by a N-terminal domain and a C-terminal extension (residues 149 - 175) (Ganea, 2001; MacRae, 2000). αB-crystallin is abundantly expressed, together with αA-crystallin and other similar sHSPs in the lens where it prevents cataract formation (Horwitz, 2003). It is also found in other tissues, with the highest level in cardiac and skeletal muscles (Iwaki et al., 1990; Sax & Piatigorsky, 1994). In these tissues, αB-crystallin is localized to the Z-disc, and its expression is induced after stress (Golenhofen et al., 2004; Lutsch et al., 1997). αB-crystallin is known to act as a molecular chaperone of desmin, actin, tubulin and several other soluble molecules (Goldfarb & Dalakas, 2009). αB-crystallin expression reduces aggregate formation, both *in vitro* and *in vivo*, and is supposed to help neosynthetized desmin proteins by avoiding their aggregation (Bennardini et al., 1992).

The first identification of a MFM case due to a heterozygous missense mutation in the αB-crystallin gene (R120G) was reported in 1998 (Vicart et al., 1998). Since then 9 other mutations have been discovered. Some patients develop also a familial cataract. The only knock-out model is deleted for both αB-crystallin and HspB2 (MKBP) genes because of their close proximity on the chromosome (Brady et al., 2001). CRYAB/HspB2 null mouse heart display poorer functional recovery, high cell death rate, increased stiffness and poor relaxation of myocardium following ischemia / reperfusion. In these mice, mitochondrial permeability transition and calcium uptake were increased in cardiomyocytes (Morrison et al., 2004). In contrast, overexpression of WT αB-crystallin delays or suppresses cardiac hypertrophic response to pressure overload (Kumarapeli et al., 2008). In addition, transgenic mice with cardiac-specific expression of R120G mutant αB-crystallin develop cardiomyopathy in three months and die of heart failure in six - seven months. Just as it is the case of the desmin mutations causing MFMs, αB-crystallinopathies present cytoplasmic aggregates that include desmin, αB-crystallin and several other proteins (Wang et al., 2001b).

2.3.3 Myotilin

Myotilin is a 57 kDa protein that is predominantly expressed in skeletal muscle and more weakly in the heart (Salmikangas et al., 1999). The human gene (NM_001135940) is located at the locus 5q31. The N-terminal region contains serine-rich and hydrophobic stretches, and the C-terminal half two immunoglobulin-(Ig)-like domains. The Ig-like domains are required for the formation of antiparallel myotilin dimers. Myotilin is located at the Z-disc where it binds to α-actinin, the main component of the Z-disc, and to filamin C at the periphery. Myotilin also cross-links actin filaments and plays a role in the alignment of myofibrils (Salmikangas et al., 2003). The involvement of myotilin was detected in the year 2000 as a missense mutation (T57I) and was identified as limb-girdle muscular dystrophy 1A (LGMD1A) (Hauser et al., 2000). Since then, six new myotilin mutations were identified in eight unrelated patients of the Mayo Clinic MFM cohort. The LGDM1A pathology is therefore a MFM (Selcen & Engel, 2004). Cardiac involvement was found in a subset of patients. While myotilin deletion in mice does not lead to obvious abnormalities, transgenic mice expressing the T57I mutant reproduce morphological and functional features of human myotilinopathies (Garvey et al., 2006). As for desmin, abnormal accumulation of many proteins occur in myotilinopathies.

2.3.4 ZASP

ZASP (Z band Alternatively Spliced PDZ motif-containing protein), also called Oracle or Cypher, is expressed predominantly in cardiac and skeletal muscles (Faulkner et al., 1999). The ZASP gene, called LDB3 (NM_001080114), situated on chromosome 10 (10q22.3-q23.2), encompasses 16 exons, and splice variants exist in cardiac and skeletal muscles, each expressing 3 distincts variants. All ZASP isoforms have a N- terminal PDZ (PSD-95/SAP90, ZO-1 proteins) domain important for interaction with other proteins, and a ZASP-like motif (ZM) needed for the interaction with α-actinin. The largest isoforms have three C-terminal LIM (LIN-11, Isl1m, MEC-3 proteins) domains that interact with Protein kinases C (PKCs) (Zhou et al., 1999). ZASP proteins were shown to localize at the Z disc (Klaavuniemi & Ylanne, 2006). The first case of ZASPopathy causing MFM was described in 2005 in 11 MFM patients carrying heterozygous missense mutations (Selcen & Engel, 2005). There was a cardiac involvement in 3 of these 11 patients. Mutations in ZASP was also shown to be responsible for dilated cardiac myopathy, and left-ventricle non compaction (Vatta et al., 2003). Knockout mice for ZASP develop skeletal and cardiac myopathy with fragmented Z-discs (Zheng et al., 2009).

2.3.5 Filamin C

Filamin C (γ-filamin or Filamin 2) belongs to a family of high molecular weight cytoskeletal proteins, expressed in skeletal and cardiac muscle, in contrast to an ubiquitous expression of filamin A and B. Filamin C (NM_001127487) is a 48-exon gene (280 aminoacids) on chromosome 7 (7q32) which belongs to the filamin family of actin-binding proteins that are involved in the reshaping of the actin cytoskeleton and it is associated to myotilin. The amino terminal domain contains an actin-binding domain, followed by a semiflexible rod comprising 24 Ig-like folds, serving as interface for interaction with numerous filamin-binding proteins (van der Flier & Sonnenberg, 2001). Homodimers of Filamin C are involved in the organization of actin filaments and serve as a scaffold for signaling proteins. They link the Z-disc to the sarcolemma by interacting with Z-disc proteins and sarcoglycans in costameres (Thompson et al., 2000). The Ig-like domain 20 also binds to myotilin, and may represent a Z disc targeting motif (van der Ven et al., 2000). The nonsense mutation W2710X was identified in 2005 in patients presenting MFM signs, associated with cardiomyopathy, respiratory insufficiency and peripheral neuropathy (Vorgerd et al., 2005). Life expectancy is shortened in patients who have mutations in the filamin C gene because of cardiomyopathy and the involvement of the respiratory muscles. Cataract and peripheral neuropathy can also occur thus demonstrating that there is a multisystem involvement. Filamin C is expressed before formation of myotubules and is required for a proper muscle development (van der Ven et al., 2000).

2.3.6 BAG3

BAG3 (Bcl-2 associated athanogen 3), which gene (NM_004281) is situated on chromosome 10 (10q25.2-q26.2), encodes a 535 aminoacid protein. It is a complex cochaperone which principally mediates interaction with Hsp70, Hsc70 and Bcl-2, an antiapoptotic protein, through its C-terminal BAG domain. The proline-rich domain interacts with the WW-domain (~35–40 amino acid residues including two highly conserved tryptophan (W) residues separated by 20–23 amino acids) that interacts with proteins implicated in signal transduction (Takayama & Reed, 2001). BAG3 forms a stable complex with HspB8 (Hsp22) and therefore participates to the degradation, via autophagy, of misfolded and aggregated proteins (Carra et al., 2008a). The first case of BAG3 mutation causing MFM was described in 2009 (P209L) in exon 3 (Selcen et al., 2009). All patients presented a childhood onset with severe progressive muscle weakness and atrophy, associated with large left atrium, pulmonary and mitral regurgitation with a restrictive cardiomyopathy pattern. There is also bilateral diaphragm paralysis, reduced forced vital capacity and respiratory insufficiency. Patients have a rigid spine and scapular winging. The progression of illness was found rapid when compared to other MFM mutations, and was linked to a significant level of apoptosis (8 % of nuclei). The function of BAG3 is to stabilize myofibril structure through F-actin. When it is mutated there is myofibril disruption and destabilization of the Z-disk structure under mechanical stress. Knockout mice for BAG3 results in a rapidly-developing myopathy with early lethality and apoptotic features, suggesting a role for BAG3 in supporting cytoskeletal connections between the Z-disc and myofibrils under mechanical stress (Homma et al., 2006).

2.4 Conclusion

MFMS are muscular dystrophies with specific, but not always identical morphologic features. All six genes causing MFMs with cardiac involvement identified so far encode proteins (Figure 1) that are related to the Z-disc. It is therefore important to study the Z-disc, which appears increasingly more complex. In fact, it is subjected to an exquisitely fine-tuned process of proteins quality control and protein turnover, and is involved in a mechanism of mechanosensing and signaling. These two important functions will be detailed in the following part.

3. Integrative biology of myofibrillar myopathies-involved genes

To understand how MFMs develop, it is necessary to describe how muscles are depending on the optimal functioning of the products of the genes described above. For that purpose, this part will develop how the different partners of the muscular structure interact with each others, in a static as well as in a dynamic point of view.

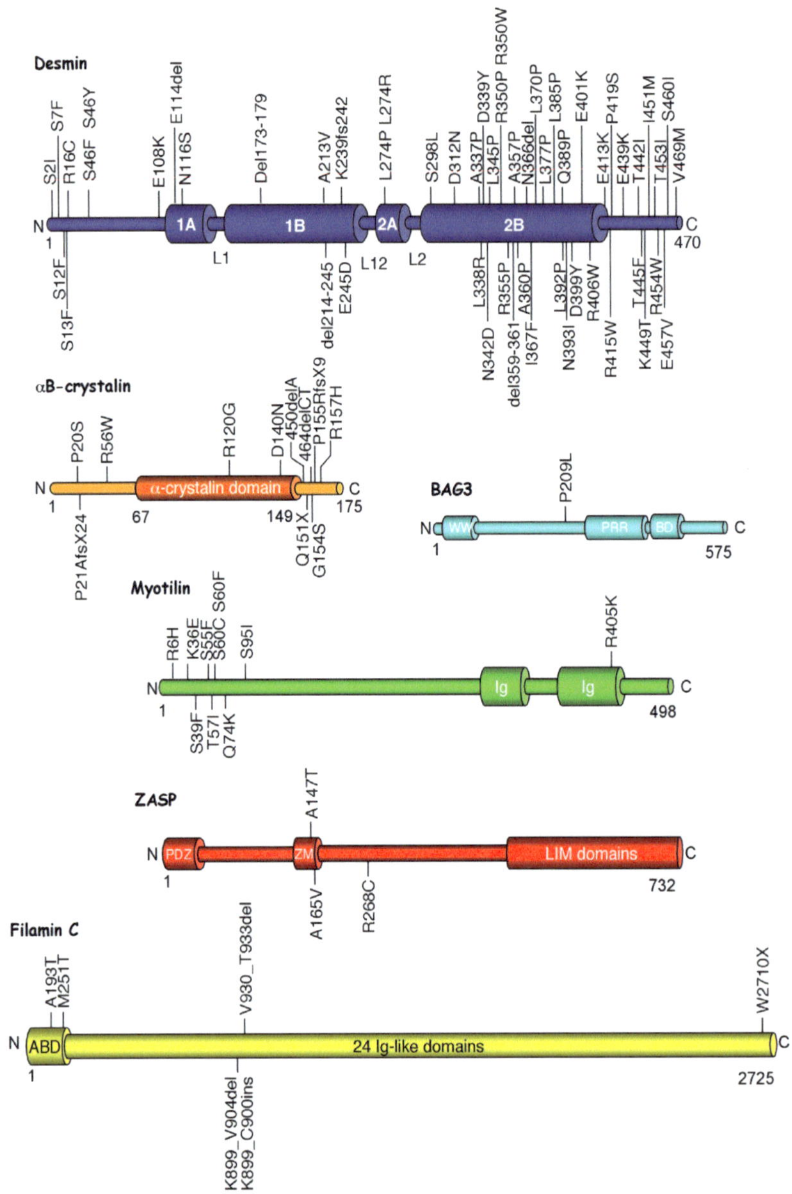

Fig. 1. Schematic representation and localization of mutations in the six proteins involved in myofibrilar myopathies.

N, C: respectively aminoterminal and carboxyterminal extremities. Numbers indicate the aminoacid position in the molecule. 1A, 1B, 2A, 2B are the helical domains of desmin. L1, L12, L2 are the non-helical linkers. WW: tryptophan-conserved domain interacting with proline-rich regions. PRR: Proline-rich region, interacting with WW domains. BD: BAG-domain. Ig: immunoglobulin-like domain. PDZ: PSD-95 / SAP90 / ZO-1 proteins common domain. ZM: ZASP-like motif. LIM domains: LIN-11 / Isl1m / MEC-3 proteins common domain. ABD: Actin-binding domain. Ig-like domains: immunoglobulin-like domain.

3.1 The smallest contractile unit: The sarcomere

The myocardium is composed of an assembly of a number of interconnecting, branching fibers, or short cells, separated at their end by the intercalated disk. The fibers contain numerous fibrils, composed of a regular repeating structure termed the "sarcomere" (Figure 2A) (Sonnenblick, 1968). The sarcomere is the basic and fundamental unit of striated muscles. Understanding the structure-function relationship linking the structure of the sarcomere to the physiology of normal or pathologic heart is therefore essential to understand myofibrillar myopathies development. Sarcomeres are distinguished by the striated distribution of their proteins, visible in light microscopy as three major bands, called A, I and Z (Figure 2B). A bands contain thick filaments of myosin and proteins that bind to myosin. The I band comprise thin actin filaments and proteins that bind actin. In the middle of the A is the "M band" also called "M line". The middle part of the I band is the "Z band", also called the "Z line" or "Z disk". The basic contractile system is the well known actin-myosin tandem. Two heavy myosin chains are associated to two light chains and form a globular part. Actin filaments, the thin structure, are composed of a double helix of G-actin (a globular molecule of 46 kDa) polymerized into a chain (Lehninger et al., 2005). αB-crystallin as chaperone molecule, myotilin and filamin C as scaffolding molecules, are known to interact with actin.

3.2 Force transmission

The first important role of Z-discs is passive transmission of tension through the Z-disc structural assembly. When a mutation occurs, like in MFM, the mechanism that maintains fixed Z-disc may go awry. In addition, Z-disc proteins allow to transmit force and ensure mechanical coupling between sarcomeres and the sarcolemma via the costameres. Three of four filaments systems of the sarcomere, filamentous F-actin, titin and nebulin/nebulette, interact with the Z-disc structure. Two proteins participate to the cardiac sacomeric cytoskeleton: titin and nebulette (Figure 2B).

Titin is a giant 3 MDa elastic protein that spans half sarcomeres from Z-disc to M-band, thus forming a continuous structure from one end of the sarcomere to the other, with consecutive titins. Titin can be considered as a giant bidirectional spring responsible for the generation of passive retraction force in mechanically stretched cardiac myocytes (Granzier & Labeit, 2004). Stiffness of titin can be adjusted during development and diseases through a shift in the expression ratio of the two main titin isoforms in cardiac sarcomeres (Lahmers et al., 2004; Opitz et al., 2004; Warren et al., 2004). Titin binds to more than 20 structural, contractile or signaling molecules, and therefore plays a role as major integrating component in the mechanosensory complexes associated to the sarcomeres.

Nebulette is a 107 kDa nebulin homologue present in the cardiac muscle Z-disc. It is composed of only 22 nebulin motifs (compared to up to 185 in nebulin), and contains a nebulin-like C terminus, mediating Z-disc localization (Moncman & Wang, 1995). At present, however, its molecular function in cardiac myocytes is still unclear.

The backbone of the Z-disc consists of layers of α-actinin aligned in an antiparallel fashion. In muscle, it cross-links actin filaments of opposite polarity originating from adjacent sarcomeres (Stromer & Goll, 1972) and provides anchors for the binding of actin thin filaments, as well as titin and nebulin/nebulette (Otey & Carpen, 2004). Myotilin and ZASP interact with α-actinin, and myotilin is linked to filamin C, thus creating a network of proteins at the Z-disc.

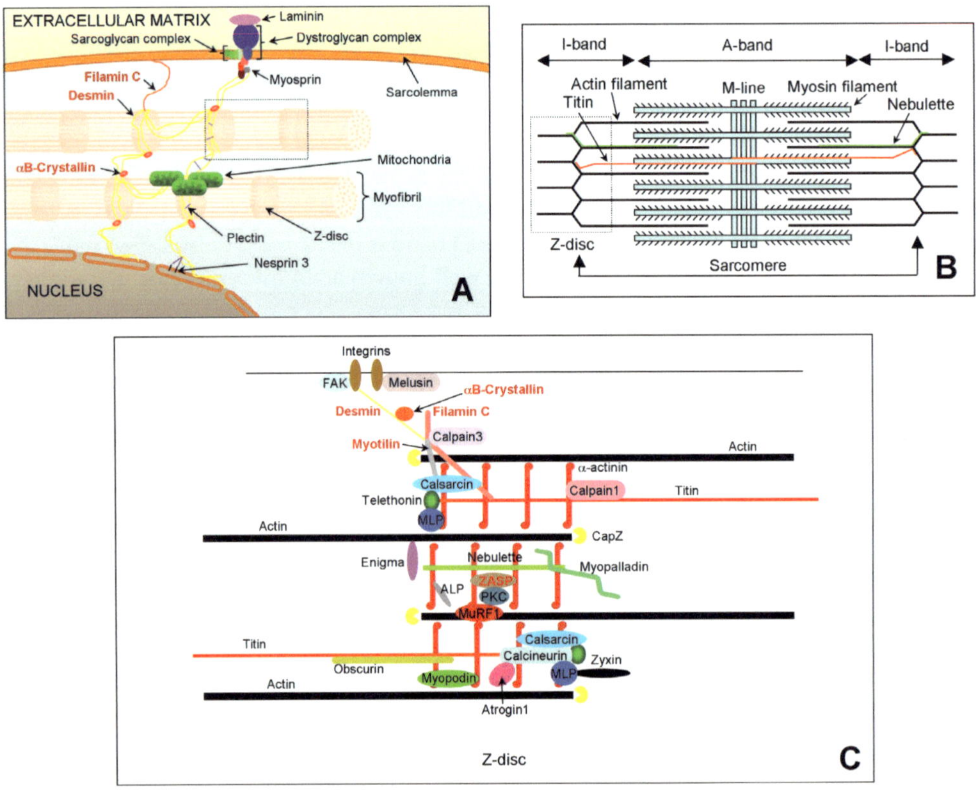

Fig. 2. Schematic representation of the general organization of muscular fibers (A), sarcomere (B) and schematic localization of the major proteins involved in the cardiac Z-disc structure (C).
Figure 2B represents the enlarged dotted rectangle in figure 2A, and Figure 2C the enlarged representation of the dotted rectangle in Figure 2B. Names in red and bold correspond to proteins involved in myofibrillar myopathies, excepted for Bag3 which is not represented. Not all proteins participating to the Z-disc structure or signaling are represented, due to the complexity of this structure. For more details, see text. Figure C is adapted from Frank et al., 2006.

Another essential component is CapZ, a heterodimer composed of α and β subunits, which caps the barbed ends of actin filaments. CapZ is proposed to regulate actin dynamics at the barbed end, thereby anchoring the thin filament system to the Z-disc (Schafer et al., 1996).

The costameres are multiproteic complexes which link the marginal Z-discs at their circumferences to the sarcolemma, the specialized membrane of the individual myofibers. Costameres have been described as transmitters of contractile force to the sarcolemma and extracellular matrix. This lateral force transmission ensures identical sarcomere length, thereby minimizing shear stress. However, desmin, filamin C, dystrophin, sarcoglycans, integrins, melusin and focal adhesion kinases have been involved in its structure (reviewed in Bloch et al., 2002).
Many other proteins (myopalladin, obscurin, Enigma, telethonin, zyxin, ...) participate to the Z-disc structure (Table 1), but their study is beyond the scope of this review (reviewed in Frank et al., 2006). The six genes held responsible for MFM are involved at various degrees in Z-disc structure and force transmission (Figure 2C). Desmin forms a continuous network that maintains a spatial relationship between the contractile apparatus and other structural elements of the cells, and is believed to provide maintenance of structural integrity, force transmission, mechanosignaling, and resistance to external mechanical stress. Myotilin constitutes the core of a network of proteins, including actin, α-actinin and filamin C, that are part of the force transmission mechanism. In turn, filamin C provides a scaffold for signaling proteins at the Z-disc, and may be part of a mechanosensing device.

3.3 Energy metabolism

In this part, we will focus on specific effects of the alteration of genes causing MFMs on energy in muscle. The main effects have been studied on the localization and function of mitochondria. Structural studies of intracellular arrangements of mitochondria into functional complexes with myofibrils and sarcoplasmic reticulum demonstrate their importance in mitochondrial oxydative activity and membrane permeability (Andrienko et al., 2003; Appaix et al., 2003). There are findings with pathological respiratory chain enzyme activities in patients with MFM (Reimann et al., 2003). Desmin intermediate filaments (IFs) might participate in mitochondrial positioning to areas of high energy demand, respiratory function, and calcium cycling in cardiac and skeletal muscle (Capetanaki, 2002).

3.4 Dynamic view of the sarcomere

While often described as a static structure, the sarcomere is actually dynamic and undergoes constant turnover, allowing to adapt to physiological changes while still maintaining its function. New factors have been identified that play a role in the regulation of protein quality control in the sarcomere, including chaperones that mediate the assembly of sarcomere components and ubiquitin ligases that control their specific degradation. The Z-disc has additional important roles as it houses or anchors many additional proteins, which have various roles, including stretch sensing and signaling or protein quality control. The Z-disc can therefore be considered as a nodal point in signaling and disease (reviewed in Frank et al., 2006). In MFMs, the Z-discs are abnormal, the arrangements of myofibrils are in disarray, or aggregates of proteins are present, often near the Z-disc. The highly ordered arrangements of proteins in the sarcomere, which persists even as contractile force is generated, suggest that binding interactions between Z-disc proteins are strong and very stable (Sanger & Sanger, 2008). Thus, the continual remodelling of the cardiac sarcomere allows efficient adaptation to physiological stresses, including exercice or metabolic variations, but also initial efficient adaptation to starting pathologies such as ischemic heart disease and myofibrillar myopathies. Since this dynamic turnover is the basis of homeostatic mechanism of sarcomere maintenance, it is essential to better understand it.

NAME	Size (kDa)	BINDING	FUNCTION	REMARKS
Obscuring	868	M-line, calmodulin, titin	Rho-GEF domain signaling	Giant protein
Myopalladin	145	Nebulette, α-actinin cadiac ankyrin repeat proteins (CARP)	Intra-Z-disc meshwork binds nebulette (directly) and titin (via α-actinin) to actin, CARP signaling ?	Palladin familly
ALP	39	Spectrin repeats of α-actinin	enhances cross-linking actin to α-actinin	PDZ and LIM domain protein 3 (PDLIM3)
Enigma	50	Ret kinase, actin, insulin receptor β tropomyosin	anchor for LIM proteins	PDLIM7
ENH	64	α-actinin 2, PKCε (brain)	hypertrophic program	PDLIM5
CLP36	36	α-actinin 2, Clik1 kinase	stress fibers control, FA	PDLIM1
Zyxin	61	binds actin to MLP α-actinin	close to Z-disc and FAK signalling / antiapoptotic	LIM protein family Nucleoplasmic shuttling
MLP	21	α-actinin, telethonin calcineurin, β spectrin	cardiac stretch receptor and mechanosignalling, negative regulator of cardiac hypertrophy	Nucleoplasmic shuttling
Telethonin	19	Titin N-terminus K+ channels, calsarcin	cardiomyocytes passive tension	negative regulator of myostatin = T-Cap
Calsarcin	27 - 32 *	Calcineurin, α-actinin telethonin, Filamin C, α-actinin	crosslinks Z-disc and Ca^{2+}/ calcineurin signalling, inhibits hypertrophic genes sensor for biomechanical stress	= synaptopodin-2
Myopodin	118 - 136 *	α-actinin colocalization	multiadaptator protein ?	nucleoplasmic shuttling

Table 1. Proteins involved in the Z-disc structure as well as in Z-disc signaling, and not detailed in the text.

Other structural and signaling molecules are described paragraphs 3.1, 3.2 and paragraph 3.4.6, respectively. ALP: Actinin-associated LIM Protein. PDZ: PSD-95 / SAP90 / ZO-1 proteins common domain. LIM domains: LIN-11 / Isl1m / MEC-3 proteins common domain. ENH: Enigma Homologue protein. MLP: Muscle LIM Protein. FA: Focal Adhesion. FAK: Focal Adhesion Kinase. PKC: Protein Kinase C.

3.4.1 Main contractile protein turnover

The following half-lives have been estimated in myocytes:
Actin: 7 to 10 days (Zak, 1977).
Myosin: 5 to 8 days (Martin et al., 1977).
Tropomyosin: 7 to 10 days (Zak, 1977).
Troponin: 3 to 5 days (Michele et al., 1999).
Titin is subjected to a "rapid" turnover, with a half-life estimated to be 3 days in myocytes (Fong et al., 1996).

3.4.2 Protein quality control: Role of chaperone molecules

Multiple endogenous pathways are engaged in restoring cellular homeostasis, among which one of the best characterized mechanism involves protein folding by the heat-shock family of stress proteins (HSP), also termed chaperones. There are several families of molecular chaperones present in the cytoplasm of mammalian cells, including Hsp90, Hsp70, TCP1 (CCT, TriC) and small HSP (sHSPs). Members of the Hsp90 family are the most abundant chaperones located in the cytosol in non-stressed cells which are inducible with stress.
Hsp70 and Hsc70 (Hsp70 cognate protein) are major players in cardiomyocyte protection: the induction of HSP70 by ischemia, and conversely, overexpression of Hsp70 or Hsc70 promotes substantial cardioprotective benefits (Donnelly et al., 1992; Hutter et al., 1994).
Chaperonin TRiC requires additional components, such as Hsp40, to stimulate the Hsc70 ATPase for protein folding, and is required for folding of actin and tubulin *in vivo*.
Unlike Hsp70, small HSPs, including αB-crystallin, Hsp27, Hsp22 and Hsp20 cannot bind nor hydrolyze ATP, and are not able to refold proteins, but can buffer them against aggregation (Merck et al., 1993). αB-crystallin represents a substantial fraction of adult heart total soluble proteins (1 to 3 %) (Kato et al., 1991). The highest level of αB-crystallin expression in muscles has been found in the cardiac conduction fibers (Leach et al., 1994). Previous studies indicate that αB-crystallin is highly soluble and localized in the cytosolic fraction in unstimulated cardiac myocytes. Heat or ischemia triggers rapid translocation of αB-crystallin into the cytoskeletal and nuclear fraction and specific interactions at the Z-disc (Neufer et al., 1998). HspB8 (Hsp22) and HspB6 (Hsp20) are also expressed in striated myogenic lineages with high oxidative capacity, such as the heart and type I skeletal muscle fibers (Depre et al., 2002).
HSP molecules are assisted by co-chaperones which perform a variety of tasks, including modulation of ATPase activity (DNAJ), substrate protein binding and release (BAG : Bcl-2 -Associated athanoGene), protein folding (Hsp40 family), assembly, and translocation or degradation (CHIP : Carboxyterminus of Hsp70 Interacting Protein). Co-chaperones also bind substrate proteins to modulate folding in a substrate-specific manner (reviewed in Willis & Patterson, 2010). Among many proteins (more than 40 Co-chaperones), only DnaJ, BAG-1, Hop and CHIP have been described in the heart. pDJA1 (DnaJ-like molecule) expression is restricted to cardiomyocytes. Its levels increase four-fold after reperfusion (Depre et al., 2003). BAG-1 is able to inhibit apoptosis and to induce autophagy by interacting with Hsc70, stimulated after ischemia / reperfusion injury (Townsend et al., 2004). The BAG-3 isoform participates in the induction of macroautophagy in association with HspB8 (Gurusamy et al., 2009). Another protein,

CHIP, plays a role as cochaperone of Hsp70 and in the ubiquitin-proteasome system as an ubiquitin ligase. CHIP may exert a critical function in shuttling damaged and oxydized proteins into autophagic pathways after ischemia / reperfusion injury (Zhang et al., 2005). Increased cochaperone expression in the heart has been found to be cardioprotective in ischemia (Benjamin & McMillan, 1998).

During assembling of the sarcomere, molecular chaperones are needed for the correct folding, assembly and prevention of aggregation. Two molecular chaperone GimC (prefoldin) and TriC (TCP-1 Ring Complex) have been found to play a synergistic role during synthesis and incorporation of actin filaments into the sarcomere. In contrast to actin, myosin cannot self-assemble without additional factors, including chaperones such as Unc45, Hsp90 and Hsp70. The assembly of desmin requires the chaperone αB-crystallin, to prevent its misfolding and aggregation (Bennardini et al., 1992). αB-crystallin also interacts with titin and actin. These data suggest a highly cooperative relationship between various chaperones during the assembly of the actin filaments in the sarcomere.

In animal models with targeted deletion of muscle-specific chaperone proteins, there is a clear evidence of sarcomere disorganization. Cardiac chaperones such as Hsp70, αB-crystallin and HspB8 levels are increased during the development of cardiac hypertrophy. Hsp27 and αB-crystallin can protect cardiomyocytes against ischemic damages (Martin et al., 1997). Increase in HspB8 expression also results in the re-expression of the foetal gene program characteristic of cardiac hypertrophy (Depre et al., 2002). The protective role of Hsp22 in ischemia / reperfusion injury appears to be due to its function in activating autophagy, which is critical during the course of this type of injury (Carra et al., 2008b).

3.4.3 The specific ubiquitin – Proteasome system in the sarcomere

The ubiquitin-proteasome system (UPS) recognizes specific proteins and target them for degradation. Ubiquitin ligases recognize proteins to be degraded and interact with E1 (activating) and E2 (conjugating) enzymes to create poly-ubiquitin chains on the substrate. Poly-ubiquitin chains are then recognized by the 20S proteasome prior to degradation. Several ubiquitin ligases integrated to the sarcomere have been identified: the MuRF family proteins (MuRF1, MuRF2 and MuRF3), MAFbx / atrogin-1 and MDM2.

MuRF1 is found mainly in the M-line of the sarcomere where it interacts with the giant protein titin. MuRF1 specifically recognizes and degrades troponin I. MuRF1 and MuRF2 are reported to interact with troponin T, myosin light chain 2, myotilin and telethonin. While single deletion of either MuRF1 or MuRF2 allows a normal development, cardiac hypertrophy develop in mice lacking both genes (Witt et al., 2008). MuRF1 and MuRF3 also interact together with the E2 enzyme to degrade β / slow myosin heavy chains in the heart. Mice lacking both proteins develop a hypertrophic cardiomyopathy and skeletal muscle myopathy (Fielitz et al., 2007). MuRF1 may preferentially poly-ubiquitinate oxydized proteins as previous results suggest it (Zhao et al., 2007). Therefore, MuRF1, in cooperation with MuRF2 and MuRF3 may ensure protein quality control by detecting damaged proteins, to allow continuous optimal functions of the cardiac sarcomere (reviewed in Willis et al., 2009).

Additional ubiquitin ligases are also playing important roles in sarcomere maintenance:
CHIP, which plays a role as co-chaperone of Hsp70 and as ubiquitin ligase has been recognized as an important factor involved in ischemia / reperfusion injury in the heart (Zhang et al., 2005).
MAFbx / atrogin-1 was first identified as an ubiquitin ligase involved in skeletal muscle atrophy (Bodine et al., 2001), possibly by regulating cardiac hypertrophy genes (Li et al., 2007).
MDM-2 is a critical regulator of apoptosis through its ubiquitin-dependent degradation of ARC (Apoptosis Repressor with Caspase recruitment domain). It interacts and mediates telethonin degradation in a proteasome-dependent manner (Tian et al., 2006). Its specific role in the maintenance of sarcomere has to be further explored.

3.4.4 Calpain degradation

The highly integrative organization of the sarcomere does not allow direct degradation of the integrated proteins. Predigestion by proteases such as calpains which are embedded in the sarcomeric structure is therefore required. Calpains are a group of calcium-dependent, non-lysosomal cystein proteases expressed ubiquitously in all cells. Calpains are involved in a variety of cellular processes such as cell-cycle control and cell fusion (Goll et al., 2003). Calpain 1 has been found tightly associated to titin in a calcium-dependent manner. It is required to allow the dissociation of sarcomere proteins from the assembled myofibrils before the ubiquitin proteasome system is able to degrade them (Dargelos et al., 2008; Jackman & Kandarian, 2004). When calpains are inhibited in the heart, protein aggregation occur, ubiquitin ligases such as MuRF1 and MAFbx / atrogin-1 are no longer efficient in mediating proteasome-dependent degradation, and autophagy is increased. However, increased levels of calpain 1 in cardiomyocytes of transgenic models lead to cell lysis, cardiac hypertrophy, inflammation and ultimately heart failure (Galvez et al., 2007). These findings are consistent with a critical role of the calpain system in protein quality control in the heart.

3.4.5 Sarcomere maintenance and autophagy

Autophagy is a process for protein degradation that uses lysosomal hydrolases working at acidic pH. Autophagy begins with the formation of isolation membrane (phagophore). The phagophore then elongates and engulfs a portion of the cytoplasm to form a mature autophagosome, which then fuses with lysosomes to form autolysosomes. Autophagy removes damaged organelles such as mitochondria and aggregates of misfolded or damaged proteins (Beau et al., 2011). Autophagy-mediated degradation also contributes to the maintenance of the sarcomere (Portbury et al., 2011). In cardiomyocytes, autophagy occurs at the basal level and can be further induced by physiological or pathological conditions such as starvation, haemodynamic stress, ischemia / reperfusion, proteotoxicity, and toxins (Gustafsson & Gottlieb, 2008). Inhibition of autophagy leads to global disorganization of the sarcomere, mitochondrial aggregation, with ventricular dilation, cardiac hypertrophy and contractile dysfunction in adult animal models (Nakai et al., 2007). When autophagy is inactivated, there is an increase in poly-ubiquitinated proteins, as well as in proteasome activity, which suggest that despite its compensatory increase in activity, the UPS may be rapidely overwhelmed by the accumulation of toxic proteins (Bennett et al., 2005). Conversely, inhibition of proteasome activity leads to the accumulation of poly-ubiquitinated proteins and activation of autophagy (Tannous et al., 2008b). These results suggest, therefore, an essential role of cooperativeness between UPS and autophagy in maintaining protein quality control in the heart. Cell signaling pathways, such as PI3K / Akt, and transcription factors like FOXO3 have just begun to be involved as essential mediators in coordinating the proteasomal and lysosomal systems. In addition, sHSP and co-chaperones, like the Hsp22 - BAG3 complex activate autophagy, while BAG1 / BAG3 ratio is important to the balance between proteasomal to autophagic degradation (reviewed in Willis et al., 2009).

3.4.6 Physiological signaling and stress signals

An essential component of cardiac signaling is a process termed mechanotransduction, which translates a mechanical stress into a transcriptional response, and may constitute one of the most important stimuli leading to cardiac hypertrophy. Z-disc-associated proteins appear to play a critical role in this process (Frank et al., 2008). Mechanosignaling results in increased rate of protein synthesis, alteration of cell shape and increased expression of genes that are normally expressed predominantly during fetal life. Nodal points of mechanotransduction are found along the cardiac sarcomere, notably in the Z-disc, I-band and M-band regions (reviewed in Frank et al., 2006). It has been found that separate directional pathways are implicated by static transverse and longitudinal forces applied to cardiomyocytes to activate distinct cell signaling pathways. The mains involved are focal adhesion kinases (FAK), proteins kinase C (PKC) and integrins:

FAK is the primary effector of integrin signaling, and is localized to costameres in myocytes (Tornatore et al., 2011). Mechanical stress leads to disruption of FAK interaction with myosin heavy chain at the A-band to Z-disc, costameres and nuclei. Cyclic stretch induces a FAK-mediated activation of JNK and c-jun as well as of MEF2 (Nadruz et al., 2005). FAK appears therefore to play a critical function in hypertrophy, triggered in biomechanical as well as pharmacological models.

PKCε is a modulator of cardiac hypertrophy that belongs to the groups of "unconventional" PKCs which do not require Ca^{2+} for their activation (Dorn & Force, 2005). PKCε translocate to the Z-disc in cardiomyocytes upon stimulation, in particular by mechanical stress, or in pressure overload (Gu & Bishop, 1994). PKCε is necessary for cardiac hypertrophy induced by G protein receptors coupled agonists (Iwata et al., 2005). CapZ also plays a role in PKC signaling, which subsequent effects on cardiac contractility. Anchors to the Z-disc for PKCε are also provided by ZASP which links them to α-actinin through binding either to PDZ or LIM domains.

Other molecules, including PDE5A (PhosphoDiEsterase 5A), PCAF (P300/CBP Associated Factor), Zyxin, myopodin and HDAC4, ArgBP2, localize to the Z-disc, A-bands and I-bands of myocardial tissue, were found to shuttle between the sarcomere and the nucleus, and modulate the signaling pathways involved in cardiomyopathies (rewieved in Frank & Frey, 2011).

Strains on cultured cardiomyocytes also increases FAK activity and PKCε, which lead to the activation of the Rho/ROCK GTPases/kinase pathway, for which substantial evidences support a role in myofibrillogenesis (Franchini et al., 2000; Torsoni et al., 2003). One of the target of PKCε is the muscle actin capping protein for the barbed end of the actin filament (Schafer et al., 1994). Myocyte contractility, through titin and T-cap may also regulate muscle LIM proteins (MLP) shuttling to and from the nucleus, that may play a further role

in myocyte remodeling and hypertrophy, and is required for adaptation to hypertrophic stimuli (Iwata et al., 2005).
Integrins are transmembrane proteins which transduce signals from the extracellular matrix to the inner cell space and conversely. In the myocardium, integrin signalling plays an important role in mediating hypertrophic signals converging on the kinases Erk 1/2, PKC (Heidkamp et al., 2003), p38 MAPK (Aikawa et al., 2002) or JNK (Zhang et al., 2003). Among the proteins binding to integrins upon signaling, were identified the Integrin-Linked Kinase (ILK), FAK and Melusin.
ILK is a serine/threonine kinase. Its specific cardiac deletion in mice leads to dilated cardiomyopathy (DCM) and sudden death, while cardiac-restricted overexpression of ILK induces cardiac hypertrophy via activation of Erk 1/2 and p38 MAPK, indicating a function in hypertrophic signaling (Bendig et al., 2006; Lu et al., 2006).
Melusin is transiently upregulated in the heart upon pressure overload. Deletion of the Melusin gene show DCM and contractile dysfunction upon stress only, while overexpression leads to pathological hypertrophy (Brancaccio et al., 2003; De Acetis et al., 2005).
The Calcineurin / NFAT pathway is modulated by proteins like CIB1/ MLP/Calsarcin/LMDC1 that play a pivotal role in the mediation of pathologic cardiac hypertrophy (Frey et al., 2004). Calcineurin is linked to the Z-disc via calsarcin and MLP, and directly binds to the L-Type Calcium Channel, the major mediator of calcium influx in cardiomyocytes. Calcineurin activates by dephosphorylation the NFAT (Nuclear Factor of Activated T cells) transcription factors family, one of the major mediators of cardiac hypertrophy and remodelling.
PKA and PKG (cGMP-dependent protein kinase-G) are bound to titin. PKA is stimulated by β-adrenergic stimulation by catecholamines, while PKG is stimulated by nitric oxide and the natriuretic peptide (Wong & Fiscus, 2010). PKA can phosphorylate troponin-I, myosin-binding protein C and titin (Yamasaki et al., 2002; Yang et al., 2001; Zakhary et al., 1999).

4. From healthy to failing heart : Etiology and studies of myofibrilar cardiomyopathies

4.1 Diagnosis

As MFM refers to a group of genetically distinct disorders, common morphologic features observed on muscles are determinant. The following clinical findings should direct the diagnosis to a myofibrillar myopathy.

4.1.1 Clinical signs

Most patients with MFM show progressive muscle weakness. A small proportion of patients show paresthesias, muscle atrophy, stiffness or aching, cramps, dyspnea or dysphagia, or mild facial weakness. In about one third of the cases, the weakness is predominantly distal, in another third it is more proximal than distal, and in the other third it is mixed. In some patients, however, the cardiomyopathy may precede the muscle weakness.
Cardiomyopathy is a "classical" feature in MFM and may precede, coincide or follow the skeletal muscle weakness. Cardiomyopathy includes arrhythmogenic type (with atrio-ventricular blocks, supraventricular and ventricular ectopic beats and tachycardia), hypertrophic, dilated or restrictive features (reviewed in Ferrer & Olive, 2008; Goldfarb & Dalakas, 2009; Schroder & Schoser, 2009; Selcen, 2011).

Serum creatine kinase (CK) is variable, sometimes elevated. Differences depending on the causal gene have been reported (Schroder & Schoser, 2009):
DES, CRYAB and MYOT: normal up to 5 fold (reported maximal 15 fold for MYOT)
FLNC: normal up to 10 fold
ZASP: normal up to 6 fold
BAG3: 3 up to 15 fold

4.1.2 Histopathology

Muscle histology is essential and reveals characteristic features:

- Amorphous, hyaline or granular materials stained by trichrome.
- hyaline structures intensely positive for Congo red staining.
- significant decrease of oxidative enzyme activity in many abnormal fibers regions.
- small vacuoles in a variable number of fibers.

Immunohistochemistry performed on frozen sections (paraformaledehyde-fixed (4%)) from biopsies show abnormal ectopic expression of desmin, αB-crystallin, myotilin and dystrophin (Claeys et al., 2009; Schroder & Schoser, 2009; Selcen, 2011).

4.1.3 Electromyography

Electromyography (EMG) should be performed to confirm the histopathological data. EMG reveals abnormal electrical irritability often with myotonic discharges. The motor unit potentials are mostly myopathic, sometimes in combination with neurogenic features (Schroder & Schoser, 2009).

4.1.4 Electron microscopy

Electron microscopy of muscles showing progressive myofibrillar degeneration reveal abnormalities starting from the Z-disc area: streaming, defects in stacking, accumulation of granulo-filamentous dense materials, sarcomere disintegration, dislocated membranous materials, autophagic vacuoles, abnormal accumulation or location of mitochondria. Ultrastructural observation may allow to differentiate between granulofilamentous accumulation, "sandwich" formation, filamentous bundles, floccular thin filaments, tubular filamentous accumulations, and early apoptotic changes, to allow to direct diagnostic efforts toward the type of gene causing the MFM (Claeys et al., 2008).

4.2 Clinical perspectives and therapeutic considerations

There is currently no specific treatment for myofibrillar myopathies, nor clinical trial investigations (to the best of our knowledge).
MFM share protein aggregation with other aggregate-prone diseases, such as Alzheimer's, Parkinson's and Huntington's diseases. Accumulation of toxic β-amyloid oligomers, impairment of the ubiquitin proteasome system, alteration of the efficiency of the autophagic process have also been reported in studies about these diseases (Aguzzi & O'Connor, 2010). Several treatments have been set up and are currently tested for clinical trials, and may possibly be studied in the case of myofibrillar myopathies. However, caution should be taken because reducing the formation of aggregates may not directly allow to the cure of the disease (Sanbe et al., 2005).
Curcumin, a polyphenol naturally occurring in plant products, has been shown to inhibit α-synuclein aggregates formation involved in Parkinson's disease (Pandey et al., 2008).

Another way to reduce aggregates formation is to activate HSP, which may favour refolding or degradation of mutant proteins, or folding of the WT proteins expressed in the normal allele. Non-steroidal anti-inflammatory drugs, prostaglandins (Amici et al., 1992), Celastrol (Westerheide et al., 2004) or Geranylgeranylacetone (Sanbe et al., 2009) have been shown to activate the heat shock response. However, it is probably not judicious to induce αB-crystallin if this gene is mutated.

Activators of the autophagic pathway of degradation have been reported and could constitute a way to clear aggregates from the cardiomyocytes. Among many compounds actually tested, one can cite starvation, rapamycin, wortmanin, trehalose, etc (Sarkar & Rubinsztein, 2008).

Antioxydant agents, such as vitamin C, N-acetyl cysteine, ROS trapping agents like phenyl-N-tert-butylnitrone may also help to reduce aggregates formation, or help to their degradation (Squier, 2001).

5. Conclusion

There has been considerable improvement in the understanding of myofibrillar myopathies since they were first reported in 1978 (Fardeau et al., 1978). New avenues of discoveries have just opened with concepts of protein quality control, involving chaperone molecules, the ubiquitine proteasome system, and macroautophagy. Moreover, the sarcomere is not only seen now as a passive force generator, but also as a mechanosensor which signals to the nucleus and to the whole muscular fiber, and activates specific programs of renewal of sarcomeric proteins, in case of damages. These new findings will help to integrate more components of the muscle physiology, and to understand how they are modified when MFM-causing genes are mutated. However, only 20 % of MFM have found a "culprit" gene, so it may be necessary to analyze other Z-disc-specific structural, quality control or signaling genes to find new candidates responsible for MFMs.

6. Acknowledgment

We thank Sabrina Pichon and Patrick Vicart for careful reading of the manuscript. This work was supported by grants from Association Française contre les Myopathies (AFM) and CNRS (A.L).

7. References

A. Aguzzi & T. O'Connor. (2010) Protein aggregation diseases: pathogenicity and therapeutic perspectives. *Nat Rev Drug Discov,* Vol.9, No.3, pp. 237-48

R. Aikawa, T. Nagai, S. Kudoh, Y. Zou, M. Tanaka, M. Tamura, H. Akazawa, H. Takano, R. Nagai & I. Komuro. (2002) Integrins play a critical role in mechanical stress-induced p38 MAPK activation. *Hypertension,* Vol.39, No.2, pp. 233-8

C. Amici, L. Sistonen, M. G. Santoro & R. I. Morimoto. (1992) Antiproliferative prostaglandins activate heat shock transcription factor. *Proc Natl Acad Sci U S A,* Vol.89, No.14, pp. 6227-31

T. Andrienko, A. V. Kuznetsov, T. Kaambre, Y. Usson, A. Orosco, F. Appaix, T. Tiivel, P. Sikk, M. Vendelin, R. Margreiter & V. A. Saks. (2003) Metabolic consequences of functional complexes of mitochondria, myofibrils and sarcoplasmic reticulum in muscle cells. *J Exp Biol,* Vol.206, No.Pt 12, pp. 2059-72

F. Appaix, A. V. Kuznetsov, Y. Usson, L. Kay, T. Andrienko, J. Olivares, T. Kaambre, P. Sikk, R. Margreiter & V. Saks. (2003) Possible role of cytoskeleton in intracellular arrangement and regulation of mitochondria. *Exp Physiol,* Vol.88, No.1, pp. 175-90

H. Bar, S. V. Strelkov, G. Sjoberg, U. Aebi & H. Herrmann. (2004) The biology of desmin filaments: how do mutations affect their structure, assembly, and organisation? *J Struct Biol,* Vol.148, No.2, pp. 137-52

I. Beau, M. Mehrpour & P. Codogno. (2011) Autophagosomes and human diseases. *Int J Biochem Cell Biol,* Vol.43, No.4, pp. 460-4

G. Bendig, M. Grimmler, I. G. Huttner, G. Wessels, T. Dahme, S. Just, N. Trano, H. A. Katus, M. C. Fishman & W. Rottbauer. (2006) Integrin-linked kinase, a novel component of the cardiac mechanical stretch sensor, controls contractility in the zebrafish heart. *Genes Dev,* Vol.20, No.17, pp. 2361-72

I. J. Benjamin & D. R. McMillan. (1998) Stress (heat shock) proteins: molecular chaperones in cardiovascular biology and disease. *Circ Res,* Vol.83, No.2, pp. 117-32

F. Bennardini, A. Wrzosek & M. Chiesi. (1992) Alpha B-crystallin in cardiac tissue. Association with actin and desmin filaments. *Circ Res,* Vol.71, No.2, pp. 288-94

E. J. Bennett, N. F. Bence, R. Jayakumar & R. R. Kopito. (2005) Global impairment of the ubiquitin-proteasome system by nuclear or cytoplasmic protein aggregates precedes inclusion body formation. *Mol Cell,* Vol.17, No.3, pp. 351-65

R. J. Bloch, Y. Capetanaki, A. O'Neill, P. Reed, M. W. Williams, W. G. Resneck, N. C. Porter & J. A. Ursitti. (2002) Costameres: repeating structures at the sarcolemma of skeletal muscle. *Clin Orthop Relat Res,* No.403 Suppl, pp. S203-10

S. C. Bodine, E. Latres, S. Baumhueter, V. K. Lai, L. Nunez, B. A. Clarke, W. T. Poueymirou, F. J. Panaro, E. Na, K. Dharmarajan, Z. Q. Pan, D. M. Valenzuela, T. M. DeChiara, T. N. Stitt, G. D. Yancopoulos & D. J. Glass. (2001) Identification of ubiquitin ligases required for skeletal muscle atrophy. *Science,* Vol.294, No.5547, pp. 1704-8

J. P. Brady, D. L. Garland, D. E. Green, E. R. Tamm, F. J. Giblin & E. F. Wawrousek. (2001) AlphaB-crystallin in lens development and muscle integrity: a gene knockout approach. *Invest Ophthalmol Vis Sci,* Vol.42, No.12, pp. 2924-34

M. Brancaccio, L. Fratta, A. Notte, E. Hirsch, R. Poulet, S. Guazzone, M. De Acetis, C. Vecchione, G. Marino, F. Altruda, L. Silengo, G. Tarone & G. Lembo. (2003) Melusin, a muscle-specific integrin beta1-interacting protein, is required to prevent cardiac failure in response to chronic pressure overload. *Nat Med,* Vol.9, No.1, pp. 68-75

Y. Capetanaki. (2002) Desmin cytoskeleton: a potential regulator of muscle mitochondrial behavior and function. *Trends Cardiovasc Med,* Vol.12, No.8, pp. 339-48

S. Carra, S. J. Seguin & J. Landry. (2008a) HspB8 and Bag3: a new chaperone complex targeting misfolded proteins to macroautophagy. *Autophagy,* Vol.4, No.2, pp. 237-9

S. Carra, S. J. Seguin, H. Lambert & J. Landry. (2008b) HspB8 chaperone activity toward poly(Q)-containing proteins depends on its association with Bag3, a stimulator of macroautophagy. *J Biol Chem,* Vol.283, No.3, pp. 1437-44

K. G. Claeys, M. Fardeau, R. Schroder, T. Suominen, K. Tolksdorf, A. Behin, O. Dubourg, B. Eymard, T. Maisonobe, T. Stojkovic, G. Faulkner, P. Richard, P. Vicart, B. Udd, T. Voit & G. Stoltenburg. (2008) Electron microscopy in myofibrillar myopathies reveals clues to the mutated gene. *Neuromuscul Disord,* Vol.18, No.8, pp. 656-66

K. G. Claeys, P. F. van der Ven, A. Behin, T. Stojkovic, B. Eymard, O. Dubourg, P. Laforet, G. Faulkner, P. Richard, P. Vicart, N. B. Romero, G. Stoltenburg, B. Udd, M. Fardeau, T. Voit & D. O. Furst. (2009) Differential involvement of sarcomeric proteins in myofibrillar myopathies: a morphological and immunohistochemical study. *Acta Neuropathol,* Vol.117, No.3, pp. 293-307

M. L. Costa, R. Escaleira, A. Cataldo, F. Oliveira & C. S. Mermelstein. (2004) Desmin: molecular interactions and putative functions of the muscle intermediate filament protein. *Braz J Med Biol Res,* Vol.37, No.12, pp. 1819-30

E. Dargelos, S. Poussard, C. Brule, L. Daury & P. Cottin. (2008) Calcium-dependent proteolytic system and muscle dysfunctions: a possible role of calpains in sarcopenia. *Biochimie,* Vol.90, No.2, pp. 359-68

M. De Acetis, A. Notte, F. Accornero, G. Selvetella, M. Brancaccio, C. Vecchione, M. Sbroggio, F. Collino, B. Pacchioni, G. Lanfranchi, A. Aretini, R. Ferretti, A. Maffei, F. Altruda, L. Silengo, G. Tarone & G. Lembo. (2005) Cardiac overexpression of melusin protects from dilated cardiomyopathy due to long-standing pressure overload. *Circ Res,* Vol.96, No.10, pp. 1087-94

C. Depre, M. Hase, V. Gaussin, A. Zajac, L. Wang, L. Hittinger, B. Ghaleh, X. Yu, R. K. Kudej, T. Wagner, J. Sadoshima & S. F. Vatner. (2002) H11 kinase is a novel mediator of myocardial hypertrophy *in vivo*. *Circ Res,* Vol.91, No.11, pp. 1007-14

C. Depre, L. Wang, J. E. Tomlinson, V. Gaussin, M. Abdellatif, J. N. Topper & S. F. Vatner. (2003) Characterization of pDJA1, a cardiac-specific chaperone found by genomic profiling of the post-ischemic swine heart. *Cardiovasc Res,* Vol.58, No.1, pp. 126-35

T. J. Donnelly, R. E. Sievers, F. L. Vissern, W. J. Welch & C. L. Wolfe. (1992) Heat shock protein induction in rat hearts. A role for improved myocardial salvage after ischemia and reperfusion? *Circulation,* Vol.85, No.2, pp. 769-78

G. W. Dorn, 2nd & T. Force. (2005) Protein kinase cascades in the regulation of cardiac hypertrophy. *J Clin Invest,* Vol.115, No.3, pp. 527-37

M. Fardeau, J. Godet-Guillain, F. M. Tome, H. Collin, S. Gaudeau, C. Boffety & P. Vernant. (1978) [A new familial muscular disorder demonstrated by the intra-sarcoplasmic accumulation of a granulo-filamentous material which is dense on electron microscopy (author's transl)]. *Rev Neurol (Paris),* Vol.134, No.6-7, pp. 411-25

G. Faulkner, A. Pallavicini, E. Formentin, A. Comelli, C. Ievolella, S. Trevisan, G. Bortoletto, P. Scannapieco, M. Salamon, V. Mouly, G. Valle & G. Lanfranchi. (1999) ZASP: a new Z-band alternatively spliced PDZ-motif protein. *J Cell Biol,* Vol.146, No.2, pp. 465-75

I. Ferrer & M. Olive. (2008) Molecular pathology of myofibrillar myopathies. *Expert Rev Mol Med,* Vol.10, e25

J. Fielitz, M. S. Kim, J. M. Shelton, S. Latif, J. A. Spencer, D. J. Glass, J. A. Richardson, R. Bassel-Duby & E. N. Olson. (2007) Myosin accumulation and striated muscle myopathy result from the loss of muscle RING finger 1 and 3. *J Clin Invest,* Vol.117, No.9, pp. 2486-95

J. Finsterer & C. Stollberger. (2008) Primary myopathies and the heart. *Scand Cardiovasc J,* Vol.42, No.1, pp. 9-24

S. Fong, S. J. Hamill, M. Proctor, S. M. Freund, G. M. Benian, C. Chothia, M. Bycroft & J. Clarke. (1996) Structure and stability of an immunoglobulin superfamily domain from twitchin, a muscle protein of the nematode Caenorhabditis elegans. *J Mol Biol,* Vol.264, No.3, pp. 624-39

K. G. Franchini, A. S. Torsoni, P. H. Soares & M. J. Saad. (2000) Early activation of the multicomponent signaling complex associated with focal adhesion kinase induced by pressure overload in the rat heart. *Circ Res,* Vol.87, No.7, pp. 558-65

D. Frank, C. Kuhn, H. A. Katus & N. Frey. (2006) The sarcomeric Z-disc: a nodal point in signalling and disease. *J Mol Med,* Vol.84, No.6, pp. 446-68

D. Frank, C. Kuhn, B. Brors, C. Hanselmann, M. Ludde, H. A. Katus & N. Frey. (2008) Gene expression pattern in biomechanically stretched cardiomyocytes: evidence for a stretch-specific gene program. *Hypertension,* Vol.51, No.2, pp. 309-18

D. Frank & N. Frey. (2011) Cardiac Z-disc signaling network. *J Biol Chem,* Vol.286, No.12, pp. 9897-904

N. Frey, T. Barrientos, J. M. Shelton, D. Frank, H. Rutten, D. Gehring, C. Kuhn, M. Lutz, B. Rothermel, R. Bassel-Duby, J. A. Richardson, H. A. Katus, J. A. Hill & E. N. Olson. (2004) Mice lacking calsarcin-1 are sensitized to calcineurin signaling and show accelerated cardiomyopathy in response to pathological biomechanical stress. *Nat Med,* Vol.10, No.12, pp. 1336-43

A. S. Galvez, A. Diwan, A. M. Odley, H. S. Hahn, H. Osinska, J. G. Melendez, J. Robbins, R. A. Lynch, Y. Marreez & G. W. Dorn, 2nd. (2007) Cardiomyocyte degeneration with calpain deficiency reveals a critical role in protein homeostasis. *Circ Res,* Vol.100, No.7, pp. 1071-8

E. Ganea. (2001) Chaperone-like activity of alpha-crystallin and other small heat shock proteins. *Curr Protein Pept Sci,* Vol.2, No.3, pp. 205-25

S. M. Garvey, S. E. Miller, D. R. Claflin, J. A. Faulkner & M. A. Hauser. (2006) Transgenic mice expressing the myotilin T57I mutation unite the pathology associated with LGMD1A and MFM. *Hum Mol Genet,* Vol.15, No.15, pp. 2348-62

L. G. Goldfarb, K. Y. Park, L. Cervenakova, S. Gorokhova, H. S. Lee, O. Vasconcelos, J. W. Nagle, C. Semino-Mora, K. Sivakumar & M. C. Dalakas. (1998) Missense mutations in desmin associated with familial cardiac and skeletal myopathy. *Nat Genet,* Vol.19, No.4, pp. 402-3

L. G. Goldfarb, P. Vicart, H. H. Goebel & M. C. Dalakas. (2004) Desmin myopathy. *Brain,* Vol.127, No.Pt 4, pp. 723-34

L. G. Goldfarb & M. C. Dalakas. (2009) Tragedy in a heartbeat: malfunctioning desmin causes skeletal and cardiac muscle disease. *J Clin Invest,* Vol.119, No.7, pp. 1806-13

N. Golenhofen, M. D. Perng, R. A. Quinlan & D. Drenckhahn. (2004) Comparison of the small heat shock proteins alphaB-crystallin, MKBP, HSP25, HSP20, and cvHSP in heart and skeletal muscle. *Histochem Cell Biol,* Vol.122, No.5, pp. 415-25

D. E. Goll, V. F. Thompson, H. Li, W. Wei & J. Cong. (2003) The calpain system. *Physiol Rev,* Vol.83, No.3, pp. 731-801

H. L. Granzier & S. Labeit. (2004) The giant protein titin: a major player in myocardial mechanics, signaling, and disease. *Circ Res,* Vol.94, No.3, pp. 284-95

X. Gu & S. P. Bishop. (1994) Increased protein kinase C and isozyme redistribution in pressure-overload cardiac hypertrophy in the rat. *Circ Res,* Vol.75, No.5, pp. 926-31

N. Gurusamy, I. Lekli, M. Gherghiceanu, L. M. Popescu & D. K. Das. (2009) BAG-1 induces autophagy for cardiac cell survival. *Autophagy,* Vol.5, No.1, pp. 120-1

A. B. Gustafsson & R. A. Gottlieb. (2008) Recycle or die: the role of autophagy in cardioprotection. *J Mol Cell Cardiol,* Vol.44, No.4, pp. 654-61

M. A. Hauser, S. K. Horrigan, P. Salmikangas, U. M. Torian, K. D. Viles, R. Dancel, R. W. Tim, A. Taivainen, L. Bartoloni, J. M. Gilchrist, J. M. Stajich, P. C. Gaskell, J. R. Gilbert, J. M. Vance, M. A. Pericak-Vance, O. Carpen, C. A. Westbrook & M. C. Speer. (2000) Myotilin is mutated in limb girdle muscular dystrophy 1A. *Hum Mol Genet,* Vol.9, No.14, pp. 2141-7

M. C. Heidkamp, A. L. Bayer, B. T. Scully, D. M. Eble & A. M. Samarel. (2003) Activation of focal adhesion kinase by protein kinase C epsilon in neonatal rat ventricular myocytes. *Am J Physiol Heart Circ Physiol,* Vol.285, No.4, pp. H1684-96

S. Homma, M. Iwasaki, G. D. Shelton, E. Engvall, J. C. Reed & S. Takayama. (2006) BAG3 deficiency results in fulminant myopathy and early lethality. *Am J Pathol,* Vol.169, No.3, pp. 761-73

J. Horwitz. (2003) Alpha-crystallin. *Exp Eye Res,* Vol.76, No.2, pp. 145-53

M. M. Hutter, R. E. Sievers, V. Barbosa & C. L. Wolfe. (1994) Heat-shock protein induction in rat hearts. A direct correlation between the amount of heat-shock protein induced and the degree of myocardial protection. *Circulation,* Vol.89, No.1, pp. 355-60

T. Iwaki, A. Kume-Iwaki & J. E. Goldman. (1990) Cellular distribution of alpha B-crystallin in non-lenticular tissues. *J Histochem Cytochem,* Vol.38, No.1, pp. 31-9

M. Iwata, A. Maturana, M. Hoshijima, K. Tatematsu, T. Okajima, J. R. Vandenheede, J. Van Lint, K. Tanizawa & S. Kuroda. (2005) PKCepsilon-PKD1 signaling complex at Z-discs plays a pivotal role in the cardiac hypertrophy induced by G-protein coupling receptor agonists. *Biochem Biophys Res Commun,* Vol.327, No.4, pp. 1105-13

R. W. Jackman & S. C. Kandarian. (2004) The molecular basis of skeletal muscle atrophy. *Am J Physiol Cell Physiol,* Vol.287, No.4, pp. C834-43

J. A. Johnston, W. C. L. & R. R. Kopito. (1998) Aggresomes: a cellular response to misfolded proteins. *J. Cell. Biol.,* Vol.143, No.7, pp. 1883-1898

K. Kato, H. Shinohara, N. Kurobe, Y. Inaguma, K. Shimizu & K. Ohshima. (1991) Tissue distribution and developmental profiles of immunoreactive alpha B crystallin in the rat determined with a sensitive immunoassay system. *Biochim Biophys Acta,* Vol.1074, No.1, pp. 201-8

T. Klaavuniemi & J. Ylanne. (2006) Zasp/Cypher internal ZM-motif containing fragments are sufficient to co-localize with alpha-actinin--analysis of patient mutations. *Exp Cell Res,* Vol.312, No.8, pp. 1299-311

B. Klauke, S. Kossmann, A. Gaertner, K. Brand, I. Stork, A. Brodehl, M. Dieding, V. Walhorn, D. Anselmetti, D. Gerdes, B. Bohms, U. Schulz, E. Zu Knyphausen, M.

Vorgerd, J. Gummert & H. Milting. (2010) De novo desmin-mutation N116S is associated with arrhythmogenic right ventricular cardiomyopathy. *Hum Mol Genet,* Vol.19, No.23, pp. 4595-607

A. R. Kumarapeli, H. Su, W. Huang, M. Tang, H. Zheng, K. M. Horak, M. Li & X. Wang. (2008) Alpha B-crystallin suppresses pressure overload cardiac hypertrophy. *Circ Res,* Vol.103, No.12, pp. 1473-82

S. Lahmers, Y. Wu, D. R. Call, S. Labeit & H. Granzier. (2004) Developmental control of titin isoform expression and passive stiffness in fetal and neonatal myocardium. *Circ Res,* Vol.94, No.4, pp. 505-13

E. Lazarides & B. D. Hubbard. (1976) Immunological characterization of the subunit of the 100 A filaments from muscle cells. *Proc Natl Acad Sci U S A,* Vol.73, No.12, pp. 4344-8

I. H. Leach, M. L. Tsang, R. J. Church & J. Lowe. (1994) Alpha-B crystallin in the normal human myocardium and cardiac conducting system. *J Pathol,* Vol.173, No.3, pp. 255-60

A. L. Lehninger, D. L. Nelson & M. M. Cox (2005) *Principles of biochemistry* (4th), W.H. Freeman, 9780716743392,

D. Li, T. Tapscoft, O. Gonzalez, P. E. Burch, M. A. Quinones, W. A. Zoghbi, R. Hill, L. L. Bachinski, D. L. Mann & R. Roberts. (1999) Desmin mutation responsible for idiopathic dilated cardiomyopathy. *Circulation,* Vol.100, No.5, pp. 461-4

H. H. Li, M. S. Willis, P. Lockyer, N. Miller, H. McDonough, D. J. Glass & C. Patterson. (2007) Atrogin-1 inhibits Akt-dependent cardiac hypertrophy in mice via ubiquitin-dependent coactivation of Forkhead proteins. *J Clin Invest,* Vol.117, No.11, pp. 3211-23

Z. Li, E. Colucci-Guyon, M. Pincon-Raymond, M. Mericskay, S. Pournin, D. Paulin & C. Babinet. (1996) Cardiovascular lesions and skeletal myopathy in mice lacking desmin. *Dev Biol,* Vol.175, No.2, pp. 362-6

Z. L. Li, A. Lilienbaum, G. Butler-Browne & D. Paulin. (1989) Human desmin-coding gene: complete nucleotide sequence, characterization and regulation of expression during myogenesis and development. *Gene,* Vol.78, No.2, pp. 243-54

J. Liu, Q. Chen, W. Huang, K. M. Horak, H. Zheng, R. Mestril & X. Wang. (2006) Impairment of the ubiquitin-proteasome system in desminopathy mouse hearts. *Faseb J,* Vol.20, No.2, pp. 362-4

H. Lu, P. W. Fedak, X. Dai, C. Du, Y. Q. Zhou, M. Henkelman, P. S. Mongroo, A. Lau, H. Yamabi, A. Hinek, M. Husain, G. Hannigan & J. G. Coles. (2006) Integrin-linked kinase expression is elevated in human cardiac hypertrophy and induces hypertrophy in transgenic mice. *Circulation,* Vol.114, No.21, pp. 2271-9

G. Lutsch, R. Vetter, U. Offhauss, M. Wieske, H. J. Grone, R. Klemenz, I. Schimke, J. Stahl & R. Benndorf. (1997) Abundance and location of the small heat shock proteins HSP25 and alphaB-crystallin in rat and human heart. *Circulation,* Vol.96, No.10, pp. 3466-76

T. H. MacRae. (2000) Structure and function of small heat shock/alpha-crystallin proteins: established concepts and emerging ideas. *Cell Mol Life Sci,* Vol.57, No.6, pp. 899-913

A. F. Martin, M. Rabinowitz, R. Blough, G. Prior & R. Zak. (1977) Measurements of half-life of rat cardiac myosin heavy chain with leucyl-tRNA used as precursor pool. *J Biol Chem,* Vol.252, No.10, pp. 3422-9

J. L. Martin, R. Mestril, R. Hilal-Dandan, L. L. Brunton & W. H. Dillmann. (1997) Small heat shock proteins and protection against ischemic injury in cardiac myocytes. *Circulation,* Vol.96, No.12, pp. 4343-8

K. B. Merck, P. J. Groenen, C. E. Voorter, W. A. de Haard-Hoekman, J. Horwitz, H. Bloemendal & W. W. de Jong. (1993) Structural and functional similarities of bovine alpha-crystallin and mouse small heat-shock protein. A family of chaperones. *J Biol Chem,* Vol.268, No.2, pp. 1046-52

D. E. Michele, F. P. Albayya & J. M. Metzger. (1999) Thin filament protein dynamics in fully differentiated adult cardiac myocytes: toward a model of sarcomere maintenance. *J Cell Biol,* Vol.145, No.7, pp. 1483-95

D. J. Milner, G. Weitzer, D. Tran, A. Bradley & Y. Capetanaki. (1996) Disruption of muscle architecture and myocardial degeneration in mice lacking desmin. *J Cell Biol,* Vol.134, No.5, pp. 1255-70

C. L. Moncman & K. Wang. (1995) Nebulette: a 107 kD nebulin-like protein in cardiac muscle. *Cell Motil Cytoskeleton,* Vol.32, No.3, pp. 205-25

L. E. Morrison, R. J. Whittaker, R. E. Klepper, E. F. Wawrousek & C. C. Glembotski. (2004) Roles for alphaB-crystallin and HSPB2 in protecting the myocardium from ischemia-reperfusion-induced damage in a KO mouse model. *Am J Physiol Heart Circ Physiol,* Vol.286, No.3, pp. H847-55

A. M. Muñoz-Marmol, G. Strasser, M. Isamat, P. A. Coulombe, Y. Yang, X. Roca, E. Vela, J. L. Mate, J. Coll, M. T. Fernandez-Figueras, J. J. Navas-Palacios, A. Ariza & E. Fuchs. (1998) A dysfunctional desmin mutation in a patient with severe generalized myopathy. *Proc Natl Acad Sci U S A,* Vol.95, No.19, pp. 11312-7

F. Muntoni, G. Bonne, L. G. Goldfarb, E. Mercuri, R. J. Piercy, M. Burke, R. B. Yaou, P. Richard, D. Recan, A. Shatunov, C. A. Sewry & S. C. Brown. (2006) Disease severity in dominant Emery Dreifuss is increased by mutations in both emerin and desmin proteins. *Brain,* Vol.129, No.Pt 5, pp. 1260-8

W. Nadruz, Jr., M. A. Corat, T. M. Marin, G. A. Guimaraes Pereira & K. G. Franchini. (2005) Focal adhesion kinase mediates MEF2 and c-Jun activation by stretch: role in the activation of the cardiac hypertrophic genetic program. *Cardiovasc Res,* Vol.68, No.1, pp. 87-97

A. Nakai, O. Yamaguchi, T. Takeda, Y. Higuchi, S. Hikoso, M. Taniike, S. Omiya, I. Mizote, Y. Matsumura, M. Asahi, K. Nishida, M. Hori, N. Mizushima & K. Otsu. (2007) The role of autophagy in cardiomyocytes in the basal state and in response to hemodynamic stress. *Nat Med,* Vol.13, No.5, pp. 619-24

P. D. Neufer, G. A. Ordway & R. S. Williams. (1998) Transient regulation of c-fos, alpha B-crystallin, and hsp70 in muscle during recovery from contractile activity. *Am J Physiol,* Vol.274, No.2 Pt 1, pp. C341-6

C. A. Opitz, M. C. Leake, I. Makarenko, V. Benes & W. A. Linke. (2004) Developmentally regulated switching of titin size alters myofibrillar stiffness in the perinatal heart. *Circ Res,* Vol.94, No.7, pp. 967-75

C. A. Otey & O. Carpen. (2004) Alpha-actinin revisited: a fresh look at an old player. *Cell Motil Cytoskeleton,* Vol.58, No.2, pp. 104-11

N. Pandey, J. Strider, W. C. Nolan, S. X. Yan & J. E. Galvin. (2008) Curcumin inhibits aggregation of alpha-synuclein. *Acta Neuropathol,* Vol.115, No.4, pp. 479-89

D. Paulin, A. Huet, L. Khanamyrian & Z. Xue. (2004) Desminopathies in muscle disease. *J Pathol,* Vol.204, No.4, pp. 418-27

D. Paulin & Z. Li. (2004) Desmin: a major intermediate filament protein essential for the structural integrity and function of muscle. *Exp Cell Res,* Vol.301, No.1, pp. 1-7

A. L. Portbury, M. S. Willis & C. Patterson. (2011) Tearin' up my heart: proteolysis in the cardiac sarcomere. *J Biol Chem,* Vol.286, No.12, pp. 9929-34

J. Reimann, W. S. Kunz, S. Vielhaber, K. Kappes-Horn & R. Schroder. (2003) Mitochondrial dysfunction in myofibrillar myopathy. *Neuropathol Appl Neurobiol,* Vol.29, No.1, pp. 45-51

P. Salmikangas, O. M. Mykkanen, M. Gronholm, L. Heiska, J. Kere & O. Carpen. (1999) Myotilin, a novel sarcomeric protein with two Ig-like domains, is encoded by a candidate gene for limb-girdle muscular dystrophy. *Hum Mol Genet,* Vol.8, No.7, pp. 1329-36

P. Salmikangas, P. F. van der Ven, M. Lalowski, A. Taivainen, F. Zhao, H. Suila, R. Schroder, P. Lappalainen, D. O. Furst & O. Carpen. (2003) Myotilin, the limb-girdle muscular dystrophy 1A (LGMD1A) protein, cross-links actin filaments and controls sarcomere assembly. *Hum Mol Genet,* Vol.12, No.2, pp. 189-203

A. Sanbe, H. Osinska, C. Villa, J. Gulick, R. Klevitsky, C. G. Glabe, R. Kayed & J. Robbins. (2005) Reversal of amyloid-induced heart disease in desmin-related cardiomyopathy. *Proc Natl Acad Sci U S A,* Vol.102, No.38, pp. 13592-7

A. Sanbe, T. Daicho, R. Mizutani, T. Endo, N. Miyauchi, J. Yamauchi, K. Tanonaka, C. Glabe & A. Tanoue. (2009) Protective effect of geranylgeranylacetone via enhancement of HSPB8 induction in desmin-related cardiomyopathy. *PLoS One,* Vol.4, No.4, pp. e5351

J. M. Sanger & J. W. Sanger. (2008) The dynamic Z bands of striated muscle cells. *Science signaling,* Vol.1, pe37

S. Sarkar & D. C. Rubinsztein. (2008) Small molecule enhancers of autophagy for neurodegenerative diseases. *Mol Biosyst,* Vol.4, No.9, pp. 895-901

C. M. Sax & J. Piatigorsky. (1994) Expression of the alpha-crystallin/small heat-shock protein/molecular chaperone genes in the lens and other tissues. *Adv Enzymol Relat Areas Mol Biol,* Vol.69, 155-201

D. A. Schafer, Y. O. Korshunova, T. A. Schroer & J. A. Cooper. (1994) Differential localization and sequence analysis of capping protein beta-subunit isoforms of vertebrates. *J Cell Biol,* Vol.127, No.2, pp. 453-65

D. A. Schafer, P. B. Jennings & J. A. Cooper. (1996) Dynamics of capping protein and actin assembly *in vitro*: uncapping barbed ends by polyphosphoinositides. *J Cell Biol,* Vol.135, No.1, pp. 169-79

R. Schroder, A. Vrabie & H. H. Goebel. (2007) Primary desminopathies. *J Cell Mol Med,* Vol.11, No.3, pp. 416-26

R. Schroder & B. Schoser. (2009) Myofibrillar myopathies: a clinical and myopathological guide. *Brain Pathol,* Vol.19, No.3, pp. 483-92

D. Selcen & A. G. Engel. (2004) Mutations in myotilin cause myofibrillar myopathy. *Neurology,* Vol.62, No.8, pp. 1363-71

D. Selcen & A. G. Engel. (2005) Mutations in ZASP define a novel form of muscular dystrophy in humans. *Ann Neurol,* Vol.57, No.2, pp. 269-76

D. Selcen, F. Muntoni, B.K. Burton, E. Pegoraro, C. Sewry, A.C. Bite & E. Engel. (2009) Mutation in BAG3 causes severe dominant chilhood muscular dystrophy. *Ann. Neurol.* Vol.65, No.3, pp. 83-89

D. Selcen. (2011) Myofibrillar myopathies. *Neuromuscul Disord,* Vol.21, No.3, pp. 161-71

E. H. Sonnenblick. (1968) Correlation of myocardial ultrastructure and function. *Circulation,* Vol.38, No.1, pp. 29-44

T. C. Squier. (2001) Oxidative stress and protein aggregation during biological aging. *Exp Gerontol,* Vol.36, No.9, pp. 1539-50

M. H. Stromer & D. E. Goll. (1972) Studies on purified -actinin. II. Electron microscopic studies on the competitive binding of -actinin and tropomyosin to Z-line extracted myofibrils. *J Mol Biol,* Vol.67, No.3, pp. 489-94

S. Takayama & J. C. Reed. (2001) Molecular chaperone targeting and regulation by BAG family proteins. *Nat Cell Biol,* Vol.3, No.10, pp. E237-41

P. Tannous, H. Zhu, J. L. Johnstone, J. M. Shelton, N. S. Rajasekaran, I. J. Benjamin, L. Nguyen, R. D. Gerard, B. Levine, B. A. Rothermel & J. A. Hill. (2008a) Autophagy is an adaptive response in desmin-related cardiomyopathy. *Proc Natl Acad Sci U S A,* Vol.105, No.28, pp. 9745-50

P. Tannous, H. Zhu, A. Nemchenko, J. M. Berry, J. L. Johnstone, J. M. Shelton, F. J. Miller, Jr., B. A. Rothermel & J. A. Hill. (2008b) Intracellular protein aggregation is a proximal trigger of cardiomyocyte autophagy. *Circulation,* Vol.117, No.24, pp. 3070-8

T. G. Thompson, Y. M. Chan, A. A. Hack, M. Brosius, M. Rajala, H. G. Lidov, E. M. McNally, S. Watkins & L. M. Kunkel. (2000) Filamin 2 (FLN2): A muscle-specific sarcoglycan interacting protein. *J Cell Biol,* Vol.148, No.1, pp. 115-26

L. E. Thornell & A. Eriksson. (1981) Filament systems in the Purkinje fibers of the heart. *Am J Physiol,* Vol.241, No.3, pp. H291-305

L. F. Tian, H. Y. Li, B. F. Jin, X. Pan, J. H. Man, P. J. Zhang, W. H. Li, B. Liang, H. Liu, J. Zhao, W. L. Gong, T. Zhou & X. M. Zhang. (2006) MDM2 interacts with and downregulates a sarcomeric protein, TCAP. *Biochem Biophys Res Commun,* Vol.345, No.1, pp. 355-61

T. F. Tornatore, A. P. Dalla Costa, C. F. Clemente, C. Judice, S. A. Rocco, V. C. Calegari, L. Cardoso, A. C. Cardoso, A. Goncalves, Jr. & K. G. Franchini. (2011) A role for focal adhesion kinase in cardiac mitochondrial biogenesis induced by mechanical stress. *Am J Physiol Heart Circ Physiol,* Vol.300, No.3, pp. H902-12

A. S. Torsoni, S. S. Constancio, W. Nadruz, Jr., S. K. Hanks & K. G. Franchini. (2003) Focal adhesion kinase is activated and mediates the early hypertrophic response to stretch in cardiac myocytes. *Circ Res,* Vol.93, No.2, pp. 140-7

P. A. Townsend, R. I. Cutress, C. J. Carroll, K. M. Lawrence, T. M. Scarabelli, G. Packham, A. Stephanou & D. S. Latchman. (2004) BAG-1 proteins protect cardiac myocytes from simulated ischemia/reperfusion-induced apoptosis via an alternate mechanism of cell survival independent of the proteasome. *J Biol Chem,* Vol.279, No.20, pp. 20723-8

A. van der Flier & A. Sonnenberg. (2001) Structural and functional aspects of filamins. *Biochim Biophys Acta,* Vol.1538, No.2-3, pp. 99-117

P. F. van der Ven, W. M. Obermann, B. Lemke, M. Gautel, K. Weber & D. O. Furst. (2000) Characterization of muscle filamin isoforms suggests a possible role of gamma-filamin/ABP-L in sarcomeric Z-disc formation. *Cell Motil Cytoskeleton,* Vol.45, No.2, pp. 149-62

K. van Spaendonck-Zwarts, L. van Hessem, J. D. Jongbloed, H. E. de Walle, Y. Capetanaki, A. J. van der Kooi, I. M. van Langen, M. P. van den Berg & J. P. van Tintelen. (2010) Desmin-related myopathy: a review and meta-analysis. *Clin Genet,* PMID: 20718792

M. Vatta, B. Mohapatra, S. Jimenez, X. Sanchez, G. Faulkner, Z. Perles, G. Sinagra, J. H. Lin, T. M. Vu, Q. Zhou, K. R. Bowles, A. Di Lenarda, L. Schimmenti, M. Fox, M. A. Chrisco, R. T. Murphy, W. McKenna, P. Elliott, N. E. Bowles, J. Chen, G. Valle & J. A. Towbin. (2003) Mutations in Cypher/ZASP in patients with dilated cardiomyopathy and left ventricular non-compaction. *J Am Coll Cardiol,* Vol.42, No.11, pp. 2014-27

L. Vernengo, O. Chourbagi, A. Panuncio, A. Lilienbaum, S. Batonnet-Pichon, F. Bruston, F. Rodrigues-Lima, R. Mesa, C. Pizzarossa, L. Demay, P. Richard, P. Vicart & M. M. Rodriguez. (2010) Desmin myopathy with severe cardiomyopathy in a Uruguayan family due to a codon deletion in a new location within the desmin 1A rod domain. *Neuromuscul Disord,* Vol.20, No.3, pp. 178-87

P. Vicart, A. Caron, P. Guicheney, Z. Li, M. C. Prevost, A. Faure, D. Chateau, F. Chapon, F. Tome, J. M. Dupret, D. Paulin & M. Fardeau. (1998) A missense mutation in the alphaB-crystallin chaperone gene causes a desmin-related myopathy. *Nat Genet,* Vol.20, No.1, pp. 92-5

M. Vorgerd, P. F. van der Ven, V. Bruchertseifer, T. Lowe, R. A. Kley, R. Schroder, H. Lochmuller, M. Himmel, K. Koehler, D. O. Furst & A. Huebner. (2005) A mutation in the dimerization domain of filamin c causes a novel type of autosomal dominant myofibrillar myopathy. *Am J Hum Genet,* Vol.77, No.2, pp. 297-304

M. C. Walter, P. Reilich, A. Huebner, D. Fischer, R. Schroder, M. Vorgerd, W. Kress, C. Born, B. G. Schoser, K. H. Krause, U. Klutzny, S. Bulst, J. R. Frey & H. Lochmuller. (2007) Scapuloperoneal syndrome type Kaeser and a wide phenotypic spectrum of adult-onset, dominant myopathies are associated with the desmin mutation R350P. *Brain,* Vol.130, No.Pt 6, pp. 1485-96

X. Wang, H. Osinska, G. W. Dorn, 2nd, M. Nieman, J. N. Lorenz, A. M. Gerdes, S. Witt, T. Kimball, J. Gulick & J. Robbins. (2001a) Mouse model of desmin-related cardiomyopathy. *Circulation,* Vol.103, No.19, pp. 2402-7

X. Wang, H. Osinska, R. Klevitsky, A. M. Gerdes, M. Nieman, J. Lorenz, T. Hewett & J. Robbins. (2001b) Expression of R120G-alphaB-crystallin causes aberrant desmin and alphaB-crystallin aggregation and cardiomyopathy in mice. *Circ Res,* Vol.89, No.1, pp. 84-91

C. M. Warren, P. R. Krzesinski, K. S. Campbell, R. L. Moss & M. L. Greaser. (2004) Titin isoform changes in rat myocardium during development. *Mech Dev,* Vol.121, No.11, pp. 1301-12

S. D. Westerheide, J. D. Bosman, B. N. Mbadugha, T. L. Kawahara, G. Matsumoto, S. Kim, W. Gu, J. P. Devlin, R. B. Silverman & R. I. Morimoto. (2004) Celastrols as inducers of the heat shock response and cytoprotection. *J Biol Chem,* Vol.279, No.53, pp. 56053-60

M. S. Willis, J. C. Schisler, A. L. Portbury & C. Patterson. (2009) Build it up-Tear it down: protein quality control in the cardiac sarcomere. *Cardiovasc Res,* Vol.81, No.3, pp. 439-48

M. S. Willis & C. Patterson. (2010) Hold me tight: Role of the heat shock protein family of chaperones in cardiac disease. *Circulation,* Vol.122, No.17, pp. 1740-51

C. C. Witt, S. H. Witt, S. Lerche, D. Labeit, W. Back & S. Labeit. (2008) Cooperative control of striated muscle mass and metabolism by MuRF1 and MuRF2. *Embo J,* Vol.27, No.2, pp. 350-60

E. S. Wong, J. M. Tan, W. E. Soong, K. Hussein, N. Nukina, V. L. Dawson, T. M. Dawson, A. M. Cuervo & K. L. Lim. (2008) Autophagy-mediated clearance of aggresomes is not a universal phenomenon. *Hum Mol Genet,* Vol.17, No.16, pp. 2570-82

J. C. Wong & R. R. Fiscus. (2010) Essential roles of the nitric oxide (NO)/cGMP/protein kinase G type-Ialpha (PKG-Ialpha) signaling pathway and the atrial natriuretic peptide (ANP)/cGMP/PKG-Ialpha autocrine loop in promoting proliferation and cell survival of OP9 bone marrow stromal cells. *J Cell Biochem,* PMID: 21190199

R. Yamasaki, Y. Wu, M. McNabb, M. Greaser, S. Labeit & H. Granzier. (2002) Protein kinase A phosphorylates titin's cardiac-specific N2B domain and reduces passive tension in rat cardiac myocytes. *Circ Res,* Vol.90, No.11, pp. 1181-8

Q. Yang, T. E. Hewett, R. Klevitsky, A. Sanbe, X. Wang & J. Robbins. (2001) PKA-dependent phosphorylation of cardiac myosin binding protein C in transgenic mice. *Cardiovasc Res,* Vol.51, No.1, pp. 80-8

R. Zak. (1977) Metabolism of myofibrillar proteins in the normal and hypertrophic heart. *Basic Res Cardiol,* Vol.72, No.2-3, pp. 235-40

D. R. Zakhary, C. S. Moravec, R. W. Stewart & M. Bond. (1999) Protein kinase A (PKA)-dependent troponin-I phosphorylation and PKA regulatory subunits are decreased in human dilated cardiomyopathy. *Circulation,* Vol.99, No.4, pp. 505-10

C. Zhang, Z. Xu, X. R. He, L. H. Michael & C. Patterson. (2005) CHIP, a cochaperone/ubiquitin ligase that regulates protein quality control, is required for maximal cardioprotection after myocardial infarction in mice. *Am J Physiol Heart Circ Physiol,* Vol.288, No.6, pp. H2836-42

S. Zhang, C. Weinheimer, M. Courtois, A. Kovacs, C. E. Zhang, A. M. Cheng, Y. Wang & A. J. Muslin. (2003) The role of the Grb2-p38 MAPK signaling pathway in cardiac hypertrophy and fibrosis. *J Clin Invest,* Vol.111, No.6, pp. 833-41

T. J. Zhao, Y. B. Yan, Y. Liu & H. M. Zhou. (2007) The generation of the oxidized form of creatine kinase is a negative regulation on muscle creatine kinase. *J Biol Chem,* Vol.282, No.16, pp. 12022-9

M. Zheng, H. Cheng, X. Li, J. Zhang, L. Cui, K. Ouyang, L. Han, T. Zhao, Y. Gu, N. D. Dalton, M. L. Bang, K. L. Peterson & J. Chen. (2009) Cardiac-specific ablation of Cypher leads to a severe form of dilated cardiomyopathy with premature death. *Hum Mol Genet,* Vol.18, No.4, pp. 701-13

Q. Zhou, P. Ruiz-Lozano, M. E. Martone & J. Chen. (1999) Cypher, a striated muscle-restricted PDZ and LIM domain-containing protein, binds to alpha-actinin-2 and protein kinase C. *J Biol Chem,* Vol.274, No.28, pp. 19807-13

17

Functional Consequences of Mutations in the Myosin Regulatory Light Chain Associated with Hypertrophic Cardiomyopathy

Priya Muthu, Wenrui Huang,
Katarzyna Kazmierczak and Danuta Szczesna-Cordary
University of Miami Miller School of Medicine, Miami, FL, USA

1. Introduction

Familial hypertrophic cardiomyopathy (FHC) is an autosomal dominant disease characterized by left ventricular wall thickening, myofilament disarray and abnormal echocardiography findings. Molecular genetic studies have defined FHC as a disease of the sarcomere caused by mutations in all major sarcomeric proteins, such as β-myosin heavy chain (44%), myosin binding protein C (35%), regulatory light chain (2%), essential light chain (1.6%), α-tropomyosin (2.5%), troponin T (7%), troponin I (5%), troponin C (~1%), α-actin (1%), and titin (<1%) (Alcalai et al., 2008).

Although mutations in the regulatory light chain (RLC) of myosin are rare, they are of great significance given the importance of RLC for muscle contraction and heart function. The RLC plays an essential structural and functional role by supporting the architecture of the myosin neck region and fine-tuning the kinetics of the actin-myosin interaction (Morano, 1999; Szczesna, 2003). As shown in **Fig. 1**, the RLC wraps around the α-helical neck region of the myosin head by binding to a 35 amino acid IQ motif in the myosin heavy chain (MHC) (Rayment et al., 1993). This domain of MHC is anticipated to act as a lever arm, amplifying small conformational changes that originate at the catalytic site into large movements thus allowing myosin to generate motion and force (Geeves & Holmes, 2005; Lowey et al., 1993). Furthermore, this neck region has been proposed to serve as the compliant element of the myosin cross-bridge with the RLC contributing to the stiffness of the lever arm (Howard & Spudich, 1996; Pant et al., 2009). Two functionally important domains of the RLC molecule include its Ca^{2+}-Mg^{2+} binding site, comprised of the N-terminal helix-loop-helix EF-hand Ca^{2+} binding motif, and a highly conserved N-terminal phosphorylatable serine constituting a myosin light chain kinase (MLCK)-dependent phosphorylation site.

The N-terminal divalent cation-binding site of the RLC is thought to be occupied by Mg^{2+} when muscles are in the relaxed state and may become partially saturated with Ca^{2+}, depending on the length of the [Ca^{2+}] transient (Robertson et al., 1981). The MLCK phosphorylation site of RLC is also of great structural and functional importance. Phosphorylation of this site in smooth muscle activates contraction (Hartshorne & Mrwa, 1982; Small & Sobieszek, 1977; Sobieszek, 1977). In skeletal and cardiac muscle, Ca^{2+}-

calmodulin (CaM) activated MLCK phosphorylation of RLC modulates contraction by increasing the Ca^{2+} sensitivity and the level of force and also by modulating the kinetics of force generating myosin cross-bridges (for review see (Kamm & Stull, 2011)). Of particular importance, the phosphorylation of RLC has been shown to regulate the function of myosin in the heart (Morano, 1999; Szczesna, 2003). Attenuation of RLC phosphorylation was demonstrated to lead to ventricular myocyte hypertrophy with histological evidence of necrosis and fibrosis (Ding et al., 2010). Recent results from Szczesna-Cordary's lab shown that RLC phosphorylation plays an essential role not only in the physiological performance of the heart, but also helps to maintain normal cardiac function in the diseased myocardium (Muthu et al., 2011). At the level of protein, the phosphorylation of RLC at Ser-15 was shown to alter the secondary structure (α-helical content) and Ca^{2+} binding affinity of the human ventricular RLC protein (Szczesna et al., 2001). At the level of myofilaments, RLC phosphorylation was demonstrated to result in a significantly decreased distance between the myosin heads and actin filaments bringing them closer to each other (Colson et al., 2010)

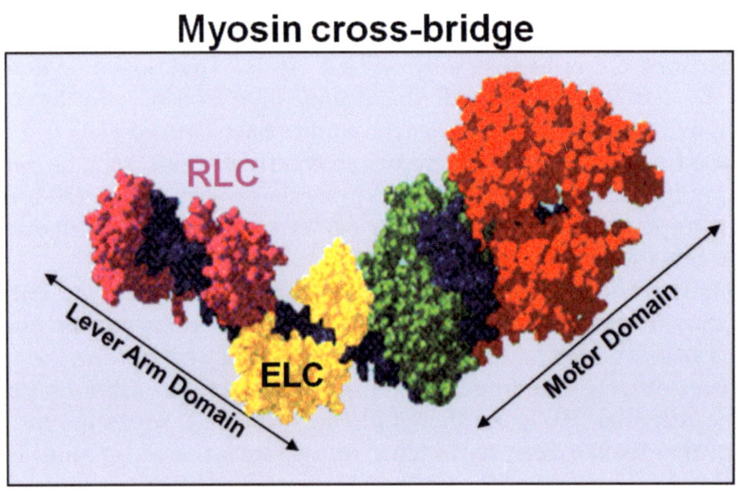

Fig. 1. Schematic representation of the myosin head (cross-bridge) containing regulatory (RLC, labeled in magenta) and essential (ELC, labeled in yellow) light chains. Indicated are 1) motor domain, and 2) lever arm (Rayment et al., 1993).

1.1 FHC-linked mutations in the regulatory light chain (RLC)

To date, eight single point mutations and two intron alternative splicing mutations in the *MYL2* gene encoding for the human ventricular RLC (Swiss-Prot: P10916) have been identified to cause FHC (**Fig. 2**). They are A13T (alanine to threonine), F18L (phenylalanine to leucine), E22K (glutamic acid to lysine), N47K (asparagine to lysine), R58Q (arginine to glutamine), P95A (proline to alanine), K104E (lysine to glutamic acid), D166V (aspartic acid to valine), IVS5-2 (a A>G transversion in intron 5 that leads to a premature termination codon), and IVS6-1 (a G>C transversion in the acceptor splice site of intron 6).

The A13T mutation arises from a replacement of alanine, an uncharged and nonpolar amino acid by threonine, an uncharged but polar amino acid. The mutation was first discovered in an American patient (Poetter et al., 1996) and was later found in a Danish proband diagnosed with hypertrophic cardiomyopathy (HCM). Two of his family members were found to be heterozygous for the mutation (Andersen et al., 2001). The proband, 42 years old, suffered from exercise-induced dyspnoea and had pronounced septal hypertrophy, diastolic filling abnormities but no significantly increased left ventricular outflow tract. One of the family members, the mother of the proband, was diagnosed with HCM late in life and died at the age of 72; while the other, 10 years old, showed no sign of HCM. In 2005, another proband carrying the A13T mutation was also identified in a Danish population (Hougs et al., 2005). Overall, this mutation is associated with a rare HCM phenotype characterized by mid left ventricular obstruction, enlarged papillary muscles and profound septal hypertrophy.

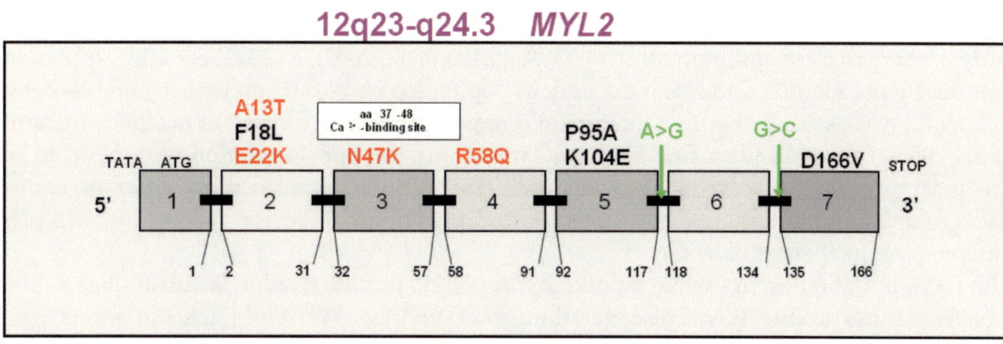

Fig. 2. Exon organization of the *MYL2* gene (chromosome 12q23-q24.3) and FHC-linked mutations in human ventricular RLC (Swiss-Prot: P10916). Labeled in red, FHC mutations described in this review; in black, other identified RLC mutations; and in green, intronic splice site mutations: A (adenine) → G (guanine) transversion in intron 5 and G → C (cytosine) transversion in intron 6.

The F18L mutation arises from a replacement of a bulky nonpolar and hydrophobic phenylalanine by the small uncharged and nonpolar leucine residue. It was found in three unrelated French families and is associated with a classic phenotype of left ventricular wall thickening and electrocardiographic (ECG) abnormities (Richard et al., 2003).

The E22K mutation results from a substitution of a negatively charged glutamate with a positively charged lysine leading to potential alterations in the net charge and polarity of the mutation-bearing domain of RLC. The mutation was first identified in three persons (two brothers and one non-related individual) from two unrelated families screened together with 399 unrelated HCM patients (Poetter et al., 1996). Subsequent studies by Kabaeva, et al. identified seven individuals in a German family carrying the mutation. However, only four patients suffered from HCM while the phenotype of the remaining individuals was defined as "uncertain" (Kabaeva et al., 2002). Based on the latest clinical reports on this mutation, it is known to be associated with moderate septal hypertrophy, late onset of clinical manifestations, and benign to severe disease outcomes.

The N47K mutation results from the replacement of a polar uncharged asparagine residue by the positively charged lysine. It was first discovered in an individual of Danish descent (Andersen et al., 2001). This mutation is associated with a late onset of the disease and a rapidly progressing phenotype. The proband was diagnosed with HCM at the age of 60, and quickly progressed to a severe hypertrophic phenotype and diastolic dysfunction. It was interesting that septal hypertrophy of this patient increased rapidly (from 31 mm to 45 mm) in the two years after diagnosis. In 2005, a Danish patient carrying both N47K and a β-cardiac myosin heavy chain mutation was identified. The proband bearing both of these mutations displayed a more severe phenotype than patients with either mutation alone (Hougs et al., 2005). However, no incidence of sudden cardiac death (SCD) associated with this mutation has yet been reported.

The R58Q mutation occurs when the bulky positively charged arginine is replaced by an uncharged but polar glutamine. It was first discovered by Flavigny, et al. in 1998 in three unrelated French families with HCM (Flavigny et al., 1998). The mutation was associated with a classic form of FHC characterized by left ventricular wall thickness, abnormal ECG findings and SCD (Flavigny et al., 1998). In 2002, Kabaeva, et al. detected this R58Q mutation in a German proband with a clinical phenotype of moderate septal hypertrophy, early onset of disease and premature SCD (Kabaeva et al., 2002). In 2003, the R58Q mutation was once more identified in two independent population studies (from France and Sweden), and again was associated with a malignant disease phenotype (Morner et al., 2003; Richard et al., 2003). Out of all identified FHC RLC mutations, the R58Q mutation was found to be the most prevalent, occurring independently in multiple families with different ethnic backgrounds. The mutation is associated with a phenotype of severe cardiac hypertrophy and multiple incidences of SCD.

The P95A mutation occurs when a bulky hydrophobic proline residue is substituted with a smaller alanine residue. It was discovered together with the A13T and E22K mutations in an American family and shares a rare clinical phenotype, similar to that of A13T and E22K positive patients (Poetter et al., 1996).

The K104E mutation results from a replacement of the positively charged lysine with the negatively charged glutamic acid. The mutation was first observed in a Danish family and was mistakenly reported as L103E (Andersen et al., 2001). The parents carrying this mutation were asymptomatic with a normal ECG pattern. However, their son was diagnosed with pronounced septal hypertrophy at the age of 17 and progressed to diastolic dysfunction. His sister, 42 years old, was also positive for the mutation, but no typical hypertrophic phenotype was observed in her case. This mutation is associated with pronounced septal hypertrophy and diastolic filling abnormalities.

The D166V mutation occurs when a negatively charged aspartic acid is substituted with a bulky polar valine residue. This mutation was identified in a French proband, with the potential to cause SCD at a young age. It was first mistakenly presented as D166L in Richard, et al., 2003 and later corrected to D166V (Richard et al., 2003; 2004). Similar to R58Q, this mutation is associated with a malignant disease phenotype and SCD.

Intron mutations: Intron 6-1 G>C mutation (IVS 6-1) was discovered along with K104E in the Danish population and is associated with pronounced septal hypertrophy (Andersen et al., 2001). The other intronic mutation 5-2 A>G, (IVS 5-2) was first discovered in the French population and is associated with a malignant form of FHC (Richard et al., 2003). The mutation is predicted to lead to a premature codon termination.

The clinical phenotype associated with FHC-linked mutations in the regulatory light chain and current to date literature citations are illustrated in **Table 1**.

This review focuses on the functional phenotypes associated with five (A13T, E22K, N47K, R58Q and D166V) RLC mutations extensively studied *in vitro* using RLC-mutant reconstituted muscle systems and *in vivo,* using cardiac muscle preparations from transgenic mice expressing FHC-RLC mutations.

Mutation in RLC	Clinical phenotype	Population	Major findings
A13T	Massive hypertrophy of cardiac papillary muscles, mid-cavity left ventricular obstruction, pronounced septal and ventricular hypertrophy and diastolic filling abnormalities	Danish (Andersen et al., 2001; Hougs et al., 2005); American (Poetter et al., 1996)	Mutation-induced changes in α-helical content and in Ca^{2+} binding properties of RLC (Szczesna et al., 2001). No change in Ca^{2+}sensitivity of myofibrillar ATPase activity (Szczesna et al., 2001). Increased force production in skinned papillary muscle fibers from Tg-A13T mice (unpublished data). Histopathological changes in left ventricles and inter-ventricular septa of Tg-A13T mice (unpublished data)
F18L	Classic form of HCM – increased left ventricular wall thickness, abnormal ECG findings, no mid left ventricular obstruction	French (Flavigny et al., 1998; Richard et al., 2003)	Decrease in Ca^{2+} binding affinity to RLC (Szczesna et al., 2001). Increase in α-helical content of RLC (Szczesna et al., 2001). Decrease in Ca^{2+} sensivity of myofibrillar ATPase activity (Szczesna-Cordary et al., 2004a). Compromised maximal tension, cooperativity and Ca^{2+} sensitivity of force (Roopnarine, 2003).
E22K	Moderate septal hypertrophy, late onset of clinical manifestation or no symptoms of FHC (Kabaeva). Also associated with massive hypertrophy of cardiac papillary muscles and adjacent venstricular tissue causing midcavity obstruction (Poetter)	German (Kabaeva et al., 2002), American (Poetter et al., 1996)	Protein non-phosphorylatable (Szczesna et al., 2001). Mutation induced changes in α-helical content and Ca^{2+} binding properties of RLC (Szczesna et al., 2001). Increase in Ca^{2+} sensitivity of force (Levine et al., 1998; Roopnarine, 2003; Szczesna-Cordary et al., 2004a) and decrease in maximal ATPase and force in skinned fibers from Tg-E22K mice (Szczesna-Cordary et al., 2007). No effect on cross-bridge kinetics (Szczesna-Cordary et al., 2007; (Dumka et al., 2006). Enlarged inter-ventricular septa and papillary muscles (Szczesna-Cordary et al., 2005). No hypertrophy detected in Tg-E22K mice (Sanbe et al., 2000). No changes in ECG (Szczesna-Cordary et al., 2005).
N47K	Pronounced interventricular (septal) and papillary musle hypertrophy; relatively high midventricular flow gradient, diastolic filling abnormalities; late onset disease with a rapidly progressing phenotype	Danish (Andersen et al., 2001; Hougs et al., 2005)	Abolished Ca^{2+} binding to RLC (Szczesna-Cordary et al., 2004a). Increased Ca^{2+} sensivity of myofibrillar ATPase activity (Szczesna-Cordary et al., 2004a). No change in pCa_{50} of force (Szczesna-Cordary et al., 2004a). Prolonged Ca^{2+} transient with no change in force transients in intact papillary muslces (Wang et al., 2006). Decreased isometric force in N47K-myosin based *in vitro* motility assays (Greenberg et al., 2009). Reduction in force and power output under loaded conditions (Greenberg et al., 2010). Decreased cardiac function in isolated perfused working hearts (Abraham et al., 2009).

Mutation in RLC	Clinical phenotype	Population	Major findings
R58Q	Malignant FHC phenotype, early onset of clinical manifestation and high incidence of premature SCD; classic form of HCM - increased left ventricular wall thickness and abnormal ECG findings	German (Kabaeva et al., 2002), French (Flavigny et al., 1998; Richard et al., 2003), Swedish (Morner et al., 2003)	Abolished Ca^{2+} binding to RLC, which was restored upon RLC phosphorylation. (Szczesna et al., 2001). Mutation induced increase in α-helical content of RLC (Szczesna et al., 2001). Increased Ca^{2+} sensitivity of force (Szczesna-Cordary et al., 2004a), and Ca^{2+} and force transient in intact papillary muscles (Wang et al., 2006). Higher ATPase rate and increased activation at submaximal Ca^{2+} (Greenberg et al., 2009). Decreased skewness and kurtosis of fluctuations during contraction (Borejdo et al., 2010). Decreased force (Abraham et al., 2009; Greenberg et al., 2010; Greenberg et al., 2009; Wang et al., 2006). Reduced level of endogenous RLC phosphorylation (Abraham et al., 2009). Decreased cardiac function in isolated perfused working hearts (Abraham et al., 2009). Alterations in diastolic transmitral velocities and increased deceleration time, indicative of diastolic dysfunction (Abraham et al., 2009).
P95A	Rare clinical phenotype, similar to E22K and A13T, of midventricular obstruction	American (Poetter et al., 1996)	Mutation-induced decrease in Ca^{2+} binding to RLC (Szczesna et al., 2001). No significant effect on tension, Ca^{2+} sensitivity, or cooperativity in P95A-reconstituted fibers (Roopnarine, 2003).
K104E	Pronounced septal hypertrophy and diastolic filling abnormalities	Danish (Andersen et al., 2001)	Impaired interaction with IQ-MHC peptide (Szczesna-Cordary et al., 2004b). Slight decrease in binding to RLC-depleted porcine myosin (Huang et al., 2011).
D166V	Malignant FHC phenotype - poor prognosis and SCD at young age	French (Richard et al., 2003; 2004)	Decrease in maximal force and large increase in Ca^{2+} sensitivity in papillary muscle fibers from Tg-D166V mice (Kerrick et al., 2009). Decrease in Ca^{2+} sensitivity of force upon phosphorylation (Muthu et al., 2011). Slower cross bridge kinetics (Borejdo et al., 2010; Mettikolla et al., 2009; Muthu et al., 2010). Reduced level of endogenous RLC phosphorylation (Kerrick et al., 2009). Severe fibrotic lesions in older Tg-D166V mouse hearts (Kerrick et al., 2009).
IVS6-1	Pronounced proximal septal hypertrophy	Danish (Andersen et al., 2001)	G>C transversion in Intron 6 (Andersen et al., 2001).
IVS5-2	Malignant prognosis	French (Richard et al., 2003)	Donor-site splice mutation (A>G) in Intron 5 predicted to lead to a premature termination codon (Richard et al., 2003).

Table 1. Summary of clinical and functional phenotypes of FHC mutations in the regulatory light chain (RLC).

2. Effect of FHC mutations on the secondary RLC structure and calcium binding properties

This review reports on the studies that were conducted to elucidate the structural and functional effects of FHC-linked RLC mutations. The RLC protein, labeled in red in **Fig. 3**, wraps around the myosin heavy chain (dark blue) and connects the myosin head with the myosin rod region. The three-dimensional (3D) structure of the RLC demonstrates the close proximity of the FHC mutations to either the phosphorylation site of RLC (Ser-15) or the Ca^{2+} binding site (amino acids 37–48 in the sequence of human ventricual RLC) (**Fig. 3**). The presence of these two important RLC domains in the RLC structure prompted the studies aimed at understanding the effects of the FHC mutations on Ca^{2+} binding to RLC and to determine how MLCK-dependent phosphorylation of RLC is affected in FHC disease. Furthermore, additional studies were conducted to determine the effect of FHC-linked RLC mutation and phosphorylation on the secondary RLC structure.

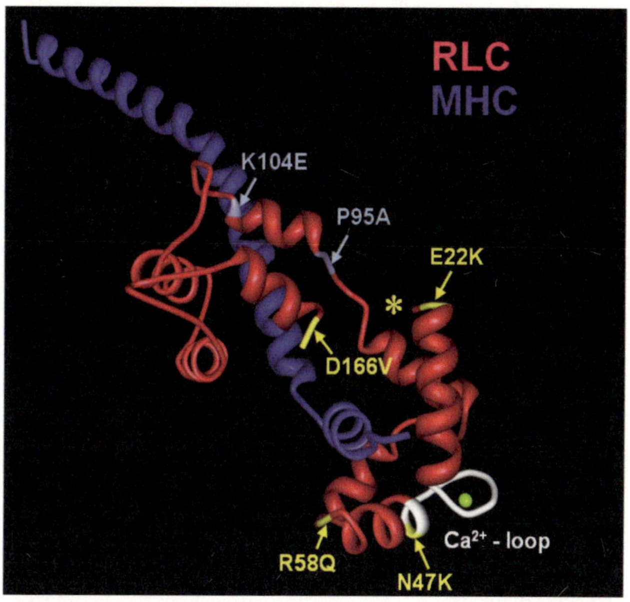

Fig. 3. Structure of the regulatory domain of scallop myosin (1WDC) (Houdusse & Cohen, 1996): Indicated are the FHC mutations, Ca^{2+}-Mg^{2+} binding site and the phosphorylation site. The MHC (myosin heavy chain) is labeled in dark blue, and the RLC (regulatory light chain) in red. Asterisks (*) depict the predicted location of A13T and F18L mutations and Ser-15 phosphorylation site (the region of RLC which is not resolved in all available vertebrate myosin crystal structures).

2.1 Circular dichroism study

In order to test the effect of RLC mutations on the secondary structure of RLC, far-UV circular dichroism (CD) spectra measurements were performed and the α-helical content determined (Szczesna-Cordary et al., 2004a; Szczesna et al., 2001). Far-UV CD spectra were obtained using a 1-mm path quartz cell in a Jasco J-720 spectropolarimeter and were recorded at 195–250 nm. Mean residue ellipticity ($[\theta]_{MRE}$, in degrees *cm^2/dmol) for the spectra were calculated using the following equation:

$$[\theta]_{MRE}=[\theta]/(10*Cr*l)$$

where [θ] is the measured ellipticity in millidegrees, *Cr* is the mean residue molar concentration, and *l* is the path length in cm.

The α-helical content for each mutant was calculated using the standard equation for [θ] at 222 nm (Chen & Yang, 1971):

$$[\theta]_{222}=-30{,}000*f_H - 2340$$

where f_H is the fraction of α-helical content (f_H * 100, expressed in %). Any change above 2% in the α -helical content was considered statistically significant.

As the mutations lie in the proximity of the phosphorylation site (Ser-15) and/or the Ca^{2+}-Mg^{2+} binding site (**Fig. 3**), the α-helical content was measured in the absence (Apo) and presence of Ca^{2+}. In addition, data were collected for phosphorylated RLC (**Table 2**).

Protein	Apo	$+Ca^{2+}$	+P	$+P +Ca^{2+}$
RLC-WT	18	23	18	18
A13T	29	25	19	18
E22K	24	20	No phosphorylation	
N47K	18.7	ND	ND	ND
R58Q	20	22	20	28
P95A	19	23	ND	ND

Table 2. Effect of phosphorylation and Ca^{2+}-binding on the α-helical content of RLC expressed in %. (ND: not determined) (Szczesna-Cordary et al., 2004a; Szczesna et al., 2001).

Based on these results, it was determined that under Apo (no metal) conditions, with the exception of the N47K and P95A mutants, the FHC-linked RLC mutation led to an increased α-helical content compared to RLC-WT (Szczesna-Cordary et al., 2004a; Szczesna et al., 2001). It was also observed that upon binding of Ca^{2+} to RLC, the α-helical content was significantly increased in all proteins including WT (**Table 2**), suggesting that binding of calcium to RLC could be conformation dependent. Interestingly, upon phosphorylation, A13T displayed a significant decrease in the α-helical content compared to non-phosphorylated A13T in the presence or absence of Ca^{2+}. Therefore, phosphorylation of the A13T mutant rescued the secondary structure of the mutant bringing the α-helical content to the level of RLC-WT. The authors concluded that phosphorylation of RLC could reverse the detrimental effect of FHC brought about by the A13T mutation (Szczesna et al., 2001).

2.2 Calcium binding study

As shown above in **Fig. 3,** the N-terminal domain of RLC contains the EF-hand Ca^{2+}-Mg^{2+} binding site, similar to the EF-hand Ca^{2+}-sites present in troponin C (TnC), parvalbumin, calmodulin (CaM) and essential light chain (ELC). To test how these mutations affect calcium binding to the RLC, flow dialysis experiments were conducted and the Ca^{2+} association/dissociation constant was determined (Szczesna et al., 2001). Radio-labeled substrate ($^{45}Ca^{2+}$) was first added into a chamber containing a fixed amount of RLC. Once the reaction reached steady-state, radio-labeled $^{45}Ca^{2+}$ was chased by unlabeled Ca^{2+}. The concentrations of bound-Ca^{2+} and free-Ca^{2+} were determined and the K_{Ca} values analyzed. Calcium association constant K_{Ca} was extrapolated from the following equation:

$$C_{Ca\text{-}bound}/C_{Ca\text{-}free}/C_p = -K_{Ca} * C_{Ca\text{-}bound}/C_p + n*K_{Ca}$$

$C_{Ca\text{-bound}}$ and $C_{Ca\text{-free}}$ represent the concentration of the bound and free metal, respectively, C_p is the concentration of the protein, n is the total number of Ca^{2+} binding sites, and K_{Ca} is the Ca^{2+} binding affinity. $1/K_{Ca}$ represents the apparent calcium dissociation constant K_d (in μM). The effect of the mutations on calcium binding to recombinant human cardiac RLC and FHC-linked mutants is summarized in **Table 3** (Szczesna et al., 2001). **Table 3** also summarizes the effect of FHC RLC mutations on calcium binding to myofibrils and skinned muscle fibers reconstituted with WT or FHC-mutant proteins (Szczesna-Cordary et al., 2004a).

RLC protein	Isolated RLC (no Mg^{2+}) (μ*M*)	Myofibrils# (2 mM Mg^{2+}) (μ*M*)	Fibers# (1 mMMg^{2+}) (μ*M*)
RLC-WT	1.50 ± 0.02	0.200 ± 0.009	2.88 ± 0.19
A13T	4.85 ± 0.31	0.191 ± 0.015	3.02 ± 0.06
E22K	25.64 ± 3.48	0.178 ± 0.001	2.63 ± 0.10
N47K	No binding	0.141 ± 0.009	2.51 ± 0.10
R58Q	No binding	0.170 ± 0.004	2.19 ± 0.10
P95A	4.74 ± 1.05	0.200 ± 0.011	2.75 ± 0.25

Table 3. Apparent K_d ($1/K_{Ca}$) of isolated RLC-WT and FHC mutants and in mutant-reconstituted myofibrils and skinned porcine muscle fibers (#K_d calculated from the pCa_{50} values ±S.E.) (Szczesna-Cordary et al., 2004a).

Flow dialysis experiments with recombinant RLC-WT and FHC-mutants showed that A13T and P95A decreased the K_{Ca} ~3-fold, whereas E22K, N47K and R58Q, changed the Ca^{2+} binding properties in a more drastic way. Compared with RLC-WT, the E22K mutation decreased the K_{Ca} value by ~17-fold, whereas both N47K and R58Q mutations eliminated Ca^{2+} binding to RLC (**Table 3**) (Szczesna et al., 2001). These three Ca^{2+} binding site mutants also showed an increase in the Ca^{2+} sensitivity of myofibrillar ATPase activity and force development, with R58Q demonstrating significantly higher K_{Ca} compared to RLC WT-reconstituted muscle preparations (**Table 3**) (Szczesna-Cordary et al., 2004a). Interestingly, flow dialysis studies showed that the restricted ability of the R58Q mutant to bind calcium was restored upon phosphorylation (Szczesna et al., 2001). These studies suggested that the phosphorylation and Ca^{2+} binding to human cardiac RLC are important for physiological function and that alteration of any of these properties may contribute to the development of hypertrophic cardiomyopathy. Results from the *in vitro* studies prompted generation of the animal models of FHC-linked RLC mutations and subsequent investigations of their functional effects *in vivo.* Studies included experiments performed at different levels of complexity; from single molecules to organized sarcomeres in muscle fibers and to the organ and organism levels. Transgenic mice carrying FHC RLC mutations were used in these experiments.

3. Animal models of FHC

3.1 Generation of transgenic mice

Transgenic (Tg) mouse models expressing wild-type (WT) and FHC-mutated human ventricular cardiac RLC (A13T, E22K, N47K, R58Q and D166V) were generated using the α-myosin heavy chain (α-MHC) promoter (clone 26, a generous gift from Dr J. Robbins, Cincinnati Children's Hospital Medical Center, Cincinnati, OH, USA). All of the founders were bred to non-transgenic (NTg) B6SJL mice. Two types of Tg-WT mice were generated as necessary controls for the transgenic mutant mice; one expressing human ventricular cardiac RLC and another expressing the human ventricular cardiac RLC along with a myc-tag sequence. The following transgenic mouse models were produced and used for the experiments described in this review: WT, A13T, E22K, N47K, R58Q and D166V.

3.2 Phenotypic characterization of FHC-RLC animal models

3.2.1 Assessment of cardiac hypertrophy by HW/BW ratio

The heart weight to body weight (HW/BW) ratio was used to examine all generated FHC RLC animal models for heart hypertrophy. **Fig. 4** demonstrates the HW/BW ratios determined for mice carrying A13T, D166V, N47K and R58Q mutations. No evidence of hypertrophy was observed in the majority of mutant mice compared to WT (Kerrick et al., 2009; Wang et al., 2006). Differences in HW/BW were only seen between the hearts from Tg-N47K *versus* Tg-WT mice, but no statistically significant changes were observed.

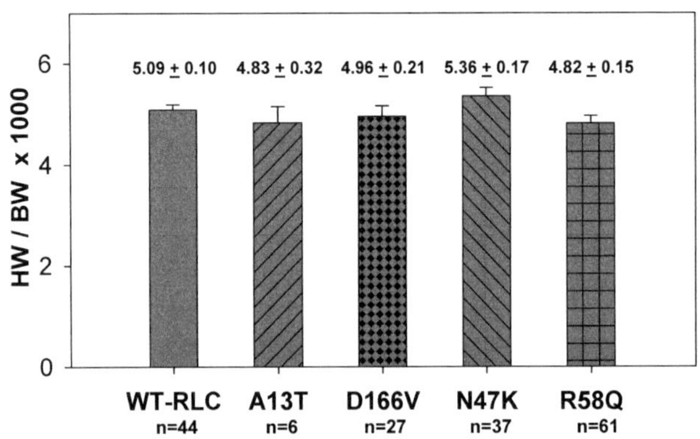

Fig. 4. Heart weight to body weight ratios in transgenic RLC animal models: P-values for all mutant mice (A13T, D166V, N47K and R58Q) *versus* WT-RLC were >0.05.

These results suggested that the histopathological and functional changes observed due to these mutations (discussed later) may be more indicative of the FHC phenotype than overall heart hypertrophy.

3.2.2 Histopathology

The most specific histological feature of hypertrophic cardiomyopathy is an extensive disorganization of the myocyte structure (myocyte disarray). Often observed are abnormally branched (Y-shaped) myocytes with adjacent myocytes arranged perpendicularly or obliquely to each other (Binder et al., 2005). Histological studies were performed to characterize the mutation specific cardiac phenotype at the level of the Tg mouse model and to establish a correlation with the phenotypes observed in patients harboring these FHC RLC mutations. Histopatological evaluation of the hearts from Tg-A13T, Tg-E22K, Tg-WT and NTg mice is presented in **Fig. 5**. The upper panel shows longitudinal sections of the whole hearts from Tg-A13T *versus* control mice and the lower panel presents Tg-E22K mouse hearts. As indicated with arrows, a significantly larger LV and inter-ventricular septal mass was observed for both Tg-A13T (unpublished data) and Tg-E22K (Szczesna-Cordary et al., 2005) mice compared with Tg-WT or NTg littermates.

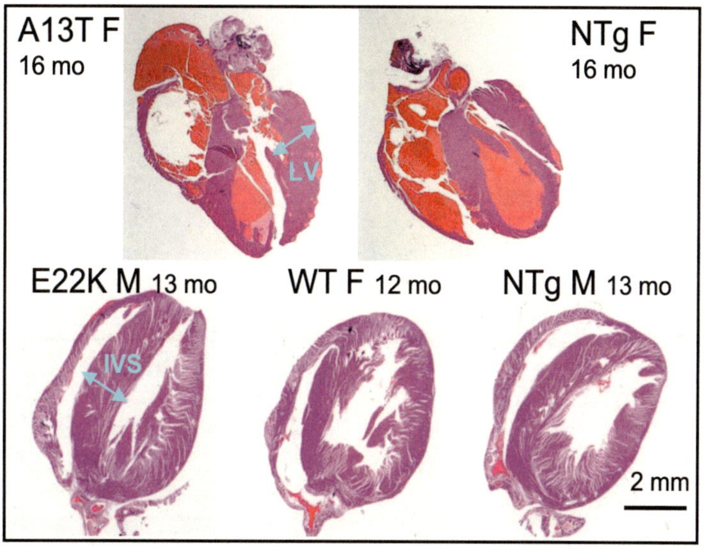

Fig. 5. Longitudinal sections of whole mouse hearts stained with hematoxylin and eosin (H & E). Upper panel: Tg-A13T *versus* NTg controls (unpublished data). Bottom panel: Tg-E22K and controls (Szczesna-Cordary et al., 2005). Abbreviations: F, female; M, male; mo, age of mice in months; LV, left ventricle; IVS, interventricular septum.

Gross morphological evaluation of the hearts from Tg-A13T and Tg-E22K mice revealed a common phenotype of enlarged inter-ventricular septa (**Fig. 6**), a phenotype observed in patients carrying the A13T and E22K mutations (Poetter et al., 1996). Interestingly, in another study transgenic mice expressing the E22K mutation did not show any features of the FHC disease despite almost total replacement of the endogenous WT RLC with mutant RLC (Sanbe et al., 2000). No hypertrophy was detected in mature adult animals either when chamber weights were determined or at the cellular level (Sanbe et al., 2000).
Other RLC FHC mutant mice were examined for histopathological abnormalities, and longitudinal ventricular sections were stained with hematoxylin and eosin to detect any tissue disorganization and with Masson's trichrome to determine the presence of abnormal collagen deposits and fibrosis. As shown in **Fig. 6**, mice carrying the malignant R58Q mutation manifested histopathological changes (myofibrillar disarray and abnormal clustering of nuclei) as early as at 4 months of age (**Fig. 6A, B**). The changes seen in older (~17 months old) mice, presented in Wang et al. were profound in both Tg-R58Q and Tg-N47K mice (Wang et al., 2006). The changes observed in Tg-N47K mice correlated with the phenotype found in humans demonstrating a late onset of disease with a rapidly progressing phenotype. Similarly, examination of the older (~17 months of age) Tg-D166V mice revealed severe fibrotic lesions present in the left ventricles compared with age matched Tg-WT and NTg littermates (**Fig. 6C**). Morphological changes found in the older Tg-D166V mice suggest that the ventricles of the FHC Tg-D166V mice undergo temporal phenotypic changes that are not present in the younger mice (~ 7 months of age) (Kerrick et al., 2009). These studies suggested that while in Tg-N47K and Tg-D166V animals the functional changes induced by the mutations (evident at 3-6 months of age in mice) may precede the development of any detrimental morphological changes; the histopathological changes observed in Tg-R58Q mice paralleled the functional abnormalities.

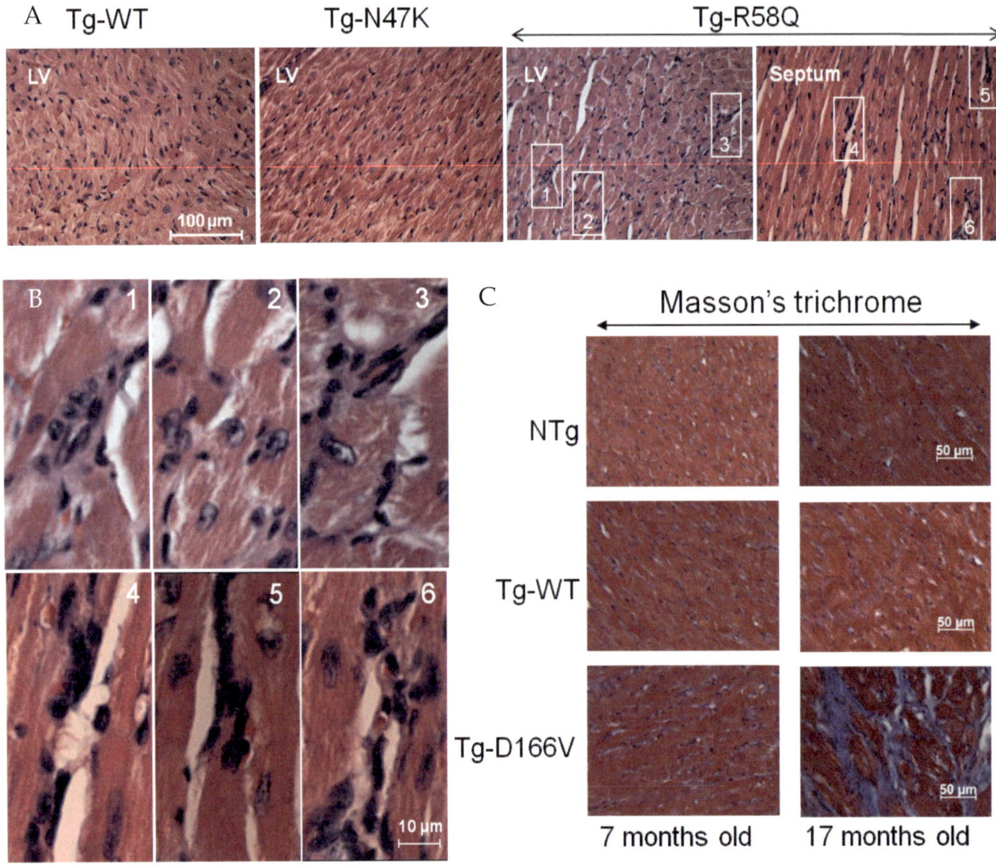

Fig. 6. Histopathology of transgenic mouse hearts. (A) The hearts of representative 4 month-old mice from Tg-WT, Tg-N47K and Tg-R58Q mice were stained with hematoxylin and eosin. Note that nuclei stain blue with hematoxylin, whereas the cells stain pink/red with eosin. Scale bar, 100 µm. (B) Enlarged views of the left ventricle and septal tissues of Tg-R58Q hearts. Scale bar, 10 µm. As indicated, clusters of nuclei could be clearly observed in Tg-R58Q tissues compared to control samples suggesting occurrences of the R58Q-mediated degeneration in Tg-R58Q myocardium. (C) Microscopic views of left ventricles from Tg-D166V and control Tg-WT and NTg mice stained with Masson's trichrome stain (Kerrick et al., 2009). Note the severe fibrotic lesions in the myocardium of older 17 months old Tg-D166V mice. Scale bar, 50 µm.

3.2.3 Echocardiography

Echocardiography, a test in which ultrasound measurements are used to examine the heart, is the least invasive method available to screen for cardiac hypertrophy. The echocardiogram allows for detailed morphological and functional assessment of the heart. Echocardiography examination performed on Tg-E22K mice did not show any major differences between transgenic E22K and control WT and/or NTg hearts (Szczesna-Cordary et al., 2005).

Doppler echocardiography, another technique of ultrasound examination is used to look at how blood flows through the heart chambers, heart valves, and blood vessels. It allows determination of the velocity and direction of blood flow by utilizing the Doppler effect.

Based on the cellular findings, Abraham et al. hypothesized that a malignant FHC phenotype associated with the R58Q mutation could be related to diastolic dysfunction of the R58Q-mutated myocardium (Abraham et al., 2009). Global diastolic haemodynamics were evaluated using transmitral Doppler velocities in Tg-R58Q and Tg-N47K mice and compared to controls (NTg and Tg-WT). An apical four-chamber view of the heart was obtained. A pulsed Doppler sample was placed at the tip of the mitral leaflets and transmitral early (E) and late (A) diastolic velocities and the deceleration time were measured and used as noninvasive indicators of global diastolic function (Abraham et al., 2009). Interestingly, alterations in diastolic transmitral velocities and prolonged deceleration time were only noted in Tg-R58Q myocardium (**Fig. 7**). The authors suggested that the malignant FHC phenotype associated with R58Q could be related to abnormal relaxation and diastolic dysfunction of the mutated myocardium. The key conclusion of this study was that diastolic function is affected earlier in the disease process in the transgenic mouse model and may likely be a more sensitive indicator of a malignant FHC phenotype than hypertrophy or systolic dysfunction (Abraham et al., 2009).

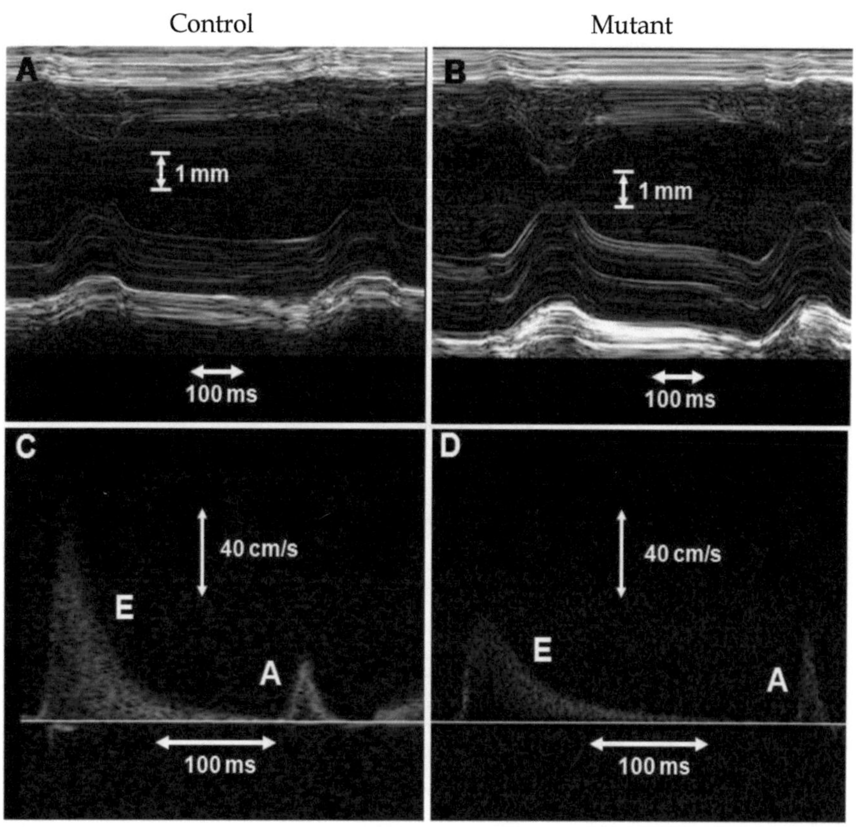

Fig. 7. Representative high resolution echocardiography B-mode images from control (A) and Tg-R58Q mice (B) show no significant difference in chamber dimensions or wall thickness. Representative pulsed Doppler tracings of the mitral valve in controls (C) and Tg-R58Q mice (D) demonstrating reduced E wave velocity and longer deceleration times in the latter group (Abraham et al., 2009).

3.2.4 Perfused working heart model

The hearts of transgenic mice carrying different RLC mutations were tested for the ability to perform work under conditions of physiologically relevant levels of metabolic demands and for glucose and fatty acid oxidation measured in isolated working hearts (Abraham et al., 2009; Szczesna-Cordary et al., 2007). Studies with Tg-E22K mice showed a similar energy metabolism pattern compared to control Tg-WT and NTg mouse hearts, but following 20 minutes of no flow ischemia, the E22K hearts demonstrated a slightly better recovery compared to WT hearts (Szczesna-Cordary et al., 2007). In another study with Tg-R58Q and Tg-N47K mice, it was shown that cardiac output, cardiac work and cardiac power were drastically compromised compared with controls, Tg-WT or NTg mice (Abraham et al., 2009). Additional data attained with Tg-R58Q mice also demonstrated significantly decreased cardiac efficiency in aerobically perfused R58Q hearts compared to controls and poor recovery after an acute ischemic episode confirming greatly compromised cardiac function in Tg-R58Q mice (Abraham et al., 2009). Results from these studies mirrored the severity of the human phenotypes associated with R58Q and N47K mutations, with less severe outcomes in N47K patients, while matching the malignant phenotype with multiple cases of SCD in R58Q-positive patients.

3.2.5 Endogenous level of RLC phosphorylation

The highly conserved Ser-15 in RLC can be reversibly phosphorylated *in vivo* by Ca^{2+}-CaM-activated MLCK. Given the role that RLC phosphorylation can play in affecting thick filament structure and cardiac contractility, examining the mutation induced effect on RLC phosphorylation is important in understanding the effects of any of the FHC mutation. Mutations studied in this review can be categorized into two groups based on

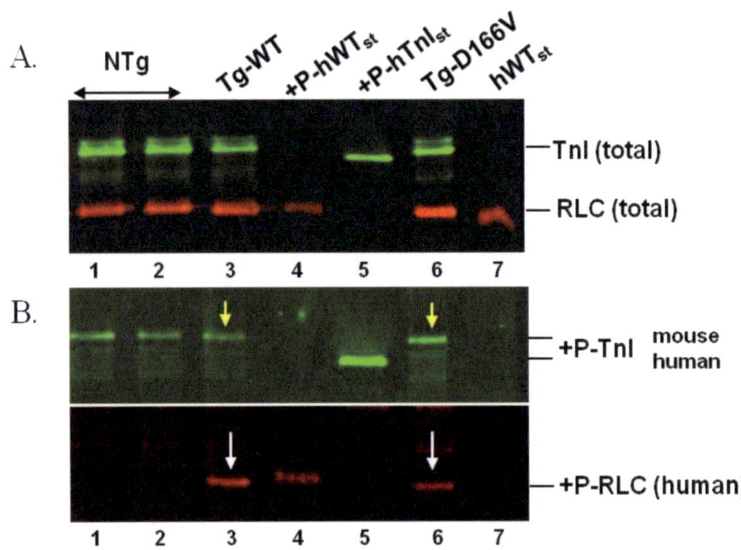

Fig. 8. The effect of the D166V mutation on the phosphorylation status of RLC and Troponin I (TnI) in transgenic mouse ventricular extracts blotted with CT-1 antibody recognizing total RLC protein and 6F9 antibody recognizing total TnI protein (A) and Mab14 MMS-418R antibody recognizing +P-TnI (top panel) and +P-human RLC antibody recognizing +P-RLC human (Tg) (bottom panel) (B) (Kerrick et al., 2009).

their location in the sequence and the 3D organization of RLC (**Fig. 3**): N47K and R58Q-located close or within the Ca^{2+} binding site, and A13T, E22K and D166V- located in close proximity to the phosphorylation site (Ser-15). The status of phosphorylation was examined for transgenic mice carrying the R58Q, N47K and D166V mutations (Abraham et al., 2009; Kerrick et al., 2009; Muthu et al., 2010; Muthu et al., 2011). Mouse extracts from ventricular tissue were rapidly frozen in liquid nitrogen and analyzed by immunoblotting. The phosphorylated Tg-RLC was detected with +P-human RLC antibodies (generously provided by Dr. Neal Epstein, NIH), specific for the phosphorylated form of the ventricular RLC; followed by a secondary goat anti-rabbit antibody conjugated with the fluorescent dye, IR red 800. It was interesting to note that the mutations in RLC associated with a malignant phenotype (R58Q and D166V) displayed a reduced level of phosphorylation compared to N47K and/or WT.

The decreased level of phosphorylation coincided with those FHC mutations that are associated with a severe phenotype (**Fig. 8**) (Abraham et al., 2009; Kerrick et al., 2009). This suggested that phosphorylation of the regulatory light chain of myosin could have an important physiological role in the regulation of cardiac muscle contraction.

4. Functional studies using cardiac muscle preparations

4.1 ATPase assays

4.1.1 Actin activated myosin ATPase activity

Myosin's ability to perform mechanical work, powered by the hydrolysis of ATP, requires that the enzymatic and mechanical cycles be coupled. Both the hydrolysis of ATP and the generation of force and motion are known to be multi-step processes. The cross-bridge cycle can be broadly divided into states where myosin is strongly or weakly bound to actin. It starts with the physiologically short-lived rigor state where myosin is bound strongly to actin in the absence of ATP. If ATP or its hydrolysis products are bound (M▫ATP, M▫ADP▫Pi), myosin shifts to the weakly bound state. Either prior to or following inorganic phosphate (Pi) release, myosin undergoes its power stroke increasing its affinity for actin.

The actin activated myosin ATPase activity, measured as a function of actin concentration was determined for FHC-linked RLC mutants using myosin purified from the mouse hearts or RLC-depleted porcine myosin reconstituted with WT or FHC RLC mutant protein. The assay consisted of titrating myosin with increasing concentrations of skeletal muscle actin. The data were analyzed with the Michaelis-Menten equation yielding the V_{max} (maximal ATPase rate) and K_m (apparent dissociation constant) parameters.

This assay was performed to understand the effect of the N47K and R58Q mutations on the cross bridge cycle (Greenberg et al., 2009). The maximal ATPase rates (V_{max}) for NTg (0.43 s^{-1}) and Tg-WT (0.43 s^{-1}) were seen to be similar to those of RLC carrying the N47K mutation (0.43 s^{-1}). However, Tg-R58Q showed a significant increase in V_{max} (0.63 s^{-1}). On the other hand, a significant decrease in V_{max} was observed in Tg-A13T mice (0.38 s^{-1}) compared to Tg-WT (0.51 s^{-1}) or NTg (0.63 s^{-1}) mice (unpublished data). The observed changes in the ATPase activity for the mutant RLC compared to controls suggest that the total amount of free ATP in the cell may vary affecting several ATP dependent processes in the heart and leading to the development of FHC phenotype. Moreover, as V_{max} represents the rate constant of the transition from the weakly to strongly bound myosin cross-bridges, the FHC mutations are expected to affect the kinetics of force generating myosin cross-bridges and muscle contraction.

4.1.2 Myofibrillar ATPase activity

To understand the effect of mutations in RLC at the myofibrillar level, assays were performed on two types of systems: porcine myofibrils reconstituted with the FHC mutant or cardiac myofibrils prepared from transgenic mice carrying the RLC mutation.

For the reconstituted myofibrillar assays, porcine cardiac myofibrils (CMF) were depleted of RLC using Triton and CDTA (Szczesna-Cordary et al., 2004a). The CDTA extraction method resulted in about 80% depletion of the endogenous RLC. These RLC depleted CMF were then reconstituted with exogenous recombinant human cardiac RLC-WT and FHC mutants (A13T, F18L, E22K, N47K and R58Q). The authors observed that myofibrils lacking the RLC demonstrated dramatic impairment of the Ca^{2+} regulation of ATPase activity at pCa 8 (low Ca^{2+}) and 4.5 (high Ca^{2+}) and also demonstrated lower Ca^{2+} sensitivity of ATPase. The latter was determined to be due to partial extraction of troponin C (TnC) that occurs during RLC extraction. Reconstitution of the RLC-depleted CMF with cardiac TnC and RLC (WT or FHC mutant) recovered the Ca^{2+} regulation of ATPase activity, however; the maximal level of ATPase activation was slightly different for various FHC mutants with the highest level observed for R58Q-reconstituted CMF. As presented in **Table 3**, Ca^{2+} sensitivity of myofibrillar ATPase activity was significantly increased for N47K mutant, slightly increased for E22K and R58Q, slightly decreased for F18L whereas no change was monitored for A13T mutant. It is interesting to note that three of the mutants (N47K, E22K and R58Q) that increased the Ca^{2+} sensitivity of ATPase were seen to either decrease the affinity for Ca^{2+} or to inactivate the Ca^{2+} binding site of the human cardiac RLC (Szczesna-Cordary et al., 2004a; Szczesna et al., 2001).

Myofibrils from mouse ventricular, septal and papillary muscles of NTg, Tg-WT, Tg-E22K, Tg-R58Q and Tg-N47K mice were examined for their Ca^{2+} sensitivity of ATPase activity(Abraham et al., 2009; Szczesna-Cordary et al., 2005). Tg-WT and NTg myofibrils showed similar pCa_{50} when compared among themselves. This established that the Ca^{2+} sensitivity was not RLC-isoform (human *versus* mouse)-dependent. A statistically significant increase in the Ca^{2+} sensitivity of myofibrillar ATPase activity was observed between NTg or Tg-WT mice and Tg-E22K mice ($\Delta pCa_{50} \cong 0.14$) (Szczesna-Cordary et al., 2004a). Studies on myofibrils from Tg-N47K and Tg-R58Q showed a decrease in the cooperativity of the actin–myosin interaction with a much more dramatic effect exhibited by the R58Q mutation. Though these results reflect what was seen with porcine CMF reconstituted with FHC mutants, the effect seemed to be more pronounced in Tg mice. Recent studies also showed that the maximal ATPase activity in myofibrils from Tg-D166V mice were significantly lower when compared to WT. However, it is interesting to note that following phosphorylation, the low levels of ATPase activity observed in Tg-D166V was recovered to the level of Tg-WT (Muthu et al., 2011). The latter study brought to light the beneficial role that RLC phosphorylation may have on cardiac function. More details on the role of Ca^{2+} binding and phosphorylation of the regulatory light chain on the cross bridge cycle are discussed later in this review.

4.2 Studies on cardiac muscle fibers

To test the functional consequence of FHC mutations at higher levels of organization, cardiac papillary muscle fibers from transgenic mice or RLC-depleted and mutant reconstituted porcine cardiac papillary muscle fibers were used in steady-state force and ATPase measurements.

i. Porcine cardiac papillary muscle fibers reconstituted with mutant RLC: Endogenous RLC was depleted from porcine cardiac muscle fiber preparations using CDTA and Triton (Szczesna-Cordary et al., 2004a). Depletion of endogenous RLC resulted in partial extraction of TnC (similar to that seen in porcine CMF). Therefore, TnC was added back along with the mutant RLC during reconstitution. It was observed that depletion of RLC, which was accompanied by a partial extraction of TnC, resulted in a decrease in the maximal level of force development from 100% to ~46%. Reconstitution of RLC-depleted fibers with TnC and RLC-WT restored the maximal level of force to ~84% (Szczesna-Cordary et al., 2004a). FHC mutants (A13T, E22K, N47K and R58Q mutants) were then tested for steady-state force development and the regulation of Ca^{2+} sensitivity of force. The lowest level of recovered force was observed for the E22K mutant (66%) whereas N47K- and R58Q-reconstituted fibers demonstrated 74% and 78%, respectively. Also, The E22K mutation was shown to cause a slight increase while the two Ca^{2+} binding site mutants, N47K and R58Q, showed a significantly large increase in the Ca^{2+} sensitivity of force development (Szczesna-Cordary et al., 2004a). Interestingly, in studies performed on skinned rabbit psoas muscle fibers reconstituted with the E22K mutation, it was observed that the tension at pCa 6.0 and the pCa_{50} value were significantly increased compared to WT-reconstituted psoas fibers (Roopnarine, 2003).

These results were in accord with the previous studies by Levine et. al on human biopsy samples from patients carrying the E22K mutation. A leftward shift in the tension-pCa curve was observed signifying a mutation mediated increase in the Ca^{2+} sensitivity of force development (Levine et al., 1998). Levine's group also studied the structure of the thick filaments carrying the E22K mutation compared to normal human fibers isolated from slow skeletal muscle. The authors speculated that because the E22K mutation occurs due to the substitution of a positively charged residue for a residue that is acidic, an ordered state of myosin cross-bridges was expected in both the mutant as well as normal fibers. However, they observed a disordered state of the filaments from the mutant biopsy while the wild type filaments from the normal human sample showed an ordered relaxed state (Levine et al., 1998).

ii. Transgenic cardiac papillary muscle fibers: To avoid difficulties related to the extraction/replacement of the RLC in porcine muscle preparations, cardiac papillary muscle fibers from transgenic mice expressing RLC mutations were used. The Ca^{2+} sensitivity of force development was first examined in transgenic mice carrying the E22K mutation of RLC and the results compared to WT control mice (Szczesna-Cordary et al., 2005). The mutation was seen to increase the Ca^{2+} sensitivity of force development compared to WT. In addition, a slight gene-dose effect in the force development was observed and the glycerinated skinned muscle fibers from TgE22K L4 expressing 87% transgene demonstrated slightly higher Ca^{2+} sensitivity of force than in Tg-E22K L2 expressing 67% mutant protein (pCa_{50}=5.65 vs. 5.62) (Szczesna-Cordary et al., 2005). The authors concluded that the E22K-mediated structural perturbations in the RLC and altered Ca^{2+}-binding-properties were most likely responsible for the abnormal function of the mutated myocardium and initiation of hypertrophic response and FHC.

Similar force measurement studies in papillary muscle fibers from Tg-D166V mice revealed that the presence of the D166V mutation, associated with malignant clinical outcomes, caused a decrease in maximal force as well as a significant leftward shift in myofilament Ca^{2+} sensitivity compared to Tg-WT (Muthu et al., 2011). This report was also the first to demonstrate the physiological effects of RLC phosphorylation in cardiomyopathic transgenic mouse hearts. As expected, a small leftward shift in the force–pCa dependence was observed for Tg-WT papillary muscle fibers (**Fig.9**). In contrast, MLCK-treatment of Tg-D166V fibers resulted in a large decrease in myofilament Ca^{2+} sensitivity (**Fig.9**). Therefore, phosphorylation of D166V- diseased muscle reversed the increased Ca^{2+} sensitivity of force and brought it back to the level observed for Tg-WT.

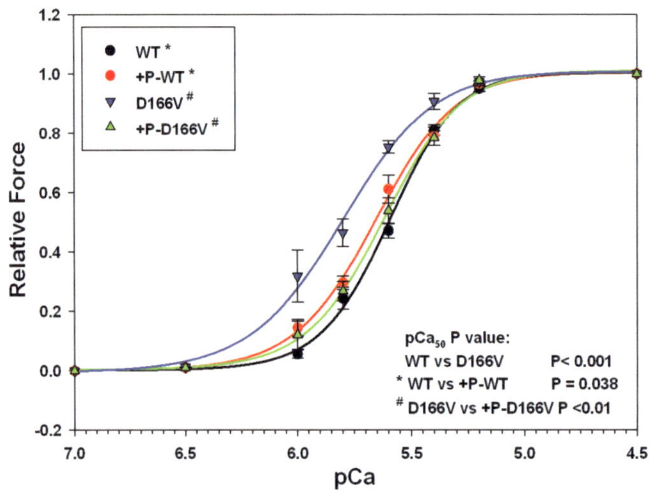

Fig. 9. Effect of RLC phosphorylation on the force–pCa relationship in skinned muscle fibers from Tg-WT mice and Tg-D166V (Muthu et al., 2011).

In addition to calcium sensitivity, the authors determined the effect of RLC phosphorylation on maximal steady-state force (Muthu et al., 2011). In contrast to Tg-WT, which displayed a phosphorylation-induced increase in force, the maximal tension in Tg-D166V papillary muscle fibers decreased upon phosphorylation. The authors concluded that phosphorylation of myosin RLC could work as a regulator of the acto–myosin interaction in both normal and cardiomyopathic hearts. A phosphorylation induced tuning of cardiac function in the diseased heart was seen to be different from the healthy heart and was anticipated to vary depending on the type and the level of cardiac insult.

Simultaneous ATPase/force-pCa relationships: Studies were designed to perform simultaneous force and ATPase measurements in freshly isolated (not glycerinated) skinned papillary muscle fibers from transgenic mice (Kerrick et al., 2009; Wang et al., 2006). ATPase activity was measured by the NADH fluorescence method (Guth & Wojciechowski, 1986). In this method, the regeneration of ATP from ADP and PEP (phospho-enol-pyruvate) by the enzyme PK (pyruvate kinase) is coupled to the oxidation of NADH (fluorescent) to NAD (non-fluorescent) by LDH (Griffiths et al., 1980; Takashi & Putnam, 1979). The decrease in NADH concentration is detected by a decrease in the fluorescence signal at 450 nm. The slope of the linear decrease in NADH concentration is used to calculate ATPase activity. In these measurements, force was recorded simultaneously with ATPase. The concentration of Ca^{2+} during ATPase/force measurements was measured with Calcium Green-2 fluorescence and the data fit to the Hill equation yielding the pCa_{50} and Hill coefficient n_H values (Kerrick et al., 2009; Wang et al., 2006).

Skinned muscle fibers from Tg-E22K mice showed a significant (20%) decrease in maximum ATPase and force compared to Tg-WT controls (Szczesna-Cordary et al., 2007). However, contrary to previously reported studies (Szczesna-Cordary et al., 2005) in glycerinated skinned muscle fibers, no significant difference in the pCa_{50} of force/ATPase-pCa relationships was observed between Tg-E22K and Tg-WT mice. Similar studies on skinned muscle fibers from Tg-D166V and Tg-R58Q mice showed that compared to Tg-WT, the mutations associated with a malignant disease phenotype (R58Q and D166V) caused large increases in the Ca^{2+} sensitivity of ATPase and force while those of benign phenotype (N47K) showed no changes in the force/ATPase-pCa dependence (Kerrick et al., 2009; Wang et al., 2006). Simultaneous ATPase/force-pCa measurements using freshly skinned papillary muscle fibers from Tg-D166V mice demonstrated a large increase in the Ca^{2+} sensitivity of force and ATPase compared to control NTg and Tg-WT mice (Kerrick et al., 2009). In addition, the maximal ATPase and force per cross-section of muscle fiber were largely decreased in the mutant Tg-D166V fibers compared to controls. The authors proceeded to calculate the rate of dissociation of the myosin heads from actin (rate of cross-bridge dissociation, "g") and showed a mutation-dependent dramatic decrease in g at all levels of force activation (Kerrick et al., 2009). Additionally, the energy cost per cross-bridge (fiber ATPase/force) was slightly higher in Tg-D166V fibers compared to controls although the difference between Tg-D166V and Tg-WT fibers was not statistically significant (Kerrick et al., 2009). The authors speculated that a slower relaxation rate of cycling myosin cross-bridges most likely triggered a series of pathological responses resulting in an abnormal regulation of cardiac muscle contraction in Tg-D166V mice.

Studies in intact papillary muscle fibers to monitor the rates and amplitudes of [Ca^{2+}] and force transients: In parallel to skinned fiber studies, the measurements of force and calcium transients were performed in electrically stimulated intact papillary muscle fibers (Kerrick et al., 2009; Wang et al., 2006). These experiments directly addressed potential abnormalities of the mutated myocardium of diastolic and systolic function observed in the FHC-mutated myocardium. Force and Ca^{2+} transients were seen to be significantly shortened in Tg-E22K intact fibers compared to Tg-WT (Szczesna-Cordary et al., 2007). The authors hypothesized that by changing the properties of the RLC Ca^{2+}-Mg^{2+} binding site, the E22K mutation could be affecting the function of RLC as a delayed Ca^{2+} buffer. Consequently, a faster Ca^{2+} reuptake by the sarcoplasmic reticulum proteins and the shorter duration of [Ca^{2+}] and force transients could be expected, both indicative of enhanced muscle relaxation. In line with this explanation, the R58Q mutation, which was seen to inactivate the RLC calcium binding site for Ca^{2+} binding, should induce an opposite effect to E22K in intact papillary muscle fibers. This was in fact observed and significantly prolonged force and [Ca^{2+}] transients were monitored in Tg-R58Q papillary muscles compared to Tg-WT (Wang et al., 2006). In parallel, intact fiber studies on Tg-N47K mutation showed no change in force transients with small changes in [Ca^{2+}] transients (Wang et al., 2006).

In the study on the D166V mutation, the authors investigated whether the slower kinetics of force generating myosin cross-bridges, as determined in Tg-D166V skinned papillary muscle fibers (above), resulted in slower relaxation measured in intact papillary muscles from Tg-D166V mice (Kerrick et al., 2009). It was observed that the rates of force relaxation in Tg-D166V muscles were significantly slower than the rates measured in Tg-WT or NTg papillary muscle fibers. However, the prolonged force transients in Tg-D166V muscle fibers were not paralleled by delayed calcium transients and no differences were observed between [Ca^{2+}] transients of Tg-D166V *versus* Tg-WT or NTg intact muscle fibers (Kerrick et al., 2009). Results of this study suggested several potential D166V-mediated factors that could contribute to FHC when placed *in vivo*. First, a large increase in Ca^{2+} sensitivity could contribute to decreased ventricular filling at high heart rates when the tail end of the first Ca^{2+} transient begins to fuse with the second. Secondly, the slow force relaxation rate of the fibers could also start to fuse with the next contraction when heart rates are high also contributing to diastolic dysfunction. If severe enough these two factors could affect diastolic filling of the heart sufficiently to result in systolic dysfunction, i.e. decrease in stroke volume. This ultimately would cause the heart to compensate by increasing wall thickness (hypertrophy). Finally, the prediction of decreased twitch force caused by a decrease in the time constant for the rate of rise of force would also result in systolic dysfunction that could only be compensated for by increases in heart rates.

Overall, studies in skinned and intact muscle fibers from FHC transgenic animals revealed a correlation between the mutant-mediated course of the disease in humans and the extent of physiological changes observed in the studies with muscle fibers. Prolonged [Ca^{2+}] and force transients in intact Tg-R58Q and Tg-D166V papillary muscles as well as increased Ca^{2+} sensitivity of ATPase/force observed in skinned fibers correlated with a poor prognosis in R58Q and D166V mutated patients whose phenotype included SCD. Likewise, the slightly prolonged [Ca^{2+}] transient with no alterations in force transient, and no change in Ca^{2+} sensitivity of ATPase/force observed in Tg-N47K mice, correlated with the phenotype of hypertrophic cardiomyopathy described for N47K patients, including lack of SCD.

5. Studies with single molecules

5.1 *In vitro* motility assays

In vitro motility assays were utilized to examine the effects of FHC RLC mutations on the biochemical and mechanical properties of myosin isolated from the hearts of transgenic mice or reconstituted with the recombinant human cardiac WT or FHC mutant. In the study by Greenberg et al., myosin was purified from Tg-N47K and Tg-R58Q mouse hearts and used in *in vitro* motility assays with Tg-WT myosin as a control (Greenberg et al., 2009). Unregulated motility assays were used to determine whether the mutations caused any changes in the duty cycle and/or actin filament sliding velocity. The principle behind this assay was that the actin filament moves at its maximal velocity when incubated with enough myosin to ensure that at least one myosin head is interacting with the actin filament at all times. Therefore, the amount of myosin required to achieve maximal velocity would give a qualitative measurement of the duty cycle. The authors observed a significant increase in velocity caused by the R58Q mutation while no major change in actin sliding velocity was observed for Tg-N47K myosin compared to Tg-WT (Greenberg et al., 2009).

Additionally, the isometric force of the mutant myosins was studied using a frictional loading assay (Greenberg et al., 2009). A low affinity actin binding protein, α-actinin, was introduced in the assay and the concentration of α-actinin needed to stop the filament motility was used as a measurement of myosin isometric force. Tg-N47K myosin showed a dramatic reduction in isometric force while a less pronounced decrease in force was seen for Tg-R58Q compared to Tg-WT myosins. The authors also determined the effect of RLC mutation on the velocity-pCa dependence using actin complexed with the regulatory proteins, troponin and tropomyosin (Greenberg et al., 2009). While Tg-R58Q myosin showed a significant leftward shift in the calcium sensitivity of velocity, Tg-N47K and Tg-

WT myosins showed no difference in the velocity-pCa curve. This result was consistent with the earlier (Wang et al., 2006) and more recent (Mettikolla et al., 2011) fiber studies using papillary muscles from these mice, where a significant increase in the Ca^{2+} sensitivity of force was observed for Tg-R58Q mice. Though both Tg-R58Q and Tg-N47K myosins displayed a reduction in isometric force, the authors concluded that the more extreme phenotype for R58Q could stem from an increase in myosin ATPase activity (discussed above in "Actin activated myosin ATPase assays") (Greenberg et al., 2009). On the other hand, study results with myosin isolated from transgenic E22K mice showed no effect of the mutation on actin sliding velocity or the velocity-pCa dependence (Szczesna-Cordary et al., 2007).

The effect of R58Q and N47K mutations was further tested using porcine myosin depleted of endogenous RLC and reconstituted with the mutant (R58Q or N47K) RLC proteins (Greenberg et al., 2010). The authors examined the effects of these mutations on the mechanical properties of myosin under both unloaded and loaded conditions. They found that, whereas the mutant myosins were indistinguishable from the controls (WT or native myosin) under unloaded conditions, both R58Q- and N47K-exchanged myosins showed reductions in force and power output compared with WT or native myosin. They also showed that the changes in loaded kinetics resulted from mutation-induced loss of myosin strain sensitivity of ADP affinity (Greenberg et al., 2010). The authors concluded that the R58Q and N47K mutations alter the mechanical properties of the myosin neck region, leading to altered load dependent kinetics that may explain the observed mutant-induced FHC phenotypes (Greenberg et al., 2010).

5.2 Single molecule detection (SMD)

The advances in single molecule detection (SMD) by fluorescence techniques were employed to study some of the earlier discussed FHC-linked RLC mutations. The advantage of SMD includes studying the motion of a small population of myosin cross bridges while working in their native environment of the sarcomere. Another advantage of this approach is the ability to unambiguously determine the behavior (kinetics, orientation, etc.) of the normal *versus* mutated muscle by observing a few molecules (myosin cross-bridges). Since humans are heterozygous for FHC mutations, the distribution of the healthy and diseased molecules is random and any collection containing more than a few molecules carries a high probability of containing a mixture of healthy and diseased moieties. It is therefore essential to use a technique such as SMD which is capable of monitoring properties of single molecules without averaging over ensembles of molecules with different properties.

The E22K substitution was the first FHC-associated mutation in RLC studied by SMD (Dumka et al., 2006). Mechanical events were measured by monitoring the anisotropy of actin labeled with rhodamine phalloidin. The measurements were done on a small population of cross bridges in contracting Tg-WT and Tg-E22K cardiac myofibrils. The results showed that the mutation did not significantly affect the time of cross-bridge dissociation and had no major effect on the mechanical performance of the cross bridges. Another mutation that was studied using SMD was the D166V mutation associated with a malignant FHC phenotype (Borejdo et al., 2010; Mettikolla et al., 2009; Muthu et al., 2010). In one experiment, myofibrils from Tg-D166V mice were labeled with Alexa 488-phalloidin and the measurements of the fluorescence lifetime (average rate of decay of a fluorescent species from its excited state) of the actin attached fluorophores were performed. No differences between lifetimes of Tg-WT and Tg-D166V muscle were observed (Mettikolla et al., 2009).

In addition to fluorescence lifetime, a meaningful indicator of the state of muscle that can be studied with SMD is the cross-bridge duty cycle (Mettikolla et al., 2009; Muthu et al., 2010). It was assumed that a cross-bridge is in its strongly attached to actin state for a period of time t_s, while it remains in a dissociated or a weakly attached state for a period of time, t_d. The ratio $\Psi=t_s/(t_d + t_s)$, was defined as the duty cycle. To measure Ψ, one can follow the changes in the environment of a cross-bridge while it undergoes a cycle of association and dissociation from actin. In the study by Muthu et al. the authors derived the myosin cross-bridge kinetic rates by tracking the orientation of a fluorescently labeled single actin molecule (Muthu et al., 2010). Orientation (measured by polarized fluorescence) oscillated between two states, corresponding to the actin-bound (t_s) and actin-free (t_d) states of the myosin cross-bridge. The rate of cross-bridge attachment during isometric contraction decreased from 3 s^{-1} in myofibrils from Tg-WT to 1.4 s^{-1} in myofibrils from Tg-D166V. The rate of detachment decreased from 1.3 s^{-1} (Tg-WT) to 1.2 s^{-1} (Tg-D166V). In addition, the average value of the duty cycle in isometrically contracting myofibrils from Tg-WT and Tg-D166V mice was 30% and 50%, respectively (Muthu et al., 2010). The authors hypothesized that the slower kinetics of Tg-D166V myosin cross-bridges could be the result of a mutation-mediated decrease in endogenous phosphorylation of myosin RLC, as was observed in the hearts of Tg-D166V mice (Kerrick et al., 2009). Indeed, the authors showed that the level of RLC phosphorylation was largely decreased in Tg-D166V myofibrils compared to Tg-WT (Muthu et al., 2010). They concluded that the D166V-induced change in the cross-bridge kinetics could further lead to abnormalities in diastolic and/or systolic function that in the long term would result in a compensatory hypertrophy and sudden cardiac death, as observed in patients harboring the D166V mutation in RLC.

The SMD technique was further refined in the study by Borejdo et al. (Borejdo et al., 2010). The authors analyzed the probability distribution of polarized intensity fluctuations and measured fluctuations by recording the parallel and perpendicular components of fluorescent light emitted by an actin-bound fluorophore (Borejdo et al., 2010). The histograms of fluctuations of fluorescent actin molecules in Tg-WT hearts in rigor were represented by perfect Gaussian curves. In contrast, histograms of contracting heart muscle were peaked and asymmetric, suggesting that contraction in the heart driven by the interaction of myosin cross-bridges with actin occurred in at least two steps (Borejdo et al., 2010). Importantly, there were statistically significant differences between the histograms of contracting FHC-linked R58Q and D166V cardiac muscle preparations *versus* corresponding contracting WT hearts. On the basis of these results, the authors suggested a simple new method of distinguishing between healthy and FHC R58Q and D166V hearts by analyzing the probability distribution of polarized fluorescence intensity fluctuations of sparsely labeled actin molecules (Borejdo et al., 2010).

Further studies using SMD were performed on cardiac myofibrils from Tg-R58Q mice (Mettikolla et al., 2011). The results showed that the R58Q mutation resulted in a decrease in the rate of cross-bridge binding to actin, dissociation from actin and a decreased rate at which the cross-bridge undergoes the power stroke (Mettikolla et al., 2011). The authors hypothesized that slower R58Q cross-bridge kinetics were most likely responsible for the lower force measured in Tg-R58Q skinned muscle fibers. The combined data on the R58Q mutation led the authors to conclude that the R58Q hearts may be subject to inefficient energy utilization and compromised heart performance.

6. Concluding remarks and future directions

With the advent of molecular biology and the ability to clone, express and purify myosin RLC and the FHC-linked mutations, it has been possible to begin to reconstruct muscle with various RLC mutants to learn about their function in increasingly more complex systems. The advance of transgenesis has catapulted the researchers to a new era of research where the function of FHC-linked RLC mutations could be studied *in vivo* in transgenic mouse hearts. Using various innovative approaches applied at the single molecule, skinned fiber, and intact muscle levels, it has been possible to begin to understand the effect of FHC mutations on cardiac function. The presented results indicate that RLC phosphorylation and Ca^{2+} binding to the RLC EF-hand calcium binding site may play important roles not only in the physiological performance of the heart, but also in muscle contraction of the diseased heart. The MLCK-dependent phosphorylation of RLC was shown to be critical to maintain normal cardiac function and was suggested to be especially important in the adaptive responses of the heart to pathophysiological injury. Unraveling the molecular basis of RLC-mediated cardiac dysfunction can ultimately open new possibilities for an effective treatment(s) and efforts should be directed towards developing phosphorylation-mediated rescue strategies. Collectively, the results presented in this review provided insight into the mechanisms underlying the development of FHC disease caused by the mutations in the cardiac RLC. Future investigations should be focused on the preventive treatments to alleviate or reverse the detrimental effects of all identified RLC mutations.

7. Acknowledgments

This work was supported by grants from the National Institutes of Health (HL071778 and HL090786) to Danuta Szczesna-Cordary and the American Heart Association (10POST3420009) to Priya Muthu.

8. References

Abraham, T.P.; Jones, M.; Kazmierczak, K.; Liang, H.-Y.; Pinheiro, A.C.; Wagg, C.S.; Lopaschuk, G.D. & Szczesna-Cordary, D. (2009). Diastolic dysfunction in familial hypertrophic cardiomyopathy transgenic model mice. *Cardiovasc Res*. 82:84-92.

Alcalai, R.; Seidman, J.G. & Seidman, C.E. (2008). Genetic basis of hypertrophic cardiomyopathy: from bench to the clinics. *J Cardiovasc Electrophysiol*. 19:104-10.

Andersen, P.S.; Havndrup, O.; Bundgaard, H.; Moolman-Smook, J.C.; Larsen, L.A.; Mogensen, J.; Brink, P.A.; Borglum, A.D.; Corfield, V.A.; Kjeldsen, K.; Vuust, J. & Christiansen, M. (2001). Myosin light chain mutations in familial hypertrophic cardiomyopathy: phenotypic presentation and frequency in Danish and South African populations. *J Med Genet*. 38:E43.

Binder, W.D.; Fifer, M.A.; King, M.E. & Stone, J.R. (2005). Case records of the Massachusetts General Hospital. Case 26-2005. A 48-year-old man with sudden loss of consciousness while jogging. *N Engl J Med*. 353:824-32.

Borejdo, J.; Szczesna-Cordary, D.; Muthu, P. & Calander, N. (2010). Familial hypertrophic cardiomyopathy can be characterized by a specific pattern of orientation fluctuations of actin molecules. *Biochemistry*. 49:5269-77.

Chen, Y.H. & Yang, J.T. (1971). A new approach to the calculation of secondary structures of globular proteins by optical rotatory dispersion and circular dichroism. *Biochem Biophys Res Commun*. 44:1285-91.

Colson, B.A.; Locher, M.R.; Bekyarova, T.; Patel, J.R.; Fitzsimons, D.P.; Irving, T.C. & Moss, R.L. (2010). Differential roles of regulatory light chain and myosin binding protein-C phosphorylations in the modulation of cardiac force development. *J Physiol*. 588:981-93.

Ding, P.; Huang, J.; Battiprolu, P.K.; Hill, J.A.; Kamm, K.E. & Stull, J.T. (2010). Cardiac myosin light chain kinase is necessary for myosin regulatory light chain phosphorylation and cardiac performance in vivo. *J Biol Chem*. 285:40819-29.

Dumka, D.; Talent, J.; Akopova, I.; Guzman, G.; Szczesna-Cordary, D. & Borejdo, J. (2006). E22K mutation of RLC that causes familial hypertrophic cardiomyopathy in heterozygous mouse myocardium: effect on cross-bridge kinetics. *Am J Physiol Heart Circ Physiol*. 291:H2098-2106.

Flavigny, J.; Richard, P.; Isnard, R.; Carrier, L.; Charron, P.; Bonne, G.; Forissier, J.F.; Desnos, M.; Dubourg, O.; Komajda, M.; Schwartz, K. & Hainque, B. (1998). Identification of two novel mutations in the ventricular regulatory myosin light chain gene (MYL2) associated with familial and classical forms of hypertrophic cardiomyopathy. *J Mol Med*. 76:208-14.

Geeves, M.A. & Holmes, K.C. (2005). The molecular mechanism of muscle contraction. *Adv Protein Chem*. 71:161-93.

Greenberg, M.J.; Kazmierczak, K.; Szczesna-Cordary, D. & Moore, J.R. (2010). Cardiomyopathy-linked myosin regulatory light chain mutations disrupt myosin strain-dependent biochemistry. *Proc Natl Acad Sci U S A*. 107:17403-8.

Greenberg, M.J.; Watt, J.D.; Jones, M.; Kazmierczak, K.; Szczesna-Cordary, D. & Moore, J.R. (2009). Regulatory light chain mutations associated with cardiomyopathy affect myosin mechanics and kinetics. *J Mol Cell Cardiol*. 46:108-115.

Griffiths, P.J.; Guth, K.; Kuhn, H.J. & Ruegg, J.C. (1980). ATPase activity in rapidly activated skinned muscle fibres. *Pflugers Arch*. 387:167-73.

Guth, K. & Wojciechowski, R. (1986). Perfusion cuvette for the simultaneous measurement of mechanical, optical and energetic parameters of skinned muscle fibres. *Pflugers Arch*. 407:552-7.

Hartshorne, D.J. & Mrwa, U. (1982). Regulation of smooth muscle actomyosin. *Blood Vessels*. 19:1-18.

Houdusse, A. & Cohen, C. (1996). Structure of the regulatory domain of scallop myosin at 2 A resolution: implications for regulation. *Structure*. 4:21-32.

Hougs, L.; Havndrup, O.; Bundgaard, H.; Kober, L.; Vuust, J.; Larsen, L.A.; Christiansen, M. & Andersen, P.S. (2005). One third of Danish hypertrophic cardiomyopathy patients have mutations in MYH7 rod region. *Eur J Hum Genet*. . 13:161-165.

Howard, J. & Spudich, J.A. (1996). Is the lever arm of myosin a molecular elastic element? *Proc Natl Acad Sci U S A*. 93:4462-4.

Huang, W.; Muthu, P.; Kazmierczak, K. & Szczesna-Cordary, D. (2011). FHC-Linked Myosin Regulatory Light Chain Mutations A13T and K104E Do Not Generate Major Structural Changes Sufficient to Affect Binding of Myosin to Actin. *Biophysical journal*. 100:110a-111a.

Kabaeva, Z.T.; Perrot, A.; Wolter, B.; Dietz, R.; Cardim, N.; Correia, J.M.; Schulte, H.D.; Aldashev, A.A.; Mirrakhimov, M.M. & Osterziel, K.J. (2002). Systematic analysis of the regulatory and essential myosin light chain genes: genetic variants and mutations in hypertrophic cardiomyopathy. *Eur J Hum Genet.* 10:741-8.

Kamm, K.E. & Stull, J.T. (2011). Signaling to Myosin Regulatory Light Chain in Sarcomeres. *Journal of Biological Chemistry.* 286:9941-9947.

Kerrick, W.G.L.; Kazmierczak, K.; Xu, Y.; Wang, Y. & Szczesna-Cordary, D. (2009). Malignant familial hypertrophic cardiomyopathy D166V mutation in the ventricular myosin regulatory light chain causes profound effects in skinned and intact papillary muscle fibers from transgenic mice. *FASEB J.* 23:855-865.

Levine, R.J.; Yang, Z.; Epstein, N.D.; Fananapazir, L.; Stull, J.T. & Sweeney, H.L. (1998). Structural and functional responses of mammalian thick filaments to alterations in myosin regulatory light chains. *J Struct Biol.* 122:149-61.

Lowey, S.; Waller, G.S. & Trybus, K.M. (1993). Skeletal muscle myosin light chains are essential for physiological speeds of shortening. *Nature.* 365:454-6.

Mettikolla, P.; Calander, N.; Luchowski, R.; Gryczynski, I.; Gryczynski, Z.; Zhao, J.; Szczesna-Cordary, D. & Borejdo, J. (2011). Cross-bridge kinetics in myofibrils containing familial hypertrophic cardiomyopathy R58Q mutation in the regulatory light chain of myosin. *J Theor Biol.* 284:71-81.

Mettikolla, P.; Luchowski, R.; Gryczynski, I.; Gryczynski, Z.; Szczesna-Cordary, D. & Borejdo, J. (2009). Fluorescence Lifetime of Actin in the Familial Hypertrophic Cardiomyopathy Transgenic Heart. *Biochemistry.* 48:1264-1271.

Morano, I. (1999). Tuning the human heart molecular motors by myosin light chains. *J Mol Med.* 77:544-55.

Morner, S.; Richard, P.; Kazzam, E.; Hellman, U.; Hainque, B.; Schwartz, K. & Waldenstrom, A. (2003). Identification of the genotypes causing hypertrophic cardiomyopathy in northern Sweden. *J Mol Cell Card.* 35:841-849.

Muthu, P.; Kazmierczak, K.; Jones, M. & Szczesna-Cordary, D. (2011). The effect of myosin RLC phosphorylation in normal and cardiomyopathic mouse hearts. *J Cell Mol Med.*

Muthu, P.; Mettikolla, P.; Calander, N.; Luchowski, R.; Gryczynski, I.; Gryczynski, Z.; Szczesna-Cordary, D. & Borejdo, J. (2010). Single molecule kinetics in the familial hypertrophic cardiomyopathy D166V mutant mouse heart. *J Mol Cell Cardiol.* 48:989-998.

Pant, K.; Watt, J.; Greenberg, M.; Jones, M.; Szczesna-Cordary, D. & Moore, J.R. (2009). Removal of the cardiac myosin regulatory light chain increases isometric force production. *FASEB J.* 23:3571-3580.

Poetter, K.; Jiang, H.; Hassanzadeh, S.; Master, S.R.; Chang, A.; Dalakas, M.C.; Rayment, I.; Sellers, J.R.; Fananapazir, L. & Epstein, N.D. (1996). Mutations in either the essential or regulatory light chains of myosin are associated with a rare myopathy in human heart and skeletal muscle. *Nat Genet.* 13:63-9.

Rayment, I.; Rypniewski, W.R.; Schmidt-Base, K.; Smith, R.; Tomchick, D.R.; Benning, M.M.; Winkelmann, D.A.; Wesenberg, G. & Holden, H.M. (1993). Three-dimensional structure of myosin subfragment-1: a molecular motor. *Science.* 261:50-8.

Richard, P.; Charron, P.; Carrier, L.; Ledeuil, C.; Cheav, T.; Pichereau, C.; Benaiche, A.; Isnard, R.; Dubourg, O.; Burban, M.; Gueffet, J.-P.; Millaire, A.; Desnos, M.; Schwartz, K.; Hainque, B.; Komajda, M. & for the EUROGENE Heart Failure Project (2003). Hypertrophic cardiomyopathy: Distribution of disease genes, spectrum of mutations, and implications for a molecular diagnosis strategy. *Circulation.* 107:2227-2232.

Richard, P.; Charron, P.; Carrier, L.; Ledeuil, C.; Cheav, T.; Pichereau, C.; Benaiche, A.; Isnard, R.; Dubourg, O.; Burban, M.; Gueffet, J.-P.; Millaire, A.; Desnos, M.; Schwartz, K.; Hainque, B.; Komajda, M. & for the EUROGENE Heart Failure Project (2004). Correction to: "Hypertrophic cardiomyopathy: distribution of disease genes, spectrum of mutations, and implications for a molecular diagnosis strategy". *Circulation*. 109:3258.

Robertson, S.P.; Johnson, J.D. & Potter, J.D. (1981). The time-course of Ca^{2+} exchange with calmodulin, troponin, parvalbumin, and myosin in response to transient increases in Ca2+. *Biophys J*. 34:559-69.

Roopnarine, O. (2003). Mechanical Defects of Muscle Fibers with Myosin Light Chain Mutants that Cause Cardiomyopathy. *Biophys. J*. 84:2440-2449.

Sanbe, A.; Nelson, D.; Gulick, J.; Setser, E.; Osinska, H.; Wang, X.; Hewett, T.E.; Klevitsky, R.; Hayes, E.; Warshaw, D.M. & Robbins, J. (2000). In vivo analysis of an essential myosin light chain mutation linked to familial hypertrophic cardiomyopathy. *Circ Res*. 87:296-302.

Small, J.V. & Sobieszek, A. (1977). Ca-regulation of mammalian smooth muscle actomyosin via a kinase-phosphatase-dependent phosphorylation and dephosphorylation of the 20 000-Mr light chain of myosin. *Eur J Biochem*. 76:521-30.

Sobieszek, A. (1977). Ca-linked phosphorylation of a light chain of vertebrate smooth-muscle myosin. *Eur J Biochem*. 73:477-83.

Szczesna-Cordary, D.; Guzman, G.; Ng, S.S. & Zhao, J. (2004a). Familial hypertrophic cardiomyopathy-linked alterations in Ca^{2+} binding of human cardiac myosin regulatory light chain affect cardiac muscle contraction. *J Biol Chem*. 279:3535-42.

Szczesna-Cordary, D.; Guzman, G.; Zhao, J.; Hernandez, O.; Wei, J. & Diaz-Perez, Z. (2005). The E22K mutation of myosin RLC that causes familial hypertrophic cardiomyopathy increases calcium sensitivity of force and ATPase in transgenic mice. *J Cell Sci*. 118:3675-83.

Szczesna-Cordary, D.; Jones, M. & Guzman, G. (2004b). Interaction of Myosin Regulatory Light Chain Mutants Implicated in Familial Hypertrophic Cardiomyopathy with IQ-Myosin Heavy Chain Peptides. *Biophys J*. 86:393a.

Szczesna-Cordary, D.; Jones, M.; Moore, J.R.; Watt, J.; Kerrick, W.G.L.; Xu, Y.; Wang, Y.; Wagg, C. & Lopaschuk, G.D. (2007). Myosin regulatory light chain E22K mutation results in decreased cardiac intracellular calcium and force transients. *FASEB J*. 21:3974-3985.

Szczesna, D. (2003). Regulatory light chains of striated muscle myosin. Structure, function and malfunction. *Curr Drug Targets Cardiovasc Haematol Disord*. 3:187-97.

Szczesna, D.; Ghosh, D.; Li, Q.; Gomes, A.V.; Guzman, G.; Arana, C.; Zhi, G.; Stull, J.T. & Potter, J.D. (2001). Familial hypertrophic cardiomyopathy mutations in the regulatory light chains of myosin affect their structure, Ca^{2+} binding, and phosphorylation. *J Biol Chem*. 276:7086-92.

Takashi, R. & Putnam, S. (1979). A fluorimetric method for continuously assaying ATPase: application to small specimens of glycerol-extracted muscle fibers. *Anal Biochem*. 92:375-82.

Wang, Y.; Xu, Y.; Kerrick, W.G.L.; Wang, Y.; Guzman, G.; Diaz-Perez, Z. & Szczesna-Cordary, D. (2006). Prolonged Ca^{2+} and force transients in myosin RLC transgenic mouse fibers expressing malignant and benign FHC mutations. *J Mol Biol*. 361:286-299.

18

Role of Genetic Factors in Dilated Cardiomyopathy

Cieslewicz Artur and Jablecka Anna
Karol Marcinkowski Medical University in Poznan, Department of Clinical Pharmacology
Poland

1. Introduction

Dilated cardiomyopathy (DCM) is a heart muscle disease characterized by cardiac chamber enlargement and impaired systolic (and almost always diastolic) function. It is usually associated with heart failure, arrhythmias and/or conduction system disease and thromboembolic disease but may also be asymptomatic. DCM is diagnosed in the presence of left ventricular enlargement and systolic dysfunction (left ventricular ejection fraction less than 50% or fractional shortening of less than 25-30%). It is considered one of the most common causes of heart failure, resulting in considerable morbidity and mortality. Patients with DCM suffer from heart failure, arrhythmia and are at risk of premature death. The prevalence of dilated cardiomyopathy is one case out of 2500 patients with an incidence of 7/100 000/year and it is 3 times more frequent in blacks and males than whites and females (Bender et al., 2011, Hershberger et al., 2007, Taylor et al., 2006).
DCM may appear sporadic in a single member of family and is called then idiopathic DCM (IDC). Dilated cardiomyopathy may be also inherited and is termed familial DCM (FDC), contributing for 20-48 % of DCM. According to Mestroni et al. (1999), the diagnosis of FDC is made in the presence of two or more affected individuals in a single family or in the presence of a first-degree relative of a dilated cardiomyopathy patient with well documented unexplained sudden death at < 35 years of age. The principle causes of FDC are genetic mutations affecting cardiac myocytes (Taylor et al., 2006). Knowledge about genes involved in development of dilated cardiomyopathy can be used to create genetic tests for assessing the risk of DCM.
As DCM is a multigenic disorder, there are many genes contributing to development of this disease. More than 30 genes, coding a variety of proteins such as nuclear envelope proteins, cardiac sarcomere units, ion channels, transcription factors, or dystrophin-associated cytoskeletal complex, were identified as causes of dilated cardiomyopathy (Hershberger et al., 2009a). Some of these genes (discussed in this chapter) are presented in Table 1. For additional information see Hershberger et al. (2010) and UpToDate® website.

2.Major genetic causes of DCM

2.1 Lamins A/C (LMNA)

Nuclear lamins (see Figure 1) are intermediate filament-type proteins that are major building blocks of the nuclear lamina - a meshwork underlying the inner nuclear membrane. They can also be localized in the nuclear interior. Nuclei assembled *in vitro* in the absence of lamins are fragile, indicating the role of lamins in stabilizing the cell nucleus. Lamins also take part in DNA replication, chromatin organization, spatial arrangement of nuclear pore complexes, nuclear growth and anchorage of nuclear envelope proteins (Stuurman et al., 1998). Patients carrying mutations in LMNA gene are known to be at risk of conduction disorders and arrhythmic events in addition to ventricular dilatation and heart failure (Haugaa et al., 2009).

Gene	Encoded protein	Function
Major genetic factors		
LMNA	lamins A/C	building blocks of nuclear lamina
TNNT2	cardiac troponin T (cTnT)	regulation of muscle contraction
β-MYH7	β-myosin heavy chain	conversion of chemical energy into mechanical force
Other genetic factors		
SCN5A	alpha subunit of type V voltage-gated sodium channel	control of the flow of sodium ions into cardiac muscle cells
TCAP	titin-cap (telethonin)	regulation of sarcomere assembly
HBEGF	heparin-binding epidermal growth factor	regulation of cell growth and differentiation
SRA1	steroid receptor RNA activator 1	stimulation of proliferation and apoptosis
IK	cytokine	down-regulation of expression of HLA class II antigens
TPM1	α-tropomyosin	regulation of actin-myosin interaction
PSEN 1/2	presenilin 1 / 2	multi-pass transmembrane proteins
Dnm1l	dynamin-1-like	establishing mitochondrial morphology
LDB3	LIM domain binding 3	interaction with α-actinin-2 and protein kinase C

Table 1. Genes associated with dilated cardiomyopathy

Many studies suggest that defects in LMNA gene, encoding lamins A/C, are one of the most significant genetic causes of dilated cardiomyopathy. According to Colombo et al. (2008), the LMNA gene is involved in up to 30-50% of patients with cardiac conduction disorders and DCM. Arbustini et al. (2002) were one of the first to reveal the role of LMNA mutations in developing dilated cardiomyopathy. The researchers investigated the prevalence of LMNA gene defects in familial and idiopathic DCM associated with atrioventricular block or increased serum creatine-phosphokinase (sCPK). 73 cases of DCM (15 with atrioventricular block) were analysed, revealing five LMNA mutations (K97E, E111X, R190W, E317K and 4 base pair insertion at 1713 cDNA) in five cases of familial autosomal dominant DCM with atrioventricular block (33%). The role of LMNA mutations was further confirmed by Hermida-Prieto et al. (2004) in the study on 67 consecutive patients with DCM (18 with FDC, 17 with possible FDC and 32 with idiopathic DCM). The researchers observed two disease-causing mutations in LMNA gene, a novel R349L substitution and R190W (the same as in Arbustini et al. study). Both mutations were associated with severe forms of familial DCM. Another discovery concerning lamins was brought by Kärkkäinen et al. (2006). The study was carried out on 66 DCM patients, who received heart transplant. DNA sequencing revealed 6 mutations in LMNA gene (A132P, S143P, R190W, T1085 deletion, G1493 deletion, and R541S) which explained DCM in 9% patients. Moreover, one of these mutations (S143P) explained 7 % of all cases in an unselected DCM population.

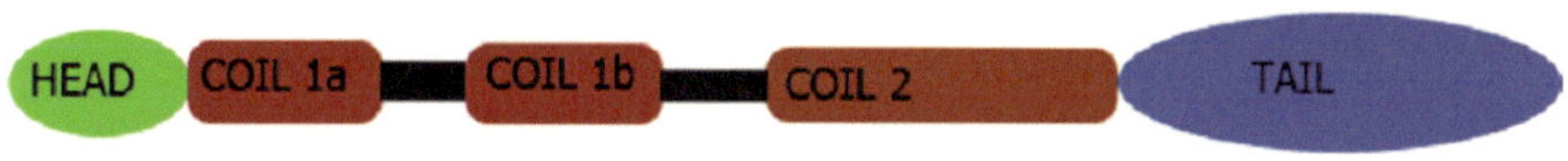

Fig. 1. Structure of human lamin.

In order to investigate mechanism responsible for electrophysiologic and myocardial phenotypes caused by dominant human LMNA mutations, an experiment was carried out on heterozygous *Lmna* +/- mice (Wolf et al., 2008). Cardiac function and electrophysiology were examined in heterozygous mice which underwent a targeted deletion of LMNA gene resulting in reduced level of lamin A/C protein in hearts. The researchers found out that despite normal structure and function in young *Lmna* +/- mice, older mice had altered atrioventricular nodal architecture, functional electrophysiological deficits and arrhythmias. Moreover, aged *Lmna* +/- mice, similar to humans with LMNA mutations, developed DCM, sometimes without overt conductions system disease. 50-week old *Lmna* +/- mice had enlarged ventricular chambers in systole ($p=0.01$) and diastole ($p=0.002$) corresponding to significantly decreased fractional shortening ($p=0.02$). Cardiac sections of these mice also showed more fibrosis than wildtype mice. Cell and sarcomere shortening were decreased in *Lmna* +/- myocytes compared to wildtype ($p<0.001$) with ventricular dilatation and depressed cardiac contractility consistent with DCM in aged *Lmna* +/- mice. These findings confirmed lamin A/C haploinsufficency as a possible mechanism leading to DCM.

Parks et al. (2008) were one of the first to carry out a research concerning lamins A/C mutation on a large group of patients. DNA from 324 patients with DCM (187 with FDC) was sequenced for nucleotide alterations in LMNA gene. 18 protein-altering variants (14 novel) were identified in 5.9% cases (7.5% of FDC and 3.6% of IDC). 11 alterations were missense mutations (which changed conserved amino acid), three were nonsense, another three were insertion/deletion and one was a splice site alteration. Conduction system disease and DCM were common among the carriers of these LMNA variants. These findings were further investigated by Cowan et al. (2010), who expressed in COS7 cells GFP-prelamin A constructs including 13 LMNA variants identified by Parks et al. (see Table 2). Confocal immunofluorescence microscopy was then used to characterize GFP-lamin A localization and nuclear morphology. Abnormal phenotypes were observed for 10 out of 13 analyzed variants, providing evidence which supported pathogenicity of these variants.

Recently, Botto et al. (2010) described additional novel LMNA mutation in FDC. Sequencing of the patient's LMNA coding exons revealed heterozygous missense mutation cytosine to thymine at nucleotide 565 in exon 3 which caused a substitution of arginine to hydrophobic tryptophan (R189W mutation) in a conserved residue located in the coil 1b of the alpha-helical rod domain. This mutation was located near the most prevalent lamin A/C mutation R190W, suggesting a "hot-spot" region at exon 3 and was not identified in a group of 50 healthy volunteers. Moreover, the mutation was identified in 3 relatives of patient, who will then benefit from regular clinical cardiac follow-up and early treatment.

LMNA variant	Mutation type	Pathogenicity of mutation (+/-)
R89L	substitution: Arg to Leu	+
R101P	substitution: Arg to Pro	+
R166P	substitution: Arg to Pro	+
R190Q	substitution: Arg to Gln	+
E203K	substitution: Glu to Lys	+
I210S	substitution: Ile to Ser	+
L215P	substitution: Leu to Pro	+
A318T	substitution: Ala to Thr	-
R388H	substitution: Arg to His	+
R399C	substitution: Arg to Cys	-
S437Hfsx1	substitution: Ser to His, frameshift, STOP codon (nonsense)	+
R471H	substitution: Arg to His	-
R654X	STOP codon (nonsense)	+

Table 2. LMNA variants inspected in patients with DCM (Cowan et al., 2010).

2.2 Cardiac troponin T (TNNT2)

Troponin T is the tropomyosin-binding protein in the troponin regulatory complex located on the thin filament of the contractile apparatus (see Figure 2). There are three isotype forms of troponin T: fast skeletal muscle, slow skeletal muscle and cardiac troponin T. These muscle-specific isoforms are expressed by different genes. Further diversity of troponin T comes from alternative splicing of RNA molecule (Katus et al., 1992).

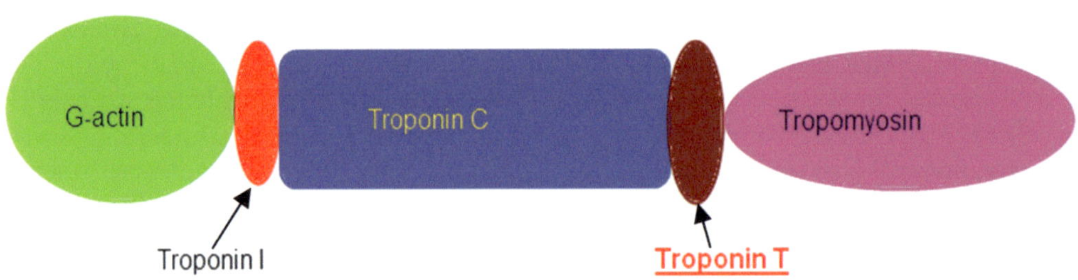

Fig. 2. Location of troponin T in the troponin regulatory complex.

Cardiac troponin T is encoded by TNNT2 gene, which alterations significantly contribute to dilated cardiomyopathy. Kamisago et al. (2000) were one of the first to show the role of TNNT2, identifying a deletion of AGA triplet resulting in deletion of lysine in residue 210 (K210 deletion) of troponin T protein chain in samples from two unrelated families suffering DCM. K210 mutation is one of the most frequent variants observed in patients suffering DCM. Otten et al. (2010) carried out a study, identifying 6 DCM patients carrying K210 deletion from 4 Dutch families. These patients showed severe form of DCM with early disease manifestation (mean age of DCM manifestation was 33 years). Moreover, heart transplantation was required in three patients at ages 12, 18 and 19 years.

The evidence from large cohort of patients was further provided by Mogensen et al. (2004). The researchers performed the study on 235 patients suffering DCM (102 with FDC). Mutation analysis of TNNT2 resulted in identification of three novel mutations (R131W, R205L and D270N) and one reported previously(K210 deletion) in 13 patients from 4 families. Three out of 13 patients received cardiac transplants, three died of heart failure, another three died suddenly and four remained stable on conventional heart failure therapy. All mutations segregated with the disease in each family and were absent in the control group and in the group of patients with hypertrophic cardiomyopathy (HCM). Identified mutations were considered disease-causing, because they co-segregated with disease in each family, were absent in control and HCM groups and were localized in conserved and functionally important regions of gene. Moreover, functional studies of mutated protein revealed altered troponin protein-protein interactions.

Additional data concerning the role of TNNT2 mutations in DCM was delivered by Hershberger et al. (2009b). The researchers carried out bidirectional sequencing of TNNT2 using DNA samples from 313 unrelated probands with DCM (183 with FDC and 130 with IDC). Six protein-altering mutations were identified in 9 probands (2.9% of all patients). None of these variants were present in control group (253 patients). Five variants were missense mutations altering highly conserved amino acids (four novel mutations: R134G, R151C, R159Q, R205W and one previously reported in HCM:E244D)and one was K210 deletion. All of these mutations were considered possibly or likely disease-causing based on the clinical, pedigree and molecular genetic data (see Table 3). Additional functional studies of these mutations, carried out in cardiac myocytes reconstituted with mutant troponin T proteins revealed decreased Ca^{2+} sensitivity of force development (a hallmark of DCM), supporting disease-causing potential of these genetic variants.

TNNT2 variant	Mutation type	Disease-causing
R134G	substitution: Arg to Gly	yes (segregated with disease in other affected family members)
R151C	substitution: Arg to Cys	yes (homozygous mutation associated with aggresive disease)
R159Q	substitution: Arg to Gln	yes (replacement of conserved amino acid)
R205W	substitution: Arg to Trp	yes (similar to disease-causing R205L mutation reported by Mogensen et al., 2004)
E244D	substitution: Glu to Asp	yes (reported as disease-causing in patient with HCM)
K210del	deletion of lysine	yes (reported as disease-causing in several cases)

Table 3. Disease-causing TNNT2 variants observed in patients with DCM (Hershberger et al., 2009b)

Mutations in TNNT2 may be also associated with more than one type of cardiomyopathy. For example, Menon et al. (2008) study conducted on a family with autosomal dominant heart disease variably expressed as restrictive cardiomyopathy (RCM), HCM and DCM revealed cosegregation of TNNT2 mutation with disease phenotype. Sequencing of TNNT2 identified a heterozygous missense mutation resulting in I79N substitution inherited by all 9 affected family members but none of the six unaffected relatives. Mutation carriers were diagnosed with RCM (2 patients), HCM (3 patients), DCM (2 patients), mixed cardiomyopathy (1 patient) and mild concentric left ventricular hypertrophy (1 patient).

An experiment on mice, carried out by Ahmad et al. (2008) revealed the role of cardiac troponin T quantity and function in development of heart and in dilated cardiomyopathy. The researchers created heterozygous TNNT2$^{+/-}$ mice (i.e. lacking one TNNT2 allele) and then crossbred them to obtain homozygous null TNNT2$^{-/-}$ embryos. Moreover, transgenic mice overexpressing wildtype (TG^{WT}) or mutant (TG$^{K210\Delta}$: K210 deletion) TNNT2 were also generated and used to create individuals lacking one allele of TNNT2 and carrying wildtype (TNNT2$^{+/-}$/ TG^{WT}) or mutant (TNNT2$^{+/-}$/ TG$^{K210\Delta}$) transgenes. The scientists found out that TNNT2$^{+/-}$ mice compared to wildtype had significantly reduced transcript but not protein. Moreover, TNNT2$^{+/-}$ mice had normal hearts. On the other hand TNNT2$^{+/-}$/ TG$^{K210\Delta}$ mice had severe DCM whileTG$^{K210\Delta}$ only mild DCM, suggesting the role of greater ratio of mutant to wildtype TNNT2 transcript in TNNT2$^{+/-}$/ TG$^{K210\Delta}$ mice compared to TG$^{K210\Delta}$ individuals. TNNT2$^{+/-}$/ TG$^{K210\Delta}$ also showed muscle Ca2+ desenization but no difference in maximum force generation. The TNNT2$^{-/-}$ embryos had normally looped hearts but thin ventricular walls, large pericardial effusions, noncontractile hearts and severely disorganized sarcomers.

2.3 β-myosin heavy chain (MYH7)

Myosin is a protein that converts chemical energy into mechanical force through hydrolysis of ATP. Within the cell, it is organized as a pair of heavy chains and two pairs of light chains. The myosin heavy chain is a highly asymmetric molecule with a predominantly globular head and a rod-like tail, which is formed of two α-helices and accounts for the formation of the thick filament backbone (see Figure 3). The globular head contains a light-chain-binding domain and a catalytic domain with actin and ATP-binding sites (Kabaeva 2002).

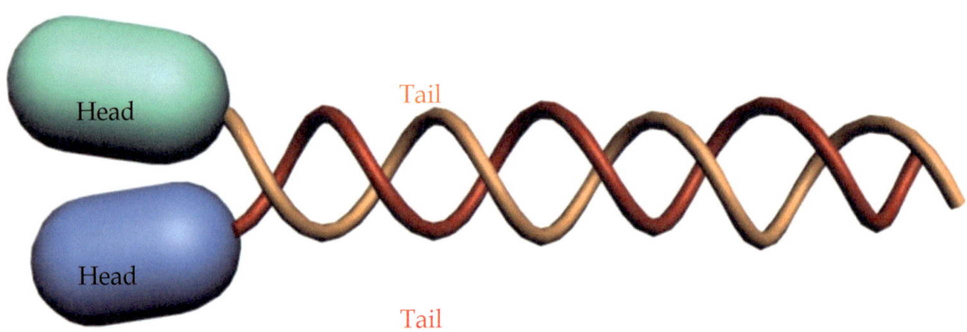

Fig. 3. A pair of myosin heavy chains.

Currently, more than 70 different mutations have been identified in MYH7 gene in association with DCM (Tanjore et al., 2010). Moreover, mutations in MYH7 have been reported in 4.2% cases of dilated cardiomyopathy (Hershberger et al., 2008). Clinical evaluations carried out in 21 kindreds with FDC delivered first data suggesting the role of MYH7 mutations in dilated cardiomyopathy (Kamisago et al., 2000). A genome-wide linkage study revealed genetic locus for mutations associated with DCM located at chromosome 14q11.2-13, encoding the gene for

cardiac β-myosin heavy chain. Disease-causing dominant mutations of MYH7 (S532P and F764L) were identified in 4 kindreds, resulting in early-onset ventricular dilatation (average age: 24 years) and diminished contractile function.
Two novel mutations were identified in the study conducted by Kärkkäinen et al. (2004), carried out on 52 DCM Finnish patients. Screening of MYH7 coding regions resulted in identification of R1053Q and R1500W mutations in two patients. The R1500W mutation was associated with typical DCM phenotype. On the other hand, patient with R1053Q variant had dilated left ventricle and impaired systolic function, but other family members carrying this mutation had septal hypertrophy, suggesting that this variant was primarily an HCM mutation which could also lead to DCM.
Additional MYH7 mutations were identified by Villard et al. (2005). The researchers screened all coding regions of MYH7 and TNNT2 gene in 96 independent patients (54 with FDC and 42 with IDC), identifying seven new mutations in MYH7 gene (see Table 4). Moreover, contrasting clinical features were observed between MYH7 and TNNT2 mutation carriers: mean age at diagnosis was late, penetrance was incomplete in adults and mean age at major cardiac event was higher in MYH7 mutation carriers compared to TNNT2.

MYH7 variant	Mutation type	Affected part of myosine heavy chain
I201T	substitution: Ile to Thr	head
T412N	substitution: Thr to Asn	head
A550V	substitution: Ala to Val	head
T1019N	substitution: Thr to Asn	tail
R1193S	substitution: Arg to Ser	tail
E1426K	substitution: Glu to Lys	tail
R1634S	substitution: Arg to Ser	tail

Table 4. Disease-causing MYH7 variants observed in patients with DCM (Villard et al., 2005)

Hershberger et al. (2008) in a study carried out on a cohort of 313 patients identified 12 mutations in MYH7 gene (9 novel): R237W, V964L, A970V, R1045C, D1096Y, R1359C, R1500W, E1619K, V1692M, G1808A, H1901Q and R1863Q. These variants were observed in 13 out of 313 probands (4.2%), revealing that MYH7 was the most commonly mutated gene in studied group. All observed variants were considered possibly or likely disease-causing.
Additional two mutations were described by Boda et al. (2009) in the group of 100 DCM patients. Screening of MYH7 gene revealed a substitution G377R in one DCM patient, diagnosed at the age of 11 years and R787H substitution in another patient, diagnosed at the age of 7 years. Møller et al. (2009) identified three MYH7 mutations (K637E, resulting in charge change in actin cleft, L1038P introducing helix-breaking proline in the rod and R1832C resulting in loss of plus charge in light meromyosin and introduction of reactive cysteine) in one-quarter of studied DCM patients.
Tanjore et al. (2010) in the study carried out on 292 individuals (100 healthy controls, 95 HCM and 92 DCM) revealed common genetic variation (5 SNPs) in exons 7, 12, 19 and 20 of MYH7 gene for DCM and HCM patients. However, three out of 5 variants were heterozygous in HCM, whereas the same SNPs were found to be homozygous in DCM patients, revealing the dose effect of the protein with the gross anatomical variations in the ventricles leading to heart failure in DCM cases.

Rare mutations explain only a small percentage of DCM cases. Rampersaud et al. (2009) assumed that more common variants may also play a role in increasing susceptibility to DCM, similarly to observations in other common complex diseases. To verify that hypothesis, case-control analyses were performed on all DNA polymorphic variation identified in a resequencing study of six genes associated with DCM carried out on 477 individuals (289 probands with DCM and 188 controls). Multivariate analyses revealed that a block of 9 MYH7 variants was strongly associated with DCM.

3. Other genes involved in development of DCM

Variation in three genes discussed above is considered to explain abut 10% of DCM cases. There are however other genetic factors that can also play role in development of dilated cardiomyopathy.

SCN5A gene encodes alpha subunit of type V voltage-gated sodium channel (see Figure 4), which is abundant in cardiac muscle and controls the flow of sodium ions into cardiac muscle cells, playing major role in signalling start of each heartbeat, coordinating the contractions of the upper and lower chambers of heart and maintaining normal heart rhythm.

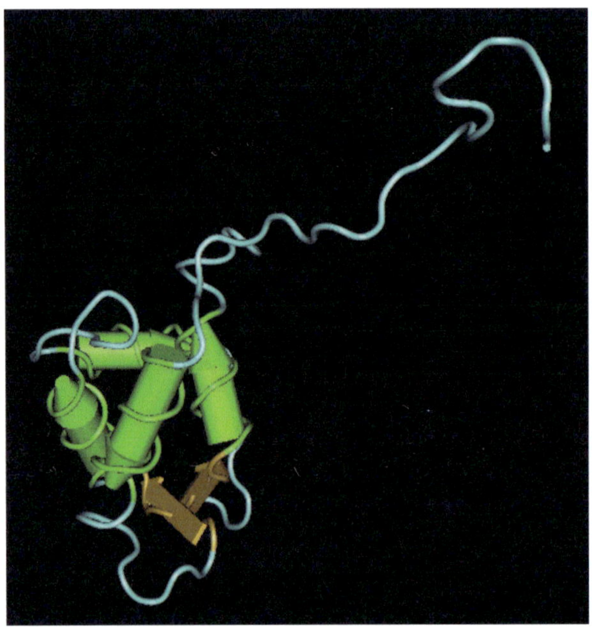

Fig. 4. Structure of the C-terminal Ef-hand domain of human cardiac sodium channel. Available from http://www.ncbi.nlm.nih.gov/Structure/mmdb/mmdbsrv.cgi?uid=68594 (Chagot et al., 2009).

Mutations in SCN5A has been described as causative in long QT syndrome and dilated cardiomyopathy. McNair et al. (2004) carried out a research on a large family affected by an autosomal cardiac conduction disorder associated with sinus node dysfunction, arrhythmia and ventricular dilatation and dysfunction. Linkage analyses mapped the disease phenotype to a region on chromosome 3p22-p25, containing cardiac sodium channel gene SCN5A. SCN5A gene was screened in 21 subjects, revealing a heterozygous G to A substitution at position 3823, changing aspartic acid to asparagine (D1275N) in highly conserved residue. The mutation was present in all affected family members (19 patients), while being absent in 300 control chromosomes, and predicted a change of charge within the S3 segment of protein domain III. All of mutations changed conserved amino acids. Two novel variants segregated with FDC in families and were considered likely disease-causing. On the other hand, two variants associated also with Brugada syndrome (R526H) and long QT-syndrome (A572D) did not segregate with DCM.

SCN5A variant	Mutation type	Pathogenicity of mutation (+/-)	Also associated with
S216L	substitution: Ser to Leu	+	LQT syndrome
R222Q	substitution: Arg to Gln	+	-
R526H	substitution: Arg to His	-	Brugada syndrome
A572D	substitution: Ala to Asp	-	LQT syndrome
P648L	substitution: Pro to Leu	+	LQT syndrome
I1835T	substitution: Ile to Thr	+	-
P2005A	substitution: Pro to Ala	+	LQT syndrome

Table 5. SCN5A variants observed in patients with DCM (Hershberger et al., 2008)

A study performed on 338 DCM patients from Familial Cardiomyopathy Registry revealed 5 missense SCN5A mutations, including novel E446K, F1520L, V1279I and already described D1275 and R222Q. Mutations were detected in 1.7% of DCM families. Most of them were localized to the highly conserved homologous S3 and S4 transmembrane segments , suggesting a shared mechanism of disruption of the voltage-sensing mechanism of this channel leading to DCM. Patients carrying SCN5A mutations showed strong arrhythmic pattern that had clinical and diagnostic implications (McNair et al., 2011).

Titin-cap (or telethonin), encoded by **TCAP** gene, is a protein regulating sarcomere assembly. It has kinase activity and serves as attachment for myofibrils and other muscle-related proteins (Valle et al., 1997). Mutations in TCAP gene were described in association with cardiomyopathies. Hayashi et al. (2004) analyzed TCAP genotype in 346 patients with HCM and 136 with DCM (34 FDC, 102 IDC), revealing two mutations in patients with HCM and one (E132Q substitution) in patient with DCM. Moreover, the researchers demonstrated that HCM-associated mutations augmented the ability of titin-cap to interact with titin and calsarcin-1, whereas DCM-associated mutations impaired the interaction of titin-cap with muscle LIM protein, titin and calsarcin-1. The role of TCAP in development of DCM was also confirmed by Hershberger et al. (2008), who found three protein-altering variants of TCAP in 3 out of 313 DCM patients (with two variants segregating with disease).

LDB3 (LIM domain binding 3), also known as ZASP or CYPHER is another gene associated with DCM. It encodes a protein containing PDZ domain which interacts with α-actinin-2 through its N-terminal PDZ domain and with protein kinase C through C-terminal LIM domains (a cysteine-rich motif containing two zinc-binding modules). It also interacts with myozenin family members.

First data revealing the role of LDB3 in DCM was delivered by Vatta et al. (2003). The research was carried out on 100 DCM probands and resulted in identification of 5 mutations (substitutions: S196L, I352M, D117N, K136M and T213I) in 6 patients (two families and four sporadic cases). None of these mutations were identified in the control group (200 individuals). 5 out of 6 mutations resulted in substitutions in conserved regions and all lied within the linker between PDZ and LIM domains. *In vitro* studies showed cytoskeleton disarray in cells transfected with mutated LDB3. One additional mutation in LDB3 was discovered by Arimura et al. (2004) in the study carried out on 96 unrelated Japanese patients with DCM. D626N substitution located within the LIM domain was identified in a familial case but not in the unrelated controls. A family study showed that all affected siblings had the same mutation, associated with late onset cardiomyopathy. A yeast two-hybrid assay demonstrated that described mutation increased the affinity of LIM domain for protein kinase C, suggesting a novel biochemical mechanism of the pathogenesis of DCM. Hershberger et al. (2008) identified two mutations in the LIM domain of LDB3 (A371T and A698T). Second mutation was identified in two unrelated probands and was predicted to change highly conserved amino acid; therefore it was considered disease-associated.

TPM1 is a gene encoding tropomyosin α-1 protein and another candidate gene for DCM. Tropomyosines are highly conserved actin-binding proteins involved in the contractile system of striated and smooth muscles and cytoskeleton of non-muscle cells. TPM1 forms predominant tropomyosine of striated muscle and functions in association with troponin complex to regulate calcium-dependent interaction of actin and myosin during muscle contraction. Mutations in this gene are associated with HCM and also DCM. Lakdawala et al. (2010) performed direct sequencing of 6 sarcomere genes on 334 probands with DCM, revealing D230N missense mutation in TPM1 gene, which segregated with DCM in two large unrelated families. Additional *in vitro* studies demonstrated major inhibitory effects on sarcomere function with reduced Ca^{2+} sensitivity, maximum activation and Ca^{2+} affinity compared to wildtype TPM1.

A role of **presenilin** genes in dilated cardiomyopathy was described by Li et al. (2006). Presenilins are multi-pass transmembrane proteins which function as a part of γ-secretase intramembrane protease complex. There are two presenilin genes in human genome: **PSEN1** and **PSEN2**, both showing conservation between species. Mutations in these genes are the most common cause of Alzheimer's disease. They are also expressed in the heart and play critical role in cardiac development. The researchers analyzed sequence variation of PSEN1 and PSEN2 in 315 patients with DCM, revealing novel PSEN1 mutation D333G in one family and a single PSEN2 mutation S130L in two other families. Both mutations segregated with DCM and heart failure. PSEN1 mutation was associated with complete penetrance and progressive disease that resulted in the necessity of cardiac transplantation or in death, whereas carriers of PSEN2 mutation showed partial penetrance, milder disease and more favourable prognosis. Moreover, calcium signalling was altered in cultured fibroblasts from mutation carriers.

Genes that are associated with complex diseases can also be organized as linkage disequilibrium clusters that are often inherited together. Friedriechs et al. (2009) described such 600-kb region of linkage disequilibrium on 5q31.2-3 chromosome, harboring multiple genes to be associated with DCM in three independent Caucasian populations. Functional assessments in zebrafish demonstrated that at least three genes from this region (**HBEGF** – heparin-binding epidermal growth factor, **IK** cytokine and **SRA1** – steroid receptor RNA activator 1) resulted independently in a phenotype of myocardial contractile dysfunction under the condition of reduced expression.

Most of the genes associated with DCM phenotype are present in nuclear genome. There are however examples of mitochondrial genes that can also contribute to development of dilated cardiomyopathy. Ashrafian et al. (2010) described C452F mutation in highly conserved region of the M domain of **Dnm1l** (dynamin1-like gene) in mice, resulting in reduced levels of mitochondria enzyme complexes in hearts, which then suffered from ATP depletion (energy deficiency that might contribute to DCM).

4. Conclusions

It is always difficult to find genetic cause of multigenic disorders, such as dilated cardiomyopathy, especially if it is considered that mutations in genome are only one of factors contributing to disease. Nevertheless, knowledge about genetic basis underlying such diseases proves to be very useful both in diagnostics and treatment, providing the possibility of early diagnosis and thus increasing the chance of successful therapy.

5. References

Ahmad F, Banerjee SK, Lage ML, Huang XN, Smith SH, Saba S, Rager J, Conner DA, Janczewski AM, Tobita K, Tinney JP, Moskowitz IP, Perez-Atayde AR, Keller BB, Mathier MA, Shroff SG, Seidman CE & Seidman JG (2008). The role of cardiac troponin t quantity and function in cardiac development and dilated cardiomyopathy. *PLoS ONE*, Vol.3, No.7, pp. e2642

Arbustini E, Pilotto A, Repetto A, Grasso M, Negri A, Diegoli M, Campana C, Scelsi L, Baldini E, Gavazzi A & Tavazzi L (2002). Autosomal dominant dilated cardiomyopathy with atrioventricular block: a lamin A/C defect-related disease. *J Am Coll Cardiol*, Vol.39, No.6, pp. 981-90

Arimura T, Hayashi T, Terada H, Lee SY, Zhou Q, Takahashi M, Ueda K, Nouchi T, Hohda S, Shibutani M, Hirose M, Chen J, Park JE, Yasunami M, Hayashi H & Kimura A (2004). A Cypher/ZASP mutation associated with dilated cardiomyopathy alters the binding affinity to protein kinase C. *J Biol Chem*, Vol.279, No.8, pp. 6746-52.

Ashrafian H, Docherty L, Leo V, Towlson C, Neilan M, Steeples V, Lygate CA, Hough T, Townsend S, Williams D, Wells S, Norris D, Glyn-Jones S, Land J, Barbaric I, Lalanne Z, Denny P, Szumska D, Bhattacharya S, Griffin JL, Hargreaves I, Fernandez-Fuentes N, Cheeseman M, Watkins H & Dear TN (2010). A mutation in the mitochondrial fission gene dnm1l leads to cardiomyopathy. *PLoS Genet*, Vol.6, No.6, pp. e1001000

Bender JR, Russel KS, Rosenfeld L & Chaudry S (Eds.). (2011) *Oxford American handbook of Cardiology*. Oxford University Press, Inc., ISBN 978-0-19-538969-2, New York

Boda U, Vadapalli S, Calambur N & Nallari P (2009). Novel mutations in beta-myosin heavy chain, actin and troponin-I genes associated with dilated cardiomyopathy in Indian population. *J Genet*, Vol.88, No.3, pp. 373-7

Botto N, Vittorini S, Colombo MG, Biagini A, Paradossi U, Aquaro G & Andreassi MG (2010). A novel LMNA mutation (R189W) in familial dilated cardiomyopathy: evidence for a 'hot spot' region at exon 3: a case report. *Cardiovasc Ultrasound*, Vol.8, No.9, available from http://www.cardiovascularultrasound.com/content/8/1/9

Chagot B, Potet F, Balser JR & Chazin WJ (2009). Solution NMR structure of the C-terminal EF-hand domain of human cardiac sodium channel NaV1.5. *J Biol Chem*, Vol.284, No.10, pp. 6436-45

Colombo MG, Botto N, Vittorini S, Paradossi U & Andreassi MG (2008). Clinical utility of genetic tests for inherited hypertrophic and dilated cardiomyopathies. *Cardiovasc Ultrasound*, Vol.6, No.62, available from http://www.cardiovascularultrasound.com/content/6/1/62

Cowan J, Li D, Gonzalez-Quintana J, Morales A & Hershberger RE (2010). Morphological analysis of 13 LMNA variants identified in a cohort of 324 unrelated patients with idiopathic or familial dilated cardiomyopathy. *Circ Cardiovasc Genet*, Vol.3, No.1, pp. 6–14

Friedrichs F, Zugck C, Rauch GJ, Ivandic B, Weichenhan D, Müller-Bardorff M, Meder B, El Mokhtari NE, Regitz-Zagrosek V, Hetzer R, Schäfer A, Schreiber S, Chen J, Neuhaus I, Ji R, Siemers NO, Frey N, Rottbauer W, Katus HA & Stoll M (2009). HBEGF, SRA1, and IK: Three cosegregating genes as determinants of cardiomyopathy. *Genome Res*, Vol.19, No.3, pp. 395–403

Genes associated with nonsyndromic dilated cardiomyopathy. UpToDate.com Available from http://www.uptodate.com/contents/image?imageKey=CARD%2F29266&topicKey=CARD%2F4911&source=see_link

Haugaa KH, Leren TP & Amlie JP (2009). Genetic testing in specific cardiomyopathies. *F1000 Med Rep*, Vol1, No.52, available from http://f1000.com/reports/m/1/52

Hayashi T, Arimura T, Itoh-Satoh M, Ueda K, Hohda S, Inagaki N, Takahashi M, Hori H, Yasunami M, Nishi H, Koga Y, Nakamura H, Matsuzaki M, Choi BY, Bae SW, You CW, Han KH, Park JE, Knöll R, Hoshijima M, Chien KR & Kimura A (2004). Tcap gene mutations in hypertrophic cardiomyopathy and dilated cardiomyopathy. *J Am Coll Cardiol*, Vol.44, No.11, pp. 2192-201

Hermida-Prieto M, Monserrat L, Castro-Beiras A, Laredo R, Soler R, Peteiro J, Rodríguez E, Bouzas B, Alvarez N, Muñiz J & Crespo-Leiro M (2004). Familial dilated cardiomyopathy and isolated left ventricular noncompaction associated with lamin A/C gene mutations. *Am J Cardiol*, Vol.94, No.1, pp. 50-4

Hershberger RE, Kushner JD & Parks SB (2007). Dilated cardiomyopathy overview, In: *Gene Reviews* (1993-2011), Pagon RA, Bird TD, Dolan CR & Stephens K (Ed.). Available from http://www.ncbi.nlm.nih.gov/books/NBK1309/?&log$=disease6_name

Hershberger RE, Parks SB, Kushner JD, Li D, Ludwigsen S, Jakobs P, Nauman D, Burgess D, Partain J & Litt M (2008). Coding sequence mutations identified in MYH7, TNNT2, SCN5A, CSRP3, LBD3, and TCAP from 313 patients with familial or idiopathic dilated cardiomyopathy. *Clin Transl Sci*, Vol.1, No.1, pp. 21–26

Hershberger RE, Cowan J, Morales A & Siegfried JD (2009a). Progress with genetic cardiomyopathies: Screening, counseling, and testing in dilated, hypertrophic and arrhythmogenic right ventricular dysplasia/cardiomyopathy. *Circ Heart Fail*, Vol.2, No.3, pp. 253–261

Hershberger RE, Pinto JR, Parks SB, Kushner JD, Li D, Ludwigsen S, Cowan J, Morales A, Parvatiyar MS & Potter JD (2009b). Clinical and functional characterization of TNNT2 mutations identified in patients with dilated cardiomyopathy. *Circ Cardiovasc Genet*, Vol.2, No.4, pp. 306–313

Hershberger RE, Morales MS & Siegfried MS (2010). Clinical and genetic issues in dilated cardiomyopathy: A review for genetics professionals. *Genet Med*, Vol.12, pp: 655-67

Kamisago M, Sharma SD, DePalma SR, Solomon S, Sharma P, McDonough B, Smoot L, Mullen MP, Woolf PK, Wigle ED, Seidman JG & Seidman CE (2000). Mutations in sarcomere protein genes as a cause of dilated cardiomyopathy. *N Engl J Med*, Vol.343, No.23, pp. 1688-96

Kärkkäinen S, Heliö T, Jääskeläinen P, Miettinen R, Tuomainen P, Ylitalo K, Kaartinen M, Reissell E, Toivonen L, Nieminen MS, Kuusisto J, Laakso M & Peuhkurinen K (2004). Two novel mutations in the beta-myosin heavy chain gene associated with dilated cardiomyopathy. *Eur J Heart Fail*, Vol.6, No.7, pp. 861-8

Kärkkäinen S, Reissell E, Heliö T, Kaartinen M, Tuomainen P, Toivonen L, Kuusisto J, Kupari M, Nieminen MS, Laakso M & Peuhkurinen K (2006). Novel mutations in the lamin A/C gene in heart transplant recipients with end stage dilated cardiomyopathy. *Heart*, Vol.92, No.4, pp. 524-6

Katus HA, Looser S, Hallermayer K, Remppis A, Scheffold T, Borgya A, Essig U & Geuss U (1992). Development and in vitro characterization of a new immunoassay of cardiac troponin T. *Clin Chem*, Vol.38, No.3, pp. 386-93.

Khabaeva Z. Genetic analysis in hypertrophic cardiomyopathy: missense mutations in the ventricular myosin regulatory light chain gene. Humboldt University, Berlin, 2002

Lakdawala N, Dellefave L, Redwood CS, Sparks E, Cirino AL, Depalma S, Colan SD, Funke B, Zimmerman RS, Robinson P, Watkins H, Seidman CE, Seidman JG, McNally EM & Ho CY (2010). Familial dilated cardiomyopathy caused by an alpha-tropomyosin mutation: the distinctive natural history of sarcomeric dcm. *J Am Coll Cardiol*, Vol.55, No.4, pp. 320–329

Li D, Parks SB, Kushner JD, Nauman D, Burgess D, Ludwigsen S, Partain J, Nixon RR, Allen CN, Irwin RP, Jakobs PM, Litt M & Hershberger RE (2006). Mutations of presenilin genes in dilated cardiomyopathy and heart failure. *Am J Hum Genet*, Vol.79, No.6, pp. 1030–1039

McNair WP, Ku L, Taylor MR, Fain PR, Dao D, Wolfel E & Mestroni L (2004). SCN5A mutation associated with dilated cardiomyopathy, conduction disorder, and arrhythmia. *Circulation*, Vol.110, No.15, pp. 2163-7

McNair WP, Sinagra G, Taylor MR, Di Lenarda A, Ferguson DA, Salcedo EE, Slavov D, Zhu X, Caldwell JH & Mestroni L (2011). SCN5A mutations associate with arrhythmic dilated cardiomyopathy and commonly localize to the voltage-sensing mechanism. *J Am Coll Cardiol*, Vol.57, No.21, pp. 2160-8

Menon SC, Michels VV, Pellikka PA, Ballew JD, Karst ML, Herron KJ, Nelson SM, Rodeheffer RJ & Olson TM (2008). Cardiac troponin T mutation in familial cardiomyopathy with variable remodeling and restrictive physiology. *Clin Genet*, Vol.74, No.5, pp. 445-54

Mestroni L, Maisch B, McKenna WJ, Schwartz K, Charron P, Rocco C, Tesson F, Richter A, Wilke A & Komajda M (1999). Guidelines for the study of familial dilated cardiomyopathies. Collaborative Research Group of the European Human and Capital Mobility Project on Familial Dilated Cardiomyopathy. *Eur Heart J*, Vol.20, No.2, pp. 93-102

Mogensen J, Murphy RT, Shaw T, Bahl A, Redwood C, Watkins H, Burke M, Elliott PM & McKenna WJ (2004). Severe disease expression of cardiac troponin C and T mutations in patients with idiopathic dilated cardiomyopathy. *J Am Coll Cardiol*, Vol.44, No.10, pp. 2033-40

Møller DV, Andersen PS, Hedley P, Ersbøll MK, Bundgaard H, Moolman-Smook J, Christiansen M & Køber L (2009). The role of sarcomere gene mutations in patients with idiopathic dilated cardiomyopathy. *Eur J Hum Genet*, Vol.17, No.10, pp. 1241-9

Otten E, Lekanne dit Deprez RH, Weiss MM, van Slegtenhorst M, Joosten M, van der Smagt JJ, de Jonge N, Kerstjens-Frederikse WS, Roofthooft MTR, Balk AHMM, van den Berg MP, Ruiter JS & van Tintelen JP (2010). Recurrent and founder mutations in the Netherlands: mutation p.K217del in troponin T2, causing dilated cardiomyopathy. *Neth Heart J*, Vol.18, No.10, pp. 478–485

Parks SB, Kushner JD, Nauman D, Burgess D, Ludwigsen S, Peterson A, Li D, Jakobs P, Litt M, Porter CB, Rahko PS & Hershberger RE (2008). Lamin A/C mutation analysis in a cohort of 324 unrelated patients with idiopathic or familial dilated cardiomyopathy. *Am Heart J*, Vol.156, No.1, pp. 161–169

Parks SB, Kushner JD, Nauman D, Burgess D, Ludwigsen S, Peterson A, Li D, Jakobs P, Litt M, Porter CB, Rahko PS & Hershberger RE (2008). Lamin A/C mutation analysis in a cohort of 324 unrelated patients with idiopathic or familial dilated cardiomyopathy. *Am Heart J*, Vol.156, No.1, pp. 161-9

Rampersaud E, Kinnamon DD, Hamilton K, Khuri S, Hershberger RE, & Martin ER (2010). Common susceptibility variants examined for association with dilated cardiomyopathy. *Ann Hum Genet*, Vol.74, No.2, pp. 110–116

Stuurman N, Heins S & Aebi U (1998). Nuclear lamins: their structure, assembly, and interactions. *J Struct Biol*, Vol.122, pp. 42-66

Tanjore R, RangaRaju A, Vadapalli S, Remersu S, Narsimhan C & Nallari P (2010). Genetic variations of β-MYH7 in hypertrophic cardiomyopathy and dilated cardiomyopathy. *Indian J Hum Genet*, Vol.16, pp. 67-71

Taylor MRG, Carniel E & Mestroni L (2006). Cardiomyopathy, familial dilated. *Orph J Rare Dis*, Vol.1, No.27, available from http://www.ojrd.com/content/1/1/27

Valle G, Faulkner G, De Antoni A, Pacchioni B, Pallavicini A, Pandolfo D, Tiso N, Toppo S, Trevisan S & Lanfranchi G (1997). Telethonin, a novel sarcomeric protein of heart and skeletal muscle. *FEBS Lett*, Vol.415, No.2, pp. 163-8

Vatta M, Mohapatra B, Jimenez S, Sanchez X, Faulkner G, Perles Z, Sinagra G, Lin JH, Vu TM, Zhou Q, Bowles KR, Di Lenarda A, Schimmenti L, Fox M, Chrisco MA, Murphy RT, McKenna W, Elliott P, Bowles NE, Chen J, Valle G & Towbin JA (2003). Mutations in Cypher/ZASP in patients with dilated cardiomyopathy and left ventricular non-compaction. *J Am Coll Cardiol*, Vol.42, No.11, pp. 2014-27

Villard E, Duboscq-Bidot L, Charron P, Benaiche A, Conraads V, Sylvius N & Komajda M (2005). Mutation screening in dilated cardiomyopathy: prominent role of the beta myosin heavy chain gene. *Eur Heart J*, Vol.26, No.8, pp. 794-803

Wolf CM, Wang L, Alcalai R, Pizard A, Burgon PG, Ahmad F, Sherwood M, Branco DM, Wakimoto H, Fishman GI, See V, Stewart CL, Conner DA, Berul CI, Seidman CE & Seidman JG (2008). Lamin A/C haploinsufficiency causes dilated cardiomyopathy and apoptosis-triggered cardiac conduction system disease. *J Mol Cell Cardiol*, Vol.44, No.2, pp. 293-303

Part 3

Cardiomyopathies and Imaging Methods

19

Role of Advanced Cardiac Magnetic Resonance Imaging in Atypical Cardiomyopathies such as Stress-Induced Cardiomyopathie and Left-Ventricular Non-Compaction Cardiomyopathy

Oliver Strohm[1,2], Abdullah Shehab[3] and Anwer Qureshi[4]
[1]*University of Calgary,*
[2]*Center for Cardiology and Pediatric Cardiology Baden-Baden,*
[3]*UAE University,*
[4]*Tawam Hospital, Al Ain,*
[1]*Canada*
[2]*Germany*
[3,4]*United Arab Emirates*

1. Introduction

Magnetic Resonance Imaging (MRI) is a medical imaging technique that has been in clinical use since the 1980's, and has advanced significantly in the last decade.

MRI scans are usually performed at magnetic field strengths of 1.5 to 3.0 Tesla. Such a magnetic field is at least 25,000 times stronger than that of the earth and is required to align and modify the behaviour of unevenly charged protons in the patient's body. Brief radio frequency pulses with specific properties are applied, which change the axis of rotation (precession) in the protons. The protons rapidly resume their original precession angle and emit a small signal, which is used to compute images. Importantly, the behaviour of resuming their previous state is strongly dependent on the molecular environment; in other words: different tissue composition creates different image contrasts (14-16)

The main advantages of MRI techniques include their completely non-invasive nature, lack of any harmful radiation or radioactivity, and the lack of need for Iodine-based contrast agents. It is considered to be free of any harm to patients, but - since metal is affected in a magnetic field - it may not be performed if the patient carries certain magnetic material such as specific electronic devices or some metallic implants. The most commonly performed MRI scans are of the head, brain, spine, large joints and abdomen (15).

Cardiac applications of MRI have been applied since the late 1980's and have evolved into a robust, clinically valid application due to recent advances in both hardware and software. CMR provides a variety of valuable diagnostic information including anatomy and function of the heart, flow of blood, and perfusion and viability of the myocardium. Its most unique advantage is the ability to visualize tissue characteristics selectively based on molecular environments, adding a new and valuable piece of information to medical testing

Contrast-enhanced cardiac magnetic resonance imaging (CMR) allows for a non-invasive assessment of the tissue composition using contrast-free (T2, e.g. STIR) and contrast-enhanced techniques (early and late Gadolinium enhancement). Together with a functional assessment, it can be used to determine the acuity of e.g. inflammatory diseases and provide a non-invasive follow-up tool.

1.1 CMR techniques used

Functional imaging with high-resolution sequences such as SSFP cines allow to assess the whole left and right ventricles and calculate volumes, ejection fraction and mass. Myocardial wall stress can be calculated from these.

Assessment of valvular function is needed and may require additional flow studies for the calculation of regurgitation fraction of aortic and mitral valve. Assessment of the pericardium can be done on the functional images, too.

T2-weighted images with fat suppression allow assessing myocardial water content, thus allowing to assess the stage of disease. To provide an "internal standard", skeletal muscle is used as control; an SI-ratio of more than 2.0 is considered abnormal.

T1-weighted images allow to demonstrate acute inflammatory changes including increased extracellular volume and membrane integrity. As in T2-weighted imaging a skeletal muscle is used as "internal standard"; an enhancement - ratio (myocardial enhancement / muscle enhancement) of more than 4.0 is considered abnormal. The body-coil is used to obtain homogenous SI through the images, short axis or axial images are selected to optimize image quality.

Newer sequences may improve image quality and allow for the use of multi-element coils.

Late Gadolinium enhancement allows to non-invasively diagnose irreversible damage in the myocardium (e.g. fibrosis, infarcts). Due to the specific location in ischemic damages (starts at the subendocardial layer), it is easy to distinguish non-ischemic damages (as in myocarditis) from ischemic problems. Combining T2-information, early and late enhancement, CMR is able to safely assess the acuity and reversibility of the disease process in non-ischemic Cardiomyopathies and inflammatory processes (16).

2. Left ventricular non-compaction

2.1 Introduction

Left ventricular non-compaction (LVNC) is a distinct cardiomyopathy resulting from arrest of fetal development of the heart (1). This leads to altered myocardial architecture that is seen as a two layered myocardium with a thin, compacted epicardial layer and a thick, non-compacted endocardial region. The non-compacted myocardial region is comprised of prominent trabeculations and deep intertrabecular recesses that directly communicate with the left ventricular cavity (2, 3) .The condition may present without any associated cardiac malformation and is then labelled isolated left ventricular non compaction (LVNC). Non compacted myocardium is also seen in conjunction with other cardiac abnormalities including cyanotic congenital heart disease, Ebstein's anomaly and other cardiomyopathies. Clinical presentation in LVNC is seen with congestive heart failure, ventricular arrhythmia and systemic thromboembolism. The condition is listed as an unclassified cardiomyopathy in the WHO and European Society of Cardiology classification of cardiomyopathies (4, 5) and as a primary genetic cardiomyopathy in the American Heart Association classification (6).

2.2 Pathophysiology

Early intrauterine myocardial perfusion is through direct diffusion of nutrients from the left ventricular (LV) cavity to the myocardium. The presence of deep trabecular recesses filled with blood facilitates this process. Development of coronary circulation in the second trimester provides direct blood supply to the myocardium with consequent compaction of extensive intrauterine trabeculations of the myocardial wall. Failure in this process results in a non-compacted myocardium (1). The exact mechanism for this is not known.

2.3 Inheritance

Both sporadic and familial forms are described. In the latter an autosomal dominant or X-linked inheritance with genetic heterogeneity is reported. Mutations in *MYH7* encoding β-myosin heavy chain is seen in patients with Ebstein's anomaly and LVNC (7). In X-linked inheritance mutation of G4.5 TAZ gene with abnormality of tafazzin is reported (8, 9). This can be seen with or without Barth syndrome.

2.4 Prevalence

The presence of significant non compaction is estimated at 1:2.000 in the general population (10). The condition is, however, more prevalent in heart failure patients. More frequent use of cardiac imaging in clinical practice has increased recognition of this condition.

2.5 Clinical presentation

This is variable from asymptomatic individuals to those with severe disease presenting with heart failure, ventricular arrhythmia and systemic thromboembolism (9, 11-13). Non cardiac features may include facial dysmorphism and neuromuscular disorders.

2.6 Diagnostic criteria

Trabeculation in the LV wall is seen even in healthy volunteers. To separate benign LV trabeculation from pathological LVNC following diagnostic criteria is proposed.

- Echo: ratio of non-compacted to compacted myocardium in end-systole of > 2:1 (14)
- Cardiac MRI: ratio of non-compacted to compacted myocardium in end-diastole of > 2.3:1 (15)

2.7 Cardiac MRI in the diagnosis of LVNC

Cardiovascular imaging is central to the diagnosis of left ventricular non compaction. Compared to echocardiography better resolution of cardiac MRI makes it a preferred imaging modality particularly in those with limited echo windows. Additionally, non-compacted segment may be confined to the LV apex where echo has inherent imaging problems. Cardiac MRI is also reliable in distinguishing LVNC from other causes of LV apical deformity including apical variant of hypertrophic cardiomyopathy, endomyocardial fibrosis and apical thrombus.

2.8 Cardiac MRI imaging protocol

LV morphology and function is evaluated with cine images using a steady-state free precession (SSFP) technique. Images are usually displayed in three to six long axes and in contiguous short axis projections.

After baseline imaging post Gadolinium delayed enhancement (LGE) is performed to assess myocardial fibrosis.

2.9 Myocardial morphology on cardiac MRI

Besides pathological LVNC myocardial trabeculation is also seen in normal healthy individuals as well as in patients with hypertrophic and dilated cardiomyopathies. In LVNC distribution of non-compacted myocardium can be accurately assessed by MRI. There is involvement of the LV apex along with more frequent non compaction of the mid and apical segments of inferior and lateral wall. Non-compaction of the right ventricular wall is seen in some of these individuals. However, it is the severity of non-compaction rather than the distribution that distinguishes pathological LVNC from other disorders (15). A ratio of non-compacted to compacted myocardium of > 2.3 in diastole has as a sensitivity of 86% with a very high specificity of 99% and positive and negative predictive values of 75% and 99% respectively.

In contrast to echocardiography where systolic frame images are used to measure the relationship of non-compacted to compacted myocardium, diastolic frame images are used in MRI. This is possible because of improved spatial resolution of MRI. In systole, thickening of compacted myocardium may account for the altered relationship of compacted and non-compacted myocardium and this may explain the lower ratio of non-compacted to compacted myocardium of > 2:1 used in echocardiography (15).

Others have suggested that a trabeculated LV mass of > 20% of the total LV mass separates LVNC from other causes of LV trabeculation both benign and that seen in dilated and hypertrophic cardiomyopathy with a sensitivity and specificity of > 90%(16).

2.10 Myocardial kinetics and function

Cine short-axis images are used for calculation of ejection fraction (EF) using Simpson's method by tracing end diastolic and end systolic volumes in all imaging planes.

The spectrum of myocardial function may range from normal to severe systolic dysfunction. Quantitative assessment of left ventricular function by cardiac MRI is the current reference standard and can be compared longitudinally. However, in patients with LVNC interobserver and intraobserver reproducibility may be affected, depending on whether the inner contour (interface between the LV cavity and non-compacted myocardium) or outer contour (interface between the compacted and non-compacted myocardium) are used to calculate LV volumes. Latter may have the effect of increasing left ventricular end-diastolic volume and falsely overestimating volumetric EF (17). Therefore, additional qualitative information of LV function from review of myocardial kinetics on cine images is suggested.

2.11 Tissue characterization-late gadolinium enhancement

Late Gadolinium enhancement (LGE), a marker of myocardial fibrosis, was seen in 23 out of 42 patients (55%) in a study conducted by Nucifora, et al. The degree of LGE in their study correlated with clinical symptoms, LV systolic dysfunction and arrhythmia (18). In another study Dodd et al. demonstrated a correlation between trabecular LGE and LV dysfunction (19).

2.12 Clinical management

This is largely supportive with standard heart failure therapy. Heart transplantation remains an option in patients with advanced disease. Ventricular arrhythmia is not directly related to severity of LV dysfunction and a prophylactic ICD is recommended. Anticoagulation to prevent thromboembolic complications is recommended, particularly in patients with severe contractile dysfunction. Family members of affected individual should be screened and counseled.

2.13 Summary

Left ventricular non-compaction is a rare cardiomyopathy arising from developmental arrest of the left ventricular myocardium. It has distinct morphometric appearance with a two layer myocardium-a compacted and a non-compacted zone. Sporadic and familial forms are described. The triad of heart failure, arrhythmia and systemic thromboembolism are feared complications. In milder forms the patient may be completely asymptomatic. Increased awareness of this disorder and improvement in cardiovascular imaging has contributed to greater recognition of this condition. Cardiac MRI with its improved spatial resolution can conclusively establish the diagnosis and the unique property of LGE on cardiac MRI can identify severe forms of this disorder which may have both therapeutic and prognostic implications.

3. Stress-induced or "Tako-Tsubo" cardiomyopathy

3.1 Introduction

This cardiomyopathy is a transient and reversible cardiomyopathy that was first reported in Japan by Dote, et al., in 1991 (1). Clinical presentation may be indistinguishable from acute coronary syndrome, invariably necessitating coronary angiography for exclusion of obstructive coronary artery disease. Prevalence is in 1-2% of patients undergoing coronary angiography for acute coronary syndrome. Complimentary imaging modalities including echocardiography and cardiac MRI are helpful in diagnosis and in monitoring clinical recovery. Absence of delayed hyperenhancement on cardiac MRI is particularly important in differentiating this condition from ischemic and other types of non-ischemic cardiomyopathy and acute myocarditis (2). Based on morphologic features of the left ventricle, presumed causative role of stress and catecholamine excess and transient nature of the contractile dysfunction, other nomenclature used to describe this cardiomyopathy include ampulla cardiomyopathy, stress cardiomyopathy or catecholamine cardiotoxicity and transient left ventricular apical ballooning syndrome.

3.2 Pathophysiology

Distinct pattern of contractile abnormality is noted in the left ventricle. In the typical case the LV apex is dyskinetic and expanded and may be associated with hyperdynamic contractility of the basal LV segments. The shape of left ventricle in systole resembles a Japanese octopus trap (Takotusbo), which has a narrow neck and a wide base (1).

The condition is associated with markedly elevated circulating catecholamine, which is assumed to be central in the pathophysiology of this condition though exact mechanism at the cellular level is not fully understood. In a report by Wittstein, et al., two to three times higher plasma catecholamine concentrations were found in 13 patients with transient LV apical ballooning syndrome compared with 7 controls hospitalized for acute MI with Killip class III heart failure (3). Other proposed mechanisms include neurogenic stunned myocardium, coronary vasospasm, microvasculature dysfunction and altered cellular metabolism (4, 8-11). Preponderance of females afflicted by this condition is unclear. Estrogen deficiency in the post-menopausal state may play a role. Of particular interest, in other conditions with elevated catecholamine levels like subarachnoid hemorrhage, segmental wall motion abnormality is also predominantly seen in women (12). A reverse pattern of contractile abnormality with apical sparing has also been reported (13).

3.3 Clinical features

The presentation is typically following intense emotional or physical stress. The condition is predominantly seen in post-menopausal female with more than 80% of patients being female and more than 90% above the age of 50 years. Presentation may be clinically indistinguishable from ACS including ST segment elevation on ECG and rise in cardiac biomarkers. Chest pain and mild dyspnea are most common features encountered in more than 70% of patients. More significant heart failure and some degree of LVOT tract obstruction from hyperdynamic contraction of basal LV segments may be encountered in 15-20% of patients. Complications including cardiogenic shock may complicate the clinical course in up to 5% of patients. This may be secondary to either severe LV systolic dysfunction or obstruction of LVOT or both. Systemic thromboembolism from apical LV thrombus is reported. Ventricular arrhythmia is seen in 1-2% of patients (1-14).

Although presentation is typically encountered in the setting of profound emotional or physical stress, this characteristic trigger can be absent in up to a third of patients (14). Right ventricular involvement in takotsubo is seen in 25-30% of patients and is associated with a more complicated clinical course (15). It is encountered in patients with more severe LV involvement (16). However, isolated right ventricular takotsubo has been reported (17).

3.4 Diagnosis

History of intense emotional or physical stress and a typical pattern of left ventricular contractile dysfunction on cardiac imaging are suggestive of the diagnosis. Invariably, however, coronary angiography is required in the acute setting to exclude obstructive coronary artery disease. Both echocardiography and cardiac MRI provide information on the distinct morphologic and contractile dysfunction of takotsubo cardiomyopathy. However, cardiac MRI is instrumental in conclusively distinguishing takotsubo cardiomyopathy from other conditions.

3.5 Cardiac MRI in the diagnosis of Takotsubo cardiomyopathy

3.5.1 Assessment of myocardial morphology and contractility

Imaging sequence includes Standard TrueFISP (fast imaging with steady-state precession) cine images acquisition in 3 long-axis slices and 11 to 15 short-axis slices, 7 mm in thickness with a 3-mm interslice gap, achieving full ventricular coverage. Apical ballooning with or without mid myocardial contractile dysfunction and with basal sparing can be easily appreciated. In addition hyperdynamic contraction of basal segments with LVOT obstruction can be identified. The above-described pattern of contractile dysfunction in takotsubo cardiomyopathy does not fit a coronary artery distribution and is helpful in differentiating this condition from acute coronary syndrome. Left ventricular apical thrombus, which can complicate the clinical course, can be diagnosed using the long axis cine projections and LGE images.

Right ventricular involvement is seen in some patients. Because of the difficulty in assessing RV morphology and function by echocardiography, cardiac MRI is a preferred modality for identification of right ventricular involvement (15-17) and in quantification of RV dysfunction. However, cautious interpretation of RV dysfunction by MRI is advised in view of some degree of projection dependent contractile dysfunction seen even in normal subjects (18-19).

Sequential cardiac imaging study will show normalization of contractile dysfunction within a few days to weeks.

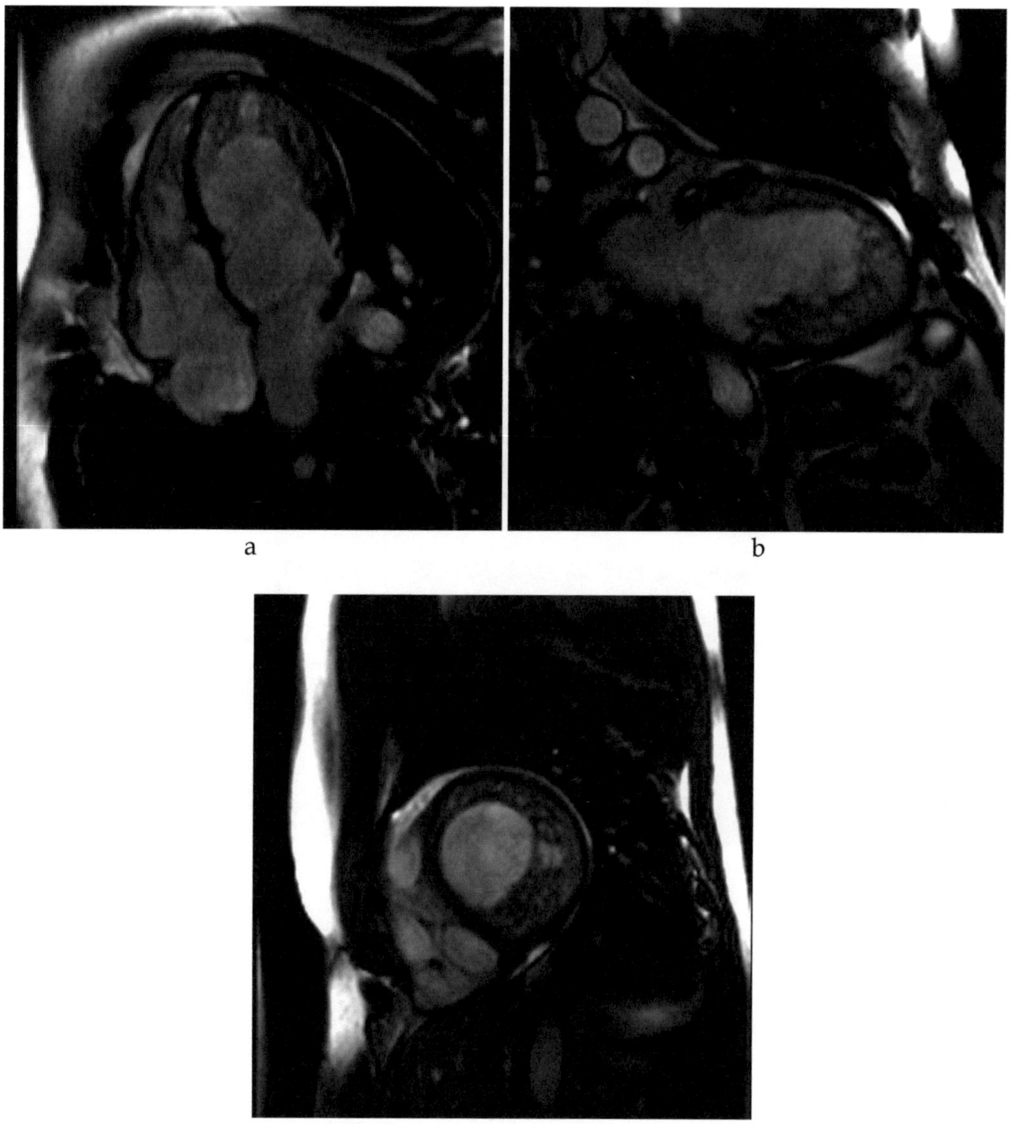

a b

c

Fig. 1. Long axis and short axis SSFP images in diastole (a: 4-chamber view long axis; b: 2-chamber view long axis; c: short axis at mid ventricular level) in a patient with genetically proven non-compaction cardiomyopathy. Note increased end-diastolic volume and increased

3.5.2 First pass myocardial perfusion

In contrast to apical myocardial infarction rest first-pass contrast enhanced myocardial perfusion on cardiac MRI is usually normal in takotsubo cardiomyopathy providing another feature to distinguish between the two conditions.

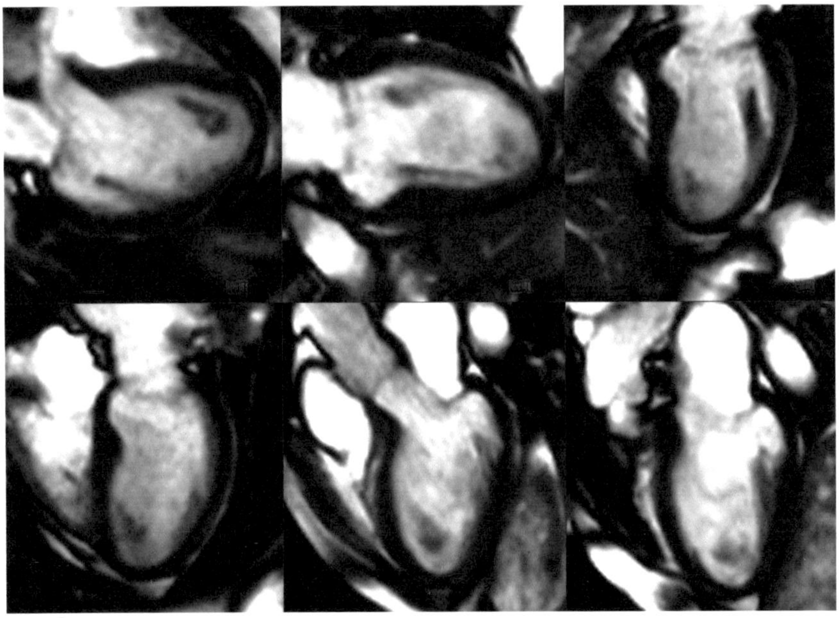

a

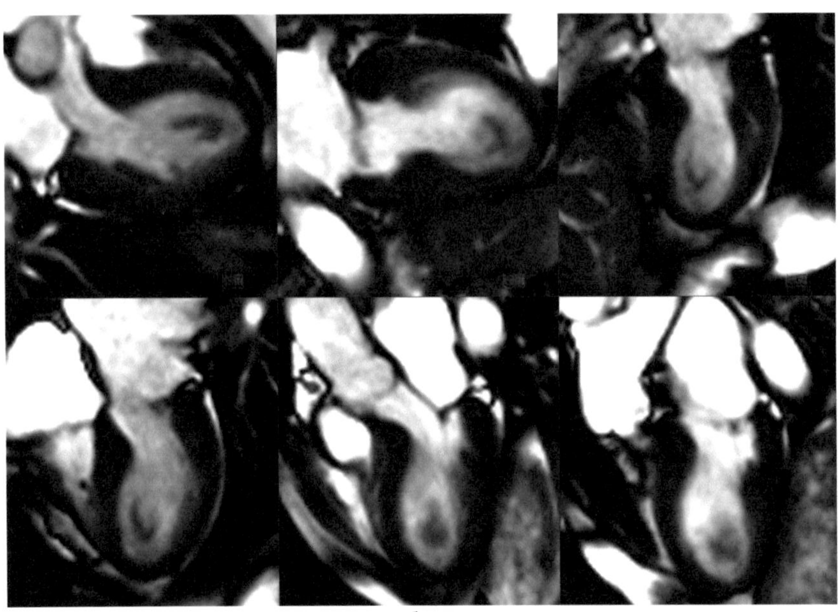

b

Fig. 2. Set of mulitple long axis SSFP cines in diastole (2-a) and systole (2-b). Note hypo- to akinetic mid ventricular and apical segments in this apical ballooning syndrome.

3.5.3 Tissue characterization – Myocardial edema on t2-weighted images

Myocardial edema following myocardial injury, ischemic or non-ischemic, can be detected using T2-weighted short tau inversion recovery (T2-STIR) images obtained in basal, mid, and apical short-axis, vertical long-axis, 3-chamber, and horizontal long-axis planes (20). Elevated T2- signal consistent with myocardial edema is seen in patients with takotsubo cardiomyopathy. T2 signal is highest in myocardium with the most impaired function and resolves over time (21-22). Myocardial edema on T2-STIR sequence is also a hallmark of ischemic myocardium prior to irreversible myocardial injury (23). In contrast to ischemic myocardium, myocardial edema in patients with takotsubo cardiomyopathy may represent catecholamine-induced myocardial stunning due to microvascular dysfunction (2).

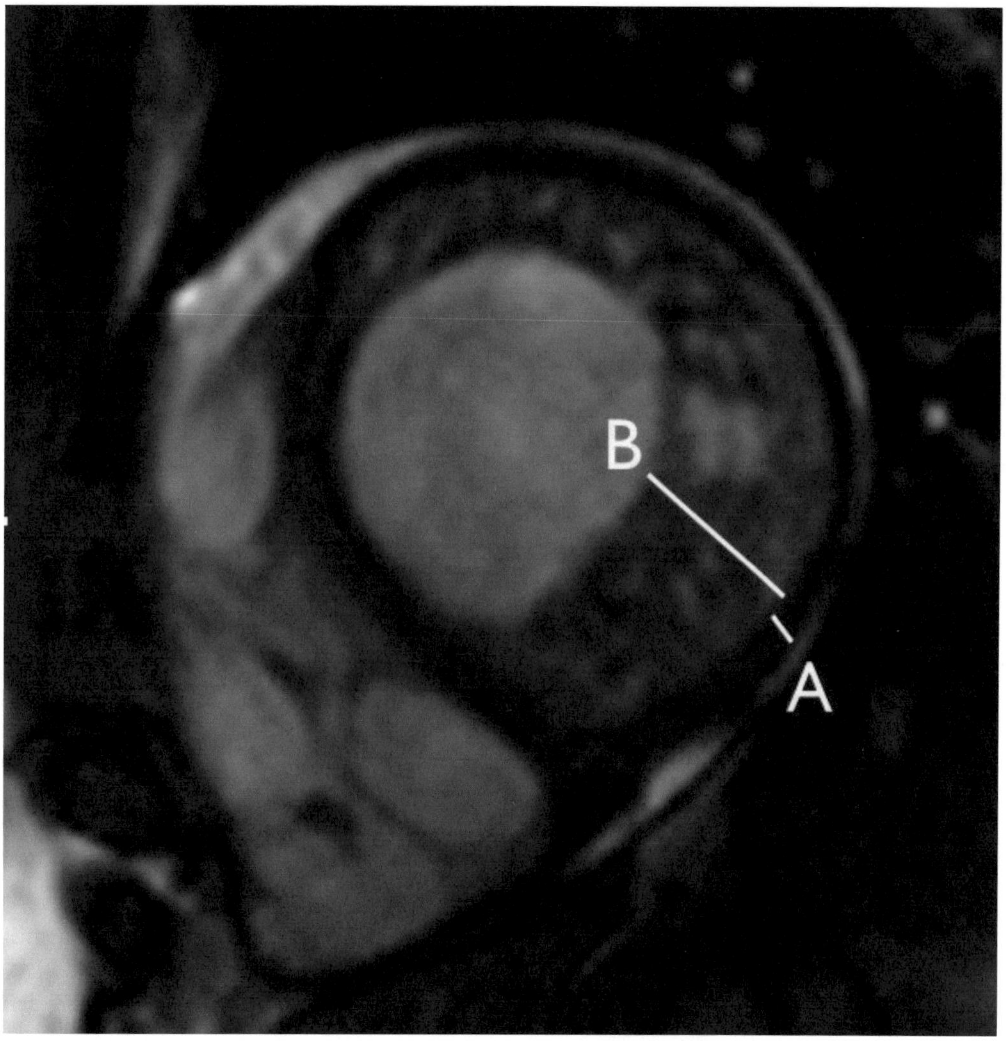

Fig. 3. Short axis SSFP cine image in diastole in a patient with non-compaction cardiomyopathy. Line A denotes the thickness of the compacted myocardium, line B denotes the non-compacted myocardium.

3.5.4 Tissue characterization – Late gadolinium enhancement (LGE) on T1-weighted Images

Gadolinium concentrates in region of damaged myocardium and appears bright on T1-weighted images (24). Cine images using a segmented gradient-echo sequence (6-mm slice thickness) is obtained in multiple short-axis views every 10 mm covering the whole left ventricle (LV). Ten to 15 min after injection of a Gadolinium-based contrast agent, images are acquired in the same orientation as the cine images using a segmented inversion-recovery gradient-echo pulse sequence. Abnormal myocardium is usually bright on T1-weighted images. LGE is absent in patients with takotsubo cardiomyopathy (2, 3, 5, 25). This indicates viable myocardium and is particularly useful in distinguishing it from myocardial infarction, other types of non-ischemic cardiomyopathy and myocarditis.

In a prospective study using CMR conducted by Eitel, et al., 6.100 patients presenting with ACS underwent coronary angiography and left ventriculography. In 59 patients with normal coronary angiography and typical contractile pattern of takotsubo cardiomyopathy, cardiac MRI was performed. Using strict criteria of absence of any late Gadolinium enhancement, takotsubo cardiomyopathy was diagnosed in 38. In the remaining 21 patients, based on the pattern of delayed hyperenhancement, a diagnosis of ischemic heart disease was made in 13 and of myocarditis in 8 patients (2). However, in a study of 15 patients with takotsubo cardiomyopathy, low intensity, patchy, mid-myocardial LGE was seen in 5 out of 15 patients. Increase in extracellular collagen was reported to be a plausible mechanism for this finding (26).

3.5.5 Coronary magnetic resonance angiography (MRA)

Coronary MRA though quite helpful in delineating the course of proximal coronary arteries (27), is not feasible for assessment of obstructive coronary artery disease and hence cannot be substituted for invasive or CT angiography (28).

3.6 Management

Treatment is supportive. ß-blockers are the mainstay in blunting catecholamine cardiotoxicity. This should be used cautiously to avoid worsening of heart failure. In patients with cardiogenic shock inotropic and IABP support may be required. However, the possibility of exacerbating LVOT obstruction with these measures requires careful monitoring and appropriate adjustment of therapy including discontinuation of inotropes and IABP support (29). ACE-I are beneficial and warfarin is recommended till left ventricular recovery is complete. In addition to these therapeutic measures, emotional or physical precipitating factors should be addressed. Prognosis is usually very good with complete or near complete recovery of LV contractile dysfunction. For prevention of rare recurrent episodes of takotsubo even after removal of initial trigger, indefinite neurohormonal modulation with ß-blockers and ACE-I merits consideration (30).

3.7 Summary

Takotsubo cardiomyopathy presents with clinical features that can be indistinguishable from acute coronary syndrome. However, distinct myocardial contractile dysfunction on echocardiography or cardiac MRI, absence of obstructive CAD on invasive angiography and exposure to an emotional or physical stressor is helpful in initially distinguishing it from ACS. Furthermore, cardiac MRI with normal first-pass contrast enhanced rest myocardial perfusion, reversible myocardial edema in regions of contractile dysfunction and absence of late gadolinium enhancement is strongly indicative of the diagnosis of takotsubo cardiomyopathy. Resolution of contractile dysfunction, days to weeks after initial presentation, is confirmatory of the diagnosis.

4. References

4.1 Part one references

[1] Sedmera D, Pexieder T, Vuillemin M, Thompson RP,Anderson RH. Developmental patterning of the myocardium. *Anat Rec* 2000; 258: 319–337.

[2] Chin TK, Perloff JK, Williams RG, Jue K, Mohrmann R. Isolated noncompaction of left ventricular myocardium. A study of eight cases. Circulation 1990;82:507-513.

[3] Dusek J, Ostadal B, Duskova M. Postnatal persistence of spongy myocardium with embryonic blood supply. Arch Pathol 1975;99:312-317.

[4] *Richardson P, McKenna W, Bristow M, Maisch B, Mautner B, O'Connell J, Olsen E, Thiene G, Goodwin J.*Report of the 1995 World Health Organisation/International Society and Federation of Cardiology Task Force on the definition and classification of cardiomoypathies. Circulation 1996; 93:841–842.

[5] Perry Elliott, Bert Andersson, Eloisa Arbustini, Zofia Bilinska, Franco Cecchi, Philippe Charron, Olivier Dubourg, Uwe Kühl, Bernhard Maisch, William J. McKenna, Lorenzo Monserrat, Sabine Pankuweit, Claudio Rapezzi, Petar Seferovic, Luigi Tavazzi, Andre Keren. Classification of the cardiomyopathies: a position statement from the European society of cardiology working group on myocardial and pericardial diseases. *Eur Heart J* (2008) 29 (2): 270-276

[6] Barry J. Maron, MD, Chair; Jeffrey A. Towbin, MD, FAHA; Gaetano Thiene, MD; Charles Antzelevitch, PhD, FAHA; Domenico Corrado, MD, PhD; Donna Arnett, PhD, FAHA; Arthur J. Moss, MD, FAHA; Christine E. Seidman, MD, FAHA; James B. Young, MD, FAHA. Contemporary Definitions and Classification of the Cardiomyopathies. An American Heart Association Scientific Statement from the Council on Clinical Cardiology, Heart Failure and Transplantation Committee; Quality of Care and Outcomes Research and Functional Genomics and Translational Biology Interdisciplinary Working Groups; and Council on Epidemiology and Prevention. *Circulation.* 2006;113:1807-1816.

[7] Mutations in the Sarcomere Gene *MYH7* in Ebstein Anomaly / Clinical Perspective.Alex V. Postma, Klaartje van Engelen, Judith van de Meerakker, Thahira Rahman, Susanne Probst, Marieke J.H. Baars, Ulrike Bauer, Thomas Pickardt, Silke R. Sperling, Felix Berger, Antoon F.M. Moorman, Barbara J.M. Mulder, Ludwig Thierfelder, Bernard Keavney, Judith Goodship, and Sabine Klaassen. Circ Cardiovasc Genet. *2011;4:43-50*

[8] Ichida F, Tsubata S, Bowles KR, Haneda N, Uese K, Miyawaki T, Dreyer WJ, Messina J, Li H, Bowles NE, Towbin JA. Novel Gene Mutations in Patients with Left Ventricular Noncompaction or Barth Syndrome. Circulation 2001;103;1256-1263.

[9] Pignatelli RH, McMahon CJ, Dreyer WJ, Denfield SW, Price J, Belmont JW, et al. Clinical characterization of left ventricular noncompaction in children: a relatively common form of cardiomyopathy. Circulation 2003;108:2672–8

[10] Ritter M, Oechslin E, Sutsch G, Attenhofer C, Schneider J, Jenni R. Isolated noncompaction of the myocardium in adults. Mayo Clin Proc 1997;72:26-31.

[11] Oechslin EN, Attenhofer Jost CH, Rojas JR, Kaufmann PA, Jenni R. Long-term follow-up of 34 adults with isolated left ventricular noncompaction: a distinct cardiomyopathy with poor prognosis. *J Am Coll Cardiol* 2000; 36: 493–500.
[12] Ichida F, Hamamichi Y, Miyawaki T, Ono Y, Kamiya T, Akagi T, et al., Clinical features of isolated noncompaction of the ventricular myocardium. *J Am Coll Cardiol* 1999; 34: 233–240.
[13] Murphy RT, Thaman R, Blanes JG, Ward D, Sevdalis E, Papra E, Kiotsekolglou A, Tome MT, Pellerin D, McKenna WJ, Elliott PM. Natural history and familial characteristics of isolated left ventricular non-compaction. European Heart Journal (2005) 26, 187–192.
[14] Jenni R, Oechslin E, Schneider J,Attenhofer Jost C, Kaufmann PA. Echocardiographic and pathoanatomical characteristics of isolated left ventricular non-compaction: a step towards classification as a distinct cardiomyopathy. Heart 2001;86:666-671.
[15] Petersen SE, Selvanayagam JB, Wiesmann F, Robson, MD, Francis JM, Anderson RH, Watkins H, Neubauer S. Left ventricular non-compaction: insights from cardiovascular magnetic resonance imaging J Am Coll Cardiol 2005;46:101-105
[16] Jacquier A, Thuny F, Jop B, Giorgi R, Cohen F, Gaubert J, Vidal V, Bartoli JM, Habib G, Moulin G. Measurement of trabeculated left ventricular mass using cardiac magnetic resonance imaging in the diagnosis of left ventricular non-compaction. *Eur Heart J* (2010) 31 (9): 1098-1104.
[17] Papavassiliu T, Kuhl HP, Schroder M, Suselbeck T, Bondarenko O, Bohm CK, Beek A, Hofman MM, van Rossum AC. Effect of endocardial trabeculae on left ventricular measurements and measurement reproducibility at cardiovascular MR imaging. Radiology 2005;236:57–64.
[18] Nucifora G, Aquaro GD, Pingitore A, Masci PG, Lombardi M: Myocardial fibrosis in isolated left ventricular non-compaction and its relation to disease severity. *Eur J Heart Fail* (2011) 13 (2): 170-176.
[19] Dodd JD, Holmvang G, Hoffmann U, et al. Quantification of left ventricular noncompaction and trabecular delayed hyperenhancement with cardiac MRI: correlation with clinical severity. Am J Roentgenol 2007;189:974-980.

4.2 Part two references

[1] Dote K, Sato H, Tateishi H, Uchida T, Ishihara M. Myocardial stunning due to simultaneous multivessel coronary spasms: a review of 5 cases. J Cardiol 1991;21: 203–214.
[2] Eitel I, Behrendt F, Schindler K, Kivelitz D, Gutberlet M, Schuler G, Thiele H. Differential diagnosis of suspected apical ballooning syndrome using contrast-enhanced magnetic resonance imaging. Eur Heart J (2008) 29 (21): 2651-2659.
[3] Wittstein IS, Thiemann DR, Lima JA, Baughman KL, Schulman SP, Gerstenblith G, et al. Neurohumoral features of myocardial stunning due to sudden emotional stress. N Engl J Med. 2005;352:539–548.
[4] Abe Y, Kondo M, Matsuoka R, Araki M, Dohyama K, Tanio H. Assessment of clinical features in transient left ventricular apical ballooning. J Am Coll Cardiol. 2003;41:737–742.

[5] Sharkey SW, Lesser JR, Zenovich AG, Maron MS, Lindberg J, Longe TF, Maron BJ. Acute and Reversible Cardiomyopathy Provoked by Stress in Women From the United States. Circulation 2005;111:472-479.

[6] Bybee KA, Prasad A. Stress-related cardiomyopathy syndromes Circulation 2008;118:397-40.

[7] Sharkey SW, Windenburg DC, Lesser JR, Maron MS, Hauser RG, Lesser JN, Haas TS, Hodges JS, Maron BJ. Natural History and Expansive Clinical Profile of Stress (Tako-Tsubo) Cardiomyopathy. J. Am. Coll. Cardiol., January 26, 2010; 55(4): 333 - 341.

[8] Bybee KA, Prasad A, Barsness GW, et al. Clinical characteristics and thrombolysis in myocardial infarction frame counts in women with transient left ventricular apical ballooning syndrome. Am J Cardiol 2004;94:343-346.

[9] Sansen V, Holvoet G. Takotsubo cardiomyopathy presenting as multivessel coronary spasm syndrome: case report and review of the literature. Acta Cardiol 2007;62:507-511.

[10] Afonso L, Bachour K, Awad K, Sandidge G. Takotsubo cardiomyopathy: pathogenetic insights and myocardial perfusion kinetics using myocardial contrast echocardiography Eur J Echocardiogr 2008;9:849-854

[11] Kurisu S, Inoue I, Kawagoe T, Ishihara M, Shimatani Y, Nishioka K, Umemura T, Nakamura S, Yoshida M, Sato H. Myocardial perfusion and fatty acid metabolism in patients with tako-tsubo-like left ventricular dysfunction. J Am Coll Cardiol. 2003 Mar 5;41(5):743-8.

[12] Mayer SA, Lin J, Homma S, et al. Myocardial injury and left ventricular performance after subarachnoid hemorrhage Stroke 1999;30:780-786.

[13] Hurst RT, Prasad A, Askew III JW, Sengupta PP, Tajik AJ. Takotsubo Cardiomyopathy: A Unique Cardiomyopathy with Variable Ventricular Morphology. J. Am. Coll. Cardiol. Img., June 1, 2010; 3(6): 641 - 649.

[14] Gianni M, Dentali F, Grandi AM, Sumner G, Hiralal R, Lonn E. Apical ballooning syndrome or takotsubo cardiomyopathy: a systematic review. European Heart Journal (2006) 27, 1523–1529.

[15] Elesber AA, Prasad A, Bybee KA, Valeti U, Motiei A, Lerman A, Chandrasekaran K, Rihal CS, Transient Cardiac Apical Ballooning Syndrome: Prevalence and Clinical Implications of Right Ventricular Involvement. J Am Coll Cardiol, 2006; 47:1082-1083.

[16] Haghi D, Athanasiadis A, Papavassiliu T, Suselbeck T, Fluechter S, Mahrholdt H, Borggrefe M, Sechtem U. Right ventricular involvement in Takotsubo Cardiomyopathy. Eur Heart J (2006) 27, 2433–2439.

[17] Mrdovic I, Kostic J, Perunicic J, Asanin A, Vasiljevic Z, and Ostojic M. Right Ventricular Takotsubo Cardiomyopathy. J. Am. Coll. Cardiol., April 20, 2010; 55(16): 1751 - 1751.

[18] Sievers B, Addo M, Franken U, Trappe HJ. Right ventricular wall motion abnormalities found in healthy subjects by cardiovascular magnetic resonance imaging and characterized with a new segmental model. J Cardiovasc Magn Reson 2004;6:601–608.

[19] Fritz J, Solaiyappan M, Tandri H, MD, Bomma C, Genc A, Claus D. Claussen CD, Lima JAC, Bluemke DA.Right Ventricle Shape and Contraction Patterns and Relation to Magnetic Resonance Imaging Findings. J Comput Assist Tomogr 2005;29:725–733.

[20] Simonetti OP, Finn JP, White RD, Laub G, Henry DA. 'Black blood' T2-weighted inversion-recovery MR imaging of the heart. Radiology 1996;199:49–57.

[21] Abdel-Aty H, Cocker M, Friedrich MG. Myocardial edema is a feature of Tako-Tsubo cardiomyopathy and is related to the severity of systolic dysfunction: Insights from T2-weighted cardiovascular magnetic resonance. Int J Cardiol. 2009 Feb 20;132(2):291-3.

[22] Joshi SB, Chow T, Herzka DA, Zeman PR, Cooper HA, Lindsay J, Fuisz AR. Cardiovascular magnetic resonance T2 signal abnormalities in left ventricular ballooning syndrome. Int J Cardiovasc Imaging: Vol. 26, No. 2, 227-232.

[23] Abdel-Aty H, Cocker M, Meek C, Tyberg JV, Friedrich MG. Edema as a very early marker for acute myocardial ischemia: a cardiovascular magnetic resonance study J Am Coll Cardiol 2009;53:1194-120.

[24] Saeed M, Wendland MF, Yu KK, Lauerma K, Li HT, Derugin N, Cavagna FM, Higgins CB. Identification of myocardial reperfusion with echoplanar magnetic resonance imaging: discrimination between occlusive and reperfused infarction. Circulation 1994; 90:1492–1501.

[25] Teraoka K, Kiuchi S, Takada N, Hirano M, Yamashina A. Images in cardiovascular medicine. No delayed enhancement on contrast magnetic resonance imaging with Takotsubo cardiomyopathy. Circulation. 2005;111:e261–e262

[26] Rolf A, Nef HM, Mollmann H, et al. Immunohistological basis of the late gadolinium enhancement phenomenon in tako-tsubo cardiomyopathy. *Eur Heart J*. 2009;30:1635-1642.

[27] Taylor AM, Thorne SA, Rubens MB, Jhooti P, Keegan J, Gatehouse PD,Wiesmann F, Grothues F, Somerville J, Pennell DJ. Coronary artery imaging in grown up congenital heart disease: complementary role of magnetic resonance and x-ray coronary angiography. *Circulation*. 2000;101:1670 –1678.

[28] Bluemke DA, Achenbach S, Budoff M, Gerber TC, Gersh B, Hillis LD, Hundley WG, Manning WJ, Printz BF, Stuber M, Woodard PK. Noninvasive coronary artery imaging: magnetic resonance angiography and multidetector computed tomography angiography: a scientific statement from the American Heart Association Committee on Cardiovascular Imaging and Intervention of the Council on Cardiovascular Radiology and Intervention, and the Councils on Clinical Cardiology and Cardiovascular Disease in the Young. *Circulation*. 2008;118:586–606.

[29] Echocardiographic Guidance in Treatment of Cardiogenic Shock Complicating Transient Left Ventricular Apical Ballooning Syndrome. Good CW, Hubbard CR, Harrison TA, Qureshi A: J Am Coll Cardiol Img 2009 March 2; (3):372-374.

[30] Dec, GW. Recognition of the Apical Ballooning Syndrome in the United States. Circulation: 2005;111:388-390.

20

The Use of Contrast-Enhancement Cardiovascular Magnetic Resonance Imaging in Cardiomyopathies

Marlon A.G.M. Olimulder, Michel A. Galjee, Jan van Es, Lodewijk J. Wagenaar and Clemens von Birgelen
Medisch Spectrum Twente
The Netherlands

1. Introduction

The clinical applications of cardiovascular magnetic resonance imaging (CMR), are expanding as the result of the development in hardware, pulse sequence and the ability of post-processing techniques. As the result of the flexibility of CMR to use different pulse-sequences, with or without the use of Gadolinium, CMR has developed as a powerful tool for clinical relevant tissue characterization. CMR in combination with the contrast-enhancement (CE) technique was initially developed to distinguish viable from non-viable myocardium following myocardial infarction. Nowadays, CE-CMR is increasingly used for tissue characterization in ischemic as well as non-ischemic cardiomyopathies to determine the exact etiology, guide proper treatment, and predict outcome and prognosis. In this chapter, we would like to discuss and illustrate the value of CE-CMR imaging in various cardiomyopathies.

2. Utility of different CMR acquisition modes in cardiomyopathy

CMR imaging includes several techniques that can be used in various combinations to assess left ventricular functional parameters, morphology, as well as myocardial disorders (such as edema, scar/fibrosis, microvascular obstruction, myocardial salvage) within one examination. Therefore, it is increasingly used in clinical practice for the diagnosis and management of cardiac diseases. In this respect, recent reviews concerning this aspect have been published (Marcu et al., 2007; Olimulder et al. 2011; Vogel-Claussen et al. 2006; Vohringer 2007; Weinsaft et al. 2007). Some technical aspect of cine - and CE imaging but also T2-weighted imaging (increasingly used when CE imaging is applied) are shortly discussed below.

2.1 Cine CMR for quantitative assessment of ventricular dimension, function and mass

By application of ECG-gated, breath-holding, cine-bright blood sequences, a stack of contiguous left ventricular short-axis slices (5-10 mm thick) are made from basal to apical (figure 1a) (Marcu et al. 2006). CMR is a tomographic technique that uses volumetric quantification based on Simpson's rule. Each separate slice is distributed approximately in 30 phases (simplified in figure 1b; from 1 separate slice, 8 phases from end-diastolic to end-systolic are shown); the endocardium is traced manually in the end-diastolic and end-systolic phase. Left ventricular end-diastolic and end-systolic volume is then calculated by summation of the endocardial surfaces and multiplication by the slice thickness of each separate slice.

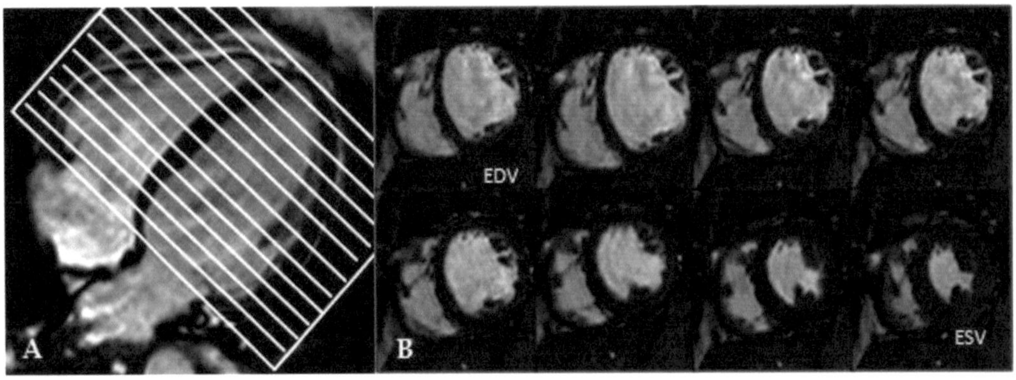

Fig. 1. Schematic figure for A: multiple short axis slices from basal to apical are made from a four chamber view, B: from 1 separate short axis slice, phases from end-diastolic to end-systolic are illustrated.

Left ventricular ejection fraction is calculated by the formula: ((end-diastolic volume – end-systolic volume)/end-diastolic volume) × 100%.
Left ventricular mass can be calculated by 1. tracing the epicardium in the end-diastolic phase in each separate slice; 2. obtaining a myocardial volume by summation of the surfaces between the epicardial and endocardial lines and multiplication by the slice thicknesses; and 3. multiplication of the myocardial volume with weight density (1.05 g/cm^3) of muscle.

2.2 CE-CMR imaging for assessment of damaged myocardium

The technique of CE-CMR imaging involves an intravenous injection of a contrast agent (e.g., gadolinium at a preferred dose of 0.2 mmol/kg body weight) followed by an ECG-gated T1-weight pulse sequence 10-15 minutes after injection (5 minutes after injection if microvascular obstruction is assessed). (Jackson et al. 2007) The timing of the image acquisition is of paramount importance, as too early image acquisition reduces the difference in contrast between normal and damaged myocardium (such as scar or fibrosis) because of an insufficient washout of contrast medium from the normal myocardium; too late image acquisition, on the other hand, may result in an excessive washout from damaged myocardial tissue that leads to an inferior signal-to-noise ratio. (Vogel-Claussen et al. 2006) The typical pulse sequence for CE-CMR imaging is a segmented T1-weighted inversion-recovery-prepared fast gradient-echo sequence. An inversion-recovery pulse is used to null the signal of normal myocardium in order to optimize the difference between normal and damaged myocardial areas (which still contain contrast medium) (Figure 2).

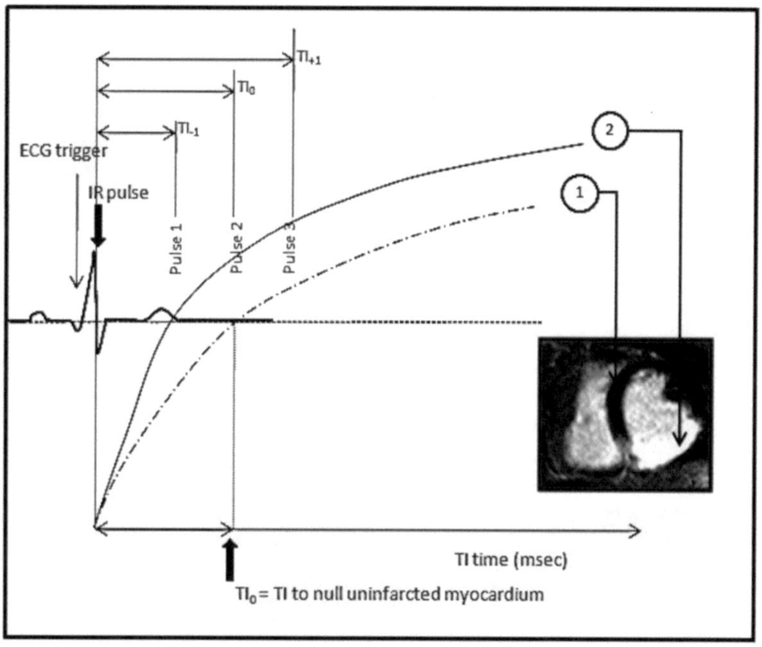

Fig. 2. Schematic figure for inversion time (TI) mapping. Following the ECG trigger, an inversion recovery (IR) pulse is applied. Before image acquisition, low-resolution TI scout images at mid-ventricular level with increasing TI (interval TI 30 msec) are performed. The optimal time to inversion (TI_0) is defined visually as the inversion time at which the uninfarcted myocardium (1) is nulled. (2) = infarcted myocardium.

The optimal inversion time depends on the contrast clearance from the normal myocardium which may show considerable inter-patient variability, depending on several factors such as the patient weight, left ventricular or renal function. Therefore, just before image acquisition, the inversion time is optimized on a per-patient basis using low-resolution scout images at mid-ventricular level with increasing inversion times at intervals of 30ms, from which the optimal inversion time can be derived (Jackson et al. 2007). The process is synchronized to the *R*-wave of the ECG and mid-diastolic images are acquired every other heart beat during breath-hold (Marcu et al. 2007).

2.3 T2-weighted CMR imaging for assessment of myocardial edema

T2-weighted CMR imaging is a pulse sequence sensitive to regional or global increases of myocardial water (a substantial feature of inflammatory responses) (Zagrosek et al. 2008; bdel-Aty et al. 2005). Therefore very useful in the (sub) acute phase of myocardial infarction and myocarditis. The long T2 relaxation times of water-bound protons are used to generate a water-specific contrast when applying T2-weighted sequences resulting in a high signal intensity of edematous tissue. Standard T2-weighted imaging of myocardial edema typically utilizes turbo spin-echo readouts with or without fat saturation pulses (to separate fat from water), mostly combined with dark-blood preparation (Eitel et al. 2011). An alternative acquisition mode can be the T2-prepared steady state free precession technique, which may be more reliable in imaging edema as it provides fewer artifacts and has better diagnostic accuracy than conventional darkblood acquisitions (Kellman et al. 2007).

3. CE-CMR findings in the different cardiomyopathies

3.1 CE-CMR after myocardial infarction

Myocardial infarction occurs after coronary occlusion of at least 20-30 minutes (without sufficient collateral blood supply to the affected myocardium) (Edelman, 2004). In the early phase of myocardial infarction, cellular degradation in the infarcted myocardium results in an increase in the permeability and enlargement of the extravascular space (edema), and thus, an increased distribution volume for the CMR contrast agent. Later on, due to different wash-in and wash-out kinetics, myocardial scars retain contrast agents longer than normal myocardium. The net result of both mechanisms is that infarcted myocardium appears bright on CE-T1-weighted images.

CE in patients with MI generally shows a typical pattern that is related to the perfusion area of the culprit vessel. Myocardial changes (and thus CE) of the subendocardium can generally be found which may extend to a transmural distribution in cases with prolonged coronary occlusion (Figure 3a,b).

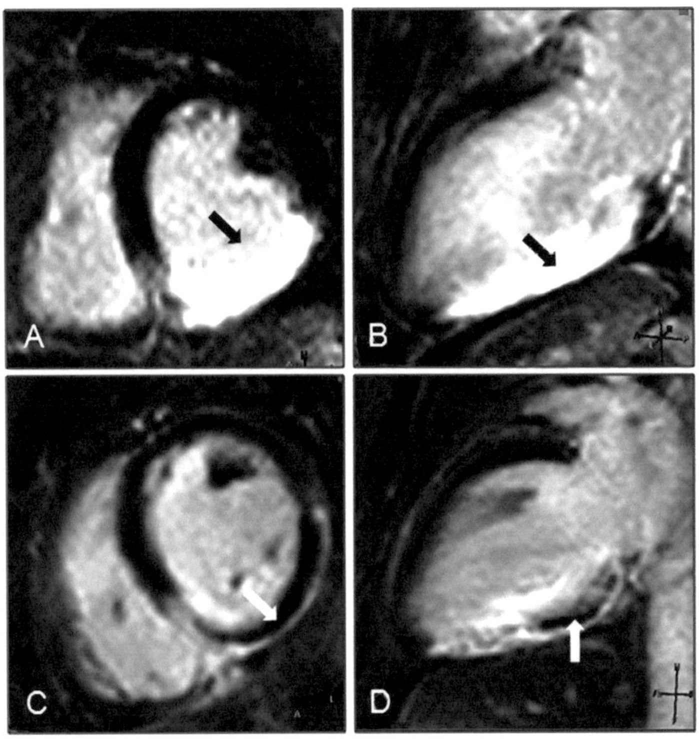

Fig. 3. CE-CMR patterns post myocardial infarction. A,B: CE short axis and long axis view showing transmural inferior infarction (black arrow). C,D: Short axis and long axis view showing an inferior infarction with microvascular obstruction (white arrow).

In patients after MI, the assessment of myocardial viability can provide clinically important information to guide further treatment because only viable myocardium may benefit from revascularization (Kim et al., 2005). Generally, a standardized 17 myocardial segment-model is used to report the results of viability assessment by CE-CMR (Figure 4) (Cerquira et al., 2002).

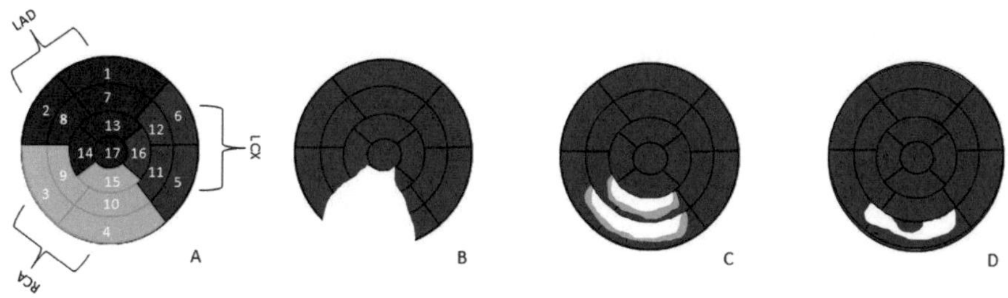

Fig. 4. Bulls eye scheme according to the 17 segmental model, demonstrating CE characteristics post myocardial infarction. A: assignment of the 17 segments to one of the 3 major coronary arteries, with segment 1, 2, 7,8, 13, 14, and 17 corresponding to the left anterior descending coronary artery ; segments 3, 4, 9, 10 and 15 corresponding to the right coronary artery when it is dominant; and segments 5, 6, 11, 12, and 16 are assigned to the left circumflex artery. B: Transmural inferior MI. C: Inferoseptal MI with a core zone (white area) and a peri infarction zone (gray area). D: Inferior MI with microvascular obstruction (black area in myocardial infarction area).

In addition, quantification of infarcted tissue helps to prognosticate left ventricular remodeling (Orn et al., 2007). In this respect, the transmural extent of infarcted tissue as determined by CE-CMR has been shown to be a powerful predictor of the contractile response to both medical therapy and myocardial revascularization (Weinsaft et al., 2007).
Primary coronary intervention with stent implantation is meanwhile the standard for treatment of all acute ST-segment elevation myocardial infarctions, even in cases with a very challenging anatomy (Basalus et al., 2009). The early intervention rapidly restores the patency of the epicardial coronary vessels and often improves the prognosis, as is early indicated by ST-segment resolution on the electrocardiogram (van der Zwaan et al., 2010). Nowadays, aspiration of thrombi is often performed prior to stent implantation in thrombus-containing lesions in order to minimize distal embolization (Hermens et al. 2010; Stoel et al., 2009) that contributes to the development of left ventricular dysfunction after MI. In our recent CMR study, we also found that left ventricular wall motion abnormalities were significantly better in patients who underwent successful early revascularization for acute myocardial infarction (Olimulder et al., 2011).
Increasing interest is also laid on the assessment of characteristics of infarcted myocardial tissue as potential predictor of life-threatening ventricular arrhythmias. Recently, a highly significant relation between inferior MI and ventricular arrhythmias has been observed (Pascale et al. 2009). Multivariate analysis of data from 91 patients suggested that the heterogeneity of infarcted tissue (also called peri infarct zone or border zone), can be an important predictor of spontaneous ventricular arrhythmias (Roes et al., 2009).
The area of CE tends to be larger during the acute phase of MI (first week) and progressively decreases in size during the healing phase (1-4 weeks), until it reaches the state of a healed myocardial infarction (after 4 weeks) (Thygesen et al. 2007). These observations are consistent with the established pathological understanding of remodeling after MI: during the acute phase, there is myocardial edema which subsequently regresses while the necrotic myocardium is replaced by scar tissue (Marcu et al., 2007). Experimental studies have revealed that final MI size is strongly influenced by the extent of the edema in the acute phase, which is also called *area at risk*. By combining T2-weighted images to visualize myocardial edema (and thus the area at risk) and CE-CMR imaging to visualize scar (the *final infarct size*), a *myocardial salvage index* can be calculated by subtracting the infarct size from the area at risk (Aletras et al.,

2006). The myocardial salvage index has recently shown to be independently associated with adverse left ventricular remodeling and early ST-segment resolution, and may represent an interesting parameter for the assessment of novel reperfusion strategies in patients with myocardial infarction (trial registration number: NL19151.044.07).

In addition, some patients develop microvascular obstruction within the ischemic myocardial region in the acute phase of a myocardial infarction (Masci et al. 2010). Microvascular obstruction is represented by a dark zone within the infarcted region, usually located in the subendocardium because the contrast medium does not reach this area (Figure 3c,d). Its presence is associated with greater left ventricular remodeling and inferior clinical outcome. (Nijveldt et al. 2008).

3.2 CE-CMR in nonischemic cardiomyopathies

3.2.1 Hypertrophic cardiomyopathy

Hypertrophic cardiomyopathy is a primary myocardial disease characterized by focal (mostly septal) or diffuse left ventricular wall thickening (with or without left ventricular outflow obstruction). Myofibrillar hypertrophy and disarray and myocardial fibrosis have been described histologically. Inadequate capillary density and intimal hyperplasia of intramural coronary arteries, which were also seen in such patients, may contribute to myocardial ischemia (Marcu et al., 2007). There are predilection patterns of CE in patients with hypertrophic cardiomyopathies: more than 80% of patients exhibit patchy fibrosis at the right ventricular insertion points and in the anteroseptal wall in the region of characteristic septal thickening (Figure 5ab; Figure 6a) (Moon et al., 2003; Choudhury et al., 2002).

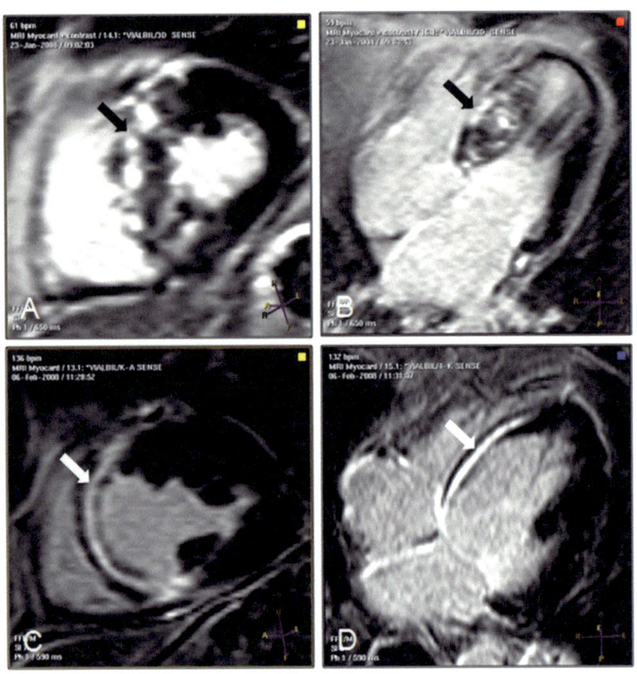

Fig. 5. CE-CMR patterns in nonischemic cardiomyopathies. A,B: CE short axis and long axis view showing hypertrophic cardiomyopathy with patchy CE septal and in the right ventricular insertion points. (black arrow). C,D: Short axis and long axis view showing dilated cardiomyopathy with CE having septal midwall predominance (white arrow).

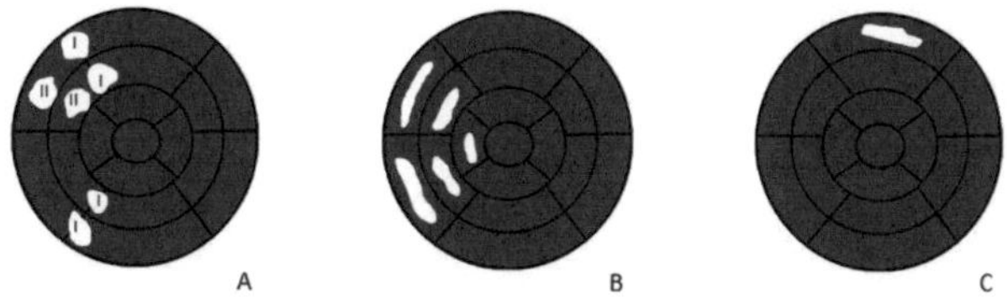

Fig. 6. Bulls eye scheme according to the 17 segmental model, demonstrating typical CE patterns in nonischemic cardiomyopathies. A: Hypertrophic cardiomyopathy with predilection CE (i.e., fibrosis) pattern at the right ventricular insertion points (I) and anteroseptal (II). Myocardial fibrosis is also located in non-hypertrophic segments. B: Idiopathic dilated cardiomyopathy with CE predominantly located in the midwall with septal predominance. C: Arrhythmogenic right ventricular cardiomyopathy with midwall CE found in the basal anterior region. CE is also found in the right ventricular outflow tract.

Myocardial fibrosis, however, is also located in non-hypertrophic segments (Bohl et al., 2008). As the amount of CE in hypertrophic cardiomyopathies often corresponds with functional parameters and the frequency of cardiac events, CE-CMR may potentially be useful for risk stratification and selection for implantable cardioverter defibrillator implantation (Rubinstein et al., 2010). Presence and extent of CE following percutaneous alcohol septal ablation for the treatment of significant left ventricular outflow tract obstruction indicates the location and extent of therapeutic myocardial tissue destruction. (Sievers et al., 2002).

3.2.2 Idiopathic dilated cardiomyopathy

Idiopathic dilated cardomyopathy is characterized by dilation and impaired contractility of the left ventricle or both ventricles in the absence of abnormal loading conditions (e.g., arterial hypertension; valvular disease), and/or a cardiomyopathy with a distinct cause (e.g., ischemic heart disease; peripartum cardiomyopathy; toxin, chemotherapy or tachycardia induced cardiomyopathy; certain endocrinopathies) (Mueller & Attili, 2008). Histology is nonspecific and a variety of myocardial tissue alterations may occur or coexist, including myocyte hypertrophy and segmental or diffuse interstitial fibrosis. Current CE-CMR techniques are unlikely to detect diffuse fibrosis due to limited voxel resolution (Vohringer et al., 2006). Myocardial fibrosis in idiopathic dilated cardiomyopathy is mostly seen in the left ventricular midwall with septal predominance and a linear pattern (Figure 5c,d; Figure 6b); however, it has occasionally been described at subendocardial and subepicardial locations with a more patchy pattern. (Bohl et al., 2008). Of note, in various studies the prevalence of myocardial fibrosis varied from 13% to 62% (Yokokawa et al., 2009; Isbell et al., 2006). It has been suggested that the degree of CE may correlate with functional impairment of the left ventricle (Koito et al., 1996). There are preliminary data demonstrating that the presence of CE is associated with an unfavorable clinical outcome and may be a predictor of sudden death in patients with idiopathic dilated cardiomyopathy (Yokokawa et al., 2009, 2009; Assomull et al., 2009).

3.2.3 Arrhythmogenic right ventricular cardiomyopathy

The arrhythmogenic right ventricular cardiomyopathy is characterized by structural and functional abnormalities, with progressive fibrous and fatty infiltration involving variable regions of the right and left ventricular myocardium. This process finally leads to progressive right ventricular failure and ventricular tachyarrhythmia (Bohl et al., 2008). Diagnosis of this condition remains a challenge, with nonspecific abnormalities on echocardiographic and angiographic examinations. Endomyocardial biopsy has a low sensitivity, as samples are usually taken from the septum, a region that is infrequently involved (Bohl et al., 2008). Further, endomyocardial biopsy is potential a dangerous procedure.

Information from CE-CMR may help to guide targeted endomyocardial biopsies. Predilection patterns with midwall CE are found in the basal anterior region (Figure 6c) and/or the right ventricular outflow tract. These patterns of fibrosis correlate with fibro-fatty replacement of the myocardium at histologic assessment and predict induction of ventricular tachycardia during electrophysiological studies. As the presence of arrhythmogenic right ventricular cardiomyopathy cannot be ruled out based on CMR findings alone, standardized guidelines have been proposed which define major and minor criteria, including morphological, histological, electrocardiographic, functional, and genetic characteristics (McKenna et al., 1994).

3.3 CE-CMR in myocarditis

3.3.1 Myocarditis

Myocarditis is an acute or chronic inflammatory disease of the myocardium, which can be caused by viruses or initiated by post-infectious immune or primarily organ-specific autoimmune responses. (Caforio et al., 2002). Patients generally recover or infrequently develop dilated cardiomyopathy, sometimes even with life-threatening complications including severe heart failure and malignant arrhythmias (Zagrosek et al., 2008). Diagnosis of myocarditis is challenging because of a diverse clinical presentation and a limited sensitivity of endomyocardial biopsies, but may be facilitated by use of CE-CMR or myocardial global relative enhancement CMR (bdel-Aty et al., 2005; Gutberlet et al., 2008). Diagnosis of acute myocarditis is more important nowadays because of the therapeutic medical options in selected patients. (Corsten et al., 2010). Presence of CE has been reported in 44-95% of patients with myocarditis, (Mahrholdt et al., 2004, 2006) indicating areas of myocardial damage with a sensitivity of 100% and a specificity of 90% (compared to histopathology) (Mahrholdt et al., 2004). In acute myocarditis, CE is frequently located in the lateral wall, originating from the epicardium. The subendocardium is generally not involved, with the exception of eosinophilic myocarditis, which frequently involves the endomyocardium (Figure 7a). (Bohl et al., 2008; Deb et al., 2008).

In chronic myocarditis, besides an increased edema on T2-weighted imaging, an increased global relative enhancement is a common finding as confirmed in immunohistological analyses. (Gutberlet et al., 2008). CE-CMR identified areas of myocardial damage in 70% of patients with biopsy-proven chronic myocarditis and showed a predilection pattern (left ventricular midwall and/or subepicardial). In myocarditis, CE may provide additional information that could help to differentiate between viral origins, as in the majority of parvovirus B19 patients, CE is found in the lateral free wall, while in patients with human herpes virus 6 myocarditis CE frequently involves the interventricular septal midwall (Yelgec et al;2007). In addition, we recently studied a limited number of patients with chronic fatigue syndrome and concomitant ebstein barr virus or cytomegalovirus myocarditis who showed in the presence of CE a certain predilection of the septal region. Inflammatory activity on T2-weighted imaging and myocardial fibrosis on CE-CMR may have relevant prognostic implications in acute and chronic myocarditis and may ultimatively serve as a tool to triage patients. In addition, cardiac function and regression of myocardial changes can be well observed with CMR.

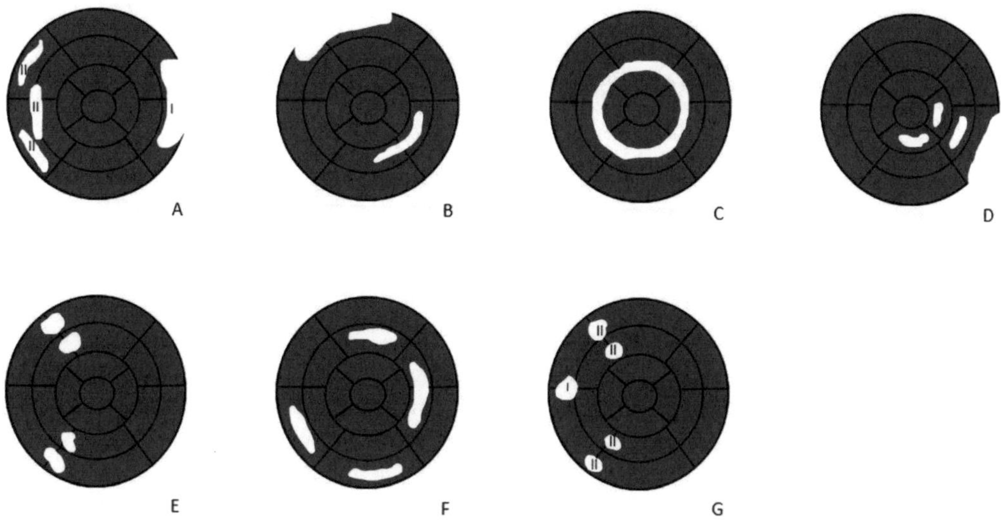

Fig. 7. Bulls eye scheme according to the 17 segmental model, demonstrating typical CE patterns in myocarditis and cardiac involvement of other diseases.
A: Myocarditis with CE frequently located in the lateral wall originating from the epicardium (I). CE patterns in myocarditis differ according to viral origin, with parvovirus B19 having CE in the lateral free wall (I), HHV6 having CE frequently in the interventricular septal midwall (II), and chronic fatigue syndrome myocarditis having CE anteroseptal and inferoseptal (III). B: Sarcoidosis with CE midwall or epicardial; however subendocardial or transmural CE may be observed. C: Amyloidosis , usually with a global diffuse CE pattern, frequently involving the subendocardium. D: Chagas' disease with CE epicardial or midwall, with a predilection pattern inferolateral. E. Pulmonary hypertension with CE involving the right ventricular insertion points and the interventricular septum. F: Muscular dystrophy with CE observed in the midwall. G: Chloroquine induced cardiomyopathy with hypertrophy and accompanying CE in the basal septum (I) and the right ventricular insertion points (I).

3.4 CE-CMR in systemic diseases inducing cardiomyopathy

3.4.1 Sarcoidosis

Cardiac involvement in sarcoidosis, a multisystem granulomatous disorder of unknown etiology, is clinically often asymptomatic (95%) while autopsy revealed cardiac manifestation in up to 60% (Patel et al., 2009). *Advanced* sarcoidosis leads to septal thinning, systolic and diastolic dysfunction, and pericardial effusion which can be detected with echocardiography (Jackson et al., 2007). *Early* sarcoidosis, however, is more challenging to diagnose, and CMR can be very useful in this context. During the acute stage of this disease, regions of active inflammation and edema are visible on T2-weighted images as areas of increased signal intensity. During the chronic stage, CE will typically appear as a midwall or epicardial nonischemic pattern (Figure 7b; figure 8).

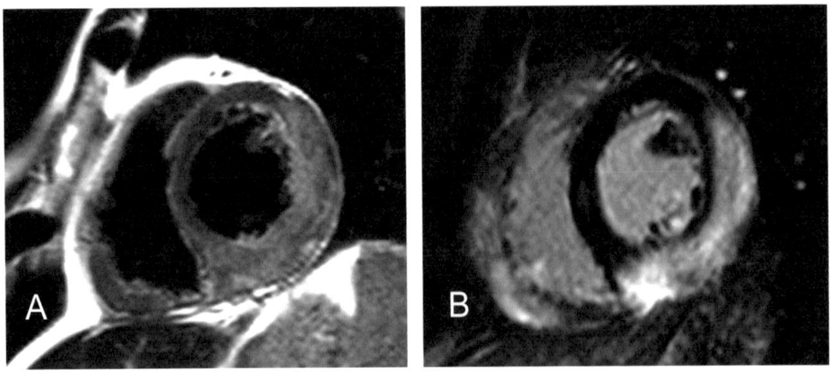

Fig. 8. CMR in a patient with sarcoidosis. A: T2 weighted imaging shorta axix view showing Figure 8 hyperenhancement epicardial inferior, inferolateral and anterolateral.
B: Short axis view showing CE epicardial inferior, inferolateral and anterolateral.

But occasionally subendocardial or transmural CE may be observed, mimicking a pattern of post-MI. CE has been found in 50% of all patients diagnosed with sarcoidosis (Shimada et al., 2001). CE-CMR may also be useful to evaluate the response to therapy. In a CMR study of patients with sarcoidosis, CE was markedly diminished 1 month after the initiation of steroid therapy (Shimada et al., 2001). CE in sarcoidosis patients may be associated with future adverse events (including cardiac death) but confirmation in larger patient cohorts is required (Patel et al., 2009).

3.4.2 Amyloidosis

Both primary and secondary amyloidosis are characterized by extracellular deposition of fibrillar proteins (Mueller et al, 2008), which may lead to restrictive cardiomyopathy with an initially preserved systolic left ventricular function (Wynne et al., 2005). In cardiac amyloidosis, CE is commonly found as a result of the expansion of interstitial space and some endomyocardial fibrosis (Maceira et al., 2008), leading to a usually global and diffuse CE pattern (Jackson et al., 2007). Although the subendocardium is commonly involved (as in ischemic heart disease), the distribution of CE is not related to a particular coronary perfusion area (Figure 7c; figure 9) (Jackson et al., 2007).

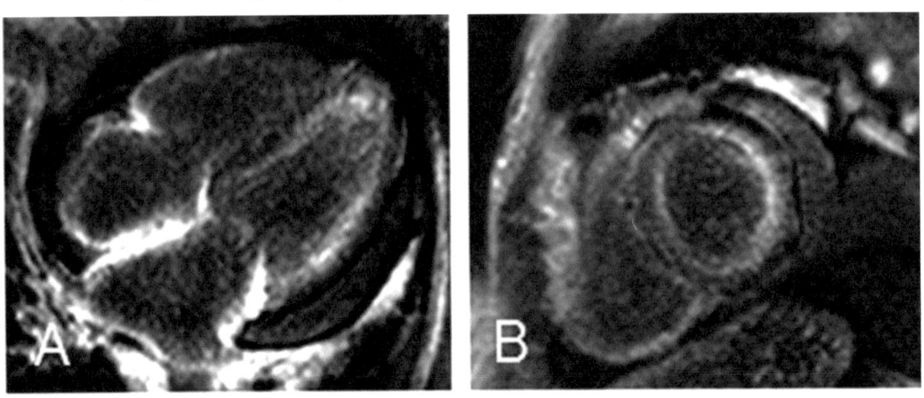

Fig. 9. CMR in a patient with amyloidosis.
A,B: four chamber and short axis view showing diffuse subendocardial CE.

3.4.3 Chagas' disease

The parasitic protozoan Trypanosoma cruzi causes Chagas' disaese, which is endemic in the Latin American region (Jackson et al., 2007). During chronic disease, the heart is the most frequently affected organ, and patients present with refractory heart failure, disorders of the conduction system, or ventricular tachycardia (Marcu et al., 2007; Rochitte et al., 2005). The fundamental pathological processes include an inflammatory response, cellular damage with a broad variation of intensity (minimal alterations up to extensive necrosis), and fibrosis (Rochitte et al., 2007). Early cardiac involvement may be detected by CE-CMR before the onset of symptoms (Rochitte et al., 2003). CE is often located epicardial or in the left ventricle midwall with a inferolateral predilection pattern (Figure 7d), but other regions - including the apex - may also sometimes be affected (Jackson et al., 2007).

3.4.4 Pulmonary hypertension

Pulmonary arterial hypertension, both primary and secondary, is characterized by an increased pulmonary vascular resistance that results in pressure overload on the right ventricle (Kovacs et al., 2008). Cine CMR permits accurate assessment of right ventricular mass and volumes which is often difficult to accomplish with other imaging modalities (Marcu et al., 2007). Myocardial CE is frequently observed in patients with severe symptomatic pulmonary artery hypertension with predilection patterns involving both right ventricular septal insertion points and the interventricular septum (Figure 7e). CE in the interventricular septum was found to be associated with septal bowing (on cine CMR), and the extent of CE correlated inversely with right ventricular systolic function (Blyth et al., 2005).

3.4.5 Muscular dystrophy

Both Becker and Duchenne muscular dystrophies are progressive X chromosome-linked recessive neuromuscular diseases with myocardial involvement in up to 72% of patients showing a mildly reduced left ventricular function up to severe left ventricular impairment and dilated cardiomyopathy. Cardiac myocyte dystrophin deficiency leads to necrosis causing replacement of damaged myocardium by connective tissue and fat in both ventricles. On CE-CMR, hyperenhancement is predominantly seen in left ventricular midwall (Figure 7f) and has been described in 73-100% of patients (Yilmaz et al., 2008). Early diagnosis of myocardial involvement as assessed with CE-CMR may permit an earlier treatment of heart failure which could increase life expectancy.

3.4.6 Chloroquine-induced cardiomyopathy

Chloroquine-induced cardiomyopathy is a rare iatrogenic disease that is associated with long-term intake of chloroquine, which is most frequently prescribed for treatment of rheumatoid arthritis and malaria prophylaxis (Reffelman et al., 2006). This cardiomyopathy is characterized by ineffective lysosomal metabolism because of an increase in pH that leads to accumulation of lysosomal glycosphingolipids and finally thickening of cardiac walls (Pieroni et al., 2007). The time interval between the start of chloroquine therapy and disease manifestation varies greatly, ranging from several months to more than 20 years (Reffelman et al., 2006). CMR may demonstrate the presence of left ventricular hypertrophy with accompanying areas of CE in the basal septum and at the insertion point of the right ventricle (Figure 7g).

Fabry disease, an X chromosome-linked lysosomal storage disease caused by a deficient activity of the enzyme α-galactosidase A, can also result in the accumulation of glycosphingolipids in multiple organs, including the heart (Pieroni et al., 2007; Gange et al.,2009). Fabry disease cardiomypathy should therefore always be considered in the differential diagnosis of "idiopathic" left ventricular hypertrophy (in the absence of arterial hypertension or valvular disease).

3.5 CE-CMR in other diseases inducing cardiomyopathy

3.5.1 Tsako Tsubo cardiomyopathy

This relatively 'novel' cardiomyopathy is characterized by acute but rapidly reversible distinctive regional left ventricular dysfunction, in the absence of significant coronary artery disease. Japanese investigators were intrigued by the unusual end-systolic shape of the left ventricle, resembling the original Japanese octupus trap (figure 10a) (Sharkey et al., 2011).

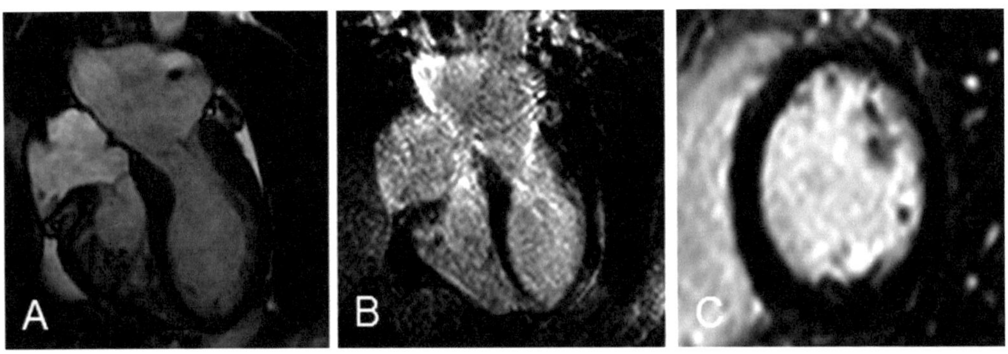

Fig. 10. CMR of a patient with tsako tsubo. A: cine four chamber view with characteristic end-systolic apical ballooning. B,C: four chamber and short axis view with no presence of CE in the myocardium.

Consequently, the term tsako tsubo cardiomyopathy was introduced in 1990. Several pathofysiological mechanisms have been proposed, including multivessel coronary spasm, catecholamine induced myocardial stunning, coronary emboli with spontaneous fibrinolysis, and myocardial inflammation (Eitel et al., 2010). Recently, variant forms are described, including inverted tako-tsubo and mid-ventricular ballooning cardiomyopathy (Marti et al., 2009; Yasu et al., 2006).

In the setting of tako tsubo cardiomyopathy, CMR may identify increased myocardial mass and myocardial edema (using T2-weighted imaging) as well as the normalization of these parameters as the left ventricular dysfunction improves. (Stensaeth et al. 2011). Of important note, (with only a few exceptions, reported in literature) (Koeth et al. 2008) no CE is present in this disease, consistent with preserved myocardial viability, as reflected by the transient nature of left ventricular dysfunction (figure10b) (Eitel et al, 2010; Deetjen et al., 2006) .At follow up, there is complete normalization of left ventricular function, in the absence of CE, edema and pericardial effusion (Eitel et al., 2010; Koeth et al., 2008). The lack of CE (initial and follow up) allows thus for distinction between different causative aetiologies including MI, infiltrative diseases and cases of myocarditis.

Therefore, CMR in combination with T2 weighted imaging and CE may provide valuable additional information for the differential diagnoses and therapeutic decision-making in patients with suspected tako tsubo cardiomyopathy.

3.5.2 Noncompaction cardiomyopathy

Left ventricular noncompaction cardiomyopathy is characterized by a thin, compacted epicardial layer and a thick endocardial layer with prominent trabeculation and deep recessesm (figure 11) (Jacuier et al,).

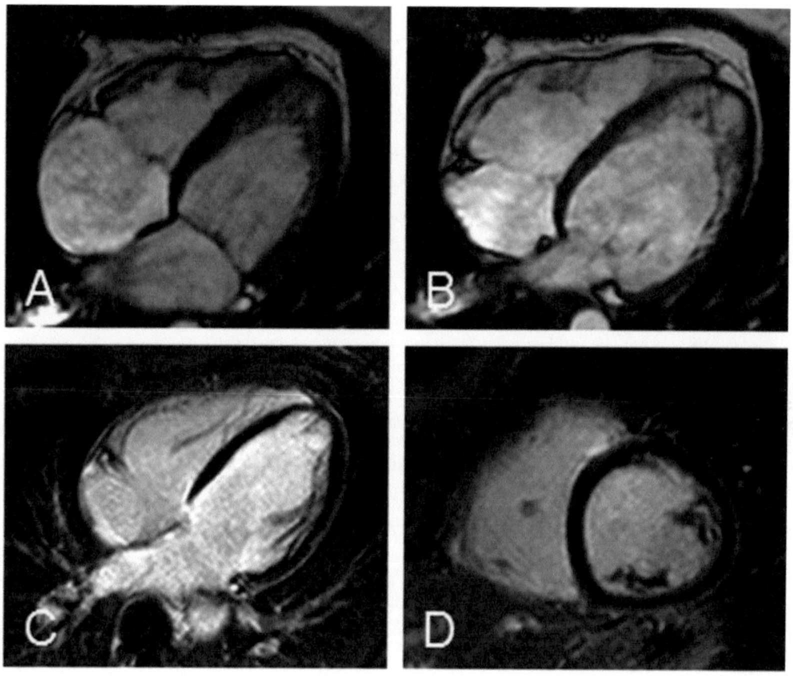

Fig. 11. Patient with noncompaction cardiomyopathy. A,B: end-systolic and end-diastolic four chamber view with characteristic prominent trabeculation and deep recessesm. C,D: four chamber and short axis view with no presence of CE.

It can occur isolated or in association with numerous congenital cardiac malformations, including atrial and ventricular septal defects, aortic stenosis, and aortic calcification. It is usually diagnosed in pediatric age. Accurate diagnostic criteria are clinically important as it is associated with severe left ventricular dysfunction, thrombo-embolism, and ventricular arrhythmia. According to Jacuier et al., a CMR-assessed trabeculated left ventricular mass above 20% of the global left ventricular mass is highly sensitive and specific for the diagnosis of left ventricular noncompaction. Right ventricular noncompaction which can be easily assessed with CMR, is reported in up to 60% op patients (Dursun et al., 2010). Recently, Dursun et al. found that presence of CE (fibrosis) was found in 70% of the investigated patients with left ventricular noncompaction. Dodd et al, showed that the amount of CE in patients with left ventricular noncompaction is inversely related with left ventricular ejection fraction (Dodd et al., 2007). The presence of CE is thus probably of bad prognosis in this disease (Jacquier et al., 2010).

3.5.3 CE-CMR imaging in chemotherapy induced cardiomyopathy

Several chemotherapeutic therapies in the setting of malignant diseases have been associated with the development of cardiac failure. Chemotherapies with a high incidence of cardiac failure are anthracyclines (doxorubicin) 3-26%, and monoclonal antibodies (trastuzumab) 2-28% (Yeh et al., 2009). The cumulative dose (especially doxorubicin; cumulative dose 550 mg/m^2), the administration schedule, concomitant use of other cardiotoxic therapies, and a history of cardiovascular disease, determines the likelihood of inducing cardiomyopathy.
Little is known about the utility of CE-CMR in the assessment of chemotherapy induced cardiomyopathy. Fallah-Rad et al. reported in 10 out of 160 breast cancer patients with trastuzumab induced cardiomyopahty (left ventricular ejection fraction < 40%), presence of epicardial CE. Recently, Kirthy et al. studied (using CE-CMR) 12 breast cancer patients with adjuvant trastuzumab; whereas left ventricular dysfunction was observed, no evidence of necrosis or fibrosis was found in any of the patients (Kirthy et al., 2011). Data on other chemotherapy induced cardiomypathy assessed with CE-CMR are scarce (Lightfoot et al., 2010; Wassmuth et al., 2001; Wu et al., 2009). Therefore, further studies are needed to validate the usefulness of CE-CMR as a marker for (irreversible) left ventricular dysfunction and development as well as prevention of cardiac failure when chemotherapy is given.

4. Guided endomyocardial biopsy

CE patterns on CMR imaging may also help to guide endomyocardial biopsies as scar/fibrosis patterns on CE-CMR may serve as a map for the exact location to accomplish endomyocardial biopsies if necessary; thus enhancing the diagnostic accuracy. A small study has indeed confirmed that the diagnostic performance of endomyocardial biopsies is increased when biopsies are obtained from the region of CE in the case of myocarditis (Mahrholdt et al., 2004, 2006). However, according to Yilmaz et al. who where unable to confirm the value of CE-CMR for guiding endomyocardial biopsies, endomyocardial biopsies exactly obtained from the region of CE may sometimes be impracticle as the area of CE may be small and as a consequence cannot exactly be reached by the bioptome because of the limited steerability of the bioptome (Yilmaz et al., 2010).

5. Screening for cardiomyopathy

Cardiomyopathy can occur as part of inherited syndromes. In the case of hypertrophic cardiomyopathy, over 900 gene mutations have been linked. The gene mutations predominantly encode for contractile proteins, such as cardiac myosin-binding protein C (MYBPC3) and beta-myosin heavy chain (MYH7) (thick filament of the sarcomere), and troponin T and troponin I (encoding for thin filament of the sarcomere; accounting for ≈ 6% of the hypertrophic cardiomyopathy-causing mutations). Next to sarcomeric mutations, several metabolic disorders are linked to the hypertrophic cardiomyopathy phenotype, such as Fabry disease (as mentioned above), an X chromosome-linked lysosomal storage disease (Brouwer et al., 2011). Thus, there is currently no consensus of a definitive screening test based on genetic studies for hypertrophic cardiomyopathy. Additionally, genetic screening can not differentiate between gene carriers who express the disease and those who do not (Devlin et al., 2000). As a consequence, the heterogeneous expression includes patients suffering from severe symptomatic hypertrophic cardiomyopathy (diminished left ventricular function and fibrosis of the myocardium) as well as asymptomatic individuals.

CE-CMR imaging is able to provide accurate assessment of functional parameters and myocardial disorders in one single examination. Therefore, familial screening (especially in autosomal dominant disorders) with CE-CMR may be of utmost importance as individual findings may have significant therapeutic consequences.
As an example, in our tertiary centre, an 18 year old female patient was diagnosed with familiar hypertrophic cardiomyopathy (cardiac myosin-binding protein C). CE-CMR imaging revealed assymmetrical septal hypertrophy (septal thickness 38 mm) and presence of fibrosis (figure 12).

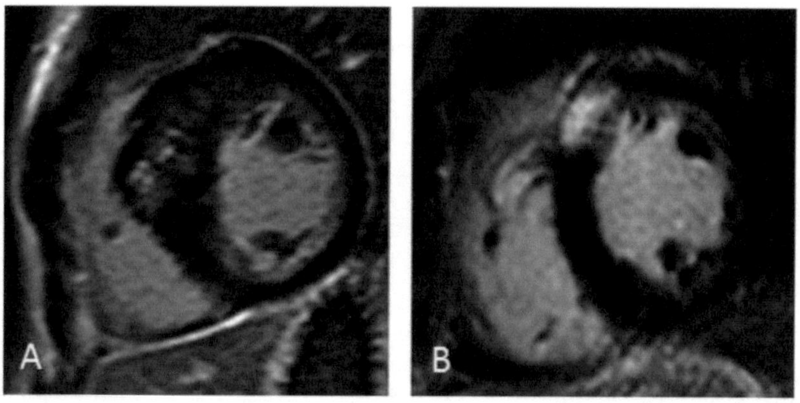

Fig. 12. Screening a relative for cardiomyopathy A. 18 year old female patient with genetic disorder cardiac myosin-binding protein C. Short axis view showing assymetrical septal hypertrophy with CE anteroseptal. B. 56 year old male patient (father) with the same genetic disorder. Short axis view showing identical CE anteroseptal.

Following the guidelines (septal thickness >30 mm) in addition with a medical history of a collapse, she was selected for implantable cardioverter defibrillator therapy (Maron et al., 2003). Her father, (familiar screened and having the same genetic disorder) showed the same pattern of assymetrical septal hypertrophy (septal thickness 24 mm) and presence of fibrosis with CE-CMR imaging, following the guidelines not an indication for implantable cardioverter defibrillator therapy. As mentioned earlier, the amount of CE in hypertrophic cardiomyopathies often corresponds with functional parameters and the frequency of cardiac events, therefore CE-CMR may potentially be useful for risk stratification and selection for implantable cardioverter defibrillator implantation.

6. Future developments

Several new strategies for the treatment of the various forms of cardiomypathy are currently subject of research, including the transplantation of primitive cell types (e.g., stem cells or myoblasts) into damaged myocardium in an attempt to promote trans-differentiation into functional myocardial cells. CE-CMR imaging can be used to monitor such studies and to evaluate the results of novel therapeutic strategies such as direct injection of primitive cell types into segments with transmural infarction. (Orlic et al., 2002). In animal models, mesenchymal stem cells have been labeled with iron-based contrast agents to examine the process of "homing" of such cells in the myocardium (Hill et al., 2003; Kraitchman et al., 2003; Garot et al., 2003).

Recently, 3.0 T CMR imaging with a 3D inversion-recovery gradient-echo sequence was compared to standard 2D imaging. The 3D technique showed superior spatial image resolution, shorter image acquisition time, preserved contrast-to-noise ratio, and similar intra and interobserver variabilities (compared to the 2D approach), which could improve the clinical utility of CE-CMR in the future (Bauner et al., 2009). At higher heart rates, though, motion artifacts can be seen.

7. Conclusion

CE-CMR is increasingly used to establish the etiology, monitor therapeutic strategies (follow up), and obtain prognostic information in a variety of cardiomyopathies. While CE-CMR can provide valuable information, there is considerable overlap in CE patterns. For that reason, CE-CMR findings should always be considered in the light of the clinical history and presentation as well as findings obtained from other diagnostic modalities. Development in CMR hardware and software are required for the ability to perform tissue characterization which fully corresponds with histopathological findings.

8. References

Aletras, AH.; Tilak, GS.; Natanzon, A.; Hsu, LY.; Gonzalez, FM.; Hoyt, RF. & Arai AE. (2006). Retrospective determination of the area at risk for reperfused acute myocardial infarction with T2-weighted cardiac magnetic resonance imaging: histopathological and displacement encoding with stimulated echoes (DENSE) functional validations. *Circulation*, Vol.113, No.15, (April 2006), pp. 1865-1870.

Amado, LC.; Gerber, BL.; Gupta, SN.; Rettman, DW.; Szarf, G.; Schock, B.; Nasir K.; Kraitchman, DL.; & Lima, JA. (2004). Accurate and objective infarct sizing by contrast-enhanced magnetic resonance imaging in a canine myocardial infarction model. *J Am Coll Cardiol* , Vol.44, No.12, (December 2004), pp.2383-2389.

Assomull ,RG.; Prasad, SK.; Lyne, J.; Smith, G.; Burman, ED.; Khan, M.; Sheppard MN.; Poole-Wilson, PA. & Pennell DJ. (2006). Cardiovascular magnetic resonance, fibrosis, and prognosis in dilated cardiomyopathy. *J Am Coll Cardiol*, Vol.48, No10, (November 2006), pp. 1977-1985.

Basalus, M.; Louwerenburg, JW.; van Houwelingen, KG.; Stoel, MG. & von Birgelen, C. (2009). Primary percutaneous coronary intervention in the left main stem of a monocoronary artery. *Neth Heart J* , Vol.17 No.7-8, (Augustus 2009), pp. 274-276.

Bauner, KU.; Muehling, O.; Theisen, D.; Hayes, C.; Wintersperger, BJ.; Reiser, MF. & Huber, AM. (2009). Assessment of Myocardial Viability with 3D MRI at 3 T. AJR *Am J Roentgenol*, Vol.192, No.6, (Juny 2009), pp. 1645-1650.bdel-Aty, H.; Boye, P.; Zagrosek, A.; Wassmuth, R.; Kumar, A.; Messroghli, D.; Bock, P.;

Dietz, R.; Friedrich, MG. & Schulz-Menger J. (2005). Diagnostic performance of cardiovascular magnetic resonance in patients with suspected acute myocarditis: comparison of different approaches. *J Am Coll Cardiol*, Vol.45, No11, (Juny 2005), pp. 1815-1822.

Bello, D.; Fieno, DS.; Kim, RJ.; Pereles, FS.; Passman, R.; Song, G.; Kadish, AH. & Goldberger, JJ. (2005). Infarct morphology identifies patients with substrate for sustained ventricular tachycardia. *J Am Coll Cardiol* , Vol.45, No7, (April 2005), pp. 1104-1108.

Blyth, KG.; Groenning, BA.; Martin, TN.; Foster, JE.; Mark, PB.; Dargie, HJ. & Peacock, AJ. (2005). Contrast enhanced-cardiovascular magnetic resonance imaging in patients with pulmonary hypertension. *Eur Heart J*, Vol.26, No.19, (Oktober 2005), pp. 1993-1999.

Bohl, S.; Wassmuth, R.; bdel-Aty, H.; Rudolph, A.; Messroghli, D.; Dietz, R. & Schulz-Menger, J. (2008). Delayed enhancement cardiac magnetic resonance imaging reveals typical patterns of myocardial injury in patients with various forms of non-ischemic heart disease. *Int J Cardiovasc Imaging*, Vol.24, No.6, (Augustus 2008), pp. 597-607.

Brouwer, WP.; van Dijk, SJ.; Stienen, GJ.; van Rossum, AC.; van der Velden, J. & Germans T. (2011). The development of familial hypertrophic cardiomyopathy: from mutation to bedside. *Eur J Clin Invest*, Vol.41, No.5, (May 2011), pp. 568-578.

Caforio, AL.; Mahon, NJ.; Tona, F. & McKenna, WJ. (2002). Circulating cardiac autoantibodies in dilated cardiomyopathy and myocarditis: pathogenetic and clinical significance. *Eur J Heart Fail*, Vol.4, No.4 (Augustus 2002), pp. 411-417.

Cerqueira, MD.; Weissman, NJ.; Dilsizian, V.; Jacobs, AK.; Kaul, S.; Laskey, WK.; Pennell, DJ.; Rumberger, JA.; Ryan, T. & Verani MS. (2002). Standardized myocardial segmentation and nomenclature for tomographic imaging of the heart: a statement for healthcare professionals from the Cardiac Imaging Committee of the Council on Clinical Cardiology of the American Heart Association. *Circulation*, Vol.105, No.4, (January 2002), pp. 539-542.

Choudhury, L.; Mahrholdt, H.; Wagner, A.; Choi, KM.; Elliott, MD.; Klocke, FJ.; Bonow, RO.; Judd, RM. & Kim, RJ. (2002). Myocardial scarring in asymptomatic or mildly symptomatic patients with hypertrophic cardiomyopathy. *J Am Coll Cardiol*, Vol.40, No.12 (December 2002), pp. 2156-2164.

Corsten, MF.; Dennert, R.; Jochems, S.; Kuznetsova, T.; Devaux, Y.; Hofstra, L.; Wagner, DR.; Staessen, JA.; Heymans, S. & Schroen B. (2010). Circulating MicroRNA-208b and MicroRNA-499 reflect myocardial damage in cardiovascular disease. *Circ Cardiovasc Genet*, Vol.3, No.6 (December 2010), pp. 499-506.

Deb, K.; Djavidani, B.; Buchner, S.; Poschenrieder, F.; Heinicke, N.; Feuerbach, S.; Riegger, G. & Luchner A. (2008). Time course of eosinophilic myocarditis visualized by CMR. *J Cardiovasc Magn Reson*, Vol.10, No.1, (2008), pp. 21.

Deetjen, AG.; Conradi, G.; Mollmann, S.; Rad, A.; Hamm, CW. & Dill T. (2006). Value of gadolinium-enhanced magnetic resonance imaging in patients with Tako-Tsubo-like left ventricular dysfunction. *J Cardiovasc Magn Reson*, Vol.8, No.2, (2006), pp. 367-372.

Devlin, AM. & Ostman-Smith, I. (2000). Diagnosis of hypertrophic cardiomyopathy and screening for the phenotype suggestive of gene carriage in familial disease: a simple echocardiographic procedure. *J Med Screen 2000*, Vol.7, No.2, (2000), pp. 82-90.

Dodd, JD.; Holmvang, G.; Hoffmann Ferencik, M.; Abbara, S.; Brady, TJ. & Cury RC. (2007). Quantification of left ventricular noncompaction and trabecular delayed hyperenhancement with cardiac MRI: correlation with clinical severity. *AJR Am J Roentgenol* , Vol.189, No.4, (Oktober 2007), pp. 974-980.

Dursun, M.; Agayev, A.; Nisli, K.; Ertugrul, T.; Onur, I.; Oflaz, H. & Yekeler E. (2010). MR imaging features of ventricular noncompaction: emphasis on distribution and pattern of fibrosis. *Eur J Radiol* 2010, Vol.74, No.1, (April 2010), pp. 147-151.

Edelman, RR. (2004) Contrast-enhanced MR imaging of the heart: overview of the literature. *Radiology*, Vol.232, No.3, (September 2004), pp. 653-668.

Eitel, I.; Lucke, C.; Grothoff, M.; Sareban, M.; Schuler, G.; Thiele, H. & Gutberlet M. (2010). Inflammation in takotsubo cardiomyopathy: insights from cardiovascular magnetic resonance imaging. *Eur Radiol*, Vol.20, No.2 (February 2010), pp. 422-431.

Eitel, I. & Friedrich, MG. (2011) T2-weighted cardiovascular magnetic resonance in acute cardiac disease. *J Cardiovasc Magn Reson*, Vol.13, (2011), pp. 13.

Gange, CA.; Link, MS. & Maron MS. (2009). Utility of cardiovascular magnetic resonance in the diagnosis of Anderson-Fabry disease. *Circulation*, Vol.120, No.13, (September 2009), pp. 96-97.

Garot, J.; Unterseeh, T.; Teiger, E.; Champagne, S.; Chazaud, B.; Gherardi, R.; Hittinger, L.; Gueret, P. & Rahmouni A. (2003). Magnetic resonance imaging of targeted catheter-based implantation of myogenic precursor cells into infarcted left ventricular myocardium. *J Am Coll Cardiol*, Vol.41, No.10, (May 2003), pp. 1841-1846.

Gutberlet, M.; Spors, B.; Thoma, T.; Bertram, H.; Denecke, T.; Felix, R.; Noutsias, M.; Schultheiss, HP. & Kuhl U. (2008). Suspected chronic myocarditis at cardiac MR: diagnostic accuracy and association with immunohistologically detected inflammation and viral persistence. *Radiology*, Vol.246, No.2, (February 2008), pp. 401-409.

Hermens, JA.; van Houwelingen, GK.; de Man, FH.; Louwerenburg, HW. & von Birgelen C. (2010). Thrombus aspiration in a series of patients with stable or unstable angina pectoris and lesion-site thrombus formation. *Neth Heart J*, Vol. 18, No.9 (September 2010), pp. 423-429.

Hill, JM.; Dick, AJ.; Raman, VK.; Thompson, RB.; Yu, ZX.; Hinds, KA.; Pessanha, BS.; Guttman, MA.; Varney, TR.; Martin, BJ.; Dubar, CE.; McVeigh, ER. & Lederman RJ. (2003). Serial cardiac magnetic resonance imaging of injected mesenchymal stem cells. *Circulation*, Vol.108, No.8, (Augustus 2003), pp. 1009-1014.

Hsu, LY.; Natanzon, A.; Kellman, P.; Hirsch, GA.; Aletras, AH. & Arai AE. (2006). Quantitative myocardial infarction on delayed enhancement MRI. Part I: Animal validation of an automated feature analysis and combined thresholding infarct sizing algorithm. *J Magn Reson Imaging*, Vol.23, No.3 (March 2006), pp. 298-308.

Isbell, DC. & Kramer, CM. (2006). The evolving role of cardiovascular magnetic resonance imaging in nonischemic cardiomyopathy. *Semin Ultrasound CT MR*, Vol.27, No.1 (February 2006), pp. 20-31.

Jackson, E. Bellenger, N.; Seddon, M.; Harden, S. & Peebles C. (2007). Ischaemic and non-ischaemic cardiomyopathies--cardiac MRI appearances with delayed enhancement. *Clin Radiol*, Vol.62, No.5 (May 2007), pp. 395-403.

Jacquier, A.; Thuny, F.; Jop, B.; Giorgi, R.; Cohen, F.; Gaubert, JY.; Vidal, V.; Bartoli, JM.; Habib, G. & Moulin G. (2010). Measurement of trabeculated left ventricular mass using cardiac magnetic resonance imaging in the diagnosis of left ventricular non-compaction. *Eur Heart J*, Vol.31, No.9, (May 2010), pp. 1098-1104.

Kellman, P.; Aletras, AH.; Mancini, C.; McVeigh, ER. & Arai, AE. (2007) T2-prepared SSFP improves diagnostic confidence in edema imaging in acute myocardial infarction compared to turbo spin echo. *Magn Reson Med*, Vol.57, No.5, (May 2007), pp.891-897.

Kim, RJ.; Wu, E.; Rafael, A.; Chen, EL.; Parker, MA.; Simonetti, O.; Klocke, FJ.; Bonow, RO. & Judd, RM. (2000). The use of contrast-enhanced magnetic resonance imaging to identify reversible myocardial dysfunction. *N Engl J*, Vol.343, No.20, (November 2000), pp. 1445-1453.

Kirthy, V.; Schultz, C. & Davies S. (2011). Cardiac Imaging of trastuzumab-induced cardiomyopathy. *European Journal of Heart Failure Supplements*, Vol.10, (2011) Koeth,

O.; Mark, B.; Kilkowski, A.; Layer, G.; Cornelius, B.; Kouraki, K.; Bauer, T.; Zahn, R.;

Senges, J. & Zeymer U. (2008). Clinical, angiographic and cardiovascular magnetic resonance findings in consecutive patients with Takotsubo cardiomyopathy. *Clin Res Cardiol,* Vol.97, No.9, (September 2008), pp. 623-627.

Koito, H.; Suzuki, J.; Ohkubo, N.; Ishiguro, Y.; Iwasaka, T. & Inada M. (1996). Gadolinium-diethylenetriamine pentaacetic acid enhanced magnetic resonance imaging of dilated cardiomyopathy: clinical significance of abnormally high signal intensity of left ventricular myocardium. *J Cardiol,* Vol.28, No1. (July 1996), pp. 41-49.

Kovacs, G.; Reiter, G.; Reiter, U.; Rienmuller, R.; Peacock, A. & Olschewski H. (2008). The emerging role of magnetic resonance imaging in the diagnosis and management of pulmonary hypertension. *Respiration,* Vol.76, No.4, (2008), pp. 458-470.

Kraitchman, DL.; Heldman, AW.; Atalar, E.; Amado, LC.; Martin, BJ.; Pittenger, MF.; Hare, JM. & Bulte JW. (2003). In vivo magnetic resonance imaging of mesenchymal stem cells in myocardial infarction. *Circulation,* Vol.107, No.18, (May 2003), pp. 2290-2293.

Lightfoot, JC.; D'Agostino, RB.; Jr., Hamilton, CA.; Jordan, J.; Torti, FM.; Kock, ND.; Jordan, J.; Workman, S. & Hundley WG. (2010). Novel approach to early detection of doxorubicin cardiotoxicity by gadolinium-enhanced cardiovascular magnetic resonance imaging in an experimental model. *Circ Cardiovasc Imaging* 2010, Vol.3, No.5, (September 2010), pp. 550-558.

Maceira, AM.; Prasad, SK.; Hawkins, PN.; Roughton, M. & Pennell DJ. (2008). Cardiovascular magnetic resonance and prognosis in cardiac amyloidosis. *J Cardiovasc Magn Reson,* Vol.10, No.1, (2008), pp. 54.

Mahrholdt, H.; Goedecke, C.; Wagner, A.; Meinhardt, G.; Athanasiadis, A.; Vogelsberg, H.; Fritz, P.; Klingel, K.; Kandolf, R. & Sechtem U. (2004). Cardiovascular magnetic resonance assessment of human myocarditis: a comparison to histology and molecular pathology. *Circulation,* Vol.109, No.10, (March 2004), pp. 1250-1258.

Mahrholdt, H.; Wagner, A.; Deluigi, CC.; Kispert, E.; Hager, S.; Meinhardt, G.; Vogelsberg, H.; Fritz, P.; Dippon, J.; Bock, CT.; Klingel, K.; Kandolf, R. & Sechtem U. (2004). Presentation, patterns of myocardial damage, and clinical course of viral myocarditis. *Circulation,* Vol.114, No.15, (Oktober 2006), pp. 1581-1590.

Marcu, CB.; Beek, AM. & van Rossum, AC. (2006). Clinical applications of cardiovascular magnetic resonance imaging. *CMAJ,* Vol.175,No.8, (Oktober 2006), pp. 911-917.

Marcu, CB.; Nijveldt, R.; Beek, AM. & van Rossum, AC. (2007). Delayed contrast enhancement magnetic resonance imaging for the assessment of cardiac disease. *Heart Lung Circ,* Vol.16, No.2, (April 2007), pp70-78

Maron, BJ.; McKenna, WJ.; Danielson, GK.; Kappenberger, LJ.; Kuhn, HJ.; Seidman, CE.; Shah, PM.; Spencer. WH.; Spirito, P.; Ten Cate, FJ. & Wigle ED. (2002). American College of Cardiology/European Society of Cardiology clinical expert consensus document on hypertrophic cardiomyopathy. A report of the American College of Cardiology Foundation Task Force on Clinical Expert Consensus Documents and the European Society of Cardiology Committee for Practice Guidelines. *J am Coll Cardiol,* Vol.42, No.9, (March 2003), pp. 1687-1713

Orlic, D.; Hill, JM. & Arai AE. (2002). Stem cells for myocardial regeneration. *Circ Res,* Vol.91, No.12, (December 2002), pp. 1092-1102.

Marti, V.; Carreras, F.; Pujadas, S. & De Rozas JM. (2009). Transient left ventricular basal ballooning-"inverted" Tako-tsubo. *Clin Cardiol,* Vol.32. No.7, (September 2009), pp. 20-21.

Masci, PG.; Ganame, J.; Strata, E.; Desmet, W.; Aquaro, GD.; Dymarkowski, S.; Valenti, V.; Janssens, S.; Lombardi, M.; Van de Werf.; L'Abbate, A. & Bogaert J. (2010). Myocardial salvage by CMR correlates with LV remodeling and early ST-segment resolution in acute myocardial infarction. *JACC Cardiovasc Imaging* , Vol.3, No.1, (January 2010), pp. 45-51.

McKenna, WJ.; Thiene, G.; Nava, A.; Fontaliran, F.; Blomstrom-Lundqvist, C.; Fontaine, G. & Camerini F. (1994). Diagnosis of arrhythmogenic right ventricular dysplasia/cardiomyopathy. Task Force of the Working Group Myocardial and Pericardial Disease of the European Society of Cardiology and of the Scientific Council on Cardiomyopathies of the International Society and Federation of Cardiology. *Br Heart J* , Vol.71, No.3, (March 1994), pp. 215-218.

Moon, JC.; McKenna, WJ.; McCrohon, JA.; Elliott, PM.; Smith, GC,. & Pennell DJ. (2003). Toward clinical risk assessment in hypertrophic cardiomyopathy with gadolinium cardiovascular magnetic resonance. *J Am Coll Cardiol*, Vol.41, No.9 (May 2003), pp. 1561-1567.

Mueller, GC. & Attili A. Cardiomyopathy: magnetic resonance imaging evaluation. *Semin Roentgenol* , Vol.43, No.3, (July 2008), pp. 204-222.

Nijveldt, R.; Beek, AM.; Hirsch, A.; Stoel, MG.; Hofman, MB.; Umans, VA.; Algra, PR.; Twisk, JW. & van Rossum AC. (2008). Functional recovery after acute myocardial infarction: comparison between angiography, electrocardiography, and cardiovascular magnetic resonance measures of microvascular injury. *J Am Coll Cardiol*, Vol.52, No3. (July 2008), pp. 181-189.

Olimulder, MA.; Galjee, MA.; van Es, J.; Wagenaar, LJ.; von Birgelen, C. (2011). Contrast-enhancement cardiac magnetic resonance imaging beyond the scope of viability. *Neth Heart J*, Vol.19, No.5 (May 2011), pp. 236-245.

Olimulder, MA.; Kraaier, K.; Galjee, MA.; Scholten, MF.; van Es, J.; Wagenaar, LJ.; van der Palen, J. & von Birgelen, C. (2011). Infarct tissue characteristics of patients with versus without early revascularization for acute myocardial infarction: a contrast-enhancement cardiovascular magnetic resonance imaging study. *Heart Vessels*, (May 2011).

Orn, S.; Manhenke, C.; Anand, IS.; Squire, I.; Nagel, E.; Edvardsen, T. & Dickstein K. (2007). Effect of left ventricular scar size, location, and transmurality on left ventricular remodeling with healed myocardial infarction. *Am J Cardiol*, Vol.99, No.8 (April 2007), pp. 1109-1114.

Pascale, P.; Schlaepfer, J.; Oddo, M.; Schaller, MD.; Vogt, P. & Fromer M. (2009). Ventricular arrhythmia in coronary artery disease: limits of a risk stratification strategy based on the ejection fraction alone and impact of infarct localization. *Europace*, Vol.11, No.12, (December 2009), pp. 1639-1646.

Patel, MR.; Cawley, PJ.; Heitner, JF.; Klem, I.; Parker, MA.; Jaroudi, WA.; Meine, TJ.; White', JB.; Elliott, MD.; Kim, HW.; Judd, RM. & Kim RJ. (2009). Detection of myocardial damage in patients with sarcoidosis. *Circulation*, Vol.120, No.20, (November 2009), pp. 1969-1977.

Pieroni, M.; Bellocci, F. & Crea F. (2007). Letter by Pieroni et al regarding article, "Contrast-enhanced magnetic resonance imaging of a patient with chloroquine-induced cardiomyopathy confirmed by endomyocardial biopsy". *Circulation*, Vol.115, No.5 (February 2007), pp. 67.

Reffelmann, T.; Naami, A.; Spuentrup, E. & Kuhl HP. (2006). Images in cardiovascular medicine. Contrast-enhanced magnetic resonance imaging of a patient with chloroquine-induced cardiomyopathy confirmed by endomyocardial biopsy. *Circulation*, Vol.114, No.8 (Augustus 2006), pp. 357-358.

Rochitte, CE.; Oliveira, PF.; Andrade, JM.; Ianni, BM.; Parga, JR.; Avila, LF.; Kalil-Filho, R.; Mady, C.; Meneghetti, JC.; Lima, JA. & Ramires, JA. (2005). Myocardial delayed enhancement by magnetic resonance imaging in patients with Chagas' disease: a marker of disease severity. *J Am Coll Cardiol*, Vol.46, No.8, (Oktober 2005), pp. 1553-1558.

Rochitte, CE.; Nacif, MS.; de Oliveira Junior, AC.; Siqueira-Batista, R.; Marchiori, E.; Uellendahl, M. & de Lourdes HM. (2007). Cardiac magnetic resonance in Chagas' disease. *Artif Organs*, Vol.31, No.4 (April 2007) pp. 259-267.

Rochitte, CE.; Olivera, PF. & Joalbo M. (2003). Chagas disease is characterised by specific pattern and location of myocardial delayed enhancement MRI. *J Cardiovasc Magn Reson*, Vol. 5 (2003), pp. 113

Roes, SD.; Borleffs, C.; van der Geest, RJ.; Westenberg, JJM.; Marsan, NA.; Kaandorp, TAM.; Reiber, JHC.; Zeppenfeld, K.; Lamb, HJ. & de Roos. (2009). Infarct Tissue Heterogeneity Assessed With Contrast-Enhanced MRI Predicts Spontaneous Ventricular Arrhythmia in Patients With Ischemic Cardiomyopathy and Implantable Cardioverter-Defibrillator. *Circulation: Cardiovascular imaging*, Vol.2, No.3, (2009), pp.183

Thygesen, K.; Alpert, JS. & White HD. (2007). Universal definition of myocardial infarction. *Eur Heart J*, Vol.28, No.20, (Oktober 2007), pp. 2525-2538.

Rubinshtein, R.; Glockner, JF.; Ommen, SR.; Araoz, PA.; Ackerman, MJ.; Sorajja, P.; Bos, JM.; Tajik. AJ.; Valeti, US.; Nishimura, A. & Gersh BJ. (2010). Characteristics and clinical significance of late gadolinium enhancement by contrast-enhanced magnetic resonance imaging in patients with hypertrophic cardiomyopathy. *Circ Heart Fail*, Vol.3, No.1, (January 2010), pp. 51-58.

Sharkey, SW.; Lesser, JR.; Maron, MS. &Maron BJ. (2011). Why not just call it tako-tsubo cardiomyopathy: a discussion of nomenclature. *J Am Coll Cardiol*, Vol.57, No.13 (March 2011), pp. 1496-1497.

Shimada, T.; Shimada, K.; Sakane, T.; Ochiai, K.; Tsukihashi, H.; Fukui, M.; Inoue, S.; Katoh, H.; Murakami, Y.; Ishibashi, Y. & Maruyama, R. (2001). Diagnosis of cardiac sarcoidosis and evaluation of the effects of steroid therapy by gadolinium-DTPA-enhanced magnetic resonance imaging. *Am J Med*, Vol.110, No.7 (May 2001), pp. 520-527.

Sievers, B.; Moon, JC. & Pennell DJ. (2002). Images in cardiovascular Medicine. Magnetic resonance contrast enhancement of iatrogenic septal myocardial infarction in hypertrophic cardiomyopathy. *Circulation* , Vol. 105, No.8, (February 2002), pp. 1018.

Stensaeth, KH.; Fossum, E.; Hoffmann, P.; Mangschau, A.; Skretteberg, PT. & Klow, NE. (2011).Takotsubo cardiomyopathy in acute coronary syndrome; clinical features and contribution of cardiac magnetic resonance during the acute and convalescent phase. *Scand Cardiovasc J*, Vol.45, No.2, (April 2011), pp. 77-85.

Stoel, MG.; von Birgelen, C. & Zijlstra F. (2009). Aspiration of embolized thrombus during primary percutaneous coronary intervention. *Catheter Cardiovasc Interv*, Vol.73. No.6 (May 2009), pp. 781-786.

Van der Zwaan, HB.; Stoel, MG.; Roos-Hesselink, JW.; Veen, G.; Boersma, E. & von Birgelen C. (2010). Early versus late ST-segment resolution and clinical outcomes after percutaneous coronary intervention for acute myocardial infarction. *Neth Heart J*, Vol.18. No.9 (September 2010), pp. 416-422.

Vogel-Claussen, J.; Rochitte, CE.; Wu, KC.; Kamel, IR.; Foo, TK, Lima, JA.; Bluemke, DA. (2006). Delayed enhancement MR imaging: utility in myocardial assessment. *Radiographics, Vol.26, No.3 (May* 2006) pp. 795-810.

Vohringer, M.; Mahrholdt, H.; Yilmaz, A. & Sechtem U. (2007) Significance of late gadolinium enhancement in cardiovascular magnetic resonance imaging (CMR). *Herz* Vol. 32, No.2, (March 2007), pp. 129-137.

Wassmuth, R.; Lentzsch, S.; Erdbruegger, U.; Schulz-Menger, J.; Doerken, B.; Dietz, R. & Friedrich MG. (2001). Subclinical cardiotoxic effects of anthracyclines as assessed by magnetic resonance imaging-a pilot study. *Am Heart J*, Vol.141, No.6, (Juny 2001), pp. 1007-1013.

Weinsaft, JW.; Klem, I. & Judd RM. (2007). MRI for the assessment of myocardial viability. *Cardiol Clin*, Vol.25, No.1 (February 2007), pp. 35-56.

Wu, CF.; Chuang, WP.; Li, AH. & Hsiao CH. (2009). Cardiac magnetic resonance imaging in sunitinib malate-related cardiomyopathy: no late gadolinium enhancement. *J Chin Med Assoc*, Vol.72, No.6, (Juny 2009), pp. 323-327.

Wynne, J. & Braunwald E. (2005). Restrictive and infiltrative cardiomyopathies. In: Zipes, DP.; Libby, P.; Bonow, RO. & Braunwald E, editors. *Braunwald's heart disease: a textbook of cardiovascular medicine*. p. 1682-1692. Elsevier Saunders, Pilalphia, Pennsylvania.

Yasu, T.; Tone, K.; Kubo, N. & Saito M. (2009). Transient mid-ventricular ballooning cardiomyopathy: a new entity of Takotsubo cardiomyopathy. *Int J Cardiol*, Vol.110, No.1, (Juny 2006), pp. 100-101.

Yeh, ET. & Bickford CL. (2009). Cardiovascular complications of cancer therapy: incidence, pathogenesis, diagnosis, and management. *J Am Coll Cardiol*, Vol.53, No.24, (Juny 2009), pp. 2231-2247.

Yelgec, NS.; Dymarkowski, S.; Ganame, J. & Bogaert J. (2007). Value of MRI in patients with a clinical suspicion of acute myocarditis. *Eur Radiol*, Vol.17, No.9, (September 2007), pp. 2211-2217.

Yilmaz, A.; Gdynia, HJ.; Baccouche, H.; Mahrholdt, H.; Meinhardt, G.; Basso, C.; Thiene, G.; Sperfeld, AD.; Ludolph, AC. & Sechtem U. (2008). Cardiac involvement in patients with Becker muscular dystrophy: new diagnostic and pathophysiological insights by a CMR approach. *J Cardiovasc Magn Reson*, Vol.10, No.1, (2008), pp. 50.

Yilmaz, A.; Kindermann, I.; Kindermann, M.; Mahfoud, F.; Ukena, C.; Athanasiadis, A.; Hill, S.; Mahrholdt, H.; Voehringer, M.; Schieber, M.; Klingel, K.; Kandolf, R.; Bohm, M. & Sechtem U. (2010). Comparative evaluation of left and right ventricular endomyocardial biopsy: differences in complication rate and diagnostic performance. *Circulation*, Vol.122, No.9, (Augustus 2010), pp. 900-909.

Yokokawa, M.; Tada, H.; Koyama, K.; Ino, T.; Hiramatsu, S.; Kaseno, K.; Naito, S.; Oshima, S. & Taniguchi, K. (2009). The characteristics and distribution of the scar tissue predict ventricular tachycardia in patients with advanced heart failure. *Pacing Clin Electrophysiol*, Vol.32, No.3, (March 2009), pp. 314-322.

Yokokawa, M.; Tada, H.; Koyama, K.; Naito, S.; Oshima, S. & Taniguchi, K. (2009). Nontransmural scar detected by magnetic resonance imaging and origin of ventricular tachycardia in structural heart disease. *Pacing Clin Electrophysiol*, Vol.32, No1. (March 2009), pp. 52-56.

Zagrosek, A.; Wassmuth, R.; bdel-Aty, H.; Rudolph, A.; Dietz, R. & Schulz-Menger, J. (2008). Relation between myocardial edema and myocardial mass during the acute and convalescent phase of myocarditis--a CMR study. *J Cardiovasc Magn Reson*, Vol.10, No.1, (2008), pp. 19.

Part 4

Metabolic and Drug-Induced Cardiomyopathies

21

The Evolving Face of Heart Failure Associated with Elevated Cardio-Metabolic Risk Factors

Chaitanya Dutt, Vijay Chauthaiwale, Anookh Mohanan, KumarPrafull Chandra, Shitalkumar Zambad, Ram Gupta and Siralee Parikh
Torrent Pharmaceuticals Limited
India

1. Introduction

1.1 Evolving profile of heart failure

There have been many definitions of Heart Failure and yet the most recent definitions rely heavily on clinical manifestations: dyspnoea or undue fatigue on exertion, along with the evidence of fluid retention, supported by objective evidence of structural or functional abnormalities of the heart at rest. A more recent classification also recognizes and emphasizes the need for the above signs and symptoms for both the development and progression of heart failure (Dickstein et al., 2008). The 2009 update of the AHA guideline identifies patients at higher risk of developing or progressing more rapidly to heart failure as traditionally defined. Table 1.

The presence of cardio-metabolic risk factors (hypertension, diabetes, obesity and metabolic syndrome) in addition to atherosclerotic disease puts the patient at twice greater risk of developing and/or progressing to heart failure as currently defined i.e. with structural or functional heart disease at rest. Studies across the world, particularly in India, China and Latin America suggest that overweight, metabolically challenged individuals are at greater risk of heart failure at a younger age and are also twice as likely to have heart failure linked events such as hospitalization or mortality (Clarke et al., 2010).

Echocardiography and Doppler imaging of the heart are the current gold standards for identification of structural and to extent also functional abnormalities. Advances in Echocardiography and Doppler imaging have enabled the identification of an under-diagnosed entity described as diastolic dysfunction, an additional handicap for a failing heart. Prognosis of patients with predominant diastolic dysfunction (Heart Failure with Preserved Ejection Fraction: HFPEF) has been reported to be similar to those who have predominant systolic dysfunction. In some population surveys, up to 50% of patients fall in this category (Paulus, 1998). Many have co-morbidities identified as risk factors in Stage A of the AHA classification. It is therefore pertinent to understand why and how these additional risk factors influence the development and progression of heart failure as different from and often in addition to Atherosclerotic Coronary Artery Disease.

Diabetes, hypertension, dyslipidemia and thyroid dysfunction affecting heart are often considered as factors contributing to coronary artery disease. However, there is evidence to suggest that diabetes and hypertension may affect myocardial function largely independent of significant epicardial coronary artery disease. The main objective of this chapter is to explain holistic effects of cardio-metabolic risk factors on heart failure. We urge the reader to consider factors beyond the myocardium, such as vascular responsiveness, neuroendocrine maladaptation and renal function and correlate it with clinical manifestations. This chapter elucidates and correlates recent advances in understanding of etiological factors affecting the myocardial function, the mechanisms which could be influencing overall progression and presentation of heart failure, current diagnostic approaches, their limitations and emerging concepts, current medical therapies, their limitations and newer emerging therapeutic approaches.

Subjects at Risk for Heart Failure

STAGE A
High risk for HF
Non symptomatic
No structural defects

PATIENTS WITH
- Hypertension
- Atherosclerotic disease
- Diabetes
- Obesity
- Metabolic syndrome

  or
- Using cardiotoxins
- With FHx CM

THERAPY

Goals
- Treat hypertension
- Encourage smoking cessation
- Treat lipid disorder
- Encourage regular exercise
- Discourage alcohol intake
- Control metabolic syndrome

Drugs
- ACEI or ARB in appropriate patients for vascular disease or diabetes

STAGE B
Non symptomatic
Structural defects present

PATIENTS WITH
- Previous MI
- LV remodeling including LVH & low EF
- Asymptomatic valvular disease

THERAPY

Goals
- All measures under stage A

Drugs
- ACEI or ARB
- β blockers

Devices
- In selected patients: Implantable defibrillators

Table 1. Stages in the development of heart failure and recommended therapy by stage. ACEI, angiotensin-converting enzyme inhibitors; ARB, angiotensin II receptor blocker; EF, ejection fraction; FHx CM, family history of cardiomyopathy; HF, heart failure; LVH, left ventricular hypertrophy; and MI, myocardial infarction. Modified from Jessup M, Abraham WT, Casey DE et al. 2009 focused update: ACCF/AHA guidelines for the diagnosis and management of heart failure in adults (Jessup et al., 2009).

2. Cardio-Metabolic Cardiomyopathy (CMCM)

The etiology of cardiomyopathy associated with diabetes is widely debated. While hyperglycemia is regarded as a sole culprit in causation of diabetic cardiomyopathy, there is a cluster of associated risk factors - obesity, hyperlipidemia, prothrombotic state, hypertension, activation of multiple hormone and cytokine systems etc, which are commonly seen in most patients presenting with diabetes of more than five years and these in turn have intricate effects in causation of cardiomyopathy. More and more researchers are now focusing on the overall impact of diabetes and cluster of these observable conditions on altered metabolism and energetics at cellular level of the target end organs, which are known to be most vulnerable to such altered conditions. Increasing evidence are now available which suggest that altered myocyte functioning is more a function of altered cellular metabolism. It is seen that simultaneous over-activation of renin-angiotensin-aldosterone system (RAAS), increased oxidative stress and compromised endothelial function, contributed by each individual component adds to overall dysfunction of myocardium. Effect on peripheral vasculature adds on to the already stressed myocardium and predispose to an early compromise in over all cardiovascular functions.

Many of the changes described occur in predisposed individuals even before the onset of diabetes, often at the stage when they may be diagnosed as having pre-hypertension or impaired glucose tolerance. There is therefore a need for holistic terminology which could represent contribution of not only of diabetes and associated hyperglycemia but equally of other factors - obesity, dyslipidemia, hypertension, in the pathogenesis of cardiomyopathy, for which the term "Cardio-metabolic Cardiomyopathy (CMCM)" seems appropriate (Fig. 1). The terminology CMCM is based on available evidence of altered

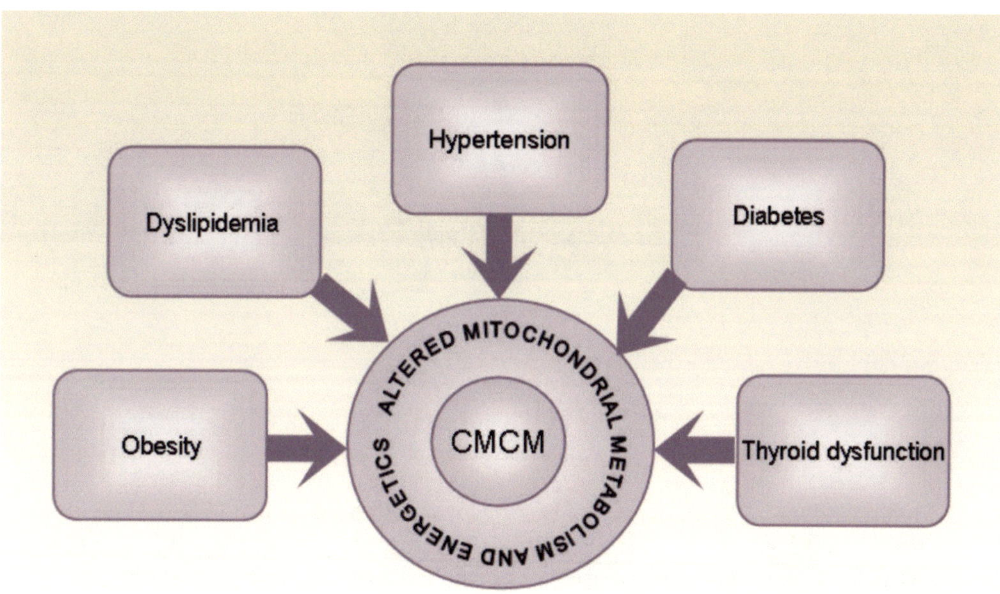

Fig. 1. Various possible risk factors that could contribute to the development of Cardio-metabolic Cardiomyopathy (CMCM).

myocytes metabolism and energetics leading to cardiomyopathy. This would need further support from ongoing and future research to consolidate itself as a new class of cardiomyopathy representing cluster of metabolic derangement and altered energetics of myocytes with a common underlying derangement - diminishing flexibility to use the appropriate fuel to provide adequate energy, resulting in dysfunctional mitochondria.

2.1 Mechanisms of CMCM

2.1.1 Myocardial metabolism in normal heart

A normal healthy heart uses free fatty acid (FFA) as its preferred fuel source and to a lesser extent, circulating glucose (Fig 2). In case of severe starvation it can also utilize lactate,

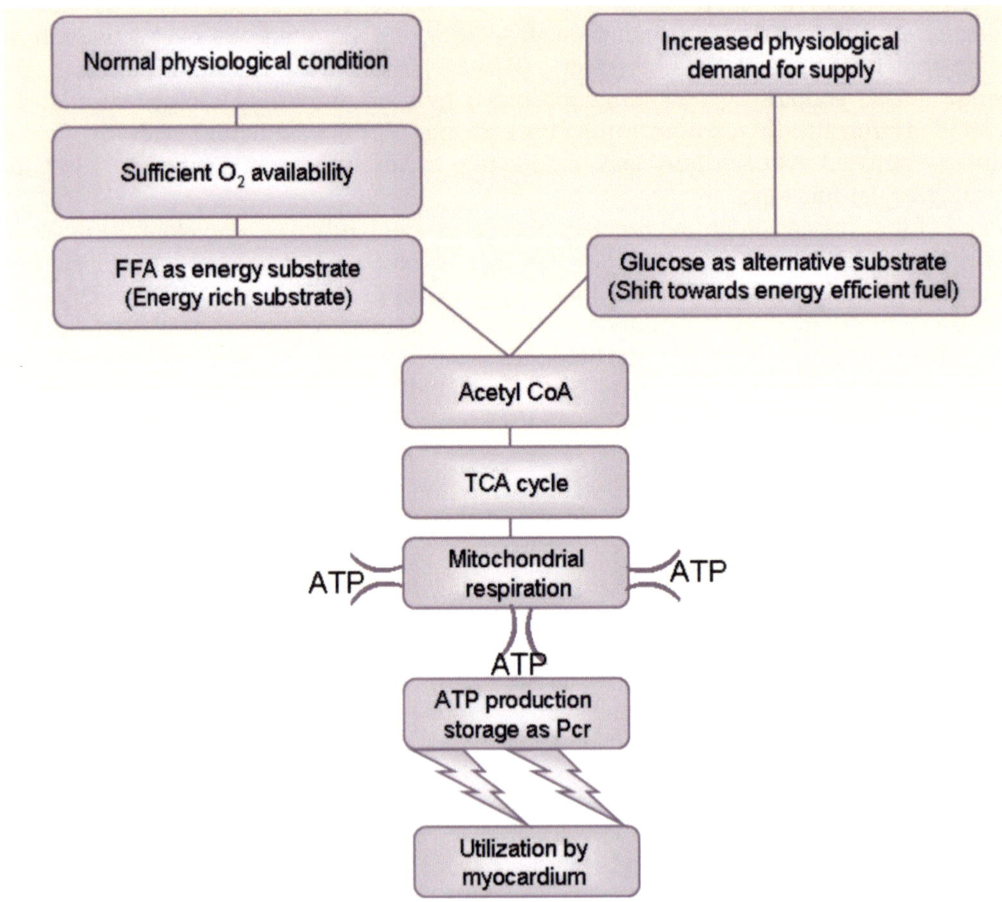

Fig. 2. Myocardial metabolism in normal heart. Normal myocardium at resting state uses FFA as a preferred fuel source, which is energy rich substrate but yield less ATP per mol of O_2. While in the state of increased peripheral physiological demand (e.g. exercise) myocardium uses glucose as energy source which is more efficient energy source and yield more ATP per mol of O_2.. ATP, Adenosine triphosphate; FFA, Free fatty acid; O_2, oxygen; Pcr, Phospho creatinine.

ketone bodies and amino acids. The regulation of myocardial metabolism is dependent on the availability and abundance of substrate, hormone levels, coronary blood flow and oxygenation and inotropic state of the tissue. With ageing, relative contribution of glucose as myocardial substrate increases as seen in elderly. The levels of FFA determine its uptake by myocytes. Following uptake and conjugation with acetyl CoA (FA-CoA), FA-CoA enters the mitochondria, via the carnitine acyl transferase shuttle (CPT-1 and CPT-2). CPT-1 is subject to allosteric regulation by malonyl CoA and effective transfer to the mitochondria requires adequate amounts of carnitine (Abel & Doenst, 2011). Upon entering the mitochondrial matrix, FA-CoA undergoes β-oxidation. Post prandial, higher levels of insulin in blood increases muscle glucose uptake by increasing glucose transporters (GLUT-1 and GLUT-4) translocation and by suppressing FFA release from adipose tissues thereby removing FFA mediated inhibition of glycolysis and pyruvate oxidation.

2.1.2 Metabolic disturbances in cardio-metabolic cardiomyopathy (CMCM)

There are many factors considered as initiators to the functional and structural alterations which contribute to the development and progression of CMCM. Most of these evidence are from animal experimental studies. Though development of CMCM is multi-factorial, metabolic disturbance is the major culprit.

2.1.2.1 Altered fuel supply and altered substrate utilization

Increasing evidence suggests that altered substrate supply and utilization by cardiac myocytes could be the initial trigger in the pathogenesis of CMCM. Under deranged metabolic milieu, inclusive of diabetes, heart use relatively more fat than normal heart (Herrero et al., 2006; Carley & Severson, 2005). The shift towards increased fatty acids and decreased glucose utilization is linked to elevated circulating levels of FFA and triglycerides as a consequence of enhanced adipose tissue lipolysis, increased FFA uptake as well as high tissue FFAs caused by hydrolysis of augmented myocardial triglyceride stores. Animal studies in db/db mice, (a model of type II diabetes with obesity and hyperglycemia), have shown increased cell membrane fatty acid (FA) transporters (FAT/CD36) and FA binding proteins leading to increased FA uptake in db/db mice hearts (Carley & Severson, 2008). To handle this increased FA, there is upregulation of mitochondrial enzymes involved in fat metabolism.

The reduced glucose utilization seen in such condition is partly accounted for by the slow rate of glucose transport across the sarco-lemmal membrane into the myocardium, which is probably due to the cellular depletion/reduced translocation of GLUT-4 caused by insulin resistance (Garvey et al., 1993). High circulating FFA and increased FA oxidation inhibits pyruvate dehydrogenase complex thereby reducing glucose oxidation.

Exercise influences myocardial glucose utilization, perhaps independent of insulin levels. Graded exercise in all cases of heart failure has been documented to be beneficial. It is likely that exercise has a beneficial effect in maintaining the substrate flexibility of the myocardium.

2.1.2.2 Lipotoxicity associated with excessive accumulation of intracellular lipids

When FA uptake exceeds FA oxidation capabilities, lipid accumulation occurs resulting in lipotoxicity. This is evident in diabetics and obese patients but not seen in non-obese. High circulating and cellular FFA necessitates abnormal higher oxygen demand during FFA metabolism in addition to enhancing peripheral insulin resistance. This results in accumulation of toxic intermediates of FFA metabolism leading to impaired functional performance. Fuel surplus is likely to activate peroxisome proliferators-activated receptor (PPAR-α) with subsequent increase in FA oxidation. Accumulation of palmitate results in increased free radical production and endoplasmic reticular stress which leads to apoptosis (Borradaile et al., 2006). Palmitate accumulation can also promote denovo ceramide production which is also an inducer of apoptosis. Carnitine, an essential substrate for myocardial FFA metabolism is reduced along with abnormal appearing mitochondria (Ashrafian et al., 2007).

Thus, impaired substrate flexibility and inefficient adenosine triphosphate (ATP) generation, resulting in inability in fulfillment of myocardial energy demand, initially on exertion, progressing to inadequacy at rest, is the hallmark of CMCM.

2.1.2.3 Increased generation of advanced glycation and lipoxidation end products along with reactive oxygen species affecting heart in altered metabolic conditions

Advanced glycation end products (AGEs) and advanced lipoxidation end products (ALEs) are formed when carbohydrate- or lipid-derived intermediates react with the amino group of proteins to form covalently modified, stable protein adducts. AGEs/ALEs formation results from a combination of hyperglycemia, hyperlipidemia, oxidative/carbonyl stress and/or decreased renal clearance (Miyata et al., 2001). These modifications may be a single change on the peptide chain or multiple modifications that can produce crosslinks within or between proteins. Long-lived proteins like collagen and elastin are highly vulnerable for crosslink formation with AGEs and ALEs. These modifications lead to impaired collagen degradation and thereby increased collagen accumulation and subsequent fibrosis.

AGEs accumulation exert their detrimental effect on cardiac structure and function by different mechanisms. Firstly, structural modification/crosslinkage of myocardial proteins involved in cardiac contraction or relaxation may occur, resulting in impaired systolic or diastolic function and structural alteration. By disrupting intra- and inter-domain tertiary structures of Sarcoplasmic/endoplasmic reticulum Ca2+-ATPase (SERCA2a), AGE complexes have shown to compromise structural movements required for translocating calcium ions from the cytosol to the lumen of the sarcoplasmic reticulum. Secondly, AGEs promote trans-differentiation of epithelial cells to myofibroblasts via their specific receptors (e.g., RAGE). Finally, activation of RAGE promotes inflammation and oxidative stress, which can decrease the bioavailability of nitric oxide. This may result in further increased oxidative stress and attenuated contribution of nitric oxide during myocardial relaxation (Goldin et al., 2006). Thus, AGE-RAGE interaction can have a direct functional impact on myocardial relaxation. There is also increased free radical generation and oxidative stress with subsequent activation of many deleterious pathways which lead to apoptosis and cell death. Effects of AGEs leading to increased stiffness of connective tissue, increased permeability and pro-coagulant state due to effects on endothelial functions, increased vascular matrix through mononuclear cell activation and defective vascular relaxation due to decreased nitrous oxide (NO) release, run hand in hand, with direct effects on heart and contribute to overall patho-physiology of CMCM.

Although many studies have not been reported with ALEs, yet, recent evidence suggests that ALEs induce inflammatory pathways and network similar to AGEs leading to vascular complications (Shanmugam et al., 2008). ALEs and AGEs go hand in hand from their generation to effect on different end organs and are not limited to diabetes. Effects of ALEs on myocardium in isolation, could be similar to AGEs, however, need further studies for better understanding.

2.1.3 Dysfunctional calcium homeostasis

Calcium, essential for the process of excitation–contraction, is the primary ionic regulator in the heart. In Type 2 rodent models of diabetes, altered expression, activity and function of many regulatory and contractile proteins/transporters involved in excitation–contraction coupling; SERCA, Na^+/Ca^{2+} exchange (NCX), ryanodine receptors (RyR) and plasma membrane Ca^{2+}-ATPase (PMCA), as well as dysfunctional intracellular calcium signaling, have been reported (Pereira et al., 2006; Vetter et al., 2002). These alterations have been attributed to accumulation of toxic molecules such as long-chain acylcarnitines, free radicals and abnormal membrane lipid content as well as to AGEs altering the structure and function of several proteins described above. The consequences of these changes include alterations to the calcium sensitivity of regulatory proteins involved in the regulation of the cardiac actomyosin system, possibly due to phosphorylation of sarcomeric protein troponin I. The diminished calcium sensitivity and altered activity of regulatory and contractile proteins may all contribute to impaired left ventricular (LV) function.

2.1.4 Altered thyroid hormone status

Recent evidence indicates that heart failure can lead to down-regulation of the thyroid hormone signaling system in the heart. In the failing heart, there is decrease in thyroid hormone receptor expression; in addition, serum levels of T4 and T3 are decreased with heart failure in the frame of the non-thyroidal illness syndrome (Kinugawa et al., 2001). Thyroid hormone levels have a profound impact on mitochondria, the organelles responsible for the majority of cellular ATP production. The hypermetabolic effects of thyroid hormones are partially due to an increased demand for ATP and partially due to increased uncoupling. In addition, thyroid hormones are potent activators of mitochondriogenesis. Key events in thyroid-hormone-induced mitochondriogenesis include the increased expression of the mitochondrial transcription factors, nuclear respiratory factor-1 (NRF-1) and peroxisome-proliferator-activated receptor gamma co-activator-1a (PGC-1a). In addition, transcriptional and post-transcriptional mechanisms are important for the effects of T3, for example, in the synthesis of cytochrome c oxidase subunits. Thus, thyroid hormones are key regulator of mitochondrial energetics. In animal models, it has been shown that in pressure overload-induced cardiac hypertrophy a decrease of thyroid hormone receptor level occurs. The decrease in T3 serves as an indicator for a bad prognosis in the heart failure patient being linked to increased mortality (Dillmann, 2010).

2.1.5 Up regulated renin-angiotensin-aldosterone and sympathetic system

RAAS and sympathetic system are profoundly dysregulated in metabolic deranged conditions and adipose tissue has a full local renin-angiotensin system that is active at local and systemic level (Sarzani et al., 2008). RAAS is considered to have a prime role in hypertensive cardiomyopathy even though several growth factors influence initiation and maintenance of myocardial hypertrophy. Both angiotensin II and aldosterone are shown to contribute to myocardial fibrosis (Sopel et al., 2011; Struthers & Unger, 2011). Correlation between circulating renin–angiotensin levels and left ventricular mass have long been established and same has been proved by the study showing regression of hypertensive left ventricular hypertrophy upon targeting RAAS (Solomon et al., 2009). Though synergistic effects of angiotensin II and aldosterone are well established with regard to perivascular and interstitial fibrosis of the ventricle; angiotensin-independent effect of aldosterone on myocardial fibrosis has also been demonstrated. Current evidence shows that aldosterone has some role in the transition of left ventricular hypertrophy to cardiac failure. In addition, aldosterone also has a role in fluid retention. Altered RAAS has implication in chronic kidney disease and impaired kidney function resulting in volume overload which results in exacerbation of symptoms of heart failure and disease progression.

In addition to high RAAS drive, sympathetic hyperactivity present in patients with deranged metabolic profile contributes not only to high blood pressure, but seems to have further adverse metabolic effects also, such as insulin resistance, hyperinsulinaemia and hyperlipidaemia. Experimental evidence has indicated that heightened sympathetic nervous system activity facilitates the development of myocardial hypertrophy in animals and humans. Antihypertensive vasodilators (hydralazine and minoxidil) which are known to have some stimulating effect on sympathetic nervous system fail to reduce left ventricular hypertrophy despite their well-documented antihypertensive effects (Elliott et al., 2008). Thus, if such a relationship between RAAS, sympathetic activation and left ventricular hypertrophy exists, there are all possibilities that cardiomyopathy in hypertensive patients may be resultant of this interaction. This becomes more evident especially since neuroendocrine activation is found in hypertensive cardiomyopathy, with activation of the RAAS and the sympathetic system. All these components are hypothesized to be constituent part of CMCM as both RAAS and sympathetic systems are up-regulated in them.

2.1.6 Diastolic dysfunction, systolic dysfunction and ventricular hypertrophy in CMCM

Ventricular diastolic function is dependent on an active relaxation process in conjunction with passive elastic properties of the myocardium. In diastolic dysfunction, there is impairment in ventricular relaxation and passive filling. About 75% of diabetics show this dysfunction which is more pronounced when other metabolic abnormalities co-exist. In diastolic heart failure, though the ejection fraction may be normal, there is diastolic dysfunction along with elevated end diastolic pressure.

Functional abnormalities occur as a result of structural remodeling. In diastolic dysfunction a moderate increase in left ventricular mass and an elevated ventricular wall thickness to chamber radius is seen (Ozasa et al., 2008). The end diastolic volume is nearly normal. Increase in AGE crosslinks of cardiac SERCA impairs the ability or capacity of SERCA to translocate calcium and thus slows the rate of cardiac relaxation. The reduction in elasticity of the myocardium is due to myocardial collagen deposition and AGE crosslinks with elastin (Van et al., 2008). This early cardiac dysfunction, along with other exacerbating risk factors accelerates the decline in cardiac function.

Under conditions of hyperinsulinemia, a basic component of increased cardio-metabolic risks, insulin stimulates hypertrophy in cardiomyocytes by several pathways, mainly by activation of Akt and ERK. Increased circulating angiotensin II induces cardiomyocyte hypertrophy and interstitial fibrosis (He et al., 2005). Angiotensin II is also reported to increase reactive oxygen species (ROS) production and excess ROS produces cardiomyocyte death and results in replacement fibrosis. Sympathetic activation, in addition to effects on blood pressure, seems to have adverse metabolic effects. Hence, the interstitial fibrosis, protein glycosylation and myocyte hypertrophy are likely factors contributing to reduced diastolic compliance and ventricular hypertrophy in CMCM patients.

In the presence of predominant diastolic dysfunction, supervening reduced systolic reserve is often overlooked by diagnostic imaging at rest. Increased intracellular fatty acids and its metabolites are toxic to the mitochondria and induce apoptosis and damage the contractile apparatus. Many studies have demonstrated that the inhibitory cardiac troponin-I (cTnI) expression is markedly raised in the heart of diabetic rats and in cardiac hypertrophy. GATA binding protein 4 (GATA-4) binding site in the proximal region of cTnI gene is necessary for the transcriptional activation of this gene. GATA-4 found in cardiac myocytes regulates many other cardiac-specific gene expressions, like angiotensin II (AT_{1A}) and endothelin-1 (ET_A) receptors, atrial natriuretic factor (ANF), beta-type natriuretic peptide (BNP), myosin heavy chain (MHC) etc. Studies have shown that activation of MEK/ERK pathway by hyperglycemia-induced ROS or by direct adrenergic stimulation, increase GATA-4 phosphorylation and nuclear translocation, in addition MEK/ERK activation also causes GSK3β phosphorylation, thereby lowering the export of GATA-4 from nucleus, leading to GATA-4 preservation in the nucleus, which finally leads to an increase in the expression level of cTnI resulting in reduced cardiac contractility (Ku et al., 2011).
The longitudinal fibres responsible for long-axis contraction lie in the sub-endocardium and are particularly susceptible to the effects of fibrosis, ischemia or hypertrophy. Initially the long-axis systolic dysfunction is associated with a compensatory increase in radial thickening and mass, thus preserving left ventricular ejection fraction (LVEF). The preservation of ejection fraction is directly related to the presence of LV hypertrophy and the effect of increased muscle mass. However, reserve systolic functions are reduced and these patients show enhanced systolic functional abnormalities only during stress or exercise. Clinical studies have demonstrated that diabetic patients have an increased end-systolic diameter and volume, a diminished ejection fraction and a decreased minor axis shortening and velocity of circumferential fiber shortening in the absence of coronary artery disease. This is exaggerated when exposed to stress like exercise. These dysfunctions coupled with dysfunction in peripheral vasculature in CMCM translate into profound compromise in overall exercise reserve.

2.2 A central role for mitochondrial dysfunction in CMCM

2.2.1 Normal role of mitochondria

Myocardial contractile function is energy (ATP) dependent. Mitochondria are the major site of substrate oxidation and ATP production in cardiomyocytes. In addition, mitochondria also contribute to intracellular ROS generation. It is by oxidative phosphorylation in the mitochondrial system through which the oxidation of energy substrates in a cell is coupled to the activity of ATP synthase in the mitochondrial inner membrane. The activity of ATP synthase is powered by the electrochemical gradient existing across the mitochondrial inner membrane. The ATP produced drives energy demanding reactions not only in the mitochondrion but also in the cytoplasm.

2.2.2 Abnormal mitochondrial morphology and function

Lines of evidence have shown that mitochondrial dysfunction contributes to the development of insulin resistance and metabolic syndrome. The causes of mitochondrial dysfunction are complex, but over-nutrition and sedentary life style are among the best known causes of mitochondrial dysfunction (Kim et al., 2008). The cardio-metabolic conditions such as insulin resistance, diabetes, hypertension, dyslipidemia and sub-clinical hypothyroidism are characterized by altered mitochondrial function. Visceral obesity and related cardio-metabolic disorders are linked to defective mitochondrial biogenesis and oxidative metabolism with decreased ATP production. The hypertrophy-related changes in myocardium are likely related to mitochondrial structural and functional alterations that leads to altered mitochondrial efficiency for substrate oxidation and ATP production. Studies have revealed distinct patterns in mitochondrial structural and functional alterations in pathological and physiological cardiac hypertrophy. Among many signaling pathways that conspire to impair mitochondrial function include, decreased expression or activity of transcriptional regulators that govern mitochondrial biogenesis and oxidative capacity (i.e. PGC-1α, ERRα, and PPAR-α) and decreased transcription of mitochondrial DNA. Increased G-protein-coupled receptor signaling activates Class1B PI3Kγ that leads to constitutive activation of Akt, which may repress mitochondrial function. Activation of HIF-1α leads to a PPAR-α mediated increase in FA uptake and lipogenesis that may promote lipotoxicity, which could further impair mitochondrial function. Reduced cardiolipin content and remodeling of the mitochondrial proteome also contribute to mitochondrial dysfunction. Mitochondrial dysfunction promotes oxidative stress that leads to a vicious cycle of progressive mitochondrial damage.

At functional level, activities of mitochondrial complex I and III reduce at the stage of compensated cardiac hypertrophy, but this is accompanied by reduced mitochondrial ROS and oxidative damage that only becomes evident after the transition to heart failure. Hypertrophied hearts do not lose mitochondrial membrane potential in the context of ischemia and re-perfusion injury. However, the increase in mitochondrial membrane potential correlates with an increased risk of arrhythmias. By the time compensated hypertrophy progresses to pathological LV hypertrophy, altered mitochondrial morphology and function are evident. Pathological hypertrophic cardiomyopathy displays swollen cardiac mitochondria with disrupted cristae and substantial mitochondrial DNA depletion.

Mitochondrial membrane permeabilization is a rate limiting step of apoptosis and is mediated by the mitochondrial permeability transition pore (mtPTP). mtPTP is a nonspecific pore, permeable to all molecules of less than 1.5 kDa and is formed by the voltage-dependent anion channel (VDAC), members of the pro- and anti-apoptotic Bax/Bcl2 protein family, cyclophilin D and adenine nucleotide translocase (ANT). The ANT mediates nucleotide transfer from mitochondria to cytosol. The ATP synthesized in the mitochondria is exchanged for cytosolic adenosine diphosphate (ADP) by ANT to provide a continuous supply of ADP to mitochondria. ATP/ADP exchange by ANT is essential for the maintenance of ATP synthase activity.

On the other hand, in states of impaired function of ATP/ADP exchange, ANT plays a major role in generating ROS and inducing cell apoptosis (Kim et al., 2010). Thus, impaired ANT activity could contribute to deficient energy availability in pathological cardiac hypertrophy. Reduced level of cardiac ANT has been reported in some, but not all models of pressure overload cardiac hypertrophy. Additional proteins that were proposed to be part of the mtPTP complex are hexokinase, creatine kinase, and peripheral benzodiazepine receptor. mtPTP opening causes swelling of the mitochondrial matrix and rupture of outer membrane.

Cardiolipin, an important component and one of the most abundant phospholipid of the inner mitochondrial membrane, is essential for the optimal function of numerous enzymes that are involved in mitochondrial energy metabolism, where it regulates the activity of the mitochondrial electron transport chain, ATP synthesis and mitochondrial bioenergetics (Abel & Doenst, 2011). Abundance of linoleic acid and close proximity to the site of ROS production, i.e. the inner mitochondrial membrane make cardiolipin particularly more susceptible to damage by oxidative stress. Cardiolipin is identified as the only phospholipid in mitochondria that undergoes early oxidation during apoptosis (Kagan et al., 2005). Cardiolipin peroxidation by ROS thus affects its binding with cytochrome c and affects the activity of complex I, III, and IV of the mitochondrial respiratory chain (Paradies et al., 2004). Mitochondrial cardiolipin content is reduced in heart failure and ischemia/reperfusion and correlates with reduced electron transport chain activities. Patients with obesity and insulin resistance have poorer outcomes after myocardial infarction compared with lean subjects. These changes are associated with reduced myocardial cardiolipin content (Sparagna et al., 2007). Thus, reduced myocardial cardiolipin content contributes to the reduced mitochondrial efficiency in diabetes and metabolic syndrome and may exacerbate the progression of CMCM.

3. Diagnosis

Cardiac dysfunction caused by a constellation of metabolic abnormality may have variety of presentations. On one hand it includes myocardial dysfunction and coronary artery disease and on the other hand it may be arrhythmias and sudden death. When a patient presents with features of heart failure like, exercise intolerance, fatigue, and dyspnea with exertion as prominent symptoms in background of metabolic abnormalities like impaired glucose metabolism, dyslipidemia and hypertension with or without subclinical hypothyroidism then CMCM should be considered.

Clinical assessment of patients of heart failure with metabolic disorder should start with a thorough history followed by evaluation of pulmonary function to rule out non cardiac causes of dyspnoea. This should be followed by evaluation of functional limitations and status of the structural defect in the heart. Thereafter, causes of heart failure and extent of compromise in hemodynamic (perfusion and volume) status should be assessed. Because progression of heart failure is relatively rapid in metabolically challenged patients, it is very important to identify defects early in asymptomatic patients in order to prevent progression to symptomatic disease.

Laboratory evaluation of patients should start with complete blood count, urinalysis, serum electrolytes, blood urea nitrogen, serum creatinine, fasting blood glucose (glycohemoglobin), lipid profile and liver function tests. Thyroid dysfunctions may be subclinical with normal serum free T4 (fT4), free T3 (fT3) levels but deranged serum thyroid stimulating hormone (TSH) levels. Use of biomarkers for diagnosis of heart failure includes a number of neuroendocrine hormones, including norepinephrine, angiotensin II, renin, aldosterone, vasopressin and most recently BNP. Association of abnormal levels of these biomarkers with abnormal myocardial function and the unfavorable prognostic significance are increasingly being recognized and used. Patients with history of diabetes and elderly patients who are at high risk of developing myocardial dysfunction have a high prevalence of elevated plasma BNP levels. Thus, these high risk populations with elevated plasma levels of BNP or NT-proBNP can be identified for detailed evaluation of cardiac functions by echocardiography and/or cardiopulmonary exercise testing (CPET).

Insulin resistance can be an important etiologic factor in the development of heart failure with metabolic disorder as adaptive responses of myocardium to different stress are compromised in presence of insulin resistance. Insulin resistance has strong correlation with development of hypertension, left ventricular hypertrophy and left ventricular dysfunction and subsequent development of heart failure. There is also increased prevalence of myocardial ischemia in patients with insulin resistance and heart failure itself causes insulin resistance (Wilson, 2001; Nikolaidis et al., 2004). Evidence of insulin resistance should be evaluated by measuring fasting insulin levels.

Assessment of myocardial wall thickness, LV size and pericardium by comprehensive two-dimensional Echocardiography along with Doppler imaging are useful diagnostic tests in the evaluation of patients of heart failure. The most common abnormality associated with insulin resistance and diabetes mellitus is abnormality in diastolic function which is independent of ischemic heart disease (Fang et al., 2004; Schannwell et al., 2002). Evaluation of ventricular filling pattern by color Doppler imaging evaluating diastolic dysfunction becomes important for diagnosing such symptomatic patients who have preserved ejection fraction. A comprehensive echocardiographic examination helps in these distinctions when more than one abnormality affects the cardiac functions.

Most of the above mentioned methods of evaluation examine patients at rest, thus have limitations. Physical limitations during exercise, like shortness of breath and fatigue are caused by dynamic dysfunctions in myocardium occurring under stress and may not manifest at rest. Thus, markers of diminished cardiac reserve often go undetected by echocardiography. Stress echocardiography can detect ventricular dysfunction including wall motion abnormalities (hypokinesia, akinesia, dyskinesia or diastolic dysfunction) when exposed to stress either by dobutamin or exercise. This can pick up early cases with compromsied ventricular functions, however, peripheral components of heart failure may still not be factored in it.

CPET is a well-established method of evaluating cardiopulmonary functions in heart failure. This is highly reproducible measurement and helps in differentiation of cause of symptoms associated with heart failure. Using CPET for evaluation of limitation in cardiac functions in the patients with heart failure associated with metabolic disorder will not only evaluate dynamic response of heart to physiological stress but also peripheral component of hemodynamics which often coexists. Symptoms such as fatigue and disproportionate dyspnoea may be explained by inadequate and inappropriate vascular responsiveness (capillary recruitment) to demand generated by exercising skeletal muscles (Joshi et al., 2010). Maximal aerobic capacity (peak VO_2), Ve/VCO_2 and oxygen uptake efficiency slope (OUES) parameters obtained from CPET aids in early diagnosis of subtle pathology and helps in following the progression of the disease. These have important prognostic value also.

Impedance cardiography can be used non-invasively to measure hemodynamic parameters to diagnose covert cases of CMCM. Experimental studies in diabetic patients measuring stroke volume and cardiac output by impedance cardiography at the time of rest and exercise suggest, compromise in cardiac reserve even in the absence of any clinical symptoms of heart failure (Joshi et al., 2010). Compromise in cardiac reserve was contributed to, by an inappropriate increase in stroke volume due to diastolic compromise exaggerated by increase in heart rate. There was decrease in stroke volume and it had to be compensated for, by further increase in heart rate to maintain cardiac output. This "inflexion point", the heart rate at which the stroke volume starts decreasing, occurred at a relatively low heart rate. Recent evidence that limiting heart rate increase has favorable outcome in heart failure independent of beta blockade suggests ways of managing this dysfunction (Swedberg et al., 2010). There is speculation as to what should be the target heart rate to be achieved with such therapy. Perhaps studies such as done by Joshi et al., may provide the answer.

4. Treatment

Routine management of heart failure depending upon the status of decompensation, should be integral part of any case of CMCM. Along with this, therapy directed to pathophysiology like insulin resistance, hypothyroid state, lipid abnormality and therapies modulating the metabolic properties of myocytes should be considered.

4.1 Improving insulin resistance

Therapies which reduce insulin resistance improves outcome. There are evidence to support that therapies directed to treat heart failure also reduce insulin resistance even in non-heart failure population. Similarly, exercise improves both heart failure outcome and insulin sensitivity in non-ischemic heart failure (Kemppainen et al., 2003). Angiotensin converting enzyme inhibitor and angiotensin receptor blockers also improve insulin sensitivity in addition to their effect on heart failure (Yusuf et al., 2000; Pfeffer et al., 2003).

Drug therapy improving insulin resistance in CMCM can be at multiple levels. Different approaches consisting of lowering circulating FFA levels, facilitating glucose uptake and metabolism have been identified. These can be both anti-diabetic medication and metabolic modulator.

Drugs improving insulin sensitivity like metformin and thiazolidinediones are expected to improve outcome in cardiomyopathy associated with insulin resistance. Metformin can also improve calcium handling in myocytes (Ren et al., 1999), however, potential of causing lactic acidosis limits its utility in heart failure, especially in the context of renal dysfunction. Insulin or insulin-secretagogues could be another option as they directly promote glucose metabolism and decrease circulating FFAs but they have also failed in different animal models (Ren et al., 1996). Insulin therapy is expected to reduce catecholamine-induced myocardial damage in the heart however like with thizolidinediones, there is danger of fluid retention and hypoglycemia that may be detrimental. Several studies attempting to demonstrate the beneficial effects of tight glycemic control with insulin and secretagogues have failed to show any superiority and in fact have resulted in higher cardiovascular events.

Under the circumstances of insulin resistance, the body's compensatory mechanisms (hyperinsulinemia, up-regulation of the RAAS, catecholamines, vasopressin) are maladaptive and can further worsen the cardiomyopathy. Many counter-regulatory hormones like epinephrine, norepinephrine, glucagon, cortisol, growth hormone are upregulated and increases insulin resistance and alter glucose disposition (Nikolaidis et al., 2004). They also contribute to the pathogenesis of cardiomyopathy. Adrenergic blockade with carvedilol, long acting metoprolol and nebivolol improves myocardial efficiency by reducing consumption of FFA by myocardium and increasing preference to glucose as fuel (Nikolaidis et al., 2006) because chronic stimulation of beta-receptor seen in cardiac decompensation is known to inhibit insulin-mediated glucose uptake and insulin receptor

activation (Morisco et al., 2005). These patients are expected to achieve dramatic responses to angiotensin converting enzyme inhibition and beta-adrenergic blocking therapy, often with recovery of LVEF to normal or near-normal levels.
Limiting increase in heart rate independent of beta blockade has been shown to be of benefit in heart failure; ivabradine therapy in patients with systolic dysfunction and resting sinus rhythm of more than 70 bpm despite beta blockers or in beta blocker intolerant patients (Swedberg et al., 2010).

4.2 Metabolic modulators

Metabolic modulators target molecular metabolism within the myocardium and decrease consumption of FFA while increasing metabolism of glucose. Currently these drugs are used as antianginals as they increase energy efficiency in myocardium. Inhibitor of final enzyme in β-oxidation of FFA trimetazidine improves myocardial energy stores by increasing myocardial ATP/phosphocreatine levels (Aussedat et al., 1993). Trimetazidine improved LVEF and NYHA class in a study in 65 heart failure patients (Fragasso et al., 2006). Notably, benefits were more in nonischemic cardiomyopathy than the ischemic cardiomyopathy subgroup. Similarly perhexiline inhibit FFA metabolism and has demonstrated substantial improvements in LVEF, VO_2max and quality of life in a clinical trial with 56 heart failure patients (Lee et al., 2005). However, hepatotoxicity and peripheral neuropathy associated with perhexiline limits its clinical utility. Ranolazine is a third metabolic modulator which can potentially be used in CMCM to switch from FFA to glucose.
Although role of thyroid hormone therapy in treatment of heart failure is still not clear, its role in improvement of LV function, remodeling and microcirculation are being investigated. Use of l-thyroxin both in frank cases of hypothyroid and subclinical hypothyroid has shown reversal of structural abnormalities detected by echocardiography and is accompanied by clinical improvement. Gene therapies to modify thyroid hormone receptor or deiodinase expression and activity along with thyroid hormone replacement with T3 and/or T4, use of thyroid hormone analogs (e.g. diiodothyropropionic acid) will need further studies for proving its efficacy and safety in management of such cases (Gerdes & Iervasi, 2010).

4.3 Emerging therapies

4.3.1 AGE inhibitors and breakers

It is well established that AGEs, a heterogeneous group of molecules formed by the non-enzymatic reaction of reducing sugars with free amino groups of proteins, lipids and nucleic acids contribute significantly to diabetic complications, both macro- and micro-vascular.

4.3.1.1 Pharmacological intervention against AGE formation in vivo

Classically, efforts to target AGE-related complications had been approached either with intentions to inhibit the ongoing process of AGE formation or to cleave already formed AGE protein-protein crosslinks.

4.3.1.2 Pharmacological approach to inhibition of AGE crosslink formation

Accumulation of substantial evidence indicating AGEs as one of the culprits for diabetic complications, triggered active search for intervention in the process "by pharmacological approaches. Careful study of structural aspects lead researchers to target ketone group of the 1-amino-1-deoxyfructose residue in the amadori product, which was the key to subsequent AGE-forming reactions and that chemical deactivation of this ketone group would prevent AGE formation (Ulrich & Cerami, 2001).

Aminoguanidine was one such compound identified having desirable features to be studied for its ability to inhibit AGE crosslink formation. Prior to be explored for its AGE inhibition capabilities, some published reports existed for its experimental use in humans for unrelated purposes, without significant side-effects. During subsequent years, several researchers demonstrated effectiveness of aminoguanidine in inhibiting AGE formation in vivo in a wide variety of systems and tissues.

Usefulness of aminoguanidine has also been demonstrated in improving left ventricular end-diastolic (LVED) compliance in streptozotocin induced diabetic rats. Simultaneous administration of aminoguanidine with AGE-modified albumin prevented consequent glomerular hypertrophy (Bucala & Vlassara, 1995). Clinical utility with aminoguanidine was limited by its side effect potential, which was due to its inhibitory effect on diamine oxidase. This inhibition of diamineoxidase, results in an increase in histamine levels with attendant risk of vascular and respiratory complications. Aminoguanidine being a hydrazine derivative, its association with antihistone and antinuclear cytoplasmic antibody results in a clinical situation similar to lupus.

Few other less talked inhibitors of AGE formation have been reported, however none of them have reached advanced trials in humans. Pyridoxamine, a derivative of vitamin B6 has been suggested to prevent the degradation of protein-amadori intermediates to protein-AGE products. It is shown to reduce hyperlipidemia and prevents AGE formation in rats (Wu et al., 2011; Degenhardt et al., 2002; Stitt et al., 2002). Some preliminary clinical trials evaluating effect in diabetic nephropathy with this agent have been performed (Williams et al., 2007).

OPB-9195, a thiazolidine derivative has shown to be inhibitor of advanced glycation and to produce some benefits in attenuating progression of nephropathy in spontaneous diabetic rats (Nakamura et al., 1997). There is no current clinical experience with this compound nor is there any evidence for planned clinical trials.

LR-90, yet another compound capable of inhibiting AGE formation is being studied for its usefulness pre-clinically. Evidence are available for evaluating this compound in diabetic nephropathy and retinopathy (Figarola et al., 2008; Bhatwadekar et al., 2008). The compound has also shown to possess some anti-inflammatory properties (Figarola et al., 2007) with the potential for additional protective effects against diabetic vascular complications. However, future developmental strategy for this compound is not yet fully disclosed.

4.3.1.3 Pharmacological approach to cleave preformed AGE cross-linkages

Although attractive, approach to prevent AGE formation suffers from limitation of being unable to break preformed AGE crosslinkages. Thus, AGE breaker compounds are more desirable, as they open possibility for restoration of AGE damaged tissue to their original functionality, without relying on the body's much-slower, removal and repair mechanisms. Two such molecules, a thiazolium compound alagebrium (ALT-711) and pyridinium derivative TRC4186 are being evaluated for the treatment of heart failure in patients who are metabolically challenged.

Algebrium: Upon administration to various animal models of diabetes, it has resulted in an improvement in large-vessel elasticity, decrease in stiffness and peripheral resistance

(Wolffenbuttel et al., 1998; Candido et al., 2003), an attenuation in several functional and structural manifestations of diabetes related nephropathy (Peppa et al., 2006). Clinical studies with alagebrium in patients having uncontrolled systolic hypertension, of whom only an insignificant number were diabetic, found that the data did not indicate a treatment-related benefit (Zieman et al., 2007). Pulse wave velocity and arterial pressures, indicators of conduit vessel stiffness, were unchanged; however, brachial flow mediated dilatation, an indicator of endothelial function, was improved. In the DIAMOND study in elderly and PEDESTAL in adults with diastolic heart failure, alagebrium significantly decreased left ventricular mass, improved left ventricular diastolic filling and improved effort tolerance assessed by the 6-minute walk test. However, the trials did not meet the primary endpoint of improvement in ejection fraction. Here again, diabetes or impaired control of glycemia was not a precondition for inclusion of patients. Subsequently, further development of this compound is terminated.

TRC4186: TRC4186/TRC4149 is shown to act via multiple mechanisms, which include breaking of pre-formed AGE cross-links, reducing accumulation of carbohydrate as well as lipid derived AGEs and a potent free radical scavenging activity. Treatment of diabetic spontaneously hypertensive (SHR) rats, with TRC4149 resulted in a reduced AGE burden as evident by reduced immunochemical staining for AGE and significant reduction in VCAM expression in aorta. Ultimately, the combined actions translate into better preservation of endothelial function as well as an improved cardiac function (Pathak et al., 2008). Evaluation of TRC4186 in a more complex animal model of metabolic syndrome, ob-ZSF1 rats, demonstrated its capability to attenuate overall disease progression. The compound successfully prevented rise in blood pressure following salt loading and preserved ventricular functions. Although the exact mechanism of AGE breaking is not very clear, reduction in AGE load and all ensuing downstream events, including attenuation of the associated inflammatory response, likely contributed to the improvement observed on treatment with TRC4186. These outcomes are substantially supported by suitable histopathological and immunohistochemical findings (Joshi et al., 2009).

AGE breakers are likely to be beneficial in diabetic heart failure patients in whom there is usually a significant component of diastolic dysfunction and vascular unresponsiveness, when assessed for meaningful clinical endpoints such as physical attributes of Minnesota Living with Heart Failure Questionnaire and OUES, that are able to assess not only myocardial reserve but also vascular (nutritive perfusion) reserve. Other measures such as NT pro-BNP would be useful to assess diastolic dysfunction and fluid retention that could be exaggerated in patients with compromised renal function, a common co-morbidity in these patients. TRC4186, currently under investigation for use in diabetic patients has successfully completed phase 1 clinical trial and results of its phase 2 clinical trial Prospective Evaluation of AGE Breaker in Heart Failure (PEACH-F) are awaited.

Researchers have also focus on the possibility of preventing AGE-RAGE interaction thereby preventing subsequent deleterious downstream events contributing to AGEs related pathophysiology. Conceptually this has been attained by infusing soluble RAGE (sRAGE), and by RAGE antibodies. Though it is clear that blocking AGE receptors using antibodies would prevent AGE-RAGE interaction; it remains yet to be elucidated as to whether sRAGE acts as an antagonist inhibiting RAGE dependent signaling pathways, or scavenge AGEs and AGE precursor from circulation (Zieman & Kass, 2004). There are presently no small molecule inhibitors of RAGE, and this approach has yet to be tested in clinical studies.

Finally, intracellular signalling pathways upregulated by AGEs can be inhibited by AGE signal transduction inhibitors (e.g. PK-C inhibitors incadronate disodium, cerivastatin, and curcumin) (Peyroux & Sternberg, 2006).

4.3.2 Emerging therapy targeting mitochondrial energetics

Visceral obesity and related cardiometabolic disorders are linked to defective mitochondrial biogenesis and oxidative metabolism with a decreased ATP production. The defective mitochondrial function, a common pathophysiologic feature of these cardiometabolic disorders is a key etiopathological factor exacerbating the CMCM.

The effectiveness of beta-adrenergic blockers and angiotensin-converting enzyme inhibitors to improve ventricular function in patients with heart failure, may be, due in part to the action of these agents in decreasing energy demand. Other compounds that may also have beneficial effects in hypertrophied hearts include vanadyl sulfate, which improves tolerance of ischemia by stimulating membrane glucose transport, and propionyl-L-carnitine, which prevents myocardial mechanical alterations associated with pressure overload. There is evidence that administration of propionyl-L-carnitine increases both glucose and palmitate oxidation in hypertrophied hearts and improves the efficiency of translating ATP production into cardiac work.

On this basis, a restoration of metabolic demand by restoring mitochondrial energy efficiency may have potential as a new therapeutic treatment of the hypertensive heart and heart failure (Fujii et al., 2004). Although as yet no agent exists that promote mitochondrial biogenesis, PGC-1 alpha has generated interest. Sirt1 activators have also shown potential to increase mitochondrial biogenesis. The nitric oxide-cGMP–dependent pathway may also control mitochondrial biogenesis and may ameliorate energy deficiency in heart failure. Indeed, phosphodiesterase 5 inhibitors such as sildenafil that increase cGMP have, in preliminary studies, improved LV function and exercise capacity in heart failure.

The implications for thyroid hormones on the efficiency of energy expenditure and the handling of ROS are important. One of the thyroid hormone analog, DIPTA has been tested for heart failure in early clinical trials; however agents with greater therapeutic margin are yet desirable. Thus, there is still much scope for research into the energetic effects of thyroid hormones. The preclinical evidence of TRC150094 has shown potential to improve mitochondrial substrate oxidation capacity and mitochondrial efficiency as well as improve various cardiometabolic risks with acceptable safety (Cioffi et al., 2010; Zambad et al., 2011). However this molecule is yet to be proven in a clinical setting. The discovery of such newer agents improving mitochondrial energetics will help to explore the role of these agents in the treatment of CMCM. It would be interesting to follow the progress of some investigational drugs such as TRC150094 which are in early clinical development.

5. Conclusion and key learning

- Diabetes, hypertension, dyslipidemia and thyroid dysfunction often occur concomitantly in metabolically challenged individuals who are overweight. When present together, their effect on myocardium as well as on the vasculature contribute significantly to the clinical manifestations of patients diagnosed with heart failure not predominantly due to epicardial Coronary Artery Disease (cardio-metabolic cardiomyopathy).

- Impairment in mitochondrial energetics resulting in inflexibility in fuel utilization has a significant role in development and progression of CMCM.
- Currently recommended diagnostic methods such as Echocardiography and tissue Doppler imaging are carried out at rest and may result in underestimation of heart failure in the absence of a suitable provocative diagnostic method capable of assessing the ability of the heart to augment cardiac output (cardiac reserve) on exertional demand.
- Dynamic assessment of cardiac response during exercise with assessment of peripheral flow, distribution and nutritive perfusion such as CPET may provide an objective and sensitive measure of cardiac and microvascular correlates of the composite with better correlation to clinical manifestation and possibly also help in more accurately assessing the onset and progress of cardiovascular malfunction.
- Some of the newer emerging non-conventional diagnostic methods and therapies may offer a solution for the management of CMCM.

6. References

Abel, E. D. & Doenst, T. (2011). Mitochondrial adaptations to physiological vs. pathological cardiac hypertrophy. *Cardiovascular Research,* Vol.90, No.2, pp. 234-242, ISSN 1755-3245.

Ashrafian, H.; Frenneaux, M. P. & Opie, L. H. (2007). Metabolic mechanisms in heart failure. *Circulation,* Vol. 16, No.4, pp. 434-448, ISSN 0009-7322.

Aussedat, J.; Ray, A.; Kay, L.; Verdys, M.; Harpey, C. & Rossi, A. (1993). Improvement of long-term preservation of isolated arrested rat heart: beneficial effect of the antiischemic agent trimetazidine. *Journal of Cardiovascular Pharmacology,* Vol.21, No.1, pp. 128-135, ISSN 1533-4023.

Bhatwadekar, A.; Glenn, J. V.; Figarola, J. L.; Scott, S.; Gardiner, T. A.; Rahbar, S. & Stitt, A. W. (2008). A new advanced glycation inhibitor, LR-90, prevents experimental diabetic retinopathy in rats. *British Journal of Ophthalmology,* Vol.92, No.4, pp. 545-547, ISSN 1468-2079.

Borradaile, N. M.; Han, X.; Harp, J. D.; Gale, S. E.; Ory, D. S. & Schaffer, J. E. (2006). Disruption of endoplasmic reticulum structure and integrity in lipotoxic cell death. *Journal of Lipid Research,* Vol.47, No.12, pp. 2726-2737, ISSN 1539-7262.

Bucala, R. & Vlassara, H. (1995). Advanced glycosylation end products in diabetic renal and vascular disease. *American Journal of Kidney Disease,* Vol.26, No.6, pp. 875-888, ISSN 0272-6386.

Candido, R.; Forbes, J. M.; Thomas, M. C.; Thallas, V.; Dean, R. G.; Burns, W. C.; Tikellis, C.; Ritchie, R. H.; Twigg, S. M.; Cooper, M. E. & Burrell, L. M. (2003). A breaker of advanced glycation end products attenuates diabetes-induced myocardial structural changes. *Circulation Research,* Vol.92, No.7, pp. 785-792, ISSN 1524-4571.

Carley, A. N. & Severson, D. L. (2008). What are the biochemical mechanisms responsible for enhanced fatty acid utilization by perfused hearts from type 2 diabetic db/db mice? *Cardiovascular Drugs and Therapy,* Vol.22, No.2, pp. 83-89, ISSN 1573-7241.

Carley, A. N. & Severson, D. L. (2005). Fatty acid metabolism is enhanced in type 2 diabetic hearts. *Biochimica et Biophysica Acta,* Vol.1734, No.2, pp.112-126, ISSN 0006-3002.

Cioffi, F.; Zambad, S. P.; Chhipa, L.; Senese, R.; Busiello, R. A.; Tuli, D.; Munshi, S.; Moreno, M.; Lombardi, A.; Gupta, R. C.; Chauthaiwale, V.; Dutt, C.; de Lange, P.; Silvestri, E.; Lanni, A. & Goglia, F. (2010). TRC150094, a novel functional analog of iodothyronines, reduces adiposity by increasing energy expenditure and fatty acid oxidation in rats receiving a high-fat diet. *The FASEB Journal*, Vol.24, No.9, pp. 3451-3461, ISSN 1530- 6860.

Clarke, P. M.; Glasziou, P.; Patel, A.; Chalmers, J.; Woodward, M.; Harrap, S. B. & Salomon, J. A. (2010). Event rates, hospital utilization, and costs associated with major complications of diabetes: a multicountry comparative analysis. *PLoS Med*, Vol.7, No.2, pp. e1000236, ISSN 1549-1676.

Degenhardt, T. P.; Alderson, N. L.; Arrington, D. D.; Beattie, R. J.; Basgen, J. M.; Steffes, M. W.; Thorpe, S. R. & Baynes, J. W. (2002). Pyridoxamine inhibits early renal disease and dyslipidemia in the streptozotocin-diabetic rat. *Kidney International*, Vol.61, No.3, pp. 939-950, ISSN 1523-1755.

Dillmann, W. (2010). Cardiac hypertrophy and thyroid hormone signaling. *Heart Failure Reviews*, Vol.15, No.2, pp. 125-132, ISSN 1573-7322.

Dickstein, K.; Cohen-Solal, A.; Filippatos, G.; McMurray, J. J.; Ponikowski, P.; Poole-Wilson, P. A.; Stromberg, A.; van Veldhuisen, D. J.; Atar, D.; Hoes, A. W.; Keren, A.; Mebazaa, A.; Nieminen, M.; Priori, S. G.; Swedberg, K.; Vahanian, A.; Camm, J.; De, C. R.; Dean, V.; Dickstein, K.; Filippatos, G.; Funck-Brentano, C.; Hellemans, I.; Kristensen, S. D.; McGregor, K.; Sechtem, U.; Silber, S.; Tendera, M.; Widimsky, P. & Zamorano, J. L. (2008). ESC Guidelines for the diagnosis and treatment of acute and chronic heart failure 2008: the Task Force for the Diagnosis and Treatment of Acute and Chronic Heart Failure 2008 of the European Society of Cardiology. Developed in collaboration with the Heart Failure Association of the ESC (HFA) and endorsed by the European Society of Intensive Care Medicine (ESICM). *European Heart Journal*, Vol.29, No.19, pp. 2388-2442, ISSN 1522-9645.

Elliott, P.; Andersson, B.; Arbustini, E.; Bilinska, Z.; Cecchi, F.; Charron, P.; Dubourg, O.; Kuhl, U.; Maisch, B.; McKenna, W. J.; Monserrat, L.; Pankuweit, S.; Rapezzi, C.; Seferovic, P.; Tavazzi, L. & Keren, A. (2008). Classification of the cardiomyopathies: a position statement from the European Society Of Cardiology Working Group on Myocardial and Pericardial Diseases. *European Heart Journal*, Vol.29, No.2, pp. 270-276, ISSN 1522-9645.

Fang, Z. Y.; Prins, J. B. & Marwick, T. H. (2004). Diabetic cardiomyopathy: evidence, mechanisms, and therapeutic implications. *Endocrine Reviews*, Vol.25, No.4, pp. 543-567, ISSN 0163-769X.

Figarola, J. L.; Shanmugam, N.; Natarajan, R. & Rahbar, S. (2007). Anti-inflammatory effects of the advanced glycation end product inhibitor LR-90 in human monocytes. *Diabetes*, Vol.56, No.3, pp. 647-655, ISSN 1939-327X.

Figarola, J. L.; Loera, S.; Weng, Y.; Shanmugam, N.; Natarajan, R. & Rahbar, S. (2008). LR-90 prevents dyslipidaemia and diabetic nephropathy in the Zucker diabetic fatty rat. *Diabetologia*, Vol.51, No.5, pp. 882-891, ISSN 1432-0428.

Fragasso, G.; Palloshi, A.; Puccetti, P.; Silipigni, C.; Rossodivita, A.; Pala, M.; Calori, G.; Alfieri, O. & Margonato, A. (2006). A randomized clinical trial of trimetazidine, a partial free fatty acid oxidation inhibitor, in patients with heart failure. *Journal of American College of Cardiology*, Vol.48, No.5, pp. 992-998, ISSN 0735-1097.

Fujii, N.; Nozawa, T.; Igawa, A.; Kato, B.; Igarashi, N.; Nonomura, M.; Asanoi, H.; Tazawa, S.; Inoue, M. & Inoue, H. (2004). Saturated glucose uptake capacity and impaired fatty acid oxidation in hypertensive hearts before development of heart failure. *American Journal of Physiology Heart and Circulatory Physiology,* Vol.287, No.2, pp. H760-H766, ISSN 1522-1539.

Garvey, W. T.; Hardin, D.; Juhaszova, M. & Dominguez, J. H. (1993). Effects of diabetes on myocardial glucose transport system in rats: implications for diabetic cardiomyopathy. *American Journal of Physiology Heart and Circulatory Physiology,* Vol.264, No.3, pp. H837-H844, ISSN 1522-1539.

Gerdes, A. M. & Iervasi, G. (2010). Thyroid replacement therapy and heart failure. *Circulation,* Vol.122, No.4, pp. 385-393, ISSN 0009-7322.

Goldin, A.; Beckman, J. A.; Schmidt, A. M. & Creager, M. A. (2006). Advanced glycation end products: sparking the development of diabetic vascular injury. *Circulation,* Vol.114, No.6, pp. 597-605, ISSN 0009-7322.

He, Z.; Way, K. J.; Arikawa, E.; Chou, E.; Opland, D. M.; Clermont, A.; Isshiki, K.; Ma, R. C.; Scott, J. A.; Schoen, F. J.; Feener, E. P. & King, G. L. (2005). Differential regulation of angiotensin II-induced expression of connective tissue growth factor by protein kinase C isoforms in the myocardium. *The Journal of Biology and Chemistry,* Vol.280, No.16, pp. 15719-15726, ISSN 1083-351X.

Herrero, P.; Peterson, L. R.; McGill, J. B.; Matthew, S.; Lesniak, D.; Dence, C. & Gropler, R. J. (2006). Increased myocardial fatty acid metabolism in patients with type 1 diabetes mellitus. *Journal of American College of Cardiology,* Vol.47, No.3, pp. 598-604, ISSN 0735-1097.

Jessup, M.; Abraham, W. T.; Casey, D. E.; Feldman, A. M.; Francis, G. S.; Ganiats, T. G.; Konstam, M. A.; Mancini, D. M.; Rahko, P. S.; Silver, M. A.; Stevenson, L. W. & Yancy, C. W. (2009). 2009 focused update: ACCF/AHA Guidelines for the Diagnosis and Management of Heart Failure in Adults: a report of the American College of Cardiology Foundation/American Heart Association Task Force on Practice Guidelines: developed in collaboration with the International Society for Heart and Lung Transplantation. *Circulation,* Vol.119, No.14, pp. 1977-2016, ISSN 0009-7322.

Joshi, D.; Gupta, R.; Dubey, A.; Shiwalkar, A.; Pathak, P.; Gupta, R. C.; Chauthaiwale, V. & Dutt, C. (2009). TRC4186, a novel AGE-breaker, improves diabetic cardiomyopathy and nephropathy in Ob-ZSF1 model of type 2 diabetes. *Journal of Cardiovascular Pharmacology,* Vol.54, No.1, pp. 72-81, ISSN 1533-4023.

Joshi, D.; Shiwalkar, A.; Cross, M. R.; Sharma, S. K.; Vachhani, A. & Dutt, C. (2010). Continuous, non-invasive measurement of the haemodynamic response to submaximal exercise in patients with diabetes mellitus: evidence of impaired cardiac reserve and peripheral vascular response. *Heart,* Vol.96, No.1, pp. 36-41, ISSN 1468-201X.

Kagan, V. E.; Tyurin, V. A.; Jiang, J.; Tyurina, Y. Y.; Ritov, V. B.; Amoscato, A. A.; Osipov, A. N.; Belikova, N. A.; Kapralov, A. A.; Kini, V.; Vlasova, I. I.; Zhao, Q.; Zou, M.; Di, P.; Svistunenko, D. A.; Kurnikov, I. V. & Borisenko, G. G. (2005). Cytochrome c acts as a cardiolipin oxygenase required for release of proapoptotic factors. *Nature Chemical Biology,* Vol.1, No.4, pp. 223-232, ISSN 1552-4450.

Kemppainen, J.; Tsuchida, H.; Stolen, K.; Karlsson, H.; Bjornholm, M.; Heinonen, O. J.; Nuutila, P.; Krook, A.; Knuuti, J. & Zierath, J. R. (2003). Insulin signalling and resistance in patients with chronic heart failure. *The Journal of Physiology,* Vol.550, No.1, pp. 305-315, ISSN 1469-7793.

Kim, J. A.; Wei, Y. & Sowers, J. R. (2008). Role of mitochondrial dysfunction in insulin resistance. *Circulation Research,* Vol.102, No.4, pp. 401-414, ISSN 1524-4571.

Kim, E. H.; Koh, E. H.; Park, J. Y. & Lee, K. U. (2010). Adenine nucleotide translocator as a regulator of mitochondrial function: implication in the pathogenesis of metabolic syndrome. *Korean Diabetes Journal,* Vol.34, No.3, pp. 146-153, ISSN 2093-2650.

Kinugawa, K.; Minobe, W. A.; Wood, W. M.; Ridgway, E. C.; Baxter, J. D.; Ribeiro, R. C.; Tawadrous, M. F.; Lowes, B. A.; Long, C. S. & Bristow, M. R. (2001). Signaling pathways responsible for fetal gene induction in the failing human heart: evidence for altered thyroid hormone receptor gene expression. *Circulation,* Vol.103, No.8, pp. 1089-1094, ISSN 0009-7322.

Ku, P. M.; Chen, L. J.; Liang, J. R.; Cheng, K. C.; Li, Y. X. & Cheng, J. T. (2011). Molecular role of GATA binding protein 4 (GATA-4) in hyperglycemia-induced reduction of cardiac contractility. *Cardiovascular Diabetology,* Vol.10, No.1, pp. 57, ISSN 1475 - 2840.

Lee, L.; Campbell, R.; Scheuermann-Freestone, M.; Taylor, R.; Gunaruwan, P.; Williams, L.; Ashrafian, H.; Horowitz, J.; Fraser, A. G.; Clarke, K. & Frenneaux, M. (2005). Metabolic modulation with perhexiline in chronic heart failure: a randomized, controlled trial of short-term use of a novel treatment. *Circulation,* Vol.112, No.21, pp. 3280-3288, ISSN 0009-7322.

Miyata, T.; Saito, A.; kurokawa, K. & van Ypersele de S.C. (2001). Advanced glycation and lipoxidation end products: reactive carbonyl compounds-related uraemic toxicity. *Nephrology Dialysis Transplantation,* Vol.16, No.4, pp. 8-11, ISSN 1460-2385.

Morisco, C.; Condorelli, G.; Trimarco, V.; Bellis, A.; Marrone, C.; Condorelli, G.; Sadoshima, J. & Trimarco, B. (2005). Akt mediates the cross-talk between beta-adrenergic and insulin receptors in neonatal cardiomyocytes. *Circulation Research,* Vol.96, No.2, pp. 180-188, ISSN 1524-4571.

Nakamura, S.; Makita, Z.; Ishikawa, S.; Yasumura, K.; Fujii, W.; Yanagisawa, K.; Kawata, T. & Koike, T. (1997). Progression of nephropathy in spontaneous diabetic rats is prevented by OPB-9195, a novel inhibitor of advanced glycation. *Diabetes,* Vol.46, No.5, pp. 895-899, ISSN 1939-327X.

Nikolaidis, L. A.; Sturzu, A.; Stolarski, C.; Elahi, D. Shen, Y. T. & Shannon, R. P. (2004). The development of myocardial insulin resistance in conscious dogs with advanced dilated cardiomyopathy. *Cardiovascular Research,* Vol.61, No.2, pp. 297-306, ISSN 1755-3245.

Nikolaidis, L. A.; Poornima, I.; Parikh, P.; Magovern, M.; Shen, Y. T. & Shannon, R. P. (2006). The effects of combined versus selective adrenergic blockade on left ventricular and systemic hemodynamics, myocardial substrate preference, and regional perfusion in conscious dogs with dilated cardiomyopathy. *Journal of American College of Cardiology,* Vol.47, No.9, pp. 1871-1881, ISSN 0735-1097.

Ozasa, N.; Furukawa, Y.; Morimoto, T.; Tadamura, E.; Kita, T. & Kimura, T. (2008). Relation among left ventricular mass, insulin resistance, and hemodynamic parameters in type 2 diabetes. *Hypertension Research,* Vol.31, No.3, pp. 425-432, ISSN 0916-9636.

Paradies, G.; Petrosillo, G.; Pistolese, M.; Di, V. N.; Federici, A. & Ruggiero, F. M. (2004). Decrease in mitochondrial complex I activity in ischemic/reperfused rat heart: involvement of reactive oxygen species and cardiolipin. *Circulation Research,* Vol.94, No.1, pp. 53-59, ISSN 1524-4571.

Pathak, P.; Gupta, R.; Chaudhari, A.; Shiwalkar, A.; Dubey, A.; Mandhare, A. B.; Gupta, R. C.; Joshi, D. & Chauthaiwale, V. (2008). TRC4149 a novel advanced glycation end product breaker improves hemodynamic status in diabetic spontaneously hypertensive rats. *European Journal of Medical Research,* Vol.13, No.8, pp. 388-398, ISSN 0949-2321.

Paulus, W. J. European Study Group on Diastolic Heart Failure. (1998). How to diagnose diastolic heart failure. *European Heart Journal,* Vol.19, No.7, pp. 990-1003, ISSN 1468-201X.

Peppa, M.; Brem, H.; Cai, W.; Zhang, J. G.; Basgen, J.; Li, Z.; Vlassara, H. & Uribarri, J. (2006). Prevention and reversal of diabetic nephropathy in db/db mice treated with alagebrium (ALT-711). *American Journal of Nephrology,* Vol.26, No.5, pp. 430-436, ISSN 1421-9670.

Pereira, L.; Matthes, J.; Schuster, I.; Valdivia, H. H.; Herzig, S.; Richard, S. & Gomez, A. M. (2006). Mechanisms of [Ca2+]i transient decrease in cardiomyopathy of db/db type 2 diabetic mice. *Diabetes,* Vol.55, No.3, pp. 608-615, ISSN 1939-327X.

Peyroux, J. & Sternberg, M. (2006). Advanced glycation endproducts (AGEs): Pharmacological inhibition in diabetes. *Pathol Biol (Paris),* Vol.54, No.7, pp. 405-419, ISSN 0369-8114.

Pfeffer, M. A.; Swedberg, K.; Granger, C. B.; Held, P.; McMurray, J. J.; Michelson, E. L.; Olofsson, B.; Ostergren, J.; Yusuf, S. & Pocock, S. (2003). Effects of candesartan on mortality and morbidity in patients with chronic heart failure: the CHARM-Overall programme. *Lancet,* Vol.362, No.9386, pp. 759-766, ISSN 0140-6736.

Ren, J.; Dominguez, L. J.; Sowers, J. R. & Davidoff, A. J. (1996). Troglitazone attenuates high-glucose-induced abnormalities in relaxation and intracellular calcium in rat ventricular myocytes. *Diabetes,* Vol.45, No.12, pp. 1822-1825, ISSN 1939-327X.

Ren, J.; Dominguez, L. J.; Sowers, J. R. & Davidoff, A. J. (1999). Metformin but not glyburide prevents high glucose-induced abnormalities in relaxation and intracellular Ca2+ transients in adult rat ventricular myocytes. *Diabetes,* Vol.48, No.10, pp. 2059-2065, ISSN 1939-327X.

Sarzani, R.; Salvi, F.; ssi-Fulgheri, P. & Rappelli, A. (2008). Renin-angiotensin system, natriuretic peptides, obesity, metabolic syndrome, and hypertension: an integrated view in humans. *Journal of Hypertension,* Vol.26, No.5, pp. 831-843, ISSN1473-5598.

Schannwell, C. M.; Schneppenheim, M.; Perings, S.; Plehn, G. & Strauer, B. E. (2002). Left ventricular diastolic dysfunction as an early manifestation of diabetic cardiomyopathy. *Cardiology,* Vol.98, No.1-2, pp. 33-39.

Shanmugam, N.; Figarola, J. L.; Li, Y.; Swiderski, P. M.; Rahbar, S. & Natarajan, R. (2008). Proinflammatory effects of advanced lipoxidation end products in monocytes. *Diabetes,* Vol.57, No.4, pp. 879-888, ISSN1939-327X.

Solomon, S. D.; Appelbaum, E.; Manning, W. J.; Verma, A.; Berglund, T.; Lukashevich, V.; Cherif, P. C.; Smith, B. A. & Dahlof, B. (2009). Effect of the direct Renin inhibitor aliskiren, the Angiotensin receptor blocker losartan, or both on left ventricular mass in patients with hypertension and left ventricular hypertrophy. *Circulation,* Vol.119, No.4, pp. 530-537, ISSN 0009-7322.

Sopel, M. J.; Rosin, N. L.; Lee, T. D. & Legare, J. F. (2011). Myocardial fibrosis in response to Angiotensin II is preceded by the recruitment of mesenchymal progenitor cells. *Laboratory Investigation,* Vol.91, No.4, pp. 565-578, ISSN 0023-6837.

Sparagna, G. C.; Chicco, A. J.; Murphy, R. C.; Bristow, M. R.; Johnson, C. A.; Rees, M. L.; Maxey, M. L.; McCune, S. A. & Moore, R. L. (2007). Loss of cardiac tetralinoleoyl cardiolipin in human and experimental heart failure. *Journal of Lipid Research,* Vol.48, No.7, pp. 1559-1570, ISSN 1539-7262.

Stitt, A.; Gardiner, T. A.; Alderson, N. L.; Canning, P.; Frizzell, N.; Duffy, N.; Boyle, C.; Januszewski, A. S.; Chachich, M.; Baynes, J. W. & Thorpe, S. R. (2002). The AGE inhibitor pyridoxamine inhibits development of retinopathy in experimental diabetes. *Diabetes,* Vol.51, No.9, pp. 2826-2832, ISSN 1939-327X.

Struthers, A. D. & Unger, T. (2011). Physiology of aldosterone and pharmacology of aldosterone blockers. *European Heart Journal Suppl,* Vol.13 (suppl B), B27-B30 ISSN 1554-2815.

Swedberg, K.; Komajda, M.; Bohm, M.; Borer, J. S.; Ford, I.; Dubost-Brama, A.; Lerebours, G. & Tavazzi, L. (2010). Ivabradine and outcomes in chronic heart failure (SHIFT): a randomised placebo-controlled study. *Lancet,* Vol.376, No.9744, pp. 875-885, ISSN ISSN 0140-6736.

Ulrich, P. & Cerami, A. (2001). Protein glycation, diabetes, and aging. *Recent Progress in Hormone Research,* Vol.56, pp. 1-21, ISSN 0079-9963.

Van, H. L.; Hamdani, N.; Handoko, M. L.; Falcao-Pires, I.; Musters, R. J.; Kupreishvili, K.; Ijsselmuiden, A. J.; Schalkwijk, C. G.; Bronzwaer, J. G.; Diamant, M.; Borbely, A.; van, d., V; Stienen, G. J.; Laarman, G. J.; Niessen, H. W. & Paulus, W. J. (2008). Diastolic stiffness of the failing diabetic heart: importance of fibrosis, advanced glycation end products, and myocyte resting tension. *Circulation,* Vol.117, No.1, pp.43-51, ISSN ISSN 0009-7322.

Vetter, R.; Rehfeld, U.; Reissfelder, C.; Weiss, W.; Wagner, K. D.; Gunther, J.; Hammes, A.; Tschope, C.; Dillmann, W. & Paul, M. (2002). Transgenic overexpression of the sarcoplasmic reticulum Ca2+ATPase improves reticular Ca2+ handling in normal and diabetic rat hearts. *The FASEB Journal,* Vol.16, No.12, pp. 1657-1659, ISSN 1530-6860.

Williams, M. E.; Bolton, W. K.; Khalifah, R. G.; Degenhardt, T. P.; Schotzinger, R. J. & McGill, J. B. (2007). Effects of pyridoxamine in combined phase 2 studies of patients with type 1 and type 2 diabetes and overt nephropathy. *American Journal of Nephrology,* Vol.27, No.6, pp. 605-614, ISSN 1421-9670.

Wolffenbuttel, B. H.; Boulanger, C. M.; Crijns, F. R.; Huijberts, M. S.; Poitevin, P.; Swennen, G. N.; Vasan, S.; Egan, J. J.; Ulrich, P.; Cerami, A. & Levy, B. I. (1998). Breakers of advanced glycation end products restore large artery properties in experimental diabetes. *Proceedings of the National Academy of Sciences U. S. A.,* Vol.95, No.8, pp. 4630-4634, ISSN 0027-8424.

Wilson, P. W. (2001). Diabetes mellitus and coronary heart disease. *Endocrinology Metabolism Clinics of North America,* Vol.30, No.4, pp. 857-881, ISSN 0889-8529.

Wu, E. T.; Liang, J. T.; Wu, M. S. & Chang, K. C. (2011). Pyridoxamine prevents age-related aortic stiffening and vascular resistance in association with reduced collagen glycation. *Experimental Gerontology,* Vol.46, No.6, pp. 482-488, ISSN 1873-6815.

Yusuf, S.; Sleight, P.; Pogue, J.; Bosch, J.; Davies, R. & Dagenais, G. (2000). Effects of an angiotensin-converting-enzyme inhibitor, ramipril, on cardiovascular events in high-risk patients. The Heart Outcomes Prevention Evaluation Study Investigators. *New England Journal of Medicine,* Vol.342, No.3, pp. 145-153. ISSN 1533-4406.

Zambad, S. P.; Munshi, S.; Dubey, A.; Gupta, R.; Busiello, R. A.; Lanni, A.; Goglia, F.; Gupta, R. C.; Chauthaiwale, V. & Dutt, C. (2011). TRC150094 attenuates progression of nontraditional cardiovascular risk factors associated with obesity and type 2 diabetes in obese ZSF1 rats. *Diabetes, Metabolic Syndrome and Obesity: Targets and Therapy,* Vol. 6, No. 4, pp. 5-16, ISSN 1178-7007.

Zieman, S. & Kass, D. (2004). Advanced glycation end product cross-linking: pathophysiologic role and therapeutic target in cardiovascular disease. *Congestive Heart Failure,* Vol.10, No.3, pp. 144-149, ISSN 1751-7133.

Zieman, S. J.; Melenovsky, V.; Clattenburg, L.; Corretti, M. C.; Capriotti, A.; Gerstenblith, G. & Kass, D. A. (2007). Advanced glycation endproduct crosslink breaker (alagebrium) improves endothelial function in patients with isolated systolic hypertension. *Journal of Hypertension,* Vol.25, No.3, pp. 577-583, ISSN 1473-5598.

22

Diabetic Cardiomyopathy: Cardiac Changes, Pathophysiological Mechanisms, Biologic Markers, and the Available Therapeutic Armamentarium

Michael F. Hill
Department of Medicine, Division of Cardiovascular Medicine, Vanderbilt University Medical Center, Nashville, Tennessee United States of America

1. Introduction

Patients with diabetes mellitus (DM) exhibit greatly increased cardiovascular morbidity and mortality. The increased mortality of patients with DM stems from the more frequent development of heart failure (HF) (Bell, 2003a; Jaffe et al., 1984; Kamalesh, 2007; Marwick, 2006; Solomon et al., 2002). In the past, the high incidence and poor prognosis of HF in diabetic patients was attributed to the concurrent presence of hypertension and/or myocardial ischemia. However, follow-up studies have shown that the increased risk for developing HF persists in DM patients even after adjusting for concomitant risks such as coronary artery disease and blood pressure (Ho et al., 1993; Kannel & McGee, 1979). It is now well established that DM increases the risk of cardiovascular morbidity and mortality by promoting cardiomyopathy, a distinct entity independent of coronary artery disease, hypertension or other known cardiac risk factors with origins in diabetic cardiac muscle (Bell, 1995; Cohen, 1995; Hamby et al., 1974; Regan et al., 1977; Spector, 1998).
According to a new study commissioned by the Centers for Disease Control and Prevention, 25.8 million children and adults in the United States, or 8.3% of the population, have DM, with about 1.9 million new cases of DM being diagnosed annually (Centers for Disease Control and Prevention, 2011). Worldwide, the number of people with DM has more than doubled since 1980 to 347 million (Danaei et al., 2011). With the global burden of DM rising, it is likely that the incidence of diabetes-induced cardiomyopathy and subsequent HF will continue to increase in this high-risk population. The goal of this chapter is to review the structural and functional changes in the diabetic heart and the pathophysiological mechanisms involved in the development of diabetic cardiomyopathy, taking into account the most recent developments in basic and clinical research. An overview of the latest advances in therapeutic approaches to treat diabetic cardiomyopathy will also be presented. Particular attention is given to the role of oxidative stress in the pathogenesis of diabetic cardiomyopathy and the potential of anti-oxidative therapy. The value of newly identified candidate biomarker proteins in assessing disease presence and progression, prognosis, and efficacy of therapies in the setting of diabetic cardiomyopathy will also be discussed.

2. Cardiomyopathy in diabetes

Sustained DM leads to a deterioration of heart function that is independent of any of the known concomitant risk factors and pathologies that are frequently seen in DM patients such as dyslipidemia, coronary artery disease, thrombosis, myocardial infarction (MI), and hypertension. The clinical presentation of cardiac dysfunction in DM patients without evidence of any of these other risk factors was first reported by Rubler et al. in 1972 (Rubler et al., 1972) based on postmortem findings of HF in diabetic patients free of coronary disease. These and similar findings have been reported in numerous other clinical studies (Bell, 2003a; Boyer et al., 2004; Devereux et al., 2000; Fang et al., 2003, 2005; Galderisi et al., 1991; Hamby et al., 1974; Kannel et al., 1974; Regan et al., 1977; Zabalgoitia et al., 2001) and animal models (Borges et al., 2006; Hamblin et al., 2007a; Kaul et al., 1995, 1996; Kralik et al., 2005; Loganathan et al., 2006; Mihm et al., 2001; Shen et al., 2005, 2006). This has led to the increased recognition that DM produces damage to cardiac muscle without depending on the co-existence of other cardiovascular risk factors. This unique form of heart disease in the absence of clinically detectable atherosclerosis and/or coronary artery disease has been termed "diabetic cardiomyopathy". This diabetes-related cardiomyopathy affects the myocardium secondary to DM and is accompanied by a prolonged decline in cardiac function. This unique cardiac phenomenon has been documented to progress to HF in both type 1 and type 2 DM patients.

2.1 Contemporary clinical epidemiology of diabetic cardiomyopathy

Older cardiovascular epidemiological studies showed that 30% of diabetic subjects without overt cardiac disease had LV dysfunction (Beljic & Miric, 1994; Di Bonito et al., 1996; Nicolino et al., 1995). However, this prevalence was based on standard echocardiography testing which frequently was not able to detect mild and early diastolic dysfunction (Bell, 2003b). Contemporary assessments of the epidemiology of diabetic cardiomyopathy using more rigorous Doppler methods demonstrate that the prevalence of diabetic cardiomyopathy is much higher than was previously believed, and in addition, emphasize the ominous impact of DM on myocardial function by highlighting the high prevalence of pre-clinical diabetic cardiomyopathy in the diabetic population and its strong association with an adverse prognosis (Kiencke et al., 2010; Van Den Hurk et al., 2010). In an ambulatory clinic-based sample of middle-aged, overweight-to-obese individuals with prevalent DM for an average duration of over 10 years, diabetic cardiomyopathy was present in 48% of patients as assessed by Doppler echocardiography (Kiencke et al., 2010). Of note, diastolic function was abnormal in 38% of the DM patients studied (Kiencke et al., 2010). The use of flow and tissue Doppler techniques suggests an even higher prevalence of diastolic dysfunction (as high as 40% to 60%) in individuals with type 1 and type 2 DM without discernable coronary heart disease (Boudina & Abel, 2007; Di Bonito et al., 2005; Poirier et al., 2001; Shivalkar et al., 2006). The high incidence of such diastolic dysfunction and its association with HF and with mortality (From et al., 2010) underscore the existence of diabetic cardiomyopathy as a very serious clinical condition.

2.2 Diagnostic indices

Cardiomyopathy in type 1 or type 2 DM is associated with a cluster of common cardiac abnormalities (Table 1). The most frequent and earliest detectable functional abnormality in diabetic cardiomyopathy is impaired diastolic function (Fang et al., 2003, 2005; Karamitsos et al., 2007), owing to reduced elasticity of the diabetic myocardium as a result of interstitial collagen deposition. The reduced diastolic function early in the time course of DM is followed by late decreases in systolic performance (Devereux et al., 2000; Fang et al, 2003; Mildenberger et al., 1984; Raev, 1994; Von Bibra et al., 2005). Diabetic cardiomyopathy in humans is also manifested by left ventricular hypertrophy (LVH) (Devereux et al., 2000; Kannel et al., 1974; Ozasa et al., 2008). Although no single diagnostic test for diabetic cardiomyopathy exists, the use of different imaging modalities (echocardiography, cardiac MRI) makes it possible to detect the phenotypic features of this condition (Asghar et al., 2009). Echocardiography is the diagnostic method that can achieve early detection of diabetic cardiomyopathy since it can detect structural myocardial changes (LVH and increased cardiac mass) in addition to evaluation of diastolic and systolic heart dysfunction (Mytas et al., 2009). As a result, echocardiography based methods currently stand as the preferred diagnostic approach for diabetic cardiomyopathy in clinical practice (Maya & Villarreal, 2010).

Abnormality	Manifestation (Stage of Disease)
Diastolic Dysfunction	Early
Systolic Dysfunction	Late
Left Ventricular Hypertrophy	Late
Myocardial Fibrosis	Late

Table 1. Diagnosis of Diabetic Cardiomyopathy

Although brain natriuretic peptide (BNP), a hormone secreted by the ventricles of the heart in response to ventricular volume and pressure overload, is both sensitive and specific for HF, research has shown that BNP is of limited diagnostic utility for diagnosing diabetic cardiomyopathy (Fang et al., 2005; Valle et al., 2006). This is due in part to the fact that BNP cannot reliably distinguish between systolic and diastolic HF, which limits its use in diabetic cardiomyopathy (Asghar et al., 2009; Fang et al., 2005; Maisel et al., 2003). Furthermore, the triggers for BNP secretion (increased intraventricular volume and pressure) does not occur in patients with subclinical, asymptomatic diabetic cardiomyopathy (Mytas et al., 2009; Stevanovic et al., 2006). In light of these findings, it is recommended that BNP not be used in isolation to diagnose or exclude diabetic cardiomyopathy (Fang et al., 2005; Kamalesh, 2007).

3. Cardiac changes

3.1 Structural remodeling

3.1.1 LVH

Data from the Framingham Heart Study (Kannel et al., 1974) as well as the Strong Heart Study (Devereux et al., 2000) indicated a disproportionate increase in LV mass and wall thickness among DM patients as compared to non-DM patients, even after adjusting for other cardiac risk factors (Devereux et al., 2000). In a recent multi-ethnic population study, the presence of type 2 DM, independent of body size, was associated with a 1.5-fold increase in risk of having LV mass >75th percentile of the general population (Eguchi et al., 2008). While LVH has consistently been linked to the increased incidence of cardiovascular events in a variety of high-risk patient groups, several studies have demonstrated that this cardiovascular risk is further enhanced by the presence of DM and thereby portends an especially poor prognosis (Boner et al., 2005; Struthers & Morris, 2002; Valensi et al., 1997). Emerging evidence has implicated the diabetic milieu of hyperinsulinemia, insulin resistance, hyperglycemia, and increased non-esterified fatty acids in the pathophysiology of LVH in DM patients. In addition, higher circulating levels of the hormone leptin have been linked to the development of LVH in obese diabetic humans. Disruption of downstream leptin signaling leading to leptin excess and resistance has been implicated as a novel pathophysiological mechanism by which leptin contributes to adverse remodeling. The consistency of results demonstrate a clear impact of DM *per se* on increased LV mass that encompasses the development of diabetes-related LVH.

3.1.2 Increased connective tissue collagen deposition and fibrosis

Diabetic cardiomyopathy has been documented to be characterized by myocardial fibrosis. A significant increase in collagen deposition has frequently been observed in heart biopsy samples from DM patients without significant coronary artery disease (Regan et al., 1977; Shimizu et al., 1993; Van Heerebeek et al., 2008). Similar to humans, increased cardiac collagen deposition has also been observed in animal models of DM (Bhimji et al., 1986; Spiro & Crowley, 1993). In addition, an increase in the formation of advanced glycation end products (AGEs) has also been reported to occur in the myocardium of DM patients (Van Heerebeek et al., 2008) which cross-link with collagen and increase its tensile strength. The excess deposition of collagen as well as AGE cross-linking of collagen induced by DM has been shown to augment LV stiffness of the failing diabetic heart in the absence of coronary artery disease (Van Heerebeek et al., 2008). Because excessive LV stiffness of the diabetic heart is an important contributor to worsening HF in patients with DM, increased myocardial collagen and AGEs are thought to be important therapeutic targets for modulating the development of diabetic cardiomyopathy and subsequent HF.

3.2 Functional alterations

3.2.1 Diastolic dysfunction

LV diastolic dysfunction has been reported to be the earliest detectable functional defect in diabetic cardiomyopathy (Fang et al., 2003, 2005; Karamitsos et al., 2007; Valle et al., 2006) and is characterized by increased LV end-diastolic pressure and a decreased LV end-diastolic volume (Hamblin et al, 2007a; Regan et al., 1977). The higher filling pressures are a result of reduced diastolic ventricular compliance which thereby alters diastolic filling and HF ensues. Diastolic dysfunction is a common functional abnormality in diabetic cardiomyopathy that has been related to myocardial fibrosis occurring in response to hyperglycemia. The early reductions in diastolic performance have been found to be followed by progressive reductions in systolic function during the later stages of diabetic cardiomyopathy. Therefore, diastolic dysfunction may not necessarily exist in isolation in the setting of diabetic cardiomyopathy.

3.2.2 Systolic dysfunction

In both human and animal models of type 1 and type 2 DM, systolic functional disorders have been shown to be associated with a reduction in ejection fraction (EF), fractional shortening (FS), and cardiac output (CO) (Mihm et al., 2001; Mildenberger et al., 1984; Mytas et al., 2009). *In vivo* animal studies using invasive catheterization have revealed load-dependent and -independent indices of systolic dysfunction in diabetic hearts (Hamblin et al., 2007a; Van Den Bergh et al., 2006). Comparative investigation of cardiac dysfunction in rodent models of type 1 and type 2 DM suggest that systolic dysfunction may be more pronounced in type 1 diabetic cardiomyopathy (Radovits et al., 2009).

4. Mechanisms of diabetes-induced cardiomyopathy

4.1 Derangements in cardiac energy metabolism

The primary metabolic defect observed in diabetic hearts is an exaggerated reliance on fatty acid metabolism due to reduced insulin production or insulin resistance. As a result, cardiac glucose uptake and utilization declines while free fatty acid use and oxidation by the diabetic heart increases. The augmented fatty acid metabolism of the diabetic heart leads to intracellular lipid accumulation, energy deprivation and ultimately cardiomyopathy (An & Rodrigues, 2006). Accumulation of lipids can result in increased non-oxidative production of toxic lipid products that precipitate cell death and decrease myocardial contractile dysfunction, thereby inducing myocardial lipotoxicity. In addition, the metabolic switch to increased usage of free fatty acids impairs cardiac energy efficiency in the diabetic heart due partly to the fact that glucose utilization is about 10% more efficient at generating ATP per O_2 consumed (2.58 vs. 2.33 ATP/ oxygen atom) (Wang et al., 2006a).

We and others have shown that type 1 DM alters the protein composition of cardiac mitochondria to accommodate the increased oxidation of fatty acids (Hamblin et al., 2007a; Shen et al., 2004). In-depth mining of the type 1 diabetic myocardial proteome by proteomic analysis revealed that half of the altered proteins were localized to the mitochondria (Hamblin et al., 2007a; Shen et al., 2004). Most of the cardiac protein changes were due to increased content of enzymes required for fatty acid metabolism and oxidation (e.g. acyl coenzyme A thioester hydrolase, acyl CoA dehydrogenase) (Hamblin et al., 2007a; Shen et al., 2004). These findings identify a specific 'type 1 diabetic' pattern of cardiac proteome changes indicative of diabetic cardiomyopathy and its attendant altered metabolic phenotype of enhanced fatty acid utilization.

4.2 Advanced Glycation End products (AGEs)

AGEs are a heterogeneous group of molecules formed from the non-enzymatic reaction of reducing sugars with free amino groups of proteins, lipids, and nucleic acids (Peppa et al., 2003). The formation of these sugar-derived substances is markedly accelerated in DM because of the increased availability of glucose (Peppa et al., 2003). A common consequence of their formation is covalent cross-link formation with proteins such as collagen which decrease the compliance of the extracellular matrix (ECM) (Brownlee, 2000; Singh et al., 2001). In the myocardium, this may lead to ventricular stiffness (Bell, 1995; Spiro & Crowley, 1993) with resultant impaired diastolic function. Increased activation of the diacylglycerol (DAG)-protein kinase C (PKC) signal transduction pathway has been shown in hearts of streptozotocin (STZ)-diabetic animals (Inoguchi et al., 1992) and activation of this pathway has been documented as a mechanism linking AGEs to diabetic complications (Mamputu & Renier, 2002; Way et al., 2001). AGEs are not only directly damaging through covalent modification of proteins but they also contribute to the increased production of reactive oxygen species (ROS) by binding to the receptor for advanced glycation end products, RAGE (Wang et al., 2006a). The resulting RAGE activation by AGEs has been shown to lead to an increased generation of intracellular ROS (Brownlee, 2001).

4.3 Renin-Angiotensin-Aldosterone System (RAAS)

It is well recognized that DM is characterized by enhanced up-regulation of the local and systemic RAAS. Although the basis for dysfunction of the RAAS system in the setting of DM remains incompletely understood, its activation during DM has been demonstrated to be associated with increased oxidative damage which in turn activates the death pathways implicated in myocardial cell apoptosis and necrosis (Frustaci et al., 2000; Privratsky et al., 2003). These myocyte and non-myocyte alterations in diabetic hearts resulting from increased activation of RAAS induces impairment of ventricular function. The benefits of RAAS blockade in preventing and reversing diabetic cardiomyopathy in DM patients (Asghar et al., 2009) underscore the importance of dysregulated RAAS in the pathogenesis of diabetic cardiomyopathy.

4.4 Mitochondrial dysfunction

Abnormalities in myocardial mitochondrial function have been reported in human as well as animal models of DM. Morphological study of diabetic cardiomyopathy in OVE26 mice, a chronic model of type 1 DM, revealed a significant increase in mitochondrial area and number as well as focal regions with severe damage to mitochondria (Shen et al., 2004). Mitochondria isolated from these OVE26 diabetic hearts exhibited a reduced respiratory control ratio due to lower state 3 respiration (Shen et al., 2004), indicating impaired mitochondrial function. Similar observations have also been reported in STZ and other animal models of DM (Kuo et al., 1983; Pierce & Dhalla, 1985; Tomita et al., 1996). Impairment in mitochondrial respiratory capacity has also been shown to occur in diabetic human hearts. The most comprehensive and direct evidence to date for the presence of myocardial mitochondrial dysfunction in human diabetes comes from a recent study examining mitochondrial respiration in the atrium of type 2 diabetic human myocardium (Anderson et al., 2009). This study demonstrated decreased mitochondrial respiratory capacity with palmitoyl-carnitine and glutamate in atrial tissue of type 2 DM individuals. Collectively, these findings provide solid evidence of impairment of mitochondrial function in both type 1 and type 2 diabetic hearts which may contribute to or amplify derangements in cardiac energetics that have been linked to contractile dysfunction in diabetic cardiomyopathy over time.

4.5 Myocardial fibrosis

Interstitial and perivascular fibrosis has been described in the myocardia of patients and animals with DM. Most of this has been documented to be composed of collagen fibers (Shimizu et al., 1993). In that regard, the percentage of type III collagen in the perimysium and perivascular region has been reported to be significantly higher in the hearts of patients with DM, indicating the occurrence of collagen remodeling (Shimizu et al., 1993). It has been suggested that although collagen is a major determinant of ventricular stiffness, alterations in collagen phenotype may play an important role in the impaired LV diastolic filling that is typical of diabetic cardiomyopathy (Shimizu et al., 1993).

As indicated earlier in this chapter, it has been demonstrated that collagen is particularly susceptible to AGE cross-linking (Susic et al., 2004). The cross-linking of collagen molecules to each other not only leads to loss of elasticity but also impairment of collagen degradation, leading to further collagen accumulation or fibrosis (Wang et al., 2006a). As a result, the cross-linking of collagen molecules due to accelerated AGEs formation in the diabetic heart is thought to be an important mechanism that contributes to the myocardial fibrosis and resulting decreased myocardial compliance characteristic of diabetic cardiomyopathy.

4.6 Myocardial oxidative stress: A key contributor to diabetic cardiomyopathy

Oxidative stress is defined as an imbalance between the generation of free oxygen radicals (FORs) and the antioxidant defense system. In the simplest of terms, a free radical is any atom or molecule that has an unpaired electron in their outer orbit making that atom or molecule a highly reactive species. Free radical production occurs via the addition of an electron or by its removal in a reduction/oxidation reaction. Due to its unique diradical configuration, oxygen is a major intracellular source of radical species. A sequential univalent reduction of oxygen gives rise to reactive intermediate products (Kaul et al., 1993; Singal et al., 1988). A single electron reduction of oxygen gives rise to superoxide anion (O_2^-), which can act as both a reducing and an oxidizing agent. The relatively short half life of superoxide anion limits its diffusion away from the site of its generation. The divalent reduction of oxygen yields the nonradical species, hydrogen peroxide (H_2O_2). H_2O_2 has a relatively long half life and therefore can travel significant distances, causing damage at sites distant from its origin. A three electron reduction of oxygen yields the hydroxyl radical (OH^-), which is the most reactive and potent of all the FORs. Addition of a fourth electron results in the formation of water.

FORs are neutralized by various cellular defense mechanisms consisting of enzymatic [(superoxide dismutase (SOD), catalase (CAT), and glutathione peroxidase (GSHPx)] and non-enzymatic (vitamin E, β-carotene, vitamin C) antioxidants (Palace et al., 1999). However, during pathological conditions, the delicate balance between FOR production and the protective antioxidant defense system may shift in favor of a relative increase in free-radical production and resultant FOR-induced tissue injury via lipid peroxidation of polyunsaturated fatty acids located in the cell membrane. Hyperglycemia can elevate levels of FORs by increasing mitochondrial superoxide anion production or by the process of glucose auto-oxidation (Eriksson & Borg, 1993; Nishikawa et al., 2000).

Early experimental evidence implicating myocardial oxidative stress in diabetic cardiomyopathy was mainly derived from reports evaluating the rate of lipid peroxidation. Increased cardiac levels of thiobarbituric acid reactive substances (TBARS) and lipid peroxides were observed in rats with STZ-induced diabetic cardiomyopathy (Jain & Levine, 1995; Kaul et al., 1996; Nishio et al., 1998). More recently, F_2-isoprostanes (F_2-IsoPs), a novel class of prostaglandin F_2-like compounds formed *in vivo* by non-enzymatic free radical-catalyzed peroxidation of arachidonic acid (Montuschi et al., 2004; Morrow et al., 1990), have emerged as one of the most reliable approaches to assess oxidative stress status *in vivo* (Montuschi et al., 2004). Of these, 8-*iso*-prostaglandin $F_{2\alpha}$ (8-*iso* $PGF_{2\alpha}$) has recently been shown to be a specific and sensitive quantitative index of oxidative stress *in vivo* (Delanty et al., 1997). We and others have found that in STZ rats with type 1 diabetic cardiomyopathy, LV levels of 8-*iso* $PGF_{2\alpha}$ were significantly increased *in vivo* (Hamblin et al. 2007a, 2007b; Xia et al., 2007). Collectively, these experimental animal studies demonstrate that diabetic cardiomyopathy is associated with greater myocardial oxidative stress burden.

Intermediates in the pathway of formation of IsoPs are endoperoxides, which are reduced to form F_2-IsoPs but also undergo rearrangement to form isomeric ketoaldehydes termed isoketals (IsoKs) (Roberts et al., 1999). IsoKs are remarkably reactive compounds that adduct almost instantaneously and irreversibly with lysine (Lys) residues on proteins and cross-link proteins (Iyer et al., 1989; Jirousek et al., 1990; Salomon et al., 1987) and as such, would be expected to profoundly alter protein function. Because myocardial ischemia can induce oxidative stress and the high incidence and poor prognosis of post-MI HF in DM patients has been linked in part to the presence of an underlying diabetic cardiomyopathy, we have recently performed a preliminary study in which we measured the levels of IsoK-lysyl-lactam adducts in STZ-diabetic post-MI rat hearts at 4 weeks after induction of MI using liquid chromatography electrospray tandem mass spectrometry (LC/MS) methods (Fukuda et al., 2005). Levels of IsoK-lysyl-lactam adduct were increased strikingly in the viable LV myocardium of diabetic infarcted rats compared with the same LV region in non-diabetic infarcted hearts (Fig. 1). These results clearly demonstrate that IsoK adducts are selectively increased in diabetic post-MI hearts. Protection of diabetic hearts from the downstream effects of these novel products formed via the IsoP pathway of free radical-mediated lipid peroxidation deserves evaluation as a new therapeutic approach for the prevention and treatment of oxidative-dependent cardiac complications of DM, including cardiomyopathy.

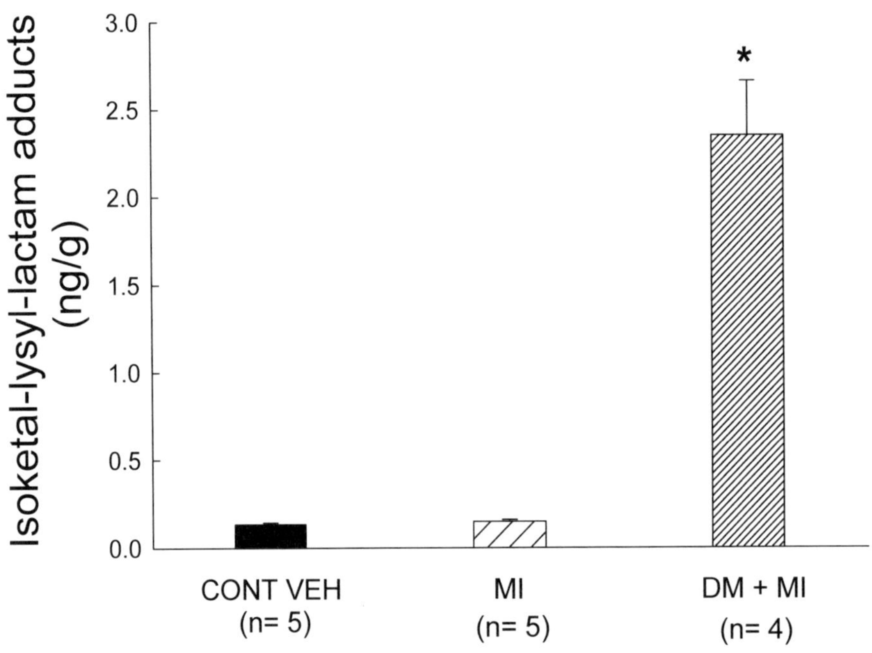

Fig. 1. Myocardial isoketal-lysyl-lactam adducts increase in DM + MI.

Myocardial isoketal-lysyl-lactam adducts in control vehicle (CONT VEH), MI, and DM + MI rats at 4 weeks post-MI. The levels of isoketal-lysyl-lactam adducts were measured in the surviving myocardium remote from the site of infarction. *Significantly different (P<0.05) from CONT VEH and MI groups.

Increased FOR production has also been shown to be involved in triggering cardiomyocyte apoptosis associated with diabetic cardiomyopathy (Cai et al., 2002). In addition, recent investigations have suggested that DM induces an inflammatory response by oxidative mechanisms, which may contribute to the development of diabetic cardiomyopathy (Garcia-Bailo et al., 2011). These synergistic impacts of myocardial oxidative stress in the presence of DM suggest that it is a major player in the pathogenesis of diabetic cardiomyopathy.

5. Candidate cardiac-specific biologic markers of diabetic cardiomyopathy

Proteomics (the concept of characterizing global alterations in protein expression of cells, tissues, and organs in health and disease) has become a powerful tool in the search for clinically useful biomarkers of disease and treatment response. Since the sum of the temporal alterations in proteins ultimately promotes or reflects the particular disease state, proteins represent an array of potential disease-specific markers and drug targets (Chaurand et al., 2004). Until recently, information concerning alterations that occur in the diabetic myocardial proteome and in the cardiac proteome of hearts with diabetic cardiomyopathy was lacking because proteomics had not been used to examine global cardiac protein changes that occur in diabetic cardiac complications. In an effort to bridge this gap, we recently performed proteomic analysis of diabetic cardiomyopathy utilizing two-dimensional difference gel electrophoresis and mass spectrometry (DIGE/MS) techniques (Hamblin et al., 2007a). Employing this technology, we established a specific 'type 1 diabetic' pattern of cardiac proteome changes indicative of diabetic cardiomyopathy (Hamblin et al., 2007a). We found that a high proportion (50%) of the altered proteins that could be identified by MS were localized to the mitochondria, many of which were up-regulated and involved in fatty acid metabolism. Specifically, protein expression levels for acyl coenzyme A thioester hydrolase and acyl CoA dehydrogenase, both of which are involved in fatty acid oxidation (J.J. Kim & Battaile, 2002), were found to be elevated 2-to 2.5-fold in the LV myocardium of rats with STZ-induced diabetic cardiomyopathy (Hamblin et al., 2007a). Our finding by proteomic analysis that these fatty acid utilization proteins are significantly more abundant in type 1 diabetic cardiomyopathy has been confirmed in proteomics-based studies of diabetic cardiomyopathy in OVE26 mice (Shen et al., 2004). Taken together, these consistent proteomic results show that elevated cardiac fatty acid utilization proteins are associated with diabetic cardiomyopathy and, hence, could serve as candidate markers and indicators of diabetic cardiomyopathy. As such, these results represent a starting point for the identification and development of a panel of cardiac biomarkers able to delineate diabetic cardiomyopathy. Continued proteomics-based studies of diabetic cardiomyopathy are essential to rapidly expand the range of biomarkers that is required for the emergence of new and successful protein diagnostics of diabetic cardiomyopathy.

6. Therapeutic strategies for the treatment of diabetic cardiomyopathy

6.1 Glycemic control

Until recently, clinical trials examining the effectiveness of good glycemic control in reducing cardiovascular events in diabetics has produced mixed results. The publication of 2 randomized intervention trials, Action in Diabetes and Vascular Disease: Preterax and Diamicron Modified Release Controlled Evaluation (ADVANCE) trial and the Action to Control Cardiovascular Risk in Diabetes Study Group (ACCORD) trial, showed that lowering of blood glucose in type 2 diabetics to near-normal levels did not significantly reduce cardiovascular events and actually increased mortality (Gerstein et al., 2008; Patel et al., 2008). However, these results were obtained from middle-aged and older patients with a long duration of DM and a high risk of cardiovascular disease. A recent epidemiologic analysis of the cardiovascular effect of glucose lowering in patients with type 2 DM revealed that patients with high levels of co-morbidity may receive diminished cardiovascular benefit from intensive blood glucose control (Greenfield et al., 2009). Furthermore, the ACCORD trial was not designed to test whether patients with HbA_{1c} levels below 7.5% receive greater benefit from intensive glucose lowering (Gerstein et al., 2008). Examination of the hazard ratios for the primary outcome and death from any cause in relation to glycated hemoglobin levels at baseline in the ACCORD trial showed a fewer number of events in type 2 DM patients with HbA_{1c} levels at baseline < 8%, suggesting a better response to therapy than patients with higher HbA_{1c} levels. This hypothesis is supported by a recent epidemiologic analysis of the cardiovascular effect of glucose lowering in type 2 DM patients whereby HbA_{1c} levels of 7.0% or less at baseline was associated with a lower 5-year incidence of cardiovascular events (Greenfield et al., 2009).

A series of recent reports have also established that improved glycemic control reduces the subsequent risk of any cardiovascular disease event in type 1 DM. The most convincing clinical evidence in support of this paradigm stems from the Diabetes Control and Complications Trial (DCCT) in which the DCCT randomly assigned 1441 patients with type 1 DM to receive either intensive diabetes therapy (three or more daily injections of insulin or insulin treatment with an external pump) or conventional diabetes therapy (one or two daily injections of insulin) for a mean of 6.5 years (DCCT, 1993). After treating them for a mean of 6.5 years, mean HbA_{1c} was 7.2% in the intensive therapy arm and 9.0% in the conventional treatment arm. Although a reduction in the risk for macrovascular events was observed in the intensive diabetes therapy arm, it did not achieve statistical significance (DCCT, 1993). After completion of this component of the DCCT, ninety-three percent of the 1441 patients were continued to be followed up as part of an ongoing observational study (Epidemiology of Diabetes Interventions and Complications [EDIC] study). After a mean follow-up of 17 years, intensive diabetes therapy, as compared to conventional therapy, reduced the risk of a cardiovascular event by 42% (Nathan et al., 2005). These beneficial effects were observed despite non-significant differences in mean HbA_{1c} concentrations between the previous intensive and conventional therapy groups at year 11 of the EDIC study, indicating intensive diabetes therapy has long-term, sustained beneficial effects on the risk of cardiovascular disease in patients with type 1 DM (Nathan et al., 2005).

The recent publication of an observational study involving type 1 DM patients has demonstrated the benefits of optimum glycemic control in reducing specifically the risk of HF in type 1 DM (Lind et al., 2011). The positive association between glycated hemoglobin and risk of HF in fairly young patients with type 1 DM together with the finding that tight control of glycemia in type 1 diabetes can prevent HF besides other aspects of cardiovascular disease (Lind et al., 2011) indicates a potential for prevention of HF with improved glycemic control. Given that patients with poorly controlled type 1 DM, as in those included in this recent observational study, have a high probability of diabetic cardiomyopathy, these results suggest that intensive glucose control be initiated as early as possible in people with type 1 DM to reduce the risk of cardiovascular complications, including cardiomyopathy and HF. In that regard, evidence that diabetic cardiomyopathy does not develop in patients with tightly controlled type 1 DM (Konduracka et al., 2007) supports the use of anti-hyperglycemic agents as part of the treatment regime for diabetic cardiomyopathy.

6.1.1 Sulfonylureas

Sulfonylureas are agents that act to increase insulin release from the beta cells in the pancreas and thus are almost exclusively used in the management of type 2 DM. Clinical studies examining the use of sulfonylureas in diabetic HF are rather limited but have produced conflicting results due in large part to the fact that the subjects included in these studies either had pre-existing cardiovascular disease or were at high risk of cardiovascular events (Simpson et al., 2006). In animal models of STZ-induced diabetic cardiomyopathy that are devoid of cardiovascular co-morbidities, chronic treatment with glyburide, the most widely used sulfonylurea, ameliorated the decline in myocardial function associated with diabetic cardiomyopathy (Mozaffari et al., 1989). Clearly, further studies are needed to determine the benefits of these drugs in patients with DM and HF.

6.1.2 Metformin

Metformin is a member of the insulin-sensitizing drugs that was previously contraindicated in patients with HF due to concerns over lactic acidosis. Although its use is still strongly cautioned, recent evidence from three cohort studies in which metformin therapy was compared with other anti-hyperglycemic agents demonstrated that metformin treatment was associated with a lower risk of all-cause mortality and all-cause hospital admissions (Eurich et al., 2007). In addition, metformin therapy has been reported to improve outcomes in older patients with DM and HF (Masoudi et al., 2005). Metformin has also been demonstrated to have favorable actions on the development of diabetic cardiomyopathy in Zucker diabetic rats (ZDF) (Forcheron et al., 2009).

6.1.3 Thiazolidinediones (TZDs)

The TZDs [PPARγ (peroxisome-proliferator-activated receptor γ) receptor agonists] are primarily insulin-sensitizing agents that have been shown to exert beneficial effects on the myocardium. However, due to their propensity for fluid retention, their use is limited to patients in New York Heart Association (NYHA) functional class I-II HF. The PROspective pioglitAzone Clinical Trial In macroVascular Events (PROactive) is currently the only completed cardiovascular (CV) outcomes study with a thiazolidinedione and remains the only large-scale, prospective, secondary prevention trial carried out entirely in patients with type 2 DM (Betteridge et al., 2008). The results from this study demonstrated that the TZD pioglitazone does not increase the risk of macrovascular events or worsen outcomes in those who develop signs of heart failure in a high-risk population with type 2 DM with macrovascular disease (Betteridge et al., 2008). Even when the increased incidence of signs of HF (with a normal ejection fraction) was taken into account, the overall CV benefit of pioglitazone remained (Betteridge et al., 2008). These results suggest that from a safety perspective, the favorable cardiovascular effects of pioglitazone treatment outweigh any inherent risks (Betteridge et al., 2008).

6.1.4 Incretins: A new line of therapy

Incretins are hormones produced by the gastrointestinal tract in response to nutrient entry that act to regulate postprandial glucose homeostasis. Among several incretin hormones, glucagon-like peptide-1 (GLP-1) stimulates insulin secretion in a glucose dependent fashion. As a result, an important safety advantage of incretin-based therapy is the abolishment of risk for hypoglycemia. Currently, there are two types of incretin-based drugs that have been developed to improve the effects of glucagon-like peptide-1 (GLP-1): incretin mimetics such as GLP-1 receptor agonists and the dipeptidyl peptidase-4 (DPP-4) inhibitors, which potentiate the incretin hormones by inhibiting the enzyme responsible for their degradation.

The GLP-1 receptor agonists mimic the actions of endogenous GLP-1 and are currently marketed as exenatide and liraglutide. Clinical trials of GLP-1 analogues have demonstrated improved LV function in patients with LV dysfunction after acute MI (Nikolaidis et al., 2004) and in patients with chronic advanced HF (Sokos et al., 2006). In an observational study involving patients with DM and HF, administration of GLP-1 over a period of three days improved the glycemic state and caused a trend towards improvement of parameters expressing LV function in DM patients with stable HF (Thrainsdottir et al., 2004). The beneficial actions on cardiac function reported so far with GLP-1 analogues provide a rationale for their use in DM patients with cardiomyopathy (Jax, 2009).

The DPP-4 inhibitors are newer drugs and currently marketed products include sitagliptin, saxagliptin, and vildagliptin. Cardiovascular outcomes as well as safety trials using this class of incretin-based drugs in patients with DM is underway to determine their efficacy and safety.

6.2 RAAS blockade

6.2.1 Renin inhibitors

The discovery that the binding of prorenin or renin to the prorenin/renin or (pro)renin receptor results in the augmented formation of angiotensin I has led to the development of direct renin inhibitors. Cardiac (pro)renin receptor expression has recently been documented to be increased in experimental diabetic cardiomyopathy (Connelly et al., 2011). Blockade of RAAS via administration of the direct renin inhibitor, aliskiren (10 mg/kg per day for 6 weeks duration), reduced cardiac over-expression of both (pro)renin mRNA and protein in diabetic TGR (mRen2)-27 rats, a transgenic rodent model that following the induction of STZ-diabetes develops diabetic cardiomyopathy (Connelly et al., 2011). Just as importantly, the reduced cardiac pro(renin) receptor expression with aliskiren treatment was associated with improved cardiac structure/function (Connelly et al., 2011). Given these exciting findings, direct renin inhibitors, particularly aliskiren, are ripe for further evaluation as novel therapeutics to modulate/prevent diabetic cardiomyopathy.

6.2.2 Angiotensin Converting Enzyme (ACE) inhibitors

Treatment with ACE inhibitors has been shown to exert an ameliorative effect on diabetic cardiomyopathy in both diabetic animals and diabetic patients. Administration of ramipril (2.5 mg/day) for 3 months to asymptomatic type 2 DM patients with echocardiographic indices of early diabetic cardiomyopathy improved echocardiographic indices of LV diastolic function in these patients (Symeonides et al., 2007). The reversal of indices of diabetic cardiomyopathy in these type 2 DM patients with ramipril was accompanied by a reduction of plasma BNP levels (Symeonides et al., 2007). In an experimental rat model of diabetic cardiomyopathy, administration of captropril (13 mg/kg) for 8 weeks in rats with clear cardiomyopathy improved the myocardial structure and cardiac function (C.H. Zhang et al., 2008). Taken together, these results suggest that treatment with ACE inhibitors can exert a beneficial effect on the development of diabetic cardiomyopathy.

6.2.3 Angiotensin Receptor Blockers (ARBs)

ARBs have emerged as a promising treatment modality for diabetic cardiomyopathy. Damage to the myocardial ultrastructure of rats with diabetic cardiomyopathy has been shown to be reduced by the type 1 angiotensin II receptor blocker (AT_1RB) valsartan (C.H. Zhang et al., 2008). In DM patients with cardiomyopathy as assessed by Doppler echocardiography, the administration of the ARB telmisartan resulted in improved echocardiographic and biochemical indices of diabetic cardiomyopathy (Symeonides et al., 2007). Since a majority of patients develop dry cough with ACE inhibitors, the cardioprotection afforded by ARBs offer the distinct advantage of having better compliance.

6.3 β-blockers

Until recently, patients with DM were less likely to be prescribed β-blockers due in part over fears of worsening insulin resistance and lipid metabolism. However, the realization of the importance of the sympathetic nervous system in the release of vasoactive substances (Murarka & Movahed, 2010) and the demonstrated benefit of β-blockers in other forms of HF has led to β-blockers being accepted as a mainstay in the treatment of DM patients with HF. The utility of β-blockade has also been demonstrated in experimental models of diabetic cardiomyopathy. Chronic treatment with the β-blocker metoprolol (β1-selective inverse agonist) has been shown to improve cardiac function in STZ-induced diabetic cardiomyopathy in rats as evidenced by significant increases in cardiac output (Sharma et al., 2008). Treatment with bisoprolol (β1-selective antagonist) for 3 months reversed myocardial hypertrophy and changes in diabetic cardiomyopathy rats (J.N. Zhang et al., 2003). Clinical trials to evaluate β-blocker intervention in patients specifically with diabetic cardiomyopathy are lacking and should be conducted to exploit this recent experimental data.

6.4 Antioxidants

As the pathogenesis of diabetic cardiomyopathy involves oxidative stress, antioxidants have received considerable interest as a therapeutic strategy. Several different approaches, such as dietary supplementation, administration of pharmacological agents with antioxidant properties, and over-expression of antioxidant enzymes to augment antioxidant defense mechanisms, have proven to be effective in reversing diabetic cardiomyopathy in animal models of both type 1 and type 2 DM.

Vitamin E, a lipid-soluble and potent antioxidant, has been shown in diabetic rats to evoke cardioprotective effects against diabetic cardiomyopathy. We have previously reported that dietary supplementation with vitamin E (2000 IU of tocopherol acetate/kg of feed) beginning early after the onset of type 1 DM in rats and continuing for a period of 8 weeks improved LV function as evidenced by a significant improvement in LVSP, LVEDP, and +dP/dt compared with un-supplemented DM rats (Hamblin et al., 2007b). The improved LV hemodynamic function of type 1 diabetic cardiomyopathy rats supplemented with vitamin E was accompanied by significantly reduced levels of myocardial oxidative stress (Hamblin et al., 2007b). Specifically, vitamin E blunted the diabetes-induced amplification of myocardial 8-*iso* $PGF_{2\alpha}$ and oxidized glutathione (GSSG) formation (Hamblin et al., 2007b). Vitamin E administration has also been documented to be associated with a significant decline in apoptosis, lipid peroxidation, protein oxidation, and enhancement of the antioxidant defense system, suggesting that this antioxidant may promote a convalescing effect on diabetic cardiomyopathy through the attenuation of oxidative stress and abrogation of apoptotic signals (Shirpoor et al., 2009). These findings demonstrate the usefulness of vitamin E as a protective anti-oxidative agent against cardiac sequel of DM involving cardiomyopathy.

Resveratrol, the principal effector constituent of red wine, has been shown to improve cardiac function in diabetic cardiomyopathy (Huang et al., 2010; Sulaiman et al., 2010). Oral administration of resveratrol (2.5 mg/kg body wt/day) to STZ-diabetic rats for 15 days has been shown to result in a direct cardioprotective effect on the diabetic myocardium (Thirunavukkarasu et al. 2007). Resveratrol treatment of chronic diabetic mice resulted in a tremendous improvement of all functional parameters to the extent that cardiac function was comparable to age-matched controls (Sulaiman et al., 2010). These data demonstrate that resveratrol can prevent diabetes-induced decline in cardiac function and resultant cardiomyopathy. Studies have revealed that resveratrol treatment improves cardiac dysfunction of diabetic myocardium in part via modulation of oxidative stress proteins (Dekkers et al., 2008). The recognition that resveratrol treatment up-regulates the protein expression of the antioxidant enzyme catalase in diabetic hearts (Dekkers et al., 2008) is further evidence of its ability to increase protection against oxidative stress.

Tempol is a membrane-permeable SOD mimetic that has been shown to attenuate the effects of FORs (Thiemermann et al., 2001). *In vivo* treatment with the antioxidant tempol (1 mmol/l in drinking water) for a period of 4-weeks to mice rendered insulin-resistant by deficiency of the insulin-sensitive GLUT4 transporter significantly and potently attenuated cardiac hypertrophy in concert with tempol up-regulated ventricular expression of thioredoxin-2 (confirming an antioxidant action) (Ritchie et al., 2007). Since the pre-diabetic insulin-resistant heart exhibits many features of diabetic cardiomyopathy, including both left ventricular dysfunction and structural abnormalities such as cardiac hypertrophy and fibrosis (Ritchie et al., 2007), these results indicate that tempol should be considered for preventing oxidative stress and cardiomyopathy in the diabetic heart.

Metallothionein (MT), a cysteine-rich protein, is a potent antioxidant owing to its high thiol content. Using a cardiac-specific, MT-overexpressing transgenic (MT-TG) mouse model, MT has been shown to be effective in preventing diabetic cardiomyopathy through the suppression of oxidative damage (Cai et al., 2005, 2006; Liang et al., 2002). Supplementation with Zinc (Zn), a potent inducer of MT, prevented the increases in cardiac morphological impairment, fibrosis, and dysfunction observed in diabetic mice without Zn supplementation (Wang et al., 2006b). Silencing of MT expression with small-interfering RNA abolished the prevention of diabetic cardiomyopathy by Zn supplementation (Wang et al., 2006b). These results demonstrate that Zn supplementation protects against diabetic cardiomyopathy via cardiac MT induction and suggest Zn supplementation, with cardiac MT induction, as a potential therapeutic approach to prevent diabetic cardiomyopathy.

Targeted over-expression of the antioxidant proteins SOD and catalase to the heart has been shown to be effective in reducing diabetic cardiomyopathy (Shen et al., 2006; Ye et al., 2004). Chronic over-expression of catalase has been documented to eliminate excess FOR production in diabetic cardiomyocytes concomitant with preservation of normal cardiac morphology and contractile function (Ye et al., 2004). Over-expression of the mitochondrial antioxidant protein manganese SOD (Mn SOD) has been reported to protect against the formation of exogenous oxidants and also completely normalize contractile function in both type 1 and type 2 models of diabetic cardiomyopathy (Shen et al., 2006).

Although a number of previous large randomized placebo-controlled clinical trials have failed to show any beneficial effects of antioxidants (in particular vitamin E) on cardiovascular events, recently published literature suggests that these clinical trials of antioxidants and cardiovascular diseases may be fatally flawed (Blumberg & Frei, 2007; Roberts et al., 2007; Traber et al., 2008). Implicit in the majority of randomized placebo-controlled clinical trials that have previously explored the benefits of antioxidants is that the antioxidants tested effectively suppressed oxidative stress status but this was never determined (Roberts et al., 2007). Furthermore, not including elevated oxidative stress in patient eligibility criteria substantially reduces statistical power to detect antioxidant or cardiovascular effects (Block et al., 2008; Roberts et al., 2009). To that end, it has recently been reported that *"the negative evidence regarding vitamin E supplements from previous randomized clinical trials is more a reflection of inadequate study design and methods of analysis than proof of failure of vitamin E in primary prevention"*(Blumberg & Frei, 2007). Data obtained in experimental animals must obviously be extrapolated to the clinical arena with caution. Nevertheless, the present findings suggest that vitamin E and other antioxidants may confer cardiovascular benefit in select patients who are diabetic and in greater oxidative stress. Indeed, support for this paradigm has recently been demonstrated in a retrospective analysis of the Heart Outcomes Prevention Evaluation (HOPE) trial where vitamin E administration to diabetic individuals homozygous for the haptoglobin (Hp) 2 allele, which confers markedly less antioxidant protection against hemoglobin-induced oxidation, was shown to result in a 50% reduction in non-fatal MI and cardiovascular death (Levy et al., 2004). The validity of these findings have subsequently been confirmed in Hp 2-2 DM individuals in a prospective, double-blind, placebo-controlled trial of vitamin E (Milman et al., 2008). These positive results impel future clinical trials to study the efficacy of antioxidants specifically in patients with diabetic cardiomyopathy.

6.5 Cell transplantation

Transplantation of stem cells has emerged as an alternative therapeutic approach to improve cardiac function in the post-MI setting as well as in ischemic cardiomyopathic hearts. However, until recently, stem cell therapy studies had not been evaluated in the diabetic heart. In the past few years, cell transplantation has begun to be examined in the setting of diabetic cardiomyopathy. Transplantation of bone marrow mesenchymal stem cells (MSCs) into the hearts of STZ-diabetic rats via injection into the femoral vein has been shown to improve the cardiac function of diabetic cardiomyopathy through increased angiogenesis and attenuation of cardiac remodeling (N. Zhang et al., 2008). Bone marrow MSC transplantation has also been reported to improve cardiac function in the rat diabetic cardiomyopathy model through an anti-apoptotic effect (Li et al., 2008). Treatment combining smooth muscle cell (SMC) transplantation via intramyocardial injection and insulin therapy has been shown to result in the preservation of heart function in STZ-diabetic rats with cardiomyopathy as assessed by echocardiographic and hemodynamic techniques (B.O. Kim et al., 2008). Although the clinical significance of these studies will require further testing and confirmation in other animal models of DM, cell transplantation holds great promise for the treatment of diabetic cardiomyopathy.

7. Conclusions and future directions

The full spectrum of diabetic cardiomyopathy encompasses a progression from subclinical LV diastolic and systolic dysfunction to clinically overt symptomatic HF. Recognition and treatment of diabetes-induced myocardial dysfunction in its infancy is paramount for the prophylaxis of ensuing cardiomyopathy and HF. Thus, there is an eminent need for early detection of this clinical entity. In that regard, the knowledge that structural and functional alterations of a particular disease state are preceded by changes in proteins has led to the recent application of proteomics to the field of DM. The use of proteomic technologies, such as mass spectrometry, provides an ideal vehicle into this arena. Analysis of protein expression profiles in serum and tissues from diabetic animals and humans is now underway and will increase our power to identify early and subtle abnormalities of cardiac dysfunction in DM. One can also foresee the use of this technology to help establish biomarkers that are predictive for risk of developing diabetic cardiomyopathy. The potential capability of proteomics to elucidate protein changes occurring in response to pharmacological therapeutics is a particularly exciting application of this technology. Studies of drug-induced proteomic changes will be required to determine the ability of this molecular technology to correlate changes in protein expression with efficacy of established and novel therapies for cardiomyopathy in DM. The recent development of more sensitive and sophisticated echocardiographic techniques such as tissue Doppler, strain, strain rate, and ultrasonic tissue characterization appears helpful in identifying early myocardial dysfunction in asymptomatic patients with DM. Integration of proteomics with sensitive diagnostic imaging modalities holds tremendous potential for the comprehensive detection of preclinical cardiac dysfunction in patients with DM and thus should facilitate earlier therapeutic intervention to prevent cardiomyopathy and subsequent HF in this high-risk patient population.

8. Acknowledgments

Supported by National Heart, Lung, and Blood Institute grant 5 R01 HL089385-02 (to M.F. Hill). I gratefully acknowledge Salisha Hill, B.Sc., for expert consultation on proteomic technologies and proteomics approaches.

9. References

An, D. & Rodrigues, B. (2006). Role of changes in cardiac metabolism in development of diabetic cardiomyopathy. *Am J Physiol Heart Circ Physiol*, 291:H1489-1506.

Anderson, E.J., Kypson, A.P., Rodriguez, E., Anderson, C.A., Lehr, E.J., & Neufer, P.D. (2009). Substrate-specific derangements in mitochondrial metabolism and redox balance in the atrium of the type 2 diabetic human heart. *J Am Coll Cardiol*, 54:1891-1898.

Asghar, O., Al-Sunni, A., Khavandi, K., Khavandi, A., Withers, S., Greenstein, A., Heagerty, A.M., & Malik, R.A. (2009). Diabetic cardiomyopathy. *Clin Sci*, 116:741-760.

Beljic, T. & Miric, M. (1994). Improved metabolic control does not reverse left ventricular filling abnormalities in newly diagnosed non-insulin-dependent diabetes patients. *Acta Diabetol*, 31:147-150.

Bell, D.S. (1995). Diabetic cardiomyopathy. A unique entity or a complication of coronary artery disease? *Diabetes Care*, 18:708-714.

Bell, D.S. (2003a). Heart failure: the frequent, forgotten, and often fatal complication of diabetes. *Diabetes Care*, 26:2433-2441.

Bell, D.S. (2003b).Diabetic cardiomyopathy. *Diabetes Care*, 26:2949-2951.

Betteridge, D.J., DeFronzo, R.A., & Chilton, R.J. (2008). PROactive: time for a critical appraisal. *Eur Heart J*, 29:969-983.

Bhimji, S., Godin, D.V., & McNeill, J.H. (1986). Insulin reversal of biochemical changes in hearts from diabetic rats. *Am J Physiol*, 251:H670-H675.

Block, G., Jensen, C.D., Morrow, J.D., Holland, N., Norkus, E.P., Milne, G.L., Hudes, M., Dalvi, T.B., Crawford, P.B., Fung, E.B., Schumacher, L., & Harmatz, P. (2008). The effect of vitamins C and E on biomarkers of oxidative stress depends on baseline level. *Free Radic Biol Med*, 45:377-384.

Blumberg, J.B. & Frei, B. (2007). Why clinical trials of vitamin E and cardiovascular diseases may be fatally flawed. Commentary on "The relationship between dose of vitamin E and suppression of oxidative stress in humans". *Free Radic Biol Med*, 43:1374-1376.

Boner, G., Cooper, M.E., McCarroll, K., Brenner, B.M., de Zeeuw, D., Kowey, P.R., Shahinfar, S., Dickson, T., Crow, R.S., & Parving, H.H.; RENAAL Investigators. (2005). Adverse effects of left ventricular hypertrophy in the reduction of endpoints in NIDDM with the angiotensin II antagonist losartan (RENAAL) study. *Diabetologia*, 48:1980-1987.

Borges, G.R., de Oliveira, M., Salgado, H.C., & Fazan, R. Jr. (2006). Myocardial performance in conscious streptozotocin diabetic rats. *Cardiovasc Diabetol*, 5:26.

Boudina, S. & Abel, E.D. (2007). Diabetic cardiomyopathy revisited. *Circulation*, 115:3213-3223.

Boyer, J.K., Thanigaraj, S., Schechtman, K.B., & Pérez, J.E. (2004). Prevalence of ventricular diastolic dysfunction in asymptomatic, normotensive patients with diabetes mellitus. *Am J Cardiol*, 93:870-875.

Brownlee, M. (2000). Negative consequences of glycation. *Metabolism*, 49:9-13.

Brownlee, M. (2001). Biochemistry and molecular cell biology of diabetic complications. *Nature*, 414:813-820.

Cai, L., Li, W., Wang, G., Guo, L., Jiang, Y., & Kang, Y.J. (2002). Hyperglycemia-induced apoptosis in mouse myocardium: mitochondrial cytochrome C-mediated caspase-3 activation pathway. *Diabetes*, 51:1938-1948.

Cai, L., Wang, J., Li, Y., Sun, X., Wang, L., Zhou, Z., & Kang, Y.J. (2005). Inhibition of superoxide generation and associated nitrosative damage is involved in metallothionein prevention of diabetic cardiomyopathy. *Diabetes*, 54:1829-1837.

Cai, L., Wang, Y., Zhou, G., Chen, T., Song, Y., Li, X., & Kang, Y.J. (2006). Attenuation by metallothionein of early cardiac cell death via suppression of mitochondrial oxidative stress results in a prevention of diabetic cardiomyopathy. *J Am Coll Cardiol*, 48:1688-1697.

Centers for Disease Control and Prevention. National diabetes fact sheet: national estimates and general information on diabetes and prediabetes in the United States, 2011. Atlanta, GA: U.S. Department of Health and Human Services, Centers for Disease Control and Prevention.

Chaurand, P., Sanders, M.E., Jensen, R.A., & Caprioli, R.M. (2004). Proteomics in diagnostic pathology: profiling and imaging proteins directly in tissue sections. *Am J Pathol*, 165:1057-1068.

Cohen, A. (1995). Diabetic cardiomyopathy. *Arch Mal Coeur Vaiss*, 88:479-486.

Connelly, K.A., Advani, A., Kim, S., Advani, S.L., Zhang, M., White, K.E., Kim, Y.M., Parker, C., Thai, K., Krum, H., Kelly, D.J., & Gilbert, R.E. (2011). The cardiac (pro)renin receptor is primarily expressed in myocyte transverse tubules and is increased in experimental diabetic cardiomyopathy. *J Hypertens*, 29:1175-1184.

Danaei, G., Finucane, M.M., Lu, Y., Singh, G.M., Cowan, M.J., Paciorek, C.J., Lin, J.K., Farzadfar, F., Khang, Y-H., Stevens, G.A., Rao, M., Ali, M.K., Riley, L.M., Robinson, C.A., & Ezzati, M., on behalf of the Global Burden of Metabolic Risk Factors of Chronic Diseases Collaborating Group (Blood Glucose). (2011). National, regional, and global trends in fasting plasma glucose and diabetes prevalence since 1980: systematic analysis of health examination surveys and epidemiological studies with 370 country-years and 2·7 million participants. *Lancet*, 378:31-40.

Dekkers, D.H., Bezstarosti, K., Gurusamy, N., Luijk, K., Verhoeven, A.J., Rijkers, E.J., Demmers, J.A., Lamers, J.M., Maulik, N., & Das, D.K. (2008). Identification by a differential proteomic approach of the induced stress and redox proteins by resveratrol in the normal and diabetic rat heart. *J Cell Mol Med*, 12:1677-1689.

Delanty, N., Reilly, M.P., Pratico, D., Lawson, J.A., McCarthy, J.F., Wood, A.E., Ohnishi, S.T., Fitzgerald, D.J., & FitzGerald, G.A. (1997). 8-epi PGF2 alpha generation during coronary reperfusion. A potential quantitative marker of oxidant stress in vivo. *Circulation*, 95:2492- 2499.

Devereux ,R.B., Roman, M.J., Paranicas, M., O'Grady, M.J., Lee, E.T., Welty, T.K., Fabsitz, R.R., Robbinsm, D., Rhoades, E.R., & Howard, B.V. (2000). Impact of diabetes on cardiac structure and function: the strong heart study. *Circulation*, 101:2271-2276.

Di Bonito, P., Cuomo, S., Moio, N., Sibilio, G., Sabatini, D., Quattrin, S., & Capaldo, B. (1996). Diastolic dysfunction in patients with non-insulin-dependent diabetes mellitus of short duration. *Diabet Med*, 13:321-324.

Di Bonito, P., Moio, N., Cavuto, L., Covino, G., Murena, E., Scilla, C., Turco, S., Capaldo, B., & Sibilio, G. (2005). Early detection of diabetic cardiomyopathy: usefulness of tissue Doppler imaging. *Diabet Med*, 22:1720-1725.

Eguchi, K., Boden-Albala, B., Jin, Z., Rundek, T., Sacco, R.L, Homma, S., & Di Tullio, M.R. (2008). Association between diabetes mellitus and left ventricular hypertrophy in a multiethnic population. *Am J Cardiol*, 101:1787-1791.

Eriksson, U.J. & Borg, L.A. (1993). Diabetes and embryonic malformations. Role of substrate-induced free-oxygen radical production for dysmorphogenesis in cultured rat embryos. *Diabetes*, 42:411-419.

Eurich, D.T., McAlister, F.A., Blackburn, D.F., Majumdar, S.R., Tsuyuki, R.T., Varney, J., & Johnson, J.A. (2007). Benefits and harms of antidiabetic agents in patients with diabetes and heart failure: systematic review. *BMJ*, 335:497.

Fang, Z.Y., Yuda, S., Anderson, V., Short, L., Case, C., & Marwick, T.H. (2003). Echocardiographic detection of early diabetic myocardial disease. *J Am Coll Cardiol*, 41:611-617.

Fang, Z.Y., Schull-Meade, R., Leano, R., Mottram, P.M., Prins, J.B., & Marwick, T.H. (2005). Screening for heart disease in diabetic subjects. *Am Heart J*, 149:349-354.

Forcheron, F., Basset, A., Abdallah, P., Del Carmine, P., Gadot, N., & Beylot, M. (2009). Diabetic cardiomyopathy: effects of fenofibrate and metformin in an experimental model- the Zucker diabetic rat. *Cardiovasc Diabetol*, 8:16.

From, A.M., Scott, C.G., & Chen, H.H. (2010). The development of heart failure in patients with diabetes mellitus and pre-clinical diastolic dysfunction a population-based study. *J Am Coll Cardiol*, 55:300-305.

Frustaci, A., Kajstura, J., Chimenti, C., Jakoniuk, I., Leri, A., Maseri, A., Nadal-Ginard, B., & Anversa, P. (2000). Myocardial cell death in human diabetes. *Circ Res*, 87:1123-1132.

Fukuda, K., Davies, S.S., Nakajima, T., Ong, B.H., Kupershmidt, S., Fessel, J., Amarnath, V., Anderson, M.E., Boyden, P.A., Viswanathan, P.C., Roberts, L.J. 2nd, & Balser, J.R. (2005). Oxidative mediated lipid peroxidation recapitulates proarrhythmic effects on cardiac sodium channels. *Circ Res*, 97:1262-1269.

Galderisi, M., Anderson, K.M., Wilson, P.W., & Levy, D. (1991). Echocardiographic evidence for the existence of a distinct diabetic cardiomyopathy (the Framingham Heart Study). *Am J Cardiol*, 68:85-89.

Garcia-Bailo, B., El-Sohemy, A., Haddad, P.S., Arora, P., Benzaied, F., Karmali, M., & Badawi, A. (2011). Vitamins D, C, and E in the prevention of type 2 diabetes mellitus: modulation of inflammation and oxidative stress. *Biologics*, 5:7-19.

Gerstein, H.C., Miller, M.E., Byington, R.P., Goff, D.C. Jr., Bigger, J.T., Buse, J.B., Cushman, W.C., Genuth, S., Ismail-Beigi, F., Grimm, R.H. Jr., Probstfield, J.L., Simons-Morton, D.G., & Friedewald, W.T. (2008). Action to Control Cardiovascular Risk in Diabetes Study Group. Effects of intensive glucose lowering in type 2 diabetes. *N Engl J Med*, 358:2545- 2559.

Greenfield, S., Billimek, J., Pellegrini, F., Franciosi, M., De Berardis, G., Nicolucci, A., & Kaplan, S.H. (2009). Comorbidity affects the relationship between glycemic control and cardiovascular outcomes in diabetes: a cohort study. *Ann Intern Med*, 151:854-860.

Hamblin, M., Friedman, D.B., Hill, S., Caprioli, R.M., Smith, H.M., & Hill, M.F. (2007a). Alterations in the diabetic myocardial proteome coupled with increased myocardial oxidative stress underlies diabetic cardiomyopathy. *J Mol Cell Cardiol*, 42:884-895.

Hamblin, M., Smith, H.M., & Hill, M.F. (2007b). Dietary supplementation with vitamin E ameliorates cardiac failure in type I diabetic cardiomyopathy by suppressing myocardial generation of 8-iso-prostaglandin F2alpha and oxidized glutathione. *J Card Fail*, 13:884- 892.

Hamby, R.I., Zoneraich, S., & Sherman, L. (1974). Diabetic cardiomyopathy. *JAMA*, 23:1749-1754.

Ho, K.K., Pinsky, J.L., Kannel, W.B., & Levy, D. (1993). The epidemiology of heart failure: the Framingham Study. *J Am Coll Cardiol*, 22(4 Suppl A):6A-13A.

Huang, J.P., Huang, S.S., Deng, J.Y., Chang, C.C., Day, Y.J., & Hung, L.M. (2010). Insulin and resveratrol act synergistically, preventing cardiac dysfunction in diabetes, but the advantage of resveratrol in diabetics with acute heart attack is antagonized by insulin. *Free Radic Biol Med*, 49:1710-1721.

Inoguchi, T., Battan, R., Handler, E., Sportsman, J.R., Heath, W., & King, G.L. (1992). Preferential elevation of protein kinase C isoform beta II and diacylglycerol levels in the aorta and heart of diabetic rats: differential reversibility to glycemic control by islet cell transplantation. *Proc Natl Acad Sci U S A*, 89:11059-11063.

Iyer, R.S., Ghosh, S., & Salomon, R.G. (1989). Levuglandin E2 crosslinks proteins. *Prostaglandins*, 37:471-480, 1989.

Jaffe, A.S., Spadaro, J.J., Schechtman, K., Roberts, R., Geltman, E.M., & Sobel, B.E. (1984). Increased congestive heart failure after myocardial infarction of modest extent in patients with diabetes mellitus. *Am Heart J*, 108:31-37.

Jain, S.K. & Levine, S.N. (1995). Elevated lipid peroxidation and vitamin E-quinone levels in heart ventricles of streptozotocin-treated diabetic rats. *Free Radic Biol Med*, 18:337-341.

Jax, T. (2009). Treatment of patients with diabetes with GLP-1 analogues or DPP-4-inhibitors: a hot topic for cardiologists? *Clin Res Cardiol*, 98:75-79.

Jirousek, M.R., Murthi, K.K., & Salomon, R.G. (1990). Electrophilic levuglandin E2-protein adducts bind glycine: a model for protein crosslinking. *Prostaglandins*, 40:187-203.

Kamalesh, M. (2007). Heart failure in diabetes and related conditions. *J Card Fail*, 13:861-873.

Kannel, W.B., Hjortland, M., & Castelli ,W.P. (1974). Role of diabetes in congestive heart failure: the Framingham study. *Am J Cardiol*, 34:29-34.

Kannel, W.B. & McGee, DL. (1979). Diabetes and cardiovascular disease. The Framingham study. *JAMA*, 11:2035-2038.

Karamitsos, T.D., Karvounis, H.I., Dalamanga, E.G., Papadopoulos, C.E., Didangellos, T.P., Karamitsos, D.T., Parharidis, G.E., & Louridas, G.E. (2007). Early diastolic impairment of diabetic heart: the significance of right ventricle. *Int J Cardiol*, 114:218-223.

Kaul, N., Siveski-Iliskovic, N., Hill, M., Slezak, J., & Singal, P.K. (1993). Free radicals and the heart. *J Pharmacol Toxicol Methods*, 30:55-67.

Kaul, N., Siveski-Iliskovic, N., Thomas, T.P., Hill, M., Khaper, N., & Singal, P.K. (1995). Probucol improves antioxidant activity and modulates development of diabetic cardiomyopathy. *Nutrition*, 11:551-554.

Kaul, N., Siveski-Iliskovic, N., Hill, M., Khaper, N., Seneviratne, C., & Singal P.K. (1996). Probucol treatment reverses antioxidant and functional deficit in diabetic cardiomyopathy. *Mol. Cell. Biochem*, 160/161: 283-288.

Kiencke, S., Handschin, R., von Dahlen, R., Muser, J., Brunner-Larocca, H.P., Schumann ,J., Felix, B., Berneis, K., & Rickenbacher, P. (2010). Pre-clinical diabetic cardiomyopathy: prevalence, screening, and outcome. *Eur J Heart Fail*, 12:951-957.

Kim, B.O., Verma, S., Weisel, R.D., Fazel, S., Jia, Z.Q., Mizuno, T., & Li, R.K. (2008). Preservation of heart function in diabetic rats by the combined effects of muscle cell implantation and insulin therapy. *Eur J Heart Fail*, 10:14-21.

Kim, J.J. & Battaile, K.P. (2002). Burning fat: the structural basis of fatty acid beta-oxidation. *Curr Opin Struct Biol*, 12:721-728.

Konduracka, E., Gackowski, A., Rostoff, P., Galicka-Latala, D., Frasik, W., & Piwowarska, W. (2007). Diabetes-specific cardiomyopathy in type 1 diabetes mellitus: no evidence for its occurrence in the era of intensive insulin therapy. *Eur Heart J*, 28:2465-2471.

Kralik, P.M., Ye, G., Metreveli, N.S., Shen, X., & Epstein, P.N. (2005). Cardiomyocyte dysfunction in models of type 1 and type 2 diabetes. *Cardiovasc Toxicol*, 5:285-292.

Kuo, T.H., Moore, K.H., Giacomelli, F., & Wiener, J. (1983). Defective oxidative metabolism of heart mitochondria from genetically diabetic mice. *Diabetes*, 32:781-787.

Levy, A.P., Gerstein, H.C., Miller-Lotan, R., Ratner, R., McQueen, M., Lonn, E, & Pogue, J. (2004). The effect of vitamin E supplementation on cardiovascular risk in diabetic individuals with different haptoglobin phenotypes. *Diabetes Care*, 27:2767.

Li, J.H., Zhang, N., & Wang, J.A. (2008). Improved anti-apoptotic and anti-remodeling potency of bone marrow mesenchymal stem cells by anoxic pre-conditioning in diabetic cardiomyopathy. *Endocrinol Invest*, 31:103-110.

Liang, Q., Carlson, E.C., Donthi, R.V., Kralik, P.M., Shen, X., & Epstein, P.N. (2002). Overexpression of metallothionein reduces diabetic cardiomyopathy. *Diabetes*, 51:174-181.

Lind, M., Bounias, I., Olsson, M., Gudbjörnsdottir, S., Svensson, A-M., & Rosengren, A. (2011). Glycaemic control and incidence of heart failure in 20 985 patients with type 1 diabetes: an observational study. *Lancet*, 378: 140–146.

Loganathan, R., Bilgen, M., Al-Hafez, B., Alenezy, M.D., & Smirnova, I.V. (2006). Cardiac dysfunction in the diabetic rat: quantitative evaluation using high resolution magnetic resonance imaging. *Cardiovasc Diabetol*, 5:7.

Maisel, A.S., McCord, J., Nowak, R.M., Hollander, J.E., Wu, A.H., Duc, P., Omland, T., Storrow, A.B., Krishnaswamy, P., Abraham, W.T., Clopton, P., Steg, G., Aumont, M.C., Westheim, A., Knudsen, C.W., Perez, A., Kamin, R., Kazanegra, R., Herrmann, H.C., & McCullough, P.A.; Breathing Not Properly Multinational Study Investigators. (2003). Bedside B-Type natriuretic peptide in the emergency diagnosis of heart failure with reduced or preserved ejection fraction. Results from the Breathing Not Properly Multinational Study. *J Am Coll Cardiol*, 41:2010-2017.

Mamputu, J.C. & Renier, G. (2002). Advanced glycation end products increase, through a protein kinase C-dependent pathway, vascular endothelial growth factor expression in retinal endothelial cells. Inhibitory effect of gliclazide. *J Diabetes Complications*, 16:284-293.

Marwick, T.H. (2006). Diabetic heart disease. *Heart*, 92:296-300.

Masoudi, F.A., Inzucchi, S.E., Wang, Y., Havranek, E.P., Foody, J.M., & Krumholz, H.M. (2005). Thiazolidinediones, metformin, and outcomes in older patients with diabetes and heart failure: an observational study. *Circulation*, 111:583-590.

Maya, L. & Villarreal, F.J. (2010). Diagnostic approaches for diabetic cardiomyopathy and myocardial fibrosis. *J Mol Cell Cardiol*, 48:524-529.

Mihm, M.J., Seifert, J.L., Coyle, C.M., & Bauer, J.A. (2001). Diabetes related cardiomyopathy time dependent echocardiographic evaluation in an experimental rat model. *Life Sci*, 69:527-542.

Mildenberger, R.R., Bar-Shlomo, B., Druck, M.N., Jablonsky, G., Morch, J.E., Hilton, J.D., Kenshole, A.B., Forbath, N., & McLaughlin, P.R. (1984). Clinically unrecognized ventricular dysfunction in young diabetic patients. *J Am Coll Cardiol*, 4:234-238.

Milman, U., Blum, S., Shapira, C., Aronson, D., Miller-Lotan, R., Anbinder, Y., Alshiek, J., Bennett, L., Kostenko, M., Landau, M., Keidar, S., Levy, Y., Khemlin, A., Radan, A., & Levy, A.P. (2008). Vitamin E supplementation reduces cardiovascular events in a subgroup of middle-aged individuals with both type 2 diabetes mellitus and the haptoglobin 2-2 genotype: a prospective double-blinded clinical trial. *Arterioscler Thromb Vasc Biol*, 28:341-347.

Montuschi, P., Barnes, P.J., & Roberts, L.J. 2nd. (2004). Isoprostanes: markers and mediators of oxidative stress. *FASEB J*, 18:1791-1800.

Morrow, J.D., Hill, K.E., Burk, R.F., Nammour, T.M., Badr, K.F., & Roberts, L.J. 2nd. (1990). A series of prostaglandin F2-like compounds are produced in vivo in humans by a non- cyclooxygenase, free radical-catalyzed mechanism. *Proc Natl Acad Sci U S A*, 87:9383- 9387.

Mozaffari, M.S., Allo, S., & Schaffer, S.W. (1989). The effect of sulfonylurea therapy on defective calcium movement associated with diabetic cardiomyopathy. *Can J Physiol Pharmacol*, 67:1431-1436.

Murarka, S. & Movahed, M.R. (2010). Diabetic cardiomyopathy. *J Card Fail*, 16:971-979.

Mytas, D.Z., Stougiannos, P.N., Zairis, M.N., Foussas, S.G., Pyrgakis, V.N., & Kyriazis, I.A. (2009). Diabetic myocardial disease: pathophysiology, early diagnosis and therapeutic options. *Diabetes Complications*, 23:273-282.

Nathan, D.M., Cleary, P.A., Backlund, J.Y., Genuth, S.M., Lachin, J.M., Orchard, T.J., Raskin, P., & Zinman B; Diabetes Control and Complications Trial/Epidemiology of Diabetes Interventions and Complications (DCCT/EDIC) Study Research Group. (2005). Intensive diabetes treatment and cardiovascular disease in patients with type 1 diabetes. *N Engl J Med*, 353:2643-2653.

Nicolino, A., Longobardi, G., Furgi, G., Rossi, M., Zoccolillo, N., Ferrara, N., & Rengo, F. (1995). Left ventricular diastolic filling in diabetes mellitus with and without hypertension. *Am J Hypertens*, 8:382-389.

Nikolaidis, L.A., Mankad, S., Sokos, G.G., Miske, G., Shah, A., Elahi, D., & Shannon, R.P. (2004). Effects of glucagon-like peptide-1 in patients with acute myocardial infarction and left ventricular dysfunction after successful reperfusion. *Circulation*, 109:962-965.

Nishikawa, T., Edelstein, D., Du, X.L., Yamagishi, S., Matsumura, T., Kaneda, Y., Yorek, M.A., Beebe, D., Oates, P.J., Hammes, H.P., Giardino, I., & Brownlee, M. (2000). Normalizing mitochondrial superoxide production blocks three pathways of hyperglycemic damage. *Nature*, 404:787-790.

Nishio, Y., Kashiwagi, A., Taki, H., Shinozaki, K., Maeno, Y., Kojima, H., Maegawa, H., Haneda, M., Hidaka, H., Yasuda, H., Horiike, K., & Kikkawa, R. (1998). Altered activities of transcription factors and their related gene expression in cardiac tissues of diabetic rats. *Diabetes*, 47:1318-1325.

Ozasa, N., Furukawa, Y., Morimoto, T., Tadamura, E., Kita, T., & Kimura, T. (2008). Relation among left ventricular mass, insulin resistance, and hemodynamic parameters in type 2 diabetes. *Hypertens Res*, 31:425-432.

Palace, V., Kumar, D., Hill, M.F., Khaper, N., & Singal, P.K. (1999). Regional differences in non-enzymatic antioxidants in the heart under control and oxidative stress conditions. *J Mol Cell Cardiol*, 31:193-202.

Patel, A., MacMahon, S., Chalmers, J., Neal, B., Billot, L., Woodward, M., Marre, M., Cooper, M., Glasziou, P., Grobbee, D., Hamet, P., Harrap, S., Heller, S., Liu, L., Mancia, G., Mogensen, C.E., Pan, C., Poulter, N., Rodgers, A., Williams, B., Bompoint, S., de Galan, B.E., Joshi, R., & Travert, F. (2008). ADVANCE Collaborative Group. Intensive blood glucose control and vascular outcomes in patients with type 2 diabetes. *N Engl J Med*, 358:2560-2572.

Peppa, J., Uribarri, J., & Vlassara, H. (2003). Glucose, advanced glycation end products, and diabetes complications: what is new and what works. *Clin Diabetes*, 21: 186–187.

Pierce, G.N. & Dhalla, N.S. (1985). Heart mitochondrial function in chronic experimental diabetes in rats. *Can J Cardiol*, 1:48-54.

Poirier, P., Bogaty, P., Garneau, C., Marois, L., & Dumesnil, J.G. (2001). Diastolic dysfunction in normotensive men with well-controlled type 2 diabetes: importance of maneuvers in echocardiographic screening for preclinical diabetic cardiomyopathy. *Diabetes Care*, 24:5- 10.

Privratsky, J.R., Wold, L.E., Sowers, J.R., Quinn, M.T., & Ren, J. (2003). AT1 blockade prevents glucose-induced cardiac dysfunction in ventricular myocytes: role of the AT1 receptor and NADPH oxidase. *Hypertension*, 42:206-212.

Radovits, T., Korkmaz, S., Loganathan, S., Barnucz, E., Bömicke, T., Arif, R., Karck, M., & Szabó, G. (2009). Comparative investigation of the left ventricular pressure-volume relationship in rat models of type 1 and type 2 diabetes mellitus. *Am J Physiol Heart Circ Physiol*, 297:H125-H133.

Raev, D.C. (1994). Which left ventricular function is impaired earlier in the evolution of diabetic cardiomyopathy? An echocardiographic study of young type I diabetic patients. *Diabetes Care*, 17:633-639.

Regan ,T.J., Lyons, M.M., Ahmed, S.S., Levinson, G.E., Oldewurtel, H.A., Ahmad, M.R., & Haider, B. (1977). Evidence for cardiomyopathy in familial diabetes mellitus. *J Clin Invest*, 60:884-899.

Ritchie, R.H., Quinn, J.M., Cao, A.H., Drummond, G.R., Kaye, D.M., Favaloro, J.M., Proietto, J., & Delbridge, L.M. (2007). The antioxidant tempol inhibits cardiac hypertrophy in the insulin-resistant GLUT4-deficient mouse in vivo. *J Mol Cell Cardiol*, 42:1119-1128.

Roberts, L.J. 2nd, Salomon, R.G., Morrow, J.D., & Brame, C.J. (1999). New developments in the isoprostane pathway: identification of novel highly reactive gamma-ketoaldehydes (isolevuglandins) and characterization of their protein adducts. *FASEB J*, 13:1157-1168.

Roberts, L.J. 2nd, Oates, J.A., Linton, M.F., Fazio, S., Meador, B.P., Gross, M.D., Shyr, Y., & Morrow, J.D. (2007). The relationship between dose of vitamin E and suppression of oxidative stress in humans. *Free Radic Biol Med*, 43:1388-1393.

Roberts, L.J. 2nd, Traber, M.G., & Frei, B. (2009). Vitamins E and C in the Prevention of Cardiovascular Disease and Cancer in Men. *Free Radic Biol Med*, 46:1558.

Rubler, S., Dlugash, J., Yuceoglu, Y.Z., Kumral, T., Branwood, A.W., & Grishman, A. (1972). New type of cardiomyopathy associated with diabetic glomerulosclerosis. *Am J Cardiol*, 30:595-602.

Salomon, R.G., Jirousek, M.R., Ghosh, S., & Sharma, R.B. (1987). Prostaglandin endoperoxides 21. Covalent binding of levuglandin E2 with proteins. *Prostaglandins*, 34:643-656.

Sharma, V., Dhillon, P., Wambolt, R., Parsons, H., Brownsey, R., Allard, M.F., & McNeill, J.H. (2008). Metoprolol improves cardiac function and modulates cardiac metabolism in the streptozotocin-diabetic rat. *Am J Physiol Heart Circ Physiol*, 294:H1609-H1620.

Shen, X., Zheng, S., Thongboonkerd, V., Xu, M., Pierce, W.M. Jr., Klein, J.B., & Epstein, P.N. (2004). Cardiac mitochondrial damage and biogenesis in a chronic model of type 1 diabetes. *Am J Physiol Endocrinol Metab*, 287:E896-E905.

Shen, X., Ye, G., Metreveli, N.S., & Epstein, P.N. (2005). Cardiomyocyte defects in diabetic models and protection with cardiac-targeted transgenes. *Methods Mol Med* ,112:379-388.

Shen, X., Zheng, S., Metreveli, N.S., & Epstein, P.N. (2006). Protection of cardiac mitochondria by overexpression of MnSOD reduces diabetic cardiomyopathy. *Diabetes*, 55:798-805.

Shimizu, M., Umeda, K., Sugihara, N., Yoshio, H., Ino, H., Takeda, R., Okada, Y., & Nakanishi, I. (1993). Collagen remodelling in myocardia of patients with diabetes. *J Clin Pathol*, 46:32-36.

Shirpoor, A., Salami, S., Khadem-Ansari, M.H., Ilkhanizadeh, B., Pakdel, F.G., & Khademvatani, K. (2009). Cardioprotective effect of vitamin E: rescues of diabetes-induced cardiac malfunction, oxidative stress, and apoptosis in rat. *Diabetes Complications*, 23:310-316.

Shivalkar, B., Dhondt, D., Goovaerts, I., Van Gaal, L., Bartunek, J., Van Crombrugge, P., & Vrints, C. (2006). Flow mediated dilatation and cardiac function in type 1 diabetes mellitus. *Am J Cardiol*, 97:77-82.

Simpson, S.H., Majumdar, S.R., Tsuyuki, R.T., Eurich, D.T., & Johnson, J.A. (2006). Dose-response relation between sulfonylurea drugs and mortality in type 2 diabetes mellitus: a population-based cohort study. *CMAJ*, 174:169-174.

Singal, P.K., Petkau, A., Gerrard, J.M., Hrushovetz, S., & Foerster, J. (1988). Free radicals in health and disease. *Mol Cell Biochem*, 84:121-122.

Singh, R., Barden, A., Mori, T., & Beilin, L. (2001). Advanced glycation end-products: a review. *Diabetologia*, 44:129-146.

Sokos, G.G., Nikolaidis, L.A., Mankad, S., Elahi, D., & Shannon RP. (2006). Glucagon-like peptide-1 infusion improves left ventricular ejection fraction and functional status in patients with chronic heart failure. *J Card Fail*,12:694-699.

Solomon, S.D., St John Sutton, M., Lamas, G.A., Plappert, T., Rouleau, J.L., Skali, H., Moyé, L., Braunwald, E., & Pfeffer, M.A.; Survival And Ventricular Enlargement (SAVE) Investigators. (2002). Ventricular remodeling does not accompany the development of heart failure in diabetic patients after myocardial infarction. *Circulation*, 106, 1251-1255.

Spector, K.S. (1998). Diabetic cardiomyopathy. *Clin Cardiol*, 21:885-887.

Spiro, M.J. & Crowley, T.J. (1993). Increased rat myocardial type VI collagen in diabetes mellitus and hypertension. *Diabetologia*, 36:93-98.

Stevanovic,A., Dekleva, M., Andric, V., Sevic, L.J.,Pencic, B., Podnar, G., & Davidovic, N. (2006). Brain natriuretic peptide level could predict the late progression of left ventricular diastolic dysfunction in diabetic patients; one year follow up. *European Journal of Echocardiography*, 7 (Suppl 1):S26.

Struthers, A.D. & Morris, A.D. (2002). Screening for and treating left-ventricular abnormalities in diabetes mellitus: a new way of reducing cardiac deaths. *Lancet*, 359:1430-1432.

Sulaiman, M., Matta, M.J., Sunderesan, N.R., Gupta, M.P., Periasamy, M., & Gupta, M. (2010). Resveratrol, an activator of SIRT1, upregulates sarcoplasmic calcium ATPase and improves cardiac function in diabetic cardiomyopathy. *Am J Physiol Heart Circ Physiol*, 298:H833-H843.

Susic, D., Varagic, J., Ahn, J., & Frohlich, E.D. (2004). Collagen cross-link breakers: a beginning of a new era in the treatment of cardiovascular changes associated with aging, diabetes, and hypertension. *Curr Drug Targets Cardiovasc Haematol Disord*, 4:97-101.

Symeonides, P., Koulouris, S., Vratsista, E., Triantafyllou, K., Ioannidis, G., Thalassinos, N., & Katritsis, D. (2007).Both ramipril and telmisartan reverse indices of early diabetic cardiomyopathy: a comparative study. *Eur J Echocardiogr*, 8:480-486.

The Diabetes Control and Complications Trial Research Group. (1993). The effect of intensive treatment of diabetes on the development and progression of long-term complications in insulin-dependent diabetes mellitus. *N Engl J Med*, 329:977-986.

Thiemermann, C., McDonald, M.C., & Cuzzocrea, S. (2001). The stable nitroxide, tempol, attenuates the effects of peroxynitrite and oxygen-derived free radicals. *Crit Care Med*, 29:223-224.

Thirunavukkarasu, M., Penumathsa, S.V., Koneru, S., Juhasz, B., Zhan, L., Otani, H., Bagchi, D., Das, D.K., & Maulik, N. (2007). Resveratrol alleviates cardiac dysfunction in streptozotocin-induced diabetes: Role of nitric oxide, thioredoxin, and heme oxygenase. *Free Radic Biol Med*, 43:720-729.

Thrainsdottir, I., Malmberg, K., Olsson, A., Gutniak, M., & Rydén, L. (2004). Initial experience with GLP-1 treatment on metabolic control and myocardial function in patients with type 2 diabetes mellitus and heart failure. *Diab Vasc Dis Res*, 1:40-43.

Tomita, M., Mukae, S., Geshi, E., Umetsu, K., Nakatani, M., & Katagiri, T. (1996). Mitochondrial respiratory impairment in streptozotocin-induced diabetic rat heart. *Jpn Circ J*, 60:673-682.

Traber, M.G., Frei, B., & Beckman, J.S. (2008). Vitamin E revisited: do new data validate benefits for chronic disease prevention? *Curr Opin Lipidol*, 19:30-38.

Valensi, P., Sachs, R.N., Lormeau, B., Taupin, J.M., Ouzan, J., Blasco, A., Nitenberg, A., Metz, D., Paries, J., Talvard, O., Leutenegger, M., & Attali, J.R. (1997). Silent myocardial ischaemia and left ventricle hypertrophy in diabetic patients. *Diabetes Metab*, 23:409-416.

Valle, R., Bagolin, E., Canali, C., Giovinazzo, P., Barro, S., Aspromonte, N., Carbonieri, E., & Milani, L. (2006). The BNP assay does not identify mild left ventricular diastolic dysfunction in asymptomatic diabetic patients. *Eur J Echocardiogr*, 7:40-44.

Van Den Bergh, A., Flameng, W., & Herijgers, P. (2006). Type II diabetic mice exhibit contractile dysfunction but maintain cardiac output by favourable loading conditions. *Eur J Heart Fail*, 8:777-783.

Van Den Hurk, K., Alssema, M., Kamp, O., Henry, R.M., Stehouwer, .C.D, Diamant, M., Boomsma, F., Heine, R.J., Nijpels, G., Paulus, W.J., & Dekker, J.M. (2010). Slightly elevated B-type natriuretic peptide levels in a non-heart failure range indicate a worse left ventricular diastolic function in individuals with, as compared with individuals without, type 2 diabetes: the Hoorn Study. *Eur J Heart Fail*, 12:958-965.

Van Heerebeek, L., Hamdani, N., Handoko, M.L., Falcao-Pires, I., Musters, R.J., Kupreishvili, K., Ijsselmuiden, A.J., Schalkwijk, C.G., Bronzwaer, J.G., Diamant, M., Borbély, A., van der Velden, J., Stienen, G.J., Laarman, G.J., Niessen, H.W., & Paulus, W.J. (2008). Diastolic stiffness of the failing diabetic heart: importance of fibrosis, advanced glycation end products, and myocyte resting tension. *Circulation*, 117:43-51.

Von Bibra, H., Thrainsdottir, I.S., Hansen, A., Dounis, V., Malmberg, K., & Rydén, L. (2005). Tissue Doppler imaging for the detection and quantitation of myocardial dysfunction in patients with type 2 diabetes mellitus. *Diab Vasc Dis Res*, 2:24-30.

Wang, J., Song, Y., Wang, Q., Kralik, P.M., & Epstein, P.N. (2006a). Causes and characteristics of diabetic cardiomyopathy. *Rev Diabet Stud*, 3:108-117.

Wang, J., Song, Y., Elsherif, L., Song, Z., Zhou, G., Prabhu, S.D., Saari, J.T., & Cai, L. (2006b). Cardiac metallothionein induction plays the major role in the prevention of diabetic cardiomyopathy by zinc supplementation. *Circulation*, 113:544-554.

Way, K.J., Katai, N., & King, G.L. (2001). Protein kinase C and the development of diabetic vascular complications. *Diabet Med*, 18:945-959.

Xia, Z., Kuo, K.H., Nagareddy, P.R., Wang, F., Guo, Z., Guo, T., Jiang, J., & McNeill, J.H. (2007). N-acetylcysteine attenuates PKCbeta2 overexpression and myocardial hypertrophy in streptozotocin-induced diabetic rats. *Cardiovasc Res*, 73:770-782.

Ye, G., Metreveli, N.S., Donthi, R.V., Xia, S., Xu, M., Carlson, E.C., & Epstein, P.N. (2004). Catalase protects cardiomyocyte function in models of type 1 and type 2 diabetes. *Diabetes*, 53:1336-1343.

Zabalgoitia, M., Ismaeil, M.F., Anderson, L., & Maklady, F.A. (2001). Prevalence of diastolic dysfunction in normotensive, asymptomatic patients with well-controlled type 2 diabetes mellitus. *Am J Cardiol*, 87:320-323.

Zhang, C.H., Lu, J., Yu, X.J., Sun, L., & Zang, W.J. (2008). Ameliorative effect of Captopril and Valsartan on an animal model of diabetic cardiomyopathy. *Biol Pharm Bull*, 31:2045-2049.

Zhang, J.N., Geng, Q., Chen, X.J., Fang, W.W., Wu, X.H., & Yang, D. (2003). Alteration of endothelin system and calcium handling protein in left ventricles following drug treatment in dilated cardiomyopathy rats. *Acta Pharmacol Sin*, 24:1099-1102.

Zhang, N., Li, J., Luo, R., Jiang, J., & Wang, J.A. (2008). Bone marrow mesenchymal stem cells induce angiogenesis and attenuate the remodeling of diabetic cardiomyopathy. *Exp Clin Endocrinol Diabetes*, 116:104-111.

Insulin Resistance and Cardiomyopathy

Jiung-Pang Huang and Li-Man Hung
Department and Graduate Institute of Biomedical Sciences and Healthy Aging Research Center, College of Medicine, Chang Gung University, Tao-Yuan
Taiwan

1. Introduction

During the past two decades, a striking increase in the number of people with metabolic syndrome has taken place worldwide. With the increased risk worldwide of not only type 2 diabetes mellitus (T2DM), but also of cardiovascular disease from the metabolic syndrome, there is an urgent need for strategies to prevent the emerging global epidemic (1-4). Insulin-mediated glucose metabolism varies widely in healthy human beings, and the more insulin resistant an individual, the more insulin they must secrete in order to prevent the development of T2DM. However, the combination of insulin resistance and compensatory hyperinsulinemia increases the likelihood that an individual will be hypertensive, and have a dyslipidemia characterized by a high plasma triglyceride (TG) and low high-density lipoprotein cholesterol (HDL-C) concentration. Given the rapid increase in the number of clinical syndromes and abnormalities associated with insulin resistance/hyperinsulinemia, it is reasonable to suggest, that the cluster of these changes related to the defect in insulin action be included within the term, insulin resistant syndrome.

Under physiological conditions, insulin in the heart is for the regulation of the substrate employed in the contraction/ relaxation cycle and cell growth (5-9). Decreased insulin sensitivity reduces cardiac performance leading to left ventricular hypertrophy, diastolic dysfunction, and heart failure (10-12). Several mechanisms are known to contribute to the myocardial dysfunction including, reduced energy production due to decreased mitochondrial respiration and pyruvate dehydrogenase activity, oxidative stress, defective cardiac contractility, and intracellular Ca^{2+} regulatory proteins such as myosin, titin, sarcoendoplasmic reticulum Ca^{2+}-ATPase (SERCA), phospholamban, and Na^{+}-Ca^{2+} exchanger (13, 14). The high incidence of cardiac problems in patients with metabolic syndrome warrants a more stringent clinical management. Although a wide variety of pharmacological targets and agents have been discovered, the clinical management of cardiovascular risk associated with metabolic syndrome is still dismal.

2. Diabetic cardiomyopathy

It has been reported that diabetic patients suffer from heart failure with normal coronary arteries and with no other obvious aetiology for heart failure (3, 4). This phenomenon has led to the use of the term "diabetic cardiomyopathy" (DCM). The term now includes diabetic individuals with diastolic dysfunction, the prevalence of which may be as high as

60% in well-controlled T2DM individuals (12, 15). Thereby, subclinical left ventricular dysfunction may be a very common feature in diabetes, in addition to the increased prevalence of coronary heart disease (16-21). In experimental rodent models, myocardial contractile dysfunction independent of coronary artery disease has also been demonstrated in db/db, ob/ob, and Zucker rodent models, supporting the existence of an obesity-related cardiomyopathy and a diabetic cardiomyopathy (3, 22). In addition, mice with a selective cardiomyocyte only deletion of the insulin receptor (CIRKO mice) have reduced insulin-stimulated glucose uptake and also have a modest decrease in contractile function, thereby implicating insulin resistance as a contributing factor in the development of contractile dysfunction in the metabolic syndrome (23, 24).

3. Metabolic disturbances and cardiomyopathy

It is well recognized that insulin regulates the critical steps in intermediary metabolism of many tissues (including skeletal muscle, adipose tissue, and liver) and consequently maintains metabolic homeostasis within the body. However, many other tissues including the heart also express insulin receptors and their important functions may be regulated by insulin. Insulin resistance is an important risk factor for the development of hypertension, atherosclerotic heart disease, left ventricular hypertrophy and dysfunction, and heart failure. It reflects a disturbance of insulin-mediated glucose metabolism and can potentially worsen metabolic efficiency of both skeletal and cardiac muscle. Recently, the relationship between insulin resistance and cardiac contractile dysfunction has been investigated by generating a new insulin resistant animal rat model on a high cholesterol-fructose (HCF) diet. The HCF diet-induced insulin resistance not only occurred in metabolic-response tissues but also in the heart as well. These results indicate cardiac insulin resistance-associated metabolic alterations may consequently lead to the development of cardiomyopathy and contractile dysfunction (25).

Diabetes causes metabolic dysregulation and contains numerous risk factors which are associated with cardiomyopathy and heart failure. Extensive cellular and molecular studies have elucidated putative process of metabolic disturbances in the pathogenesis of cardiac dysfunction in diabetes (Table.1) (26). The metabolic disturbances in the development of cardiomyopathy are listed below.

3.1 Increased triglycerides (TG) and nonesterified fatty acids (NEFAs)

Hyperlipidemia is one of the features of obesity induced T2DM. When circulating NEFAs are greater than the oxidative capacity of the heart, NEFAs are stored as intramyocardial triglycerides. Both NEFAs and TG contribute to cardiac lipotoxicity and worsened heart failure (27-32). High levels of circulating NEFAs promote insulin resistance by impairment of insulin-Akt activation and compensatory hyperinsulinemia (27, 33-36). NEFAs also induce the activation of atypical protein kinase C (PKC)θ, which is a serine/threonine kinase that phosphorylates and subsequently activates IκB kinase. Then IκB kinase phosphorylates insulin receptor substrate-1 (IRS-1) serine residues which inhibit the ability of IRS-1 to bind to SH2 domains of the p85 regulatory subunit of phosphatidylinositol 3-kinase (PI3K), and consequently impair insulin signal transduction (36). NEFAs not only trigger the development of cardiac insulin resistance but also lead to the development of myocardial contractile dysfunction. NEFAs can directly alter myocardial contractility by increasing NEFA flux into the myocardium. A recent study suggests that increasing the entry of fatty acyl coenzyme A (CoA) into the cardiomyocytes may modulate the K_{ATP} channel opening during the contractile state of the myocardium (37). Activation of K_{ATP} channel contributes to shortening of the action potential and decreases trans-sarcolemmal calcium flux and subsequent myocardial contractility (37).

TRIGGERS	MEDIATORS	EFFECTORS	TARGETS
NEFA	↑ Acyl CoA	↑ K^+_{ATP} CHANNEL	↓ ACTIVATOR Ca^{++}
	↑ ATYPICAL PKC ↑ PTEN	↓ Akt-1 ACTIVATION	INSULIN RESISTANCE
	↑ TNF α	↑ CERAMIDE	MYOCYTE APOPTOSIS
HYPERGLYCEMIA		↑ PKC	CALCIUM HOMEOSTASIS
	↑ ROS → ↑ PARP	↑ HEXOAMINE	
	↓		CONTRACTILE PROTEINS
	↓ GAPDH	↑ POLYOL FLUX	
		↑ AGE	MATRIX PROTEINS
HYPERINSULINEMIA INSULIN RESISTANCE	PI3K/Akt-1	↓ GSK-3 β ↑ mTOR	MYOCYTE HYPERTROPHY
	↑ MAP KINASE	↑ Ras/ ↑ Rho	↑ PROTEIN SYNTHESIS

Table 1. The relationship between diabetic metabolic disturbances (triggers) and the mediators, effectors, and intracellular targets that lead to a diabetic cardiomyopathic phenotype. (Modified from Poornima IG, Parikh P, Shannon RP. Diabetic cardiomyopathy: the search for a unifying hypothesis. *Circ Res*. 2006; 98: 596-605.)

3.2 Hyperglycemia

Hyperglycemia leads to increasing glucose oxidation. Brownlee and colleagues have elucidated that hyperglycemia generates reactive oxygen species (ROS) and consequently mediates tissue injury (38, 39). In fact, mitochondria generate high levels of ROS which lead to damage of DNA and inhibit the activity of glyceraldehyde phosphate dehydrogenase (GAPDH) (39, 40). On the other hand, hyperglycemia also shifts the glucose glycolytic pathway into alternative pathways that are considered mediators of hyperglycemia induced cellular injury (26). The damage resulting from hyperglycemia includes elevation of advanced glycation end products (AGEs), hexosamine and polyol pathway, activation of beta 2 isoform PKC and alteration of myocardial structure and function (41-47). In addition, it has been suggested that hyperglycemia is linked to altering the expression and function of both the ryanodine receptor (RyR) and sarco/endoplasmic reticulum Ca^{2+}-ATPase (SERCA), and this alteration may contribute to impair myocardial systolic and diastolic function (26).

3.3 Insulin resistance and hyperinsulinemia

Insulin resistance is prevalent in chronic heart failure patients with idiopathic dilated cardiomyopathy (12, 48). Furthermore, insulin resistance is a primary etiology factor in the development of nonischemic heart failure (HF) (49). The cardiac insulin action and how insulin resistance leads to the development of cardiomyopathy are discussed in detail below.

4. The cardiac action of insulin

The heart is an energy-consuming organ that requires a constant supply of fuel and oxygen in order to maintain its intracellular ATP level, which is essential for the uninterrupted myocardial contraction/relaxation cycle. Oxidation of fatty acids supplies approximately 70% of the heart's energy needs, while glucose and lactate may account for up to 30% of total ATP production. The energy requirements of the heart could be covered for a short period by the breakdown of intracellular stored glycogen and lipid droplets, but a longer duration would rely on the uptake of exogenous glucose and long chain fatty acid (LCFA). Circulating insulin and increased contractile activity are the two major signals responsible for acute increases in cardiac substrate uptake, enabled by inducing transporter translocation from intracellular stores to the sarcolemma (Fig.1) (5).
Under normal physiological conditions, the main role of insulin on the heart is the regulation of substrate utilization. Insulin regulates cardiac metabolism by modulating glucose and fatty acid transport, glycolysis, glycogen synthesis, lipid metabolism, protein synthesis, growth, contractility, and apoptosis in the cardiomyocytes (5). The actions of insulin are mediated by binding to specific cell surface receptors (insulin receptor, InsR). Each cardiomyocyte is expressed at levels of about 10,000 to 100,000 receptors of InsR. The InsR is a tetrameric enzyme comprising two extracellular α-subunits and two transmembrane β-subunits (5). The binding of insulin to the extracellular domain of InsR triggers the activation of intrinsic tyrosine kinase activity of the β-subunits of the receptor. This leads to an autotransphosphorylation of the receptor where one β-subunit phosphorylates the other on several tyrosine residues. Once activated and phosphorylated, InsR binds via its phosphotyrosine residues and phosphorylates a series of downstream elements, including the insulin receptor substrate (IRS) family and Shc (5, 50). This recruitment and activation lead to the activation of two main pathways, the phosphatidylinositol 3-kinase (PI3K) and the

mitogen-activated protein kinase (MAPK) pathway respectively. PI3K is considered to be the main player of the metabolic action of insulin, whereas the MAPK pathway is principally involved in cell growth and differentiation in the heart (Fig.2) (50, 51).

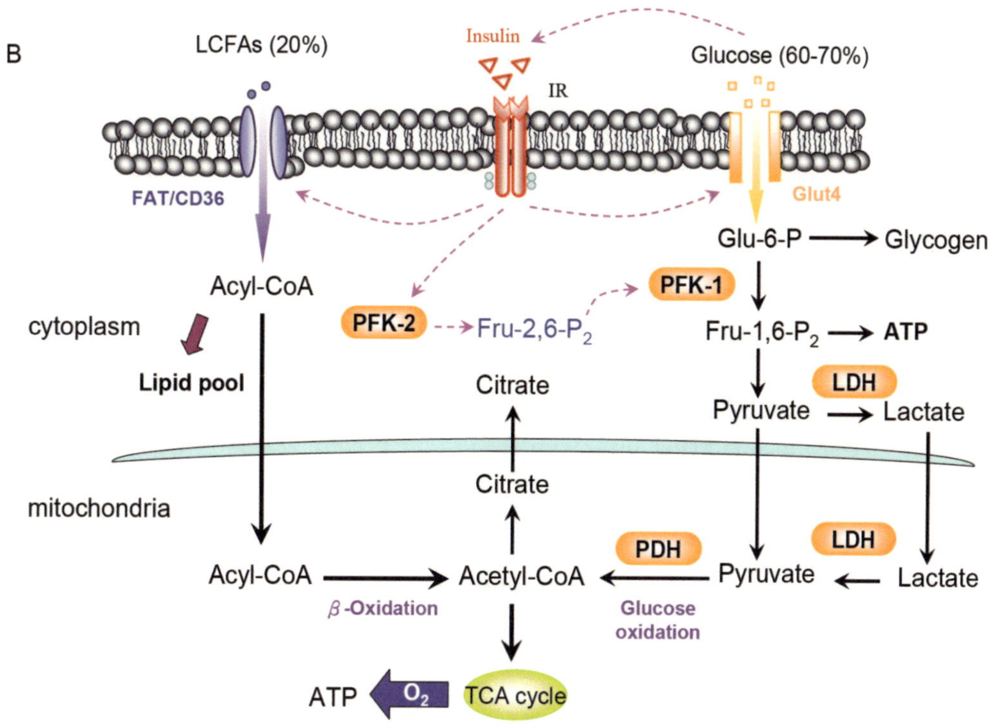

Fig. 1. Cardiac metabolism under control (A) and insulin (B) conditions. Under control conditions, ATP production comes from fatty acids and glucose oxidation. Fatty acid is the privileged substrate used by the heart, the β-oxidation inhibiting glucose oxidation via the Randle cycle. When glucose and insulin plasma levels increase, glucose becomes the main energy-providing substrate. Indeed, insulin induces Glut4 translocation and PFK-2 activation, leading to the concomitant stimulation of glucose uptake and glycolysis. (Modified from Bertrand L, Horman S, Beauloye C, Vanoverschelde JL. Insulin signalling in the heart. *Cardiovasc Res*. 2008; 79: 238-248.)

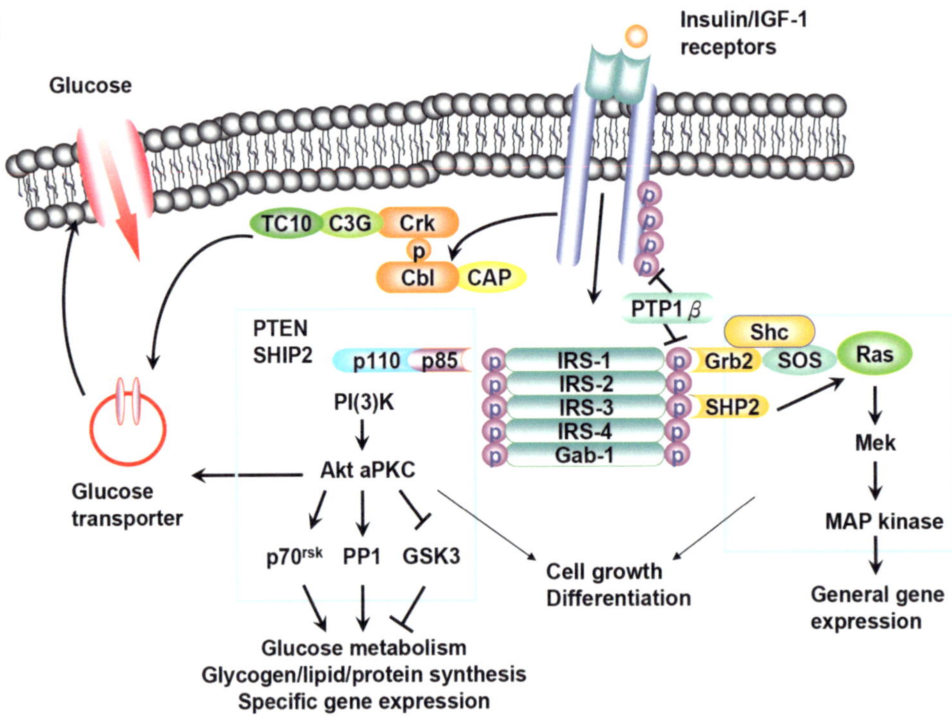

Fig. 2. Signal transduction in insulin action. The insulin receptor is a tyrosine kinase that undergoes autophosphorylation, and catalyses the phosphorylation of cellular proteins such as members of the IRS family, Shc, and Cbl. These pathways act in a concerted fashion to coordinate the regulation of vesicle trafficking, protein synthesis, enzyme activation and inactivation, and gene expression, which results in the regulation of glucose, lipid, and protein metabolism. (Modified from Saltiel AR, Kahn CR. Insulin signalling and the regulation of glucose and lipid metabolism. *Nature*. 2001; 414: 799-806.)

Insulin mediation of glucose uptake depends on the presence of glucose transporters (Gluts) at the plasma membrane. Glut1 and Glut4 are the two glucose transporters expressed in the heart; however, Glut4 is considered to be the main contributor for the insulin stimulated glucose uptake (52, 53). The role of the PI3K/PKB/Akt-signalling in the insulin-stimulated Glut4 translocation has been well established (54). Insulin not only stimulates glucose uptake, it also induces LCFA uptake in cardiomyocytes (55, 56). Insulin stimulates LCFA uptake by translocation of LCFA transporter (FAT/CD36) to the plasma membrane in the cardiomyocytes (57, 58).

Insulin also promotes protein synthesis by phosphorylation and dephosphorylation of several translational factors and ribosomal proteins through PI3K/AKT/mTOR pathway (59, 60). Activation of mTOR mainly regulates two translational factors which are 4E-binding protein-1 (4E-BP1) and the p70 ribosomal S6 protein kinase (p70S6K). Additionally, PKB/AKT also regulates GSK-3 and the forkhead transcription factor (FOXO) family, participating in the modulation of protein translation and promoting the atrogene transcriptional program (61). In addition to affecting energy metabolism, Akt activation also modulates several cellular functions which inhibit apoptosis, stimulate myocyte hypertrophy/fibrosis, and enhance nitric oxide production. Therefore, an absent insulin response can lead to less nitric oxide production, more apoptosis, and alterations in myocardial structure (62-65). Fig.3 elucidates the multiple biological functions of PKB/Akt (63).

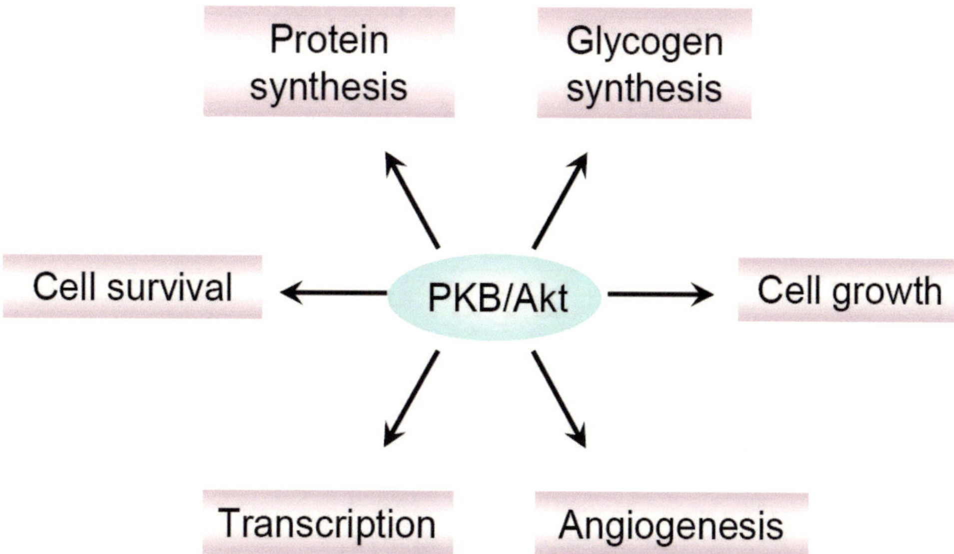

Fig. 3. Central role of protein kinase B (PKB)/Akt in multiple cellular responses. PKB/Akt control numerous of key cellular events. (Modified from Brazil DP, Hemmings BA. Ten years of protein kinase B signalling: a hard Akt to follow. *Trends Biochem Sci.* 2001; 26: 657-664.)

5. Insulin resistance induced cardiomyopathy

Insulin resistance describes an impaired biological response to insulin, and in the early stages, the plasma insulin level is increased. Although the increased insulin level may compensate for resistance to some biological actions of insulin, it may result in overexpression of actions in tissues that retain normal or slightly impaired sensitivity to insulin. In general, insulin resistance can be due to a prereceptor, receptor, or postreceptor abnormality (66). The insulin resistance induced cardiomyopathy may contain the following features.

5.1 Hypertension

Clinical studies reveal that insulin resistance and hyperinsulinemia is related to hypertension (67, 68). Mechanisms for the development of hypertension in insulin resistance and hyperinsulinemia include activation of the sympathetic nervous system, renal sodium retention, transmembrane cation transport alteration, growth-promoting effects of vascular smooth muscle cells, and vascular hyperreactivity (66, 69, 70). Fig. 4 is a schematic representation of the hypothetical relationships between obesity, insulin resistance, and hypertension (70).

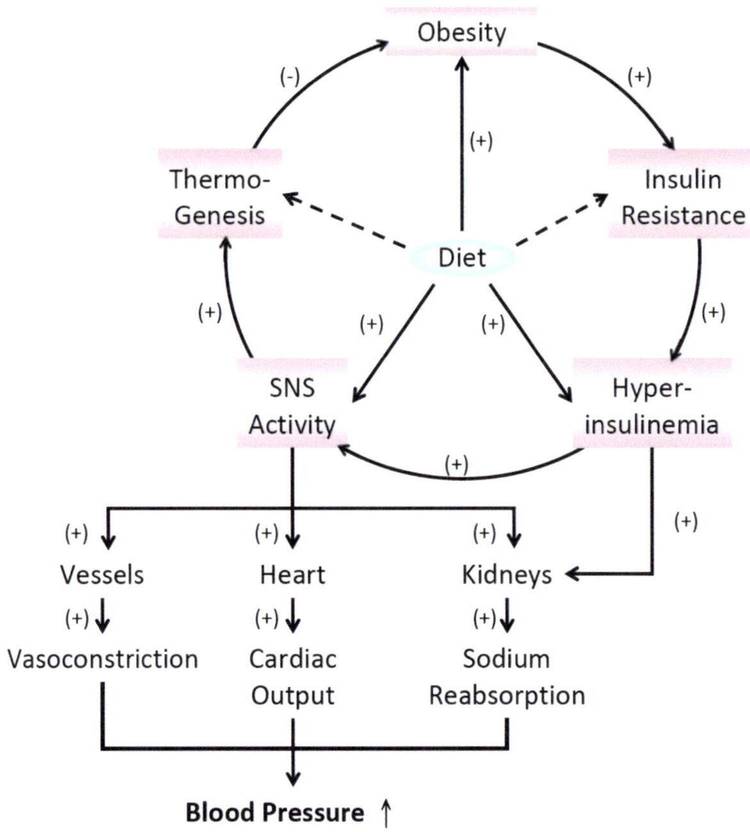

Fig. 4. Multiple role of insulin resistance to hypertension. Insulin resistance as a physiologic mechanism to restore energy balance, activate sympathetic stimulation, and leading to hypertension. The steady-state hyperinsulinemia, acting at the level of the kidney, and the consequent sympathetic stimulation of the vasculature, heart, and kidneys result in hypertension. Plus signs denote positive or stimulatory effects, the minus sign a negative or inhibitory effect, and the dotted line the direct effects of food on insulin resistance and metabolic rate. (Modified from Reaven GM, Lithell H, Landsberg L. Hypertension and associated metabolic abnormalities--the role of insulin resistance and the sympathoadrenal system. *N Engl J Med*. 1996; 334: 374-381.)

5.2 Ventricular hypertrophy

Previous studies have demonstrated that left ventricular hypertrophy and heart failure may be associated with insulin resistance (71-73). Insulin and insulin growth factor-1 (IGF-1) may exert a direct growth-promoting effect on cardiomyocytes (74, 75) and lead to cardiomyocyte hypertrophy. On the other hand, diabetes and insulin resistance are a disorder of metabolic regulation. Many acute metabolic changes alter the cellular signal transduction cascades and are believed to be involved in the adaptation of the heart to changes in its environment. PI3K, PKC and Ca^{2+}, all play a role in cardiac adaptation to regulate metabolism in the heart (76). Adrenergic activation induced hypertension may also stimulate pressure overload hypertrophy as an adaptation process (77).

5.3 Dilated cardiomyopathy and heart failure

Many studies have confirmed a strong correlation between nonischemic cardiomyopathy and diabetes, with a dramatically increased prevalence of diabetes in the dilated cardiomyopathy population (78). Additionally, abnormal glucose tolerance and insulin resistance in patients with idiopathic dilated cardiomyopathy (IDCM) has been described (49, 79). It is almost clear that insulin resistance itself is not enough to trigger dilated cardiomyopathy as the majority of patients with insulin resistance do not develop dilated cardiomyopathy. Insulin resistance is more likely to create an abnormal environment, rather than causing another stressor (e.g., pressure/volume overload, metabolic inbalance, energy defect or decreased perfusion). Insulin resistance makes the heart unable to maintain homeostasis of its energy and function, which may favor the development of cardiomyopathy and heart failure (45, 80, 81). Fig. 5 shows the relationships/mechanism between insulin resistance and heart failure (49).

5.4 Cardiac mitochondria abnormalities and ROS elevation

ROS is the one-electron reduction of O_2 to superoxide by nicotinamide adenine dinucleotide phosphate (NADPH) oxidase, which contributes to ROS generation, especially in chronic pathological states (82, 83). Mitochondria provide another significant source of cardiomyocyte ROS, particularly under acute stress. Insulin resistance impaired mitochondrial biogenesis and oxidative phosphorylation, is associated with myocardial dysfunction (84). Insulin resistance-induced hyperglycemia also directly enhances ROS generation and protein damage which leads to mitochondrial apoptosis and degradation (84). In addition, activation of the renin angiotensin aldosterone system (RAAS) is associated with increasing oxidative stress (85). The oxidative stress can impair glucose transport/utilization as well as mitochondrial ATP generation and intracellular Ca^{2+} regulatory proteins. Abnormalities in Ca^{2+} signaling/flux and myofilament functions, contribute to the cardiomyopathy changes and defective cardiac contractile function (86-87). In the 1980s, Przyklenk K et al. demonstrated that superoxide dismutase (SOD) plus catalase improve myocardial contractile function in the canine model (88). A recent study also points out that cardiac overexpression of catalase rescues insulin resistance induced myocardial contractile dysfunction (89).

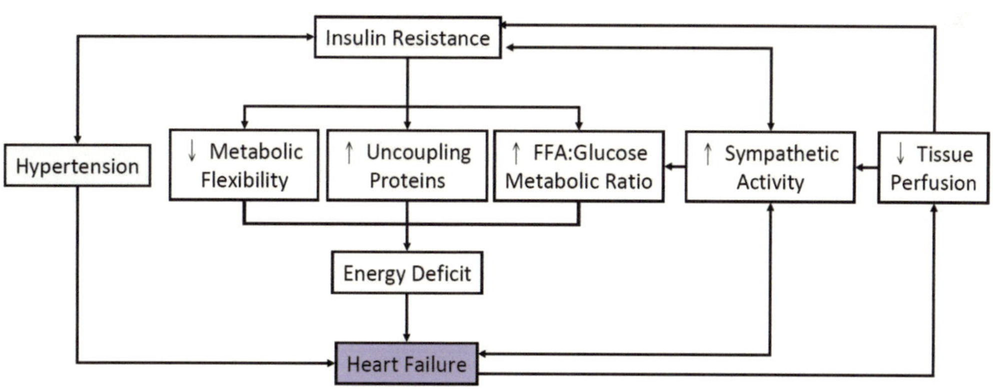

Fig. 5. Relationships/mechanism between insulin resistance to heart failure. (Modified from Witteles RM, Fowler MB. Insulin-resistant cardiomyopathy clinical evidence, mechanisms, and treatment options. *J Am Coll Cardiol.* 2008; 51: 93-102.)

6. Animal models for diabetic or insulin resistant cardiomyopathy

The impairment of glucose uptake, glycolysis, and pyruvate oxidation has been observed in both, types 1 and type 2 diabetes. In addition, attenuation of insulin function augments lipolysis and increases FFA release from adipose tissue. These abnormalities play a crucial role in the development of cardiomyopathy. Recently, several diabetic and insulin resistant animal models which include chemical (STZ-diabetes), genetic defect (*ob/ob* and *db/db* mice and Zucker diabetic fatty rats), and western diets (high fat, high fructose, high cholesterol, and high choleserol with fructose diets) diabetic induced animals, have been used to elucidate the pathophysiological processes of insulin resistance related cardiomyopathy.

6.1 Type 1 diabetes model

Streptozotocin (STZ) is a chemical generating the production of ROS which damages the pancreas with loss of function and reduced insulin production, by triggering DNA fragmentation (90, 91). The STZ-diabetic animal model can be employed for assessing the mechanisms of insulin dependent non-obese diabetes and screening potential therapies for the treatment of this condition. The characteristics of STZ-diabetes-induced cardiomyopathy include the alteration of contractile protein synthesis, abnormality of diastolic pressure-volume relationships, impairment of cardiac contractility, and incomplete relaxation of the myocardium (92, 93-97). The STZ-induced diabetics have metabolic disturbances especially, an increased plasma free fatty acid concentration (98-100). Insulin treatment reverses STZ-diabetes-induced cardiomyopathy suggesting that insulin deficiency is the major reason leading to the development of diabetic cardiomyopathy but not due to a primary cardiotoxic effect of STZ (92, 101). Resveratrol (RSV), a natural antioxidant derived from grapes, has been suggested to improve cardiac contractile function in STZ-diabetic rats (102). Moreover, the angiotensin II blocker losartan, restores cardiomyocyte functional properties in STZ-diabetic rats (103).

6.2 *Ob/ob* and *db/db* mice model

Obesity is closely associated with insulin resistance and serves as a major risk factor for the development of T2DM. Leptin or leptin receptor gene deficiency mice (*ob/ob* and *db/db* mice) are commonly used animal models for the study of T2DM. The *ob/ob* and *db/db* mice exhibit an increase of hepatic lipogenesis and gluconeogenesis resulting in increased insulin secretion by the pancreas due to the hyperglycemia and hyperlipidemia, which begins a vicious cycle of insulin resistance. Recently, contractile dysfunction independent of coronary artery disease has also been demonstrated in db/db and ob/ob mice, supporting the existence of an obesity-related cardiomyopathy and a diabetic cardiomyopathy (104-108). These genetically defective mice show a decrease in glucose oxidation rates and an increase of FFA oxidation and myocardial oxygen consumption (MVO_2), resulting in impaired cardiac efficiency (106, 108). Moreover, *ob/ob* hearts show a decrease in mitochondrial oxidative capacity, an increase of fatty acid-induced mitochondrial uncoupling, and deleterious effects on global cellular Ca^{2+} homeostasis (109, 110). As observed in STZ-diabetic rats, *db/db* mice also have excessive ROS generation, which causes cardiomyocyte damage and augmentation of apoptosis (110, 111).

6.3 Zucker diabetic fatty rat (ZDF rat)

The Zucker rat (leptin receptor gene deficient) was bred to be a genetic model for research in obesity and hypertension, and T2DM. Obese Zucker rats exhibit hyperlipidemia, hypercholesterolemia, and insulin resistance. The cardiac contractile functions and carbohydrate oxidation rates are reduced and fatty acid utilization is increased in the Zucker rat heart (28, 112-115). In contrast, several studies indicate that Zucker rats display insulin resistance without overt signs of diabetes (hyperglycemia and hyperlipidemia). These rats also show a normoglycemia phenomenon and absence of significant cardiac contractile dysfunction (116,117). Taken together, the genetic defect (leptin or leptin receptor)-induced cardiomyopathy may include several characteristics which contribute to impair myocardial contractility in diabetes mellitus. These are: (a) disturbance of substrate metabolism, (b) impairment of calcium homeostasis, (c) increased oxidative stress, (d) upregulation of the renin-angiotensin system, and (e) impairment of mitochondrial biogenesis and function (3).

6.4 Diet induced insulin resistance and cardiomyopathy

Based on previous reviews, it is widely accepted that disturbance of substrate metabolism is a key factor in the induction of insulin resistance and cardiomyopathy. Both genetic and environmental factors contribute to the development of metabolic abnormalities. Several experimental studies have demonstrated that the macronutrient composition of a diet is an important environmental determinant of the quality of insulin action (118, 119). High-fat and high-fructose intakes have been shown to contribute to conditions such as hyperlipidemia, glucose intolerance, hypertension, and atherosclerosis (120, 121). In addition, brief feeding of an excessive atherogenic diet (chow with 45% kcal from fat and 2% cholesterol) produces striking features of metabolic syndrome and coronary artery disease (122). High sugar intake is linked to an increased risk of heart disease. Simple sugars are the primary source of high triglycerides and very low-density lipoproteins (LDL), which are independent risk factors for atherosclerosis. Sugar lowers high-density lipoprotein (HDL) cholesterol and raises LDL cholesterol along with blood pressure. In addition, it has been suggested that fructose induced hyperuricemia results in endothelial dysfunction and insulin resistance, and might be a causal mechanism of the metabolic syndrome (123).

6.4.1 High fat diet (HFD)

With long term high fat intake, the response to a chronic high plasma concentration of long-chain fatty acids is that the heart is forced to increase the uptake of fatty acid. This switch in metabolic substrate uptake is accompanied by an increased presence of the fatty acid transporter FAT / CD36 at the cardiomyocyte sarcolemma. This shifts oxidation towards FA rather than glucose oxidation, and results in the development of cardiac insulin resistance and ultimately diabetic cardiomyopathy (124). It is unquestionable that chronic feeding with a high fat diet causes insulin resistance. The implication is that it decreases insulin-stimulated Akt phosphorylation, whereas cardiac basal Akt phosphorylation is elevated (124). HFD also causes cardiac lipotoxicity which may contribute to the development of diabetic cardiomyopathy (125). Additionally, hypertrophic growth and structural alterations in the context of disease is in the end maladaptive, because it will progress to, contractile dysfunction, decompensation and ultimately heart failure.

6.4.2 High fructose diet

High-fructose intake is shown to contribute to conditions such as hyperlipidemia, glucose intolerance, hypertension, and atherosclerosis (126). The preference of fructose in the lipogenesis pathway contributes to induce hyperlipidemia, in particular, a marked increase of postprandial triglyceride (TG) concentration (Fig.6) (127-129). Fructose intake is associated with an increasing incidence of insulin resistance and insulin-resistant related hypertension and cardiomyopathy (130, 131). High fructose induced insulin resistance may manifest as alterations in insulin activated PI3K/Akt pathway leading to reduced, Glut4 translocation, glucose uptake, and cardiomyocyte growth and survival. Upregulation of lipid metabolism in fructose-fed rats increases ROS production and damages the cardiomyocyte. In addition, ROS-induced dephosphorylation of Akt at Serine473 residue has been reported to participate in the insulin resistance (132).

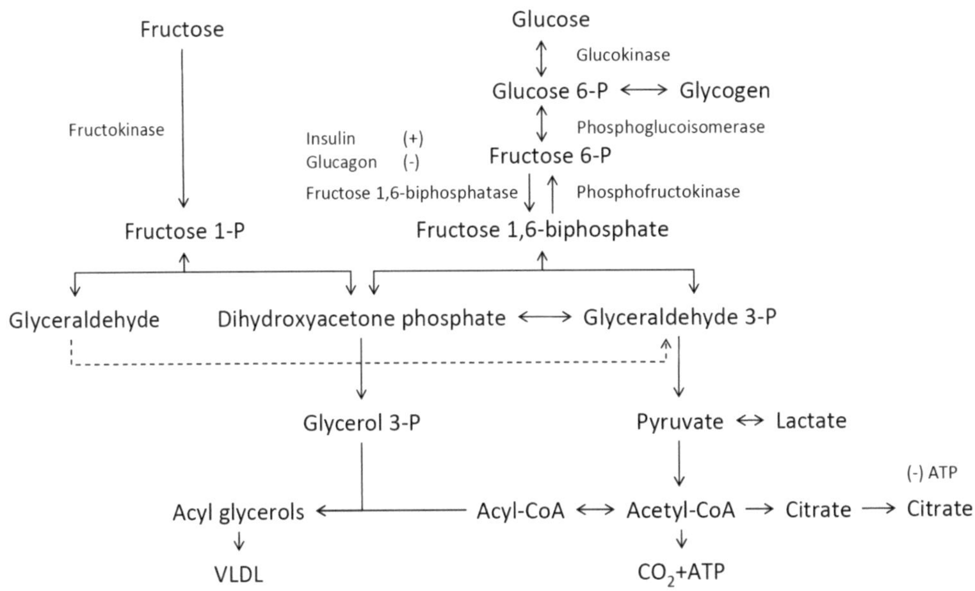

Fig. 6. Specific utilization of fructose and the glucose utilization in the liver. Hepatic fructose metabolism begins the phosphorylation by fructokinase. Fructose carbon enters the glycolytic pathway at the triose phosphate level. Thus, fructose bypasses the major control point by which glucose carbon enters glycolysis (phosphofructokinase), where glucose metabolism is limited by feedback inhibition by citrate and ATP. This allows fructose to serve as an unregulated source of both glycerol-3-phosphate and acetyl-CoA for hepatic lipogenesis. (Modified from Elliott SS, Keim NL, Stern JS, Teff K, Havel PJ. Fructose, weight gain, and the insulin resistance syndrome. *Am J Clin Nutr*. 2002; 76: 911-922.)

6.4.3 High cholesterol and fructose diet (HCF)

Brief feeding of an excessively atherogenic diet (chow with 45% kcal from fat and 2% cholesterol) produces striking features of metabolic syndrome and coronary artery disease (122). Numerous studies show that high cholesterol induces chronic inflammation. It is reported that the addition of a small amount of cholesterol to a western-type diet is associated with chronic systemic inflammation, as evidenced by an increase in atherosclerosis and circulating inflammatory protein levels (133, 134). Specifically, a study proposes the concept that, dietary cholesterol worsens adipose tissue macrophages independent of weight gain (133). This observation is consistent with the notion that adipose tissue inflammation and dysregulation of adipokines secretion contribute to the development of systemic insulin resistance (135). Our laboratory study reveals that a high cholesterol-fructose (HCF) diet also induces insulin resistance not only in metabolic-responsive tissues (i.e. liver and muscle) but also in the heart as well (25). Insulin-stimulated cardiac glucose uptake was significantly reduced after 15 weeks of HCF feeding, and cardiac insulin resistance was associated with blunted Akt-mediated insulin signaling along with GLUT4 translocation. The basal FATP1 (fatty acid transporter 1) levels were increased in HCF rat hearts. The cardiac performance of the HCF rats showed a marked reduction (25). Our results indicate that high-cholesterol food and sugar-sweetened beverages that lead to maladaptive metabolic processes may interfere with the action of insulin and increase susceptibility for the development of cardiomyopathy (25).

7. Potential therapies in insulin resistant related cardiomyopathy

Insulin resistance is an important risk factor for the development of hypertension, atherosclerotic heart disease, left ventricular hypertrophy and dysfunction, and heart failure (136-138). It reflects a disturbance of glucose metabolism and can potentially worsen the metabolic efficiency of both skeletal and cardiac muscle. The exact mechanisms of cardiac insulin resistance leading to and progression of, left ventricular contractile dysfunction are not fully elucidated. Currently, the most promising potential medical therapies for insulin resistant cardiomyopathy can be divided into 2 broad categories which are, metabolic modulators and diabetic medications (Table.2)(49).

Medication	Mechanism	Other/Side-effects
Metabolic modulators		
Trimetazidine	↓ FFA metabolism	Not approved In U.S.
Perhexiline	↓ FFA metabolism	Not approved In U.S.,liver/neuro-toxicity
Ranolazine	↑ Glu metabolism	Might not be primary mechanism, ↑ QT interval
L-carnitine	↑ FFA/Glu metabolism	
Diabetic medications		
Insulin	↑ Ins	Hypoglycemia
Sulfonylureas	↑ Ins	Hypoglycemia
Metformin	↑ Ins sensitivity	Lactic acidosis (rare)
TZDs (glitazones)	↑ Ins sensitivity	Fluid retention/edema
GLP-1	↑ Ins/ ↑ Ins sensitivity	Very short half-life (1-2 min)
Exenatide	↑ Ins/ ↑ Ins sensitivity	Nausea/weight loss, subcutaneous injection
DPP-IV inhibitor	↑ Ins/ ↑ Ins sensitivity	

Table 2. Potential treatments for insulin resistant cardiomyopathy. (Modified from Witteles RM, Fowler MB. Insulin-resistant cardiomyopathy clinical evidence, mechanisms, and treatment options. *J Am Coll Cardiol*. 2008; 51: 93-102.)

1. Metabolic modulators which increase glucose metabolism, decrease FFA metabolism, and potentially enhance myocardial contractile efficiency are e.g. Trimetazidine, Perhexiline, Ranolazine, and L-carnitine.
2. Diabetic medications enhancing insulin sensitivity (TZDs) might theoretically be the most attractive therapies to improve insulin resistant related cardiomyopathy. These agents work on the activation of PPARγ, a transcription factor that promotes insulin sensitivity and decreases circulating FFA, and increases myocardial glucose uptake (139).

Moreover, several newly developed classes of antidiabetic medications have been discovered recently. Glucagon-like peptide 1(GLP1) treatment, results in promotion of post prandial insulin secretion and improvement of insulin sensitivity (140). GLP1 infusion improves left ventricular function, hemodynamic status, and cardiac efficiency (141). In addition, angiotensin converting enzyme inhibitors (ACEI), angiotensin II receptor blockers and statins all affect glucose metabolism (142-144); although combined therapy involving a diuretic agent and a calcium-channel blocker is required (145). Interestingly, a recent study shows that RSV and insulin combination treatment has preventive effects on diabetes-associated cardiovascular dysfunction. However, when a diabetic individual has suffered an acute heart attack the synergistic actions of combination treatment were nullified and the advantage of RSV was antagonized by insulin. This study provides valuable advice for using insulin and RSV in patients with diabetes and those diabetic individuals with ischemic heart disease (102).

8. Summary and conclusion

Insulin plays an important physiological role in coupling metabolic and cardiac homeostasis under healthy conditions. Loss of normal insulin action (insulin resistance) on the heart makes the heart unable to maintain homeostasis of its energy and function, which may favor the development of cardiomyopathy and heart failure. It is almost clear that insulin resistance itself is not enough to trigger dilated cardiomyopathy as the majority of patients with insulin resistance do not develop dilated cardiomyopathy. Insulin resistance is more likely to create an abnormal environment, rather than causing another stressor.

9. References

[1] Aronson D, Rayfield EJ, Chesebro JH. Mechanisms determining course and outcome of diabetic patients who have had acute myocardial infarction. *Ann Intern Med.* 1997; 126: 296-306.

[2] Gu K, Cowie CC, Harris MI. Diabetes and decline in heart disease mortality in US adults. *JAMA.* 1999; 281:1291-1297.

[3] Boudina S, Abel ED. Diabetic cardiomyopathy revisited. *Circulation.* 2007;115: 3213–3223.

[4] Rubler S, Dlugash J, Yuceoglu YZ, Kumral T, Branwood AW, Grishman A. New type of cardiomyopathy associated with diabetic glomerulosclerosis. *Am J Cardiol.* 1972; 30: 595- 602.

[5] Bertrand L, Horman S, Beauloye C, Vanoverschelde JL. Insulin signalling in the heart. *Cardiovasc Res.* 2008; 79: 238-248.

[6] Gary D. Lopaschuk, Clifford D.L. Folmes and William C. Stanley. *Circulation Research.* 2007; 101: 335-347.

[7] Heineke J, Molkentin JD. Regulation of cardiac hypertrophy by intracellular signalling pathways. *Nat Rev Mol Cell Biol.* 2006; 7: 589–600.

[8] Wang Y. Mitogen-activated protein kinases in heart development and diseases. *Circulation.* 2007; 116: 1413-1423.

[9] Proud CG. Ras, PI3-kinase and mTOR signaling in cardiac hypertrophy. *Cardiovasc Res.* 2004; 63: 403-413.

[10] Hintz KK, Aberle NS, Ren J. Insulin resistance induces hyperleptinemia, cardiac contractile dysfunction but not cardiac leptin resistance in ventricular myocytes. *International Journal of Obesity.*2003; 27: 1196–1203.

[11] Mureddu GF, Greco R, Rosato GF, Cella A, Vaccaro O, Contaldo F, de Simone G. Relation of insulin resistance to left ventricular hypertrophy and diastolic dysfunction in obesity. *Int J Obes Relat Metab Disord.* 1998; 22: 363-368.

[12] Swan JW, Anker SD, Walton C, Godsland IF, Clark AL, Leyva F, Stevenson JC, Coats AJ. Insulin resistance in chronic heart failure: relation to severity and etiology of heart failure. *J Am Coll Cardiol.* 1997; 30: 527-532.

[13] Hayat SA, Patel B, Khattar RS, Malik RA. Diabetic cardiomyopathy: mechanisms, diagnosis, and treatment. *Clin Sci.* 2004; 107: 539–557.

[14] Voulgari C, Papadogiannis D, Tentolouris N. Diabetic cardiomyopathy: from the pathophysiology of the cardiac myocytes to current diagnosis and management strategies. *Vasc Health Risk Manag.* 2010; 6: 883-903.

[15] Poirier P, Bogaty P, Garneau C, Marois L, Dumesnil JG. Diastolic dysfunction in normotensive men with well-controlled type 2 diabetes: importance of maneuvers in echocardiographic screening for preclinical diabetic cardiomyopathy. *Diabetes Care.* 2001; 24: 5-10.

[16] Grundy SM, Benjamin IJ, Burke GL, Chait A, Eckel RH, Howard BV, Mitch W, Smith SC, Sowers JR: Diabetes and cardiovascular disease: A statement for healthcare professionals from the American Heart Association.. *Circulation.* 1999; 100: 1134–1146.

[17] Chatham JC, Forder JR, McNeill JH: *The Heart in Diabetes.* Norwell, MA: Kluwer Academic Publishers, 1996.

[18] Lagadic-Gossmann D, Buckler KJ, Le Prigent K, Feuvray D. Altered Ca2+ handling in ventricular myocytes isolated from diabetic rats. *Am J Physiol.* 1996; 270(5 Pt 2):H1529-H1537.

[19] Ren J, Davidoff AJ. Diabetes rapidly induces contractile dysfunctions in isolated ventricular myocytes. *Am J Physiol.* 1997; 272(1 Pt 2): H148-H158.

[20] Margonato A, Gerundini P, Vicedomini G, Gilardi MC, Pozza G, Fazio F. Abnormal cardiovascular response to exercise in young asymptomatic diabetic patients with retinopathy. *Am Heart J.* 1986; 112: 554-560.

[21] Mirsky I. Assessment of diastolic function: suggested methods and future considerations. *Circulation.* 1984; 69: 836-841.

[22] Pelleymounter MA, Cullen MJ, Baker MB, Hecht R, Winters D, Boone T, Collins F. Effects of the obese gene product on body weight regulation in ob/ob mice. *Science.* 1995; 28; 269: 540-543.

[23] Hu P, Zhang D, Swenson L, Chakrabarti G, Abel ED, Litwin SE. Minimally invasive aortic banding in mice: effects of altered cardiomyocyte insulin signaling during pressure overload. *Am J Physiol Heart Circ Physiol.* 2003; 285: H1261-1269.

[24] McQueen AP, Zhang D, Hu P, Swenson L, Yang Y, Zaha VG, Hoffman JL, Yun UJ, Chakrabarti G, Wang Z, Albertine KH, Abel ED, Litwin SE. Contractile dysfunction in hypertrophied hearts with deficient insulin receptor signaling: possible role of reduced capillary density. *J Mol Cell Cardiol.* 2005; 39: 882-892.

[25] Deng JY, Huang JP, Lu LS, Hung LM. Impairment of cardiac insulin signaling and myocardial contractile performance in high-cholesterol/fructose-fed rats. *Am J Physiol Heart Circ Physiol.* 2007; 293: H978-H987.

[26] Poornima IG, Parikh P, Shannon RP. Diabetic cardiomyopathy: the search for a unifying hypothesis. *Circ Res.* 2006; 98: 596-605.

[27] An D, Rodrigues B. Role of changes in cardiac metabolism in development of diabetic cardiomyopathy. *Am J Physiol Heart Circ Physiol.* 2006; 291: H1489-H1506.

[28] Chiu HC, Kovacs A, Ford DA, Hsu FF, Garcia R, Herrero P, Saffitz JE, Schaffer JE. A novel mouse model of lipotoxic cardiomyopathy. *J Clin Invest.* 2001; 107: 813-822.

[29] Christoffersen C, Bollano E, Lindegaard ML, Bartels ED, Goetze JP, Andersen CB, Nielsen LB. Cardiac lipid accumulation associated with diastolic dysfunction in obese mice. *Endocrinology.* 2003; 144: 3483-3490.

[30] Pillutla P, Hwang YC, Augustus A, Yokoyama M, Yagyu H, Johnston TP, Kaneko M, Ramasamy R, Goldberg IJ. Perfusion of hearts with triglyceride-rich particles reproduces the metabolic abnormalities in lipotoxic cardiomyopathy. *Am J Physiol Endocrinol Metab.* 2005; 288: E1229-H1235.

[31] Yagyu H, Chen G, Yokoyama M, Hirata K, Augustus A, Kako Y, Seo T, Hu Y, Lutz EP, Merkel M, Bensadoun A, Homma S, Goldberg IJ. Lipoprotein lipase (LpL) on the surface of cardiomyocytes increases lipid uptake and produces a cardiomyopathy. *J Clin Invest.* 2003; 111: 419-426.

[32] Zhou YT, Grayburn P, Karim A, Shimabukuro M, Higa M, Baetens D, Orci L, Unger RH. Lipotoxic heart disease in obese rats: implications for human obesity. *Proc Natl Acad Sci U S A.* 2000; 97: 1784-1789.

[33] Shah A, Shannon RP. Insulin resistance in dilated cardiomyopathy. *Rev Cardiovasc Med.* 2003; 4 Suppl 6: S50-S57.

[34] Shulman GI. Cellular mechanisms of insulin resistance. *J Clin Invest.* 2000; 106: 171-176.

[35] Birnbaum MJ. Turning down insulin signaling. *J Clin Invest.* 2001; 108: 655-659.

[36] Kim JK, Kim YJ, Fillmore JJ, Chen Y, Moore I, Lee J, Yuan M, Li ZW, Karin M, Perret P, Shoelson SE, Shulman GI. Prevention of fat-induced insulin resistance by salicylate. *J Clin Invest.* 2001; 108: 437-446.

[37] Liu GX, Hanley PJ, Ray J, Daut J. Long-chain acyl-coenzyme A esters and fatty acids directly link metabolism to K(ATP) channels in the heart. *Circ Res.* 2001; 88: 918-924.

[38] Du X, Matsumura T, Edelstein D, Rossetti L, Zsengellér Z, Szabó C, Brownlee M. Inhibition of GAPDH activity by poly(ADP-ribose) polymerase activates three

major pathways of hyperglycemic damage in endothelial cells. *J Clin Invest*. 2003 112: 1049-1057.

[39] Nishikawa T, Edelstein D, Du XL, Yamagishi S, Matsumura T, Kaneda Y, Yorek MA, Beebe D, Oates PJ, Hammes HP, Giardino I, Brownlee M. Normalizing mitochondrial superoxide production blocks three pathways of hyperglycaemic damage. *Nature*. 2000; 404: 787-790.

[40] Du XL, Edelstein D, Rossetti L, Fantus IG, Goldberg H, Ziyadeh F, Wu J, Brownlee M. Hyperglycemia-induced mitochondrial superoxide overproduction activates the hexosamine pathway and induces plasminogen activator inhibitor-1 expression by increasing Sp1 glycosylation. *Proc Natl Acad Sci U S A*. 2000; 97: 12222-12226.

[41] Bidasee KR, Nallani K, Yu Y, Cocklin RR, Zhang Y, Wang M, Dincer UD, Besch HR Jr. Chronic diabetes increases advanced glycation end products on cardiac ryanodine receptors/calcium-release channels. *Diabetes*. 2003; 52: 1825-1836.

[42] Candido R, Forbes JM, Thomas MC, Thallas V, Dean RG, Burns WC, Tikellis C, Ritchie RH, Twigg SM, Cooper ME, Burrell LM. A breaker of advanced glycation end products attenuates diabetes-induced myocardial structural changes. *Circ Res*. 2003; 92: 785-792.

[43] Herrmann KL, McCulloch AD, Omens JH. Glycated collagen cross-linking alters cardiac mechanics in volume-overload hypertrophy. *Am J Physiol Heart Circ Physiol*. 2003; 284: H1277-H1284.

[44] Clark RJ, McDonough PM, Swanson E, Trost SU, Suzuki M, Fukuda M, Dillmann WH. Diabetes and the accompanying hyperglycemia impairs cardiomyocyte calcium cycling through increased nuclear O-GlcNAcylation. *J Biol Chem*. 2003; 278: 44230-44237.

[45] Galvez AS, Ulloa JA, Chiong M, Criollo A, Eisner V, Barros LF, Lavandero S. Aldose reductase induced by hyperosmotic stress mediates cardiomyocyte apoptosis: differential effects of sorbitol and mannitol. *J Biol Chem*. 2003; 278: 38484-38494.

[46] Koya D, King GL. Protein kinase C activation and the development of diabetic complications. *Diabetes*. 1998; 47: 859-866.

[47] Wakasaki H, Koya D, Schoen FJ, Jirousek MR, Ways DK, Hoit BD, Walsh RA, King GL. Targeted overexpression of protein kinase C beta2 isoform in myocardium causes cardiomyopathy. *Proc Natl Acad Sci U S A*. 1997; 94: 9320-9325.

[48] Paolisso G, De Riu S, Marrazzo G, Verza M, Varricchio M, D'Onofrio F. Insulin resistance and hyperinsulinemia in patients with chronic congestive heart failure. *Metabolism*. 1991; 40: 972-977.

[49] Witteles RM, Fowler MB. Insulin-resistant cardiomyopathy clinical evidence, mechanisms, and treatment options. *J Am Coll Cardiol*. 2008; 51: 93-102.

[50] Saltiel AR, Kahn CR. Insulin signalling and the regulation of glucose and lipid metabolism. *Nature*. 2001; 414: 799-806.

[51] Deprez J, Bertrand L, Alessi DR, Krause U, Hue L, Rider MH. Partial purification and characterization of a wortmannin-sensitive and insulin-stimulated protein kinase that activates heart 6-phosphofructo-2-kinase. *Biochem J*. 2000; 347 Pt 1:305-312.

[52] Zorzano A, Sevilla L, Camps M, Becker C, Meyer J, Kammermeier H, Muñoz P, Gumà A, Testar X, Palacín M, Blasi J, Fischer Y. Regulation of glucose transport, and

glucose transporters expression and trafficking in the heart: studies in cardiac myocytes. *Am J Cardiol.* 1997; 80: 65A-76A.
[53] Abel ED. Glucose transport in the heart. *Front Biosci.* 2004; 9: 201-215.
[54] Watson RT, Pessin JE. Bridging the GAP between insulin signaling and GLUT4 translocation. *Trends Biochem Sci.* 2006; 4: 215-222.
[55] Coort SL, Bonen A, van der Vusse GJ, Glatz JF, Luiken JJ. Cardiac substrate uptake and metabolism in obesity and type-2 diabetes: role of sarcolemmal substrate transporters. *Mol Cell Biochem.* 2007; 299(1-2): 5-18.
[56] Glatz JF, Bonen A, Ouwens DM, Luiken JJ. Regulation of sarcolemmal transport of substrates in the healthy and diseased heart. *Cardiovasc Drugs Ther.* 2006; 20: 471-476.
[57] Luiken JJ, Koonen DP, Willems J, Zorzano A, Becker C, Fischer Y, Tandon NN, Van Der Vusse GJ, Bonen A, Glatz JF. Insulin stimulates long-chain fatty acid utilization by rat cardiac myocytes through cellular redistribution of FAT/CD36. *Diabetes.* 2002; 51: 3113-3119.
[58] Dyck DJ, Steinberg G, Bonen A. Insulin increases FA uptake and esterification but reduces lipid utilization in isolated contracting muscle. *Am J Physiol Endocrinol Metab.* 2001; 281: E600-E607.
[59] Hedhli N, Pelat M, Depre C. Protein turnover in cardiac cell growth and survival. *Cardiovasc Res.* 2005; 68: 186-196.
[60] Proud CG. Signalling to translation: how signal transduction pathways control the protein synthetic machinery. *Biochem J.* 2007; 403: 217-234.
[61] Sandri M, Sandri C, Gilbert A, Skurk C, Calabria E, Picard A, Walsh K, Schiaffino S, Lecker SH, Goldberg AL. Foxo transcription factors induce the atrophy-related ubiquitin ligase atrogin-1 and cause skeletal muscle atrophy. *Cell.* 2004; 117: 399-412.
[62] Asbun J, Villarreal FJ. The pathogenesis of myocardial fibrosis in the setting of diabetic cardiomyopathy. *J Am Coll Cardiol.* 2006; 47: 693-700
[63] Brazil DP, Hemmings BA. Ten years of protein kinase B signalling: a hard Akt to follow. *Trends Biochem Sci.* 2001; 26: 657-664.
[64] Lawlor MA, Alessi DR. PKB/Akt: a key mediator of cell proliferation, survival and insulin responses? *J Cell Sci.* 2001; 114(Pt 16): 2903-2910.
[65] Stühlinger MC, Abbasi F, Chu JW, Lamendola C, McLaughlin TL, Cooke JP, Reaven GM, Tsao PS. Relationship between insulin resistance and an endogenous nitric oxide synthase inhibitor. *JAMA.* 2002; 287: 1420-1426.
[66] Hunter SJ, Garvey WT. Insulin action and insulin resistance: diseases involving defects in insulin receptors, signal transduction, and the glucose transport effector system. *Am J Med.* 1998; 105: 331-345.
[67] Ferrannini E, Buzzigoli G, Bonadonna R, Giorico MA, Oleggini M, Graziadei L, Pedrinelli R, Brandi L, Bevilacqua S. Insulin resistance in essential hypertension. *N Engl J Med.* 1987; 317: 350-357.
[68] Shen DC, Shieh SM, Fuh MM, Wu DA, Chen YD, Reaven GM. Resistance to insulin-stimulated-glucose uptake in patients with hypertension. *J Clin Endocrinol Metab.* 1988; 66: 580-583.

[69] Sowers JR, Sowers PS, Peuler JD. Role of insulin resistance and hyperinsulinemia in development of hypertension and atherosclerosis. *J Lab Clin Med.* 1994; 123: 647-652.

[70] Reaven GM, Lithell H, Landsberg L. Hypertension and associated metabolic abnormalities--the role of insulin resistance and the sympathoadrenal system. *N Engl J Med.* 1996; 334: 374-381.

[71] Ingelsson E, Sundström J, Arnlöv J, Zethelius B, Lind L. Insulin resistance and risk of congestive heart failure. *JAMA.* 2005; 294: 334-341.

[72] Ho KK, Pinsky JL, Kannel WB, Levy D. The epidemiology of heart failure: the Framingham Study. *J Am Coll Cardiol.* 1993; 22(4 Suppl A): 6A-13A.

[73] Verdecchia P, Reboldi G, Schillaci G, Borgioni C, Ciucci A, Telera MP, Santeusanio F, Porcellati C, Brunetti P. Circulating insulin and insulin growth factor-1 are independent determinants of left ventricular mass and geometry in essential hypertension. *Circulation.* 1999; 100: 1802-1827.

[74] Hill DJ, Milner RD. Insulin as a growth factor. *Pediatr Res.* 1985; 19: 879-886.

[75] Ito H, Hiroe M, Hirata Y, Tsujino M, Adachi S, Shichiri M, Koike A, Nogami A, Marumo F. Insulin-like growth factor-I induces hypertrophy with enhanced expression of muscle specific genes in cultured rat cardiomyocytes. *Circulation.* 1993; 87: 1715-1721.

[76] Doenst T, Taegtmeyer H. alpha-adrenergic stimulation mediates glucose uptake through phosphatidylinositol 3-kinase in rat heart. *Circ Res.* 1999; 84: 467-474.

[77] Kariya K, Karns LR, Simpson PC. An enhancer core element mediates stimulation of the rat beta-myosin heavy chain promoter by an alpha 1-adrenergic agonist and activated beta-protein kinase C in hypertrophy of cardiac myocytes. *J Biol Chem.* 1994; 269: 3775-3782.

[78] Bertoni AG, Tsai A, Kasper EK, Brancati FL. Diabetes and idiopathic cardiomyopathy: a nationwide case-control study. *Diabetes Care.* 2003; 26: 2791-2795.

[79] Witteles RM, Tang WH, Jamali AH, Chu JW, Reaven GM, Fowler MB. Insulin resistance in idiopathic dilated cardiomyopathy: a possible etiologic link. *J Am Coll Cardiol.* 2004; 44: 78-81.

[80] Nikolaidis LA, Sturzu A, Stolarski C, Elahi D, Shen YT, Shannon RP. The development of myocardial insulin resistance in conscious dogs with advanced dilated cardiomyopathy. *Cardiovasc Res.* 2004; 61: 297-306.

[81] Dávila-Román VG, Vedala G, Herrero P, de las Fuentes L, Rogers JG, Kelly DP, Gropler RJ. Altered myocardial fatty acid and glucose metabolism in idiopathic dilated cardiomyopathy. *J Am Coll Cardiol.* 2002; 40: 271-277.

[82] Selemidis S, Sobey CG, Wingler K, Schmidt HH, Drummond GR. NADPH oxidases in the vasculature: molecular features, roles in disease and pharmacological inhibition. *Pharmacol Ther.* 2008; 120: 254-291.

[83] Lambeth JD. NOX enzymes and the biology of reactive oxygen. *Nat Rev Immunol.* 2004; 4: 181-189.

[84] Ren J, Pulakat L, Whaley-Connell A, Sowers JR. Mitochondrial biogenesis in the metabolic syndrome and cardiovascular disease. *J Mol Med* (Berl). 2010; 88: 993-1001.

[85] Cooper SA, Whaley-Connell A, Habibi J, Wei Y, Lastra G, Manrique C, Stas S, Sowers JR. Renin-angiotensin-aldosterone system and oxidative stress in cardiovascular insulin resistance. *Am J Physiol Heart Circ Physiol.* 2007; 293: H2009-H2023.

[86] Choi KM, Zhong Y, Hoit BD, Grupp IL, Hahn H, Dilly KW, Guatimosim S, Lederer WJ, Matlib MA. Defective intracellular Ca(2+) signaling contributes to cardiomyopathy in Type 1 diabetic rats. *Am J Physiol Heart Circ Physiol.* 2002; 283: H1398-H1408.

[87] Dong F, Li Q, Sreejayan N, Nunn JM, Ren J. Metallothionein prevents high-fat diet induced cardiac contractile dysfunction: role of peroxisome proliferator activated receptor gamma coactivator 1alpha and mitochondrial biogenesis. *Diabetes.* 2007; 56: 2201-2212.

[88] Przyklenk K, Kloner RA. Superoxide dismutase plus catalase improve contractile function in the canine model of the "stunned myocardium". *Circ Res.* 1986; 58: 148-156.

[89] Dong F, Fang CX, Yang X, Zhang X, Lopez FL, Ren J. Cardiac overexpression of catalase rescues cardiac contractile dysfunction induced by insulin resistance: Role of oxidative stress, protein carbonyl formation and insulin sensitivity. *Diabetologia.* 2006; 49: 1421-1433.

[90] Kakkar R, Mantha SV, Radhi J, Prasad K, Kalra J. Increased oxidative stress in rat liver and pancreas during progression of streptozotocin-induced diabetes. *Clin Sci* (Lond). 1998; 94: 623-632.

[91] Szkudelski T. The mechanism of alloxan and streptozotocin action in B cells of the rat pancreas. *Physiol Res.* 2001; 50: 537-546.

[92] Huang JP, Huang SS, Deng JY, Hung LM. Impairment of insulin-stimulated Akt/GLUT4 signaling is associated with cardiac contractile dysfunction and aggravates I/R injury in STZ-diabetic rats. *J Biomed Sci.* 2009; 16:77.

[93] Fein FS, Kornstein LB, Strobeck JE, Capasso JM, Sonnenblick EH. Altered myocardial mechanics in diabetic rats. *Circ Res.* 1980; 47: 922-933.

[94] Regan TJ, Lyons MM, Ahmed SS, et al. Evidence for cardiomyopathy in familial diabetes mellitus. *J Clin Invest.* 1977; 60: 885–899.

[95] Regan TJ, Ettinger PO, Khan MU, et al. Altered myocardial function and metabolism in chronic diabetes mellitus without ischemia in dogs. *Circ Res.* 1974; 35: 222–237.

[96] Garber DW, Neely JR. Decreased myocardial function and myosin ATPase in hearts from diabetic rats. *Am J Physiol.* 1983; 244: H586– H591.

[97] How OJ, Aasum E, Severson DL, Chan WY, Essop MF, Larsen TS. Increased myocardial oxygen consumption reduces cardiac efficiency in diabetic mice. *Diabetes.* 2006; 55: 466-473.

[98] Penpargkul S, Schaible T, Yipintsoi T, Scheuer J. The effect of diabetes on performance and metabolism of rat hearts. *Circ Res.* 1980; 47: 911-921.

[99] Ogihara M, Tokumitsu Y, Ui M. Metabolic alterations in normal and streptozotocin-diabetic rats in vivo: influence of prolonged starvation. *Jpn J Pharmacol.* 1984; 34: 307-311.

[100] Malone JI, Cuthbertson DD, Malone MA, Schocken DD. Cardio-protective effects of carnitine in streptozotocin-induced diabetic rats. *Cardiovasc Diabetol.* 2006; 19; 5: 2.

[101] Schaible TF, Malhotra A, Bauman WA, Scheuer J. Left ventricular function after chronic insulin treatment in diabetic and normal rats. *J Mol Cell Cardiol.* 1983; 15: 445-458.

[102] Huang JP, Huang SS, Deng JY, Chang CC, Day YJ, Hung LM. Insulin and resveratrol act synergistically, preventing cardiac dysfunction in diabetes, but the advantage of resveratrol in diabetics with acute heart attack is antagonized by insulin. *Free Radic Biol Med.* 2010; 49: 1710-1721.

[103] Raimondi L, De Paoli P, Mannucci E, Lonardo G, Sartiani L, Banchelli G, Pirisino R, Mugelli A, Cerbai E. Restoration of cardiomyocyte functional properties by angiotensin II receptor blockade in diabetic rats. *Diabetes.* 2004; 53: 1927-1933.

[104] Wolf G. Insulin resistance associated with leptin deficiency in mice: a possible model for noninsulin-dependent diabetes mellitus. *Nutr Rev.* 2001; 59: 177-179.

[105] Buchanan J, Mazumder PK, Hu P, Chakrabarti G, Roberts MW, Yun UJ, Cooksey RC, Litwin SE, Abel ED. Reduced cardiac efficiency and altered substrate metabolism precedes the onset of hyperglycemia and contractile dysfunction in two mouse models of insulin resistance and obesity. *Endocrinology.* 2005; 146: 5341-5349.

[106] Belke DD, Larsen TS, Gibbs EM, Severson DL. Altered metabolism causes cardiac dysfunction in perfused hearts from diabetic (db/db) mice. *Am J Physiol Endocrinol Metab.* 2000; 279: E1104-E1113.

[107] Mazumder PK, O'Neill BT, Roberts MW, Buchanan J, Yun UJ, Cooksey RC, Boudina S, Abel ED. Impaired cardiac efficiency and increased fatty acid oxidation in insulin-resistant ob/ob mouse hearts. *Diabetes.* 2004; 53: 2366-2374.

[108] Boudina S, Sena S, O'Neill BT, Tathireddy P, Young ME, Abel ED. Reduced mitochondrial oxidative capacity and increased mitochondrial uncoupling impair myocardial energetics in obesity. *Circulation.* 2005; 112: 2686-2695.

[109] Fauconnier J, Andersson DC, Zhang SJ, Lanner JT, Wibom R, Katz A, Bruton JD, Westerblad H. Effects of palmitate on Ca($^{2+}$) handling in adult control and ob/ob cardiomyocytes: impact of mitochondrial reactive oxygen species. *Diabetes.* 2007; 56: 1136-1142.

[110] Barouch LA, Gao D, Chen L, Miller KL, Xu W, Phan AC, Kittleson MM, Minhas KM, Berkowitz DE, Wei C, Hare JM. Cardiac myocyte apoptosis is associated with increased DNA damage and decreased survival in murine models of obesity. *Circ Res.* 2006; 98: 119-124.

[111] Cai L, Li W, Wang G, Guo L, Jiang Y, Kang YJ. Hyperglycemia-induced apoptosis in mouse myocardium: mitochondrial cytochrome C-mediated caspase-3 activation pathway. *Diabetes.* 2002; 51: 1938-1948.

[112] Young ME, Guthrie PH, Razeghi P, Leighton B, Abbasi S, Patil S, Youker KA, Taegtmeyer H. Impaired long-chain fatty acid oxidation and contractile dysfunction in the obese Zucker rat heart. *Diabetes.* 2002; 51: 2587-2595.

[113] Chatham JC, Seymour AM. Cardiac carbohydrate metabolism in Zucker diabetic fatty rats. *Cardiovasc Res.* 2002; 55: 104-112.

[114] Wang P, Lloyd SG, Zeng H, Bonen A, Chatham JC. Impact of altered substrate utilization on cardiac function in isolated hearts from Zucker diabetic fatty rats. *Am J Physiol Heart Circ Physiol.* 2005; 288: H2102-H2110.

[115] Rösen P, Herberg L, Reinauer H. Different types of postinsulin receptor defects contribute to insulin resistance in hearts of obese Zucker rats. *Endocrinology.* 1986; 119: 1285-1291.

[116] Coort SL, Hasselbaink DM, Koonen DP, Willems J, Coumans WA, Chabowski A, van der Vusse GJ, Bonen A, Glatz JF, Luiken JJ. Enhanced sarcolemmal FAT/CD36 content and triacylglycerol storage in cardiac myocytes from obese zucker rats. *Diabetes.* 2004; 53: 1655-1663.

[117] Carley AN, Severson DL. Fatty acid metabolism is enhanced in type 2 diabetic hearts. *Biochim Biophys Acta.* 2005; 1734: 112-126.

[118] Axen KV, Dikeakos A, Sclafani A. High dietary fat promotes syndrome X in nonobese rats. *J Nutr.* 2003; 133: 2244-2249.

[119] Bessesen DH. The role of carbohydrates in insulin resistance. *J Nutr.* 2001; 131: 2782S-2786S.

[120] Mann JI. Diet and risk of coronary heart disease and type 2 diabetes. *Lancet.* 2002; 360: 783-789.

[121] Storlien LH, Kraegen EW, Jenkins AB, Chisholm DJ. Effects of sucrose vs starch diets on in vivo insulin action, thermogenesis, and obesity in rats. *Am J Clin Nutr.* 1988; 47: 420-427.

[122] Dyson MC, Alloosh M, Vuchetich JP, Mokelke EA, Sturek M. Components of metabolic syndrome and coronary artery disease in female Ossabaw swine fed excess atherogenic diet. *Comp Med.* 2006; 56: 35-45.

[123] Nakagawa T, Tuttle KR, Short RA, Johnson RJ. Hypothesis: fructose-induced hyperuricemia as a causal mechanism for the epidemic of the metabolic syndrome. *Nat Clin Pract Nephrol.* 2005; 1: 80-86.

[124] Ouwens DM, Diamant M, Fodor M, Habets DD, Pelsers MM, El Hasnaoui M, Dang ZC, van den Brom CE, Vlasblom R, Rietdijk A, Boer C, Coort SL, Glatz JF, Luiken JJ. Cardiac contractile dysfunction in insulin-resistant rats fed a high-fat diet is associated with elevated CD36-mediated fatty acid uptake and esterification. *Diabetologia.* 2007; 50: 1938-1948.

[125] Schaffer JE. Lipotoxicity: when tissues overeat. *Curr Opin Lipidol.* 2003; 14: 281-287.

[126] Kuczmarski RJ, Flegal KM, Campbell SM, Johnson CL. Increasing prevalence of overweight among US adults. The National Health and Nutrition Examination Surveys, 1960 to 1991. *JAMA.* 1994; 272: 205-211.

[127] Bantle JP, Raatz SK, Thomas W, Georgopoulos A. Effects of dietary fructose on plasma lipids in healthy subjects. *Am J Clin Nutr.* 2000; 72: 1128-1134.

[128] Teff KL, Elliott SS, Tschöp M, Kieffer TJ, Rader D, Heiman M, Townsend RR, Keim NL, D'Alessio D, Havel PJ. Dietary fructose reduces circulating insulin and leptin, attenuates postprandial suppression of ghrelin, and increases triglycerides in women. *J Clin Endocrinol Metab.* 2004; 89: 2963-2972.

[129] Elliott SS, Keim NL, Stern JS, Teff K, Havel PJ. Fructose, weight gain, and the insulin resistance syndrome. *Am J Clin Nutr*. 2002; 76: 911-922.

[130] Hwang IS, Ho H, Hoffman BB, Reaven GM. Fructose-induced insulin resistance and hypertension in rats. *Hypertension*. 1987; 10: 512-516.

[131] Mellor KM, Bell JR, Young MJ, Ritchie RH, Delbridge LM. Myocardial autophagy activation and suppressed survival signaling is associated with insulin resistance in fructose-fed mice. *J Mol Cell Cardiol*. 2011; 50: 1035-1043.

[132] Cao J, Xu D, Wang D, Wu R, Zhang L, Zhu H, He Q, Yang B. ROS-driven Akt dephosphorylation at Ser-473 is involved in 4-HPR-mediated apoptosis in NB4 cells. *Free Radic Biol Med*. 2009; 47: 536-547.

[133] Subramanian S, Han CY, Chiba T, McMillen TS, Wang SA, Haw A 3rd, Kirk EA, O'Brien KD, Chait A. Dietary cholesterol worsens adipose tissue macrophage accumulation and atherosclerosis in obese LDL receptor-deficient mice. *Arterioscler Thromb Vasc Biol*. 2008; 28: 685-691.

[134] Lewis KE, Kirk EA, McDonald TO, Wang S, Wight TN, O'Brien KD, Chait A. Increase in serum amyloid a evoked by dietary cholesterol is associated with increased atherosclerosis in mice. *Circulation*. 2004; 110: 540-545.

[135] Berg AH, Scherer PE. Adipose tissue, inflammation, and cardiovascular disease. *Circ Res*. 2005; 96: 939-949.

[136] Ferrannini E, Iozzo P. Is insulin resistance atherogenic? A review of the evidence. *Atheroscler Suppl*. 2006; 7: 5-10.

[137] Govindarajan G, Whaley-Connell A, Mugo M, Stump C, Sowers JR. The cardiometabolic syndrome as a cardiovascular risk factor. *Am J Med Sci*. 2005; 330: 311-318.

[138] Paternostro G, Pagano D, Gnecchi-Ruscone T, Bonser RS, Camici PG. Insulin resistance in patients with cardiac hypertrophy. *Cardiovasc Res*. 1999; 42: 246-253.

[139] Hällsten K, Virtanen KA, Lönnqvist F, Janatuinen T, Turiceanu M, Rönnemaa T, Viikari J, Lehtimäki T, Knuuti J, Nuutila P. Enhancement of insulin-stimulated myocardial glucose uptake in patients with Type 2 diabetes treated with rosiglitazone. *Diabet Med*. 2004; 21: 1280-1287.

[140] Salehi M, D'Alessio DA. New therapies for type 2 diabetes based on glucagon-like peptide 1. *Cleve Clin J Med*. 2006; 73: 382-389.

[141] Nikolaidis LA, Elahi D, Hentosz T, Doverspike A, Huerbin R, Zourelias L, Stolarski C, Shen YT, Shannon RP. Recombinant glucagon-like peptide-1 increases myocardial glucose uptake and improves left ventricular performance in conscious dogs with pacing-induced dilated cardiomyopathy. *Circulation*. 2004; 110: 955-961.

[142] Freeman DJ, Norrie J, Sattar N, Neely RD, Cobbe SM, Ford I, Isles C, Lorimer AR, Macfarlane PW, McKillop JH, Packard CJ, Shepherd J, Gaw A. Pravastatin and the development of diabetes mellitus: evidence for a protective treatment effect in the West of Scotland Coronary Prevention Study. *Circulation*. 2001; 103: 357-362.

[143] Pfeffer MA, Swedberg K, Granger CB, Held P, McMurray JJ, Michelson EL, Olofsson B, Ostergren J, Yusuf S, Pocock S; CHARM Investigators and Committees. Effects of candesartan on mortality and morbidity in patients with chronic heart failure: the CHARM-Overall programme. *Lancet*. 2003; 362: 759-766.

[144] Yusuf S, Sleight P, Pogue J, Bosch J, Davies R, Dagenais G. Effects of an angiotensin-converting-enzyme inhibitor, ramipril, on cardiovascular events in high-risk patients. The Heart Outcomes Prevention Evaluation Study Investigators. *N Engl J Med.* 2000; 342: 145-153.

[145] Williams B, Poulter NR, Brown MJ, Davis M, McInnes GT, Potter JF, Sever PS, McG Thom S; British Hypertension Society. Guidelines for management of hypertension: report of the fourth working party of the British Hypertension Society, 2004-BHS IV. *J Hum Hypertens.* 2004; 18: 139-185.

24

Taurine Depletion-Related Cardiomyopathy in Animals

Takashi Ito and Junichi Azuma
Hyogo University of Health Sciences
Japan

1. Introduction

Taurine is a nontoxic β-amino acid and a normal constituent of the human diet found in animal food sources, especially fishes and shell fishes. It is found in very high concentration in cardiac tissue, and represents approximately 60% of free amino acid pool in the mammalian heart. Mammalian cardiac taurine contents vary among the spices. Cats are known to be the species most susceptible to taurine deficiency due to poor synthetic capacity. On the other hand, rats have high amount of taurine in the heart, liver and skeletal muscle. Therefore, it may be the natural providence that cats chase rats.

While biosynthesis of taurine in heart is limited, the major determinant of myocardial taurine is uptake from plasma. The concentration in myocardium is approximately 100 times higher than that in plasma, indicating active transport process from the plasma. The biochemical aspects of its transport mechanism including changes in taurine content resulting from modification of uptake into and leakage from myocardial cells by physiological (β-adrenergic stimulation), pharmacological (guanidinoethyl sulfonate or β-alanine) and pathophysiological (congestive heart failure, ischemia, hypoxia or cardiomyopathy) interventions have been quite well documented. However, these physiological and pathophysiological roles in heart remain uncertain.

Taurine is known to possess a variety of biological actions including calcium handling, osmoregulation, anti-oxidation, bile acid conjugation and so on. In heart, some physiological or pharmacological effects have been reported, as shown in Table 1. Meanwhile, it has been discovered in 1980s that taurine deficient diet causes dilated

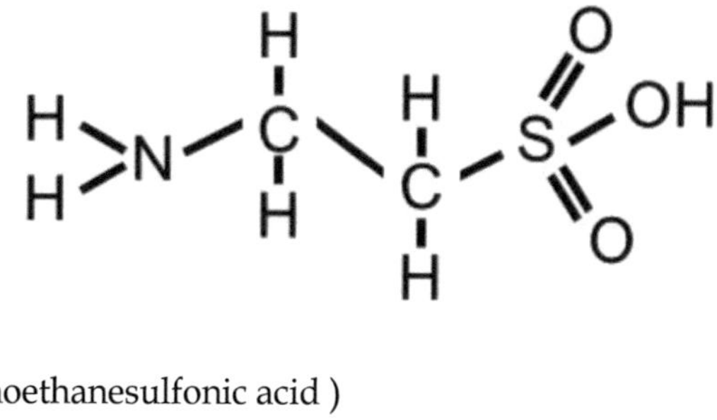

Fig. 1. Taurine (2-aminoethanesulfonic acid)

1.	Positive inotropy at low calcium concentrations
2.	Negative inotropy at high calcium concentrations
3.	Potentiation of digitalis inotropy
4.	Antagonism of negative inotropy
5.	Retardation of lesion development in calcium overload myopathy
6.	Protection against drug-induced cardiotoxicity
7.	Protection against calcium paradox- and oxygen paradox- induced myocardial injury
8.	Antiarrythmia
9.	Modulation of cardiac calcium current
10.	Antiapoptotic effect

Table 1. Action of taurine on the heart

cardiomyopathy (DCM) implicated with taurine depletion in house cats. Thereafter, taurine depletion-related cardiomyopathy has been reported in foxes and dogs. It has been reported that amount of taurine intake is widely varied among individuals in human and correlates to mortality rate caused by ischemia heart diseases in epidemiologic studies (Yamori et al., 2001, 2009), indicating taurine depletion may also occur in human. Hence, taurine depletion-induced DCM should be focused as one of the etiology of cardiomyopathy in human. In this chapter, we introduce taurine depletion-related cardiomyopathy in animals. Moreover, mechanisms underlying the pathogenesis of taurine depletion-related cardiomyopathy have been investigated, while the mechanisms remain uncertain. Studies by using β-alanine and guanidinoethane sulfonate (GES) which are the inhibitors of taurine influx into cells through taurine transporter are very useful to evaluate the molecular mechanism. Further, the genetically engineered mice knocking out taurine transporter have been recently developed. These mice also exhibited the cardiomyopathy with cardiac atrophy. We also describe recent evidences and possible mechanisms which should associate with the taurine depletion-related cardiomyopathy.

Furthermore, a lot of studies support the beneficial effect of taurine on cardiomyopathy and heart failure in animal model as well as in human. In the latter half of this chapter, we describe the pharmacological effects of taurine supplementation against heart diseases.

2. Taurine depletion-related cardiomyopathy

2.1 Cats

Taurine depletion-related DCM was firstly identified in domestic cats in 1980s. Pion et al. reported that low taurine concentration in plasma is a major causal factor of DCM in pet cats (Pion et al., 1987). They analyzed the pet cats having a diagnosis of heart failure in hospital, and found that 22 of 23 cats with echocardiographic evidence of DCM had low concentration of plasma taurine. Moreover, treatment of taurine (0.5 g administered twice daily) improved cats echocardiographically in 2-week period after treatment. At the end all cats were clinically and echocardiographically normal and were no longer receiving medication of their heart failure. In further study, the authors prospectively evaluated the long term benefits of administering taurine to cats with moderate to severe DCM (Pion et al., 1992). They compared the survival times of this prospectively evaluated population to the other population which were diagnosed as DCM before the discovery of the role of taurine deficiency in the cause of cardiomyopathy. As a result, all cats that survived more than 30 days remained clinically stable despite withdrawal of all medications except taurine. The clinical response and 1-year survival rate of 58% in the taurine treatment group represents a marked improvement compared with a 1-year survival rate of 13% in the retrospectively evaluated population.

Further, Novotny et al. examined the intrinsic contraction-relaxation properties of left ventricle using perfused hearts isolated from cats maintained by taurine-deficient diet with or without taurine supplementation (Novotny et al., 1991). They demonstrated that coronary-perfused hearts from the taurine deficient cats did not achieve isovolumic systolic pressure and ±dP/dt max values of the magnitude generated by heart from taurine-treated cats. They also identified that the pressure-volume relation curve resulted from isovolumic heart preparations of taurine-deficient cats were shifted downward and to the right of control curves, indicating inotropic depression and increased chamber compliance or distensibility. Therefore, these data illustrate the myocardial contractile dysfunction and LV chamber dilatation in hearts from taurine-deficient cats.

Subsequent control study with cats also showed the evidence that dietary taurine deficiency induces myocardial failure (Novotny et al., 1994). Novotny et al. evaluated left ventricular function using M-mode echocardiography in cats maintained on a taurine deficient diet for 6-15 months. At 4 months from the onset of the study, plasma taurine concentration of cats fed taurine-deficient diet is 12 nmol/mL, while baseline value is 227 nmol/mL. They demonstrated that 74% of taurine-deficient cats experienced greater than 25% reductions in fraction shortening values and 91% had a greater than 25% increase in LV end-systolic short axis diameter values in response to taurine deficient diet. The average reduction of fraction shortening was 37%. Moreover, the study with colony-source cats revealed that the greatest rate of change occurred during the first four months in taurine-deficient cats. The authors concluded that while DCM was observed in some cats, decreased systolic pump function and increased LV end-systolic short axis diameter were more consistent findings.

Pion reported in 2004 that in their repeated studies, approximately 25% of all (n>100) cats depleted of taurine for more than 2 years developed overt myocardial failure (Pion, 2004). He mentioned that the other factors required for taurine developed overt myocardial failure are unknown, and that nutritional taurine deficiency combined with other causes of myocardial stress, such as congenital or acquired left ventricle overload, toxic, ischemic, nutritional, endocrine or metabolic problems, may lead to synergistic complicating effects. Furthermore, he noted that taurine deficiency in cats may be a direct result of inadequate amounts of taurine in the diet, such commercial pet food, in most cases and is thus preventable.

2.2 Foxes

Foxes are also known to have low taurine synthesis capacity. Moise et al. reported the relationship between taurine deficiency and DCM in foxes (Moise et al., 1991). They found that plasma taurine concentration in foxes from farms with a history of death caused by DCM was less than that in foxes without family history of cardiac death. Furthermore, they demonstrated that the activity of hepatic cysteinesulfinic acid decarboxylase which is a rate-limiting enzyme in taurine synthesis from cysteine was less in foxes with DCM, suggesting that inadequate cysteinesulfinic acid decarboxylase activity may contribute to susceptibility to dietary taurine deficiency. Also, the therapy with taurine supplementation for 2 months in foxes with DCM reduced cardiac size, resolved pulmonary edema and improved systolic function, indicating DCM was reversed.

2.3 Dogs

Taurine is not an essential amino acid in dogs. Normal dogs fed diets with little or no taurine maintain plasma and whole blood taurine concentration similar to those found in normal cats. The activity of cysteinesulfinic acid decarboxylase is high in dog compared to the cat. Therefore, until recently, it was thought that taurine deficiency was not a clinical issue to consider when managing canine patients (Pion, 2004).

Soon after the identification of taurine deficiency myocardial failure in cats, Pion who firstly identified taurine depletion-related DCM in cats,, as mentioned above, began administering taurine to dogs with DCM (Kramer et al., 1995; Pion, 2004). Then he and his colleagues found that plasma taurine concentration was low in 17% of dogs with DCM studied, although there were no significant differences in the average of plasma taurine concentrations between dogs with DCM and the control dogs. They also identified that a certain breeds, such as American Cocker Spaniel and Golden Retriever, with DCM had low plasma taurine concentrations, while it was not decreased in the breeds that are more commonly afflicted with DCM. Recently, DCM associated with low taurine concentration has been reported in American Cocker Spaniel, Golden Retriever, Dalmatian, boxer, Newfoundland, Portuguese water dog, English setter, Alaskan malamute and Scottish terrier (Freeman et al., 1996; Kittleson et al., 1997; Pion et al., 1998; Fascetti et al., 2003; Alroy et al., 2005; Belanger et al., 2005). Additionally, Ko et al. reported that taurine biosynthesis rate was lower in large dogs than small dogs (Ko et al., 2007), which may be associated with the greater incidence of taurine deficiency-related cardiomyopathy in large dogs than in small dogs.

2.4 Rodents

In contrast to foxes and cats, the size of the intracellular taurine pool of most animal species remains fairly constant even with significant reductions in dietary taurine content. Despite resistance to depletion, tissue taurine levels can be decreased by treatment of these animals with a taurine transport inhibitors, such β-alanine or GES, which interfere with taurine uptake by the tissues. However, Mozaffari et al. reported that GES treatment for 3 weeks resulted in the decrease in cardiac taurine content from 77 to 34 micromoles/g dry wet weight, while it did not affect myocardial contraction as assessed by perfusion technique (Mozaffari et al., 1986). Thus, although taurine depletion model induced by β-alanine and GES is a good model to analyze the physiological role of taurine deficiency, as described below, treatment of these animals with a taurine transport inhibitor does not generally cause sufficient taurine deficiency to promote the development of severe, overt pathology.

2.5 Taurine transporter knockout mice

Therefore, a more effective means of producing taurine deficiency in rodents is the formation of taurine transporter- (TauT-) null animals. Recently, transgenic mice lacking TauT gene have been generated by us and the other group. A variety of disorders have been reported in various tissues, such as eye, kidney, heart, muscle and so on, accompanied with drastic taurine deficiency in TauTKO mice (Heller-Stilb et al., 2002; Warskulat et al., 2007).

We demonstrated that taurine influx was eliminated in the cells isolated from TauTKO mice, indicating loss of taurine transport activity in TauTKO mice (Ito et al., 2008). Tissue taurine level is severely decreased in several tissues. Especially, cardiac taurine could not be detected in TauTKO mice, and skeletal muscle taurine level is decreased by 96% in TauTKO mice compared with wild-type mice. Then, we determined the cardiac phenotype of TauTKO mice. TauTKO mice exhibited a decrease in heart weight concomitant with a lower body weight than their control littermates. According to histological analyses, it was found that the ventricular wall was thinning and the ventricle lumen was dilated in the TauTKO heart compared to their wild-type littermates (Fig. 2). Moreover, the size of cardiomyocyte was markedly decreased in the TauTKO heart, indicating cardiac atrophy in TauTKO mice. Based on echocardiographic analysis, ejection fraction was diminished in the old TauTKO mice, indicating that cardiac function was eventually compromised in the TauTKO mice. Moreover, detailed functional analysis on Langendorff perfused heart also demonstrated the age-dependent cardiac dysfunction, such as a decrease in peak positive dp/dt and an increase in negative dp/dt as well as decreased ejection fraction in TauTKO mice (unpublished data). It is well established that the expression of fetal genes, including atrial natriuretic peptide (ANP), brain natriuretic peptide (BNP) and β-myosin heavy chain (β-MHC), is reactivated in heart failure (Rajabi et al., 2007). These cardiac failure markers were significantly elevated in TauTKO mice. Consistent with the cardiac function, the inductions of these genes were more significant in the old TauTKO mice. Thus, these data indicate that knockout of the TauT gene leads to an age-dependent DCM. Furthermore, in contrast to the orderly myofibrillar architecture present in wild-type cardiac muscle, electron microscopy revealed pronounced myofibrillar fragmentation, disruption of the outer mitochondrial membrane and cellular vacuolization in TauTKO hearts.

On the other hand, in another TauTKO model reported by Warskulat et al., TauTKO mice exhibited a largely normal phenotype under both control and stimulated conditions, as assessed by magnetic resonance imaging, echocardiography, and isolated heart studies (Warskulat et al., 2004). Only vasodilation was enhanced in isolated perfused TauTKO hearts during dobutamine stimulation. A possible reason for the inconsistent results between two TauTKO models is the difference of genetic background, since difference of inbred strains affects the cardiovascular phenotypes and susceptibilities against pathological stressors in mice (Barrick et al., 2007; Deschepper et al., 2004). Meanwhile, Warskulat et al. also reported that biomarker genes for heart failure, including ANP, BNP and a cardiac ankyrin repeat protein (CARP), are upregulated in TauTKO hearts, which is consistent with our TauTKO model (Warskulat et al., 2006). Furthermore, they also demonstrated that the TauTKO hearts showed a switch from α-actin 1 (skeletal muscle type, α- SKA) to α-actin 2 (smooth muscle type, α-SKA) expression. α-SMA is generally expressed in developing muscle cells, and α-SKA and α-cardiac actin (α-CAA) become upregulated and replace α-SMA during final steps of myogenesis (Tondeleir et al., 2009; Woodcock-Mitchell et al., 1988). Thus, it may be due to a reactivation of fetal gene program which is observed in pathologically hypertrophied or failing heart. Indeed, induction of smooth muscle actin has been reported in heart of DCM patients and in hypertrophied or failing heart in experimental animals. Therefore, they concluded that these hearts may be more susceptible to failure under further exogenous stresses.

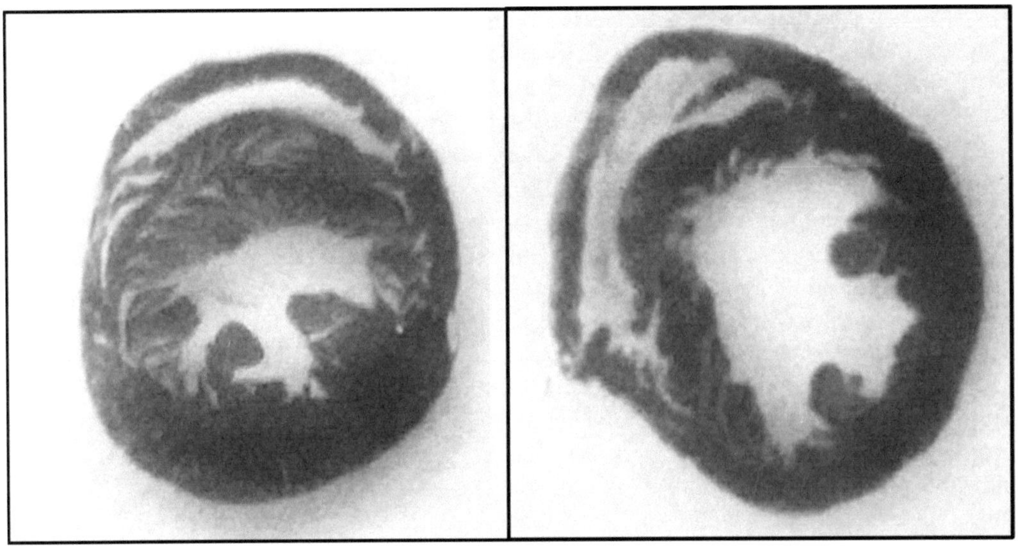

Fig. 2. Histological analysis of heart sections from WT and TauTKO mice. Heart sections were stained by hematoxylin-eosin staining method. Left: WT, Right: TauTKO. Thinning of the ventricular walls and septum and dilatation of the ventricular lumen are observed in the heart section of TauTKO mice. Ito et al. (2008)

3. Possible mechanisms for taurine depletion-related cardiomyopathy

3.1 Carbohydrate metabolism

Although the molecular mechanisms underlying the taurine depletion-related cardiomyopathy remain unclear, some potential mechanisms have been suggested.

Mozaffari et al. demonstrated that taurine depletion altered myocardial carbohydrate metabolism (Mozaffari et al., 1986). They identified that the major effect of GES treatment was stimulation in the rate of glycolysis and lactate production in rats. Furthermore, they found the activation of phosphofructokinase and a decrease in citrate in GES-treated hearts, which may relate to the activation of glycolysis. The authors concluded that taurine-depleted hearts exhibit abnormal energy metabolism and these changes may take on added importance in the stressed myocardium.

Furthermore, we reported that drug-induced taurine depletion of rat heart led to high energy phosphate metabolism due to the accumulation of free CoA, free carnitine and long-chain acylcarnitine, but a small decrease in long-chain fatty acyl-CoA (Harada et al., 1990).

Lomberdini reported the role of taurine depletion on the phosphorylation of specific protein in cardiac tissue. They demonstrated that 6-week treatment of GES in tap water increased in the phosphorylation of about 44kDa protein present in the mitochondrial fraction of the rat heart (Lombardini, 1996). Later, he identified that the 44kDa protein was pyruvate dehydrogenase which is responsible for transforming pyruvate into acetyl-CoA (Lombardini, 1998). This data suggest the role of taurine depletion in the carbohydrate metabolism through the regulation of pyruvate dehydrogenase activity. The reduction of this enzyme activity gives an explanation for the activation of lactate production in taurine-depleted hearts of GES-treated rats.

3.2 Electrophysiology and excitation-contraction coupling

Lake et al. reported the effect of GES-induced taurine depletion on electrophysiology (Lake et al., 1987). They identified an increase in the duration of ventricular action potentials in GES-treated rats and it accounted for the prolongation of QT interval by using electrocardiograms, suggesting the increased susceptibility against arrhythmias. Further, they have explored the idea that taurine deficiency may enhance vulnerability to arrhythmias in GES-treated rats operated with left coronary artery occlusion (Lake, 1992). As a result, they observed that taurine depleted animals had more and longer episodes of ventricular tachycardia and fibrillation, indicating that taurine deficient animals appear to be more susceptible to ischemia-induced arrhythmia.

Lake et al. also investigated the influence of taurine depletion to excitation-contraction coupling. They first identified that papillary muscle isolated from GES-treated rats generated tensions two third of control (Lake, 1990, 1992). Importantly, they observed small deficits in sensitivity to calcium and calcium recirculation through sarcoplasmic reticulum, but the magnitude of these change did not appear adequate to account for >40% loss in maximal calcium-activated force generation. Furthermore, Eley et al. reported that ventricular trabeculas from GES-treated rats exhibited the reductions in isometric twitch force, and demonstrated that substantial deficit in force development in taurine-depleted trabeculas was consistent with a reduced population of force generators and decreases in sarcomere proteins, but not intracellular calcium handling (Eley et al., 1994). Thus, they concluded that the inability of taurine depleted myocardium to generate the force is related to a loss of contractile proteins, which may be related to etiology of taurine depletion-related cardiomyopathy.

3.3 Osmoregulation

One of the most important biological actions of taurine is osmoregulation. In TauTKO models, compensatory induction of other organic osmolytes and osmotic stress related genes have been reported. Warskulat et al. found increases in the cytosolic concentration of various organic osmolytes, such as glutamine, alanine, glycine and glycerophosphorylcholine. Moreover, mRNA level of the system An amino acid transport protein was higher in the heart of TauTKO than of WT mice, concomitant with the increase in amino acids (Warskulat et al., 2004). Consistently, we also found increases in several genes responsive to osmotic stress, such as heat shock protein (Hsp70), amino acid transporters (Slc38a2, Slc38a4) and S100 calcium binding protein (S100A4), in TauTKO hearts (Ito et al., 2008), indicating the activation of some signal pathways responsible for regulating intracellular Osmotic balance. Thus, these data suggest that taurine depletion impairs the cellular osmotic balance, which, in turn, may activate the compensatory mechanism against osmotic stress.

Although the role of myocardial osmotic imbalance in etiology of cardiomyopathy is unknown, several possibilities are expected. First, it may be associated with ion movement in cardiac cells. When a cell is subjected to hyperosmotic stress, organic osmolytes, such as taurine, are accumulated, which minimizes the movement of water and the resulting decrease in cell volume. By contrast, hypoosmotic stress, which increases cell volume, leads to a loss of taurine and a decrease in intracellular osmolality. Although the regulatory volume change is usually transient, in the case of the cardiomyocyte of the TauTKO mouse there is a chronic decrease in cell volume. It is assumable that taurine depletion leads the accumulation of intracellular electrolytes and results in the impairment of the cell volume regulation in cardiac muscles. It may be also associated with prolongation of the QT interval observed in GES-treated rats, as mentioned above. The role of osmoregulation in ion movement has been reviewed by Schaffer et al. (Schaffer et al., 2000).

Second, organic osmolytes have been reported to play as chemical chaperones in mammalian cells, while osmotic stress and the disturbance of ion balance also impair the membrane and protein stability (Howard et al., 2003; Yancey, 2005). Based on our electron microscopic analyses, a number of organelle collapses, such as myofibril and mitochondrial breakdowns were found in TauTKO hearts. Similarly, a decrease in contractile proteins has been observed in the heart of GES-treated rats. We assume that these findings are likely associated with the loss of macromolecular stability due to osmotic imbalance which is resulted from taurine depletion.

3.4 The role of taurine in Renin-angiotensin-aldosterone system

Renin-angiotensin-aldosterone system (RAAS) plays a crucial role in the development of heart failure through the cardiac remodelling, as well as an increase in body fluid and impairment of vascular function. We previously demonstrated that taurine treatment suppressed angiotensin II-induced hypertrophic responses, including an increase in surface cell area and an induction in hypertrophic marker genes, in the cultured cardiac myocyte (Azuma et al., 2000). Moreover, while angiotensin II induced apoptosis in the cultured cardiac myocyte, Schaffer et al. have demonstrated that taurine depletion by exposure to β-alanine enhanced the angiotensin-II induced apoptosis (Schaffer et al., 2003). They also demonstrated that this effect of taurine depletion was mediated by enhanced increases in Bax and c-Jun N-terminal kinase, which are proapoptotic proteins. These beneficial actions of taurine against angiotensin II may relate to taurine depletion-related cardiomyopathy. Furthermore, taurine might prevent angiotensin II-induced oxidative stress through the inhibition of NADPH oxidase. Grishko et al. has demonstrated that angiotensin II-induced cell death is associated with the ROS production through the activation of NADPH oxidase in the cultured cardiac myocyte (Grishko et al., 2003). Recently, Li et al. have reported that treatment with taurine prevented the cardiac myocyte from the apoptosis induced by phenylephrine (Li et al., 2009). They also found that taurine treatment suppressed the oxidative stress induced by phenylephrine through the inhibition of NADPH oxidase activation. Thus, it is assumable that inhibition of NADPH oxidase may be a critical pathway of the antiapoptotic effect of taurine against angiotensin II-induced cell apoptosis.

Further studies may provide key elements on the molecular mechanism of taurine depletion-related cardiomyopathy.

4. Pharmacological effects of taurine on cardiomyopathy and heart failure

4.1 Animal models

The useful effect of taurine against cardiomyopathy was firstly reported by McBroom and Welty in cardiomyopathic hamster BIO 14.6 (McBroom & Welty, 1977). They demonstrated that taurine treatment for 4 weeks decreased calcium overload in cardiomyopathic hamsters. Subsequently, Azari et al. examined the effect of taurine in controlling calcium overload and necrotic lesion severity in advanced stages of cardiomyopathy (Azari et al.,

1980). They demonstrated that oral taurine given for 1 month was effective in decreasing in cardiac calcium concentration and subsequent severity of lesion in myopathic hamsters.
Thereafter, we and others reported that taurine has protective activity against myocardial damage in experimental models caused by massive doses of isoproterenol or doxorubicin and by calcium paradox phenomenon. We demonstrated that oral administration of taurine in chick treated with toxic dose of isoproterenol suppressed the increased lipoperoxide and the decreased phospholipid (Ohta et al., 1988), suggesting that the beneficial effect of taurine may be due to inhibition of lipid peroxidation and calcium accumulation and due to protection against the deterioration of membrane phospholipids.
Furthermore, we reported the effect of taurine on doxorubicin-induced cardiotoxicity in mice (Hamaguchi et al., 1988). Taurine administration attenuated doxorubicin-induced biochemical alterations, such as the depletion of creatine phosphokinase, glutamic oxaloacetic transaminase and lactate dehydrogenase activities, in the myocardium. Moreover, taurine significantly improved the survival rate of the mice treated with doxorubicin.
Additionally, to confirm the effect of taurine against heart failure, we tested whether daily oral treatment with taurine had any effect upon the survival rate and hemodynamics in animal model for Chronic heart failure (CHF) induced artificially by aortic regurgitation (Azuma et al., 1985b; Takihara et al., 1986). Cumulative mortality rate at 8 weeks following aortic regurgitation was 10% in taurine treated rabbits compared with 53% in non-treated rabbits. On the hemodynamic study, the mean value of max dP/dt was significantly decreased in rabbit with aortic regurgitation without taurine. Taurine produced a marked increase in max dP/dt compared to non-treated animals, indicating that taurine improved the contractility in heart failure. Therefore, we concluded that taurine prevents the rapid decline of CHF and consequently prolongs the life expectancy.

4.2 Clinical studies

In 1974, Huxtable and Bresseler have reported that the left ventricular taurine content in patients who died of CHF was twice that in patients who died of other causes and had no cardiac pathology (Huxtable and Bressler, 1974). Subsequently, increased myocardial taurine content has been also reported in experimental animals with heart failure. It is still unclear whether the increase in myocardial taurine is causal factor in heart failure or whether this is secondary to factor related to the disease process, such as compensatory mechanism. Based on the concept of replacement therapy for deficiency symptom, such as hormone or vitamin, administration of taurine to patients with heart failure was not accepted around that time in Japan. However, since many evidence has been accumulated to show that taurine exerts various beneficial actions, including positive inotropic activity, and is useful to animals with cardiomyopathy, as described above, we dared to test the effect of taurine in patients with CHF. In 1982-1992, we have reported some clinical studies in which we evaluated the usefulness of taurine administration in the treatment of CHF.
Firstly, we have observed that the administration of taurine to the patient suffering from CHF alleviated their physical signs and symptoms (Azuma et al., 1982; Azuma et al., 1983). In open pilot study, the clinical efficacy of oral taurine administration was studied in 24 patients with CHF (New York Heart Association (NYHA) functional class; II-IV) as a result from various heart diseases, including congenital heart failure, acquired valvular disease, cardiomyopathy, ischemic heart diseases and hypertension heart diseases. The severity of

heart failure was scored based on the clinical signs (diastolic gallop rhythm, pulsus alternans, positive hepatojugular reflex, pulmonary crackles, neck vein distension, hilar congestion on chest x-lay film, cardiomegaly on chest x-lay film, pleural effusion, peripheral edema, ascites, decreased urinary output, tachycardia and weight gain) and symptoms (orthopnea, paroxysmal nocturnal dyspnea, dyspnea on exertion, fatigue, anorexia, nausea, vomiting, and palpitation) and on roentgenographic data. The benefit for taurine treatment in patients was estimated by the difference between their pretreatment and post-treatment scores. In 19 of 24 patients taurine administration for 4 weeks improved the severity of CHF. Moreover, 13 of 15 patients who were designated as NYHA class III or IV before receiving taurine were designated as NYHA class II after they completed the study.

Subsequently, we conducted another clinical study to elucidate whether oral administration of taurine to conventional management could improve the systolic time intervals in 14 patients with CHF by a placebo-controlled, double blind, crossover method (Azuma et al., 1985a; Azuma et al., 1985b). As well as prior clinical study, the effect of taurine was observed in improvement of the NYHA class, pulmonary crackles and chest-film abnormality, and was superior to placebo. Importantly, pre-ejection period index was reduced after 4 weeks of treatment with taurine, indicating the improvement of left ventricular function. Thus, these studies have confirmed the clinical usefulness of taurine in CHF.

Furthermore, in an attempt to further clarify the effect of taurine on CHF and to define its clinical position as the therapeutic agent for heart failure, we conducted a double-blind comparative study using coenzyme Q10 as a control agent (Azuma et al., 1989; Azuma et al., 1992). In this study a total of 158 patients from 26 hospitals were randomized, and finally 138 patients were divided three treatment groups; daily dose of taurine 3g, taurine 6g and coenzyme Q10 30mg. Taurine were given orally daily for 8 weeks and the patients continued to receive their prescribed conventional drugs. Improvements of NYHA functional classes were observed both of 3 groups. Moreover, significant improvements compared with baseline were noted in the severity of the objective signs, including hepatomegaly and edema in 3 groups. However, no significant differences were observed in the changes of NYHA class and objective signs. We also tested the effect of taurine on the left ventricular performance using echocardiography, and significant improvements were also noted in the parameters of cardiac output in the taurine 3g group; systolic volume, cardiac output, ejection fraction (EF) and mean velocity of circumferential fiber shortening (mVcf) in the taurine 6g group, whereas coenzyme Q10 possessed no such pharmacological activity. Thus, this study confirms that the therapeutic effects of taurine compare favorably to CoQ10. Moreover, only 3.8% of patients treated with 6g of taurine experienced minor problems, including slight anorexia and soft feces, indicating the safety of taurine.

These studies illustrated that taurine is an effective agent for the treatment of heart failure without any adverse effects. Nowadays, powder of taurine is clinically used for patients with CHF in Japan.

Since RAAS plays a central role in the pathology of CHF and taurine antagonizes against angiotensin II-induced cell damage in vitro studies, as described above, a systemic clinical study is necessary to evaluate the benefit of taurine against RAAS in future.

5. Conclusion

In this chapter, we reviewed 1) the taurine depletion-related cardiomyopathy in cats, foxes, dogs, and genetically engineered mice lacking taurine transporter and 2) the pharmacological benefit of taurine in patients and experimental animal models with heart failure. In these animals, it is apparent that taurine deficient diet causes taurine depletion in plasma and heart, which in turn leads to cardiomyopathy. Urinary taurine concentration in human, which can represent the amount of taurine intake, varies by more than 10 times among individuals; therefore, taurine depletion may also occur in human. Although taurine depletion-related cardiomyopathy has not been reported so far, taurine deficiency should be considered as a potential pathogenesis of heart failure and/or cardiomyopathy. Meanwhile, whereas myocardial taurine content is increased in failing heart, taurine administration is "paradoxically" useful to patients with heart failure. Since an increment of myocardial taurine may be due to the activation of active transport of taurine, taurine supplementation might be necessary for some patients with failing heart as compensatory mechanism to maintain the cardiac function. To verify the unsolved problems, the physiological role of taurine in heart must be fully clarified.

It should be noted that the increasing rate of plasma taurine concentration after taurine administration varies widely among individuals (Brons et al., 2004). Additionally, there may be some genetic polymorphisms of taurine transporter which affects the taurine transport activity in human genome. Now it is well known that polymorphisms influence disease risk, drug efficacy and side-effect. Therefore, we suppose that the genetic polymorphisms of taurine transporter or the other molecules involved in the kinetics of taurine may contribute to the variation of plasma and tissue taurine concentrations. Thus, it will be plausible to find out the genetic polymorphisms which determine the variation of tissue taurine content and the rate of rise in plasma taurine after taurine administration, which will help us elucidate the role of taurine deficiency in the etiology of human cardiomyopathy.

6. Acknowledgment

This review work is partially supported by a research grant from Taisho Pharmaceutical Co. Ltd. (Japan).

7. References

Alroy, J.;Rush, J.E.&Sarkar, S. (2005). Infantile dilated cardiomyopathy in Portuguese water dogs: correlation of the autosomal recessive trait with low plasma taurine at infancy. *Amino Acids*, Vol.28, No.1,pp. 51-56, ISSN 0939-4451

Azari, J.;Brumbaugh, P.&Huxtable, R. (1980). Prophylaxis by taurine in the hearts of cardiomyopathic hamsters. *Journal of Molecular and Cellular Cardiology*, Vol.12, No.12,pp. 1353-1366, ISSN 0022-2828

Azuma, J.;Hasegawa, H.;Sawamura, A.;Awata, N.;Harada, H.;Ogura, K.&Kishimoto, S. (1982). Taurine for treatment of congestive heart failure. *International Journal of Cardiology*, Vol.2, No.2,pp. 303-304, ISSN 0167-5273

Azuma, J.;Hasegawa, H.;Sawamura, A.;Awata, N.;Ogura, K.;Harada, H.;Yamamura, Y.&Kishimoto, S. (1983). Therapy of congestive heart failure with orally administered taurine. *Clinical Therapeutics*, Vol.5, No.4,pp. 398-408, ISSN 0149-2918

Azuma, J.;Katsume, H.;Kagisgima, T.;Furukawa, K.;Awata, N.;Ishiyama, T.;Yamagami, T.;Ishikawa, H.;Iwata, H.;Kishimoto, S.&Yamamura, Y. (1989). Clinical evaluation of taurine in congestive heart failure - a double-blind comparative study using CoQ10 as a control drug. In *Taurine and The Heart*, H. Iwata; J.B. Lombardini&T. Segawa, eds. pp. 75-97,ISBN 0-89838-396-X,Boston, Kluwer academic publishers.

Azuma, J.;Sawamura, A.&Awata, N. (1992). Usefulness of taurine in chronic congestive heart failure and its prospective application. *Japanese Circulation Journal,* Vol.56, No.1,pp. 95-99, ISSN 0047-1828.

Azuma, J.;Sawamura, A.;Awata, N.;Ohta, H.;Hamaguchi, T.;Harada, H.;Takihara, K.;Hasegawa, H.;Yamagami, T.;Ishiyama, T.&et al. (1985a). Therapeutic effect of taurine in congestive heart failure: a double-blind crossover trial. *Clinical Cardiology,* Vol.8, No.5,pp. 276-282, ISSN 0160-9289

Azuma, J.;Takihara, K.;Awata, N.;Sawamura, A.;Ohta, H.;Hamaguchi, T.;Tanaka, Y.;Fukuda, K.&Kishimoto, S. (1985b). Taurine and failing heart: experimental and clinical aspects. *Progress in Clinical and Biological Research,* Vol.179,pp. 195-213, ISSN 0361-7742

Azuma, M.;Takahashi, K.;Fukuda, T.;Ohyabu, Y.;Yamamoto, I.;Kim, S.;Iwao, H.;Schaffer, S.W.&Azuma, J. (2000). Taurine attenuates hypertrophy induced by angiotensin II in cultured neonatal rat cardiac myocytes. *European Journal of Pharmacology,* Vol.403, No.3,pp. 181-188, ISSN 0014-2999

Barrick, C.J.;Rojas, M.;Schoonhoven, R.;Smyth, S.S.&Threadgill, D.W. (2007). Cardiac response to pressure overload in 129S1/SvImJ and C57BL/6J mice: temporal- and background-dependent development of concentric left ventricular hypertrophy. *American journal of physiology Heart and circulatory physiology,* Vol.292, No.5,pp. H2119-2130, ISSN 0363-6135

Belanger, M.C.;Ouellet, M.;Queney, G.&Moreau, M. (2005). Taurine-deficient dilated cardiomyopathy in a family of golden retrievers. *Journal of the American Animal Hospital Association,* Vol.41, No.5,pp. 284-291, ISSN 1547-3317

Brons, C.;Spohr, C.;Storgaard, H.;Dyerberg, J.&Vaag, A. (2004). Effect of taurine treatment on insulin secretion and action, and on serum lipid levels in overweight men with a genetic predisposition for type II diabetes mellitus. *European Journal of Clinical Nutrition,* Vol.58, No.9,pp. 1239-1247, ISSN 0954-3007

Deschepper, C.F.;Olson, J.L.;Otis, M.&Gallo-Payet, N. (2004). Characterization of blood pressure and morphological traits in cardiovascular-related organs in 13 different inbred mouse strains. *Journal of Applied Physiology,* Vol.97, No.1,pp. 369-376, ISSN 8750-7587

Eley, D.W.;Lake, N.&ter Keurs, H.E. (1994). Taurine depletion and excitation-contraction coupling in rat myocardium. *Circulation Research,* Vol.74, No.6,pp. 1210-1219, ISSN 0009-7330

Fascetti, A.J.;Reed, J.R.;Rogers, Q.R.&Backus, R.C. (2003). Taurine deficiency in dogs with dilated cardiomyopathy: 12 cases (1997-2001). *Journal of the American Veterinary Medical Association,* Vol.223, No.8,pp. 1137-1141, ISSN 0003-1488

Freeman, L.M.;Michel, K.E.;Brown, D.J.;Kaplan, P.M.;Stamoulis, M.E.;Rosenthal, S.L.;Keene, B.W.&Rush, J.E. (1996). Idiopathic dilated cardiomyopathy in Dalmatians: nine cases (1990-1995). *Journal of the American Veterinary Medical Association,* Vol.209, No.9,pp. 1592-1596, ISSN 0003-1488

Grishko, V.;Pastukh, V.;Solodushko, V.;Gillespie, M.;Azuma, J.&Schaffer, S. (2003). Apoptotic cascade initiated by angiotensin II in neonatal cardiomyocytes: role of DNA damage. *American Journal of Physiology Heart and circulatory physiology,* Vol.285, No.6,pp. H2364-2372, ISSN 0363-6135

Hamaguchi, T.;Azuma, J.;Awata, N.;Ohta, H.;Takihara, K.;Harada, H.;Kishimoto, S.&Sperelakis, N. (1988). Reduction of doxorubicin-induced cardiotoxicity in mice by taurine. *Research Communications in Chemical Pathology and Pharmacology,* Vol.59, No.1,pp. 21-30, ISSN 0034-5164

Harada, H.;Cusack, B.J.;Olson, R.D.;Stroo, W.;Azuma, J.;Hamaguchi, T.&Schaffer, S.W. (1990). Taurine deficiency and doxorubicin: interaction with the cardiac sarcolemmal calcium pump. *Biochemical pharmacology,* Vol.39, No.4,pp. 745-751, ISSN 0006-2952

Heller-Stilb, B.;van Roeyen, C.;Rascher, K.;Hartwig, H.G.;Huth, A.;Seeliger, M.W.;Warskulat, U.&Haussinger, D. (2002). Disruption of the taurine transporter gene (taut) leads to retinal degeneration in mice. *The FASEB journal,* Vol.16, No.2,pp. 231-233, ISSN 1530-6860

Howard, M.;Fischer, H.;Roux, J.;Santos, B.C.;Gullans, S.R.;Yancey, P.H.&Welch, W.J. (2003). Mammalian osmolytes and S-nitrosoglutathione promote Delta F508 cystic fibrosis transmembrane conductance regulator (CFTR) protein maturation and function. *The Journal of Biological Chemistry,* Vol.278, No.37,pp. 35159-35167, ISSN 0021-9258

Huxtable, R.&Bressler, R. (1974). Taurine concentrations in congestive heart failure. *Science,* Vol.184, No.142,pp. 1187-1188, ISSN 0036-8075

Ito, T.;Kimura, Y.;Uozumi, Y.;Takai, M.;Muraoka, S.;Matsuda, T.;Ueki, K.;Yoshiyama, M.;Ikawa, M.;Okabe, M.;Schaffer, S.W.;Fujio, Y.&Azuma, J. (2008). Taurine depletion caused by knocking out the taurine transporter gene leads to cardiomyopathy with cardiac atrophy. *Journal of Molecular and Cellular Cardiology,* Vol.44, No.5,pp. 927-937, ISSN 1095-8584

Kittleson, M.D.;Keene, B.;Pion, P.D.&Loyer, C.G. (1997). Results of the multicenter spaniel trial (MUST): taurine- and carnitine-responsive dilated cardiomyopathy in American cocker spaniels with decreased plasma taurine concentration. *Journal of veterinary internal medicine / American College of Veterinary Internal Medicine,* Vol.11, No.4,pp. 204-211, ISSN 0891-6640

Ko, K.S.;Backus, R.C.;Berg, J.R.;Lame, M.W.&Rogers, Q.R. (2007). Differences in taurine synthesis rate among dogs relate to differences in their maintenance energy requirement. *The Journal of nutrition,* Vol.137, No.5,pp. 1171-1175, ISSN 0022-3166

Kramer, G.A.;Kittleson, M.D.;Fox, P.R.;Lewis, J.&Pion, P.D. (1995). Plasma taurine concentrations in normal dogs and in dogs with heart disease. *Journal of Veterinary Internal Medicine / American College of Veterinary Internal Medicine,* Vol.9, No.4,pp. 253-258, ISSN 0891-6640

Lake, N. (1990). Effects of taurine depletion on excitable tissues: recent studies. *Progress in Clinical and Biological Research,* Vol.351,pp. 407-414, ISSN 0361-7742

Lake, N. (1992). Effects of taurine deficiency on arrhythmogenesis and excitation-contraction coupling in cardiac tissue. *Advances in Experimental Medicine and Biology,* Vol.315,pp. 173-179, ISSN 0065-2598

Lake, N.;de Roode, M.&Nattel, S. (1987). Effects of taurine depletion on rat cardiac electrophysiology: in vivo and in vitro studies. *Life Sciences,* Vol.40, No.10,pp. 997-1005, ISSN 0024-3205

Li, Y.;Arnold, J.M.;Pampillo, M.;Babwah, A.V.&Peng, T. (2009). Taurine prevents cardiomyocyte death by inhibiting NADPH oxidase-mediated calpain activation. *Free Radical Biology & Medicine,* Vol.46, No.1,pp. 51-61, ISSN 1873-4596

Lombardini, J.B. (1996). Taurine depletion in the intact animal stimulates in vitro phosphorylation of an approximately 44-kDa protein present in the mitochondrial fraction of the rat heart. *Journal of Molecular and Cellular Cardiology,* Vol.28, No.9,pp. 1957-1961, ISSN 0022-2828

Lombardini, J.B. (1998). Increased phosphorylation of specific rat cardiac and retinal proteins in taurine-depleted animals: isolation and identification of the phosphoproteins. *Advances in experimental medicine and biology,* Vol.442,pp. 441-447, ISSN 0065-2598

McBroom, M.J.&Welty, J.D. (1977). Effects of taurine on heart calcium in the cardiomyopathic hamster. *Journal of Molecular and Cellular Cardiology,* Vol.9, No.10,pp. 853-858, ISSN 0022-2828

Moise, N.S.;Pacioretty, L.M.;Kallfelz, F.A.;Stipanuk, M.H.;King, J.M.&Gilmour, R.F. (1991). Dietary Taurine Deficiency and Dilated Cardiomyopathy in the Fox. *American heart journal,* Vol.121, No.2,pp. 541-547, ISSN 0002-8703.

Mozaffari, M.S.;Tan, B.H.;Lucia, M.A.&Schaffer, S.W. (1986). Effect of drug-induced taurine depletion on cardiac contractility and metabolism. *Biochemicarmacology,* Vol.35, No.6,pp. 985-989, ISSN 0006-2952

Novotny, M.J.;Hogan, P.M.&Flannigan, G. (1994). Echocardiographic Evidence for Myocardial Failure Induced by Taurine Deficiency in Domestic Cats. *Canadian Journal of Veterinary Research-Revue Canadienne De Recherche Veterinaire,* Vol.58, No.1,pp. 6-12, ISSN 0830-9000.

Novotny, M.J.;Hogan, P.M.;Paley, D.M.&Adams, H.R. (1991). Systolic and Diastolic Dysfunction of the Left-Ventricle Induced by Dietary Taurine Deficiency in Cats. *American Journal of Physiology,* Vol.261, No.1,pp. H121-H127, ISSN 0002-9513.

Ohta, H.;Azuma, J.;Awata, N.;Hamaguchi, T.;Tanaka, Y.;Sawamura, A.;Kishimoto, S.&Sperelakis, N. (1988). Mechanism of the protective action of taurine against isoprenaline induced myocardial damage. *Cardiovascular research,* Vol.22, No.6,pp. 407-413, ISSN 0008-6363

Pion, P.D. (2004). Traditional and nontraditional effective and noneffective therapies for cardiac disease in dogs and cats. *Veterinary Clinics of North America-Small Animal Practice,* Vol.34, No.1,pp. 187-+, ISSN 0195-5616.

Pion, P.D.;Kittleson, M.D.;Rogers, Q.R.&Morris, J.G. (1987). Myocardial Failure in Cats Associated with Low Plasma Taurine - a Reversible Cardiomyopathy. *Science,* Vol.237, No.4816,pp. 764-768, ISSN 0036-8075.

Pion, P.D.;Kittleson, M.D.;Thomas, W.P.;Delellis, L.A.&Rogers, Q.R. (1992). Response of Cats with Dilated Cardiomyopathy to Taurine Supplementation. *Journal of the American Veterinary Medical Association,* Vol.201, No.2,pp. 275-284, ISSN 0003-1488.

Pion, P.D.;Sanderson, S.L.&Kittelson, M.D. (1998). The effectiveness of taurine and levocarnitine in dogs with heart disease. *The Veterinary clinics of North America Small animal practice,* Vol.28, No.6,pp. 1495-1514, ix, ISSN 0195-5616

Rajabi, M.;Kassiotis, C.;Razeghi, P.&Taegtmeyer, H. (2007). Return to the fetal gene program protects the stressed heart: a strong hypothesis. *Heart Failure Reviews,* Vol.12, No.3-4,pp. 331-343, ISSN 1382-4147

Schaffer, S.;Solodushko, V.;Pastukh, V.;Ricci, C.&Azuma, J. (2003). Possible cause of taurine-deficient cardiomyopathy: potentiation of angiotensin II action. *Journal of cardiovascular pharmacology,* Vol.41, No.5,pp. 751-759, ISSN 0160-2446

Schaffer, S.;Takahashi, K.&Azuma, J. (2000). Role of osmoregulation in the actions of taurine. *Amino Acids,* Vol.19, No.3-4,pp. 527-546, ISSN 0939-4451

Takihara, K.;Azuma, J.;Awata, N.;Ohta, H.;Hamaguchi, T.;Sawamura, A.;Tanaka, Y.;Kishimoto, S.&Sperelakis, N. (1986). Beneficial effect of taurine in rabbits with chronic congestive heart failure. *American Heart Journal,* Vol.112, No.6,pp. 1278-1284, ISSN 0002-8703

Tondeleir, D.;Vandamme, D.;Vandekerckhove, J.;Ampe, C.&Lambrechts, A. (2009). Actin isoform expression patterns during mammalian development and in pathology: insights from mouse models. *Cell motility and the cytoskeleton,* Vol.66, No.10,pp. 798-815, ISSN 1097-0169

Warskulat, U.;Andree, B.;Lusebrink, J.;Kohrer, K.&Haussinger, D. (2006). Switch from actin $\alpha 1$ to $\alpha 2$ expression and upregulation of biomarkers for pressure overload and cardiac hypertrophy in taurine-deficient mouse heart. *Biological chemistry,* Vol.387, No.10-11,pp. 1449-1454, ISSN 1431-6730

Warskulat, U.;Flogel, U.;Jacoby, C.;Hartwig, H.G.;Thewissen, M.;Merx, M.W.;Molojavyi, A.;Heller-Stilb, B.;Schrader, J.&Haussinger, D. (2004). Taurine transporter knockout depletes muscle taurine levels and results in severe skeletal muscle impairment but leaves cardiac function uncompromised. *The FASEB journal,* Vol.18, No.3,pp. 577-579, ISSN 1530-6860

Warskulat, U.;Heller-Stilb, B.;Oermann, E.;Zilles, K.;Haas, H.;Lang, F.&Haussinger, D. (2007). Phenotype of the taurine transporter knockout mouse. *Methods in enzymology,* Vol.428,pp. 439-458, ISSN 0076-6879

Woodcock-Mitchell, J.;Mitchell, J.J.;Low, R.B.;Kieny, M.;Sengel, P.;Rubbia, L.;Skalli, O.;Jackson, B.&Gabbiani, G. (1988). A-smooth muscle actin is transiently expressed in embryonic rat cardiac and skeletal muscles. *Differentiation; research in biological diversity,* Vol.39, No.3,pp. 161-166, ISSN 0301-4681

Yamori, Y.;Liu, L.;Ikeda, K.;Miura, A.;Mizushima, S.;Miki, T.&Nara, Y. (2001). Distribution of twenty-four hour urinary taurine excretion and association with ischemic heart disease mortality in 24 populations of 16 countries: results from the WHO-CARDIAC study. *Hypertension research,* Vol.24, No.4,pp. 453-457, ISSSN 0916-9636

Yamori, Y.;Liu, L.;Mori, M.;Sagara, M.;Murakami, S.;Nara, Y.&Mizushima, S. (2009). Taurine as the nutritional factor for the longevity of the Japanese revealed by a world-wide epidemiological survey. *Advances in experimental medicine and biology,* Vol.643,pp. 13-25, ISSN 0065-2598

Yancey, P.H. (2005). Organic osmolytes as compatible, metabolic and counteracting cytoprotectants in high osmolarity and other stresses. *The Journal of experimental biology,* Vol.208, No.Pt 15,pp. 2819-2830, ISSN 0022-0949

25

Thyrotoxic Cardiomyopathy

Alina Yu. Babenko, Alekber A. Bairamov,
Elena N. Grineva and Eugenia O. Ulupova
Almazov Federal Heart, Blood and Endocrinology Centre, St. Petersburg, Russia

1. Introduction

1.1 Thyrotoxicosis and thyrotoxic cardiomyopathy – Current state

Thyrotoxicosis is a common syndrome, and according to the Wickham Survey its prevalence is 2% among women and 0.2% in men in the areas with normal iodine consumption. Over the 20-year follow-up the incidence of thyrotoxicosis was 0.8:1000 in women and 0.6:1000 in men (Bird et al,1977).

Subclinical thyrotoxicosis (ST) is defined by low or undetectable serum thyrotropin stimulating hormone (TSH) and normal free thyroxin (FT4) and free triiodthyronin (FT3) concentrations (Biondi & Cooper, 2008). Although thyroid hormones are defined as being within normal range in patients with ST, they are often at the upper limit of the reference range, and thus sufficiently increased to suppress TSH and potentially produce abnormal tissue effects.

The prevalence of subclinical thyrotoxicosis varies from 0.6 to 16% % (Biondi et al., 2002; Wang & Crapo, 1997; Samuels, 1998) depending on such risk factors as age (it is twice higher in elderly people), iodine deficiency (5-times higher in the areas of iodine deficiency), and decreased TSH level. All authors agree that ST is more common compared to overt thyrotoxicosis.

There are exogenous (iatrogenic) and endogenous causes of thyrotoxicosis. Exogenous thyrotoxicosis usually is subclinical and mainly is caused by suppressive therapy with L-thyroxin leading to the decrease of TSH below normal values. It is commonly present in postoperative patients with differentiated thyroid cancer (papillary and follicular) as the mean of cancer recurrence prevention. This group of patients gets prolonged (2 years and longer) high-dose L-thyroxin therapy, and is considered in studies regarding side-effects of suppressive treatment. At the same time patients with benign thyroid nodules get short courses (6-12 months) of suppressive therapy, leading to a less decrease of TSH (above 0,1 mIU/l). According to the majority of data 1/2-2/3 of ST cases are exogenous (Figge et al., 1994; Canaris et al., 2002; Hoogendoorn et al., 2004).

Endogenous thyrotoxicosis can be also divided into immune (Graves' disease, "Hashitox") and non-immune (toxic (pretoxic) thyroid adenoma and toxic multinodular goiter) (Ross, 1996; Marqusee et al., 1998; Al-Abadi, 2001). Graves' disease is the most common cause of overt thyrotoxicosis.

Thyrotoxic cardiomyopathy (TCMP) is a threatening complication of thyrotoxicosis increasing risk of disability and mortality. Until recently myocardial alterations observed in

thyrotoxicosis were considered favorable regarding prognosis because of the high reversibility if euthyroid state is quickly achieved. However, long-term follow-up studies demonstrated that the involution of the changes is not always complete. Some irreversible histological alterations of myocardium are found in patients who had thyrotoxicosis in past: necrosis of the hypertrophied myocytes and fibrosis development (Ortmann et al., 1999). Myocardial fibrosis has been also detected by radioimmunoimaging with antimyosin antibodies in patients with TCMP complicated by heart failure (HF) (Martí et al., 1997).
There is a current evidence that even successfully treated thyrotoxicosis is associated with the worse prognosis. Thus, cardiovascular (hypertension, valvular diseases, heart failure, and to a lesser extent coronary artery disease) mortality is 1.2 higher in these patients, and cerebrovascular mortality is 1.4 higher than in general population (Osman et al., 2002). Persistent cardiovascular alterations are considered an evident cause of the increased mortality in thyrotoxicosis (Metso et al., 2007; Sheu et al., 2010). Health effects of subclinical thyrotoxicosis are not fully recognized, and some questions are still unsolved. However, quite large amount of publications of the last two decades verify deleterious effects of thyrotoxicosis, and uppermost, on cardiovascular system (Biondi et al., 2002). Moreover, there is evidence of the increased mortality in subclinical thyrotoxicosis (Sgarbi, 2010). Thus, in British study among patients over 60 years of age mortality (5 year follow-up) in subjects with TSH below normal values was about twice that of euthyroid subjects (Parle et al., 2001). Cardiovascular diseases were the most common cause of lethal events. Therefore, cardiovascular complications of thyrotoxicosis are of great medical importance.

2. Definition – Epidemiology of thyrotoxic cardiomyopathy and its clinical variants

Thyrotoxic cardiomyopathy defines a myocardial damage caused by the toxic effects of abundant thyroid hormones (TH) (Report of the 1995 WHO/ISFC) that result in altered energy production by myocytes (oxidative phosphorylation, glycolysis), intracellular metabolism (protein synthesis) and myofibril contractile function (Klein, 1990).
The main manifestations of thyrotoxic cardiomyopathy (TCMP) are left ventricular hypertrophy (LVH) (Ching et al., 1996, Dorr et al., 2005), heart rhythm disturbances (usually, atrial fibrillation (AF)) (Dunn et al., 1986; Frost et al., 2004), dilation of the heart chambers and heart failure (HF) (Dougherty & Craige, 1973; Siu et al., 2007), pulmonary hypertension (PH) (Chu et al., 2002; Rubin & Badesch, 2006), and diastolic dysfunction.
Epidemiology data on TCMP are currently lacking. This is due to the lack of diagnostic criteria and to the late introduction of the term "thyrotoxic cardiomyopathy" in clinical and research practice that occurred only after implementation of WHO classification of cardiomyopathies (Report of the 1995 WHO/ISFC).
Meanwhile et al. (1959) found that 4 out of 9 postmortem examinations detected no other cause for severe congestive HF but thyrotoxicosis, and that 64 out of 150 patients (43%) with thyrotoxicosis had cardiovascular complications in the absence of any known pre-existing heart disease.
The available evidence provides only data on the incidence of TCMP manifestations, including the most severe ones - AF and HF.
The incidence of heart rhythm disturbances in thyrotoxicosis varies in a wide range. Sinus tachycardia is the most common occurring in 42%-73% [Burggraaf J et al 2001, Cacciatori V, et al. 1996]. Tachycardia at rest and during sleep is a typical symptom in thyrotoxicosis.

Heart rate at rest is known to be one of the most important reserve parameters and a predictor of fatal cardiovascular complications. Elevated resting heart rate is associated with higher mortality. Risk of death from all causes is three-times higher in subjects with resting heart rate of 90-99 versus 60 beats per minute. Predictive value of heart rate is higher in hypertensive people and those with coronary artery disease. High resting heart rate might cause worsening of hypertension, increases risk of acute cardiovascular events, coronary artery disease, fatal ventricular arrhythmias as the most common causes of a sudden death, blood pressure elevation and heart failure development. Sinus bradycardia is rather rare in thyrotoxicosis.

Atrial fibrillation takes second place among heart rhythm disturbances occurring in 9%-23% of thyrotoxic patients compared to 0.4%-1.0% in general population (Petersen & Hansen, 1988; Presti & Hart, 1989; Parle et al., 1991; Frost et al., 2004). This is the most common cardiovascular complication of thyrotoxicosis), and is associated with high morbidity and mortality related to the thromboembolism (Staffurt et al., 1977). The complication rate varies widely and will be discussed later. Thus, Sandler and Wilson (1959) and Petersen and Hansen (1988) found 14% and 14.9% occurrence of atrial fibrillation, respectively, in the population of subjects without concomitant heart disease. In a study of women with different cardiac pathology atrial fibrillation was diagnosed in 67% of subjects with thyrotoxicosis (Ladenson, 1993).

Subclinical thyrotoxicosis is associated with the increased risk of atrial fibrillation (Auer et al., 2001). In the Framingham study at 20-year follow-up the incidence of AF was 25% in patients with low TSH that is 3 times as high as in euthyroid patients (7%) (Sawin et al., 1994). The prevalence of AF seems to be comparable in overt and subclinical thyrotoxicosis. According to Auer J. et al. (2001) it was 13.8% in patients with overt thyrotoxicosis, 12.7 % in subclinical thyrotoxicosis, and 2.3 % in euthyroid subjects (Auer et al., 2001). Extrasystole (5%-7%), paroxysmal tachycardia (0.2%-3.3%) and atrial flutter (approximately 1.4%) rarely occur in thyrotoxicosis. 24-hour ECG monitoring studies demonstrated that atrial heart rhythm disturbances are typical for thyrotoxicosis while ventricular ones usually occur only in severe cases and in subjects with concomitant cardiovascular diseases (table1).

Arrhythmias	Frequency (%)
Sinus tachycardia	42-73
Atrial fibrillation	9-23
Extrasystole	5-7
Atrial flutter	1,2-2,3
Paroxysmal tachycardia	0,2-3,3
AV-block	2,7-5
Sick sinus syndrome can develop in elderly people	

Table 1. Arrhythmias in thyrotoxicosis

The evidence on **left ventricular hypertrophy** (LVH) prevalence is not enough. On the one hand, some authors found the increase in left ventricular myocardium mass in both overt (Nixon et al., 1979; Auer et al., 2001; Dorr et al., 2005; Marcisz et al., 2006) and subclinical (Ching et al., 1996; Biondi, 1999, 2000; Auer, 2001) thyrotoxicosis. On the other hand, there are not enough studies considering LVH occurrence in thyrotoxicosis and factors contributing its development, geometry type (eccentric or concentric), and reversibility.

According to the epidemiology study (1510 patients over 45 years of age) by M. Dörr et al. (2005) LVH was diagnosed in 57,1% of patients with thyrotoxicosis, compared to 10.5% in euthyroid individuals. Therefore, thyrotoxicosis was considered an independent predictor of LVH (odds ratio, 13.65; 95% confidence interval, 2.83–65.75; $p < 0.01$). We have analyzed the occurrence of LVH and factors contributing its development and reversibility among in-patients with thyrotoxicosis. The LVH occurrence was 22.7% that is lower compared to the mentioned data. We included patients under 55 years of age without concomitant cardiovascular pathology, and this could be a possible reason for the lower prevalence (Babenko et al., 2011).

The increase of left ventricular myocardial mass index (LVMMI) was demonstrated in all studies regarding subclinical thyrotoxicosis (Ching et al., 1996; Auer, 2001), however, the values did not meet diagnostic criteria for left ventricular hypertrophy (Biondi, 1999, 2000).

Only women with overt thyrotoxicosis, unlike those with subclinical thyrotoxicosis, had high values of LVMMI (meeting LVH criteria) associated with the decrease of end-diastolic left ventricular volume and development of concentric LVH (CLVH), as reported by Donatelli M et al. (2003) on the other hand, the majority of studies demonstrate increase of both LVMMI and end-diastolic left ventricular volume and development of eccentric LVH (ELVH) (Levina, 1989; Marcisz et al., 2006; Babenko et al., 2007, 2008, 2011).

Concentric remodeling of left ventricle occurs in ST (Biondi et al., 2002; Donatelli et al., 2003), while eccentric remodeling is more common in overt thyrotoxicosis.

Prevalence of heart failure also widely varies - from 12% to 68% (Forfar et al., 1982; Hrnciar, 2002; Roffi et al., 2003); up to 90% of patients with thyrotoxicosis and HF develop AF (Siu et al., 2007).

Dilated TCMP as a threatening complication of thyrotoxicosis should be mentioned (Goland et al., 1999). Siu C-W. et al. (2007) reported 1% occurrence of **dilated thyrotoxic cardiomyopathy** in patients with thyrotoxicosis, and one thirds of cases is irreversible. Thyrotoxicosis accounts for 1% of the reasons of dilated TCMP (Lutton et al., 2001).

Association between thyrotoxicosis and pulmonary hypertension (PH) has been described as early as in the beginning of 1980s (Mier et al., 1989) and the linking mechanisms are discussed till nowadays (Yanai-Landau et al., 1995; Barst & Loyd, 1998; Menzel et al., 2000; Armigliato et al., 2006). Graves' (autoimmune) disease accounts for the most cases of PH: 47-65% of patients with diffuse goiter have PH (Mercé et al., 2005, Armigliato et al., 2006; Yung et al., 2006), such a high prevalence can be explained by both severe form of thyrotoxicosis and autoimmune effects (Yanai-Landau et al., 1995; Chu et al., 2002). The occurrence of PH in subclinical thyrotoxicosis is almost unknown. According to our data, the prevalence of PH was 29% in ST, and 39.6% in overt thyrotoxicosis.

The prevalence of mitral valve prolapse is 18-41% in thyrotoxicosis compared to 6-20% in general population (Brauman et al., 1985, Kahaly, 1986, Evangelopoulou et al., 1999).

3. The pathogenesis of thyrotoxic cardiomyopathy and its manifestations

3.1 Cardiovascular effects of thyroid hormones

Thyroid hormones (TH) affect cardiovascular system through three main intracellular processes in cardiomyocytes: energy production (oxidative phosphorylation, glycolysis), protein synthesis and cardiomyofibril contractility (Dillmann, 1990; Klein et al., 2000, 2001).

Alteration of energy production. Myocardial oxygen consumption increases in thyrotoxicosis. The number of mitochondria and their functional activity grows leading to the enhancement of adenosine triphosphate (ATP) production. However, in severe thyrotoxicosis, despite the increased oxygen consumption, the efficiency of its utilization decreases significantly. This follows altered oxidative phosphorylation resulted from the abnormal oxidative enzyme activity (decrease of myocardial ATP and creatine phosphate levels results in glycolysis activation) (Golber & Kandror, 1972).

Direct and indirect effects on myocardial of abundant TH **result in alteration of cardiomyofibril contractility**. **Direct effects** involve transcription of some genes regulating function of cardiomyiocytes, vascular smooth muscle cells (SMC) and other structural units (Dillmann, 1990; Klein et al., 2000, 2001)(Fig.1). Triiodothyronine (T3) is a biologically active thyroid hormone that enters cardiomyocytes through specific transporters located in the cellular membrane, and binds thyroid hormone receptor (THR) in the nucleus (Dillmann,1990; Everts et al., 1996). Nowadays two types of THR are known: homodimer (THR/THR) and heterodimer - 9-cis retinoic acid receptor (THR/RXR). Active forms of these receptors affect gene expression through binding specific DNA response elements, so called thyroid hormone-sensitive elements (TRE), located in the promoter region of T3-sensitive genes (Brent, 1994; Everts et al., 1996; Fazio et al., 2004). Gene transcription is augmented in the regions encoding alpha-myosine heavy chains (MNC-a), Ca^{2+}-ATPase of sarcoplasmatic reticulum of the cardiomyocytes, Ca^{2+}-K^{+}-ATPase Ca^{2+}- -uretic, beta1-adrenergic receptors, troponine I and Ca^{+}-uretic peptide. Three types of myosine isoforms are distinguished: V1 consisting of the MNC-alpha/alpha chains, V2 - consisting of MNC-alpha/beta chains, and V3 - consisting of MNC-beta/beta chains. High levels of TH affect myosine isoform expression and lead to the enhanced synthesis of V1 isoform and decrease of V3 isoform. ATPase being more active in MNC-alpha/alpha myosine chains compared to MNC-beta/beta chains, the velocity of myofibril contractions increases (Klein & Ojamaa, 2000, 2001) (Fig.1).

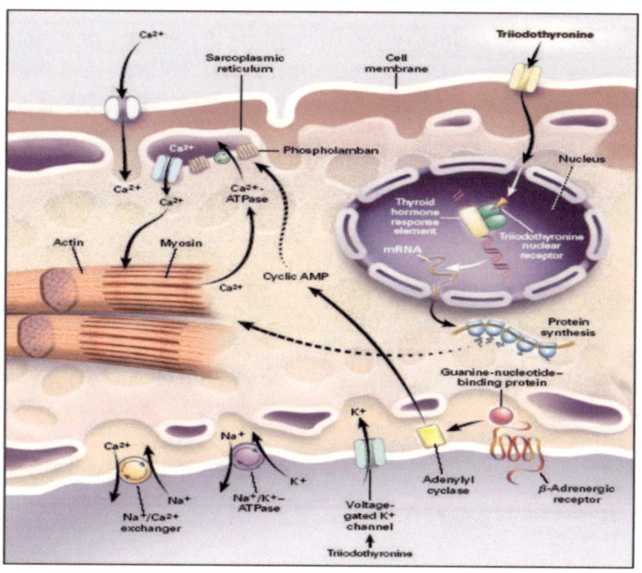

Fig. 1. Genom and nongenom effects of triiodthyronine in cardiomyocytes (from Klein& Ojamaa, 2000)

Indirect myocardial effect of abundant thyroid hormones include Ca^{2+} release from the intracellular depots and their subsequent reuptake by sarcoplasmic reticulum. The latter results from the enhanced Ca^{2+} ATPase (SERCA) expression and phospholamban suppression that are involved in the regulation of calcium intramyocyte concentration during cardiac cycle (systole and diastole). This leads to the increase of peak strain of cardiomyofibrils and shortening of the ventricular systole. Abundant thyroid hormone have been shown to induce expression of ryanodine receptors facilitating calcium (Ca2+) release from sarcoplasmic reticulum, thus amplifying contraction and myocardial hypertrophy. Moreover, high levels of TH cause intracellular calcium mobilization directly affecting L-type of Ca2+-channels (Dillmann , 1990, Kiss et al., 1994; Klein & Ojamaa, 2000, 2001)(Fig.1).

Therefore, high levels of TH contribute to the increased myocardial contractility through enhanced transcription of the genes encoding heavy chains of myocine beta-isoform and calcium-dependent ATPase, induced protein synthesis and augmented calcium and glucose myocardial consumption. In addition, thyroid hormones cause 50-70% reduction of the **systemic vascular resistance** (SVR) through direct and indirect (increase of tissue thermogenesis and lactate hyperproduction) effects on vascular smooth muscle cells leading to the decrease of diastolic blood pressure (DBP) and the increase of end-diastolic left ventricular volume. In particular, TH are known to induce nitric oxide production causing vasodilatation through direct effects on vascular smooth muscle cells (Ishikawa et al., 1989; Klein & Ojamaa, 2000, 2001; Vargas et al., 2006). Moreover, high levels of TH lead to the increase of circulating blood volume and venous return through the following mechanisms: aldosterone-renin system activation, enhancement of erythropoietin synthesis and renal sodium reabsorption (Jiménez et al., 1982; Marchant et al., 1993; Klein & Ojamaa, 2000, 2001; Vargas et al., 2006). Renal juxteglomerular complex is activated when DBP is reduced (Büssemaker et al., 2003). In addition, T3 directly stimulates rennin substrate synthesis by liver (Ganong WF. 1982). The reduction of BP and SVR induces production of rennin and aldosterone resulting in the increase of circulating blood volume and end-diastolic volume that finally amplifies workload on heart (Klein & Ojamaa, 2000, 2001; Vargas et al., 2006) (fig.2).

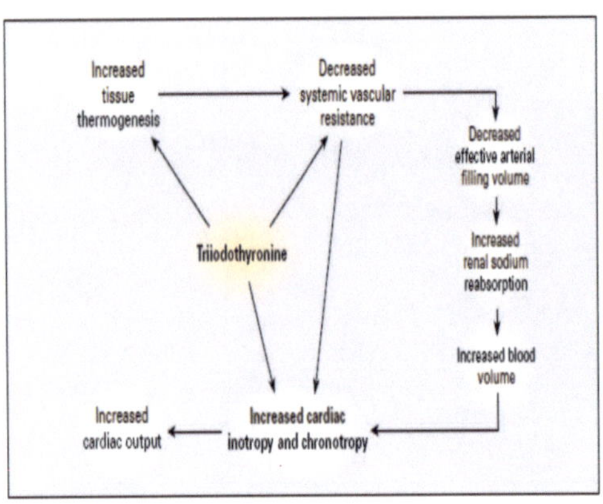

- The diagram shows the way in which triiodothyronine increases cardiac output by affecting tissue oxygen consumption (thermogenesis),
- vascular resistance, blood volume, cardiac contractility, and heart rate

(from Klein I. and Ojamaa K. 2001)

Fig. 2. Effects of Thyroid Hormone on Cardiovascular Hemodynamics

Tachycardia is a typical feature of thyrotoxicosis (Nordyke, 1988; Cacciatori, 1996; Biondi, 2000). It is caused by the faster diastolic depolarization associated with the shortening of action potential of the sinoatrial node (Osman et al., 2002). In general, the TH effects on pacemaker and conductive cardiac system include acceleration of systolic and diastolic depolarization and shortening of action potential, as well as of refractory period of atrial and atrioventricular myocytes. The latter can result in the increase of AF occurrence in thyrotoxicosis. Other mechanisms include augmentation of the pressure in left atrium, ischemia and left atrial premature ectopic heart beats (Bielecka-Dabrowa et al., 2009).

Thyroid hormones regulate some myocardial genes encoding synthesis of ion channels (K^+/Na^+-ATPase, Ca^+/Na^+- exchanger and potential-depending potassium channels) in cell membrane. These extranuclear effects involve the transport of aminoacids, glucose and calcium through cell membrane. Therefore, T3 can alter the activity of various ion channels (including sodium, potassium and calcium channels) located in cell membrane. (Bielecka-Dabrowa et al., 2009). In particular, phospholipid and Ca-dependent proteinkinase, cAMP-dependent proteinkinase, and Ca2+-calmodulin complex as the components of signal transmission system are involved in the T3 non-genomic cell effects. Thus, non-genomic actions of thyroid hormones include regulation of intracellular ion levels and their intracellular distribution. Changing transmembrane ion transport TH affect electrophysiologic features of cardiomyocytes (Kim & Smith, 1984). T3-induced expression of L-type calcium channels leads to the following: less calcium ions enter cardiomyocytes through L-type channels, and action potential gets shorter (Freedberg et al., 1970).

The occurrence of atrial rhythm disturbances (atrial fibrillation, atrial premature heart beats) is higher at thyrotoxicosis, while the rate of ventricular arrhythmias is comparable with the one in general population (Osman et al., 2002). Atrial and ventricular myocardial sensitivity to thyroid hormones is different that can be the cause of the variation in atrial and ventricular arrhythmia prevalence. High atrial sensitivity to arrhythmogenic thyroid effects is due to the high β-adrenoreceptor density at the surface of atrial cardiomyocytes and to the different autonomic innervation of atria and ventricles (Polikar et al., 1993; Lombardi et al., 1994). Golf et al. (1985) found that β-adrenoreceptor density in right atria of human heart samplings is more than twice as high as in left ventricle. Higher β-adrenoreceptor density in thyrotoxicosis is associated with the greater catecholamine myocardial sensitivity. Androgens up-regulate expression of the β-adrenoreceptor genes leading to their density increase. This can explain higher susceptibility to heart rhythm disturbances in men compared to one of women.

Expression of potential-dependent K+-channels in atria is 30% as high as in ventricles (Ojamaa et al., 1999). Expression of genes encoding both β-adrenoreceptor and potential-dependent K+-channels depends on thyroid hormones that induce heart rhythm disturbances. Experimental mice studies demonstrated that duration of atrial action potential is shorter, and atrial delayed rectifier potassium current (ultra rapid - Ikur and slow - Iss) mediating repolarization is greater in thyrotoxicosis. RNA messenger level and expression of genes of K+-channels (Kv1.5 и Kv2.1) were shown to be higher in both atria that also leads to the greater density of delayed rectifier potassium channels (Ikur и Iss) in hyperthyroidism. Thyroid effects on action potential and delayed rectifier potassium current are more expressed in right atrium compared to left one resulting in low interatrial difference of action potential duration (Bielecka-Dabrowa et al., 2009).

Shortening of atrial action potential in thyrotoxicosis is associated with the shorter duration of effective refractory period facilitating re-entry foci developing. On the other hand, normal interatrial difference of action potential is of great importance for synchronous atrial contraction (regarding right-sided location of the sinus node). Spontaneous ectopic activity, particularly in left atrium, can increase leading to atrial heart rhythm disturbances (atrial fibrillation) when the interatrial action potential difference is reduced (Bielecka-Dabrowa, 2009).
Pulmonary veins are known to initiate paroxysmal atrial fibrillation that can be due to the increased spontaneous activity of that region. Shorter action potential of the cardiomyocytes located in pulmonary veins associated with the shortening of refractory period and facilitating re-entry onset was shown in experimental thyrotoxicosis models (Chen, 2002). Incubation with thyroid hormones increased spontaneous activity in pulmonary vein cardiomyocytes similar to its effect on sinoatrial node cells. Trigger activity is supposed to underlie spontaneous activity of pulmonary veins (Bielecka-Dabrowa et al., 2009).

3.2 Pathogenesis of clinical manifestations of thyrotoxic cardiomyopathy

Tachycardia in thyrotoxicosis develops due to the faster diastolic depolarization associated with the shortening of action potential of the sinoatrial node cells [Osman F et al. 2002]. Sinus bradycardia can develop in case of congenital disorders or sick sinus syndrome. The latter, as well as abnormal heart rhythm can result from the decreased reserves of the mediator acetylcholine.
Mechanisms of arrhythmogenesis are discussed in the former chapter. Pathogenesis of heart rhythm disorders is not clear, and the following pathogenetic factors are being discussed: toxic effects of thyroid hormones, increased sympathetic activity, reduced intracellular potassium level (Table 2).

Effects of thyroid hormones	Pathogenesis of influence of thyroid hormones
Toxic influence on myocardium (amplification cardiomyofibril contractility and hypertrophy right atrium and left ventricule of heart)	Alteration oxidative phosphorylation. Increase synthesis of protein, action of enzymes, uptake of O_2 Alteration power processes and changes of K+/Na+-pump - increase velocity of diastolic depolarization
Increase sensitivity of SNS	Increase of number of β1-adrenoreceptors
Decrease of intracellular pool of potassium	Hyperfunction of heart and increase of action of simpatoadrenal influence
Change of vascular reactivity	Hyperrelaxations vascular myocites

Table 2. Pathogenesis of arrhythmias in thyrotoxicosis

Cardiac hyperfunction and increased adrenergic stimulation contribute the loss of intracellular potassium ions leading to heart rhythm disorders. Atrial dystrophic alterations associated with the structural myocardial heterogeneity are a confounding factor for atrial fibrillation. Exposure to any additional factor increasing myocardial heterogeneity can result in the complete myocardial uncoupling inducing heart rhythm disturbances. Atrial dilation, increased excitability of atria associated with the myocardial heterogeneity mediating functional conductive disorders underlie re-entry arrhythmias. Re-entry associated with the frequent focal activity are supposed to be the main mechanism of atrial fibrillation and flutter in thyrotoxicosis.

Increased cardiac output and reduced system vascular resistance (SVR) in thyrotoxicosis commonly lead to the amplification of pulse amplitude. Hemodynamics is altered in thyrotoxicosis as it has been mentioned above. The changes include elevation of heart rate, stroke and minute volumes, acceleration of blood flow, decrease of systemic vascular resistance (Fig.3), and resulting changes of blood pressure - systolic blood pressure is moderately increased, while diastolic blood pressure is within normal values or decreased. Thus pulse pressure goes up. The recent studies have demonstrated arterial stiffening and low SVR in thyrotoxicosis (Palmieri et al., 2004). Therefore, high levels of thyroid hormones cause systolic blood pressure (BP) elevation leading to **isolated systolic hypertension** in elderly patients with decreased arterial elasticity due to the atherosclerotic vascular lesion. The prevalence of isolated systolic hypertension is significantly higher in patients with thyrotoxicosis compared to euthyroid subjects (Marcisz et al., 2001). ST can resulting in an increase in nighttime systolic and mean blood pressure (Botella-Carretero et al, 2004). It appears to be one of the factors for LVH development in thyrotoxicosis.

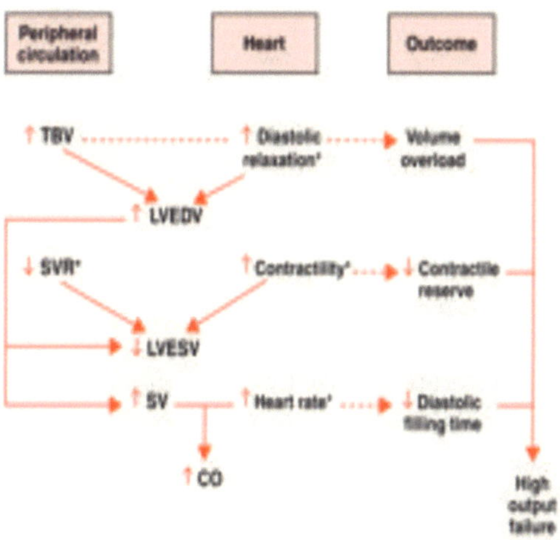

TBV- total blood volume;
LVEDV - left ventricular end diastolic volume; LVESV - left ventricular end systolic volume;
SV - stroke volume;
SVR - systemic vascular resistance;
CO - cardiac output;
↑ increase; ↓ decrease.
Solid arrows indicate direct effects, and dashed arrows potential outcomes.
*Features for which T3 is directly responsible. (from A Toft, N Boon 2000)

Fig. 3. Effects of hyperthyroidism on the cardiovascular system and the possible outcomesEccentric type of LVH, as a result of low SVR and volume overload on the heart, is a typical feature of thyrotoxicosis. However, there are data showing both normal LV geometry (Levina, 1989; Babenko, 2008), and LVH (eccentric type (Levina, 1989; Marcisz et al., 2006; Babenko et al., 2008, 2011) as well as concentric one (Donatelli et al., 2003) in patients with thyrotoxicosis. It depends on the degree of cardiovascular damage influenced by the variety of factors that will be discussed later.

Reduced **functional cardiac reserve** and physical load tolerance are also common in thyrotoxicosis because tachycardia at rest prevents from the increase of heart rate and effusion fraction and from the SVR lowering at physical load.

Pulmonary hypertension (PH) (mean pulmonary pressure more than 25 mmHg at rest and more than 30 mmHg at load) is frequently reported at overt thyrotoxicosis. Pulmonary hypertension is often associated with valvular insufficiency (of tricuspid and mitral valves) due to the papillary muscles dysfunction (Whitner et al., 2005; Mercé et al., 2005). Patients with Graves' disease are more likely to have myxomatous degeneration and prolapse of mitral valve as a consequence of endocardium involvement compared to subjects with toxic multinodular goiter (Kahaly, 1987).

There are two possible mechanisms of valve involvement in Graves' disease. First mechanism includes induction of glycosaminoglycan synthesis in endocardium (similar to one in retrobulbar space in ophthalmopathy) leading to the valve cusp thickening (Kahaly, 1987). The second one implies the reduced tone of papillary muscles and their consequent overstretching resulting in prolapse of mitral valve cusps in left atrium during ventricular systole (Brauman et al., 1985).

Pulmonary hypertension develops due to Kitaev reflex - spasm of pulmonary arterioles leading to the increase of pulmonary resistance (Okura & Takatsu, 1994). Thyroid hormones seem to affect pulmonary vessels in a rather different way compared to other vessels as they cause SVR reduction and circulating blood volume elevation. Blood pressure decreases in resistive vessels due to the vasodilatation effect of TH, and increases in pulmonary vessels. This is possibly mediated by endothelial dysfunction (Okura & Takatsu, 1994), and by the accelerated metabolism of pulmonary vasodilatation substances, such as acetylcholine, observed in patients with severe thyrotoxicosis (Okura & Takatsu, 1994; Nakchbandi et al., 1999). In addition, autonomic imbalance, in particular, sympathetic hyperactivity and lower vagal tone (Burggraaf et al., 2001), caused by hyperthyroidism facilitates further pulmonary vasoconstriction and PH development. Autoimmune mechanism might be an additional factor for PH development (Yanai-Landau et al., 1995; Barst & Loyd, 1998; James et al., 2002).

The diagnosis of heart failure in thyrotoxic patients is complex, because classic symptoms of heart failure including tachycardia and dyspnea, occur at the onset of hyperthyroidism due to both toxic effects of thyroid hormones on sinoatrial node and respiratory centre and intercostal muscles weakness. Heart failure (HF) develops in thyrotoxicosis because of the isotonic contraction (volume overload) of left ventricle and mixed overload (both volume and resistance overload) of right ventricle, thus right ventricular HF is more common for hyperthyroid state. Concomitant tricuspid valve insufficiency and regurgitation can worsen the situation (Whitner et al., 2005). Mitral valve prolapse is a common disorder in thyrotoxicosis, but it is rarely symptomatic.

Heart failure (HF) associated with thyrotoxicosis is more common in elderly rather than in young patients, and the mechanisms are better studied in aged group. Elderly subjects usually have co-existing cardiovascular diseases (coronary artery disease, valvular heart disease, arterial hypertension) leading to the functional and structural cardiac alterations, thus, myocardium contractility is easily impaired in case of increased myocardial load caused by hyperthyroidism. Elderly patients with heart rhythm disturbances, such as atrial fibrillation (AF), have the highest risk of HF development, because AF is usually associated with the increased heart rate followed by functional impairment of cardiomyocytes. Younger patients without cardiovascular pathology more often develop "high output heart failure" (Okura & Takatsu, 1994). This type of HF is characterized by the myocardial hypercontractility. HF with low output and heart chambers dilation (dilated thyrotoxic cardiomyopathy) can develop in young patients in case of the long-lasting severe thyrotoxicosis (Manger et al., 1988; Soh & Croxson, 2008). However, long duration of hyperthyroidism is not always evident, so the mechanisms are not fully understood.

Autoimmune mechanisms were considered possible (Kahaly, 1987; Koshiyama et al., 1996), but the hypothesis was denied afterwards (Fatourechi & Edwards, 2000). Two hypotheses are discussed nowadays. According to the first one two diseases are supposed to coexist in one individual - Graves' disease and idiopathic dilated cardiomyopathy (IDC). It is supported by their common pathogenesis - genetic predisposition determined by the HLA haplotypes (Limas & Limas, 1989; Olson et al., 1992) and common association of IDC and autoimmune thyroid diseases (Marković et al., 2005). According to the second hypothesis long-lasting myocardial hypertrophy can transform into dilation, and heart chamber dilation can develop in untreated prolonged overt and even subclinical thyrotoxicosis (Soh & Croxson, 2008).

Therefore, there are two main mechanisms of heart failure development in thyrotoxicosis: 1) tachycardia-induced HF with left ventricular dysfunction (left ventricular HF) is most common in patients with AF; 2) right ventricular HF resulted from volume overload of right ventricle due to the increased circulating blood volume and venous return is characterized by right ventricular dilation, enlargement of the tricuspid valve ring and tricuspid insufficiency and is frequently associated with pulmonary hypertension (Okura & Takatsu, 1994; Xenopoulos et al., 1996; Whitner et al., 2005).

Three stages of thyrotoxic cardiomyopathy are defined: hyperkinetic (with preserved left ventricular function, but at physical load left ventricular effusion fraction does not increase), normokinetic (a compensatory stage with a reversible myocardial hypertrophy and preserved cardiac output), and hypokinetic stage (decompensation stage with low cardiac output and stroke volume, either reversible or irreversible heart chamber hypertrophy and dilation).

High occurrence of thromboembolic events (higher than in general population) is typical for thyrotoxicosis, and even in absence of AF. Endothelial dysfunction is a possible explanation for high rate of thromboembolism: altered vasodilation response to acetylcholine exposure (Faber et al., 2001, Napoli et al., 2001), as well as elevated level of humoral substances Von Willebrand factor (Cucuianu et al., 1987; Squizzato et al., 2007), plasminogen activator, endothelin (Baumgartner-Parzer et al., 1997) confirm thrombogenesis activation in thyrotoxicosis (Homoncik et al., 2007). ST has been recently shown to have a prothrombogenic effects (Horne et al., 2004; Erem, 2006). Increased activity of Von Willebrand factor (Coban et al., 2006) and elevated fibrinogen level (Dörr et al., 2001) were demonstrated at ST.

4. Clinical manifestations and diagnostic tests of thyrotoxic cardiomyopathy

The most common symptoms of thyrotoxic cardiomyopathy are palpitations, chest pain (cardialgia), dyspnea, irregular heart beats. Tachycardia and heart rhythm disturbances, systolic hypertension, orthostatic hypotension, heart enlargement, systolic murmur maximal over mitral valve and bubbling rales in case of HF are the most common findings at physical examination. Tachycardia at rest and during sleep and significant increase of heart rate at minimal physical exertion are typical for thyrotoxicosis. Tachycardia is position-independent and resistant to therapy by cardiac glycosides. Usually there is a direct relation between tachycardia intensity and the severity of diffuse goiter. Heart rate increases up to 120-140 beats per minute, and up to 160 beats per minute and more on movement, at physical and emotional exertion. Patients complain of pulsation in the neck, head and abdomen. Atrial fibrillation can develop in both clinical thyrotoxicosis and subclinical and latent forms. Thus, as a potential cause thyrotoxicosis should be excluded in all patients with persistent atrial fibrillation resistant to antiarrhythmic drugs. Thyroid dysfunction is the cause of 46% of arrhythmias of this type. Paroxysmal atrial fibrillation at the onset of thyrotoxicosis usually turns into permanent form with the progression of the disease. There is a particular form of thyrotoxicosis characterized by paroxysmal atrial fibrillation with normal sinus rhythm or bradycardia without any other symptoms of thyrotoxicosis. The level of thyroid hormones is crucial to make the diagnosis in such cases. Physical examination reveals tachycardia and ascending apex beat. The cardiac borders are expanded to the left, the heart sounds are intensive, first heart sound is loud, and systolic murmur can be heard. Systolic blood pressure is increased, while diastolic blood pressure is within normal values or decreased (resulting in high pulse pressure, or pulse amplitude). Water retention is usual, and edema can be found even in patients with preserved ejection fraction. If the symptoms are persistent after successful treatment of thyrotoxicosis coexistent cardiovascular pathology should be excluded. In otherwise healthy individuals palpitations are associated with female sex and age older than 50 years, dyspnea is linked to female sex and increased level of T4>30 pmol/l. After euthyroid state restoration dyspnea can persist in smoking subjects (Osman et al., 2007).

Heart failure is associated with the pleural effusions, and right ventricular heart failure is more prevalent in diffuse goiter (Levina, 1989). Patients with dilated thyroid cardiomyopathy reveals cardiomegaly and pulmonary congestion (Soh & Croxson, *2008)* and all spectre clinical sins of heart failure.

Diagnosis. ECG changes include high, sharp P and T waves, atrial fibrillation, and extrasystole. ST segment depression and T wave inversion might be also present without angina pectoris, and are due to metabolic changes. ECG changes are reversible if the thyroid hormone levels are normalized.

Dilation of both ventricles and conus pulmonalis expansion are typical radiological signs in severe thyrotoxicosis. Conus pulmonalis expansion and right ventricle enlargement form mitral configuration of the heart. However, there is no left atrium enlargement at oblique view unlike the changes in mitral stenosis.

Pulmonary edema is another radiological sign in thyrotoxicosis. Echocardiography finds left ventricular hypertrophy including posterior wall and interventricular septum thickening, increase of end-diastolic volume and of left ventricular myocardial mass. Mitral valve prolapse is a common finding in thyrotoxicosis. The dilation of all heart chambers and decreased systolic function of left ventricle can be found in dilated thyrotoxic cardiomyopathy.

Perfusion scintigraphy of the heart with thallium chloride 201 demonstrates diffuse or small-focal decrease of cardiomyocyte metabolic activity. This diagnostic method enables assessment of the intact cardiomyocytes, and is helpful to exclude myocardial damage at early stages of the disease.

Stress-echocardiography is useful for assessment of functional myocardial reserve.

Increased levels of thyroid hormones and TSH suppression are crucial parameters to confirm the underlying cause (thyrotoxicosis) of the clinical findings.

5. The impact of various factors in clinical manifestations of thyrotoxic cardiomyopathy

5.1 Left atrial dilation and atrial fibrillation

Right atrial hypertrophy associated with dilation and verified by ECG was found in 30.5% of patients with thyrotoxicosis, left atrial hypertrophy - in 13.7%, and the hypertrophy of both atria was found in 11.8% patients.

Atrial fibrillation occurrence in thyrotoxicosis widely varies depending on the studied population. Age, sex, severity and intensity of hyperthyroidism, and concomitant cardiovascular diseases affect the incidence of atrial fibrillation.
Age-dependence is well-known: the risk of AF development increases as patients get older. Thus, at 10-year follow-up the incidence of atrial fibrillation was 25% in patients over 65 years of age with thyrotoxicosis, even its subclinical form, and this is threefold risk of patients with normal TSH (7%). The prevalence of AF was 21% in total cohort patients with clinical thyrotoxicosis (Iwasaki T et al, 1989), and 31% in subjects over 40 years old, while there was no single case of AF in individuals younger than 40 years. In another study 25% of thyrotoxic subjects over 60 years old had AF compared to 5% in younger group (Agner et al., 1984). Regression analysis performed by Nakazawa H. (2000) demonstrated a clear age-dependence of AF prevalence increasing stepwise till the maximal values in patients older than 70 years.
Male sex is another risk factor for AF (Staffurt et al., 1977). Toft A. & Boon N (2000) reported up to 50% prevalence of AF in males aged 60 years with hyperthyroidism.
The impact of the **duration of thyrotoxicosis** is less investigated. AF is quite rare (less than 2%) at onset of overt thyrotoxicosis (Nakazawa et al., 2000) and in patients under 40 years old without concomitant cardiovascular diseases Toft A. & Boon N (2000). The following factors are considered the most significant for AF development in young subjects without concomitant cardiovascular pathology: thyrotoxicosis duration ($p=0,0005$, $OR=72$ (6,6-794)), male sex ($OR=10,4$ (3,0-36,0), $p=0,0003$), and heart rate ($OR=1,07$ (1,03-1,11) $p=0,0001$) (Babenko et al., 2011). These factors are also important in case of coexistent heart pathology. Having examined 40 628 patients with thyrotoxicosis Frost (2004), showed that the highest risk of AF is associated with male sex, coronary artery disease and congestive HF. J. Mercé et al. (2005) found higher occurrence of AF in thyrotoxic patients with symptomatic insufficiency of either mitral or tricuspid valves (40% vs. 14%, $P=0,02$ in mitral regurgitation, and 86% vs. 3%,$P=0,01$ in tricuspid regurgitation).
Data on the effect of thyrotoxicosis intensity (overt or subclinical) are controversial. Auer et al.(2001) reported similar relative risk of AF in both subclinical and overt thyrotoxicosis (12,7 % and 13,8%, respectively). According to other data, AF occurrence in ST was 7% compared to 16% in clinical thyrotoxicosis (Babenko et al., 2011). There is an association between atrial fibrillation occurrence and type of predominantly elevated thyroid hormone (T3 or T4). Thus, atrial fibrillation occurs in 36% patients if T3 is elevated, in 13% - if T4 is increased, and in 21% - if the levels of both thyroid hormones are high. Therefore, the highest occurrence of atrial fibrillation was observed in the thyrotoxicosis due to isolated T3 excess. However, the difference could be explained by the different duration of the disease: isolated T3 thyrotoxicosis develops in nodal thyroid autonomy that is characterized by the long-term asymptomatic period and slow increase of thyroid hormone level at first leading to subclinical thyrotoxicosis, and then to T3 thyrotoxicosis. Conversion to sinus rhythm was reported only in 19% of patients with atrial fibrillation and at subclinical thyrotoxicosis. Risk factors for atrial fibrillation are listed in table 3.
Standard ECG could be used to identify high-risk patients at subclinical thyrotoxicosis: those with a short P-R interval who are predisposed to reentrant atrioventricular nodal tachycardia (Biondi B et al, 1998) and those with higher maximum P wave duration and P wave dispersion who are predisposed to AF (Aras D et al, 2005). In predisposed patients (those with two functionally distinct AV nodal conduction patterns), l-thyroxine (l-T4) suppressive therapy may increase the occurrence of reentrant-atrioventricular nodal

tachycardia because of the enhanced atrial excitability, which increases the number of atrial premature beats, and the shortening of the refractory period of the conducting tissue (Biondi B et al, 1998). Moreover, by measuring P maximum and P wave dispersion values, one could theoretically identify the patients with ST that are at high risk of AF (Aras D et al, 2005). Holter ECG could be performed before starting l-T4 treatment in doses that suppress TSH to potentially identify patients who may be less tolerant to l-T4 treatment.

Age
Male sex
Duration of hyperthyroidism
Heart rate
Concomitant cardiovascular diseases

Table 3. Risk factors for atrial fibrillation development.

5.2 Left ventricular hypertrophy

LVMMI is influenced by T3 level, systolic BP level and body mass index in patients with thyrotoxicosis (Marcisz et al., 2006). Eccentric left ventricular remodeling is predominant, and treatment and restoration of euthyroid state is not associated with LVMI normalization (9-month follow-up).

Sex also affects the occurrence of left ventricular hypertrophy (LVH) in thyrotoxic patients: the incidence of LVH is higher in men than in women (21,3% vs. 30,6%, respectively, OR=3,6; CI (1,8; 7,4); p=0,05). Eccentric type of LVH was present in 18,2%, and concentric one - in 4,3%, concentric remodeling occurred in 7,4% of patients (Babenko et al., 2011).

LVH rate increases in older population, however, the age-dependence is different in men and women. Correlation between LVMI and age is significant in general population (r=0,22, p=0,0007), and in females (r=0,27, p=0,0002), compared to non-significant association in males (r=0,10, p=0,58). More precise analysis showed that these parameters are related nonlinearly, and variability of LVMI increases in older subjects. Non-linear regression analysis defined an age threshold of 44 years: LVMI does not change up to this limit, and increases rapidly in older subjects for more than 10 g/m^2. It is even more evident in females: mean LVMI is 90±20 g/m^2 in women younger 44 years, and 105±25 g/m^2 - in older ones. The prevalence of left ventricular hypertrophy increases significantly from 11 up to 36% (OR=4,4; CI (2,1; 9,1), p=0,0002). Similar LVMI increase is observed in males - from 117±27 to 124±36 g/m^2, but changes of LVMI values and LVH prevalence are not significant because of the high LVMI variability (and smaller group) (p=0,63) (Babenko et al., 2011).

Atrial fibrillation is another factor associated with both LVH presence and severity (LVMI value) (Babenko et al., 2011).

The factors affecting left ventricular hypertrophy in subclinical thyrotoxicosis are not completely established. Shapiro L.C. et al. (1997) did not find LVH development in long-lasting ST (9,2±5,4 years) and very low TSH - 0,001 mIU/l in subjects with endogenous ST (mean age 45±10 years (27-63)). Biondi B. et al. (2000) reported significant increase of LVMI (162±24 g/m^2) in an age-matching group (43±9 years (27-69)) with endogenous ST but with higher TSH values (0,15 mIU/l) and shorter duration of subclinical thyrotoxicosis (6 months), however, it should be mentioned that 80% of the group were women. The same authors (Biondi et al., 1999) also demonstrated positive correlation between LVMI and duration and dozing of L-thyroxin treatment in patients with endogenous ST. There is evidence of different underlying mechanisms of LVH development in clinical and subclinical thyrotoxicosis (Donatelli et al., 2003), although the degree of LVH is comparable. LVH was shown to develop even in ST with normal heart rate, blood pressure and systolic left ventricular function that indicates the direct trophic effect of TH.

LVMI is higher in patients with subclinical thyrotoxicosis of variable etiology (iatrogenic, autoimmune hyperthyroidism caused by subclinical Graves' disease and nonimmune hyperthyroidism at pretoxic thyroid adenoma) compared to age- and sex-matching control group (p<0,005). LVH prevalence is 39% (43 patients, 45,5% in males and 38,4% in females) in ST. There was no difference in etiology and duration of ST. Male sex is a risk factor for LVH in ST as well as in clinical hyperthyroidism (Babenko et al., 2011).

Age and systolic blood pressure are two other risk factors for left ventricular hypertrophy (Babenko et al., 2007). Therefore, risk factors for left ventricular hypertrophy and atrial fibrillation development are different (Table 4)

Age
Male sex
Duration of thyrotoxicosis
Systolic blood pressure
Concomitant cardiovascular diseases

Table 4. Risk factors for left ventricular hypertrophy

5.3 Pulmonary hypertension

J. Mercé et al. (2005) analyzed data on pulmonary hypertension and its risk factors. Pulmonary hypertension (PH) occurs in 41% of thyrotoxic patients. Patients with thyrotoxicosis and symptomatic mitral or tricuspid insufficiency have higher pulmonary pressure: 53,8 vs. 34,9 mmHg, P=0,0001 in mitral insufficiency, 43,9 vs. 35,12 mmHg, P =0,07 in tricuspid insufficiency. There is no relationship between PH and following factors: age, sex, the cause of hyperthyroidism, cardiovascular or other symptoms, heart rate and type of heart rhythm disturbance, the level of thyroperoxidase antibodies, TSH, and TH. Pulmonary hypertension persisted in 16% of subjects after euthyroid state restoration. We found 39% prevalence of PH in thyrotoxicosis, and pulmonary pressure lowered till normal values in 61.5% of patients after persistent euthyroidism was achieved. The increase of pulmonary pressure was associated with free thyroxine level before treatment (r=0,5, p=0,0001), age (r=0,25, p=0,002) and endothelial vasodilatation function (the lower the response in reactive hyperemia test, the higher pulmonary pressure, r=-0,37, p=0,002). Right ventricular diameter positively correlated with pulmonary pressure (r=0,36, p=0,0001), and was considered a predictor of PH as there was 100% elevation of pulmonary pressure in patients with initial right ventricular dilation and normal pulmonary pressure.

According to our data pulmonary hypertension occurs in 29.6% of patients with subclinical thyrotoxicosis. The occurrence was highest (37,5%) in subjects with endogenous nonimmune ST (autonomic thyroid nodules). Free T3 and the degree of TSH suppression had the greatest impact. Thus, there was a positive correlation between pulmonary pressure and free T3 level (r=0,56, p<0,001), and negative - with TSH (r=-0,34, p<0,005). Higher level of T3 appears to be the reason of the greater elevation of pulmonary pressure in nonimmune endogenous ST (Babenko et al., 2008).

5.4 Heart failure

Risk factors of heart failure (HF) development in thyrotoxicosis are not well understood. As reported by Siu C-W et al. (2007), 5.8 % thyrotoxic patients developed heart failure, and AF was an independent predictor of HF (OR 37,4, (CI 9,72- 144,0, p <0,001)). 47% had left ventricular dysfunction (EF < 50%) that was more severe in patients with the lowest serum TSH level. Male sex was related with heart failure development (OR 26,6 (CI 2,6-272,5), p = 0,006). Left ventricular dysfunction and heart chamber dilation were present in one third of patients with restored euthyroidism. Patients with preserved output (ejection fraction 55% vs. 30 %, p <0.001) and lower functional class of heart failure (NYHA) demonstrate better outcome (reverse changes) (1.2 (0.1) vs. 2.5 (0.2), p <0.001).

The following main predictors of HF development in thyrotoxicosis (Babenko et al., 2011) are defined by multifactorial analysis: systolic blood pressure and free T3 level before treatment, dilation of left ventricle and to a lesser extent of other heart chambers.

To sum up, duration of hyperthyroidism, sex (male) and age are the main predictors of development of thyrotoxic cardiomyopathy and its clinical manifestations (left atrial dilation, atrial fibrillation, LVH, HF).

6. Predictive and therapeutic approach to thyrotoxic cardiomyopathy based on its risk stratification

Therapeutic approach should consider the factors affecting developing of thyrotoxic cardiomyopathy (TCMP) because persistent cardiac alterations have negative impact on cardiovascular prognosis.

European guidelines on management of toxic diffuse goiter offer the following strategy: conservative treatment by antithyroid drugs should be administered for 18 months with the following withdrawal in case of remission achieved, otherwise non-medication (irreversible) treatment is strongly recommended.

Persistent euthyroid state achievement is of great importance in management of thyrotoxic cardiomyopathy symptoms, while greater duration and older age are associated with worse cardiovascular prognosis. In our study (Babenko et al., 2011) median duration of hyperthyroidism was 10 (6; 16) months in women without left ventricular hypertrophy (LVH) and 10 (6; 15) in men, while it was up to 20 (9; 40) months in women with LVH (p=0,006) and up to 19 (12; 30) in men with left ventricular hypertrophy (p=0,09). Therefore, left ventricular hypertrophy risk is low in thyrotoxicosis lasting for less than 10 months, but it is significantly higher in more prolonged disease. In addition, left ventricular hypertrophy risk was higher in women over 44 years old, but it was age-dependent in men. Age and sex differences should be considered in clinical practice, and early non-medication treatment (after 8-10 months of antithyroid therapy) should be recommended in all male subjects and in women older 44 years. On the other hand, left ventricular hypertrophy in a newly diagnosed thyrotoxicosis is the sign of the long-lasting pathology, and its total duration is longer than mentioned periods. These subjects should undergo irreversible treatment earlier. Systolic hypertension worsens cardiovascular prognosis and it must be effective curation.

The choice of non-medication therapy- surgery or radioiodine intervention - is not easy in patients with thyrotoxic cardiomyopathy. Surgical treatment is associated with the high peri- and intraoperative risk, and radioiodine therapy is linked to the worse prognosis. The latter is due to the radioactive thyreoiditis development leading to the "leakage"

thyrotoxicosis, causing atrial fibrillation recurrence, vasospasm and cardiovascular events (myocardial infarction, stroke, pulmonary thromboembolism). I131 treatment is associated with the high early mortality at 1-2 months after intervention that coincides with the time of radioactive thyreoiditis onset.
Because increasing cardiovascular risk is present in older ST patients, treatment of endogenous ST (antithyroid drugs or radioiodine) is recommended to these patients. Restoration of euthyreoidism improves cardiovascular parameters (reduction in heart rate and the number of atrial and ventricular premature beats, LVMI and cardiac output) (Biondi and Cooper, 2008).
At older patients it is necessary to avoid whenever possible exogenous ST. Recent guidelines do not recommend suppressive therapy with l-T4 (to suppress serum TSH to below 0.1 mIU/liter) of benign thyroid nodules. Long-term suppressive therapy with serum TSH concentrations below 0.1 mIU/liter is recommended for DTC patients with persistent disease and a high risk of recurrence. Beta-blockade might be considered in high-risk thyroid cancer patients with adrenergic hyperresponsiveness to l-T4 (Biondi et al, 2005).
Symptomatic therapy of thyrotoxic cardiomyopathy should consider underlying pathogenetic mechanisms. Regarding high β-adrenoreceptor density, tachycardia due to increased adrenergic activity and volume heart load, β-blockers and diuretics should be administered. Diuretics are of great importance in patients with congestion symptoms (edema, dyspnea). Beta-blockers do not influence the release of thyroid hormones and are used to decrease sympathetic hyperactivity, thus leading to the reduction of cardiac load and myocardial oxygen demand. The choice of β-blocker is a highly debated question till nowadays. On the one hand, antithyroid activity of non-selective β-blockers (e.g. propranolol) is well-known . There is evidence that beta-blockers (propranolol) affect metabolism of thyroid hormones by inhibition of deiodinase type 2 in different tissues including cardiomyocytes and contributing transformation of T4 to inactive T3 – reversible hormone (Fig 4).

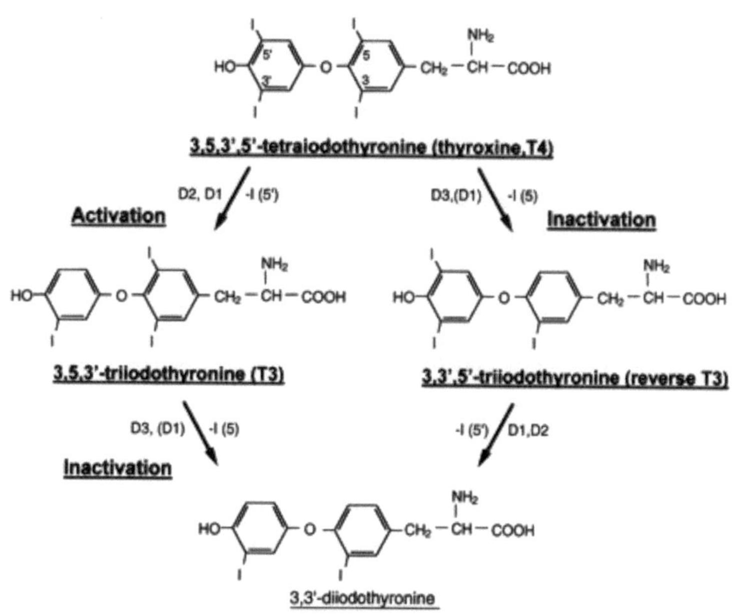

Fig. 4. Structures and interrelationships between the principal iodothyronines activated or inactivated by the selenodeiodinases (from A. Bianco, 2002)

Deiodinases are the selenoenzymes regulating thyroxine (T4) transformation into triiodothyronine (T3) (Bianco et al. 2002, Kohrle, 1999). Type 1 deiodinase (D1) is present in liver, kidneys and thyroid gland (Bianco et al. 2002, Peeters et al. 2003) and is supposed to play the key role in active circulating hormone T3 production (Kohrle, 1999). Type 2 deiodinase (D2) enables T3 production in the following tissues: central nervous system, pituitary gland, brown adipose tissue, myocardium, somatic muscles, osteocytes; and it is less expressed in liver and kidneys (Bianco et al. 2002, Kohrle, 1999, Peeters et al 2006). Thus, D2 plays the key role in local tissue T3 production, however D2 activity in somatic muscles makes a major contribution to serological markers output (Peeters et al, 2006, Maia, 2005) . Therefore, free T3 concentration in tissues depends on both T4 synthesis in thyroid gland and, correspondingly, circulating T4 concentration, and deiodinase activity in tissues. D1 contribution varies from 15-39% in the most of studies to 80% (Bianco et al. 2002, Pilo, 1990) (fig.5). T3 tissue concentration less depends on plasma thyroid hormone levels as D2 activity can contribute to a larger T3 tissue output. As a result, T3 concentration differs a lot in various organs and tissues. For example, T3 saturation usually is about 50% in liver and kidneys while it amounts to 95% in central nervous system (Bianco A et al. 2002). According to scientific data, type 2 deiodinase activity rises many times in some tissues in patients with Graves' disease. Thus, high D2 activity was revealed in thyroid tissue extracted from patient with Graves' disease at surgery (Salvatore et al, 1996). There are data showing that thyrotoxicosis clinical manifestations do not always correlate with circulating thyroid hormone concentration. B.Biondi et al. (2000) using questionnaire (with special symptoms scale) revealed manifested thyrotoxic symptoms in some patients with subclinical thyrotoxicosis. Cardiovascular examination of these patients (Echocardiography (EchoCG), bicycle ergometry, electrocardiography, etc.) also revealed severe pathologic changes (high atrial arrhythmia prevalence, left ventricular hypertrophy, diastolic dysfunction).

Heart lesions similar to ones described in thyrotoxicosis patients were revealed in experiments involving mice with induced high D2 gene expression activity in cardiomyocytes (Pachucki et al, 2001).

Based on these data it was supposed that the severity of many pathologic changes including cardiovascular abnormalities in patients with Graves' disease can be associated with both circulating hormone level and deiodinase-dependent T3 tissue production. In particularly, energy consumption in skeletal muscles was shown to correlate with free thyroxin (FT4) and TSH circulating levels, but not with free triiodothyronine level (FT3) (Canani et al, 2005). Type 2 deiodinase is assumed to play the key role in T3 tissue concentration changes, at least, in the tissues (such as myocardium, vessel wall) with high D2 gene expression.

Latter studies showed clinical impact of certain polymorphisms of deiodinase genes. One of these is found in humans and includes D2 polymorphisms characterized by threonine (Thr) changed for alanine (Ala) in codone 92 (D2 Thr92Ala).

Ala/Ala homozygous patients demonstrate lower D2 tissue activity compared to Ala/Thr heterozygous and Thr/Thr homozygous patients. Therefore, this polymorphism can decrease T3 effects in tissues with high D2 gene expression (Bianco et al. 2002, Kohrle, 1999). Therefore, this polymorphism is suggested to influence clinical manifestations and the severity of heart damage in patients with thyrotoxicosis.

Our study shows that Thr92Ala D2 polymorphism can impact clinical course of Graves' disease and heart damage (Grineva et al, 2009).

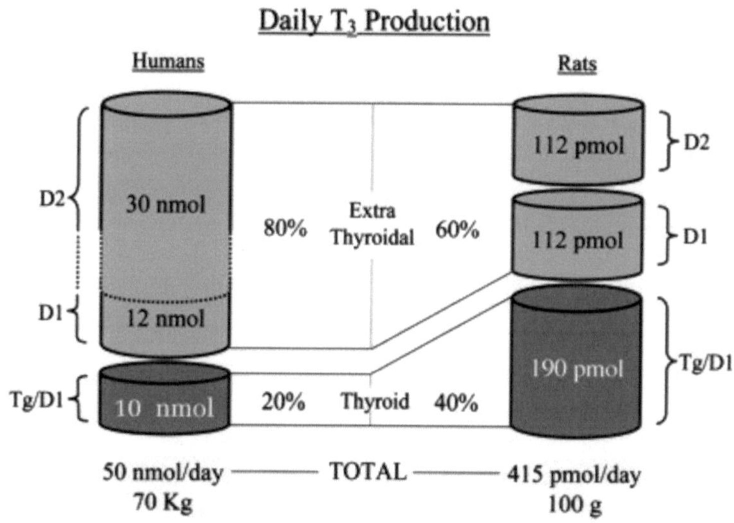

Fig. 5. Pathways of T_3 production in humans and rats. The dotted lines in the cylinder representing human extrathyroidal production reflect the uncertainty about the exact contributions of D1 and D2 to this pool. Values given are based on the studies cited in the text. Values for rats are normalized to 100 g body weight (from A. Bianco, 2002)

T3 level and T3/T4 index before treatment are considered as predictors of Graves' disease remission. We show significant differences between these parameters depending on Thr92Ala D2 polymorphism occurrence prove its role as a predictor of Graves' disease prognosis. It is confirmed by considerable difference in disease duration in groups of patients with various genotype. Thr92Ala D2 polymorphism seems to be protective as disease duration and relapse prevalence were considerably lower in Ala/Ala homozygous patients. This leads to inhibition of T3 effects in tissues with high D2 expression, such as: heart, thyroid and pituitary gland. Our data prove that Thr92Ala D2 polymorphism can impact clinical manifestations of Graves' disease including thyroid volume gain and heart rate. Ala/Ala homozygous patients reveal lower heart rate than heterozygous and Thr/Thr homozygous ones. All these clinical features (lower hormone level and heart rate, less thyrotoxicosis duration) contribute to less severe thyrotoxic cardiomyopathy in Ala/Ala homozygous patients.

Ala/Ala genotype of D2 polymorphism is also protective lowering total LVH risk and negative prognostic types of remodeling (concentric hypertrophy and dilatation of chambers), in particular. Therefore, medications leading to the decrease of deiodinase 2 activity could result in the reduced clinical manifestations of TCMP, however, no evidence is still available (Grineva et al, 2009).

However, only high doses of propranolol (more than 160 mg daily) can significantly decrease T3 plasma level (for approximately 30%), and it can result in severe reduction of blood pressure in the majority of patients (normotensive ones) as far as only some of them develop systolic hypertension.

On the other hand, β1-adrenoreceptor density is the first to be increased in thyrotoxicosis. Selective β1-blockers are supposed to be more effective. However, the advantage of any certain β-blocker in TCMP management is not evident, thus, the choice is based on the other advantages, e.g. dosage: once- or twice-daily drugs are preferred. It should be stated that elderly subjects as well as patients with low output HF and low blood pressure level are at high risk of hypotension (in particular, postural hypotension) development when treated by beta-blockers. (15)Low doses of cardioselective beta-blockers - betaxolol, atenolol, metoprolol - are preferable in this group of patients and in subjects who have relative contraindications (eg. bronchial obstruction) to beta-blockers. Beta-blockers are usually administered while euthyroid state is achieved, and then the doses are gradually diminished and withdrawn, in some cases if necessary low doses are maintained for a long time. The latter includes sustained tachycardia resistant to antithyroid therapy, heart rhythm disturbances such as extrasystole and atrial fibrillation; heart failure due to the forceful cardiac contractions. Beta-blockers are also used before the effects of antithyroid drugs or radioiodine are apparent, as well as in thyrotoxic storm and as a part of preoperative care.

Combination therapy by beta-blockers and antithyroid drugs has certain cardiovascular benefits compared to monotherapy. However, individual beta-blocker susceptibility should be assessed. Decrease of heart rate and absence of side effects are the main signs of the correct dosing. Significant positive clinical effect is usually apparent after 5-7 days of therapy by beta-blocker, including reduction of sympathetic hyperactivity and related symptoms, decrease of heart rate (in sinus rhythm as well as in atrial fibrillation), extrasystoles are less frequent or disappear, in some cases atrial fibrillation converts to sinus rhythm.

In patients with exogenous ST, the administration of a beta-blocking drug reduced the increased heart rate and left ventricular mass (Fazio et al, 1995). Therefore, beta–adrenergic blocking drugs should reduce the cardiovascular risk, and thus they might be considered for patients requiring long-term TSH suppressive therapy, especially symptomatic patients with high-risk thyroid cancer in which more aggressive TSH suppression may be required (Biondi and Cooper, 2008).

Cardiac glycosides usually are not indicated in thyrotoxicosis even in patients with severe HF. They lead to systole enhancement, diastole prolongation, being vagotropic they slow down cardiac conductivity, in particular atrioventricular conduction. Thyrotoxicosis is characterized by hyperkinetic hemodynamics, delayed atrioventricular conduction, and cardiac glycosides are even dangerous as digitalis intoxication easily develops. Thyrotoxic patients are usually resistant to antiarrhythmic drugs, and amiodarone (containing one third of iodine) can induce severe therapy-resistant thyrotoxicosis, including thyrotoxic crisis.

Efficacy of AF treatment depends on several factors. Younger age (under 50 years), absence of HF symptoms or other coexistent cardiovascular pathology, short duration (<4 month) and paroxysmal AF, normal systolic blood pressure and fast hypothyroidism achievement by antithyroid medication are the main predictors of sinus rhythm restoration that is observed in about one third of patients. **Spontaneous conversion to sinus rhythm** usually occurs at 3-month persistent euthyroid state. Otherwise standard guideline-based management of atrial fibrillation should be applied. The indirect relation between probability of successful cardioversion and duration of atrial fibrillation from any cause should be considered before the procedure (either pharmacologic or electrical cardioversion). Warfarin should be prescribed in patients with persistent AF, or aspirin should be considered in case of contraindications to anticoagulation therapy.

7. Conclusion – Up-to-date prevention of thyrotoxic cardiomyopathy and future prospects

LVH used to be considered reversible in TCMP patients as it was mentioned above. In basic animal research thyroxine induced LVH was found to be completely reversible when euthyroidism was achieved. Nixon et al. (1979) and Ching et al.(1996) demonstrated LVMI reduction after euthyroidism restoration in patients with thyrotoxicosis. However, it was not proven in more prolonged studies when thyroid function was normalized by thymasol therapy (Merillon et al.1989, Makaruk et al., 1998), According to Marcisz et al (2006) cardiac function and output, as well as systolic blood pressure were altered even after euthyroid state was restored, compared to healthy control group. It could result from TH-induced expression of the genes of contractile proteins and β-adrenoreceptors. Reversible changes might not be complete and would take longer time.

Beta-adrenergic effects have been investigated for years. Some authors confirmed beta-blocker benefits for LVH prevention in animal models, while others did not. A number of articles have been recently published regarding the impact of rennin-angiotensin system on LVH development and potential role of angiotensin converting enzyme inhibitors (ACEi) in LVH prevention and treatment in thyrotoxicosis. However, all available data are provided by experimental studies. As far as LVH is a common indication for ACEi we studied their effects in humans with TCMP. We found non-complete, but more pronounced reverse changes of LVH and left atrial dilation in patients treated by ACEi (Babenko et al. 2006).

Therefore, recent studies demonstrated high risk of irreversible LVH and left atrial dilation in AF in prolonged thyrotoxicosis and/or in elderly patients. The risk is high even after euthyroidism restoration by antithyroid medication. Beta-blockers and ACEi contribute to a better reversibility of the alterations, but complete recovery is not observed. Therefore, non-reversible (non-medication) treatment seems to be beneficial in a high-risk patients (males, women over the age of 44 years, systolic hypertension) regarding TCMP prevention.

Delayed diagnosis of thyrotoxicosis is of great medical importance as TCMP may manifest at first examination. These patients should be considered for non-medication treatment immediately after euthyroidism is restored.

8. References

Agner T. et al. (1984). A reevaluation of atrial fibrillation in thyrotoxicosis. *Dan Med Bull* 1984, 31:157-159.

Al-Abadi A. (2001). Subclinical thyrotoxicosis. *Postgrad Med J*. 2001;77:29

Aras D, et al (2005) Simple electrocardiographic markers for the prediction of paroxysmal atrial fibrillation in hyperthyroidism. Int J Cardiol 99:59–64

Armigliato M. et al. (2006). Hyperthyroidism as a cause of pulmonary arterial hypertension: a prospective study. *Angiology*. 2006 Oct-Nov;57(5):600-6.

Auer J. et al. (2001) Subclinical hyperthyroidism as a risk factor for atrial fibrillation. *Am Heart J* 2001, 142:838-842

Babenko A. et al. 2006. «Effect of ingibitors converting enzime on echocardiography parametrs at a thyrotoxicosis» poster of 31 annual meting ETA, Italy, Napoly, 2-6.09.

Babenko A. (2006). «Influence of subclinical thyrotoxicosis of varius genesis on cardiovascular system». «*Scientific notes of S-Petersburg Medical Uneversity named after Pavlov* » 2006, V.13, №4, p.65-69.

Babenko A. (2007) «Remodeling of cardiovascular system at thyreotoxicosis, its influense on vital prognosis» «Arterial hypertension» 2007 V.13, № 1 p.14-21.

Babenko A. (2008) «Character of geometry at clinical and subclinical thyrotoxicosis» «Vestnik of S-Petersburg Uneversity» s. 11 «Medicine», Vol. 4, dec. 2008 г., p.40-46.

Babenko A. et al. (2011). Analisis of contribution of various factors in development and type of remodeling left ventricule at thyreotoxicosis. *Bulleten of Almazov Federal Heart, Blood and Endocrinology Centre*. - 2011. - N 2 (в печати)

Barst RJ & Loyd JE. (1998). Genetics and immunogenetic aspects of primary pulmonary hypertension *Chest.* 1998;114;231-236.

Baumgartner-Parzer S.M. et al. (1997). Increase by triiodothyronine of endothelin-1, fibronectin and von Willebrand factor in cultured endothelial cells . *J. Endocrinol.* 1997. Vol. 154, №. 2. P. 231-239.

Bianco A et al (2002). Biochemistry, Cellular and Molecular Biology, and Physiological Roles of the Iodothyronine Selenodeiodinases. *Endocrine Reviews* 2002; 23(1): 38-89.

Bielecka-Dabrowa A et al. (2009) The mechanisms of atrial fibrillation in hyperthyroidism Review. *Thyroid Research* V.2

Biondi B, et al (1998) Clinical case seminar: reentrant atrioventricular nodal tachycardia induced by levothyroxine. *J Clin Endocrinol Metab* 83:2643–2645

Biondi B. et al. (1999). Effects of chronic subclinical hyperthyroidism from levothyroxine on cardiac morphology and function. *Cardiologia*. - 1999. Vol. 44. P. 443-449.

Biondi B. et al. (2000). Endogenous subclinical hyperthyroidism affects quality of life and cardiac morphology and function in young and middle-aged patients. *J Clin Endocrinol Metab.* 2000; 85: 4701–4705.

Biondi B. et al. (2002). Effects of Subclinical Thyroid Dysfunction on the Heart. *Ann Intern Med*, Dec. 3, 2002; 137(11): 904–914

Biondi B. et al. (2002). Effects of thyroid hormone on cardiac function: the relative importance of heart rate, loading conditions, and myocardial contractility in the regulation of cardiac performance in human hyperthyroidism. *J Clin Endocrinol Metab.* 2002; 87: 968–974.

Biondi B, Filetti S, Schlumberger M 2005 Thyroid hormone therapy and thyroid cancer: a reassessment. *Nat Clin Pract EndocrinolMetab* 1:32–40 363.

Biondi B. & Cooper D. (2008). The clinical significance of subclinical thyroid dysfunction. *Endocr Rev* 2008;29:76-131.

Bird T et al. The spectrum of thyroid disease in a community: the Whickham survey. 1977. www.feedback@ist-world.org.

Botella-Carretero JI et al. (2004) Chronic thyrotropin-suppressive therapy with levothyroxine and shortterm overt hypothyroidism after thyroxine withdrawal are associated with undesirable cardiovascular effects in patients with differentiated thyroid carcinoma. *Endocr Relat Cancer* 11:345–356

Brauman A. et al. (1985). Mitral valve prolapse in hyperthyroidism of two different origins. *Br Heart J.* 1985. Vol. 53. - P.374-377.

Brent G (1994). The molecular basis of thyroid hormone action. *N Engl J Med* 1994, 331:847-853

Burggraaf J. et al. (2001) Sympathovagal imbalance in hyperthyroidism. *Am J Physiol Endocrinol Metab.* 2001. 281: P190-195.

Büssemaker E. et al. (2003). Hyperthyroidism enhances endothelium-dependent relaxation in the rat renal artery. *Cardiovascular Research.* 2003. Vol.59. P.181–188.

Cacciatori V. et al. (1996). Power spectral analysis of heart rate in hyperthyroidism. *J Clin Endocrinol Metab.* 1996; 81: 2828–2835.

Canaris G et al. (2000). The Colorado thyroid disease prevalence study. *Arch Intern Med.* 2000;160:526-34.

Canani LH, et al (2005) The Type 2 Deiodinase A-G (Thr92Ala) Polymorphism Is Associated with Decreased Enzyme Velocity and Increased Insulin Resistance in Patients with Type 2 Diabetes Mellitus. . *J Clin Endocrinol Metab.* 2005; 90(6): 3472-3478.

Cappola A. et al. (2006). Thyroid Status, Cardiovascular Risk, and Mortality in Older Adults. JAMA. 2006. Vol. 295. P.1033-1041

Chen Y et al. (2002). Effects of thyroid hormone on the arrhythmogenic activity of pulmonary vein cardiomyocytes. *J Am Coll Cardiol* 2002, 39:366-372

Ching G. et al. (1996). Cardiac hypertrophy as a result of long-term thyroxine therapy and thyrotoxicosis. *Heart.* 1996.Vol.75. P. 363-368.

Chu J. et al. (2002). FCCP High Prevalence of Autoimmune Thyroid Disease in Pulmonary Arterial Hypertension. *Chest.* 2002;122:1668-1673

Coban E. et al. (2006) Endothelial dysfunction in subjects with subclinical hyperthyroidism. *J Endocrinol Invest* 29:197–200

Cucuianu M. et al. (1987). High levels of plasma von Willebrand factor in hyperthyroidism. *Rev Roum Med* 25:205–210

Dillmann W. (1990). Biochemical basis of thyroid hormone action in the heart. *Am J Med.* 1990. 88:626–630

Donatelli M. et al. (2003). Cardiac changes in subclinical and overt hyperthyroid women: retrospective study. *Int J Cardiol.* 2003. Vol. 90. P.:159–164.

Dorr M. et al. (2001). Low serum thyrotropin is associated with high plasma fibrinogen. *Thyroid.* 2001. Vol. 11. P. 153-160.

Dorr M. et al. (2005). The association of thyroid function with cardiac mass and left ventricular hypertrophy. *J Clin Endocrinol Metab.* 2005; 90: 673–677.

Dougherty M & Craige E. (1973). Apathetic hyperthyroidism presenting as tricuspid regurgitation. *Chest* 1973;63:767–72.

Dunn M. et al. (1989). Antithrombotic therapy in atrial fibrillation. *Chest.* 1989;95(2 Suppl):118S-127S.

Erem C (2006) Blood coagulation, fibrinolytic activity and lipid profile in subclinical thyroid disease: subclinical hyperthyroidism increases plasma factor X activity. *Clin Endocrinol (Oxf)* 64:323–329

Evangelopoulou M. et al. (1999). Mitral valve prolapse in autoimmune thyroid disease: an index of systemic autoimmunity? *Thyroid.* 1999. Vol. 9. P. 973-977

Everts M et al. (1996). Uptake of thyroid hormone in neonatal rat cardiac myocytes. *Endocrinology* 1996, 137:4235-4242

Faber J et al. (2001). Haemodynamic changes following treatment of subclinical and overt hyperthyroidism. *Eur J Endocrinol* 2001;145:391–6

Fazio S. et al. 2004. Effects of Thyroid Hormone on the Cardiovascular System. *Recent Progr Horm Res* 2004, 59:31-50

Figge J et al. (1994). The clinical evaluation of patients with subclinical hyperthyroidism and free triiodothyronine (free T_3) toxicosis. *Am J Med* 1994;96:229-234

Forfar J. et al. (1982). Abnormal left ventricular function in hyperthyroidism: evidence for a possible reversible cardiomyopathy. *N Engl J Med.* 1982. Vol. 307. P.1165-1175.

Freedberg A et al. (1970). The effect of altered thyroid state on atrial intracellular potentials. *J Physiol* 1970, 207:357-369

Frost L. et al. (2004). Hyperthyroidism and risk of atrial fibrillation or flutter: a population-based study. *Arch.Intern.Med.* 2004. Vol.164. P.1675–1678.

Ganong W (1982). Thyroid hormones and renin secretion. *Life Science.* 1982. Vol.30. P.577–584.

Gerdes A et al. (1985). Failure of propranolol to prevent chronic hyperthyroid induced cardiac hypertrophy and multifocal cellular necrosis in the rat. *Can J Cardiol.* 1985 Sep-Oct;1(5):340-5.

Goland S. et al. (1999) Dilated cardiomyopathy in thyrotoxicosis. *Heart* 1999;81:444-445.

Golber L & Kandror V 1972. *Thyreotoxic Heart.* Moscow, Russia.

Golf S et al. (1985). Beta-adrenoceptor density and relative number of beta-adrenoceptor subtypes in biopsies from human right atrial, left ventricular, and right ventricular myocard. *Cardiovasc Res* 19:636–641.

Grineva E. (2009) Type 2 deiodinase Thr92Ala polymorphism impact on clinical course and myocardial remodeling in patients with Graves' disease. *Cell Cycle.* Vol.8. Is.16 P.2565-2570.

Hoogendoorn E et al. (2004). Subclinical hyperthyroidism: to treat or not to treat? *Postgraduate Medical Journal* 2004;80:394-398

Homoncik M. et al. (2007) Altered platelet plug formation in hyperthyroidism and hypothyroidism. *J. Clin. Endocrinol.Metab.* 2007. Vol. 92, No. 8. P. 3006-3012.

Horne M et al. (2004). Is thyroid hormone suppression therapy prothrombotic? *J Clin Endocrinol Metab 2004* 89 4469–4473

Hrnciar J. (2002). Cor thyreotoxicum. Part I - new findings about its etiopathogenesis and diagnosis. Overview of the problem based on 35 years' experience. *Vntr Lek.* 2002. Vol. 48(1). P. 38-43.

Ikram H. (1977). Haemodynamic effects of beta-adrenergic blockade in hyperthyroid patients with and without heart failure. *BMJ 1977*;i:1505-7.

Ishikawa T. et al. (1989). Thyroid hormones directly interact with vascular smooth muscle strips. *Molecular Pharmaceutics.* 1989. Vol.35. P.760–765.

Iwasaki T. et al. (1989) Echocardiographic studies on the relationship between atrial fibrillation and atrial enlargement in patients with hyperthyroidism of Graves' disease. *Cardiology.* 1989. Vol.76. N 1. P.10-17.

Jiménez E. et al. (1982). Effects of hyper-and hypothyroidism on the basal levels of angiotensin I and kinetic parameters of renin angiotensin system in male rats. *Revista Española de Fisiologia.* 1982. Vol.38. P.149–154.

Kahaly G. (1987). Graves' disease and mitral valve prolapse. *JAMA.* 1987. Vol.257.-P. 22-28.

Kim D & Smith T (1984). Effect of thyroid hormone on sodium pump sites, sodium content, and contractile response to cardiac glycosides in cultured chick ventricular cells. *J Clin Invest* 1984, 74:1481-1488

Kiss E et al. (1994). Thyroid hormone induced alterations in phospholamban protein expression. Regulatory effects on sarcoplasmic reticulum calcium transport and myocardial relaxation. *Circ Res* 75:245–251.

Klein I. (1988). Thyroxine-induced cardiac hypertrophy: time course of development and inhibition by propranolol. *Endocrinology.* 1988. № 123. P.203–210.

Klein I. (1990). Thyroid hormone and the cardiovascular system. *Am. J. of Medicine.* 1990. № 88. P.631–637.

Klein I & Levey GS. (2000). The cardiovascular system in thyrotoxicosis. In: Braverman LE, Utiger RD, eds. *The thyroid,* 8th ed. Philadelphia: Lippincott-Raven, 2000;596-604.

Klein I. & Ojamaa K. (2001). Thyroid hormone and cardiovascular system. *N Engl J Med,* 2001Vol. 344, No. 7 February 15, p.501-509.

Kobori H et al. (1999). Local renin-angiotensin system contributes to hyperthyroidism-induced cardiac hypertrophy. *J. Endocrinol.* 1999. V.160, I. 1, 43-47.

Kohrle J. Local activation and inactivation of thyroid hormones: the deiodinase family. Mol Cell Endocrinol. 1999 May 25; 151(1-2):103-19.

Ladenson P. (1993). Thyrotoxicosis and the heart: something old and something new[Editorial]. *J Clin Endocrinol Metab.* 1993. Vol. 77. P. 332-333.

Levina L. (1989). *Heart at endocrine diseases.* Leningrad, Russia.

Lombardi G. et al. (1994). *Heart and Thyroid.* Wien. - P.86-91.

Lutton S. et al. (2001) *Cardiomyopathy and myocardial failure.*

Maia A et al (2005) Type 2 iodothyronine deiodinase is the major source of plasma T3 in euthyroid humans. *J.Clin. Invest.* 2005; 115: 2524–2533

Makaruk B et al. (1998). Changes of echocardiographic indices of the left cardiac ventricle systolic function during thyrostatic therapy. *Polish J Endocrinol,* 1998; 49: 307-12.

Manger J et al. (1988). Congestive heart failure and sudden death in a young woman with thyrotoxicosis. *West J Med* 1988; 149:86-91

Marchant C.et al. (1993). Renin-angiotensin system in thyroid dysfunction in rats. *J.of Cardiovascular Pharmacology.* – 1993. – Vol.22. – P.449–455.

Marcisz C et al.(2001). Influence of short-time application of a low sodium diet on blood pressure in patients with hyperthyroidism or hypothyroidism during therapy. *Am J Hypertens.* 2001; 14: 995–1002

Marcisz C. et al. (2006). Left ventricular mass in patients with hyperthyroidism. *Med Sci Monit.* 2006. 12(11) P.481-486.

Marqusee E et al. (1998). Subclinical thyrotoxicosis. Endocrinol Metab Clin North Am. 1998;27:37-49

Martí V et al. (1997). Myocardial damage does not occur in untreated hyperthyroidism unless associated with congestive heart failure. *Am Heart J.* 1997 Dec;134(6):1133-7

Menzel T et al. (2000). Pathophysiology of impaired right and left ventricular function in chronic embolic pulmonary hypertension: changes after pulmonary thromboendarterectomy. *Chest* 118: 897–903, 2000.

Mercé J. et al. (2005). Cardiovascular abnormalities in hyperthyroidism: A prospective Doppler echocardiographic study. *Am. J.Medicine* (2005) 118, 126-131.

Merillon J et al. (1981). Left ventricular function and hyperthyroidism. *Br Heart J,* 1981; 46: 137-43.

Metso, S. et al. (2007) Increased Cardiovascular and Cancer Mortality after Radioiodine Treatment for Hyperthyroidism *J Clin Endocrinol Metab* 2007;92:2190-2196

Mier A et al (1989) Reversible respiratory muscle weakness in hyperthyroidism. *Am Rev Respir Dis* 139,529-533

Nakazawa H et al. (2000). Is there a place for the late cardioversion of atrial fibrillation? A long-term follow-up study of patients with post-thyrotoxic atrial fibrillation. *Eur Heart J.* 2000; 21: 327–333.

Nakchbandi I et al. (1999) Pulmonary Hypertension Caused by Graves' Thyrotoxicosis* Normal Pulmonary Hemodynamics Restored by ^{131}I Treatment *Chest.* 1999;116:1483-1485.

Napoli R et al. (2001) Impact of Hyperthyroidism and Its Correction on Vascular Reactivity in Humans. *Circulation.* 2001;104:3076

Nordyke R et al. (1988) Graves' disease: influence of age on clinical findings. *Arch Intern Med.* 1988; 148: 626–631.

Nixon J et al. (1979). Alterations in left ventricular mass and performance in patients treated effectively for hyrotoxicosis. A comparative echocardiographic study. *Am J Med.* 1979 Aug;67(2):268-76 .

Ojamaa K et al. (1999) Regulation of rat cardiac Kv1.5 gene expression by thyroid hormone is rapid and chamber specific. *Endocrinology.* 1999.140:3170–3176.

Okura H & Takatsu Y. (1994) High-Output Heart Failure as a Cause of Pulmonary Hypertension. *Intern. Med.* Vol. 33, No. 6 June 1994

Ortmann C et al. (1999) Inflammation of the cardiac conduction system in a case of hyperthyroidism. *Int J. Legal. Med.* 1999. № 112. - P.271–274.

Osman F. et al. (2000) Cardiac rhythm abnormalities in thyrotoxicosis—the explanation for excess vascular mortality *J.Endocrinology.* - 2000. - Vol.164. -P.321.

Osman F. et al. (2002). Cardiac Dysrhythmias and Thyroid Dysfunction - The Hidden Menace? *J Clin Endocrinol Metab.* 2002 Vol. 87, No. 3 963-967.

Osman F. et al. (2007) Cardiovascular Manifestations of Hyperthyroidism Before and After Antithyroid Therapy. *J Am Coll Cardiol*, 2007; 49:71-81

Pachucki J, et al (2001) Type 2 Iodothyronine Deiodinase Transgene Expression in the Mouse Heart Causes Cardiac-Specific Thyrotoxicosis. *Endocrinology.* 2001; 142(1): 13-20.

Palmieri E et al. (2004) Myocardial contractility and total arterial stiffness in patients with overt hyperthyroidism: acute effects of beta1-adrenergic blockade. *Eur J Endocrinol.* 2004; 150: 757–762.

Paran Y et al. (2006) Pulmonary hypertension and predominant right heart failure in thyrotoxicosis. *Resuscitation.* 2006; 69: 339–341.

Parle J. et al.(2001). A single low serum thyrotrophin (TSH) concentration predicts increased all-cause and cardiovascular mortality in older persons in the community: a 10-year cohort study. *Lancet.* 2001. Vol.358. P.861–865.

Parle J. et al. (1991). Prevalence and follow-up of abnormal thyrotrophin (TSH) concentrations in the elderly in the United Kingdom. *Clin Endocrinol* (Oxf). 1991. № 34. P.77-83.

Peeters R et al (2003). Polymorphisms in Thyroid Hormone Pathway Genes Are Associated with Plasma TSH and Iodothyronine Levels in Healthy Subjects? *J Clin Endocrinol Metab.* 2003; 88(6): 2880-2888.

Peeters R et al. (2006). Genetic variation in thyroid hormone pathway genes; polymorphisms in the TSH receptor and the iodothyronine deiodinases. *Eur. J. Endocrinol.* 2006; 155(5): 655-662.

Petersen P. & Hansen J.M. (1988) Stroke in thyrotoxicosis with atrial fibrillation. *Stroke.* 1988. Vol.19. P.15–18.

Pilo A et al. (1990) Thyroidal and peripheral production of 3,5,3'-triiodothyronine in humans by multicompartmental analysis. Am J Physiol 1990; 258:715–726

Polikar R. et al. The thyroid and the heart. *Circulation.* 1993.Vol. 87. P.1435-1441.

Presti C. & Hart R. Thyrotoxicosis, atrial fibrillation, and embolism, revisited. *Am.Heart J.* 1989. Vol.117. P.976-977.

Report of the 1995 World Health Organization/International Society and Federation of Cardiology Task Force on the Definition and Classification of Cardiomyopathies. *Circulation.* 1996. Vol. 93. P. 841-842

Roffi M. et al. (2003) Thyrotoxicosis and the cardiovascular system: Subtle but serious effects. *Cleveland Clinic Journal Of Medicine.* 2003. Vol. 70.P. 57-63.

Ross D (1996) Subclinical thyrotoxicosis. In: Braverman LE, Utiger RD, eds. Werner and Ingbar's *The Thyroid*: A Fundamental and Clinical Text. 7th ed. Philadelphia: Lippincott Williams & Wilkins; 1996:1016-20.

Rubin L. & Badesch D. (2006) Thyrotoxicosis as a Risk Factor for Pulmonary Arterial Hypertension. *Ann Intern Med*, February 7, 2006; 144(3): 222 - 223.

Salvatore D, et al (1996). Type 2 iodothyronine deiodinase is highly expressed in human thyroid. *J Clin Invest* 1996; 98:962–968.

Samuels M (1998) Subclinical thyroid disease in the elderly. *Thyroid*.1998;8:803-13

Sandier G. & Wilson G. (1959)The nature and prognosis of heart disease in thyrotoxicosis: a review of 150 patients treated with I^{131}. *QJM* 1959. Vol. 28. P. 347-352.

Sawin C. T. et al.(1994) Low serum thyrotropin concentrations as a risk factor for atrial fibrillation in older persons. *N Engl J Med.* 1994. Vol. 331.-P. 1249-1254.

Scivoletto R. et al. (1986) Thyroid hormones and vascular reactivity: role of the endothelial cell. *Eur. J. Pharm.* 1986. Vol.129. P.271–278.

Shapiro L et al. (1997) Minimal cardiac effects in asymptomatic athyreotic patients chronically treated with thyrotropin-suppressive doses of l-thyroxine. *J Clin Endocrinol Metab.* 1997;82:2592-5.

Sgarbi J et al (2010) Subclinical thyroid dysfunctions are independent risk factors for mortality in a 7.5-year follow-up: the Japanese-Brazilian thyroid study.*Eur J Endocrinol* 2010;162:569-77.

Siu C-W. et al. (2007) Incidence, clinical characteristics and outcome of congestive heart failure as the initial presentation in patients with primary hyperthyroidism. *Heart* 2007;93:483-487.

Soh M & Croxson M. (2008) Fatal thyrotoxic cardiomyopathy in a young man. *BMJ.* 2008; 337: a531

Squizzato A. et al. (2007) Thyroid Dysfunction and Effects on Coagulation and Fibrinolysis: A Systematic Review. *J Clin Endocrinol Metab.*2007. Vol. 92, No. 7 2415-2420

Staffurt J et al. (1977) Arterial embolism in thyrotoxicosis with atrial fibrillation. *Br Med J* 1977, 2:688-690

Toft A & Boon N (2000) Thyroid disease and the heart. *Heart* 2000;84:455-460

Yanai-Landau H et al (1995) Autoimmune aspects of primary pulmonary hypertension. *Pathobiology*. 1995;63(2):71-5.

Yung C. et al. (2006) Hemodynamic Changes in Hyperthyroidism-Related Pulmonary Hypertension: A Prospective Echocardiographic Study. *J Clin Endocrinol Metab.* 2006 Vol. 92, No. 5 1736-1742

Vargas F et al. (2006) Vascular and renal function in experimental thyroid disorders. *Eur. J. Endocrinol.*, 2006, Vol 154, I 2, 197-212.

Wang C & Crapo L (1997)The epidemiology of thyroid disease and implications for screening. [PMID: 9074859] *Endocrinol Metab Clin North Am.* 1997;26:189-218

Whitner T. et al. (2005) Hyperthyroidism. Presenting as Isolated Tricuspid Regurgitation and Right Heart Failure. *Tex Heart Inst J.* 2005; 32(2): 244–245.

Woeber K (1992) Thyrotoxicosis and the heart. *N Engl J Med* 1992;327:94-98.

Xenopoulos NP et al.(1996) Severe right heart failure in a patient with Graves' disease. *Clin Cardiol* 1996;19:903–5.

26

Drug-Induced Cardiomyopathies

Jan Klimas
Department of Pharmacology and Toxicology, Faculty of Pharmacy, Comenius University in Bratislava, Slovak Republic

1. Introduction

Heart failure represents one of most important causes of death in Western countries. Its high mortality originates in part from severe complications like cardiac contractile dysfunction and/or sudden cardiac death caused by ventricular arrhythmias (Shin et al. 2007). Unfortunately, significant portion of heart failure stems from use (and misuse) of several drugs and medications. Indeed, the cardiac muscle is widely known as a target of injury for many drugs and many other chemical compounds. Following their cardiotoxic action, these could be divided into two relevant categories: i) drugs and cardiotoxic substances leading to heart failure in terms of abrupt contractile performance, and ii) drugs affecting ion channels or pumps and, in most cases, leading to prolongation of cardiac repolarisation (and QT interval) and to increased risk of severe cardiac arrhythmias (such as *Torsades de Pointes*) and premature death. In some cases, it is very difficult to divide them in those categories as they have both of actions. Additionally, drug-induced cardiomyopathies not only belong to the serious adverse events of drug actions but they are widely used as experimental models for studying several cardiac conditions and diseases, offering the advantage of precise control of the onset time and can often be studied in a longitudinal fashion. This chapter covers in detail certain drug groups, as for example anthracyclines or some drugs of abuse, which are clearly associated with the development of cardiomyopathy followed by heart failure. Similarly, note is made regarding experimental models of primary or secondary drug-induced cardiomyopathies, QT prolonging agents and rhythm disturbances-triggering drugs. It must be noted that some of the mentioned substances are of clinical importance, the others have their use largely limited, but some of them lost their therapeutic use because of their cardiotoxicity.

2. Drugs inducing heart failure

Some substances cause acute cardiac depression as they lower heart rate, contractility and conduction and in certain causes even cardiac arrest. These substances include barbiturates (thiopental) or halogenated hydrocarbons (halothane, metoxyflurane and enflurane), even at concentrations used in surgery. However, many of drugs are administered chronically and are cardiotoxic and may trigger the development of cardiac injury even when used appropriately. As mentioned in ESC guidelines, there are some specific drug groups and substances which are strongly related to development of heart failure. Literally, beta-blockers, calcium antagonists, antiarrhythmics, cytotoxic agents, alcohol, cocaine and some trace elements are mentioned (Dickstein et al. 2008). Several pathophysiologic mechanisms of action have been proposed how and why drugs affect the cardiac tissue. They vary depending on the inciting agent, including direct toxic effects, neurohormonal activation, altered calcium homeostasis, and oxidative stress (Figueredo 2011). Conclusively, numerous chemicals and drugs are implicated in cardiomyopathy and even many of them remain unrecognised.

Amphetamine	Ethanol
Anabolic-androgenic steroids	Idarubicin
Anthraquinone	Imatinib
Antipsychotic phenothiazine derivates	Isoproterenol
Arnica herb	Ephedrine
Arsenic	Melarsoprol
Azidothymidine	Methamphetamine
Anagrelide	Methylphenidate
Catecholamines	Minoxidil
Cytarabine	Mitomycin
Clozapine	Mitoxantrone
Cobalt	Paclitaxel
Cocaine	Pentamidine
Chloroquine	Stibogluconate
Cyclophosphamide	Sunitinib
Daunorubicin	Trastuzumab
Diazoxide	Tricyclic antidepressants
Doxorubicin	Zidovudine

Table 1. Drugs and substances implicated in cardiomyopathy (Figueredo 2011).

2.1 Anthracyclines

In the first line, anti-cancer drugs are long recognised as strong cardiotoxic substances. Predominantly, anthracyclines are the best known and the most discussed drugs which hardly affect cardiac muscle. They were discovered in the 1960s and remain one of the mainstays of modern cancer therapy. The first two members of this group - daunorubicin (also known as daunomycin and rubidomycin) and doxorubicin (also known as adriamycin), were isolated from *Streptomyces peucetius*, a species of actinobacteria (Tan et al. 1967; Arcamone et al. 1969) and are well established as highly efficacious antineoplastic agents for various hemopoietic and solid tumors (such as breast cancer, sarcoma, ovarian and bronchogenic carcinoma as well as lymphoma, and certain forms of leukemia). Newer derivates are epirubicin and idarubicin. Despite their extensive use (and despite of the fact that they are extensively studied), their precise anticancerous mechanism is not completely understood. Most probably, it is a combination of several different actions, what accounts for the high efficiency of this class of anti-cancer drugs (Gewirtz, 1999; Minotti et al. 2004). It might include inhibition of DNA replication by intercalating between the base pairs which prevents replication of rapidly growing cancer cells (Sinha et al. 1984). However, contradictory to that, some studies have shown that at clinically relevant anthracycline concentrations, intercalation is unlikely to play a major role and stressed the topoisomerase II as the key target for anthracyclines (Binaschi et al. 2001). According to this, they act by stabilizing a reaction intermediate in which DNA strands are cut and covalently linked to tyrosine residues of topoisomerase II, which blocks subsequent DNA resealing. Failure to relax the supercoiled DNA blocks DNA replication and transcription. Other important mechanisms participating in the anticancer effects should be the apoptosis of cancer cells via the p-53 dependent pathway (Ruiz-Ruiz et al. 2003) as well as modifications of cellular proteins and organelles by formation of reactive oxygen species and lipid peroxidation (Muindi et al. 1984).

The cardiotoxicity of anthracyclines, which has been recognized shortly after their introduction in clinical practice, continues to limit their therapeutic potential and to threaten the cardiac function of many patients with cancer. Its manifestation can be diverse and may range from QT interval prolongation to acutely induced cardiac arrhythmias, changes in coronary vasomotion with consecutive myocardial ischemia, myocarditis, pericarditis, severe contractile dysfunction, and potentially fatal cardiac insufficiency (Zuppinger et al. 2007). Three distinct types of anthracycline-induced cardiotoxicity have been described (Shan et al. 1996). First, acute or subacute injury can occur immediately after treatment. This rare form of cardiotoxicity may cause transient arrhythmias, infrequently a pericarditis-myocarditis syndrome, or acute failure of the left ventricle. These manifestations usually respond promptly to the cessation of anthracycline infusion and rarely preclude further continuation of anthracycline treatment. Second, anthracyclines can induce chronic cardiotoxicity resulting in cardiomyopathy. This is a more common form of damage and is clinically the most important. Finally, late-onset anthracycline cardiotoxicity causing late-onset ventricular dysfunction and arrhythmias, which manifest years to decades after anthracycline treatment has been completed, is increasingly recognized. Both, chronic or late-onset forms most frequently lead to cardiomyopathy with a bad prognosis for the affected patients. Indeed, survival of patients with anthracycline-associated heart failure is worse than that of patients with ischemic or dilated cardiomyopathy (Felker et al. 2000). Echocardiography is currently the gold standard method for diagnosis and monitoring of anthracycline-induced cardiac impairment. Abnormalities in diastolic dysfunction detected by Doppler echocardiography likely represent early cardiotoxicity that precedes the onset of apparent systolic dysfunction (Wu 2008; Carver et al. 2008). However, some data suggest that the risk of anthracycline-associated heart failure is higher than usually estimated (Swain et al. 2003).

There are several known risk factors for anthracycline-associated cardiotoxicity. The total cumulative dose has been earlier identified as to be the major risk factor (Von Hoff et al. 1979). When focused on doxorubicine in a clinical study, the estimated cumulative percentage of patients who developed congestive heart failure at a cumulative dose of 400 mg/m^2 was 3%, increasing to 7% at 550 mg/m^2 and to 18% at 700 mg/m^2. It also was shown that doxorubicin-related congestive heart failure is schedule dependent. Consequently, modern adjuvant anthracycline regimens typically contain less than the cumulative dose associated with increased risk of cardiomyopathy (Wu 2008; Carver et al. 2008). Moreover, the incidence is lower with a once-weekly schedule when compared to a once-3-weekly schedule of doxorubicin administration (Von Hoff et al. 1979). Except of dosing schedule, the age may play a critical role - childhood as well as old age seem to be of risk. Young females who were treated with high cumulative doses of anthracyclines or with regimens of high individual doses, as well as patients of both sexes who were relatively young at the time of treatment or have had long periods of follow-up since doxorubicin therapy, appear to be at the highest risk for late cardiotoxic effects (Lipshultz et al. 1995). Patients who are younger at the time of diagnosis have the greatest reductions in left ventricular mass and the most profound increases in afterload. It was suggested that this difference could be due to the inhibition of myocardial growth by anthracycline, which would be accentuated in younger children, whose left ventricular mass is smaller (Lipshultz et al. 1991). Moreover, it was evidenced that limiting the cumulative dose of doxorubicin may not suffice to prevent late cardiotoxic effects in patients treated for cancer during childhood. Similarly, patients of advanced age (over 65 years old) may be at greater risk for congestive heart failure and may benefit from the early administration of a cardioprotectant (Swain et al. 2003). Interestingly enough, female gender is associated with a higher risk of cardiotoxicity as compared to males. Other risk factors include combination cancer therapy, prior or concomitant mediastinal radiotherapy, previous cardiac disease, and hypertension (Singal and Iliskovic 1998).

2.1.1 Mechanisms of cardiotoxicity of anthracyclines

In general, the pathophysiological mechanisms leading to chemotherapy-induced cardiomyopathy are mainly associated with myocardial cell loss, either due to apoptosis or necrosis what consequently leads to mild, moderate or even severe contractile dysfunction. The same is true for anthracyclines as well, but precise identification of exact mechanisms is frequently difficult since the majority of cancer patients is not only treated with a multitude of cancer drugs but might also be exposed to potentially cardiotoxic radiation therapy.

Similarly to antineoplastic action, the main cardiotoxic mechanism of anthracyclines is extensively under debate (Wu and Hasinoff 2005; Simůnek et al. 2009). As anthracyclines and their related compounds are well characterised as substances that lead to myocardial cell loss (Bristow et al. 1978; Mackay et al. 1994), it is likely that some of their anti-cancer mechanisms are involved in cardiotoxicity as well. In other words, cardiotoxicity may be viewed as an effect of the entire class of anthracyclines, which may indicate that it is inseparable from their antitumor effect. Early works on the pathogenesis of anthracycline cardiomyopathy had focused on DNA and protein synthesis (Pigram et al. 1972; Rosenoff et al. 1975; Levey et al. 1979). Currently, at least four hypotheses explaining the cardiotoxicity of anthracyclines have been proposed (Outomuro et al. 2007). First, in the 'iron and free-radical theory' an increased oxidative stress and antioxidant deficit have been suggested to play a major role. Although the molecular basis is not still clear enough, mitochondria is accepted as the locus where progressive molecular disorder is triggered. Second, the 'metabolic hypothesis' implicates C-13 alcohol metabolites of anthracyclines as mediators. Anthracycline alcohol metabolites can affect myocardial energy metabolism, ionic gradients, and calcium movements. Third, in the 'unifying hypothesis', chronic cardiotoxicity induced by C-13 alcohol metabolite might be primed by oxidative stress generated by anthracycline redox cycling. The two main possible mechanisms of cardiac damage that have been proposed, *i.e.* an increase calcium concentration in the interior of myocardial fibers, and damage to cell and organelle membranes by doxorubicin-generated oxygen radicals that produce an increase in the rate of endogenous lipid peroxidation, can obviously be sequentially ordered: first, doxorubicin radicals are generated and secondly they would lead, through lipid peroxidation and membrane damage, to a loss of membrane-selective permeability and towards increased calcium levels in the myocardial fibers. Fourth, the 'apoptosis hypothesis' is based on findings of myocyte cell loss through apoptosis in doxorubicin cardiomyopathy. The up-regulation of proapoptic proteins (Bax, caspases and cytochrome C), with or without the down-regulation of antiapoptotic proteins (Bcl2, Akt), has been documented and mitogen-activated protein kinases have been shown to be involved in both apoptosis and cell survival. Likewise, apoptosis is related with oxidative mechanisms as increased oxidative stress has been shown to promote apoptosis and antioxidants have been shown to inhibit this process.

Notably, the currently still prevailing hypotheses based on free radical production appeared in the centre of interest, as to be a major mechanism of anthracycline-associated cardiac dysfunction, in 1970's. And, during a time, the iron-mediated formation of reactive oxygen species and promotion of myocardial oxidative stress remains by far the most frequently proposed mechanism (Simůnek et al. 2009). It was demonstrated that anti-cancer agents whose structure contained quinone moieties could function as free radicals in NADPH-dependent microsomal oxidative reaction (Handa et al. 1975). Because superoxide dismutase inhibited this enhancement, it was suggested that the reaction precedes by formation of a free radical semiquinone which presumably then acts as both a chain initiator and in the transfer of electrons from molecular oxygen to superoxide anion. It was described that anthracyclines augments electron flow from NADPH to molecular oxygen in cardiac sarcosomes (Bachur et al. 1977) and others supported this (Myers et al. 1976; Myers et al. 1977) starting a focus on oxidative stress in explanation of cardiotoxicity of these drugs. In other words, the myocyte damage has been almost exclusively attributed to a concentration-dependent increase of intracellular oxidative stress with a consecutive increase in cytosolic calcium, mitochondrial dysfunction (Tokarska-Schlattner et al. 2006), and induction of myocyte apoptosis or necrosis (Hasinoff 1998; Gille and Nohl 1997; Doroshow 1983). Moreover, it is believed that reactive oxygen species not only lead to cell death, but also directly affect excitation-contraction coupling and calcium signaling in cardiomyocytes (Zuppinger et al. 2007). In addition to reactive oxygen species, reactive nitrogen species are also referred as to be implicated in anthracycline cardiotoxicity. The influence of anthracyclines on the NO signaling pathway has been studied in several experimental models and has been extensively reviewed (Fogli et al. 2004). It is known that anthracyclines may increase the expression of the inducible NO-synthase and so massively increase the NO production. Regarding chronic cardiotoxicity, prolonged anthracycline exposure may induce a large synthesis of byproducts of the NO-synthase mediated anthracycline redox-cycling, including $ONOO^-$, which can rapidly react with manganese-superoxide dismutase, leading to an inactivation of the enzyme (Radi et al. 2002). This results to initiation a deleterious faulty mechanism that will favour further formation of $ONOO^-$ and other NO-derived reactive nitrogen species, therefore promoting cardiomyocyte damage (Fogli et al. 2004). In addition, the generation of free radical species could lead to lipid peroxidation (primarily of the cell membrane); however, such lipid peroxidation would not indicate whether free radicals were being generated intracellularly or extracellularly (Gewirtz 1999).

The question – why is the heart so much more susceptible to the oxidative stress produced by anthracyclines than other tissues – has been widely studied. As proposed, cardiac tissue has weak antioxidant activity, since it lacks catalase (Doroshow 1983) and so cardiomyocytes could be exposed to high levels of hydrogen peroxide. In addition, cardiomyocytes are rich in mitochondria, which represent up to 50% of cardiomyocyte mass and which serve as both source and target of reactive oxygen species (Simůnek et al. 2009). Moreover, an important role has been attributed to exogenous NADH dehydrogenase. Unlike cardiac mitochondria, liver mitochondria lack the NADH-related pathway of reducing equivalents from the cytosol to the respiratory chain. As a result, liver mitochondria do not generate significant amounts of anthracycline semiquinones (Nohl et al. 2003).

One of the long reported hypotheses of cardiotoxicity of anthracyclines is based on the calcium overload (Olson et al. 1974), as they disrupt cellular and mitochondrial calcium homeostasis (Solem et al. 1994). Fleckenstein's calcium theory of myocardial cell necrosis from 1970' is widely quoted in literature as a general mechanism of myocardial cell damage (Fleckenstein et al. 1974). It must be noted that intracellular calcium dysregulation is present in all types of advanced cardiomyopathy and apparently is a late stage event that represents a final common pathway for myocardial cell damage and death. Similarly to that, anthracyclines dose-dependently increase diastolic intracellular calcium in single cardiomyocytes (Mijares and López 2001). There is a variety of modes how calcium regulating mechanism can strongly disrupt the calcium handling in cardiac cells. As anthracyclines may cross the cell surface and membranes of organelles and they, and their metabolites (doxorubicinol and daunorubicinol), may alter sarcoplasmic reticulum's calcium regulation, the recent focus is shifted to this organelle (Charlier et al. 2005; Kim et al. 2005; Park et al. 2005; Ondrias et al. 1990; Dodd et al. 1993; Arai et al. 1998). Indeed, there is now increasing evidence that depression of contractility in heart failure is linked to a malfunction of sarcoplasmic reticulum calcium release (Kirchhefer et al. 2007; Kirchhof et al. 2007). Calcium release is maintained by a macromolecular protein complex that is activated by L-type calcium current. It consists of the cardiac specific ryanodine receptor 2 (calcium release channel of sarcoplasmic reticulum), calsequestrin (calcium storage protein of sarcoplasmic reticulum), FK506-binding protein FKBP12.6, triadin, and junctin (Zhang et al. 1997; Bers 2002). Aside from cytosolic calcium, ryanodine receptor activity is also regulated by luminal calcium. Its storage and release are under the control of calsequstrin (Györke et al. 2002), whereas triadin and junctin may serve as linker proteins between calsequestrin and the ryanodine receptor. The interaction between these proteins appears to be critical for the regulation of calcium release. Importantly, anthracyclines may directly affect the calcium release complex because there is a direct anthracycline binding site on cardiac specific ryanodine receptor and on cardiac calsequestrin (Saeki et al. 2002; Park et al. 2005; Charlier et al. 2005). Indeed, it was shown that anthracyclines have biphasic effect on cardiac ryanodine receptor - initially, activate the channel, whereas after a few minutes, the channel becomes irreversibly inhibited (Ondrias et al. 1990). The ability of anthracyclines to inhibit calcium release may be more important pharmacologically than their ability to stimulate calcium release, since only nanomolar to low micromolar concentrations are required to produce inhibition, whereas release requires concentrations in the micromolar range (Olson et al. 2000). In addition to calcium regulation by sarcoplasmic reticulum, anthracyclines can affect L-type calcium channels, probably via formation of reactive oxygen species (Campbell et al. 1996), as well as Na^+/Ca^{2+} exchanger activity (Goldhaber 1996).

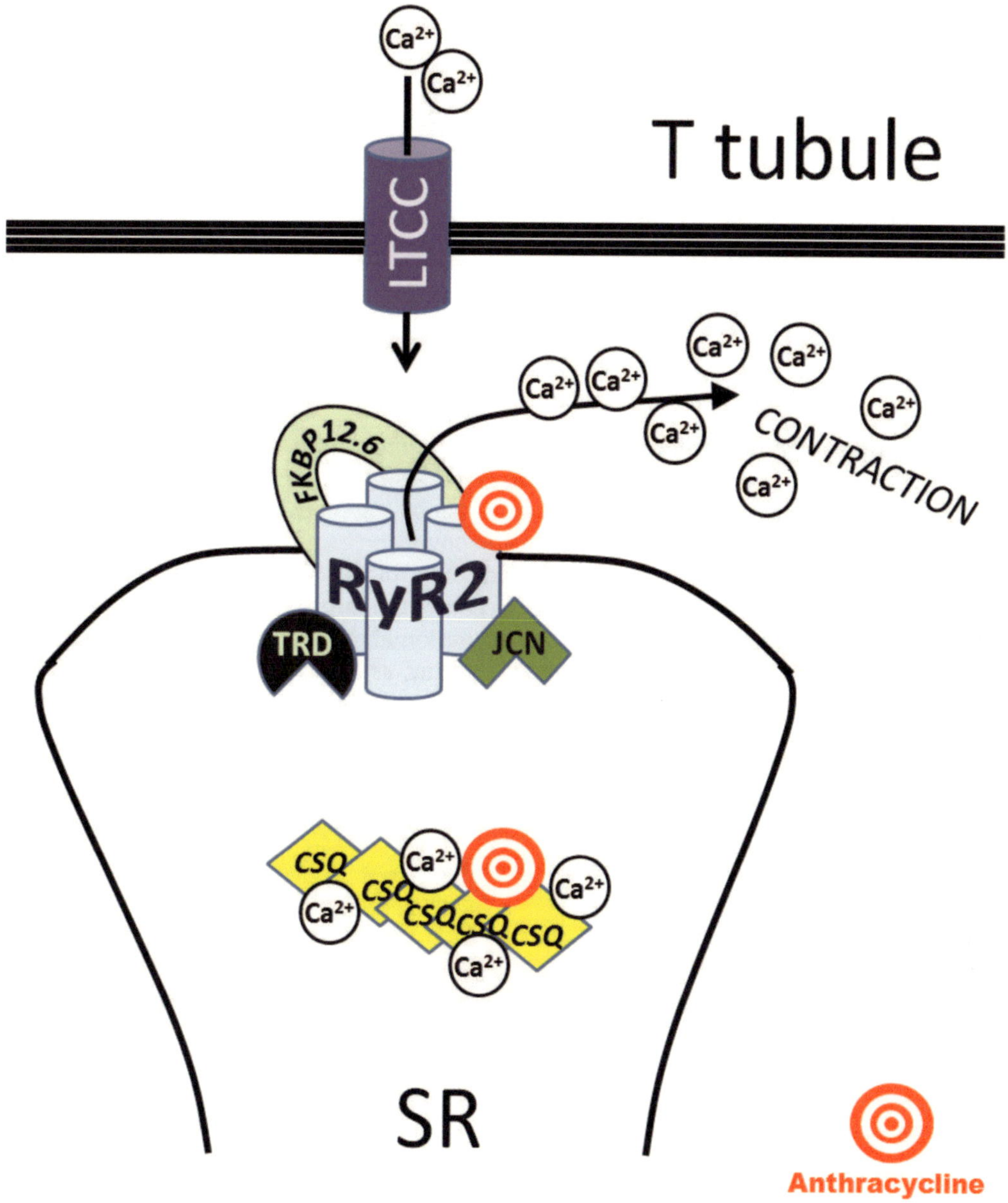

Fig. 1. Potential mechanism of anthracycline induced cardiotoxicity is based on direct binding of anthracycline on cardiac ryanodine receptor (RyR2) and/or calsequestrin (CSQ). The drug may directly modulate the calcium-induced calcium release from sarcoplasmic reticulum (SR). (Other abbreviations: LTCC - L-type Ca^{2+} channel, FKBP12.6 - FK506-binding protein 12.6, TRD - triadin, and JCN – junctin.)

Other suggested cardiotoxicity mechanisms of anthracyclines include impaired expression of various important cardiac proteins and depletion of transcription factors (Boucek et al. 1999; Aries et al. 2004), metabolism of anthracyclines into more hydrophilic and cardiotoxic substances, which subsequently accumulate in cardiomyocytes (Minotti et al. 1996), induction of mitochondrial DNA lessions (Lebrecht et al. 2005), disruption of mitochondrial bioenergetics (Tan et al. 1967), degradation of myofilamental and cytoskeletal proteins (Lim et al. 2004; Chen et al. 2006), interference with various pro-survival kinases (Peng et al. 2005) and some data suggest that the erbB2/neuregulin system might modulate anthracycline-associated cardiac toxicity, as it has been demonstrated that signaling via the erbB2 receptor can modulate doxorubicin-induced oxidative stress and myofibrillar structural damage *in vitro* (Lim t al. 2004; Sawyer et al. 2002; Pentassuglia et al. 2007). Importantly enough, all these proposed cardiotoxic pathways may contribute to cardiac cell damage, ultimately resulting in myocyte death, either by the pathway of necrosis or the pathway of apoptosis (Sawyer et al. 1999).

2.1.2 Therapy and cardioprotection against anthracycline-induced cardiotoxicity

As it is accepted that drug-induced cardiac remodelling is, similarly to other types of cardiac injury, mediated by the activation of the renin-angiotensin-aldosteron system and adrenergic system, treatment with angiotensin-converting enzyme inhibitors, angiotensin receptor blockers, aldosterone antagonists, and beta blockers are consequently used to slow the progression of disease (Mann 1999). Thus, standard treatment for systolic heart failure is indicated for treatment for both asymptomatic and symptomatic cases, with angiotensin-converting enzyme inhibitors in first line, as some trials have suggested that these drugs may reduce the incidence of left ventricular dysfunction in high risk patients after chemotherapy (Wu 2008). However, the management of such patients remains complicated.

Clinicians confront a clinical dilemma as they have to balance the efficacy of longer duration of therapy against the cardiotoxicity associated with higher cumulative doses of anthracyclines. In an effort to prevent or reduce this cardiotoxicity, numerous less cardiotoxic anthracycline analogs have been developed (epirubicin, idarubicin) such as including liposomal anthracyclines (Batist et al. 2001; Muggia and Green 1991; Muggia et al. 1997), and the cumulative and peak doses of anthracycline therapy have been diminished (Legha et al. 1982; Von Hoff et al. 1979). Another cardiotoxicity reducing strategy is based on the use of cardioprotective agents, mainly on those which might reduce oxidative stress and/or may have chelating properties. From those, dexrazoxane (also known as cardioxane) is the most investigated agent (Swain et al. 1997; Wexler et al. 1996). Moreover, it is the only approved cardioprotective agent in anthacycline chemotherapy. Interestingly, dexrazoxane prevents heart damage but there is no evidence for a difference in response rate or survival (van Dalen et al. 2011). Other agents like L-carnitine, probucol, coenzyme Q10, N-acetylcysteine, vitamin E, digoxin, enalapril, phenethylamines, deferoxamine, ethylenediaminetetraacetic acid, superoxide dismutase and monohydroxyethylrutoside are less investigated; however cardioprotective effects have been reported in numerous studies (De Leonardis et al. 1985; Elihu et al. 1998; Guthrie and Gibson 1977; Iarussi et al. 1994; Kawasaki et al. 1992; Silber et al. 2004; Singal et al. 1995; Unverferth et al. 1983; Van Acker et al. 2000). Unfortunately, none of them achieved any clinical relevance as cardioprotective agent.

2.2 Other anti-cancer agents

Several non-anthracycline based anti-cancer drugs have also been associated with significant cardiac side effects. An alkylating agent - cyclophosphamide is mainly cardiotoxic at high doses, such as those used before bone marrow or stem cell transplantation (Meinardi et al. 2000). The reported cardiotoxicity ranges from transient electrocardiographic changes and asymptomatic increases of serum levels of cardiac enzymes to more severe cardiotoxicity such as exudative pericardial effusion, ventricular hypertrophy and fatal myopericarditis and (haemorrhagic) myocardial necrosis. The onset of the latter types of cardiotoxicity is acute, with fatal consequences within 15 days. The cardiotoxic effects of cyclophosphamide probably result from direct influence on the myocardial capillaries and can probably be partly explained by damage to the endothelium with resultant increase in permeability and extravasation of plasma, red blood cells and toxic metabolites (Gottdiener et al. 1981; Fraiser et al. 1991). From the group of antimetabolites (capecitabine, cytarabine, 5-fluorouracil), the cardiotoxicity of 5-fluorouracil is the best described one. It appears to have direct toxic effects on the myocardium, although toxic effects on the coronary arteries are probably the main pathogenetic factor (Meinardi et al. 2000). Necropsy findings in humans who died from fatal myocardial infarction or cardiogenic shock after 5-fluorouracil therapy showed patchy myocardial necrosis and mononuclear inflammation unrelated to the distribution of the coronary arteries (Sasson et al. 1994). A direct interference of 5-fluorouracil with the myocardial cell metabolism leading to cellular hypoxia has been suggested from a study with an isolated perfused rat heart model (Millart et al. 1992). In addition, cases of dilated cardiomyopathy and congestive heart failure have been reported after 5-fluorouracil treatment, also suggesting a direct toxic effect on the myocardium (Schöber et al. 1993; Weidmann et al. 1995). Capecitabine may cause ischaemia and cytarabine may cause pericarditis (Wu 2008). Some risk of cardiovascular toxicity has been attributed to antimicrotubules (paclitaxel, vinca alkaloids) as well. Paclitaxel may cause hypotension or arrhythmias, both supraventricular or ventricular and atrioventricular block, and vinca alkaloids may cause ischaemia (Wu 2008).

Recently, new biological therapy opens new possibilities in the treatment of cancer. New drugs were developed with the goal to specifically inhibit selected targets and to stop cancer cell proliferation and metastasis. These targeted therapies were thought to be more effective than traditional chemotherapeutic treatments and less harmful to non-cancerous cells. However, some of the targets inhibited by these new anti-cancer drugs appear to be important also for the maintenance of cellular homeostasis of normal tissue, in particular during exposure to cytotoxic chemotherapy (Zuppinger et al. 2007). Some of the new biological anti-cancer drugs associated with myocardial contractile dysfunction are trastuzumab, imatinib, and possibly bevacizumab (Slamon et al. 2001; Tan-Chiu et al. 2005; Drímal et al. 2006; Kerkelä et al. 2006). Importantly, most of these new biological therapeutics are not cytotoxic *per se* and, therefore, need to be combined with traditional chemotherapeutics and radiation therapy. Tyrosine kinase inhibitors (sunitinib, imatinib) are small molecule agents that inhibit cellular signalling involved in tumour cell angiogenesis and proliferation. Although this targeted approach results in improved anti-tumour activity and fewer side effects, tyrosine kinases regulating non-cancer functions are also affected, leading to undesired toxic side effects, including heart failure and hypertension (Chu et al. 2007). Trastuzumab is a recombinant IgG monoclonal antibody that binds to the human epidermal growth factor receptor 2 protein and is used for treatment of breast cancer that overexpresses this growth factor. It should be noted that agents like this are still relatively new, and full understanding of long term toxicities is still evolving (Jones et al. 2007). But as expected, the combination of trastuzumab with cytotoxic agents, in particular anthracyclines, bares a significant risk of cardiotoxicity (Slamon et al. 2001; Strasser et al. 2001). Multivariate analysis for the development of cardiac dysfunction in the pivotal trastuzumab trials identified prior or concomitant anthracycline exposure, over 50 years of age, and prior cardiac disease as independent risk factors. Many of these risk factors are similar to those for doxorubicin-induced cardiac dysfunction. However, in contrast to anthracycline-induced cardiomyopathy, trastuzumab-associated cardiac dysfunction appears to be mostly reversible and non-progressive (Ewer and Lippman 2005; Ewer et al. 2005).

2.3 Stimulants

Psychomotor stimulants have a marked influence on mental function and behaviour, producing excitement and euphoria, reduced sensation of fatigue, and an increase in motor activity. Clinically, abuse of stimulants such as cocaine, ephedrine, amphetamines or methamphetamines is associated with cardiovascular action such as tachycardia, supraventricular arrhythmias, ventricular arrhythmias, impaired conduction, hypertensive crises, acute coronary syndromes, shock and cardiac arrest. A number of cellular, animal and autopsy studies, individual case reports and case series suggested that exposures of such drugs are potentially associated with structural and functional changes of myocytes, as well as clinical manifestations of cardiomyopathy and congestive heart failure (Wijetunga et al. 2003; Yeo et al. 2007). The pathogenesis is probably similar to that of catecholamine-induced cardiomyopathy, *i.e.* sympathomimetic action, as for example pathologic similarities between cocaine cardiomyopathy and those seen in pheochromocytomas suggest that chronic adrenergic stimulation may play a role in the development of cardiomyopathy. It is possible that adrenergically driven recurrent hypertensive crises ultimately result in failure of the ventricle in exactly the same way as essential hypertension, in particular when combined with inappropriate life style (Crean and Pohl 2004). Apart from that, *in vitro* experiments showed that continuous exposure to a low concentration of methamphetamine may directly facilitate the development of cellular hypertrophy (Maeno et al. 2000).

2.3.1 Amphetamines and metamphetamines

Clinically, these drugs cause central nervous system stimulation that may induce euphoria, increase alertness, intensify emotions, increase aggression, alter self-esteem, and allegedly increase sexuality. Both oral and intravenous misuses are well documented. Deaths related to intoxications from these drugs have been associated with assaults, suicides, homicides, accidents, driving impairment, and maternal-fetal and infant exposures (Albertson et al. 1999). Pharmacologically, these drugs are substrates for the neuronal uptake transporters for norepinephrine, serotonin and dopamine, and cause release of these mediators from nerve terminals in the brain. Indirectly, the hyperstimulated neurons can stimulate various other pathways. Changes in mood, excitation level, motor movement, and appetite appear to be more directly mediated by central dopaminergic alterations. Serotonin alterations may also contribute to the amphetamine-related mood changes, psychotic behavior, and aggressiveness. Cardiovascular symptoms, including chest pain, palpitations, and dyspnea,

are common. The exact frequency of such events is unknown but a clinical study showed that acute coronary syndrome is common (25%) in patients hospitalized for chest pain after methamphetamine use and the frequency of other potentially life-threatening cardiac complications is not negligible. These events occur in patients with and without underlying coronary disease and may involve multiple pathophysiologic mechanisms (Turnipseed et al. 2003). When considering cardiomyopathy, the incidence of 18% has been described in subjects abusing methamphetamine (Wijetunga et al. 2003). In other clinical study, methamphetamine use was documented in 40% of young patients with cardiomyopathy and was more severe compared to other non-ischemic cardiomyopathies. This findings support the hypothesis that methamphetamine use may be a possible cause of unexplained cardiomyopathy in young patients because its widespread use (Yeo et al. 2007).
Acute and chronic cardiomyopathy from abuse is thought to be secondary to both direct cardiac toxicity and indirect amphetamine-induced hypertension, necrosis, and ischemia (Albertson et al. 1999). The 3,4-methylenedioxymethamphetamine, commonly known as ecstasy, can cause myocardial infarction, arrhythmias, and cardiomyopathy (Mizia-Stec et al. 2008; Figueredo 2011). Animal studies showed that repeated methamphetamine administration may directly induce cellular hypertrophy of cardiomyocytes, myocarditis with inflammatory infiltrates and areas of necrosis, and consequently, may cause eccentric left ventricular dilation and diastolic dysfunction, as well as contractile dysfunction in myocytes (Shenouda et al. 2009). High dose administration may lead to cardiac function disorder with disruption of microtubules and actin (Maeno et al. 2000). It was suggested that metabolites are responsible for cardiotoxicity (Shenouda et al. 2008) as 3,4-methylenedioxymethamphetamine is metabolized to catechols that can undergo redox cycling, producing reactive oxygen and nitrogen species (Bolton et al. 2000). This suggests that potential mechanisms of 3,4-methylenedioxymethamphetamine-induced cardiomyopathy are related to oxidative stress, as well as catecholaminergic stimulation. Additionally, the recreational use of 3,4-methylenedioxymethamphetamine is often characterized by a repeated pattern of frequent drug applications (binge) followed by a period of abstinence what significantly alter cardiovascular and cardiovascular reflex function and produce cardiac toxicity (Badon et al. 2002). On the other hand, experimental as well as clinical data suggest that cardiac lessions are reversible after withdrawal of methamphetamine (Islam et al. 1995; Lopez et al. 2009).

2.3.2 Cocaine

Cocaine (benzoylmethylecgonine) is an alkaloid extracted from the leaves of the *Erythroxylon coca*, a plant native to South America. It was first used as a local anesthetics in 1884 and, interestingly, was used as an ingredient in a popular cola beverage in the early 20th century (Maraj et al. 2010). Cocaine inhibits catecholamine uptake by the norepinephrine and dopamine transporters at the presynaptic adrenergic terminals, causing an accumulation of catecholamines at the postsynaptic receptor, thereby enhancing peripheral effects of sympathetic nerve activity and producing a marked psychomotor stimulant effect. Its effects resemble those of amphetamines, although it has less tendency to produce stereotyped behaviour, delusions, hallucinations and paranoia (Johanson and Fischman 1989). It also causes the release of norepinephrine and epinephrine from the adrenal medulla and thus acting as a powerful sympathomimetic agent that can cause significant central and peripheral vasoconstriction. Cocaine has multiple cardiovascular and hematologic effects that likely contribute to the development of myocardial ischemia and/or myocardial infarction. Cocaine causes increased heart rate and blood pressure in a dose-dependent fashion, as well as increased cardiac index and dP/dt. The chronotropic effects of cocaine use are intensified in the setting of alcohol use, as well as smoking. By increasing heart rate, blood pressure, and contractility, cocaine leads to increased myocardial demand. Importantly, cocaine causes coronary vasoconstriction and thrombosis and so decreases oxygen supply and induces myocardial ischemia through a variety of mechanisms (McCord et al. 2008). Acute cellular effects include changes in calcium flux that are similar to other cardiac toxins, including digoxin. Increased intracellular concentrations of calcium have been suggested as a cause of depolarisation of the cardiac membrane and, therefore, a trigger of arrhythmias.

When misused chronically, cocaine administration can reduce left ventricular function, increase end-systolic wall stress and can cause a rare form of cardiomyopathy. The exact incidence of cocaine-induced cardiomyopathy is unknown and likely underreported. The medical literature to date consists mostly of case reports describing young men with a history of cocaine abuse and reversible cardiomyopathy (Awtry and Philippides 2010). In a review of 1278 cases of dilated cardiomyopathy patients, 10 cases were related to cocaine use (Felker et al. 1999). In a study of asymptomatic apparently healthy cocaine users, left ventricular systolic dysfunction was diagnosed in 7% by radionuclide angiography performed two weeks after cocaine use (Bertolet et al. 1990). The exact mechanism by which cocaine abuse causes cardiomyopathy is not fully understood. Furthermore, the amount and duration of cocaine use necessary to develop cocaine cardiomyopathy is currently unclear. Several pharmacologic effects of cocaine appear to be directly and indirectly related to its toxic myocardial action. Importantly, cocaine has been estimated to cause the development of cardiac hypertrophy without associated increases in arterial blood pressure, heart rate, renin, aldosterone, or cortisol, indicating a direct action on cardiac tissue remodelling and leading to heart failure. Nevertheless, whether it is a consequence of cocaine cardiomyopathy or ischemic cardiomyopathy due to cocaine vascular effects remains unclear. Finally, as direct putative pathophysiologic mechanisms of cocaine-induced cardiomyopathy and myocarditis, the following has been introduced: hyperadrenergic state produces contraction band necrosis in myocardium, direct toxic effect of cocaine on myofibrils and interstitial fibrosis, and hypersensitivity reaction of myocardium to cocaine. Other mechanisms include myocardial ischemia and infarction as a consequence of increased sympathomimetic activity with increased myocardial oxygen demand, altered calcium flux across myocyte cell membrane, altered vascular endothelium integrity (reduced prostacyclin production), increased platelet thromboxane production and increased plasminogen activator inhibitor production (Maraj et al. 2010; Awtry and Philippides 2010).

Four mechanisms have been described in more detail (Awtry and Philippides 2010). All of them alters cardiac function acutely but may lead to cardiac injury in a long-term fashion. First, promotion of intracoronary thrombus formation is widely recognised. Cocaine ingestion stimulates platelet hyperaggregability and increased thromboxane production, often in the setting of coronary vasospasm. These physiologic effects promote acute intracoronary thrombus formation and myocardial ischemic events and account, in part, for the increased incidence of myocardial infarction noted in cocaine users. Acute coronary ischemia and extensive or recurrent myocardial infarction also contribute to the left ventricular dysfunction and cardiomyopathy associated with cocaine abuse. However, many cocaine abusers with severe regional or global left ventricular dysfunction do not have a clear history of obstructive coronary disease or myocardial infarction. Thus, myocardial dysfunction can result from transient ischemic insults, perhaps in the setting of vasospasm or spontaneous coronary thrombosis. Alternatively, it is likely that nonischemic mechanisms of myocyte injury may also contribute. Second, sympathomimetic effects have to be taking into account as cocaine acts as a powerful sympathomimetic agent. Stimulation of the beta-adrenergic receptors in myocardial tissue results in increased contractility and heart rate, whereas stimulation of the alpha-adrenergic receptors in coronary and peripheral arteries results in increased coronary resistance, decreased coronary blood flow, elevated blood pressure, and increased myocardial wall stress (Kloner et al. 1992). Animal studies suggest that the increased wall stress seen in acute cocaine intoxication plays an important role in the acute depression of left ventricular function. Following cocaine infusion, ejection-phase indices of left ventricular function are reduced but the effects are attributable to increased wall stress not to reduced contractility (Mehta et al. 1995). Pathologic studies showed similarities between cocaine cardiomyopathy and chronic catecholamine stimulation (Tazelaar et al. 1987). Third, increased calcium flux into myocardial cells, and fourth, enhanced oxidative stress have been suggested as co-factors (Isabelle et al. 2007). Importantly, cocaine may alter cardiac electrophysiology what results in electrocardiological abnormalities, as evidenced in numerous experimental studies. The drug prolongs the PR, QRS, QT, and QTc durations, prolongs atrioventricular nodal conduction time and maximum sinoatrial conduction time, and may trigger frequent atrial extrasystoles and atrial fibrillation and tachycardia as well as transient ventricular tachycardia (Kloner et al. 1992).

2.3.3 Ephedra (Ma Huang)

The dietary supplement ephedra, also known as *Ma Huang* and obtained from the *Ephedra sinica* plant, contains 2 alkaloids - ephedrine and its enantiomer, pseudoephedrine. In traditional Chinese medicine this plant has been used for millennia to treat disorders such as asthma, upper respiratory illnesses and seasonal allergies. In recent years ephedra has gained tremendous popularity as a diet drug because of its biochemical activity as a stimulant and a pro-thermogenic agent. The stimulant activity of ephedra suppresses appetite while the pro-thermogenic property increases the body's metabolism, all leading to improved weight loss. However, over the past decade a number of well-documented reports of ischemic stroke and adverse cardiac events such as myocardial infarction, sudden death, and cardiomyopathy linked to ephedra have lead to a FDA ban of the drug in April 2004 as a dietary supplement (Lillegard and Porterfield 2010). Pharmacologically, ephedra increases catecholamines at synaptic areas in the brain and heart and directly stimulates alpha- and beta-adrenergic receptors. Thus, it can increase heart rate, blood pressure, cardiac output, and peripheral resistance. Coronary artery spasm and pro-arrhythmic effects can account for acute events and death. Prolonged catecholamine excess with long-term ephedra use is one likely underlying mechanism for cardiomyopathy (Figueredo 2011). Importantly, ephedra is often co-abused with anabolic-androgenic steroids (Clark and Schofield 2005; Achar et al. 2010).

2.4 Anabolic-androgenic steroids

The adrenals and the testes produce various compounds that stimulate androgen receptors. Dihydrotestosterone and testosterone are the most potent, but precursors such as dehydroepiandrosterone and androstenedione also have androgenic effects. 17-carbon androgenic precursors from either the adrenals or the gonads can be converted to testosterone by 17-hydroxysteroid dehydrogenase in the testis or ovary. In target tissues where intracellular enzymes are present, the action of testosterone is mediated by metabolism. The enzyme 5alpha-reductase produces the potent androgen dihydrotestosterone in the prostate, skin, sebaceous glands and brain. Due to this tissue-specific expression of 5alpha-reductase, androgenic effects on prostate growth and male pattern baldness are largely mediated by dihydrotestosterone. Conclusively, testosterone is irreversibly converted by the enzyme 5alpha-reductase to 5alpha-dihydrotestosterone, which binds with greater affinity to the androgen receptor, or by aromatase to oestradiol, which binds to the oestrogen receptor (Kicman 2008). All steroids that are anabolic are derivatives of testosterone (Hartgens and Kuipers 2004) and are androgenic as well as anabolic, as they stimulate growth and function of male reproductive tract. Individual drugs vary in their balance of anabolic:androgen activity but none of the currently available drugs are purely anabolic. Derivatives or structural modifications of testosterone differ by its pharmacokinetics, bioavailability, or, as mentioned above, balance of androgenic to anabolic activity. The large group of anabolic-androgenic steroids include testosterone itself, all of the derivatives that are used clinically, as well as numerous plant products that at least claim to possess anabolic actions (Kuhn 2002). Importantly, the group include many agents with chemical structures derived from cholesterol that are synthesized in the liver and then metabolized to anabolic-androgenic steroids. Their structure resembles that of corticosteroids, explaining some similarities in actions in terms of renal sodium retention and hypertension (Achar et al. 2010).

2.4.1 Therapeutic use and abuse of anabolic-androgenic steroids

Predominantly, anabolic-androgenic steroids are used in the treatment of disorders of puberty, prostatic disease and hirsutism. Testosterone replacement therapy is for hypogonal men who demonstrate clinical (reduced shaving frequency, exercise endurance, libido and testicular size) and laboratory findings (reduced free or free plus albumin-bound testosterone). Testosterone replacement therapy improves physical performance, sexual function, mood and lipid profiles within four weeks in most cases. The orally active androgens methyltestosterone and fluoxymesterone are not commonly used for androgen replacement, but are commonly abused by body builders. Other orally active androgenic steroids (testolactone, oxandrolone, stanozolol, oxymetholone) and intramuscular preparations (nandrolone) have androgenic effects and are used clinically for their anabolic actions in cancer and refractory anaemia. Newly, testosterone may have therapeutic benefit and be cardioprotective in heart failure for a number of reasons. Anabolic/catabolic imbalance, which favours catabolism, is a key pathological feature of patients with severe chronic heart failure and anabolic deficiency is an important component of the imbalance (Jankowska et al. 2006). In addition, it has been shown that pharmacological augmentation of anabolic drive can result in favourable changes in the body composition, sexual function and psychological status of aging men. Moreover, testosterone is viewed as a potential natural tonic for the failing heart (Pugh et al. 2000) and testosterone therapy has been proposed as a useful add-on treatment for men with congestive heart failure as its administration increases cardiac output acutely (Pugh et al. 2003; Pugh et al. 2004; Rauchhaus et al. 2006). Indeed, there is a clinical evidence that testosterone replacement therapy regimen in men with congestive heart failure was followed by improvement in NYHA class and functional capacity (Allan and McLachlan 2004; Malkin et al. 2006).

People have been taking testosterone to restore 'vitality' since the efficacy of some hormonal component of the testes was first described by Brown-Sequard in 1889. He reported the reversal of his own aging by self-injection of a testicular extract, thereby stimulated a flurry of experimentation into the putative anti-aging effects of testicular hormones long before the identity of testosterone was confirmed. The first use to improve athletic performance occurred shortly thereafter, in 1896. A contemporary of Brown-Sequard self-administered testicular extract, then measured his finger strength (Kuhn 2002). In modern age, anabolic-androgenic steroids, which include more than 30 natural and synthetic derivatives of testosterone, were designed in 1939 to treat conditions such as eunuchoid syndromes, impotence, depression, starvation, and cryptorchidism. The first suggestion that these drugs might enhance physical performance occurred later that same year. Mass trials conducted by Nazi Germany on their own soldiers during World War II, combined with concurrent animal studies, provided compelling data to support these theories. During the 1954 Vienna world weight lifting championships, the Russian national team introduced the use of anabolic-androgenic steroids as ergogenic aids. By the 1964 Olympics, athletes from around the world were consuming the drugs. In a survey of weight lifters at the 1968 United States Olympic Training camp, 100% had taken some form of the substance. During the 1972 Olympics held in Munich, 68% of those competing in middle or short distance and field events admitted to having taken anabolic-androgenic steroids as part of their preparation for the games. Proliferation of anabolic-androgenic steroids use throughout international competition had reached such epidemic proportions that by the 1976 Olympic games they were declared banned substances (Sullivan et al. 1998). After that, anabolic-androgenic steroids continued to be used clandestinely by Olympic athletes, and its use spread quickly to high school, intercollegiate, and professional sports. According to clinical data, self-reported rates of abuse in bodybuilders and powerlifters to enhance performance range from 29% to 67% (Curry and Wagman 1999; Achar et al. 2010). Also, there is now widespread use among non-competitive bodybuilders, recreational athletes, and those who simply desire an improved physique (Dhar et al. 2005). Thus, the risk of incidence of adverse effects in general population is relatively high. In general, anabolic-androgenic steroids are abused by athletes primarily to increase lean muscle mass, enhance appearance, and improve performance. Increased cellular protein synthesis results in build-up of tissue (anabolism), especially in muscles. A variety of anabolic-androgenic steroids are often taken simultaneously (so called 'stacking'), and in doses which result in 10–100 fold increases in androgen concentrations. Administration regimens usually involve a 6–12 week cycle and are often administered in a 'pyramidal' fashion, with doses tapering from low to high to low (Payne et al. 2004). Abused substances include testosterone, its 17-beta esters, and those based on modified steroid rings (including 17-alpha derivatives).

2.4.2 Cardiac injury

Several adverse effects of steroids have been described, predominantly when taking inappropriately. In healthy men, high-dose testosterone or synthetic androgens produce small increases in muscle mass and exercise performance, while posing the risks of aggressive mood disorder, priapism, erythrocytosis, oligospermia and worsened lipid profile. Adverse hepatic effects such as blood-filled hepatic cysts (*peliosis hepatis*), hepatic adenomas and cholestatic hepatic injury have been reported primarily with oral synthetic androgens. In elderly men, androgen supplementation increases serum concentrations of prostate-specific antigen and may worsen prostate hypertrophy.

Testosterone is a potent ligand of the human androgen receptor in muscles but also directly modulates transcription, translation, and enzymatic function in numerous other tissues (Sullivan et al. 1998). Consequently, the adverse effects from use of anabolic-androgenic steroids are widespread and affect multiple organ systems, including the heart and vessels. Several actions on cardiovascular system, and predominantly on heart, have been reported. Anabolic-androgenic steroids share with endogenous steroids influences on left ventricular hypertrophic response through direct actions on the androgen receptor (Marsh et al. 1998) what is a DNA-linked ligand-activated transcription factor with homology to mineralocorticoid and progesterone steroid receptors. Androgen receptors are ubiquitously expressed, found not only in skeletal muscle cells but also in cardiac myocytes. Anabolic-androgenic steroids can cause hypertension, dyslipidemia, and impaired fasting glucose, as well as alterations in heart structure, including left ventricular hypertrophy and dilation, and impaired contraction and relaxation. Potential sequelae include hypertension, acute myocardial infarction, sudden cardiac death, abnormal cardiac repolarisation with QT interval prolongation, ventricular fibrillation triggered by exercise, atrial fibrillation, cardiac tamponade, development of dilative cardiomyopathy, and heart failure at a dose-dependent manner (Hausmann et al. 1998; Stolt et al. 1999; Du Toit et al. 2005; Karila et al. 2003; Figueredo 2011). Several case reports have linked adverse cardiac events and anabolic-androgenic steroids abuse in healthy young athletes (Stergiopoulos et al. 2008; Ahlgrim and Guglin 2009). Recently, 49 reports describing a total of 1,467 athletes has been extensively reviewed (Achar et al. 2010). In aggregate, studies evaluated lipoprotein concentrations in 643 subjects, blood pressure in 348, left ventricular dimensions in 561, and sudden death in 102. As concluded, otherwise healthy young athletes abusing anabolic-androgenic steroids may show elevated levels of low-density lipoprotein and low levels of high-density lipoprotein. Although data are conflicting, anabolic-androgenic steroids have also been linked with elevated systolic and diastolic blood pressure and with left ventricular hypertrophy that may persist after anabolic-androgenic steroid cessation. Nevertheless, mortality appears to be significantly higher in anabolic-androgenic steroids abusers than in non-abusing athletes.

The potential pathophysiological mechanisms responsible for adverse cardiac effects are incompletely understood. Four mechanisms of anabolic-androgenic steroids-induced cardiovascular toxicity have been proposed: atherogenic, thrombotic, vasospastic, and direct myocardial injury (Melchert and Welder 1995). As already mentioned, anabolic-androgenic steroids bind to androgen receptors in the heart but in arteries as well, and physiologic levels (*e.g.*, of testosterone) may have a beneficial effect on coronary arteries via endothelial release of nitric oxide and inhibition of vascular smooth muscle tone. Conversely, animal studies show that administration of high doses of anabolic-androgenic steroids may reverse this vasodilator response and lead to growth-promoting effects on cardiac tissue, as seen in hypertrophic cardiomyopathy, followed by apoptotic cell death. These effects are likely associated with increased intracellular calcium influx and calcium release from the sarcoplasmic reticulum. This increase of intracellular calcium may be directly responsible for the development of cardiac hypertrophy as well as for the activation of apoptosis (Lieberherr and Grosse 1994; Zaugg et al. 2001). Postmortem histopathological findings of young anabolic-androgenic steroid abusers include cardiac hypertrophy, what seems to be dose-dependent and reversible (Ahlgrim and Guglin 2009). In addition, several other complications have been described, such as myocardial and endocardial fibrosis, cardiac steatosis, myocardial coagulation necrosis, decreased inotropic capacity of the myocardium, and irreversibly reduced compliance of the left ventricle, and coronary atheroma (Figueredo 2011). In other studies, endomyocardial biopsy specimens have revealed increased fibrous tissue and fat droplets in the myocardium of anabolic-androgenic steroid abusers (Nieminen et al. 1996). Direct cell injury occurs by disruption of myocardial mitochondria and induction of intrafibrillar collagen dysplasia. Cell injury ensues, and scar tissue replaces dead cells, leading to fibrosis and the potential for ventricular arrhythmias. Development of hypertension also occurs, followed by left ventricular hypertrophy and structural changes to the ventricular wall. Increased ventricular septal thickness develops rapidly and is disproportionate to the expected degree of compensatory hypertrophy from resistance training. Other studies reveal increased incidence of diastolic dysfunction, greater left ventricular posterior wall thickness, and greater left ventricular end-diastolic dimensions. In this setting, sudden death may have been caused by vasospasm potentiated by diastolic dysfunction–mediated ischemia (Dhar et al. 2005). Cardiomyopathy, cardiomegaly, and biventricular dilatation induced by anabolic-androgenic steroids can occur as a result of remodelling after myocyte injury and have been noted to be reversible after discontinuation of anabolic-androgenic steroids administration (Hausmann et al. 1998). However, it is still unclear whether such detrimental effects are directly associated with the action of anabolic-androgenic steroids or they are a consequence of co-presence of developing hypertension, hyperdynamics in cardiovascular system and dysbalance in blood lipids. Moreover, athletes abusing anabolic-androgenic steroids often exhibit left ventricular hypertrophy and because the hypertrophy may relate to increased afterload from isometric exercise, the interpretation of cardiac hypertrophy in elite athletes who admit to anabolic-androgenic steroids abuse is complex. Possible associations between anabolic-androgenic steroids and left ventricular hypertrophy may be explained as secondary to hypertension or as a direct effect on the myocardium. Notably, studies in isolated human myocytes have shown that anabolic-androgenic steroids bind to androgen receptors and may directly cause hypertrophy. It was clearly demonstrated that mammalian cardiac myocytes from hearts of different species and both sexes express the androgen receptor gene (Marsh et al. 1998). Androgens are capable of mediating a hypertrophic response of cultured adult myocytes of a magnitude nearly that of the most efficacious hypertrophic stimuli identified for heart. Consequently, androgens must be considered among the neuroeffectors, paracrine factors, and hormones that act directly on the cardiac myocyte and regulate the cardiac hypertrophic response. Indeed, a clinical study suggests a distinct form of left ventricular hypertrophy, as the abuse of anabolic-androgenic steroids in weight-lifters determines some alterations of the myocardial textural parameters when analyzed by videodensitometry (Di Bello et al. 1999). In contrast to these definite findings, studies comparing echocardiographic variables between anabolic-androgenic steroids using and nonusing strength athletes have not yielded unequivocal results (Ahlgrim and Guglin 2009). Some studies have not demonstrated any structural difference with abuse (Thompson et al. 1992) or showed that the myocardial remodeling is independent from anabolic-androgenic steroid use in power athletes (Dickerman et al. 1998). Considering the high prevalence of anabolic-androgenic steroids abuse in population, the number of cases featuring associated cardiac illness reported in current literature appears rather small. Thus the type or the intensity of training might play an important role (Ahlgrim and Guglin 2009). It remains open, whether the use of anabolic-androgenic steroids is causally related to these events or is just coincidental. Some animal studies suggest that these adverse effects cardiac muscle are causal and not coincidental. In adult rat cardiomyocytes *in vitro*, anabolic-androgenic steroids induce apoptotic cell death increasing the expression of the pro-apoptotic oncogene Bax-alpha in a dose-dependent manner (Zaugg et al. 2001). When studying the cardiac cell ultrastructure, mitochondria and myofibrils show changes similar to those observed in early heart failure, *i.e.* swollen and elongated mitochondria with sparse matrix and decreased number of cristae, and myofibrils show either disintegration and widened and twisted Z-bands or a complete dissolution of the sarcomeric units (Behrendt and Boffin 1977). Long-term testosterone administration results in myocarditis characterized by interstitial oedema, round cell infiltration, and fibrosis (Imai et al. 1978). Interestingly enough, cardiac tissue was protected from testosterone cardiotoxicity by chelating agent dexrazoxan indicating that oxidative stress might be involved (Belhani et al. 2009). Additionally, it was showed that ischemia/reperfusion injury is increased when cardiac hypertrophy develops after chronically administered nandrolone (Penna et al. 2011).

Additionally, in coronary artery disease, there is a contradiction between a documented risk and the evidence that tends to suggest just the opposite. Some short-term interventional studies show that testosterone produces a modest but consistent improvement in cardiac ischemia over placebo, comparable to the effects of existing antianginal drugs as intracoronary artery infusion of testosterone causes coronary artery dilatation and not constriction as previously thought (Liu et al. 2003). Notably, reduced testosterone levels were associated with coronary artery narrowing premature atherosclerosis, increased visceral adipose tissue, hyperinsulinemia, insulin resistance, increased body mass index, reduced high density lipoprotein levels and other risk factors for myocardial infarction (Bain 2007). Similarly in experiments, administration of testosterone significantly improves recovery from global ischemia what might be associated with an attenuation of reperfusion induced intracellular calcium overload (Callies et al. 2003). In contrast to that, testosterone overdose led to increase of apoptosis of cardiac cells after ischemia/reperfusion experiments and it was suggested that testosterone has inhibitory effects on cardioprotective Heat-Shock Protein 72 expression by modulating transcription, through testosterone receptor-mediated genomic mechanisms (Kohno et al. 2007). Similarly, testosterone decreases myocardial function after ischemia/reperfusion injury what is attributed to its proinflammatory and/or proapoptotic properties (Wang et al. 2005). It was shown that testosterone decreases the activation of cardioprotective pathway of the Signal Transducer and Activator of Transduction-3 following ischemia/reperfusion injuries (Wang et al. 2009).

3. Other cardiotoxic substances

3.1 Alcohol

Similarly to stimulants, the abuse of alcohol, as a substance affecting the central nervous system, has long recognised direct toxic effects on the heart (Bing 1978). Ethanol may induce 1) direct dose-dependent myocardial damage manifested as acute effects on rhythm and left-ventricular function, and/or 2) chronic progressive left ventricular dysfunction that may remain subclinical for a long time and is known as alcoholic cardiomyopathy.

Acute harmful drinking may induce 1) changes in cardiac contractility with systolic and diastolic dysfunction, and 2) rhythm disturbances, including sudden death (Urbano-Márquez and Fernández-Solà, 2004). The acute cardiodepressive action of ethanol is well established as it reduces the force of contraction of human heart when plasma levels exceed 75 mg per 100 ml. Such an acute intoxication causes reversible myocardial dysfunction, *i.e.* it has a direct negative inotropic action with a reversible dose-dependent decrease in myocardial contractility. Most studies of isolated myocardium have sought to explain these acute and reversible changes in the force of contraction by using pharmacologic concentrations of ethanol in the 1% (by volume) range (Knochel 1983; Guarnieri and Lakatta 1990). These studies have demonstrated that ethanol has multiple effects on the myocardium, and as such could depress the force of contraction at several points in the process of electromechanical coupling, probably at the level of the myofilaments. The effect was found to be reversible by increasing the amount of calcium presented to the myofilaments or by washing out the ethanol (Guarnieri and Lakatta 1990). This cardiodepresive action of ethanol is evidenced in experimental models designed with autonomic blockade, heart denervation, or isolated cells. On the other hand, negative inotropic action of ethanol is often masked by indirect actions resulting from an enhanced release of catecholamines *in vivo*. Remarkably, the acute cardio-depressant effect of alcohol usually has fewer clinical consequences in non-alcoholic patients with normal cardiac function, but may be more relevant in patients with previous cardiac disease or in patients with alcoholic cardiomyopathy. In these patients, episodes of heart failure may be induced by acute alcohol poisoning. When considering chronotropy, the acute negative chronotropic effect with combination of augmented release of catecholamines may induce a variety of arrhythmias, known as the 'Holiday Heart' arrhythmias, with paroxysmal atrial fibrillations and ventricular premature depolarisations (Ettinger 1984). The prolongation of conduction times and a heterogeneous increase in the refractory period may be directly associated with propensity of arrhythmias. Chronic alcoholism, acute abstinence from ethanol and coexistence of electrolyte deficiencies are strong co-factors increasing the pro-arrhythmogenicity of ethanol abuse. Moreover the presence of chronic cardiomyopathy increases the risk of arrhythmias such as ventricular fibrillation or even sudden cardiac death.

Long-standing ethanol consumption may induce more important deleterious effects on the myocardium what is usually described as alcoholic cardiomyopathy manifesting as cardiac hypertrophy, disrupting contractile function and myofibrillary architecture. When comparing alcoholics with healthy controls, the alcoholics show a lower ejection fraction, a lower mean shortening fraction, a greater mean end-diastolic diameter and left ventricular enlargement. One third of the alcoholics have an ejection fraction of 55 percent or less, and when analysed using endomyocardial biopsy specimens those patients show histologically defined changes of cardiomyopathy (Urbano-Márquez et al. 1989). The chronic ventricular dysfunction develops independently of other factors such as malnutrition or vitamin deficiencies, with both systolic and diastolic dysfunction, manifested as a decrease in left-ventricular ejection fraction and disturbances in left-ventricular relaxation, respectively. These effects may first be subclinical and, later, overt clinical alcoholic dilated cardiomyopathy with left ventricular or congestive heart failure may appear. In general, one-third to one-half of alcohol consumers, in doses higher than 100 g/day for a minimum of 10 years, is affected by progressive diastolic and systolic dysfunction.

A disproportionately large majority of reported cases of alcoholic cardiomyopathy are men. In line with this, the female gender is believed to be protected from cardiovascular morbidity because of hormones (so called 'oestrogen umbrella' effect). However, this seems to be false in the case of chronic ethanol consumption. As shown in a clinical study, a third of the alcoholic women had evidence of cardiomyopathy what is comparable to men.

Despite the fact that the mean lifetime dose of alcohol in female alcoholics is only 60% that in male alcoholics, cardiomyopathy is as common in female alcoholics as in male alcoholics. Ejection fractions in women inversely correlate with the total lifetime dose of ethanol, whereas the left ventricular mass shows a direct correlation. Similarly to women, ejection fractions also correlate inversely with the total lifetime dose of ethanol in men. However, the threshold dose for the development of cardiomyopathy is considerably less in women than in men, and the decline in the ejection fraction with increasing alcohol dose is steeper. This indicates that women are more sensitive than men to the toxic effects of alcohol on cardiac muscle (Urbano-Márquez et al. 1995).

Importantly, diastolic dysfunction is the earliest sign of subclinical alcoholic cardiomyopathy. Symptoms of alcoholic cardiomyopathy are similar to other causes of low-output dilated cardiomyopathies, with shortness of breath and early fatigue during exercise, progressing to attacks of breathlessness, orthopnea, and paroxysmal nocturnal dyspnea. Negative dromotropism and lowering of the threshold level for ventricular fibrillation have been observed in chronic drinkers, leading to ventricular fibrillation and sudden death. Alcoholism also decrease the myocardial capacity at increased cardiac activity, resulting in shortness of breath due to congestion in the pulmonary vessels. Interestingly, although the development of alcoholic cardiomyopathy is independent of liver function parameters, alcoholics with cardiomyopathy have a higher incidence of liver cirrhosis. As showed in clinical study, alcoholics with diagnosed cardiomyopathy have a higher prevalence of cirrhosis than unselected alcoholics without heart disease. Similarly, actively drinking alcoholics with cirrhosis show impaired cardiac performance, whereas abstaining alcoholics with liver disease tend to manifest normal cardiac function (Estruch et al. 1995).

As already mentioned, the long-term heavy alcohol consumption (of any beverage type) is the leading cause of a nonischemic, dilated cardiomyopathy (Piano 2002). However, there appears to be a biphasic cardiovascular effect based on the chronic dose of alcohol ingested. At low to moderate doses, studies suggest that alcohol has a favourable impact on cardiovascular outcomes, *i.e.* lower incidence of myocardial infarctions and an improved survival. At chronic high-dose intake of alcohol, there is a direct relationship to elevated blood pressure. Also, prolonged exposure to alcohol increases the likelihood of developing congestive heart failure. The exact duration and intensity of alcohol consumption preceding preclinical and symptomatic heart failure is not definitively known. It is estimated that a minimum of 10 years of exposure to excessive alcohol intake leads to the onset of heart failure. However, this link to duration and amount of alcohol consumption is weak. Some heavy users of alcohol never develop a cardiomyopathy, while others who ingest only a modest amount can be at risk for developing a cardiomyopathy. Men may be more susceptible to this risk. Concurrent smoking, hypertension, and malnutrition appear highly associated with the increased risk for developing an alcoholic cardiomyopathy. The incidence of alcohol as a major contributor to cardiomyopathy has been reported to be in the range of 20%-30%, emphasizing the clinical need to recognize the risk and contribution of alcohol in heart failure patients (Lee and Regan 2002). Some studies have observed asymptomatic cardiac dysfunction in patients reporting consumption more than 90 g/day of alcohol (8–21 standard drinks) with an average duration of drinking of 15 years. The disease is characterised by ventricular dilation and systolic dysfunction, in the absence of other causative factors such as coronary disease. In preclinical stages of alcoholic cardiomyopathy, ventricular enlargement and diastolic dysfunction can be observed on echocardiography

(Piano 2002; Wu 2008). Although alcoholic cardiomyopathy may be reversible after abstention, severe cases may still progress into congestive heart failure despite a cessation of alcohol use.
The pathophysiological mechanisms underlying alcoholic cardiomyopathy are poorly understood and diverse pathogenic theories have been postulated about the mechanisms of alcohol-induced cardiac muscle damage. Except the effects of ethanol on blood lipids and systemic blood pressure, they likely involve direct myocyte injury and several direct cellular, subcellular, and molecular derangements of cardiac tissue. In past (Bing 1978), several mechanisms have been proposed such as mitochondrial effects (decreased respiratory function, loss of mitochondrial enzymes, deterioration of ultrastructure), decreased calcium uptake by sarcoplasmic reticulum, altered myocardial lipid metabolism (triglyceride accumulation, decreased fatty acid oxidation), effects by formation of acetate and acetaldehyde, non-thrombotic myocardial infarctions and nutritional defects (thiamine deficiency, protein deficiency). It was previously supposed that malnutrition (electrolyte or vitamin deficiencies) is the main pathogenic factors. However, experimental and clinical studies have clearly demonstrated that ethanol itself is a direct noxious agent to heart in a progressive, cumulative, and dose-dependent manner, and its effects are independent of nutritional, vitamin, or mineral factors. According to current knowledge, the main relevant pathogenic mechanisms of alcohol-induced damage are due to interference in carbohydrate metabolism, protein synthesis, changes in oxidative status and mitochondrial function, disruption of transduction signals, and induction of apoptosis (Urbano-Márquez and Fernández-Solà, 2004). Alcohol alters the permeability of the sarcoplasmic reticulum to calcium ions and thus reduces the efficiency by which calcium activates muscle contraction, and it reduces the synthesis of cardiac proteins in both the contractile actin-myosin complex and in mitochondria, predominantly in alcoholics with high blood pressure. Similarly, a metabolite acetaldehyde and free radicals may contribute to decreased protein synthesis as well. In addition, there is enough evidence that alcohol can induce cardiac muscle damage by increasing the expression of a certain genes, which can promote programmed cell death, resulting in muscle cell loss (Zakhari 1997). In cell cultures, the acute alcohol exposure triggers the process of apoptosis inducing the expression of the pro-apoptotic protein Bax and increased caspase-3 enzyme activity (Chen et al. 2000). However, it is also possible that other cell types or systems are activated, such as the sympathetic nervous system, renin-angiotensin system, cytokines, and natriuretic peptides which may contribute to the overall injury. Interestingly enough, the excessive use of alcohol is not the exclusive cause of development of alcoholic cardiomyopathy *per se* as not all excessive alcohol consumers develop significant myocardial damage. When taking account the high prevalence of alcohol consumption the incidence of alcoholic cardiomyopathy is relatively low in the general population (Urbano-Márquez et al., 1995). Conclusively, in addition to the toxic effect of ethanol causing apoptosis, necrosis and cell loss, other mechanisms may influence the development of cardiac functional and structural damage.

3.2 Heavy metals

Some heavy metals, as cadmium, lead and cobalt, are known to be involved in selective cardiotoxicity. They are negatively inotropic and dromotropic and may cause structural changes. As for example, cobalt has been discovered to be the cause of an endemic cardiomyopathy in heavy beer drinkers in Canada in 1966 where it was used as an additive to stabilize the froth (Alexander 1972). The cardiac muscle of autopsied patients contained a high concentration of cobalt (Sullivan et al. 1968) but to produce the cardiac disease required a combination of: 1) protein deficient diet and 2) cobalt administration (Rona and Chappel 1973). Although the amount of ingested cobalt was lower than in certain therapies, the poor general nutritional state that is typical of chronic drinkers resulted in higher susceptibility to the cardiotoxicity of cobalt. The exact mechanism for developing of cardiomyopathy is unclear but it is known that cobalt may decrease myocardial contractility by a competitive antagonism with calcium (Hashimoto et al. 1989). Amino and sulfhydryl groups of amino acids can provide protection against cobalt effects by combining with cobalt and preventing the chelation of cobalt with sulfhydryl gropus of the myocardial tissue. One lesson to be learnt from this endemic cardiomyopathy, widely known as cobalt-beer cardiomyopathy, is that effects of any given noxious agent can be compounded and exaggerated by other coexisting metabolic defects, such as protein deficiency (Rona and Chappel 1973), thiamine and zinc depletion and prior ethanolic damage to the myocardium (Alexander 1972).

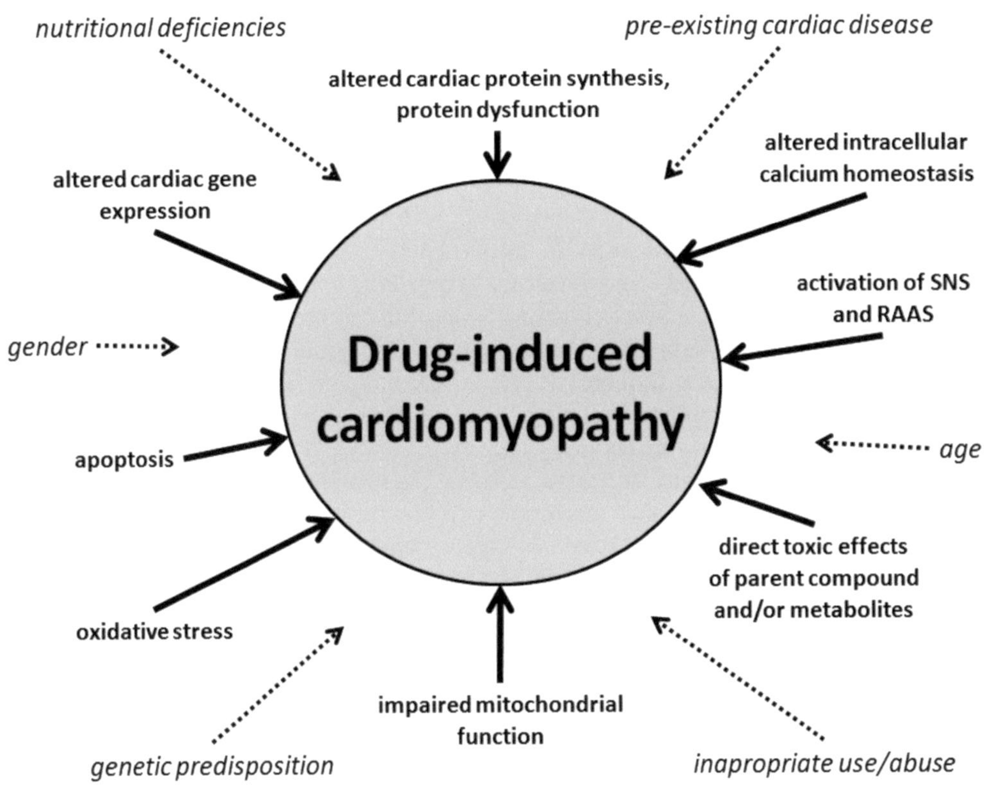

Fig. 2. Potential mechanisms (bold) and risk factors (italic) involved in drug-induced cardiomyopathies. (Abbreviations: SNS – sympathetic nervous system, RAAS – renin-angiotensin-aldosterone system.)

3.3 Experimental models of primary or secondary drug-induced cardiomyopathies

3.3.1 Catecholamines

The harmful effects of excess doses of experimentally administered catecholamines on the myocardium have been established for a long time when infarct-like lesions were produced by administration of large doses of isoproterenol (Rona et al. 1959). One of the best described models of experimental cardiomyopathies is the model of isoproterenol-induced myocardial infarction followed by cardiac hypertrophy, fibrosis and failure (Szabó et al. 1975). Similarly in clinical practice, the cardiotoxicity of catecholamines in treatment of severe asthma has been well established (Maguire et al. 1991). Moreover, catechoalmines are involved in the development of the rare 'Broken Heart Syndrome', also known as Takotsubo cardiomyopathy (Wittstein 2008). The probable mechanisms for such harmful effects of catecholamines on myocardium are not only direct effects, but also, in the case of epinephrine and isoproterenol, severe systemic hypotension with the combination producing a massive myocardial infarction. Although norepinephrine has a predominant vasopressor action, it also produces myocardial damage, which is generally of a patchy necrotic type limited to subendocardial zone occurred in patients with fatal pheochromocytoma or tetanus (Rose 1974). In past, some important mechanisms of catecholamine cardiotoxicity have been proposed: excess of calcium ions with excess excitation-contraction coupling and loss of high-energy phosphate compounds (Fleckenstein et al. 1974), increased cell membrane permeability (Rona 1985), intracellular accumulation of cyclic AMP (Lubbe et al. 1978), and increased ischemic damage (Opie et al. 1979). An important action of catecholamines is their ability to induce myocardial hypertrophy. Importantly, activation of beta-receptors induces the expression of proto-oncogenes c-fos and c-myc (Zimmer 1997). Moreover, some catecholamines induce the development of sub-endocardial fibrosis activating the proliferation of cardiac fibroblasts (Turner et al. 2003). Additionally, the role of oxidative stress (Zhang et al. 2005; Dhalla et al. 2010) and nitric oxide signalling cascade should not be neglected (Krenek et al. 2006; Krenek et al. 2009).

3.3.2 Hyperglycaemia inducing agents

Application of several drugs may lead to alterations which result in cardiac injury secondarily. One of such alteration is the long term hyperglycaemia and the development of diabetes mellitus. In experimental cardiology, two models of diabetic cardiomyopathy are widely established - streptozotocin- and alloxan-induced hyperglycaemia, diabetes and followed diabetic cardiomyopathy. Streptozotocin is a nitrosurea derivative isolated from *Streptomyces achromogenes* with broad-spectrum antibiotic and antineoplastic activity. It is a powerful alkylating agent that has been shown to interfere with glucose transport, glucokinase function and induce multiple DNA strand breaks. A single large dose of streptozotocin can produce diabetes in rodents, probably as a result of direct toxic effects characterized by a specific destruction of the pancreatic beta cells (Rees and Alcolado 2005). Streptozotocin injected rats develop severe diabetes characterized by both fasting and postprandial hyperglycemia with lack of growth in body weight and heart mass. The diabetes induced by streptozotocin can be considered as a model of both type 1 and 2 diabetes, as pancreatic islet beta cell death occurs in both types of diabetes, leading to absolute or relative insulin deficiency. Nevertheless, the model has its limits for each type. On the one hand, a single injection of streptozotocin usually does not lead to an autoimmune reaction as observed in type 1 diabetes, and on the other hand, the animals lack a significant resistance to insulin action as seen in type 2 diabetes. Nevertheless, metabolic changes typically observed in patients with diabetes, characterized by hyperglycemia and increased circulating free fatty acids, are induced. Thus, eventually the heart is exposed to the major compounds of a diabetic milieu (Dyntar et al. 2006). The developing cardiomyopathy is characterized by a decreased left ventricular performance and bradycardia under basal conditions as well as under beta-adrenergic stimulation, presence of elevated cardiac oxidative stress and changes in electrocardiograms such as the prolongation of QRS and QT interval (Howarth et al. 2005; Jankyova et al. 2009; Klimas et al. 2010). Similarly to streptozotocin, injections of alloxan induce the same blood glucose and plasma insulin responses and cause diabetes syndrome. Alloxan has two distinct pathological effects: it selectively inhibits glucose-induced insulin secretion through specific inhibition of glucokinase, the glucose sensor of the pancreatic beta cell, and it causes a state of insulin-dependent diabetes through its ability to induce reactive oxygen species formation, resulting in the selective necrosis of beta cells (Lenzen 2008). Consequently to persistent hyperglycaemia, degenerative myocardial changes are detectable in experimental settings (Mir and Darzi 2009).

3.3.3 Monocrotaline

In general, right ventricular failure is far rarer than the left ventricular failure. Experimental cardiology uses monocrotaline to induce pulmonary hypertension resulting in right ventricular hypertrophy and *cor pulmonale*. Monocrotaline is a pyrrolizidine alkaloid present in the seeds and foliage of the leguminous plant *Crotalaria spectabilis*. The administration of this alkaloid to rats produces pulmonary hypertension, hypertensive pulmonary vascular disease what results in right ventricular failure (Kay et al. 1982). The precise mechanism remains elusive but is known that to produce pulmonary insult, monocrotaline must first be activated by the liver to the putative electrophile monocrotaline pyrrole. Its stabilization by red blood cells facilitates subsequent transport to the lung where it harms the pulmonary endothelium (Lamé et al. 2000) as has been showed *in vitro* and *in vivo* as well (Boor et al. 1995).

4. Drugs inducing cardiac arrhythmias and cardiac arrest

Except of drugs inducing cellular injury or impairment resulting in depressed cardiac contractility and subsequent contractile failure, there is a number of drugs which affect ion channels and pumps and so destabilize ion homeostasis and trigger conduction defects, arrhythmias or even cardiac arrest. Importantly, these drugs do not acutely affect molecular targets but their chronic administration may affect gene expression and so change the cardiac tissue properties.

4.1 Digoxin

For more than 200 years, digoxin, a cardiotonic steroid, and its congeners have been used to treat congestive heart failure. Cardiac glycosides come from foxgloves (*Digitalis* spp.) and related plants. Nowadays, there is evidence in mammals of an endogenous digitalis-like factor closely similar to another cardiac glycoside, ouabain, and this is of potential physiological and pathological significance (Schoner 2002). Cardiotonic steroids are specific inhibitors of the the Na^+/K^+-ATP-ase of plasma membranes and this leads to an increase in the concentration of intracellular calcium via Na^+/Ca^{2+} exchanger as a secondary event. Moreover, this modulates the calcium content of the sarcoplasmic reticulum and Ca^{2+} signalling, and contributes finally to the positive inotropic effect of cardiac glycosides and an altered gene expression of proteins (Blaustein et al. 1998; Scheiner-Bobis and Schoner 2001). Because Na^+/K^+ exchange is electrogenic, inhibition of the pump by glycosides causes depolarisation, predisposing to disturbances in cardiac rhythm. Furthermore, the increased intracellular calcium causes increased after-depolarisation, leading first to bigeminy, followed eventually by ventricular tachycardia and, in certain cases, by ventricular fibrillation.

4.2 QT prolonging and Torsades de Pointes triggering drugs

The duration of QT interval measured by 12-lead electrocardiography, as a characterization of ventricular repolarisation, is one of the stable cardiac parameters widely used to describe cardiac abnormalities and safety of drugs (Klimas et al. 2008; Kmecova and Klimas 2010). The prolongation of QT interval on the surface electrocardiogram because of abnormally prolonged ventricular repolarisation is mostly referred as long QT syndrome. From a clinical perspective, it may translate into a propensity to develop syncope and sudden cardiac death. In most documented cases, death was caused by the malignant polymorphic ventricular arrhythmia called *Torsades de Pointes*. This arrhythmia is defined as a polymorphic ventricular tachycardia characterized by a 'twisting of the points' around the isoelectric line on the electrocardiogram (also formerly known as 'ballet rhythm'), and is preceded by a long QT interval (Ponte et al. 2010). Common manifestations of *Torsades de Pointes* are palpitation, symptoms of impaired cerebral circulation such as dizziness, syncope or seizures. Importantly, *Torsades de Pointes* is potentially fatal. In 20% of cases it can subsequently degenerate into ventricular fibrillation with mortality of around 10%. Predicting the development of a life-threatening arrhythmia is a hard task but, in the case of *Torsades de Pointes*, there are some useful markers. Among them, the prolongation of the QT interval is the most remarkable (Giorgi et al. 2010).

In the past few years, much attention has been focused on drugs that prolong the QT interval, potentially leading to malignant cardiac rhythm disturbances and fatal *Torsades de Pointes*. Several drugs were withdrawn from the market because they either directly caused electrocardiographic abnormality or resulted in drug-drug interactions that led to unacceptable rates of cardiotoxicity. In 1964, it was first described what would subsequently be termed drug-induced long QT syndrome with the observation that quinidine could provoke QT prolongation and arrhythmias in otherwise healthy patients (Selzer and Wray 1964). Indeed, drug administration is the most common cause of *Torsades de Pointes*. The most frequent triggers are QT-prolonging antiarrhythmics, such as quinidine, procainamide, disopyramide (class Ia) and sotalol, amiodarone, dofetilide or ibutilide (class III). With these agents, 1–8% of patients develop marked QT prolongation and *Torsades de Pointes*. On the other hand, there is a wide range of drugs developed for non-cardiovascular indications prolonging QT and inducing *Torsades de Pointes*, as well. These include high-profile drug withdrawal cases, such as terfenadine, astemizole and cisapride, as well as a variety of drugs that are in common clinical use, such as methadone, clarithromycin, erythromycin and other antibiotics, and thioridazine and other antipsychotics. An up-to-date list is maintained at the www.torsades.org website. Nevertheless, the incidence of *Torsades de Pointes* with these 'non-cardiovascular' agents is lower than with QT-prolonging antiarrhythmics (Roden 2008).

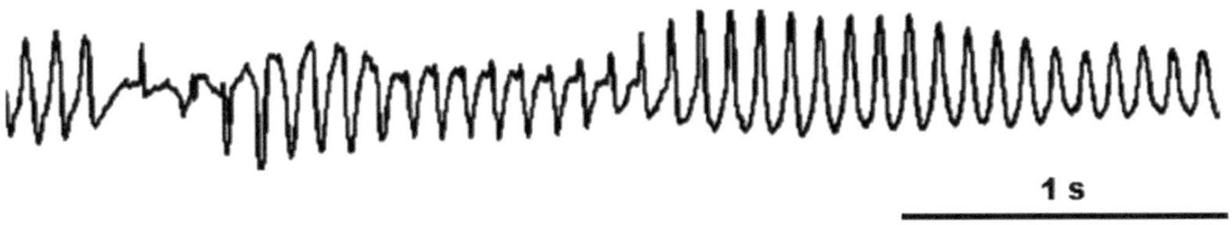

Fig. 3. The risk of *Torsades de Pointes* rises when risk factors are combined. As shown in electrocardiogram, the repeated co-administration of clarithromycin and furosemide may induce adrenergically-triggered *Torsades de Pointes* in rat (Klimas et al. 2010a).

The electrophysiological basis of QT length is the action potential of ventricular cardiomyocytes. First principles in cardiac electrophysiology dictate that an increase in QT interval must reflect an increase in action potential duration in at least some regions of the ventricle. Such increased action potential duration, in turn, must reflect an increase in inward current or a decrease in outward current (Roden 2008). Most drugs that cause *Torsades de Pointes* prolong the action potential of cardiac myocytes by blocking potassium channels (Roden 2004). Notably, the most important ionic current related to drug-induced potential of action prolongation is the delayed rectifier potassium current I_{Kr} during phase 3 of action potential. Most drugs block the I_{Kr} (Kv11.1) channel by binding to the alpha-subunits. The channel is encoded in the *human ether-a-go-go related gene* (HERG) gene. The relationship between QT prolongation and *Torsades de Pointes* has been initially supported by the fact that subjects with some forms of long QT syndrome (which have a mutation in the HERG) frequently developed *Torsades de Pointes*. Thus, extending that concept, drugs that inhibit the HERG encoded I_{Kr} channel may increase the duration of the action potential, QT interval and it might lead to *Torsades de Pointes*. In spite of this scientific evidence, the inhibition of HERG channel does not always provoke action potential and QT prolongation, mainly when the drug also blocks other ionic channels, as it happens with L-type calcium channels blockers. Moreover, some non-antiarrhythmic drugs that clearly prolong QT (as it was observed for sodium pentobarbital and ranolazine) have not been associated to *Torsades de Pointes* (Giorgi et al. 2010). However, some drugs like arsenic trioxide and pentamidine prolong the QT interval by reduced number of I_{Kr} (Kv11.1) channels on the myocardial cell membrane by causing abnormal trafficking of proteins which form the I_{Kr} (Kv11.1) channel. Importantly, only a few individuals receiving drugs that block the I_{Kr} (Kv11.1) channel develop significant QT prolongation and potentially fatal *Torsades de Pointes*. Predisposing factors include interactions with concomitantly used drugs resulting in supra-therapeutic drug levels, female gender, advanced age, bradycardia, hypokalaemia, hypomagnesaemia, ventricular hypertrophy, renal failure, central nervous system lesions, low-salt diet, congestive heart failure and nutritional disorders like prolonged starvation and anorexia nervosa. It is believed that some patients experiencing *Torsades de Pointes* may have genetic polymorphisms of genes coding for cardiac ion channels (Salvi et al. 2010).

Amiodarone	Ibutilide
Arsenic trioxide	Levomethadyl
Astemizole	Mesoridazine
Bepridil	Methadone
Chloroquine	Moxifloxacin
Chlorpromazine	Pentamidine
Cisapride	Probucol
Clarithromycin	Procainamide
Disopyramide	Quinidine
Dofetilide	Sotalol
Domperidone	Sparfloxacin
Droperidol	Terfenadine
Erythromycin	Thioridazine
Halofantrine	Vandetanib
Haloperidol	

Table 2. Drugs with a documented risk of Torsades de Pointes (Salvi et al. 2010).

5. Conclusion

The fact that drug-induced heart disease, and in particular drug-induced cardiomyopathy, does not occur more often, as would be expected from the diversity of various mechanisms, is perhaps surprising. In spite of this, cardiotoxicity remains a major problem of hundreds of pharmaceutical agents, industrial chemicals and naturally occurring products and is often a limiting factor in treatment of certain diseases. Hence, it must be taken in account in the process of clinical decision making and treatment as well as in the process of drug research and development.

6. References

Achar S, Rostamian A, Narayan SM. Cardiac and metabolic effects of anabolic-androgenic steroid abuse on lipids, blood pressure, left ventricular dimensions, and rhythm. *Am J Cardiol.* 2010;106:893-901.

Ahlgrim C, Guglin M. Anabolics and cardiomyopathy in a bodybuilder: case report and literature review. *J Card Fail.* 2009;15:496-500.

Albertson TE, Derlet RW, Van Hoozen BE. Methamphetamine and the expanding complications of amphetamines. *West J Med.* 1999;170:214-219.

Alexander CS. Cobalt-beer cardiomyopathy. A clinical and pathologic study of twenty-eight cases. *Am J Med.* 1972;53:395-417.

Allan CA, McLachlan RI. Age-related changes in testosterone and the role of replacement therapy in older men. *Clin Endocrinol (Oxf).* 2004;60:653-670.

Arai M, Tomaru K, Takizawa T, Sekiguchi K, Yokoyama T, Suzuki T, Nagai R. Sarcoplasmic reticulum genes are selectively down-regulated in cardiomyopathy produced by doxorubicin in rabbits. *J Mol Cell Cardiol.* 1998;30:243-254.

Arcamone F, Cassinelli G, Fantini G, Grein A, Orezzi P, Pol C, Spalla C. Adriamycin, 14-hydroxydaunomycin, a new antitumor antibiotic from S. peucetius var. caesius. *Biotechnol Bioeng.* 1969;11:1101-1110.

Aries A, Paradis P, Lefebvre C, Schwartz RJ, Nemer M. Essential role of GATA-4 in cell survival and drug-induced cardiotoxicity. *Proc Natl Acad Sci U S A.* 2004;101:6975-6980.

Awtry EH, Philippides GJ. Alcoholic and cocaine-associated cardiomyopathies. *Prog Cardiovasc Dis.* 2010;52:289-299.

Bachur NR, Gordon SL, Gee MV. Anthracycline antibiotic augmentation of microsomal electron transport and free radical formation. *Mol Pharmacol.* 1977;13:901-910.

Badon LA, Hicks A, Lord K, Ogden BA, Meleg-Smith S, Varner KJ. Changes in cardiovascular responsiveness and cardiotoxicity elicited during binge administration of Ecstasy. *J Pharmacol Exp Ther.* 2002;302:898-907.

Bain J. The many faces of testosterone. *Clin Interv Aging.* 2007;2:567-576

Batist G, Ramakrishnan G, Rao CS, Chandrasekharan A, Gutheil J, Guthrie T, Shah P, Khojasteh A, Nair MK, Hoelzer K, Tkaczuk K, Park YC, Lee LW. Reduced cardiotoxicity and preserved antitumor efficacy of liposome-encapsulated doxorubicin and cyclophosphamide compared with conventional doxorubicin and cyclophosphamide in a randomized, multicenter trial of metastatic breast cancer. *J Clin Oncol.* 2001;19:1444-1454.

Behrendt H, Boffin H. Myocardial cell lesions caused by an anabolic hormone. *Cell Tissue Res.* 1977;181:423-426.

Belhani D, Fanton L, Vaillant F, Descotes J, Manati W, Tabib A, Bui-Xuan B, Timour Q. Cardiac lesions induced by testosterone: protective effects of dexrazoxane and trimetazidine. *Cardiovasc Toxicol.* 2009;9:64-69.

Bers DM. Cardiac excitation-contraction coupling. *Nature.* 2002;415:198-205.

Bertolet BD, Freund G, Martin CA, Perchalski DL, Williams CM, Pepine CJ. Unrecognized left ventricular dysfunction in an apparently healthy cocaine abuse population. *Clin Cardiol.* 1990;13:323-328.

Binaschi M, Bigioni M, Cipollone A, Rossi C, Goso C, Maggi CA, Capranico G, Animati F. Anthracyclines: selected new developments. *Curr Med Chem Anticancer Agents.* 2001;1:113-130.

Bing RJ. Cardiac metabolsim: its contributions to alcoholic heart disease and myocardial failure. *Circulation.* 1978;58:965-970.

Blaustein MP, Juhaszova M, Golovina VA. The cellular mechanism of action of cardiotonic steroids: a new hypothesis. *Clin Exp Hypertens.* 1998;20:691-703.

Bolton JL, Trush MA, Penning TM, Dryhurst G, Monks TJ. Role of quinones in toxicology. *Chem Res Toxicol.* 2000;13:135-160.

Boor PJ, Gotlieb AI, Joseph EC, Kerns WD, Roth RA, Tomaszewski KE. Chemical-induced vasculature injury. Summary of the symposium presented at the 32nd annual meeting of the Society of Toxicology, New Orleans, Louisiana, March 1993. *Toxicol Appl Pharmacol.* 1995;132:177-195.

Boucek RJ Jr, Miracle A, Anderson M, Engelman R, Atkinson J, Dodd DA. Persistent effects of doxorubicin on cardiac gene expression. *J Mol Cell Cardiol.* 1999;31:1435-1446.

Bristow MR, Mason JW, Daniels JR. Monitoring of anthracycline cardiotoxicity. *Cancer Treat Rep.* 1978;62:1607-1608.

Callies F, Strömer H, Schwinger RH, Bölck B, Hu K, Frantz S, Leupold A, Beer S, Allolio B, Bonz AW. Administration of testosterone is associated with a reduced susceptibility to myocardial ischemia. *Endocrinology*. 2003;144:4478-4483.

Campbell DL, Stamler JS, Strauss HC. Redox modulation of L-type calcium channels in ferret ventricular myocytes. Dual mechanism regulation by nitric oxide and S-nitrosothiols. *J Gen Physiol*. 1996;108:277-293.

Carver JR, Ng A, Meadows AT, Vaughn DJ. Cardiovascular late effects and the ongoing care of adult cancer survivors. *Dis Manag*. 2008;11:1-6.

Charlier HA Jr, Olson RD, Thornock CM, Mercer WK, Olson DR, Broyles TS, Muhlestein DJ, Larson CL, Cusack BJ, Shadle SE. Investigations of calsequestrin as a target for anthracyclines: comparison of functional effects of daunorubicin, daunorubicinol, and trifluoperazine. *Mol Pharmacol*. 2005;67:1505-1512.

Chen DB, Wang L, Wang PH. Insulin-like growth factor I retards apoptotic signaling induced by ethanol in cardiomyocytes. *Life Sci*. 2000;67:1683-1693.

Chen Y, Daosukho C, Opii WO, Turner DM, Pierce WM, Klein JB, Vore M, Butterfield DA, St Clair DK. Redox proteomic identification of oxidized cardiac proteins in adriamycin-treated mice. *Free Radic Biol Med*. 2006;41:1470-1477.

Chu TF, Rupnick MA, Kerkela R, Dallabrida SM, Zurakowski D, Nguyen L, Woulfe K, Pravda E, Cassiola F, Desai J, George S, Morgan JA, Harris DM, Ismail NS, Chen JH, Schoen FJ, Van den Abbeele AD, Demetri GD, Force T, Chen MH. Cardiotoxicity associated with tyrosine kinase inhibitor sunitinib. *Lancet*. 2007;370:2011-2019.

Clark BM, Schofield RS. Dilated cardiomyopathy and acute liver injury associated with combined use of ephedra, gamma-hydroxybutyrate, and anabolic steroids. *Pharmacotherapy*. 2005;25:756-761.

Crean AM, Pohl JE. 'Ally McBeal heart?'-- drug induced cardiomyopathy in a young woman. *Br J Clin Pharmacol*. 2004;58:558-559.

Curry LA, Wagman DF. Qualitative description of the prevalence and use of anabolic androgenic steroids by United States powerlifters. *Percept Mot Skills*. 1999;88:224-233.

De Leonardis V, Neri B, Bacalli S, Cinelli P. Reduction of cardiac toxicity of anthracyclines by L-carnitine: preliminary overview of clinical data. *Int J Clin Pharmacol Res*. 1985;5:137-142.

Dhalla NS, Adameova A, Kaur M. Role of catecholamine oxidation in sudden cardiac death. *Fundam Clin Pharmacol*. 2010;24:539-546

Dhar R, Stout CW, Link MS, Homoud MK, Weinstock J, Estes NA 3rd. Cardiovascular toxicities of performance-enhancing substances in sports. *Mayo Clin Proc*. 2005;80:1307-1315.

Di Bello V, Giorgi D, Bianchi M, Bertini A, Caputo MT, Valenti G, Furioso O, Alessandri L, Paterni M, Giusti C. Effects of anabolic-androgenic steroids on weight-lifters' myocardium: an ultrasonic videodensitometric study. *Med Sci Sports Exerc*. 1999;31:514-521.

Dickerman RD, Schaller F, McConathy WJ. Left ventricular wall thickening does occur in elite power athletes with or without anabolic steroid Use. *Cardiology*. 1998;90:145-148.

Dickstein K, Cohen-Solal A, Filippatos G, McMurray JJ, Ponikowski P, Poole-Wilson PA, Strömberg A, van Veldhuisen DJ, Atar D, Hoes AW, Keren A, Mebazaa A, Nieminen M, Priori SG, Swedberg K; ESC Committee for Practice Guidelines (CPG). ESC guidelines for the diagnosis and treatment of acute and chronic heart failure 2008: the Task Force for the diagnosis and treatment of acute and chronic heart failure 2008 of the European Society of Cardiology. Developed in collaboration with the Heart Failure Association of the ESC (HFA) and endorsed by the European Society of Intensive Care Medicine (ESICM). *Eur J Heart Fail.* 2008;10:933-989.

Dodd DA, Atkinson JB, Olson RD, Buck S, Cusack BJ, Fleischer S, Boucek RJ Jr. Doxorubicin cardiomyopathy is associated with a decrease in calcium release channel of the sarcoplasmic reticulum in a chronic rabbit model. *J Clin Invest.* 1993;91:1697-1705.

Doroshow JH. Effect of anthracycline antibiotics on oxygen radical formation in rat heart. *Cancer Res.* 1983;43:460-472.

Drímal J, Zúrová-Nedelcevová J, Knezl V, Sotníková R, Navarová J. Cardiovascular toxicity of the first line cancer chemotherapeutic agents: doxorubicin, cyclophosphamide, streptozotocin and bevacizumab. *Neuro Endocrinol Lett.* 2006;27 Suppl 2:176-179.

Du Toit EF, Rossouw E, Van Rooyen J, Lochner A. Proposed mechanisms for the anabolic steroid-induced increase in myocardial susceptibility to ischaemia/reperfusion injury. *Cardiovasc J S Afr.* 2005;16:21-28.

Dyntar D, Sergeev P, Klisic J, Ambühl P, Schaub MC, Donath MY. High glucose alters cardiomyocyte contacts and inhibits myofibrillar formation. *J Clin Endocrinol Metab.* 2006;91:1961-1967.

Elihu N, Anandasbapathy S, Frishman WH. Chelation therapy in cardiovascular disease: ethylenediaminetetraacetic acid, deferoxamine, and dexrazoxane. *J Clin Pharmacol.* 1998;38:101-105.

Estruch R, Fernández-Solá J, Sacanella E, Paré C, Rubin E, Urbano-Márquez A. Relationship between cardiomyopathy and liver disease in chronic alcoholism. *Hepatology.* 1995;22:532-538.

Ettinger PO. Holiday heart arrhythmias. *Int J Cardiol.* 1984;5:540-542.

Ewer MS, Lippman SM. Type II chemotherapy-related cardiac dysfunction: time to recognize a new entity. *J Clin Oncol.* 2005;23:2900-2902.

Ewer MS, Vooletich MT, Durand JB, Woods ML, Davis JR, Valero V, Lenihan DJ. Reversibility of trastuzumab-related cardiotoxicity: new insights based on clinical course and response to medical treatment. *J Clin Oncol.* 2005;23:7820-7826.

Felker GM, Hu W, Hare JM, Hruban RH, Baughman KL, Kasper EK. The spectrum of dilated cardiomyopathy. The Johns Hopkins experience with 1,278 patients. *Medicine (Baltimore).* 1999;78:270-283.

Felker GM, Thompson RE, Hare JM, Hruban RH, Clemetson DE, Howard DL, Baughman KL, Kasper EK. Underlying causes and long-term survival in patients with initially unexplained cardiomyopathy. *N Engl J Med.* 2000;342:1077-1084.

Figueredo VM. Chemical cardiomyopathies: the negative effects of medications and nonprescribed drugs on the heart. *Am J Med.* 2011;124:480-488.

Fleckenstein A, Janke J, Döring HJ, Leder O. Myocardial fiber necrosis due to intracellular Ca overload-a new principle in cardiac pathophysiology. *Recent Adv Stud Cardiac Struct Metab.* 1974;4:563-580.

Fogli S, Nieri P, Breschi MC. The role of nitric oxide in anthracycline toxicity and prospects for pharmacologic prevention of cardiac damage. *FASEB J.* 2004;18:664-675.

Fraiser LH, Kanekal S, Kehrer JP. Cyclophosphamide toxicity. Characterising and avoiding the problem. *Drugs.* 1991;42:781-795.

Gewirtz DA. A critical evaluation of the mechanisms of action proposed for the antitumor effects of the anthracycline antibiotics adriamycin and daunorubicin. *Biochem Pharmacol.* 1999;57:727-741.

Gille L, Nohl H. Analyses of the molecular mechanism of adriamycin-induced cardiotoxicity. *Free Radic Biol Med.* 1997;23:775-782.

Giorgi MA, Bolaños R, Gonzalez CD, Di Girolamo G. QT interval prolongation: preclinical and clinical testing arrhythmogenesis in drugs and regulatory implications. *Curr Drug Saf.* 2010;5:54-57.

Goldhaber JI. Free radicals enhance Na+/Ca2+ exchange in ventricular myocytes. *Am J Physiol.* 1996;271(3 Pt 2):H823-H833.

Gottdiener JS, Appelbaum FR, Ferrans VJ, Deisseroth A, Ziegler J. Cardiotoxicity associated with high-dose cyclophosphamide therapy. *Arch Intern Med.* 1981;141:758-763.

Guarnieri T, Lakatta EG. Mechanism of myocardial contractile depression by clinical concentrations of ethanol. A study in ferret papillary muscles. *J Clin Invest.* 1990;85:1462-1467.

Guthrie D, Gibson AL. Doxorubicin cardiotoxicity: possible role of digoxin in its prevention. *Br Med J.* 1977;2:1447-1449.

Györke S, Györke I, Lukyanenko V, Terentyev D, Viatchenko-Karpinski S, Wiesner TF. Regulation of sarcoplasmic reticulum calcium release by luminal calcium in cardiac muscle. *Front Biosci.* 2002;7:d1454-d1463.

Handa K, Sato S. Generation of free radicals of quinone group-containing anti-cancer chemicals in NADPH-microsome system as evidenced by initiation of sulfite oxidation. *Gann.* 1975;66:43-47.

Hartgens F, Kuipers H. Effects of androgenic-anabolic steroids in athletes. *Sports Med.* 2004;34:513-554.

Hashimoto H, Yanagisawa T, Taira N. Differential antagonism of the negative inotropic effect of gentamicin by calcium ions, Bay K 8644 and isoprenaline in canine ventricular muscle: comparison with cobalt ions. *Br J Pharmacol.* 1989;96:906-912.

Hasinoff BB. Chemistry of dexrazoxane and analogues. *Semin Oncol.* 1998;25(Suppl 10):3-9.

Hausmann R, Hammer S, Betz P. Performance enhancing drugs (doping agents) and sudden death--a case report and review of the literature. *Int J Legal Med.* 1998;111:261-264.

Howarth FC, Jacobson M, Shafiullah M, Adeghate E. Long-term effects of streptozotocin-induced diabetes on the electrocardiogram, physical activity and body temperature in rats. *Exp Physiol.* 2005;90:827-835.

Iarussi D, Auricchio U, Agretto A, Murano A, Giuliano M, Casale F, Indolfi P, Iacono A. Protective effect of coenzyme Q10 on anthracyclines cardiotoxicity: control study in children with acute lymphoblastic leukemia and non-Hodgkin lymphoma. *Mol Aspects Med.* 1994;15 Suppl:s207-s212.

Imai K, Hayashi Y, Kono M. Testosterone-induced focal myocarditis in rats. I. Morphological and biochemical studies with special reference to pathogenetical mechanism and species differences. *J Toxicol Sci.* 1978;3:215-228.

Isabelle M, Vergeade A, Moritz F, Dautréaux B, Henry JP, Lallemand F, Richard V, Mulder P, Thuillez C, Monteil C. NADPH oxidase inhibition prevents cocaine-induced up-regulation of xanthine oxidoreductase and cardiac dysfunction. *J Mol Cell Cardiol.* 2007;42:326-232.

Islam MN, Kuroki H, Hongcheng B, Ogura Y, Kawaguchi N, Onishi S, Wakasugi C. Cardiac lesions and their reversibility after long term administration of methamphetamine. *Forensic Sci Int.* 1995;75:29-43.

Jankowska EA, Biel B, Majda J, Szklarska A, Lopuszanska M, Medras M, Anker SD, Banasiak W, Poole-Wilson PA, Ponikowski P. Anabolic deficiency in men with chronic heart failure: prevalence and detrimental impact on survival. *Circulation.* 2006;114:1829-1837.

Jankyova S, Kucera P, Goldenberg Z, Yaghi D, Navarova J, Kyselova Z, Stolc S, Klimas J, Racanska E, Matyas S. Pycnogenol efficiency on glycaemia, motor nerve conduction velocity and markers of oxidative stress in mild type diabetes in rats. *Phytother Res.* 2009;23:1169-1174.

Johanson CE, Fischman MW. The pharmacology of cocaine related to its abuse. *Pharmacol Rev.* 1989;41:3-52.

Jones LW, Haykowsky MJ, Swartz JJ, Douglas PS, Mackey JR. Early breast cancer therapy and cardiovascular injury. *J Am Coll Cardiol.* 2007;50:1435-1441.

Karila TA, Karjalainen JE, Mäntysaari MJ, Viitasalo MT, Seppälä TA. Anabolic androgenic steroids produce dose-dependant increase in left ventricular mass in power atheletes, and this effect is potentiated by concomitant use of growth hormone. *Int J Sports Med.* 2003;24:337-343.

Kawasaki S, Akiyama S, Kurokawa T, Kataoka M, Dohmitsu K, Kondoh K, Yamauchi M, Ito K, Watanabe T, Sugiyama S, et al. Polyoxyethylene-modified superoxide dismutase reduces side effects of adriamycin and mitomycin C. *Jpn J Cancer Res.* 1992;83:899-906.

Kay JM, Keane PM, Suyama KL, Gauthier D. Angiotensin converting enzyme activity and evolution of pulmonary vascular disease in rats with monocrotaline pulmonary hypertension. *Thorax.* 1982;37:88-96.

Kerkelä R, Grazette L, Yacobi R, Iliescu C, Patten R, Beahm C, Walters B, Shevtsov S, Pesant S, Clubb FJ, Rosenzweig A, Salomon RN, Van Etten RA, Alroy J, Durand JB, Force T. Cardiotoxicity of the cancer therapeutic agent imatinib mesylate. *Nat Med.* 2006;12:908-916.

Kicman AT. Pharmacology of anabolic steroids. *Br J Pharmacol.* 2008;154:502-521.

Kim E, Tam M, Siems WF, Kang C. Effects of drugs with muscle-related side effects and affinity for calsequestrin on the calcium regulatory function of sarcoplasmic reticulum microsomes. *Mol Pharmacol.* 2005;68:1708-1715.

Kirchhefer U, Klimas J, Baba HA, Buchwalow IB, Fabritz L, Hüls M, Matus M, Müller FU, Schmitz W, Neumann J. Triadin is a critical determinant of cellular Ca cycling and contractility in the heart. *Am J Physiol Heart Circ Physiol.* 2007;293:H3165-H3174.

Kirchhof P, Klimas J, Fabritz L, Zwiener M, Jones LR, Schäfers M, Hermann S, Boknik P, Schmitz W, Breithardt G, Kirchhefer U, Neumann J. Stress and high heart rate provoke ventricular tachycardia in mice expressing triadin. *J Mol Cell Cardiol.* 2007;42:962-971.

Klimas J, Kmecova J, Jankyova S, Yaghi D, Priesolova E, Kyselova Z, Musil P, Ochodnicky P, Krenek P, Kyselovic J, Matyas S. Pycnogenol improves left ventricular function in streptozotocin-induced diabetic cardiomyopathy in rats. *Phytother Res.* 2010;24:969-974.

Klimas J, Kmecova J, Mackovicova K, Vavrinec P, Krenek P, Kyselovic J, Ochodnicky P. Administration of clarithromycin and furosemid alters cardiac ion channel gene expression and induces beta-adrenergically evoked Torsades de Pointes in rat. *casopis.* Basic Clin Pharmacol Toxicol. 2010a;107(Suppl 1):380.

Klimas J, Stankovicova T, Kyselovic J, Bacharova L. Prolonged QT interval is associated with blood pressure rather than left ventricular mass in spontaneously hypertensive rats. *Clin Exp Hypertens.* 2008;30:475-485.

Kloner RA, Hale S, Alker K, Rezkalla S. The effects of acute and chronic cocaine use on the heart. *Circulation.* 1992;85:407-419.

Kmecova J, Klimas J. Heart rate correction of the QT duration in rats. *Eur J Pharmacol.* 2010 1;641:187-192.

Knochel JP. Cardiovascular effects of alcohol. *Ann Intern Med.* 1983;98(5 Pt 2):849-854.

Kohno H, Takahashi N, Shinohara T, Ooie T, Yufu K, Nakagawa M, Yonemochi H, Hara M, Saikawa T, Yoshimatsu H. Receptor-mediated suppression of cardiac heat-shock protein 72 expression by testosterone in male rat heart. *Endocrinology.* 2007;148:3148-3155.

Krenek P, Klimas J, Kroslakova M, Gazova A, Plandorova J, Kucerova D, Fecenkova A, Svec P, Kyselovic J. Increased expression of endothelial nitric oxide synthase and caveolin-1 in the aorta of rats with isoproterenol-induced cardiac hypertrophy. *Can J Physiol Pharmacol.* 2006;84:1245-1250.

Krenek P, Kmecova J, Kucerova D, Bajuszova Z, Musil P, Gazova A, Ochodnicky P, Klimas J, Kyselovic J. Isoproterenol-induced heart failure in the rat is associated with nitric oxide-dependent functional alterations of cardiac function. *Eur J Heart Fail.* 2009;11:140-146.

Kuhn CM. Anabolic steroids. *Recent Prog Horm Res.* 2002;57:411-434.

Lamé MW, Jones AD, Wilson DW, Dunston SK, Segall HJ. Protein targets of monocrotaline pyrrole in pulmonary artery endothelial cells. *J Biol Chem.* 2000;275:29091-29099.

Lebrecht D, Kokkori A, Ketelsen UP, Setzer B, Walker UA. Tissue-specific mtDNA lesions and radical-associated mitochondrial dysfunction in human hearts exposed to doxorubicin. *J Pathol.* 2005;207:436-444.

Lee WK, Regan TJ. Alcoholic cardiomyopathy: is it dose-dependent? *Congest Heart Fail.* 2002;8:303-306.

Legha SS, Benjamin RS, Mackay B, Ewer M, Wallace S, Valdivieso M, Rasmussen SL, Blumenschein GR, Freireich EJ. Reduction of doxorubicin cardiotoxicity by prolonged continuous intravenous infusion. *Ann Intern Med.* 1982;96:133-139.

Lenzen S. The mechanisms of alloxan- and streptozotocin-induced diabetes. *Diabetologia.* 2008;51:216-226.

Levey GS, Levey BA, Ruiz E, Lehotay DC. Selective inhibition of rat and human cardiac guanylate cyclase in vitro by doxorubicin (adriamycin): possible link to anthracycline cardiotoxicity. *J Mol Cell Cardiol.* 1979;11:591-599.

Lieberherr M, Grosse B. Adrogens increase intracellular calcium concentration and inositol 1,4,5-trisphosphate and diacylglycerol formation via a pertussis toxin-sensitive G-protein. *J Biol Chem*. 1994;269:7217-7223.

Lillegard JB, Porterfield Jr JR. Ephedra-Induced Gastric Mucosal Injury. *Case Rep Gastroenterol*. 2010;4:79-83.

Lim CC, Zuppinger C, Guo X, Kuster GM, Helmes M, Eppenberger HM, Suter TM, Liao R, Sawyer DB. Anthracyclines induce calpain-dependent titin proteolysis and necrosis in cardiomyocytes. *J Biol Chem*. 2004;279:8290-8299.

Lipshultz SE, Colan SD, Gelber RD, Perez-Atayde AR, Sallan SE, Sanders SP. Late cardiac effects of doxorubicin therapy for acute lymphoblastic leukemia in childhood. *N Engl J Med*. 1991;324:808-815.

Lipshultz SE, Lipsitz SR, Mone SM, Goorin AM, Sallan SE, Sanders SP, Orav EJ, Gelber RD, Colan SD. Female sex and drug dose as risk factors for late cardiotoxic effects of doxorubicin therapy for childhood cancer. *N Engl J Med*. 1995;332:1738-1743.

Liu PY, Death AK, Handelsman DJ. Androgens and cardiovascular disease. *Endocr Rev*. 2003;24:313-340.

Lopez JE, Yeo K, Caputo G, Buonocore M, Schaefer S. Recovery of methamphetamine associated cardiomyopathy predicted by late gadolinium enhanced cardiovascular magnetic resonance. *J Cardiovasc Magn Reson*. 2009;11:46.

Lubbe WF, Podzuweit T, Daries PS, Opie LH. The role of cyclic adenosine monophosphate in adrenergic effects on ventricular vulnerability to fibrillation in the isolated perfused rat heart. *J Clin Invest*. 1978;61:1260-1269.

Mackay B, Ewer MS, Carrasco CH, Benjamin RS. Assessment of anthracycline cardiomyopathy by endomyocardial biopsy. *Ultrastruct Pathol*. 1994;18:203-211.

Maeno Y, Iwasa M, Inoue H, Koyama H, Matoba R, Nagao M. Direct effects of methamphetamine on hypertrophy and microtubules in cultured adult rat ventricular myocytes. *Forensic Sci Int*. 2000;113:239-243.

Maguire JF, O'Rourke PP, Colan SD, Geha RS, Crone R. Cardiotoxicity during treatment of severe childhood asthma. *Pediatrics*. 1991;88:1180-1186.

Malkin CJ, Pugh PJ, West JN, van Beek EJ, Jones TH, Channer KS. Testosterone therapy in men with moderate severity heart failure: a double-blind randomized placebo controlled trial. *Eur Heart J*. 2006;27:57-64.

Mann DL. Mechanisms and models in heart failure: A combinatorial approach. *Circulation*. 1999;100:999-1008.

Maraj S, Figueredo VM, Lynn Morris D. Cocaine and the heart. *Clin Cardiol*. 2010;33:264-269.

Marsh JD, Lehmann MH, Ritchie RH, Gwathmey JK, Green GE, Schiebinger RJ. Androgen receptors mediate hypertrophy in cardiac myocytes. *Circulation*. 1998;98:256-261.

McCord J, Jneid H, Hollander JE, de Lemos JA, Cercek B, Hsue P, Gibler WB, Ohman EM, Drew B, Philippides G, Newby LK; American Heart Association Acute Cardiac Care Committee of the Council on Clinical Cardiology. Management of cocaine-associated chest pain and myocardial infarction: a scientific statement from the American Heart Association Acute Cardiac Care Committee of the Council on Clinical Cardiology. *Circulation*. 2008;117:1897-1907.

Mehta PM, Grainger TA, Lust RM, Movahed A, Terry J, Gilliland MG, Jolly SR. Effect of cocaine on left ventricular function. Relation to increased wall stress and persistence after treatment. *Circulation*. 1995;91:3002-3009.

Meinardi MT, Gietema JA, van Veldhuisen DJ, van der Graaf WT, de Vries EG, Sleijfer DT. Long-term chemotherapy-related cardiovascular morbidity. *Cancer Treat Rev.* 2000;26:429-447.

Melchert RB, Welder AA. Cardiovascular effects of androgenic-anabolic steroids. *Med Sci Sports Exerc.* 1995;27:1252-1262.

Mijares A, López JR. L-carnitine prevents increase in diastolic [CA2+] induced by doxorubicin in cardiac cells. *Eur J Pharmacol.* 2001;425:117-120.

Millart H, Brabant L, Lorenzato M, Lamiable D, Albert O, Choisy H. The effects of 5-fluorouracil on contractility and oxygen uptake of the isolated perfused rat heart. *Anticancer Res.* 1992;12:571-576.

Minotti G, Mancuso C, Frustaci A, Mordente A, Santini SA, Calafiore AM, Liberi G, Gentiloni N. Paradoxical inhibition of cardiac lipid peroxidation in cancer patients treated with doxorubicin. Pharmacologic and molecular reappraisal of anthracycline cardiotoxicity. *J Clin Invest.* 1996;98:650-661.

Minotti G, Menna P, Salvatorelli E, Cairo G, Gianni L. Anthracyclines: molecular advances and pharmacologic developments in antitumor activity and cardiotoxicity. *Pharmacol Rev.* 2004;56:185-229.

Mir SH, Darzi MM. Histopathological abnormalities of prolonged alloxan-induced diabetes mellitus in rabbits. *Int J Exp Pathol.* 2009;90:66-73.

Mizia-Stec K, Gasior Z, Wojnicz R, Haberka M, Mielczarek M, Wierzbicki A, Pstraś K, Hartleb M. Severe dilated cardiomyopathy as a consequence of Ecstasy intake. *Cardiovasc Pathol.* 2008;17:250-253.

Muggia FM, Green MD. New anthracycline antitumor antibiotics. *Crit Rev Oncol Hematol.* 1991;11:43-64.

Muggia FM, Hainsworth JD, Jeffers S, Miller P, Groshen S, Tan M, Roman L, Uziely B, Muderspach L, Garcia A, Burnett A, Greco FA, Morrow CP, Paradiso LJ, Liang LJ. Phase II study of liposomal doxorubicin in refractory ovarian cancer: antitumor activity and toxicity modification by liposomal encapsulation. *J Clin Oncol.* 1997;15:987-993.

Muindi JR, Sinha BK, Gianni L, Myers CE. Hydroxyl radical production and DNA damage induced by anthracycline-iron complex. *FEBS Lett.* 1984;172:226-230.

Myers CE, McGuire W, Young R. Adriamycin: amelioration of toxicity by alpha-tocopherol. *Cancer Treat Rep.* 1976;60:961-962.

Myers CE, McGuire WP, Liss RH, Ifrim I, Grotzinger K, Young RC. Adriamycin: the role of lipid peroxidation in cardiac toxicity and tumor response. *Science.* 1977;197:165-167.

Nieminen MS, Rämö MP, Viitasalo M, Heikkilä P, Karjalainen J, Mäntysaari M, Heikkilä J. Serious cardiovascular side effects of large doses of anabolic steroids in weight lifters. *Eur Heart J.* 1996;17:1576-1583.

Nohl H, Gille L, Kozlov A, Staniek K. Are mitochondria a spontaneous and permanent source of reactive oxygen species? *Redox Rep.* 2003;8:135-141.

Olson HM, Young DM, Prieur DJ, LeRoy AF, Reagan RL. Electrolyte and morphologic alterations of myocardium in adriamycin-treated rabbits. *Am J Pathol.* 1974;77:439-454.

Olson RD, Li X, Palade P, Shadle SE, Mushlin PS, Gambliel HA, Fill M, Boucek RJ Jr, Cusack BJ. Sarcoplasmic reticulum calcium release is stimulated and inhibited by daunorubicin and daunorubicinol. *Toxicol Appl Pharmacol.* 2000;169:168-176.

Ondrias K, Borgatta L, Kim DH, Ehrlich BE. Biphasic effects of doxorubicin on the calcium release channel from sarcoplasmic reticulum of cardiac muscle. *Circ Res.* 1990;67:1167-1174.

Opie LH, Thandroyen FT, Muller C, Bricknell OL. Adrenaline-induced "oxygen-wastage" and enzyme release from working rat heart. Effects of calcium antagonism, beta-blockade, nicotinic acid and coronary artery ligation. *J Mol Cell Cardiol.* 1979;11:1073-1094.

Outomuro D, Grana DR, Azzato F, Milei J. Adriamycin-induced myocardial toxicity: new solutions for an old problem? *Int J Cardiol.* 2007;117:6-15.

Park IY, Kim EJ, Park H, Fields K, Dunker AK, Kang C. Interaction between cardiac calsequestrin and drugs with known cardiotoxicity. *Mol Pharmacol.* 2005;67:97-104.

Payne JR, Kotwinski PJ, Montgomery HE. Cardiac effects of anabolic steroids. *Heart.* 2004;90:473-475.

Peng X, Chen B, Lim CC, Sawyer DB. The cardiotoxicology of anthracycline chemotherapeutics: translating molecular mechanism into preventative medicine. *Mol Interv.* 2005;5:163-171.

Penna C, Tullio F, Perrelli MG, Moro F, Abbadessa G, Piccione F, Carriero V, Racca S, Pagliaro P. Ischemia/reperfusion injury is increased and cardioprotection by a postconditioning protocol is lost as cardiac hypertrophy develops in nandrolone treated rats. *Basic Res Cardiol.* 2011;106:409-420.

Pentassuglia L, Timolati F, Seifriz F, Abudukadier K, Suter TM, Zuppinger C. Inhibition of ErbB2/neuregulin signaling augments paclitaxel-induced cardiotoxicity in adult ventricular myocytes. *Exp Cell Res.* 2007;313:1588-1601.

Piano MR. Alcoholic cardiomyopathy: incidence, clinical characteristics, and pathophysiology. *Chest.* 2002;121:1638-1650.

Pigram WJ, Fuller W, Hamilton LD. Stereochemistry of intercalation: interaction of daunomycin with DNA.*Nat New Biol.* 1972;235:17-19.

Ponte ML, Keller GA, Di Girolamo G. Mechanisms of drug induced QT interval prolongation. *Curr Drug Saf.* 2010;5:44-53.

Pugh PJ, English KM, Jones TH, Channer KS. Testosterone: a natural tonic for the failing heart? *QJM.* 2000;93:689-694.

Pugh PJ, Jones RD, West JN, Jones TH, Channer KS. Testosterone treatment for men with chronic heart failure. *Heart.* 2004;90:446-447.

Pugh PJ, Jones TH, Channer KS. Acute haemodynamic effects of testosterone in men with chronic heart failure. *Eur Heart J.* 2003;24:909-915.

Radi R, Cassina A, Hodara R, Quijano C, Castro L. Peroxynitrite reactions and formation in mitochondria. *Free Radic Biol Med.* 2002;33:1451-1464.

Rauchhaus M, Doehner W, Anker SD. Heart failure therapy: testosterone replacement and its implications. *Eur Heart J.* 2006;27:10-12.

Rees DA, Alcolado JC. Animal models of diabetes mellitus. *Diabet Med.* 2005;22:359-370.

Roden DM. Cellular basis of drug-induced torsades de pointes. *Br J Pharmacol.* 2008;154:1502-1507.

Roden DM. Drug-induced prolongation of the QT interval. *N Engl J Med.* 2004;350:1013-1022.

Rona G, Chappel CI, Balazs T, Gaudry R. An infarct-like myocardial lesion and other toxic manifestations produced by isoproterenol in the rat. *AMA Arch Pathol.* 1959;67:443-455.

Rona G, Chappel CI. Pathogenesis and pathology of cobalt cardiomyopathy. *Recent Adv Stud Cardiac Struct Metab.* 1973;2:407-422.

Rona G. Catecholamine cardiotoxicity. *J Mol Cell Cardiol.* 1985;17:291-306.

Rose AG. Catecholamine-induced myocardial dammage associated with phaeochromocytomas and tetanus. *S Afr Med J.* 1974;48:1285-1289.

Rosenoff SH, Brooks E, Bostick F, Young RC. Alterations in DNA synthesis in cardiac tissue induced by adriamycin in vivo-relationship to fatal toxicity. *Biochem Pharmacol.* 1975;24:1898-1901.

Ruiz-Ruiz C, Robledo G, Cano E, Redondo JM, Lopez-Rivas A. Characterization of p53-mediated up-regulation of CD95 gene expression upon genotoxic treatment in human breast tumor cells. *J Biol Chem.* 2003;278:31667-31675.

Saeki K, Obi I, Ogiku N, Shigekawa M, Imagawa T, Matsumoto T. Doxorubicin directly binds to the cardiac-type ryanodine receptor. *Life Sci.* 2002;70:2377-2389.

Salvi V, Karnad DR, Panicker GK, Kothari S. Update on the evaluation of a new drug for effects on cardiac repolarization in humans: issues in early drug development. *Br J Pharmacol.* 2010;159:34-48.

Sasson Z, Morgan CD, Wang B, Thomas G, MacKenzie B, Platts ME. 5-Fluorouracil related toxic myocarditis: case reports and pathological confirmation. *Can J Cardiol.* 1994;10:861-864.

Sawyer DB, Fukazawa R, Arstall MA, Kelly RA. Daunorubicin-induced apoptosis in rat cardiac myocytes is inhibited by dexrazoxane. *Circ Res.* 1999;84:257-265.

Sawyer DB, Zuppinger C, Miller TA, Eppenberger HM, Suter TM. Modulation of anthracycline-induced myofibrillar disarray in rat ventricular myocytes by neuregulin-1beta and anti-erbB2: potential mechanism for trastuzumab-induced cardiotoxicity. *Circulation.* 2002;105:1551-1554.

Scheiner-Bobis G, Schoner W. A fresh facet for ouabain action. *Nat Med.* 2001;7:1288-1289.

Schöber C, Papageorgiou E, Harstrick A, Bokemeyer C, Mügge A, Stahl M, Wilke H, Poliwoda H, Hiddemann W, Köhne-Wömpner CH, et al. Cardiotoxicity of 5-fluorouracil in combination with folinic acid in patients with gastrointestinal cancer. *Cancer.* 1993;72:2242-2247.

Schoner W. Endogenous cardiac glycosides, a new class of steroid hormones. *Eur J Biochem.* 2002;269:2440-2448.

Selzer A, Wray HW. Quinidine syncope paroxysmal ventricular fibrillation occuring during treatment of chronic atrial arrhythmias. *Circulation.* 1964;30:17-26.

Shan K, Lincoff AM, Young JB. Anthracycline-induced cardiotoxicity. *Ann Intern Med.* 1996;125:47-58.

Shenouda SK, Lord KC, McIlwain E, Lucchesi PA, Varner KJ. Ecstasy produces left ventricular dysfunction and oxidative stress in rats. *Cardiovasc Res.* 2008;79:662-670.

Shenouda SK, Varner KJ, Carvalho F, Lucchesi PA. Metabolites of MDMA induce oxidative stress and contractile dysfunction in adult rat left ventricular myocytes. *Cardiovasc Toxicol.* 2009;9:30-38.

Shin DD, Brandimarte F, De Luca L, Sabbah HN, Fonarow GC, Filippatos G, Komajda M, Gheorghiade M. Review of current and investigational pharmacologic agents for acute heart failure syndromes. *Am J Cardiol.* 2007;99:4A-23A.

Silber JH, Cnaan A, Clark BJ, Paridon SM, Chin AJ, Rychik J, Hogarty AN, Cohen MI, Barber G, Rutkowski M, Kimball TR, Delaat C, Steinherz LJ, Zhao H. Enalapril to prevent cardiac function decline in long-term survivors of pediatric cancer exposed to anthracyclines. *J Clin Oncol.* 2004;22:820-828.

Simůnek T, Stérba M, Popelová O, Adamcová M, Hrdina R, Gersl V. Anthracycline-induced cardiotoxicity: overview of studies examining the roles of oxidative stress and free cellular iron. *Pharmacol Rep.* 2009;61:154-171.

Singal PK, Iliskovic N. Doxorubicin-induced cardiomyopathy. *N Engl J Med.* 1998;339:900-905.

Singal PK, Siveski-Iliskovic N, Hill M, Thomas TP, Li T. Combination therapy with probucol prevents adriamycin-induced cardiomyopathy. *J Mol Cell Cardiol.* 1995;27:1055-1063.

Sinha BK, Trush MA, Kennedy KA, Mimnaugh EG. Enzymatic activation and binding of adriamycin to nuclear DNA. *Cancer Res.* 1984;44:2892-2896.

Slamon DJ, Leyland-Jones B, Shak S, Fuchs H, Paton V, Bajamonde A, Fleming T, Eiermann W, Wolter J, Pegram M, Baselga J, Norton L. Use of chemotherapy plus a monoclonal antibody against HER2 for metastatic breast cancer that overexpresses HER2. *N Engl J Med.* 2001;344:783-792.

Solem LE, Henry TR, Wallace KB. Disruption of mitochondrial calcium homeostasis following chronic doxorubicin administration. *Toxicol Appl Pharmacol.* 1994;129:214-222.

Stergiopoulos K, Brennan JJ, Mathews R, Setaro JF, Kort S. Anabolic steroids, acute myocardial infarction and polycythemia: a case report and review of the literature. *Vasc Health Risk Manag.* 2008;4:1475-1480.

Stolt A, Karila T, Viitasalo M, Mäntysaari M, Kujala UM, Karjalainen J. QT interval and QT dispersion in endurance athletes and in power athletes using large doses of anabolic steroids. *Am J Cardiol.* 1999;84:364-366.

Strasser F, Betticher DC, Suter TM. Trastuzumab and breast cancer. *N Engl J Med.* 2001;345:996.

Sullivan J, Parker M, Carson SB. Tissue cobalt content in "beer drinkers' myocardiopathy". *J Lab Clin Med.* 1968;71:893-911.

Sullivan ML, Martinez CM, Gennis P, Gallagher EJ. The cardiac toxicity of anabolic steroids. *Prog Cardiovasc Dis.* 1998;41:1-15.

Swain SM, Whaley FS, Ewer MS. Congestive heart failure in patients treated with doxorubicin: a retrospective analysis of three trials. *Cancer.* 2003;97:2869-2879.

Swain SM, Whaley FS, Gerber MC, Weisberg S, York M, Spicer D, Jones SE, Wadler S, Desai A, Vogel C, Speyer J, Mittelman A, Reddy S, Pendergrass K, Velez-Garcia E, Ewer MS, Bianchine JR, Gams RA. Cardioprotection with dexrazoxane for doxorubicin-containing therapy in advanced breast cancer. *J Clin Oncol.* 1997;15:1318-1332.

Szabó J, Csáky L, Szegi J. Experimental cardiac hypertrophy induced by isoproterenol in the rat. *Acta Physiol Acad Sci Hung.* 1975;46:281-285.

Tan C, Tasaka H, Yu KP, Murphy ML, Karnofsky DA. Daunomycin, an antitumor antibiotic, in the treatment of neoplastic disease. Clinical evaluation with special reference to childhood leukemia. *Cancer*. 1967;20:333-353.

Tan-Chiu E, Yothers G, Romond E, Geyer CE Jr, Ewer M, Keefe D, Shannon RP, Swain SM, Brown A, Fehrenbacher L, Vogel VG, Seay TE, Rastogi P, Mamounas EP, Wolmark N, Bryant J. Assessment of cardiac dysfunction in a randomized trial comparing doxorubicin and cyclophosphamide followed by paclitaxel, with or without trastuzumab as adjuvant therapy in node-positive, human epidermal growth factor receptor 2-overexpressing breast cancer: NSABP B-31.*J Clin Oncol*. 2005;23:7811-7819.

Tazelaar HD, Karch SB, Stephens BG, Billingham ME. Cocaine and the heart. *Hum Pathol*. 1987;18:195-199.

Thompson PD, Sadaniantz A, Cullinane EM, Bodziony KS, Catlin DH, Torek-Both G, Douglas PS. Left ventricular function is not impaired in weight-lifters who use anabolic steroids. *J Am Coll Cardiol*. 1992;19:278-282.

Tokarska-Schlattner M, Zaugg M, Zuppinger C, Wallimann T, Schlattner U. New insights into doxorubicin-induced cardiotoxicity: the critical role of cellular energetics. *J Mol Cell Cardiol*. 2006;41:389-405.

Turner NA, Porter KE, Smith WH, White HL, Ball SG, Balmforth AJ. Chronic beta2-adrenergic receptor stimulation increases proliferation of human cardiac fibroblasts via an autocrine mechanism. *Cardiovasc Res*. 2003;57:784-792.

Turnipseed SD, Richards JR, Kirk JD, Diercks DB, Amsterdam EA. Frequency of acute coronary syndrome in patients presenting to the emergency department with chest pain after methamphetamine use. *J Emerg Med*. 2003;24:369-373.

Unverferth DV, Jagadeesh JM, Unverferth BJ, Magorien RD, Leier CV, Balcerzak SP. Attempt to prevent doxorubicin-induced acute human myocardial morphologic damage with acetylcysteine. *J Natl Cancer Inst*. 1983;71:917-920.

Urbano-Márquez A, Estruch R, Fernández-Solá J, Nicolás JM, Paré JC, Rubin E. The greater risk of alcoholic cardiomyopathy and myopathy in women compared with men. *JAMA*. 1995;274:149-154.

Urbano-Márquez A, Estruch R, Navarro-Lopez F, Grau JM, Mont L, Rubin E. The effects of alcoholism on skeletal and cardiac muscle. *N Engl J Med*. 1989;320:409-415.

Urbano-Márquez A, Fernández-Solà J. Effects of alcohol on skeletal and cardiac muscle. *Muscle Nerve*. 2004;30:689-707.

van Acker FA, van Acker SA, Kramer K, Haenen GR, Bast A, van der Vijgh WJ. 7-monohydroxyethylrutoside protects against chronic doxorubicin-induced cardiotoxicity when administered only once per week. *Clin Cancer Res*. 2000 Apr;6(4):1337-41.

van Dalen EC, Caron HN, Dickinson HO, Kremer LC. Cardioprotective interventions for cancer patients receiving anthracyclines. *Cochrane Database Syst Rev*. 2011 Jun 15;6:CD003917.

Von Hoff DD, Layard MW, Basa P, Davis HL Jr, Von Hoff AL, Rozencweig M, Muggia FM. Risk factors for doxorubicin-induced congestive heart failure. *Ann Intern Med*. 1979;91:710-717.

Wang M, Tsai BM, Kher A, Baker LB, Wairiuko GM, Meldrum DR. Role of endogenous testosterone in myocardial proinflammatory and proapoptotic signaling after acute ischemia-reperfusion. *Am J Physiol Heart Circ Physiol*. 2005;288:H221-H226.

Wang M, Wang Y, Abarbanell A, Tan J, Weil B, Herrmann J, Meldrum DR. Both endogenous and exogenous testosterone decrease myocardial STAT3 activation and SOCS3 expression after acute ischemia and reperfusion. *Surgery*. 2009;146:138-144.

Weidmann B, Jansen W, Heider A, Niederle N. 5-Fluorouracil cardiotoxicity with left ventricular dysfunction under different dosing regimens. *Am J Cardiol*. 1995;75:194-195.

Wexler LH, Andrich MP, Venzon D, Berg SL, Weaver-McClure L, Chen CC, Dilsizian V, Avila N, Jarosinski P, Balis FM, Poplack DG, Horowitz ME. Randomized trial of the cardioprotective agent ICRF-187 in pediatric sarcoma patients treated with doxorubicin. *J Clin Oncol*. 1996;14:362-372.

Wijetunga M, Seto T, Lindsay J, Schatz I. Crystal methamphetamine-associated cardiomyopathy: tip of the iceberg? *J Toxicol Clin Toxicol*. 2003;41:981-986.

Wittstein IS. Acute stress cardiomyopathy. *Curr Heart Fail Rep*. 2008;5:61-68.

Wu AH. Cardiotoxic drugs: clinical monitoring and decision making. *Heart*. 2008;94:1503-1509.

Wu X, Hasinoff BB. The antitumor anthracyclines doxorubicin and daunorubicin do not inhibit cell growth through the formation of iron-mediated reactive oxygen species. *Anticancer Drugs*. 2005;16:93-99.

Yeo KK, Wijetunga M, Ito H, Efird JT, Tay K, Seto TB, Alimineti K, Kimata C, Schatz IJ. The association of methamphetamine use and cardiomyopathy in young patients. *Am J Med*. 2007;120:165-171.

Zakhari S. Alcohol and the cardiovascular system: molecular mechanisms for beneficial and harmful action. *Alcohol Health Res World*. 1997;21:21-29.

Zaugg M, Jamali NZ, Lucchinetti E, Xu W, Alam M, Shafiq SA, Siddiqui MA. Anabolic-androgenic steroids induce apoptotic cell death in adult rat ventricular myocytes. *J Cell Physiol*. 2001;187:90-95.

Zhang GX, Kimura S, Nishiyama A, Shokoji T, Rahman M, Yao L, Nagai Y, Fujisawa Y, Miyatake A, Abe Y. Cardiac oxidative stress in acute and chronic isoproterenol-infused rats. *Cardiovasc Res*. 2005;65:230-238.

Zhang L, Kelley J, Schmeisser G, Kobayashi YM, Jones LR. Complex formation between junctin, triadin, calsequestrin, and the ryanodine receptor. Proteins of the cardiac junctional sarcoplasmic reticulum membrane. *J Biol Chem*. 1997;272:23389-23397.

Zimmer HG. Catecholamine-induced cardiac hypertrophy: significance of proto-oncogene expression. *J Mol Med (Berl)*. 1997;75:849-859.

Zuppinger C, Timolati F, Suter TM. Pathophysiology and diagnosis of cancer drug induced cardiomyopathy. *Cardiovasc Toxicol*. 2007;7:61-66.

27

Anthracycline Cardiotoxicity

Giuseppe Visani[1], Alessandro Isidori[1] and Giorgio Minotti[2]
[1]*Hematology and Stem Cell Transplant Center, Marche Nord Hospital, Via Lombroso, Pesaro,*
[2]*Center for Integrated Research and Drug Sciences, Campus Bio-Medico University, Via Alvaro del Portillo, Rome, Italy*

1. Introduction

Cancer patients who are undergoing chemotherapy have an increased risk of developing cardiovascular complications, and the risk is even greater if there is a known history of heart disease. A wide range of chemotherapy agents have been associated with cardiotoxicity. Among the serious cardiac complications related to chemotherapy, there are arrhythmias, myocardial necrosis causing a dilated cardiomyopathy and vasoocclusion or vasospasm resulting in angina or myocardial infarction.

The anthracyclines and related compounds (doxorubicin, idarubicin, epirubicin, and the anthraquinone mitoxantrone) are some of the most frequently implicated agents. Anthracyclines, including doxorubicin, are widely used in the treatment of cancer. Although topoisomerase II inhibition remains the most persuasive mechanism to explain the antitumor activity of anthracyclines, clinically relevant concentrations of anthracyclines were shown to induce apoptosis through additional mechanisms that were not bound to the topoisomerase II - p53 machinery.

However, their use is limited by cardiotoxicity and increasing survivors' susceptibility to treatment-related complications that can remarkably affect their quality of life. Surviving patients have an increased rate of heart failure, coronary artery disease, and cerebrovascular accidents compared to the general population. The specific mechanisms of anthracycline cardiotoxicity are complex and still remain unclear. Hence, determining the factors that may increase propensity to cardiotoxicity is of great importance, as is monitoring patients during and after treatment. Additionally, treatment and prevention options, such as limiting cumulative dosage, liposomal anthracyclines, and dexrazoxane, continue to be explored.

Liposomal doxorubicin has been developed with the aim of improving the therapeutics index of doxorubicin by reducing the drug's cardiotoxicity. Two liposomal formulations are currently available: non-pegylated liposomal doxorubicin (NPLD) (Myocet®, Cephalon, USA) and pegylated liposomal doxorubicin (PLD) (Caelix®/Doxil®, Schering-Plough/Orto Biothech, USA).

In this chapter, we will analyze the cardiac complications caused by the use of anthracyclines, and the potential benefit of substituting these drugs with their liposomal counterpart. Acute and chronic cardiac toxicities, together with risk factors will also be discussed. Guidelines for monitoring and drug discontinuation will be another point to be analyzed in this chapter.

2. Pharmacology

The anthracyclines represent a broad family of antibiotics that exhibit activity in numerous tumours. The first anthracyclines, doxorubicin (DOX) and daunorubicin (DNR), were isolated from Streptomyces var. Peucetius; they were shown to be composed of a tetracyclic ring system with adjacent quinone-hydroquinone moieties, a short side chain with a carbonyl group, and an aminosugar bound to the C-7 of the four-ring system. DOX and DNR only differed in the side chain terminus (-CH_2OH in DOX vs -CH_3 in DNR). Second generation anthracyclines, like epirubicin (EPI) and idarubicin (IDA), were obtained after minor chemical modifications of DOX or DNR, respectively.

When injected by standard i.v. infusion, anthracyclines show a rapid distribution phase, a high distribution volume at steady state (~15 l/kg), a slow elimination phase (successive plasma half-lives of ~ 5 minutes, ~1 hour and ~30 hours). Anthracyclines are excreted mostly through bile, which imposes special care in patients with hepatic dysfunction (Robert & Gianni, 1993). In comparison with DOX, EPI is characterized by an unique glucuronidation that accelerates its systemic body clearance and imposes administering EPI at doses 1.5 times higher than those of DOX (Innocenti F et al., 2001).

Anthracyclines have long been known to kill tumor cells by inhibiting topoisomerase II. Anthracyclines act by stabilizing a reaction intermediate in which DNA strands are cut and covalently linked to topoisomerase II, eventually impeding DNA resealing. Anthracycline intercalation into DNA plays a role in this reaction; in fact, anthracycline rings that do not intercalate into DNA probably stabilize the complex between topoisomerase II and the DNA that it has nicked (Menna et al., 2008). Anthracycline- and topoisomerase II-mediated DNA damage is followed by growth arrest in G1 and G2 and apoptosis. This is usually, but not always, relayed by p53 and the consequent induction of the WAF1/CIP1 p21 gene product, a strong inhibitor of cyclin-dependent kinases that favour cell cycle progression through the G1 to S transition (Minotti et al., 2008).

Although topoisomerase II inhibition remains the most persuasive mechanism to explain the antitumor activity of anthracyclines, clinically relevant concentrations of anthracyclines were shown to induce apoptosis through additional mechanisms that were not bound to the topoisomerase II - p53 machinery. These mechanisms include, among others, i) the activation of neutral sphingomyelinases, followed by ceramide formation and converse activation of cell death effectors (c-Jun N-terminal kinase) or down-regulation of survival pathways (Akt/protein kinase B) ii), mitochondrial dysfunction, followed by cytochrome c release and apoptosome formation iii), induction of lipid peroxidation and formation of malondialdehyde-DNA adducts, followed by the reduced activity of cyclin E- and cyclin B-associated kinase activities and growth arrest in both p53-proficient and p53-deficient cells iv), inhibition of the proteasome, followed by an accumulation of undegraded ubiquinated proteins which signal apoptosis. The mechanisms i-iii) are triggered by reactive oxygen species (ROS), that are major byproducts of anthracycline metabolism. ROS may also enable anthracyclines to damage and shorten telomeres, long sequences of base repeats that otherwise would delay cell senescence and apoptosis by preventing the degradation and ligation of the end of chromosomes; however, anthracycline-induced telomere damage and dysfunction would be relayed to apoptosis through p53 (Minotti et al, 2004).

Anthracycline treatment may be accompanied by the acquisition of a resistance phenotype through a combination of pharmacokinetic and pharmacodynamic mechanisms. On pharmacokinetic grounds, tumor resistance is caused by the reduced accumulation and/or an altered distribution of anthracyclines in tumor cells, usually mediated by overexpression of drug transporters that belong to the ATP-binding cassette family of proteins and are collectively referred to as ABC proteins (P-glycoprotein/Pgp, multidrug resistance protein 1/MRP1, breast cancer resistance protein/BCRP). On pharmacodynamic grounds, tumor resistance may be caused by such diverse mechanisms as topoisomerase II mutation or redundancy, overexpression and preferred nuclear localization of proteasome α-type subunits (leading to a anomalous degradation of topoisomerase II), genetic deletion or loss-of-function mutations of p53, overexpression of ROS-detoxifying enzymes, overexpression of Bcl-2 (leading to a diminished cytochrome c release), etc. When taken in isolation, however, none of these factors would universally predict anthracycline-resistance in a given tumor or another (Minotti et al., 2008).

3. How do anthracyclines damage the heart

The problem of anthracycline-induced cardiomyopathy and congestive heart failure (CHF) has been around for some 40 years. On ultrastructural grounds, all of the approved anthracyclines share a pattern of damage that is characterized by loss of myofibrils, dilation of the sarcoplasmic reticulum, cytoplasmic vacuolization, swelling of mitochondria, and increased number of lysosomes; however, safety threshold may differ from one anthracyclines to another. In the case of DOX, the incidence of cardiomyopathy and congestive heart failure (CHF) averages below 5% if the cumulative dose did not exceed 400-450 mg/m^2 (Swain et al., 2003) ; EPI induces CHF at doses slightly higher than equiactive to DOX (~800-900 mg/m^2). Safety limits for DNR and IDA are less firmly established because of different regimens and schedules adopted in induction or consolidation treatment of myeloproliferative disorders. With that said, cardiac events may develop at reportedly safe cumulative doses if patients presented with hypertension, arrhythmias, valvular or coronary disease, or metabolic disorders; Moreover, children and the elderly are more vulnerable than the young-adult (Minotti et al., 2010). Perhaps more importantly, we now know that subthreshold doses of anthracyclines, as commonly adopted in many oncologic settings, may cause the development of cardiotoxicity months to years after completing chemotherapy, as if "safe doses" of anthracyclines primed the heart to a subclinical damage liable to a delayed clinical manifestation (Minotti et al., 2010). Mechanisms of anthracycline cardiotoxicity should therefore be reconciled with the concept of a lifetime risk of cardiotoxicity.

Anthracycline cardiotoxicity correlates directly with drug's peak plasma concentration (Minotti et al., 2004) but correlates inversely to the levels and activity of ABC proteins that eject drugs from endothelial cells of the blood-heart barrier (Sissung et al., 2011). Once inside cardiomyocytes, much of anthracycline toxicity seems to depend on bioactivation events.

The quinone moiety of anthracyclines undergoes one-electron reduction by a number of reductases, primarily located to mitochondria; oxidation of the so-formed semiquinone with molecular oxygen regenerates the parent quinone and exposes the cell to higher than physiological levels of ROS like superoxide anion ($O_2^{\cdot-}$), hydrogen peroxide (H_2O_2), and hydroxyl radical ($\cdot OH$). Bimolecular reaction of $O_2^{\cdot-}$ with nitric oxide also generates peroxynitrite endowed with noticeable prooxidant activities. In comparison to other cell types cardiomyocytes are very rich in mitochondria, but relatively poor in ROS-detoxifying enzymes; it follows that cardiomyocytes would readily succumb to a sustained generation of ROS that eventually induced sarcomere degradation, mitochondrial dysfunction and DNA damage, disruption of cardiac-specific gene expression programs, necrotic or apoptotic death (Minotti et al., 2004). This "oxidative stress" hypothesis of cardiotoxicity gained popularity over the years and was successfully probed in transgenic mice that overexpressed antioxidant defense systems like catalase, mitochondrial manganese-dependent superoxide dismutase, metallothioneins; Interestingly, however, robust doses of antioxidants like vitamin E or N-acetylcysteine neither delayed nor mitigated cardiotoxicity induced in patients by cumulative doses of DOX (Minotti et al., 2004). The only compound consistently found to be cardioprotective in clinical settings is the iron chelator, dexrazoxane. Iron chelation would mitigate free radical reactions that otherwise caused cardiotoxicity. Another caveat in the "oxidative stress hypothesis" is the lack of a clear-and-cut relation with the lifetime risk of cardiotoxicity. Once inside cardiomyocytes anthracyclines can diffuse back toward extracellular fluids, making the intracellular drug levels decrease to below a threshold of toxic concern (Salvatorelli et al., 2009). Some investigators suggested that DOX caused an oxidative mitochondriopathy that self-maintained after DOX had been cleared from cardiomyocytes; however, self-maintaining mitochondriopathy was documented with DOX but not EPI (Lebrecht & Walker, 2007), in spite of that EPI clearly retained a potential for inducing cardiotoxicity. On balance, anthracyclines do form ROS in the relatively unprotected cardiac tissue, but compelling evidence for a cause-and-effect relationship between oxidative stress and chronic cardiomyopathy is lacking.

The lifetime risk of cardiotoxicity from anthracyclines could be better reconciled with their conversion to secondary alcohol metabolites, formed after two electron reduction of their side chain carbonyl group. Being more polar than their parent drugs, secondary alcohol metabolites are poorly cleared from cardiomyocytes and accumulate to become a long-lasting anthracycline toxic signature in the heart (Menna et al., 2008); times more potent than their parent anthracyclines at inactivating Ca^{2+}-handling proteins of the contraction-relaxation cycle or key regulators of energy metabolism and redox balance, such as cytoplasmic aconitase. Therefore, secondary alcohol metabolites may cause cardiotoxicity both during and well after the course of chemotherapy.

In clinical settings, a retrospective study of patients enrolled in the Childhood Cancer Survivor Study suggests that the V244M polymorphism of carbonyl reductase 3 associated with a higher risk to develop CHF, presumably because the methionine244 isoform of carbonyl reductase 3 shows a greater catalytic specificity toward carbonyl substrates (Blanco et al., 2008). Most recent reports suggest that gain of function CBR polymorphisms could be invoked to particularly explain CHF development in patients exposed to subthreshold cumulative doses of anthracyclines .

There are, of course, some caveats in the alcohol metabolite hypothesis of cardiotoxicity. EPI forms fewer amounts of its alcohol metabolite as compared to DOX, which is consistent with CHF developing at cumulative doses of EPI higher than equiactive to DOX (Salvatorelli et al., 2007). In contrast, DNR and IDA generate more alcohol metabolites than DOX in spite of that their cardiotoxicity was ranked similar to or less severe than that of DOX, respectively (Minotti et al., 2004). Once again, the different modalities of administration of DNR or IDA in the settings of myeloproliferative disease could be invoked to explain such discrepancy.

4. How to prevent anthracycline induced cardiotoxicity

Anthracycline cardiotoxicity coud be prevented by replacing bolus administration with slow infusions that generate lower anthracycline plasma peaks and thus mitigate a pharmacokinetic determinant of cardiotoxicity. The benefit of replacing bolus administration (5-15 min infusion) with slow infusions (24-48 h) is quite evident in adult settings but not in pediatric settings. The current thinking is that children are more vulnerable by anthracyclines; the protective benefit obtained by lowering plasma peak concentrations would therefore be offset by damage due to the longer cardiac exposure to anthracyclines (Lipshultz et al., 2002).

The notion that anthracycline-related cardiotoxicity may develop long after completing chemotherapy suggests that drugs used to treat clinically evident cardiotoxicity should be used much earlier to protect the heart against subclinical cardiotoxicity. Unfortunately, active cardiac prevention by beta-blockers, angiotensin I-converting enzyme inhibitors, or angiotensin II receptor blockers, has been explored in only few limited studies. Prophylactic commencement of angiotensin I-converting enzyme inhibitors prevented decrements of Left Ventricular Ejection Fraction (LVEF) in patients receiving high-dose chemotherapy (Cardinale et al, 2006), while prophylactic commencement of angiotensin II receptors blockers prevented transient elevations of brain natriuretic peptide in patients receiving one cycle of standard-dose chemotherapy for non-Hodgkin lymphoma (Nakamae et al., 2005). Unfortunately, prophylactic commencement of cardiovascular medications was not prospectively assessed in patients scheduled to receiving multiple cycles of standard-dose chemotherapy. The reported protective efficacy of carvedilol, mixed a1-2-b1 blocker, was observed in patients treated with anthracycline cumulative doses higher than recommended (Kalay et al., 2006) this likely amplified the protective signal of any drug that had been administered (Florenzano & Salman, 2007). Outside of these limited exploratory studies, prophylactic commencement of cardiovascular medications is uncommon or disregarded because of concerns about class-related effects such as hypotension, bradicardia, fluid retention, cough, or other discomfort.

As already mentioned, dexrazoxane was the only compound that consistently proved effective in preventing anthracycline-related cardiotoxicity. The chemical structure of dexrazoxane consists of a *bis*-ketopiperazine that diffuses in cardiomyocytes and then undergoes stepwise hydrolysis of the two piperazine rings to form one-ring open intermediates. This one-ring intermediate hydrolyses to give a diacid-diamide (code-named ADR 925) which is structurally reminiscent of EDTA and chelates iron bound to low molecular weight cellular ligands or coordinated within 3:1 anthracycline:Fe complexes (Minotti et al., 2004). When administered by intravenous push or slow infusion some 15 to 30 min before DOX at dose ratios up to 10:1 to DOX, dexrazoxane did not interfere with DOX distribution or metabolism or excretion, but reduced the incidence of cardiotoxicity. In a randomized clinical trial, women with metastatic breast cancer who received dexrazoxane prior to DOX could be treated with more cycles and higher cumulative doses of DOX (700-1,000 mg/m^2 or more) than patients in the control group. Moreover, cardiac protection was observed in patients with or without risk factors such as e.g., prior chest wall irradiation (reviewed in Minotti et al., 2004). As a matter of fact, the pharmacological properties and clinical readouts of dexrazoxane have been widely challenged. In the pharmacological field, there have been reports that dexrazoxane could protect by mechanisms other than iron chelation, like e.g., inhibition of topoisomerase II-mediated formation of DNA double-strand breaks in cardiomyocytes (Lyu et al., 2007). Accordingly, preclinical studies showed little or no cardiac protection by dexrazoxane analogues that chelated iron but failed to inhibit toposomerase II (Sterba et al. J Pharmacol Exp Ther 2006). In the clinical setting, the risk/benefit ratio of dexrazoxane was questioned in terms of hemathologic toxicities and interference with anthracycline activity. An exacerbation of anthracycline-related myelotoxicity (usually in the form of grade 3 or 4 neutropenia) is a well- known complication of the use of dexrazoxane, but other studies raised a concern that children treated with dexrazoxane were at a higher risk for second malignancies including, among others, acute myelogenous leukaemia and myelodysplastic syndrome. This latter concern was dispelled by two authoritative studies of childhood cancer survivors who had been randomized to receive anthracyclines with or without dexrazoxane as cardioprotectant (Barryet al., J Clin Oncol. 2008; Vrooman et al., Eur J Cancer. 2011). Other concerns were raised in relation to a possible interference of dexrazoxane with anthracycline activity. One single study suggested that dexrazoxane reduced response rates in women who received DOX for the treatment of advanced breast cancer (Swain et al., J Clin Oncol 1997) but many other clinical studies showed that this was not the case in either pediatric or adult settings (Swain and Vici, J Cancer Res Clin Oncol. 2004; van Dalen et al., Cochrane Database Syst Rev. 2011). In spite of the overwhelming evidence for its safety and preventative activity in a number of oncologic settings, the American Society of Clinical Oncology, Chemotherapy, and Radiotherapy Expert Panel maintained and recommended using dexrazoxane only in patients who had received more than 300 mg of DOX/m^2 and could benefit from continuing on DOX or EPI (Schuchter et al., 2002). It is our opinion that dexrazoxane should be used with less restrictions; current limitations to using it in a prophylactic manner are not supported by available evidence.

In a similar manner, oncologists should be encouraged to use liposomal formulations of DOX. These formulations approach very high peak plasma levels and longer circulating time than conventional DOX but release little or no free anthracycline in the bloodstream. Moreover, the liposomes are small enough to diffuse through the discontinuous "leaky" endothelium of tumors, but they are big enough not to diffuse through the normal microvasculature of the heart. Liposomal formulations therefore deliver high amounts of DOX in tumors but not in the heart. One liposomal DOX (Caelyx®) has polyethylene glycol embedded in the lipid layers; another formulation (Myocet®) adopts an uncoated liposome. Regardless of obvious pharmacokinetic and toxicokinetic differences between the two formulations, both proved remarkably cardiac tolerable and allowed administering high to very high cumulative doses of anthracycline. in a number of clinical settings. A recent Cochrane Intervention Review raises caution against using liposomal doxorubicin in pediatric settings or in patients diagnosed with leukaemia, but it is quite strong in concluding that liposomal formulations should be favoured in adults with a solid tumor (van Dalen et al., 2010). Despite this authoritative recommendation, clinical use of liposomal anthracycline formulations remains quite limited, primarily because of cost-related concerns. It is our opinion that liposomal doxorubicin should remain a must in certain approved settings (like e.g., ovary cancer in the case of Caelyx) and first choice in any other patients presenting with cardiovascular risk factors (as it is the case for Myocet in high risk or older patients with non Hodgkin lymphoma) (Visani & Isidori, 2011).

Preventing the risk of anthracycline-related cardiotoxicity during the lifetime means to reshape the pharmacological management of cancer survivors. Preexisting comorbidities or unfavorable lifestyle choices (hypertension, diabetes, hyperlipidemia, reduced physical activity) had long been known to increase the risk of cardiotoxicity in patients scheduled to receiving anthracyclines. The available evidence suggests that this picture should also be viewed the other way around. In comparison to siblings or age-matched subjects from the general population, previously healthy cancer survivors tend in fact to develop more comorbidities or to reduce physical activity (De Bruin et al., 2009; Jones et al., 2007). It follows that sublinical cardiotoxicity from "safe doses" of anthracyclines may progress to symptomatic events by overlapping with risk factors that matured after ending chemotherapy. This is the so-called multiple-hit hypothesis, according to which late onset cardiotoxicity originates from pharmacological and non pharmacological sequential injuries (Minotti et al, 2010). These concepts call for a new dimension of preventative cardiology, in a sense that in cancer survivors any comorbidity or unfavourable lifestyle choice should be treated earlier or more vigorously than in the general population.

5. Monitoring

There is no universally accepted guideline for monitoring patients receiving anthracyclines. Table I provides a tentative schedule that follows on suggestions by Ewer and colleagues mainly based on widely used criteria such as cumulative dose, time elapsed after chemotherapy, presence or absence of cardiovascular risk factors or preexisting cardiac disease, concerns (or symptoms) calling for unscheduled visits and cardiological inspection, dosability in any clinical center (measurements of LVEF only).

Planned Cumulative Dose (mg/m^2)	**During treatment**		**After treatment**	
	No risk factors or Preexisting Cardiac Disease	One or more risk factors, Preexisting Cardiac disease	No risk factors or Preexisting Cardiac Disease	One or more risk factors, Preexisting Cardiac disease
Baseline	yes	yes		
<300	At the physician's discretion	Recommended after two-three cycles	Approx 1, 6, and 12 months after ending therapy, and then every two years unless symptoms occur	Approx 1, 6, and 12 months after ending therapy, and then every year unless symptoms occur
300-450	At the physician discretion; recommended anytime patients report on symptoms	Recommended every two cycles	Approx 1, 6, and 12 months after ending therapy, and then every year unless symptoms occur	Approx 1 month after ending therapy, and then every six months unless symptoms occur
>450	Recommended at midtherapy or earlier if symptoms occur	Recommended every two cycles or more often if symptoms occur	Approx 1 month after ending therapy, and then every six months unless symptoms occur	Approx 1 month after ending therapy, and then every six months unless symptoms occur

Table 1. General principles for monitoring LVEF in patients receiving doxorubicin. Modified after Ewer and Benjamin (2006).

Whereas the reported timetable is intrinsically correct and doable in everyday clinical practice, there are at least two disturbing points that need to be kept in mind if one wished to improve the caring of cancer patients and survivors. First, we now know that as little as 100 mg of DOX/m^2 may cause an increased risk of asymptomatic abnormalities at non-invasive cardiac tests, whereas 270 mg of DOX/m^2 introduces a measurable 4.5-fold excess risk of such abnormalities (Hudson et al, 2007). The second point is that dilative cardiomyopathy and systolic failure (reduced LVEF) have been considered for long time the only (or prevailing) clinical phenotypes of chronic cardiotoxicity from anthracyclines. Therefore, serial measurements of LVEF (whether by echocardiography or MUGA) have been adopted to measure the cardiac function of patients treated with anthracyclines. Keeping this in mind, we now know that asymptomatic diastolic dysfunction is seen in many cancer survivors with a history of prior exposure to anthracyclines. Anthracyclines, in fact, could cause diastolic elevated $[Ca^{2+}]_I$ and impaired left ventricle relaxation (stiffness) by a number of mechanisms (inhibition and/or reduced expression levels of the Ca^{2+}-ATPase that sequesters Ca^{2+} in sarcoplasmic reticulum, inhibition of the energy build-up that assists Ca^{2+} loading in mitochondria, inappropriate opening of the Ca^{2+}-gated Ca^{2+} release channel of the sarcoplasmic reticulum (ryanodine receptor 2) (Minotti et al, 2004). Long lasting diastolic dysfunction eventually increases interstitial pressure, thereby diminishing coronary conductance and causing ischemia that further aggravates Ca^{2+} overload and left ventricle wall tension (Hale et al., 2008). Reciprocal interactions between diastolic dysfunction and ischemia may remain asymptomatic for many years but eventually surface in the form of symptomatic ischemic disease and myocardial infarction. The risk of myocardial infarction in previously nonischemic Hodgkin's lymphoma survivors therefore correlated with their prior exposure to anthracyclines (Swerdlow et al., 2007). Furthermore, diastolic dysfunction and reduced coronary conductance would render the heart more vulnerable by comorbidities that diminish coronary flow or increased oxygen demand, like e.g. premature atherosclerosis or hypertension. All such concepts call for reshaping current modalities of follow up of cancer survivors. Serial measurements of LVEF should no longer be considered adequate to identify patients at risk for symptomatic cardiac events. Moreover, careful inspection of diastolic function (e.g., transmitral flow) is equally important and much needed, not to mention myocardial perfusion imaging techniques that show hypoperfusion under stress conditions. These approaches are less doable in clinical practice, leaving many patients with normal LVEF at risk for sudden or slowly developing cardiac events.

Current limitations in the monitoring of patients at risk for anthracycline related cardiotoxicity could be obviated by measuring pre- and post- infusional levels of circulating troponin (TnI), marker of toxic or ischemic cardiomyocyte necrosis. Persistent elevations of TnI were shown to anticipate LVEF decrements and other cardiac events in otherwise asymptomatic childhood cancer patients (Lipshultz et al., 1997) or in adults receiving high-dose chemotherapy (Cardinale et al., 2006). More recently, elevations of TnI were shown to anticipate LVEF decrements in women who had received sequential adjuvant chemotherapy and immunologic treatment with the anti-Erbb2 monoclonal antibody trastuzumab for the treatment of $Erbb2^+$ early breast cancer (J Clin Oncol., 2010, 28:3910-6). Unfortunately, TnI measurements are uncommon outside of limited exploratory studies; there is a lack of studies that prospectively evaluated TnI in large cohort of patients and firmly established laboratory ranges that should guide the physicians in making decisions such as adjusting the dose of anthracycline or commencing prophylactic cardiovascular medications. Similarly uncommon is the measurement of circulating natriuretic peptides, markers of left ventricular diastolic tension. On treatment elevations of natriuretic peptides were reported to anticipate chemotherapy-induced diastolic dysfunction, but such elevations were seen in patients treated with high-dose chemotherapy or in patients receiving just one cycle of standard-dose chemotherapy (Gianni et al., 2008, J. Clin. Oncol. 26; Nakamae et al., 2005). There is little information on the prognostic value of natriuretic peptides elevations during the course of cumulative standard-dose chemotherapy and at follow-up.

6. Liposomal formulations of doxorubicin

Daunorubicin (DNR) as the cell cycle non-specific anthracycline antibiotics is highly effective in treating a wide range of cancer diseases [5-7]. Its antineoplastic mechanisms are through DNA topoisomerase II inhibition, DNA intercalation, RNA synthesis inhibition, cell membranes interaction, free radicals production and induction of apoptosis [8-10]. However, the clinical use of daunorubicin is hampered by two major problems: cardiotoxicity [11] and drug resistance, as daunorubicin is a substrate for P-glycoprotein (MDR1; ABCB1) [12] and breast cancer resistance protein (BCRP;ABCG2) [13]. This limits of standard doxorubicin have moved forward the development of new liposomal formulations of the drug, which gained increasing interest in the therapy of onco-hematological malignancies and, in particular, for the treatment of breast cancer and B-cell lymphomas. In the early 1980s, liposomes were discovered to be good anthracycline carriers, reducing toxicity while retaining potent antitumor activity and therefore improving the therapeutic index of anthracyclines [14]. Liposomal formulations of doxorubicin have indeed been developed with the aim of improving the therapeutic index of doxorubicin by reducing the drug's cardiotoxicity. Nevertheless, liposomal conjugation of doxorubicin results in preferential distribution of the drug in the tumor compared with normal tissue.

Two liposomal formulations are currently available: non-pegylated liposomal doxorubicin (NPLD) (Myocet®, Cephalon, USA) and pegylated liposomal doxorubicin (PLD) (Caelix®/Doxil®, Schering-Plough/Orto Biothech, USA)

NPLD is a liposome encapsulated formulation of doxorubicin, which differs from pegylated liposomal doxorubicin, as well as from unencapsulated, conventional doxorubicin, resulting in an alteration in the pharmacokinetics and biodistribution. This results in a higher area under the curve, a smaller volume of distribution and a preferential distribution to liver, spleen, and lymphatics, when compared with conventional doxorubicin. Pre-clinical studies comparing equal doses of liposome-encapsulated doxorubicin and conventional doxorubicin showed that the use of nonpegylated liposomal doxorubicin resulted in a significantly lower cardiac and gastrointestinal toxicity, with similar anti-tumor efficacy.

The other liposomal compound, pegylated liposomal doxorubicin (PLD) (Caelix®/Doxil®, Schering-Plough/Orto Biothech, USA), is a liposomal formulation with a distinct pharmacokinetic profile characterized by an extended circulation time and a reduced volume of distribution [22]. Biodistribution animal studies indicate superior accumulation of PLD into various implanted mouse-human tumors, with an augmentation of liposomal drug tumor levels compared with free drugs [22]. The extended circulation time of pegylated liposomes and their ability to extravasate through the leaky vasculature of tumors results in the increased delivery of liposomal drug and/or radiotracers to the tumor site in patients with cancer. Pegylated liposomal doxorubicin has been approved for clinical use in a variety of cancer types due to its antitumor efficacy. However, the safety profile needs further improvement, as long as hand-foot syndrome remains a dose-limiting toxic effect of Doxil, maybe due to the considerable amount of drug being delivered to the skin owing to the drug's long circulation in the bloodstream.

7. Non-Pegylated Liposomal Doxorubicin (NPLD)

NPLD is a doxorubicin citrate complex encapsulated in a liposome, an aqueous dispersion of egg Phosphatydilcholine
and cholesterol, sterile, non-pyrogenous that traps doxorubicin by pulling it into the interior of the vesicle (TLC D-99 model) by the generation of an electropotential across the liposome membrane. This mechanism for remote loading involves the generation of a pH gradient between the inside and the extraliposomal buffer. At the end of the encapsulation process, the ratio of doxorubicin:lipid in NPLD is approximately 1:4 and the pH is in the range of 5.5–6.5. The maximum activity of doxorubicin and other anthracyclines manifests itself in the S phase of the cellular cycle.
The encapsulation of a cytostatic agent within a macromolecular vector such as a liposome reduces drastically its distribution volume, diminishing its diffusion in the organism and thus the toxicity for healthy tissues while increasing the concentration within the neoplastic tissue. In ideal conditions the drug can be transported in the circulatory system within the liposome's aqueous space and arrives to the site of the tumor in active form. Encapsulation in a liposome means the drug is protected from inactivation while in the blood stream and furthermore its diffusion through the healthy endothelium is limited, while it can diffuse through tumoral endothelium which would present discontinuities. Thus, NPLD should preferentially direct doxorubicin away from sites of potential toxicity, but leaves the tumor exposed.

7.1 Non-pegylated liposomal doxorubicin in breast cancer

NPLD was designed to reduce the cardiotoxicity of doxorubicin while preserving its antitumor efficacy. In the early 2000, the safety and efficacy of NPLD was tested in cancer patients, after the demonstration of a significantly lower cardiac and gastrointestinal toxicity, with similar anti-tumor efficacy showed by NPLD in pre-clinical studies.
The first studies were conduced in breast cancer patients. These phase III, randomized, multicenter trials were designed to test the hypothesis that NPLD, alone or in combination with other drugs, would result in significantly less cardiac toxicity than the same dose and schedule of conventional doxorubicin and other drugs, while providing comparable antitumor efficacy in first-line treatment of metastatic breast cancer.
Batist et al (Batist et al., 2001) randomized 297 patients with MBC and no prior chemotherapy for metastatic disease were randomized to receive either 60 mg/m^2 of NPLD or conventional doxorubicin (A), in combination with 600 mg/m^2 of cyclophosphamide (C), every 3 weeks until disease progression or unacceptable toxicity. Antitumor efficacy of MC versus AC was comparable: objective response rates, 43% versus 43%; median time to progression, 5.1% versus 5.5 months; median time to treatment failure, 4.6 versus 4.4 months; and median survival, 19 versus 16 months (Batist et al., 2001).
Cardiotoxicity was a primary end point parameter in all treated patients (Batist et al., 2001). Cardiac toxicity, sufficient for removal of a patient from study, was defined as a decrease in

resting LVEF of ≥ 20 ejection fraction (EF) units from baseline to a final value of ≥ 50%, or a decrease of ≥ 10 EF units from baseline to a final value of less than 50%, or clinical evidence of CHF. LVEFs were assessed using serial Multigated blood-pool imaging (MUGA) scans, which have been shown to be a reliable and serially reproducible method of evaluating cardiac function in patients receiving anthracycline therapy.

To ensure accuracy and objectivity, each center was required to have its equipment and methodology used for MUGA scans reviewed and certified by a cardiologist at the Core Laboratory at Yale University before enrolling patients. During the trial, all MUGA scans were sent to the Core Laboratory at Yale, where they were read by the same cardiologist blinded to the patient's treatment (Batist et al., 2001). To minimize the risk of CHF, all scans were read in real time and results provided to the site before the next scheduled dose of anthracycline therapy. CHF was determined on the basis of a treatment-blinded review of records from patients for whom the investigator had made a diagnosis of CHF, as well as patients who had a LVEF of ≤ 30%. LVEF ≤ 30% was selected as the cutoff because these patients are at significant risk for CHF (Batist et al., 2001). The blinded review was conducted by a second cardiologist at Yale University noted for his expertise in doxorubicin-induced cardiotoxicity. All MUGA scan data were interpreted and LVEF values were estimated at a core laboratory on a blinded basis. Nine patients (6%) treated with MC developed protocol-defined cardiotoxicity compared with 33 patients (21%) treated with AC (log-rank $P = .0001$). Five cases of CHF, all in the AC arm (log-rank $P = .02$), were observed after cumulative lifetime doses ranging from 360 to 480 mg/m^2. Four of the five patients with CHF were anthracycline-naive before this study; one patient had 240 mg/m^2 of prior adjuvant doxorubicin. All other patients with cardiotoxicity had an asymptomatic decrease in LVEF of ≥ 10 EF units from baseline to a final value less than 50%. The estimated (Kaplan-Meier) median cumulative lifetime dose of doxorubicin at the first occurrence of protocol-defined cardiac toxicity was more than 2,220 mg/m^2 for the MC arm versus 480 mg/m^2 for the AC arm. The hazard ratio of 4.8 shows that patients treated with MC were 80% less likely to develop cardiotoxicity with respect to patients treated with AC.

Similarly, there was a highly significant difference in the time to onset of cardiotoxicity when measured from the start of protocol therapy. The estimated median onset of protocol-defined cardiotoxicity was more than 22 months for MC versus 10 months for AC (log-rank P = .0003). There was a gradual increase in the median change from baseline LVEF to the last posttreatment LVEF among patients treated with either regimen, but this was more pronounced in the AC-treated group (Batist et al., 2001).

In the subset of patients with recognized risk factors for cardiac toxicity, the hazard ratio was increased to 16, indicating that these patients were more than 90% less likely to develop cardiac toxicity with MC relative to AC. Four percent of MC-treated patients developed a protocol-defined cardiac event versus 22% of AC-treated patients (Batist et al., 2001). The median lifetime cumulative dose of doxorubicin at onset was 480 mg/m2 for AC versus more than 2,220 mg/m2 for MC (P = .0001) (Batist et al., 2001). Four of the five patients with CHF were in this subgroup with increased risk of cardiac toxicity (Batist et al., 2001).

In conclusion, the improved therapeutic index for NPLD predicted by the preclinical data and indicated by the phase I/II clinical trials was confirmed in this phase III, randomized, multicenter trial. Statistically significantly fewer patients treated with NPLD in combination with cyclophosphamide experienced cardiac toxicity defined by reductions in LVEF or clinical CHF (Batist et al., 2001).

Another interesting study was carried on by Harris et al (Harris et al, 2002). Two hundred twenty-four patients with MBC and no prior therapy for metastatic disease were randomized to receive either TLC D-99 (75 mg/m2) or doxorubicin (75 mg/m2) every 3 weeks, in the absence of disease progression or unacceptable toxicity. The primary efficacy endpoint was response rate. The primary safety endpoint was cardiotoxicity.

Electrocardiograms and MUGA scans were done at baseline, and after reaching a lifetime cumulative doxorubicin dose of 300, 400, 500 mg/m^2, and before each subsequent dose, at off-study, and at 3-month follow-up. All MUGA scan data were transferred electronically to a core laboratory for blinded interpretation and estimation of LVEF (Harris et al, 2002). Before the first interim analysis, endomyocardial biopsies were performed at a selected number of institutions after lifetime cumulative doxorubicin dose of 425 mg/m^2. All patients whose LVEF declined by greater than 10% to a value of greater than or equal to 50%, or by greater than 6% to a value of less than 50% were to have cardiac biopsies regardless of lifetime cumulative doses (Harris et al, 2002). All biopsies were read by a core pathologist, and the results were scored according to the Billingham scale. The purpose of biopsies was to validate the results of MUGA scans. After the first interim analysis, it was determined that MUGA scans were adequate to monitor cardiac function and cardiac biopsies were discontinued (Harris et al, 2002). All MUGA scan data were sent to an independent central laboratory for estimation and interpretation of LVEF values without knowledge of treatment arm.

Cardiac events, sufficient for removal of a patient from study, were more than twice as frequent in doxorubicin-treated patients than TLC D-99–treated patients (29% vs. 13%, log-rank P = 0.0001) (Harris et al, 2002). With the increasing lifetime cumulative dose of doxorubicin and TLC D-99, there was a gradual increase in the median change from baseline LVEF to the first post-treatment LVEF among patients treated with either agent, but this was more pronounced in the doxorubicin group (Harris et al, 2002). A Kaplan–Meier estimate of the probability of the first onset of a cardiac event as related to the lifetime cumulative dose of doxorubicin or TLC D-99 showed that risk of cardiotoxicity was much higher with doxorubicin treatment than TLC D-99 (HR = 3.56) (P = 0.0001) (Harris et al, 2002). Two patients (2%) on TLC D-99 developed clinical CHF. One patient, after 13 cycles of TLC D-99 and a cumulative dose of 1110 mg/m^2, had a decrease of 14 EF units in her LVEF to 46% and was taken off-study. Two months after the last dose she presented with shortness of breath and bilateral pleural effusions and was hospitalized for CHF. Another patient, with prior adjuvant doxorubicin dose of 290 mg/m^2 and prior chest wall irradiation, received five cycles of TLC D-99 for a total lifetime doxorubicin dose of 785 mg/m^2, and went off-study for PD. Four months after the last dose, a MUGA scan showed a LVEF of 46% (a 16-point decrease from baseline). Later, the patient received five cycles of a mitomycin plus mitoxantrone, and 11 months after the last study treatment she received a diagnosis of CHF (Harris et al, 2002). Nine patients (8%) on doxorubicin developed clinical CHF at lifetime doses of 525–765 mg/m^2. Three patients had CHF within 30 days of the last dose of study treatment, including one who died of CHF after 585 mg/m^2. All nine cases were attributed to study drug treatment (Harris et al, 2002).

Before the first interim analysis, 51 patients were treated at 8 participating institutions performing endomyocardial biopsies. Of those, 36 patients qualified for the procedure, and all 36 patients had cardiac biopsies. All biopsies were read by a core pathologist, blinded to treatment assignment, and the results were scored according to the Billingham scale. There was a significant difference between the two treatment groups favoring TLC D-99 and the number of patients who had a score of greater than or equal to 2.5 (26% vs. 71%; *P* = 0.02) (Harris et al, 2002).

Regarding efficacy, the overall response rate was 26% in both treatment groups. The median TTP was 2.9 months on TLC D-99 versus 3.1 months on doxorubicin. Median survival was 16 versus 20 months with a non significant trend in favor of doxorubicin (P = 0.09).

In another randomized study, Chan et al tried to ascertain the efficacy and tolerability of NPLD and epirubicin combined with cyclophosphamide in the first-line treatment of patients with metastatic breast cancer (Chan et al., 2004). One hundred and sixty anthracycline-naïve metastatic breast cancer patients were randomised to receive NPLD (M; 75 mg/m2) or epirubicin (E; 75 mg/m2) in combination with cyclophosphamide (C; 600 mg/m2), every 3 weeks for up to eight cycles. Cardiotoxicity was low in both treatment groups: nine patients on MC and eight on EC had asymptomatic LVEF reductions at comparable cumulative doses . For MC there were two cases at 100–299 mg/m2, four at 300–399 mg/m2 and three at 500–599 mg/m2; for EC there was one case at 200–299 mg/m2, four at 300–399 mg/m2 and three at 400–499 mg/m2. There was no clinical evidence of CHF in any patient. Overall response rates were 46% and 39% for MC and EC treatment, respectively (P=0.42). MC was superior to EC with respect to median time to treatment failure (5.7 versus 4.4 months; P=0.01) and median time to disease progression (7.7 versus 5.6 months; P=0.02). Median survival times were 18.3 and 16.0 months for MC and EC, respectively (P=0.504). Unsurprisingly, the results from this study (Chan et al., 2004) suggested that, at equimolar doses, in combination with cyclophosphamide, NPLD has modest but significant advantages over epirubicin for some efficacy end points and a non-significant trend towards improvement in others. Given the well established correlation between dose and therapeutic effect for doxorubicin, and in light of the uncertainty surrounding the optimal therapeutic dose of epirubicin, NPLD offers clinicians the opportunity to make clinical use of a drug that combines the dose/effect reliability of doxorubicin with the level of safety provided by epirubicin.

In conclusion, two studies (Batist et al., 2001; Harris et al., 2002; Chan et al, 2004) clearly demonstrated reduced cardiotoxicity of NPLD when compared to standard doxorubicin, with a superimposable antitumor efficacy of the two drugs. The third study showed a trend of higher efficacy fot NPLD with respect to epirubicin, with equal cardiotoxicity.

7.2 Non-pegylated liposomal doxorubicin in non-Hodgkin lymphoma

The first study testing the safety and efficacy of NPLD in non-Hodgkin lymphoma NHL (AIDS-related) was conducted by Alexandra Levine and coworkers in 2004 (Levine et al., 2004). The study enrolled 24 patients with newly diagnosed AIDS-related NHL (median age: 43 years). Sixty-seven percent of patients had a high or high-intermediate International Prognostic Index (IPI) scores at diagnosis. Serum LDH was high in 17 patients (71%). A total of 21 patients (88%) had extranodal disease, and 12 patients (50%) had 2 or more sites of extranodal involvement.

The primary objective of the study was to evaluate the safety and efficacy of NPLD when substituted for doxorubicin in the CHOP in patients with newly diagnosed AIDS-related non-Hodgkin's lymphoma (AIDS-NHL). NPLD at doses of 40, 50, 60, and 80 mg/m2 was given with fixed doses of cyclophosphamide (750 mg/m2), vincristine (1.4 mg/m2) and prednisone (40 mg/m2) every 21 days. The maximum tolerated dose (MTD) of NPLD was defined as the dose at which less than half of the patients on a cohort experienced a dose-limiting toxicity. No dose escalations were allowed in individual patients. The MTD of NPLD was not reached at the 80 mg/m2 dose. As a high complete response (CR) rate was seen at all dose levels, a dose of 50 mg/m2 of NPLD was chosen for the phase II portion of the trial, which was expanded to a total of 24 patients, including 10 on the initial phase I dose-escalation portion. All patients received highly active antiretroviral therapy while on chemotherapy.

The results of the study were encouraging. No dose-limiting toxicities were observed at any level, with myelosuppression being the most frequent toxicity (grade 4 neutropenia in 75% of patients, neutropenic fever in 12% and neutropenic sepsis in 8%). Overall response rate was 88%, with a CR rate of 75%, and a partial response (PR) rate of 13%. The median duration of CR was 15.6 months (range, 1.7 to 43.5 months).

Moreover, 16 out of 24 AIDS-related NHL patients were evaluated for multidrug resistance (MDR-1) expression on their hystological samples. The Authors demonstrated that this NPLD-based regimen was equally effective in both MDR-1–positive and MDR-1–negative cases. The Authors postulated that the efficacy of this regimen was eventually related to the ability of NPLD to overcome excessive drug efflux due to P-gp (MDR-1) overexpression. The MDR-1 expression did not correlate with response in this study, suggesting that NPLD might evade this resistance mechanism.

In terms of potential cardiac toxicity, left ventricular ejection fraction (LVEF) was obtained at baseline and at study termination in 19 patients. No patient developed a decline in LVEF to below normal (45%). Fourteen patients had no significant change in LVEF over time, while 5 patients (26%) experienced a 10% or greater decline, though their LVEF values still remained within normal range. None of these five patients had any signs or symptoms of cardiac dysfunction, and the values returned to baseline levels in the two patients who had follow-up cardiac studies performed, 3 months after completion of chemotherapy.

Starting from that background, the same group of the Keck School of Medicine designed in 2006 a phase I-II trial to evaluate the safety of the same regimen (NPLD, cyclophosphamide, vincristine, and prednisone every 21 days) in the treatment of newly diagnosed aggressive NHL patients (Tulpule et al., 2006).

Forty-seven patients (median age: 55 years) were enrolled in the study. The vast majority of the patients had diffuse large B-cell NHL (37/47). Liposomal doxorubicin at doses of 40 mg/m2, 50 mg/m2, 60 mg/m2, and 80 mg/m2 was given with fixed doses of cyclophosphamide (750 mg/m2), vincristine (1.4mg/m2) and prednisone (40 mg/m2). Chemotherapy cycles were repeated every 21 days.

No dose-limiting toxicities were observed at any level. Reversible grade 3/4 neutropenia was the most common toxicity (95.8%). Most non-hematologic side effects were nausea, vomiting fatigue and fever and were primarily grade 1/2 in severity. Stomatitis of mild or moderate severity was reported in 23% of patients.

Two out of 47 patients (4%) developed clinically silent cardiac toxicity, with a decline in LVEF of 20% each. None of the patients presented any symptoms of cardiotoxicity. The decline in LVEF occurred in one patient after a cumulative NPLD dose of 240mg/m2 and in the other one after a cumulative NPLD dose of 640 mg/m2. In both patients the declines returned to baseline 2 months and 6 months from discontinuation of NPLD, respectively.

Complete remissions were documented in 31 of 46 evaluable patients (67.4%) and partial remissions in 7 (15.2%), for an overall major response rate of 82.6%. Responses were attained after a median of 4 cycles of therapy. Patients with T-cell lymphomas fared poorly with this regimen, with none of them achieving a CR lasting more than 6 months.
The median duration of complete remission was 27.7 months (range, 2.4 months to 59.8 months). Reported median follow-up was 3.1 years. Median survival was not reached at the time of publication. The 2-year estimated overall suvival (OS) probability was 65% (95% CI, 50-77%), with a 3-year estimated OS probability of 59% (95%CI, 44%-73%). Nineteen patients had died at the time of publication.
Regarding the relationship between MDR-1 expression and outcome, MDR-1-related p-glycoprotein expression was assessed in lymphoma tissues from 27 patients. Eight patients (30%) was MDR-1 positive at diagnosis. No difference in CR rates were observed when comparing patients whose tumors expressed MDR-1 versus those who did not (63% in MDR-1-positive and 74% in the MDR-1-negative lymphomas, P = 0.66), indicating that NPLD might overcome MDR-1 in vivo.
Rigacci and collaborators (Rigacci et al., 2007) designed a prospective study to assess the efficacy and safety of the combination of NPLD with cyclophosphamide, vincristine, prednisone and Rituximab (R-COMP) in patients with aggressive non-Hodgkin's B-cell lymphomas and concurrent cardiac disease or pre-treated with anthracyclines.
Twenty-one patients were selected for the presence of cardiac comorbidity and/or previous treatment with anthracycline-based regimens. NPLD at a dose of 50 mg/m2 was administered in association with cyclophosphamide (750 mg/m2), vincristine (1.4mg/m2), prednisone (40 mg/m2) and rituximab (375 mg/m2) every 21 days for 4 to 6 cycles unless progression or unacceptable toxicity occurred. CR rate was 76%, whereas PR rate was 14%, with an overall response rate (ORR) of 90%. Two patients (10%) did not respond to therapy. After a median follow-up of 13 months (range 2–36 months), 2/16 CR patients relapsed, with a cumulative disease-free survival (DFS) rate of 78%.
Regarding toxicities, the Authors observed only a congestive heart failure (CHF) in one patient, among a total of 115 chemotherapy cycles administered. LVEF was evaluated after the 3rd cycle and at the end of treatment in all but one patient, who developed CHF with LVEF 20% after the first cycle of R-COMP. Between the 20 evaluable patients, median LVEF was 60% (range 38%–74%) after three cycles and 60% (range 40%–69%) at the end of the treatment. There was no significant difference between LVEF at baseline, after the 3rd cycle, and at the end of study in patients with cardiac comorbidity (52, 58 and 60%, respectively), in those without cardiac diseases (62, 61 and 60%, respectively) and in those previously treated with anthracyclines. Patients were evaluated every 6 months after the end of the study. Among the 15 patients who were followed-up for at least 12 months after the end of therapy, none of them presented any cardiac dysfunction or significant decrease of LVEF.
The Authors stated that Rituximab plus NPLD-based regimen was well tolerated and highly effective in inducing clinical responses in this group of patients at high risk for cardiac toxicity or previously treated with anthracyclines. The tolerability profile was favorable, with a low incidence of cardiac events (1/21 patients).
Visani and coworkers (Visani et al., 2008) conduced a pilot study to assess the toxicity and efficacy of the combination of NPLD with cyclophosphamide, vincristine, prednisone and

Rituximab (R-COMP) in frail and elderly patients with aggressive non-Hodgkin's B-cell lymphomas.

NPLD at a dose of 50 mg/m2 was administered in association with cyclophosphamide (750 mg/m2), vincristine (1.4mg/m2), prednisone (40 mg/m2) and rituximab (375 mg/m2) every 21 days for 4 to 6 cycles unless progression or unacceptable toxicity occurred.

Twenty frail patients (median age: 73 years), as defined by Balducci & Extermann (Balducci & Extermann,2000) with diffuse large B cell or grade IIIb follicular lymphoma, either at diagnosis (15 patients) or relapsed (5 patients), were prospectively enrolled.

Thirteen out of 20 NHL patients (65%) had a complete response (CR) and an additional 5 patients (25%) achieved a partial response (PR), with an overall response rate of 90% (ORR). Notably, the median age of the study population (73 years) was the oldest ever reported in literature of patients treated with this combinations. As a matter of fact, this population consisted of particularly elderly and frail patients with advanced disease at the time of study entry. These patients had indeed an extremely high probability of being unable to complete one of the standard anthracyclines-based regimens or to suffer from cardiotoxicity.

The treatment was relatively well-tolerated. Grade 3 or 4 neutropenia occurred in 26% of cycles and febrile neutropenia in 5%. There was no significant difference between LVEF at baseline, after the 3rd cycle, and at the end of study in 16/19 patients. Notably, 2 patients presented a CHF (NYHA 3) after 1 and 3 cycles of R-COMP, respectively and were shifted to receive an anthracycline-free regimen while in CR after R-COMP. In these 2 patients, the Authors observed a 20% decrease of the LVEF which partially recovered after medical therapy. The cumulative percentage of cardiovascular complications was 15%, higher than that reported for elderly patients treated with R-CHOP 21 or 14. However, this patient population consisted only of frail patients having a poor WHO performance status and important comorbidities.

This study demonstrated for the first time the safety and efficacy of the R-COMP 21 regimen in frail and elderly patients with aggressive NHL. Cardiotoxicity was low and a promising response rate was observed in this setting patients.

Another interesting study regarding the safety and the efficacy of the R-COMP combination was recently published (Luminari et al., 2010). Seventy-five elderly patients with diffuse large B-cell lymphoma (DLBCL) were studied. Only patients with left ventricular ejection fraction (LVEF) > or =50% were allowed. R-COMP regimen was administered every 3 weeks for three cycles, followed by additional five cycles in case of complete response (CR) or partial response.

Seventy-five patients with a median age of 72 years were registered, and 72 were evaluable for response assessment. Fifty-six percent of patients had high or high-intermediate International Prognostic Index score. Median LVEF at baseline was 61%. Thirty-eight patients had history of abnormal cardiovascular conditions. The overall response rate was 71%, with a CR rate of 57%. After a median follow-up of 33 months, the 3-year overall survival, failure-free survival, and progression-free survival rates were 72%, 39%, and 69%, respectively. Neutropenia (54%) was the most frequent grade 3-4 adverse event; 21% of patients experienced cardiac adverse events, graded as 3-4 in 4% of the cases.

8. Pegylated Liposomal Doxorubicin (PLD)

Pegylated liposomal doxorubicin (PLD) is doxorubicin confined in liposomes that have been sterically stabilized by grafting polyethylene glycol onto the surface (Stealth Liposome"). PLD has a circulation half-life of approximately 73.9 h, whereas doxorubicin has a half-life of <10 min. Prolonged circulation facilitates greater uptake of PLD liposomes by tumor tissue. PLD accumulates selectively in metastatic breast carcinoma tissue, resulting in 10-fold higher intracellular drug concentrations compared with adjacent normal tissue (Symon et al., 1999). Pegylated liposomal encapsulation also reduces plasma levels of free doxorubicin and may reduce drug delivery to normal tissue, which may reduce toxicity. Studies of PLD suggest that a dose of 45 to 50 mg/m2 every 4 weeks is well tolerated with little nausea or vomiting, mild myelosuppression, minimal alopecia, and very little cardiotoxicity.

8.1 Pegylated liposomal doxorubicin in breast cancer

The first randomized, multicenter, phase III study was designed to demonstrate that efficacy in terms of progression-free survival of pegylated liposomal doxorubicin HCl (PLD) was non-inferior to doxorubicin with significantly less cardiotoxicity in first-line treatment of women with metastatic breast cancer (MBC) (O'Brien et al., 2004). Women (n = 509) with MBC and normal cardiac function were randomized to receive either PLD 50 mg/m^2 (every 4 weeks) or doxorubicin 60 mg/m^2 (every 3 weeks). Cardiac event rates were based on reductions in left ventricular ejection fraction as a function of cumulative anthracycline dose.

In this open-label, multicenter trial, patients were randomized in a 1:1 ratio by an independent central third party according to a computer-generated randomization program. Patients received either PLD [50 mg/m2 intravenous (i.v.) infusion for up to 60 min every 4 weeks] or doxorubicin [60 mg/m2 i.v. infusion for 60 min every 3 weeks]. Patients were prospectively stratified based on three criteria to balance major prognostic risk factors between treatment groups: prior adjuvant anthracycline exposure; presence of bone metastases as only site of disease; presence of at least one cardiac risk factor (O'Brien et al., 2004). Cardiac risk factors were defined as prior mediastinal irradiation, age ≥65 years, history of heart disease (previous myocardial infarction, arrhythmia or angina, not requiring treatment) or hypertension, or diabetes requiring medical treatment.

Regarding cardiotoxicity, MUGA scans were performed to measure LVEF before onset of treatment, after 300 mg/m2 cumulative anthracycline exposure, and after every additional 100 mg/m2 of PLD and every 120 mg/m2 of doxorubicin. Compliance with the protocol on performing MUGA evaluations was high. Of the 283 patients who reached doses ≥300 mg/m2 cumulative anthracyclines, all but 20 patients (nine PLD, 11 doxorubicin) had a baseline MUGA evaluation and at least one follow-up MUGA evaluation during treatment (O'Brien et al., 2004).

Overall, 339 patients (152 PLD and 187 doxorubicin) had electronic MUGA scan data for evaluation of cardiotoxicity (baseline and at least one scan during treatment) and were included in the analysis. Patients in the PLD arm had a median cumulative anthracycline dose of 398 mg/m2 (including prior anthracycline exposure). Patients in the conventional doxorubicin arm had a median cumulative anthracycline dose of 421 mg/m2 (including prior anthracycline exposure). Fifty-eight patients (10 PLD, 48 doxorubicin) met the protocol-defined LVEF criteria for cardiotoxicity during treatment and/or follow-up. The risk of developing cardiotoxicity was significantly higher for patients receiving doxorubicin than for those receiving PLD (P <0.001, HR = 3.16 for comparison of cumulative anthracycline dose at the first, protocol-specified, cardiac event) (O'Brien et al., 2004). The increase in risk of developing cardiotoxicity on doxorubicin versus PLD was observed in all subgroups analyzed, including those at high risk for developing CHF. In the subgroup that received prior adjuvant anthracycline therapy, the risk of developing cardiotoxicity was seven-fold higher with doxorubicin than with PLD. None of the 10 PLD-treated patients who had cardiotoxicity by LVEF criteria developed clinical signs or symptoms of CHF, whereas 10 of 48 doxorubicin-treated patients who had cardiotoxicity by LVEF criteria developed signs or symptoms of CHF. Two patients in each group developed clinical CHF but did not have a corresponding decrease in LVEF. As expected with doxorubicin, the mean percentage change from baseline in LVEF was positively correlated with the increase in cumulative anthracycline dose. However, with PLD, only a 2–3% mean decrease in LVEF was observed as the cumulative anthracycline dose increased. At cumulative doses at or above 450 mg/m2, a seven-fold greater mean percentage decrease in LVEF was observed with doxorubicin versus PLD (–17.2% versus– 2.3%; mean percentage change from baseline in LVEF in doxorubicin-treated and PLD-treated patients, respectively) (O'Brien et al., 2004).

Regarding efficacy, PLD and doxorubicin were comparable with respect to PFS (6.9 versus 7.8 months, respectively) and to OS (21 and 22 months for PLD and doxorubicin, respectively. Palmar-plantar erythrodysesthesia (48% versus 2%), stomatitis (22% versus 15%) and mucositis (23% versus 13%) were more often associated with PLD than doxorubicin. In conclusion, in first-line therapy for MBC, PLD provides comparable efficacy to doxorubicin, with significantly reduced cardiotoxicity (O'Brien et al., 2004).

Another multicentric, randomized trial was published on the same year (Keller et al., 2004). This trial was designed to compare the efficacy of pegylated liposomal doxorubicin (PLD) with that of a common salvage regimen (comparator) in patients with taxane-refractory advanced breast cancer. Following failure of a first- or second-line taxane-containing regimen for metastatic disease, 301 women were randomly assigned to receive PLD (50 mg/m2 every 28 days); or comparator-vinorelbine (30 mg/m2 weekly) or mitomycin C (10 mg/m2 day 1 and every 28 days) plus vinblastine (5 mg/m2 day 1, day 14, day 28, and day 42) every 6 to 8 weeks (Keller et al., 2004). Changes in LVEF values were only assessed in patients receiving PLD. Cardiac toxicity was defined as either a decrease of ≥ 15 points from baseline or a ≥ 5-point decrease from baseline with a level below the lower limit of normal for the institution. Twenty-two patients developed LVEF changes consistent with cardiac toxicity. However, decreases in LVEF did not correlate with cumulative anthracycline dose and none of these patients developed clinical congestive heart failure. The majority (n = 14) discontinued due to progressive disease. There were four patients who discontinued treatment due to cardiac toxicity (LVEF decrease), three patients who discontinued due to noncardiac adverse events, and one patient who discontinued due to noncompliance. Progression-free survival (PFS) and overall survival (OS) were similar for PLD and comparator (Keller et al., 2004).

8.2 Pegylated liposomal doxorubicin in non-Hodgkin lymphoma

Pegylated liposomal doxorubicin has been substituted for conventional doxorubicin in the CHOP regimen in a number of trials. In phase II studies in elderly patients with diffuse large B-cell lymphoma, ORR of approximately 65% was achieved: 50% CR and 15% PR, an estimated 1-year OS of 55%, and an estimated 2-year event-free survival of 45%. Neutropenia was the only grade III-IV toxicity observed [23,24].

Cutaneous T-cell lymphoma (CTCL) is a specific niche in which PLD has proven to be very active at low doses in a similar fashion to Kaposi sarcoma [25]. A response rate of 88% (44% CR) with mean OS of 18 months was observed in a retrospective analysis of 31 patients receiving PLD at doses varying from 20-40 mg/m2 every 4 weeks. These patients had recurrent or unresponsive disease, or rapidly progressive disease [25].

Indeed, PLD has been shown to have equal efficacy and a better safety profile in the treatment of multiple myeloma, when compared with conventional doxorubicin combinations. In controlled clinical trials, PLD combined with vincristine and dexamethasone provided response rates comparable with the doxorubicin-based standard vincristine/doxorubicin/dexamethasone) therapy, but the former required less hospitalization, no central venous catheter, with a reported lower toxicity in terms of alopecia and severe leukopenia [26]. There are ongoing studies trying to establish the usefulness of newer compounds in combination with liposomal anthracyclines for the therapy of multiple myeloma.

9. Conclusions

New acquisitions, particularly in terms of pathogenetical mechanisms, have considerably changed the perception of anthracycline cardiotoxicity in patients cured after a cancer diagnosis. From a " cumulative dose" era, where caution to further treatments with anthracyclines was linked more to a mere calculation of global administered dose, we are now shifting to a more prudential approach, that considers a persistent biological damage due to anthracycline administration, and prompts us toward a better definition of measures able to control, in particular, late cardiac toxicity. One item is becoming evident: a strict cohoperation between cardiologists and oncologists/hematologists could significantly improve the life expectancy and reduce the risks of major CHF in anthracycline pretreated patients, simply not underevaluating concurrent risk factors for CHF, that must be addressed early and consistently with adequate "cardiological" therapies.

On the other hand, the pharmacological research has in some way met the challenge to reduce the toxicity of the therapy with anthracyclines, both designing new, safer, anthracycline analogues, such as liposomal compounds, and reshaping the way to use protective compounds, such as dexrazoxane, during anthracycline therapy. The possible role (and optimal way of use) of iron chelators, such as deferasirox, is still under evaluation.

Cost related issues have up to now limited the use of liposomal derivatives, except for niches of fragile patients; it should be considered, anyway, if the global,high impact on costs of cardiotoxicity in cancer survivors(in terms of disability and related treatments) could justify,expecially in the long run, the costs of an optimized treatment,with modified anthracyclines or with cardioprotectants, potentially able to reduce, in particular, the frequency of late cardiac toxicity.

10. Acknowledgments

Supported in part by AIL PESARO ONLUS.

11. References

Balducci L. & Extermann, M. (2000) Management of cancer in the older person: a practical approach. *Oncologist*, Vol 5, No3,pp 224-237.

Barry EV et al.. (2008). Absence of second malignant neoplasms in children with high risk acute lymphoblastic leukemia treated with dexrazoxane. *Journal of Clinical Oncology*,Vol 26, pp. 1106-1111

Batist, G. "et al" (2001). Reduced cardiotoxicity and preserved antitumor efficacy of liposome-encapsulated doxorubicin and cyclophosphamide compared with conventional doxorubicin and cyclophosphamide in a randomized, multicenter trial of metastatic breast cancer. *Journal of Clinical Oncology*, Vol.19, pp.1444-1454.

Blanco, J.G. "et al". (2008) Genetic polymorphisms in the carbonyl reductase 3 gene CBR3 and the NAD(P)H:quinine oxidoreductase 1 gene NQO1 in patients who developed anthracycline-related congestive heart failure after childhood cancer. *Cancer*, Vol. 112, pp. 2789–2795

Cardinale, D. "et al". (2006) Prevention of high-dose chemotherapy-induced cardiotoxicity in high-risk patients by angiotensin-converting enzyme inhibition. *Circulation*, Vol.114, pp.2474-2481.

Cowens, J.W. "et al" (1993). Initial clinical (Phase I) trial of Myocet (doxorubicin encapsulated in liposomes). *Cancer Research*, Vol.53, pp. 2796-2802.

Dean, M.; Fojo, T. & Bates, S. (2005). Tumour stem cells and drug resistance. *Nature Reviews Cancer*, Vol.5, No.4, pp.275-84.

De Bruin, M.L. "et al". (2009). Increased risk of stroke and transient ischemic attack in 5-year survivors of Hodgkin lymphoma. *Journal of the National Cancer Institute*, Vol. 101, pp 928-937.

Endicott, J.A. & Ling, V. (1989). The biochemistry of P-glycoprotein-mediated multidrug resistance. Annual Reviews of Biochemistry, Vol.58, pp.137-71.

Ewer MS and Benjamin RS (2006). Doxorubicin cardiotoxicity: clinical aspects, recognition, monitoring, treatment, and prevention, in: *Cancer and the Heart (Ewer MS and Yeh E eds)*: pp 9–32, BC Decker, Hamilton, ON, Canada. Florenzano, F. & Salman, P. (2007) Carvedilol for anthracycline cardiomyopathy prevention. *Journal of the American College of Cardiology*, Vol.49,pp. 2142-2143.

Gianni, L. " et al.". Anthracycline cardiotoxicity: from bench to bedside. *Journal of Clinical. Oncology*, Vol. 26, pp. 3777-3784.

Gabizon, A.A. (1994). Liposomal anthracyclines. *Hematology/Oncology Clinics of North America* , Vol. 8, pp. 431-50.

Hale, S.L. "et al". (2008) Late sodium current inhibition as a new cardioprotective approach. *Journal of Molecular and Cellular Cardiology*, Vol.44, pp. 954-967.

Harris, L. "et al". (2002) Liposome-encapsulated doxorubicin compared with conventional doxorubicin in a randomized multicenter trial as first-line therapy of metastatic breast carcinoma. *Cancer*, Vol.94, No.1, pp 25-36.

Hudson, M.M. "et al". (2007) Noninvasive evaluation of late anthracycline cardiac toxicity in childhood cancer survivors. *Journal of Clinical Oncology*, Vol.25. pp. 3635–3643.

Innocenti, F. "et al". (2001) Epirubicin glucuronidation is catalyzed by human UDP glucuronosyltransferase 2B7. *Drug Metab Dispos*, Vol. 29, pp 686-692.

Jones, L.W. "et al". (2007). Early breast cancer therapy and cardiovascular injury. *Journal of the American College of Cardiology*, Vol. 50, pp.1435-1441.

Kalay, N. "et al". (2006) Protective effects of carvedilol against anthracycline-induced cardiomyopathy. *Journal of the American College of Cardiology*, Vol.48, pp.2258-2264.

Lasic, D.D. (1993). Liposomes: from physics to applications, p. 575. Amsterdam: Elsevier.

Lebrecht, D. & Walker, U.A. (2007). Role of mtDNA lesions in anthracycline cardiotoxicity. *Cardiovascular Toxicology* Vol.7, pp.108-113.

Levine, A.M. "et al". (2004) Liposome-encapsulated doxorubicin in combination with standard agents (cyclophosphamide, vincristine, prednisone) in patients with newly diagnosed AIDS-related non-Hodgkin's lymphoma: results of therapy and correlates of response. *Journal of Clinical Oncology*, Vol. 22, No.13, pp.2662-2670.

Lipshultz, S.E. "et al". (2002) Doxorubicin administration by continuous infusion is not cardioprotective: the Dana-Farber 91-01 Acute Lymphoblastic Leukemia protocol. *Journal of Clinical Oncology*, Vol. 20, pp. 1677-1682.

Lipshultz, S.E. "et al". (1997). Predictive value of cardiac troponin T in pediatric patients at risk for myocardial injury. *Circulation*, Vol. 96, pp. 2641-2648

Lotfi, K.; Zackrisson, A.L. & Peterson, C. (2002) Comparison of idarubicin and daunorubicin regarding intracellular uptake, induction of apoptosis, and resistance. *Cancer Letters*, Vol. 25, No.178 (2), pp.141-9.

Luminari, S. "et al". (2010). Nonpegylated liposomal doxorubicin (MyocetTM) combination (R-COMP) chemotherapy in elderly patients with diffuse large B-cell lymphoma (DLBCL): results from the phase II EUR018 trial. *Annals of Oncology*; Vol.21, No.7, pp.1492-9.

Lyu, Y.L., "et al". (2007) Topoisomerase IIbeta mediated DNA double-strand breaks: implications in doxorubicin cardiotoxicity and prevention by dexrazoxane. Cancer Res 2007;67:8839-46; Martin E, Thougaard AV, Grauslund M, et al. Evaluation of the topoisomerase II-inactive bisdioxopiperazine ICRF-161 as a protectant against doxorubicin-induced cardiomyopathy. *Toxicology*, Vol. 255, pp.72-79.

Martino R, "et al". (2002). Cyclophosphamide, pegylated liposomal doxorubicin (Caelyx), vincristine and prednisone (CCOP) in elderly patients with diffuse large B-cell lymphoma: results from a prospective phase II study. *Haematologica*, Vol.87, pp.822-7.

Menna, P. " et al". (2008) Anthracycline Cardiotoxicity. *Topics in Current Chemistry*, Vol. 283, pp 21-44.

Minotti G, "et al". (2004). Anthracyclines: molecular advances and pharmacologic developments in antitumor activity and cardiotoxicity. Pharmacological Reviews, Vol.56, No.2, pp.185-229.

Minotti G, "et al". (2008) Anthracyclines. In: Encyclopedic Reference of Molecular Pharmacology (S. Offermanns and W. Rosenthal, eds.). Springer.

Minotti, G.; Salvatorelli, E. & Menna, P. (2010). Pharmacological Foundations of Cardio-Oncology. *Journal of Pharmacology and Experimental Therapeutics*, Vol. 334, pp. 2-8.

Muthu, M.S. & Feng, S.S. (2010). Nanopharmacology of liposomes developed for cancer therapy. *Nanomedicine*, Vol.5, No.7, pp.1017-1019.

Nakamae, H. "et al". (2005) Notable effects of angiotensin II receptor blocker, valsartan, on acute cardiotoxic changes after standard chemotherapy with cyclophosphamide, doxorubicin, vincristine, and prednisolone. *Cancer*, Vol. 104, pp. 2492-2498.

Rabbani, A.; Finn, R.M. & Ausió, J. (2005) The anthracycline antibiotics: antitumor drugs that alter chromatin structure. *Bioassays*, Vol. 27, No.1, pp.50-6.

Rifkin, R.M. "et al". (2006) Pegylated liposomal doxorubicin, vincristine, and dexamethasone provide significant reduction in toxicity compared with doxorubicin, vincristine, and dexamethasone in patients with newly diagnosed multiple myeloma: a Phase III multicenter randomized trial. *Cancer*, Vol.106, pp. 848-58.

Rigacci L., "et al". (2007). Liposome-encapsulated doxorubicin in combination with cyclophosphamide, vincristine, prednisone and rituximab in patients with lymphoma and concurrent cardiac diseases or pre-treated with anthracyclines. *Hematological Oncology*, Vol. 25, No.4, pp 198-203.

Robert, J. & Gianni, L. (1993) Pharmacokinetics and metabolism of anthracyclines. *Cancer Surv*, Vol.17, pp 219-252.

Salvatorelli, E. "et al". (2009) Doxorubicinolone formation and efflux: a salvage pathway against epirubicin accumulation in human heart. *Journal of Pharmacology and Experimental Therapeutics*, vol. 329, pp 175-184.

Salvatorelli, E. "et al". (2007). Defective taxane stimulation of epirubicinol formation in the human heart: Insight into the cardiac tolerability of epirubicin-taxane chemotherapies *Journal of Pharmacology and Experimental Therapeutics*, Vol.320, pp. 790-800.

Schuchter, L.M. "et al". (2002) American Society of Clinical Oncology Chemotherapy and Radiotherapy Expert Panel. 2002 update of recommendations for the use of chemotherapy and radiotherapy protectants: clinical practice guidelines of the American Society of Clinical Oncology. *Journal of Clinical Oncology*, Vol.20, pp.2895–2903.

Sissung, T.M. "et al". Impact of ABCB1 allelic variants on QTc interval prolongation. *Clinical Cancer Research*, Vol. 17, pp. 937-946.

Soloman, R. & Gabizon, A.A. (2008). Clinical pharmacology of liposomal anthracyclines: focus on pegylated liposomal Doxorubicin. *Clinical Lymphoma Myeloma*, Vol.8, No.1, pp. 21-32.

Symon, Z. "et al". (1999) Selective delivery of doxorubicin to patients with breast carcinoma metastases by stealth liposomes. *Cancer*, Vol. 86, pp. 72–78.

Sterba, M "et al". (2006). Cardio protective effects of a novel iron chelator, pyridoxal 2-chlorobenzoylhydrazone, in the rabbit model of daunorubicin-induced cardiotoxicity. *Journal of Pharmacology and Experimental Therapy*, Vol. 319,No. 3, pp. 1336-1347

Swain, S.M. "et al". (1997). Cardioprotection with dexrazoxane for doxorubicin-containing therapy in advanced breast cancer. *Journal of Clinical Oncology*, Vol. 15,pp. 1318-1332.

Swain, S.M. Whaley, F.S. & Ewer, M.S. (2003) Congestive heart failure in patients treated with doxorubicin: a retrospective analysis of three trials. *Cancer*, Vol.97, pp. 2869–2879.

Swain, S.M. and Vici, P. (2004). The current and future role of dexrazoxane as a cardioprotectant in anthracycline treatment: expert panel review. *Journal of Cancer Research in Clinical Oncology*, vol.130,pp.1-7

Swerdlow, A.J. "et al". (2007). Myocardial infarction mortality risk after treatment for Hodgkin disease: a collaborative British cohort study. *Journal of the National Cancer Institute*, Vol.99, pp. 206-214.

Tulpule, A. "et al". (2006). Phase I/II trial of nonpegylated liposomal doxorubicin, cyclophosphamide, vincristine, and prednisone in the treatment of newly diagnosed aggressive non-Hodgkin's lymphoma. *Clinical Lymphoma Myeloma*, Vol.7, No.1, pp. 59-64.

van Dalen, E.C. "et al". (2010). Different anthracycline derivates for reducing cardiotoxicity in cancer patients. *Cochrane Database Syst Rev*, Vol 12, CD005006.

van Dalen, E.C. "et al". (2011). Cardioprotective interventions for cancer patients receiving anthracyclines. *Cochrane Database Systematic Reviews*, Vol.6: CD003917

Visani, G. "et al". (2008). R-COMP 21 for frail elderly patients with aggressive B-cell non-Hodgkin lymphoma: a pilot study. *Leukemia & Lymphoma*, Vol.49, No.6, pp.1081-6.

Visani, G. "et al". (2005) Cyclophosphamide, pegylated liposomal doxorubicin, vincristine and prednisone (CDOP) plus rituximab is effective and well tolerated in poor performance status elderly patients with non-Hodgkin's lymphoma. *Leukemia & Lymphoma*, Vol.46, No.3, pp.477-479.

Visani, G. & Isidori, A. (2009). Nonpegylated liposomal doxorubicin in the treatment of B-cell non-Hodgkin's lymphoma: where we stand. *Expert Reviews on Anticancer Therapy*, Vol.9, No.3, pp.357-63.

Vrooman, L.M. " et al". (2011). The low incidence of secondary acute myelogenous leukaemia in children and adolescents treated with dexrazoxane for acute lymphoblastic leukaemia: a report from the Dana-Farber Cancer Institute ALL Consortium. *European Journal of Cancer*, Vol. 47, pp.1373-1379.

Weiss, R.B. (1992). The anthracyclines: will we ever find a better doxorubicin? *Semin Oncol.* 19(6):670-86.

Wollina, U. "et al". (2003) Multicenter study of pegylated liposomal doxorubicin in patients with cutaneous T-cell lymphoma. *Cancer*, Vol. 98, pp. 993-1001.

Zucchi, R. & Danesi, R. (2003) Cardiac toxicity of antineoplastic anthracyclines. *Current Medicinal Chemistry - Anti-Cancer Agents*, Vol.3, No.2, pp.151-71.

28

Cardiotonic Steroids and Cardiac Fibrosis

Sandeep Vetteth, Deepak Malhotra and Joseph I. Shapiro
University of Toledo
United States of America

1. Introduction

It is well known and has been shown that patients who have chronic renal failure tend to develop and die of cardiac causes. These patients are known to develop a cardiomyopathy that is characterized by left ventricular hypertrophy and significant diastolic dysfunction. It has also been shown that the chronic renal failure condition is characterized by significant sodium pump inhibition due to increases in the circulating levels of cardiotonic steroids (CTS) such as marinobufagenin (MBG). In this review we will try to elucidate the mechanisms involved in the pathogenesis of uremic cardiomyopathy and the role of CTS in the pathogenesis as well as the possible areas of therapeutic interventions.

2. Renal failure and cardiotonic steroids

The current treatment of patients with end stage renal failure is complicated by the tremendous cardiovascular mortality associated with it. Such patients tend to develop a cardiomyopathy characterized by marked diastolic dysfunction and left ventricular hypertrophy (LVH). These patients also have substantial increases in the circulating levels of CTS (Mohmand, Malhotra et al. 2005). Perhaps of greater importance, it has more recently been shown that patients with more modest degrees of chronic renal insufficiency have markedly worse outcomes in high cardiovascular risk settings as well as a substantial worsening of cardiovascular risk (Alsheikh-Ali, Trikalinos et al. 2011; Kreuz, Horlbeck et al. 2011)

It was proposed nearly 4 decades ago that there is accumulation of CTS in chronic renal failure that causes the inhibition of the Na/K ATPase. The patients with chronic renal failure developed some antibodies to digoxin and had false positive digoxin levels even though these patients had not been treated with digitalis (Graves 1986; Graves and Williams 1987). More recently using more definitive analytical techniques several of these CTS have been characterized. These include ouabain (Hamlyn, Blaustein et al. 1991) which is a cardenolide and marinobufagenin (MBG) and telocinobufagin (TBG) (Bagrov and Fedorova 1998; Komiyama, Dong et al. 2005) which are bufadienolides. These CTS have been considered only as drugs until recently as studies now indicate that these compounds are secreted in the body and regulated by multiple physiological stimuli such as ACTH and angiotensin II (Fedorova, Agalakova et al. 2005; Bagrov, Shapiro et al. 2009). They have also been found to play an important role in renal salt handling as well as the regulation of cardiac contractility and vascular tone (Hamlyn, Blaustein et al. 1991; Fedorova, Doris et al.

1998). Recently, many other functions of these endogenous ligands of the Na/K-ATPase have been proposed.
The mechanism of elevation of these CTS possibly includes a combination of decreased elimination and increased production, but one would anticipate an elevation as it was initially thought that the these hormones functioned as natriuretic hormones since the Na/K ATPase comprises a major sodium transporting mechanism in the kidney (de Wardener, Clarkson et al. 1971). Increases in sodium levels would be caused by decreased renal elimination due to loss of renal function. It has also been thought that the increases in the CTS effect vasoconstriction by inhibition of Na/K ATPase causing coupled activation of the Na/Ca exchanger in the vascular smooth muscles (Jaitovich and Bertorello 2010). Bricker and colleagues postulated that in order to maintain sodium homeostasis in renal failure, increases in circulating CTS were necessary, but the effects of CTS on other tissues other than the kidneys explained many of the clinical features seen in renal failure. This was termed as the trade off hypothesis for the pathogenesis of the 'uremic syndrome' (Bricker and Fine 1978) and is illustrated in figure 1. Now it is well known that the reduced pump activity has been seen in red cells, white blood cells, transporting epithelia, muscle cells, adipocytes and the cardiomyocytes (Stokes, Willcocks et al. 1986; Okamoto 1988; Takahashi, Nishimura et al. 1989; Mimura, Makino et al. 1992; Periyasamy, Chen et al. 2001).

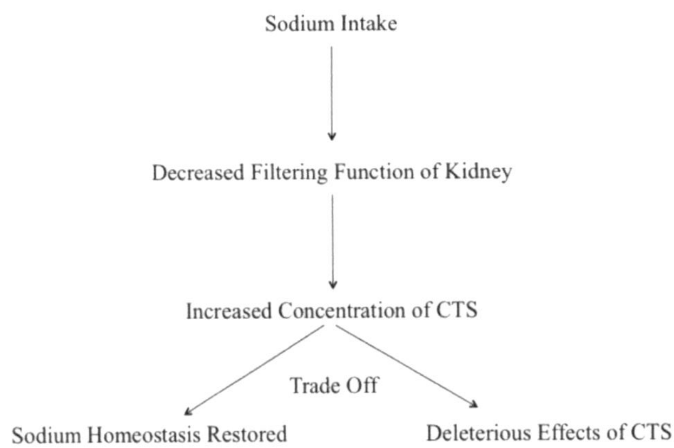

Fig. 1. Illustration of the role of cardiotonic steroids (CTS) in "trade off." With decreased filtering function, CTS concentrations increase to maintain sodium homeostasis, but these elevated hormone levels have adverse effects on different tissues.

Ouabain the prototypical CTS described in 1991 by Hamlyn and colleagues (Hamlyn, Blaustein et al. 1991) was initially thought to function as the natriuretic peptide responsible for the effects seen. However it is well known now that ouabain has high affinity to the alpha 2 and 3 isoforms of Na/K ATPase where as rat tubular cells mainly express the alpha 1 isoform which is relatively insensitive to ouabain (Sweadner 1989). However in humans the sensitivity of the different isoforms to ouabain seems to be not that significant (Croyle, Woo et al. 1997; Lingrel 2010). It is now known that ouabain probably has a more neuro-hormonal function and has been isolated from the hypothalamus and the hippocampus (Kawamura, Guo et al. 1999; Fedorova, Zhuravin et al. 2007). A new body of evidence is emerging that brain ouabain may play important role in pathogenesis of salt sensitive hypertension (Fedorova, Zhuravin et al. 2007).

More recently other CTS have been described such as MBG and TBG, which has a structure very similar to that of MBG (Bagrov, Roukoyatkina et al. 1993; Komiyama, Dong et al. 2005). They were seen to be elevated significantly in plasma of ESRD patients. The bufadienolides were first described from the skin of amphibians such as the marine toad (Bufo marinus) (Bagrov, Shapiro et al. 2009) and MBG emerged as the most important contender since it has the affinity towards the alpha 1 isoform which is the isoform present almost exclusively in the mammalian tubules. MBG at low doses also causes vasoconstriction in isolated human blood vessels (Bagrov, Roukoyatkina et al. 1995). Bagrov and colleagues have demonstrated that the levels of MBG are elevated in response to both salt loading and in the presence of experimental renal failure (Fedorova, Agalakova et al. 2005). They have also demonstrated the role of ouabain as a neuro-hormone by intra-hippocampal administration of ouabain and demonstrating an increase in the plasma and urine concentration of MBG as well as increased natriuresis from this (Fedorova, Agalakova et al. 2005). Also it has been shown that the synthesis of these CTS occurs in the mammalian adrenal cells; however the specific metabolic steps in this biosynthesis are still unknown (Dmitrieva, Bagrov et al. 2000).

3. Signaling though the sodium pump

Signaling though the sodium pump has been studied extensively in the recent years and our knowledge about the process has considerably increased. It is well known that there is more than just the 'classical enzymatic inhibition' causing increases in cytosolic sodium (Jaitovich and Bertorello 2010). One concern is that the circulating levels of CTS seen in pathological conditions do not appear to cause extensive inhibition of the pump in vitro and in vivo (Bagrov, Shapiro et al. 2009). In fact, the growth regulatory effects of CTS are seen even at nano and sub-nano molar concentrations, which do not cause any demonstrable inhibition of the pump activity (Aydemir-Koksoy, Abramowitz et al. 2001; Aydemir-Koksoy and Allen 2001; Saunders and Scheiner-Bobis 2004; Khundmiri, Metzler et al. 2006; Qiu, Gao et al. 2007). Another concern is that it has been difficult if not impossible to demonstrate changes in cytosolic sodium caused by physiological and even pharmacological concentrations of CTS. Perhaps more troubling, small increases in the cytosolic sodium levels caused by pump inhibition would be expected to minimize effects on net Na/K-ATPase activity by mass action as cytosolic Na is generally maintained at concentrations where it can actually regulate pump activity. Last but most significantly, sodium ionophores do not cause the biological effects of CTS (Liu, Tian et al. 2000; Oweis, Wu et al. 2006).

While the classical pathway of pump inhibition may still explain some of the effects of CTS, a novel signal cascade involving the Na/K-ATPase residing in specific membrane environments has been proposed and documented by Xie and others (Li and Xie 2009). This research performed on neonatal rat cardiac myocytes showed that ouabain caused the Na/K ATPase to interact with neighboring membrane proteins and caused cytosolic cascades of signaling. The administration of ouabain to the cardiomyocytes caused an increase in reactive oxygen species (ROS) (Liu, Tian et al. 2000). It was seen from the experiments that first there was phosphorylation of Src and leading to the activation of Ras. This trans-activated the EGFR and triggered a signaling cascade that led to the production of ROS (Haas, Askari et al. 2000; Liu, Tian et al. 2000; Kometiani, Askari et al. 2001; Haas, Wang et al. 2002; Wang, Haas et al. 2004; Tian, Cai et al. 2006). Also it has been shown that these ROS were key in the signaling function of Na/K ATPase. The administration of N Acetyl Cysteine (NAC) or green tea extract which act as ROS quenchers blocked the gene transcription effects of CTS (Xie, Kometiani et al. 1999; Liu, Tian et al. 2000; Priyadarshi, Valentine et al. 2003; Elkareh, Kennedy et al. 2007). At present it is unclear as to how ROS effect downstream signaling. One possibility albeit unproven is that the Na/K ATPase itself may serve as a receptor for the ROS enhancing its sensitivity by conformational change. Further work in this exciting area is currently underway. Development of ROS in response to sodium pump signaling is shown in figure 2.

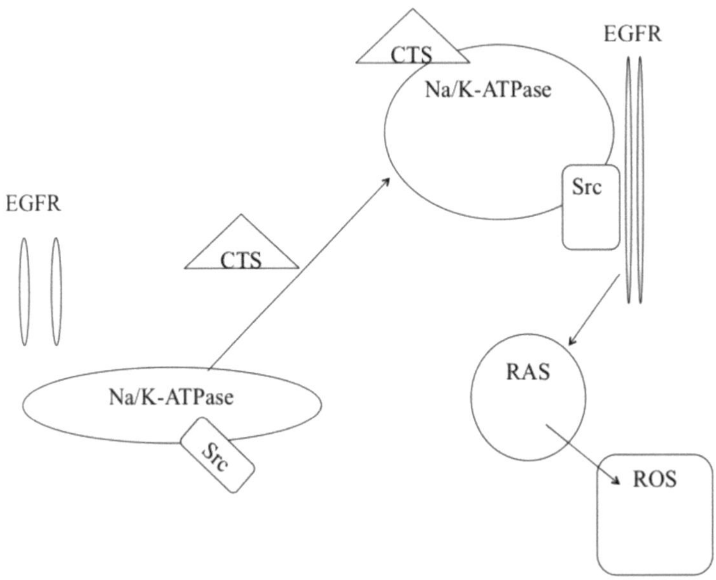

Fig. 2. Schematic showing how cardiotonic steroids (CTS) change the conformation of the Na/K-ATPase residing in caveolae or lipid rafts, allowing Src to transactivate the EGFR and cause signal transduction through RAS resulting in the generation of reactive oxygen species (ROS).

Several studies have shown that low concentrations of ouabain have stimulated tyrosine phosphorylation of several proteins in a variety of cells including cardiac myocytes, HeLa and LLC-PK1 cells (Kometiani, Li et al. 1998; Contreras, Shoshani et al. 1999; Haas, Askari et al. 2000; Aydemir-Koksoy, Abramowitz et al. 2001; Kometiani, Liu et al. 2005; Kotova, Al-Khalili et al. 2006; Kotova, Galuska et al. 2006). Importantly the addition of tyrosine kinase inhibitors like herbimycin A and genistein, blocked ouabain induced tyrosine phosphorylation and subsequently the downstream effects in these cultured cells (Haas, Askari et al. 2000; Aydemir-Koksoy, Abramowitz et al. 2001). Tyrosine phosphorylation can occur in one of two ways, either by activation of tyrosine kinases or by inhibition of tyrosine phosphatases or a combination of both. The Na/K ATPase does not have intrinsic tyrosine kinase activity. It is interesting that even though the alpha subunit has a phosphatase activity, preliminary studies suggest that it does not have significant tyrosine phosphatase activity (Li and Xie 2009). However, it has clearly been shown that ligands extrinsic to the Na/K-ATPase signal cascade can stimulate tyrosine kinase activity by employing receptors without any intrinsic tyrosine kinase activity (Ihle and Kerr 1995; McGarrigle and Huang 2007). One such demonstrated pathway is the G protein coupled receptors (GPCRs) that employ the Src family of kinases (McGarrigle and Huang 2007). It was hence postulated that

the Src family of kinases could play a role in the ouabain induced tyrosine phosphorylation (McGarrigle and Huang 2007).
Studies done by Haas et al. have indeed shown that Src is involved in the phosphorylation of proteins in CTS signaling. These studies showed that ouabain caused stimulation of Src in cardiac myocytes as well as LLC-PK1 cells. Inhibition of Src blocked the ouabain-induced phosphorylation and abolished the downstream signaling including the activation of ERK (Haas, Askari et al. 2000; Haas, Wang et al. 2002). Furthermore there is sufficient evidence for the fact the Na/K ATPase interacts with Src and forms a functional receptor complex. These workers observed that the pump and Src could be co-localized in the caveolar fractions in several different types of cells. Also immunofluorescence showed the co-localization of these two in the plasma membrane. Both the proteins could also be co-immunoprecipitated by using antibodies to either alpha 1 and to Src. Fluorescence resonance energy transfer (FRET) has also shown these two proteins to be in close proximity (Liu, Mohammadi et al. 2003; Wang, Haas et al. 2004; Liang, Cai et al. 2006; Tian, Cai et al. 2006). They have also showed that the interaction between the Na/K ATPase and Src keeps Src in an inactive state. It was seen that when ouabain binds to the sodium pump it reduced the binding of the Src Kinase domain. This freeing of the Src kinase domain possibly results in the activation of the Na/K ATPase associated Src kinase (Tian, Cai et al. 2006). Additionally experiments were done to see if the loss or knockdown of Na/K ATPase would release the interacting Src and increase in tyrosine kinase activity. Graded knockdown of LLC-PK1 cells with alpha 1 specific siRNA was achieved and Src activity was studied. It was seen that the knockdown of the pump resulted in an increase in basal Src activity in an alpha 1 amount dependent manner. Tyrosine phosphorylation of several protein molecules was also increased secondary to this. Moreover stimulation of these cells with ouabain failed to stimulate Src and ERK 1 and 2 any further. When these knockdown cells were rescued with rat alpha 1, it restored Src to its basal levels and allowed for stimulation of the complex at higher levels of Ouabain as would be expected with the differences in sensitivity of rat versus pig alpha 1 (Liang, Cai et al. 2006).
It is also known that the binding of ouabain to the receptor complex leads to the recruitment and transactivation of the EGFR. This was due to the Src dependent phosphorylation of the EGFR at sites other than the major auto-phosphorylation site Y1173. The transactivated EGFR in turn recruited Shc to the complex and resulted in the activation of the Ras/Raf/MEK/ERK cascade (Haas, Askari et al. 2000; Aydemir-Koksoy, Abramowitz et al. 2001; Haas, Wang et al. 2002; Kotova, Al-Khalili et al. 2006). Further studies have shown that once the Src Na/K ATPase complex has been activated it leads to the synthesis of ROS, which has been thought of as a second messenger. It has been demonstrated by Xie and coworkers that exposure of myocytes to ouabain causes a rapid increase in the generation of ROS. These ROS were demonstrated with the help of a fluorescence dye CMDCF. The generation of the ROS was prevented by pre-treatment of the cells to anti-oxidants such as N Acetyl Cysteine (NAC) and Vitamin E. By studying the blockade of the downstream signaling it was seen that ROS is involved with the signaling causing stimulation of Ras, activation of p42/44 mitogen-activated protein kinases, induction of genes for skeletal muscle actin and atrial natriuretic peptide and the activation and translocation of the transcription factor NF-κB among several other effects (Xie, Kometiani et al. 1999). Since a lot of these are calcium dependent steps further experiments were done to see if the ROS production was calcium dependent as well. Ouabain caused the production of ROS in

myocytes that were stimulated in culture media that were calcium deficient. This indicated that the production of ROs was calcium independent and possibly the increases in calcium was due to a parallel mechanism from the inhibition of the sodium pump activity (Liu, Tian et al. 2000)

Sites of generation and targets of ROS are currently being worked out, with clues in favor of Ras activation induced mitochondrial production (Liu, Tian et al. 2000)however other components of the downstream signaling including the involvement of PLC, PI3K and PKC have been established. Src activation led to the stimulation of PLC gamma and subsequently the activation of PKC and PI3 mediated calcium signaling. Moreover it was seen that ouabain also stimulates PI3K which works with PKC to cause endocytosis of this sodium pump complex. This probably is the explanation for how the signal transduction is eventually terminated. (Tian, Liu et al. 2003; Liu, Liang et al. 2005; Yuan, Cai et al. 2005; Pierre, Yang et al. 2007; Chen, Cai et al. 2008; Elkareh, Periyasamy et al. 2009).

This signaling pathway may link to Bricker's concept of CTS as a natriuretic hormone. Specifically, our group has noted that CTS induce endocytosis of the Na/K-ATPase in kidney tissues. In chronically salt loaded Sprague-Dawley rats, renal MBG excretion was significantly elevated and anti-MBG antibody reduced natriuresis and restored sodium pump activity in the renal cortex (Periyasamy, Liu et al. 2005). The same study demonstrated that in addition to the direct inhibition of the Na/K-ATPase, MBG is capable to exhibit its natriuretic via internalization of the sodium pump in the proximal tubule (Periyasamy, Liu et al. 2005). The endocytosis of the proximal tubular Na/K-ATPase induced by CTS has been shown to proceed through clathrin coated pits and require PI3K activation as well as the plasmalemmal pump being in the context of caveolae as well as signaling through the Src-EGFR pathway (Liu, Kesiry et al. 2004; Liu, Liang et al. 2005). Further work demonstrated that CTS could induce decreases in the apical expression of one of the plasma membrane Na^+/H^+ exchanger, NHE3 (Oweis, Wu et al. 2006; Liu and Shapiro 2007). Taken together, these data suggest that increases in the circulating levels of MBG accompany salt loading, which, in turn, may induce decreases in both basolateral and apical sodium transport in the proximal tubule.

4. Uremic cardiomyopathy

It is a well-known fact that cardiovascular mortality accounts for more that 50% of all deaths in patients with renal failure. It is seen that this mortality is more attributed to cardiac failure and sudden cardiac death than coronary events (Sarnak, Levey et al. 2003; Weiner, Tighiouart et al. 2004). Available data also suggests that pre end stage renal disease (ESRD) patients have cardiac mortality rates very similar to that of ESRD patients (Stack and Bloembergen 2001; Paparello, Kshirsagar et al. 2002; Sarnak 2003; Sarnak, Levey et al. 2003). Echocardiography has shown that diastolic dysfunction and LVH are both very common in ESRD patients on dialysis and other patients with chronic kidney disease (Harnett, Parfrey et al. 1988; Mitsnefes, Daniels et al. 2001; Stack and Saran 2002). Systolic dysfunction in these patients is less uniformly demonstrable (Raj, D'Mello et al. 1997) and it has been shown that development of LVH may be a predictor of higher mortality in dialysis patients (Nakazato, Kawada et al. 2002; Tyralla and Amann 2003) as this correlates with the development of cardiac arrhythmias.

Of late myocardial fibrosis that was described in uremia as early as 1943 by Rossle and then described again by Ritz et al. seems to play a very important role in the pathogenesis (Mall, Huther et al. 1990). It has been shown by the same group that the fibrosis occurred early after subtotal nephrectomy without myocardial necrosis suggesting a reactive fibrosis rather than a reparative fibrosis. It was seen that the interstitial volume density increased at the expense of capillary volume and this caused the swelling of the cytoplasm and nuclei of the interstitial cells where as the endothelial cells remained unchanged (Mall, Rambausek et al. 1988). The cardiac fibrosis can explain the abnormalities in the left ventricular compliance causing diastolic dysfunction as well as inhomogeneity in the electrical conduction causing arrhythmias. The factors thought to be involved in the genesis of myocardial fibrosis and LVH include anemia, hypertension, hyperparathyroidism, cardiotonic steroids, oxidative stress and the activation of the RAS aldosterone system.

Of the above-mentioned factors anemia seems to be the weakest to be implicated in uremic cardiomyopathy. Only a very modest improvement in LVH to the tune of 10-20% has been seen with sustained increases in hematocrit (Foley, Parfrey et al. 2000). Also the LVH seen is concentric in nature which is not what would be expected with anemia (Harnett, Parfrey et al. 1988). Interestingly erythropoietin therapy worsened LVH possibly because of worsening BP control (Minagawa, Hirano et al. 1994).

Among the several implicated factors hypertension seems to be the factor in chronic renal failure that is best linked to LVH (Huting and Alpert 1992; Morduchowicz, Zabludowski et al. 1993; Harnett and Parfrey 1994). Although there is sufficient evidence to prove that hypertension causes LVH, it does not account for the frequency and severity of LVH seen in ESRD patients (Huting and Alpert 1992; Foley and Parfrey 1998; Nishikimi, Minami et al. 2001). Hence this points to the presence of other factors in the pathogenesis. However hypertension must be aggressively pursued in patients with renal failure as treatment has resulted in a modest amelioration of LVH (Dyadyk, Bagriy et al. 1997).

It also seems that the activation of the renin angiotensin aldosterone axis seems to be a factor independent of hypertension. Experimental studies by Diez et al. and Ritz et al. have shown that the activation of this system in involved in the genesis of cardiac fibrosis (Amann, Simonaviciene et al. 2001; Diez, Lopez et al. 2001; Diez 2004; Gonzalez, Lopez et al. 2004). In conjunction with this Pirola et al. have also shown that angiotensin II also stimulated the release of PTH (Pirola, Wang et al. 1993; Okano, Wu et al. 1994) and in the next section we will discuss how PTH seems to be an important factor in causing fibrosis and LVH. It has been shown that treatment with ACE inhibitors causes regression of LVH independent of hypotensive effects (Cannella, Paoletti et al. 1997; Dyadyk, Bagriy et al. 1997; Vlahakos, Hahalis et al. 1997). This lends more credibility to the idea that cardiac fibrosis may be an important factor in the pathogenesis of uremic cardiomyopathy.

Hyperparathyroidism has been proposed to be a factor as it causes abnormalities in cardiac energy metabolism and growth. Calcium ions are very important for the myocardial excitation contraction coupling and the cardiac contraction and relaxation. The release of calcium from the sarcoplasmic reticulum is the key step in the initiation of the coupling. Dissociation and sequestration of the calcium by an energy dependent pump like SERCA produces relaxation. The intracellular calcium homeostasis seems to be maintained by the membrane bound Na/Ca exchanger and SERCA which in turn is dependent on Na/K ATPase and Na/H exchanger (Morgan 1991). Both parathyroid hormone (PTH) and Parathyroid hormone related peptide (PTHrP) have been shown to acutely increase the force of contraction in isolated beating rat cardiac myocytes (Wang, Wu et al. 1993; Smogorzewski 1995). PTH excess in uremic patients has also been shown to increase cytosolic calcium levels that were correlated with the plasma PTH concentrations. These were also shown to be corrected with parathyroidectomy (PTX) (Raine, Bedford et al. 1993). Even though increased calcium entry has been thought to be the most important step in sustaining high intra myocyte calcium concentrations reductions in the NA/K ATPase and Na/H exchange rates suggesting impaired calcium extrusion may contribute to altered cellular calcium homeostasis (Smogorzewski 1995). Parathyroid hormone (PTH) now is known to cause increased endocytosis of Na/K ATPase and this may amplify CTS mediated signaling through the sodium pump (Khundmiri, Bertorello et al. 2004). Baczynski el al. have also reported that there is uncoupling of the oxidative phosphorylation and inhibited myocardial energy production in isolated myocardial mitochondria which may further this problem (Baczynski, Massry et al. 1985).

In humans with ESRD the presence of secondary hyperparathyroidism has been shown to be associated with increased myocardial calcium content and impaired systolic and diastolic functions. However these changes have not consistently been seen to improve with PTX suggesting that in the long term these changes induced by PTH become irreversible or there are other factors contributing to the myocardial dysfunction that are more important than just PTH excess (Drueke, Fauchet et al. 1980; Rostand, Sanders et al. 1988; Coratelli, Buongiorno et al. 1989; Ohara, Hiramatsu et al. 1995; Rostand and Drueke 1999). In reference to this the presence of 1,25 (OH)2 D3 receptors have been confirmed on the myocardial cells and the administration of Vitamin D in ESRD patients seems to correct the cardiac dysfunction either by correcting the excessive secretion of PTH or by a Vitamin D dependent process in the cardiac cells (Coratelli, Petrarulo et al. 1984; Shane, Mancini et al. 1997).

Our group has focused attention on CTS in the pathogenesis of uremic cardiomyopathy. Along with acute impairment of relaxation in normal adult rat cardiomyocytes when exposed to MBG (Periyasamy, Chen et al. 2001) experimental chronic renal failure induced in rats by 5/6th nephrectomy (Kennedy, Elkareh et al. 2008) causes a cardiomyopathy that is very similar to clinical chronic renal failure. It has been observed that LVH develops quite early and this is accompanied by impaired myocyte relaxation causing diastolic dysfunction. It seems that this impaired relaxation is associated with a significant down regulation of SERCA2a mRNA (Kennedy, Omran et al. 2003; Kennedy, Vetteth et al. 2006), which is known to be responsible for the rapid reduction of cytosolic calcium after systole (Bassani, Bassani et al. 1995; Bers, Bassani et al. 1996; Kennedy, Vetteth et al. 2006). Left ventricular catheterization in 5/6th nephrectomized rats at 4 weeks and calculation of dP/dT for relaxation indicated the presence of significant diastolic dysfunction (Kennedy, Vetteth et al. 2006). LVH was also demonstrated in these hearts by echocardiography as well as increases in heart weights and left ventricular end systolic volumes. There were also increases in the posterior wall thickness. Interestingly the LVH and diastolic dysfunction were also present in rats that were just infused MBG using an intra-peritoneal pump, and tended to resolve in animals immunized with an MBG-BSA conjugate that resulted in high titer specific response to MBG (Kennedy, Vetteth et al. 2006).

The animal studies done to reproduce the phenotype of cardiomyopathy by infusing with MBG so as to achieve plasma levels of MBG consistent with renal failure as well as induction of experimental renal failure by 5/6th nephrectomy, both interestingly revealed a significant amount of cardiac fibrosis in both the rat and the mouse. Also active immunization against the

MBG as discussed above as well as reduction of MBG levels by adrenalectomy prevented the onset of cardiac fibrosis seen in these animals. The heart tissue from these animals also showed evidence of activation of Na/K ATPase signaling as seen by increases in Src and MAPK phosphorylation. It was also demonstrated that there was significant increases in oxidant stress in the heart and other tissues (Kennedy, Vetteth et al. 2006). This noted fibrosis seems to play a significant role in the pathogenesis of uremic cardiomyopathy.

The above studies prompted in-vitro studies on fibroblast in order to see the effects of MBG and other CTS such as ouabain. It was seen that in fibroblast cultures grown to confluence there was increased proline incorporation as well as increased collagen production. There was also evidence of activation of Na/K ATPase signaling as there was increased Src and MAPK activation. Interestingly there was evidence of increases in oxidant stress and the scavenging of these ROS resulted in the inhibition of the Src pathway as well as prevented the increases in proline incorporation and collagen synthesis (Elkareh, Kennedy et al. 2007).

It has been further established that this fibrosis is dependent on the down regulation of Fli-1, which is a negative regulator of collagen synthesis (Czuwara-Ladykowska, Shirasaki et al. 2001). MBG was seen to induce decreases in Fli-1 expression in cardiac and renal fibroblasts, which was dependent on the nuclear translocation of PKC delta from the cytoplasm. This translocation seems to be necessary for the phosphorylation and degradation of the Fli-1 (Elkareh, Periyasamy et al. 2009). This is illustrated in figure 3.

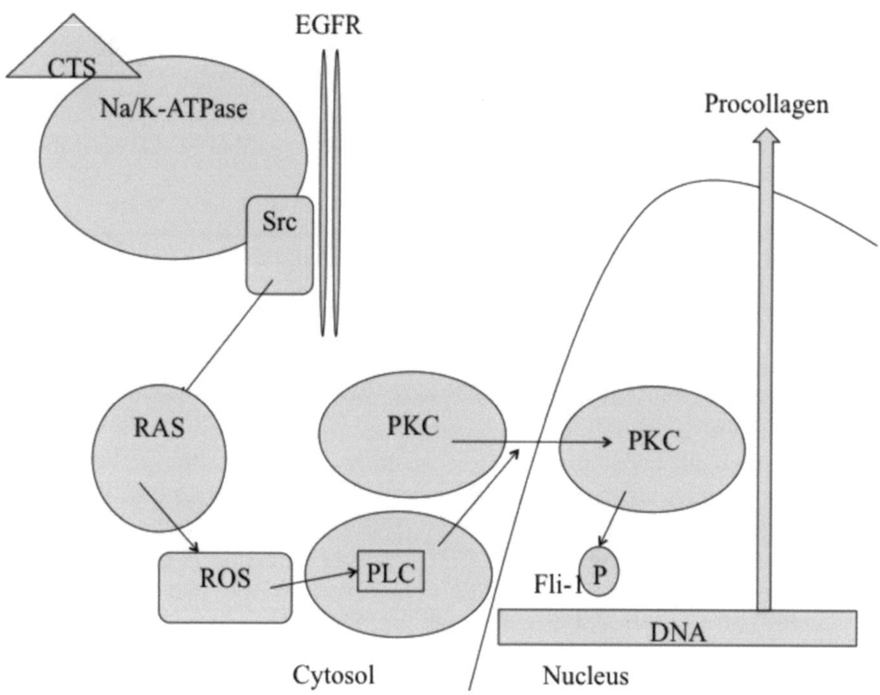

Fig. 3. Schematic showing how the signal cascade caused by cardiotonic steroids (CTS) causes the activation of phospholipase C (PLC) which then causes the translocation of protein kinase C (PKC, delta isoform) to the nucleus where it phosphorylates Fli-1. The phosphorylated Fli-1 is then rapidly degraded allowing for the disinhibition of procollagen synthesis and tissue fibrosis.

Since mineralocorticoid antagonists have been shown to ameliorate cardiac fibrosis, studies using spironolactone and canrenone have shown that both cause significant attenuation of fibrosis in-vivo as caused by experimental renal failure. Both these compounds also seemed to act as competitive inhibitors of CTS binding to Na/K ATPase and hence prevent MBG signaling (Tian, Shidyak et al. 2009). The role of CTS is thus clear in the pathogenesis of cardiac dysfunction with respect to calcium handling and the genesis of fibrosis.

The presence of oxidative stress in the ESRD patients has been well documented (Fiorillo, Oliviero et al. 1998; Tetta, Biasioli et al. 1999). Most of the reactive oxygen species are produced by the mitochondria and a dysfunction in the mitochondria has been discussed above. Oxidative stress has been well known to affect cardiovascular function, cause endothelial dysfunction and hence promote atherosclerosis as well as cause increases in sympathetic activity (Miyazaki, Matsuoka et al. 2000; Wolf 2000; Zanzinger and Czachurski 2000; Himmelfarb, Stenvinkel et al. 2002). Reactive aldehydes measured as carbonyl compounds can be formed as the end product of various oxidative reactions and have been shown to be elevated in uremia. These result in the formation of advanced glycation end products (AGE). These reactive aldehydes and AGE have been demonstrated in the pathogenesis of vascular dysfunction as well as fibrosis (Uchida 2000; Amann, Tornig et al. 2002). The interaction of the AGE with specific receptors have also shown to increase the production of IL-6 and thus increasing the production of CRP in the liver and thereby propagating inflammation (Himmelfarb, Stenvinkel et al. 2002). Increases in CRP have a strong negative correlation with the levels of plasma tocopherol as shown by Thevenin et al. (Nguyen-Khoa, Massy et al. 2001) further showing that antioxidants are decreased in inflammation. Importantly it has been shown that tocopherol decreased fibrosis in the hearts of nephrectomized rats (Amann, Tornig et al. 2002). Hence chronic oxidative stress and damage seems to be an important mechanism in the pathogenesis of chronic inflammation and uremic cardiomyopathy.

5. Conclusion

Chronic renal failure is complicated by a cardiomyopathy that is characterized by LVH and diastolic dysfunction. CTS such as MBG are found in higher concentrations in the plasma of such patients. It is clear form several studies that these CTS are involved via signaling through Na/K ATPase in causing cardiomyocyte hypertrophy, impairing relaxation and inducing fibrosis by increased collagen synthesis, which seems to be dependent on increased oxidant stress. Other major factors possibly involved in the pathogenesis of this cardiomyopathy include hyperparathyroidism, chronic oxidant stress and the activation of the RAS aldosterone system.

However mechanisms involving CTS and PTH and the interaction of the two systems seem to be emerging as the foremost candidate involved in the pathogenesis of uremic cardiomyopathy and may present prime targets for therapeutic interventions in the future.

6. References

Alsheikh-Ali, A. A., T. A. Trikalinos, et al. (2011). "Risk of arrhythmic and nonarrhythmic death in patients with heart failure and chronic kidney disease." *American heart journal* 161(1): 204-209 e201.

Amann, K., A. Simonaviciene, et al. (2001). "Blood pressure-independent additive effects of pharmacologic blockade of the renin-angiotensin and endothelin systems on progression in a low-renin model of renal damage." *Journal of the American Society of Nephrology : JASN* 12(12): 2572-2584.

Amann, K., J. Tornig, et al. (2002). "Effect of antioxidant therapy with dl-alpha-tocopherol on cardiovascular structure in experimental renal failure." *Kidney international* 62(3): 877-884.

Aydemir-Koksoy, A., J. Abramowitz, et al. (2001). "Ouabain-induced signaling and vascular smooth muscle cell proliferation." *The Journal of biological chemistry* 276(49): 46605-46611.

Aydemir-Koksoy, A. and J. C. Allen (2001). "Low concentrations of ouabain induce vascular smooth muscle cell proliferation." *Cellular and molecular biology* 47(2): 341-345.

Baczynski, R., S. G. Massry, et al. (1985). "Effect of parathyroid hormone on myocardial energy metabolism in the rat." *Kidney international* 27(5): 718-725.

Bagrov, A. Y. and O. V. Fedorova (1998). "Effects of two putative endogenous digitalis-like factors, marinobufagenin and ouabain, on the Na+, K+-pump in human mesenteric arteries." *Journal of hypertension* 16(12 Pt 2): 1953-1958.

Bagrov, A. Y., N. I. Roukoyatkina, et al. (1993). "Digitalis-like and vasoconstrictor effects of endogenous digoxin-like factor(s) from the venom of Bufo marinus toad." *Eur J Pharmacol* 234(2-3): 165-172.

Bagrov, A. Y., N. I. Roukoyatkina, et al. (1995). "Effects of two endogenous Na+,K(+)-ATPase inhibitors, marinobufagenin and ouabain, on isolated rat aorta." *Eur J Pharmacol* 274(1-3): 151-158.

Bagrov, A. Y., J. I. Shapiro, et al. (2009). "Endogenous cardiotonic steroids: physiology, pharmacology, and novel therapeutic targets." *Pharmacol Rev* 61(1): 9-38.

Bassani, R. A., J. W. Bassani, et al. (1995). "Relaxation in ferret ventricular myocytes: role of the sarcolemmal Ca ATPase." *Pflugers Archiv : European journal of physiology* 430(4): 573-578.

Bers, D. M., J. W. Bassani, et al. (1996). "Na-Ca exchange and Ca fluxes during contraction and relaxation in mammalian ventricular muscle." *Annals of the New York Academy of Sciences* 779: 430-442.

Bricker, N. S. and L. G. Fine (1978). "Uremia: formulations and expectations. The trade-off hypothesis: current status." *Kidney international. Supplement*(8): S5-8.

Cannella, G., E. Paoletti, et al. (1997). "Prolonged therapy with ACE inhibitors induces a regression of left ventricular hypertrophy of dialyzed uremic patients independently from hypotensive effects." *American journal of kidney diseases : the official journal of the National Kidney Foundation* 30(5): 659-664.

Chen, Y., T. Cai, et al. (2008). "Regulation of inositol 1,4,5-trisphosphate receptor-mediated calcium release by the Na/K-ATPase in cultured renal epithelial cells." *J Biol Chem* 283(2): 1128-1136.

Contreras, R. G., L. Shoshani, et al. (1999). "Relationship between Na(+),K(+)-ATPase and cell attachment." *Journal of cell science* 112 (Pt 23): 4223-4232.

Coratelli, P., E. Buongiorno, et al. (1989). "Pathogenetic aspects of uremic cardiomyopathy." *Mineral and electrolyte metabolism* 15(4): 246-253.

Coratelli, P., F. Petrarulo, et al. (1984). "Improvement in left ventricular function during treatment of hemodialysis patients with 25-OHD3." *Contributions to nephrology* 41: 433-437.

Croyle, M. L., A. L. Woo, et al. (1997). "Extensive random mutagenesis analysis of the Na+/K+-ATPase alpha subunit identifies known and previously unidentified amino acid residues that alter ouabain sensitivity--implications for ouabain binding." *European journal of biochemistry / FEBS* 248(2): 488-495.

Czuwara-Ladykowska, J., F. Shirasaki, et al. (2001). "Fli-1 inhibits collagen type I production in dermal fibroblasts via an Sp1-dependent pathway." *J Biol Chem* 276(24): 20839-20848.

de Wardener, H. E., E. M. Clarkson, et al. (1971). "Evidence for a hormone other than aldosterone which controls urinary sodium excretion." *Adv Nephrol Necker Hosp* 1: 97-111.

Diez, J. (2004). "Profibrotic effects of angiotensin II in the heart: a matter of mediators." *Hypertension* 43(6): 1164-1165.

Diez, J., B. Lopez, et al. (2001). "Clinical aspects of hypertensive myocardial fibrosis." *Current opinion in cardiology* 16(6): 328-335.

Dmitrieva, R. I., A. Y. Bagrov, et al. (2000). "Mammalian bufadienolide is synthesized from cholesterol in the adrenal cortex by a pathway that Is independent of cholesterol side-chain cleavage." *Hypertension* 36(3): 442-448.

Drueke, T., M. Fauchet, et al. (1980). "Effect of parathyroidectomy on left-ventricular function in haemodialysis patients." *Lancet* 1(8160): 112-114.

Dyadyk, A. I., A. E. Bagriy, et al. (1997). "ACE inhibitors captopril and enalapril induce regression of left ventricular hypertrophy in hypertensive patients with chronic renal failure." *Nephrology, dialysis, transplantation : official publication of the European Dialysis and Transplant Association - European Renal Association* 12(5): 945-951.

Elkareh, J., D. J. Kennedy, et al. (2007). "Marinobufagenin stimulates fibroblast collagen production and causes fibrosis in experimental uremic cardiomyopathy." *Hypertension* 49(1): 215-224.

Elkareh, J., S. M. Periyasamy, et al. (2009). "Marinobufagenin induces increases in procollagen expression in a process involving protein kinase C and Fli-1: implications for uremic cardiomyopathy." *Am J Physiol Renal Physiol* 296(5): F1219-1226.

Fedorova, O. V., N. I. Agalakova, et al. (2005). "Brain ouabain stimulates peripheral marinobufagenin via angiotensin II signalling in NaCl-loaded Dahl-S rats." *J Hypertens* 23(8): 1515-1523.

Fedorova, O. V., P. A. Doris, et al. (1998). "Endogenous marinobufagenin-like factor in acute plasma volume expansion." *Clinical and experimental hypertension* 20(5-6): 581-591.

Fedorova, O. V., I. A. Zhuravin, et al. (2007). "Intrahippocampal microinjection of an exquisitely low dose of ouabain mimics NaCl loading and stimulates a bufadienolide Na/K-ATPase inhibitor." *J Hypertens* 25(9): 1834-1844.

Fiorillo, C., C. Oliviero, et al. (1998). "Oxidative stress and antioxidant defenses in renal patients receiving regular haemodialysis." *Clinical chemistry and laboratory medicine : CCLM / FESCC* 36(3): 149-153.

Foley, R. N. and P. S. Parfrey (1998). "Cardiovascular disease and mortality in ESRD." *Journal of nephrology* 11(5): 239-245.

Foley, R. N., P. S. Parfrey, et al. (2000). "Effect of hemoglobin levels in hemodialysis patients with asymptomatic cardiomyopathy." *Kidney international* 58(3): 1325-1335.

Gonzalez, A., B. Lopez, et al. (2004). "Fibrosis in hypertensive heart disease: role of the renin-angiotensin-aldosterone system." *The Medical clinics of North America* 88(1): 83-97.

Graves, S. W. (1986). "Endogenous digitalis-like factors." *Critical reviews in clinical laboratory sciences* 23(3): 177-200.

Graves, S. W. and G. H. Williams (1987). "Endogenous digitalis-like natriuretic factors." *Annual review of medicine* 38: 433-444.

Haas, M., A. Askari, et al. (2000). "Involvement of Src and epidermal growth factor receptor in the signal-transducing function of Na+/K+-ATPase." *J Biol Chem* 275(36): 27832-27837.

Haas, M., H. Wang, et al. (2002). "Src-mediated inter-receptor cross-talk between the Na+/K+-ATPase and the epidermal growth factor receptor relays the signal from ouabain to mitogen-activated protein kinases." *J Biol Chem* 277(21): 18694-18702.

Hamlyn, J. M., M. P. Blaustein, et al. (1991). "Identification and characterization of a ouabain-like compound from human plasma." *Proc Natl Acad Sci U S A* 88(14): 6259-6263.

Harnett, J. D. and P. S. Parfrey (1994). "Blood pressure control and regression of LV hypertrophy in dialysis patients." *Contributions to nephrology* 106: 110-113.

Harnett, J. D., P. S. Parfrey, et al. (1988). "Left ventricular hypertrophy in end-stage renal disease." *Nephron* 48(2): 107-115.

Himmelfarb, J., P. Stenvinkel, et al. (2002). "The elephant in uremia: oxidant stress as a unifying concept of cardiovascular disease in uremia." *Kidney international* 62(5): 1524-1538.

Huting, J. and M. A. Alpert (1992). "Progression of left ventricular hypertrophy in end-stage renal disease treated by continuous ambulatory peritoneal dialysis depends on hypertension and hypercirculation." *Clinical cardiology* 15(3): 190-196.

Ihle, J. N. and I. M. Kerr (1995). "Jaks and Stats in signaling by the cytokine receptor superfamily." *Trends in genetics : TIG* 11(2): 69-74.

Jaitovich, A. and A. M. Bertorello (2010). "Salt, Na+,K+-ATPase and hypertension." *Life Sci* 86(3-4): 73-78.

Kawamura, A., J. Guo, et al. (1999). "On the structure of endogenous ouabain." *Proceedings of the National Academy of Sciences of the United States of America* 96(12): 6654-6659.

Kennedy, D., E. Omran, et al. (2003). "Effect of chronic renal failure on cardiac contractile function, calcium cycling, and gene expression of proteins important for calcium homeostasis in the rat." *Journal of the American Society of Nephrology : JASN* 14(1): 90-97.

Kennedy, D. J., J. Elkareh, et al. (2008). "Partial nephrectomy as a model for uremic cardiomyopathy in the mouse." *Am J Physiol Renal Physiol* 294(2): F450-454.

Kennedy, D. J., S. Vetteth, et al. (2006). "Central role for the cardiotonic steroid marinobufagenin in the pathogenesis of experimental uremic cardiomyopathy." *Hypertension* 47(3): 488-495.

Kennedy, D. J., S. Vetteth, et al. (2006). "Ouabain decreases sarco(endo)plasmic reticulum calcium ATPase activity in rat hearts by a process involving protein oxidation." *American journal of physiology. Heart and circulatory physiology* 291(6): H3003-3011.

Khundmiri, S. J., A. M. Bertorello, et al. (2004). "Clathrin-mediated endocytosis of Na+,K+-ATPase in response to parathyroid hormone requires ERK-dependent phosphorylation of Ser-11 within the alpha1-subunit." *The Journal of biological chemistry* 279(17): 17418-17427.

Khundmiri, S. J., M. A. Metzler, et al. (2006). "Ouabain induces cell proliferation through calcium-dependent phosphorylation of Akt (protein kinase B) in opossum kidney proximal tubule cells." *American journal of physiology. Cell physiology* 291(6): C1247-1257.

Kometiani, P., A. Askari, et al. (2001). "Downregulation of cardiac myocyte Na(+)-K(+)-ATPase by adenovirus-mediated expression of an alpha-subunit fragment." *American journal of physiology. Heart and circulatory physiology* 280(3): H1415-1421.

Kometiani, P., J. Li, et al. (1998). "Multiple signal transduction pathways link Na+/K+-ATPase to growth-related genes in cardiac myocytes. The roles of Ras and mitogen-activated protein kinases." *The Journal of biological chemistry* 273(24): 15249-15256.

Kometiani, P., L. Liu, et al. (2005). "Digitalis-induced signaling by Na+/K+-ATPase in human breast cancer cells." *Molecular pharmacology* 67(3): 929-936.

Komiyama, Y., X. H. Dong, et al. (2005). "A novel endogenous digitalis, telocinobufagin, exhibits elevated plasma levels in patients with terminal renal failure." *Clin Biochem* 38(1): 36-45.

Kotova, O., L. Al-Khalili, et al. (2006). "Cardiotonic steroids stimulate glycogen synthesis in human skeletal muscle cells via a Src- and ERK1/2-dependent mechanism." *The Journal of biological chemistry* 281(29): 20085-20094.

Kotova, O., D. Galuska, et al. (2006). "Metabolic and signaling events mediated by cardiotonic steroid ouabain in rat skeletal muscle." *Cellular and molecular biology* 52(8): 48-57.

Kreuz, J., F. Horlbeck, et al. (2011). "An impaired renal function: a predictor of ventricular arrhythmias and mortality in patients with nonischemic cardiomyopathy and heart failure." *Pacing and clinical electrophysiology : PACE* 34(7): 894-899.

Li, Z. and Z. Xie (2009). "The Na/K-ATPase/Src complex and cardiotonic steroid-activated protein kinase cascades." *Pflugers Archiv : European journal of physiology* 457(3): 635-644.

Liang, M., T. Cai, et al. (2006). "Functional characterization of Src-interacting Na/K-ATPase using RNA interference assay." *The Journal of biological chemistry* 281(28): 19709-19719.

Lingrel, J. B. (2010). "The physiological significance of the cardiotonic steroid/ouabain-binding site of the Na,K-ATPase." *Annual review of physiology* 72: 395-412.

Liu, J., R. Kesiry, et al. (2004). "Ouabain induces endocytosis of plasmalemmal Na/K-ATPase in LLC-PK1 cells by a clathrin-dependent mechanism." *Kidney Int* 66(1): 227-241.

Liu, J., M. Liang, et al. (2005). "Ouabain-induced endocytosis of the plasmalemmal Na/K-ATPase in LLC-PK1 cells requires caveolin-1." *Kidney Int* 67(5): 1844-1854.

Liu, J. and J. I. Shapiro (2007). "Regulation of sodium pump endocytosis by cardiotonic steroids: Molecular mechanisms and physiological implications." *Pathophysiology*.

Liu, J., J. Tian, et al. (2000). "Ouabain interaction with cardiac Na+/K+-ATPase initiates signal cascades independent of changes in intracellular Na+ and Ca2+ concentrations." *J Biol Chem* 275(36): 27838-27844.

Liu, L., K. Mohammadi, et al. (2003). "Role of caveolae in signal-transducing function of cardiac Na+/K+-ATPase." *American journal of physiology. Cell physiology* 284(6): C1550-1560.
Mall, G., W. Huther, et al. (1990). "Diffuse intermyocardiocytic fibrosis in uraemic patients." *Nephrology, dialysis, transplantation : official publication of the European Dialysis and Transplant Association - European Renal Association* 5(1): 39-44.
Mall, G., M. Rambausek, et al. (1988). "Myocardial interstitial fibrosis in experimental uremia--implications for cardiac compliance." *Kidney international* 33(4): 804-811.
McGarrigle, D. and X. Y. Huang (2007). "GPCRs signaling directly through Src-family kinases." *Science's STKE : signal transduction knowledge environment* 2007(392): pe35.
Mimura, M., H. Makino, et al. (1992). "Reduction of erythrocyte (Na(+)-K+) ATPase activities in non-insulin-dependent diabetic patients with hyperkalemia." *Metabolism: clinical and experimental* 41(4): 426-430.
Minagawa, T., T. Hirano, et al. (1994). "The effect of recombinant human erythropoietin (r-HuEPO) on left ventricular mass and left ventricular hemodynamics in hemodialysis patients." *Nippon Jinzo Gakkai shi* 36(8): 934-941.
Mitsnefes, M. M., S. R. Daniels, et al. (2001). "Changes in left ventricular mass in children and adolescents during chronic dialysis." *Pediatric nephrology* 16(4): 318-323.
Miyazaki, H., H. Matsuoka, et al. (2000). "Hemodialysis impairs endothelial function via oxidative stress: effects of vitamin E-coated dialyzer." *Circulation* 101(9): 1002-1006.
Mohmand, B., D. K. Malhotra, et al. (2005). "Uremic cardiomyopathy: role of circulating digitalis like substances." *Front Biosci* 10: 2036-2044.
Morduchowicz, G., J. Zabludowski, et al. (1993). "Ambulatory blood pressure monitoring assessment of blood pressure control in hypertension associated with chronic renal failure." *Nephrology, dialysis, transplantation : official publication of the European Dialysis and Transplant Association - European Renal Association* 8(10): 1169-1171.
Morgan, J. P. (1991). "Abnormal intracellular modulation of calcium as a major cause of cardiac contractile dysfunction." *The New England journal of medicine* 325(9): 625-632.
Nakazato, T., T. Kawada, et al. (2002). "Left ventricular hypertrophy was infrequent in patients starting dialysis after undergoing a strict blood pressure control in the pre-dialytic period." *Internal medicine* 41(11): 925-930.
Nguyen-Khoa, T., Z. A. Massy, et al. (2001). "Oxidative stress and haemodialysis: role of inflammation and duration of dialysis treatment." *Nephrology, dialysis, transplantation : official publication of the European Dialysis and Transplant Association - European Renal Association* 16(2): 335-340.
Nishikimi, T., J. Minami, et al. (2001). "Left ventricular mass relates to average systolic blood pressure, but not loss of circadian blood pressure in stable hemodialysis patients: an ambulatory 48-hour blood pressure study." *Hypertension research : official journal of the Japanese Society of Hypertension* 24(5): 507-514.
Ohara, N., K. Hiramatsu, et al. (1995). "Effect of parathyroid hormone on left ventricular diastolic function in patients with primary hyperparathyroidism." *Mineral and electrolyte metabolism* 21(1-3): 63-66.
Okamoto, S. (1988). "[Endogenous digitalis-like substance and Na-K-ATPase inhibitor in cardiovascular and renal disease]." *Nippon Naibunpi Gakkai zasshi* 64(1): 39-50.
Okano, K., S. Wu, et al. (1994). "Parathyroid hormone (PTH)/PTH-related protein (PTHrP) receptor and its messenger ribonucleic acid in rat aortic vascular smooth muscle

cells and UMR osteoblast-like cells: cell-specific regulation by angiotensin-II and PTHrP." *Endocrinology* 135(3): 1093-1099.

Oweis, S., L. Wu, et al. (2006). "Cardiac glycoside downregulates NHE3 activity and expression in LLC-PK1 cells." *Am J Physiol Renal Physiol* 290(5): F997-1008.

Paparello, J., A. Kshirsagar, et al. (2002). "Comorbidity and cardiovascular risk factors in patients with chronic kidney disease." *Seminars in nephrology* 22(6): 494-506.

Periyasamy, S. M., J. Chen, et al. (2001). "Effects of uremic serum on isolated cardiac myocyte calcium cycling and contractile function." *Kidney international* 60(6): 2367-2376.

Periyasamy, S. M., J. Liu, et al. (2005). "Salt loading induces redistribution of the plasmalemmal Na/K-ATPase in proximal tubule cells." *Kidney Int* 67(5): 1868-1877.

Pierre, S. V., C. Yang, et al. (2007). "Ouabain triggers preconditioning through activation of the Na+,K+-ATPase signaling cascade in rat hearts." *Cardiovasc Res* 73(3): 488-496.

Pirola, C. J., H. M. Wang, et al. (1993). "Angiotensin II regulates parathyroid hormone-related protein expression in cultured rat aortic smooth muscle cells through transcriptional and post-transcriptional mechanisms." *The Journal of biological chemistry* 268(3): 1987-1994.

Priyadarshi, S., B. Valentine, et al. (2003). "Effect of green tea extract on cardiac hypertrophy following 5/6 nephrectomy in the rat." *Kidney Int* 63(5): 1785-1790.

Qiu, J., H. Q. Gao, et al. (2007). "Proteomics analysis of the proliferative effect of low-dose ouabain on human endothelial cells." *Biological & pharmaceutical bulletin* 30(2): 247-253.

Raine, A. E., L. Bedford, et al. (1993). "Hyperparathyroidism, platelet intracellular free calcium and hypertension in chronic renal failure." *Kidney international* 43(3): 700-705.

Raj, D. S., S. D'Mello, et al. (1997). "Left ventricular morphology in chronic renal failure by echocardiography." *Renal failure* 19(6): 799-806.

Rostand, S. G. and T. B. Drueke (1999). "Parathyroid hormone, vitamin D, and cardiovascular disease in chronic renal failure." *Kidney international* 56(2): 383-392.

Rostand, S. G., C. Sanders, et al. (1988). "Myocardial calcification and cardiac dysfunction in chronic renal failure." *The American journal of medicine* 85(5): 651-657.

Sarnak, M. J. (2003). "Cardiovascular complications in chronic kidney disease." *American journal of kidney diseases : the official journal of the National Kidney Foundation* 41(5 Suppl): 11-17.

Sarnak, M. J., A. S. Levey, et al. (2003). "Kidney disease as a risk factor for development of cardiovascular disease: a statement from the American Heart Association Councils on Kidney in Cardiovascular Disease, High Blood Pressure Research, Clinical Cardiology, and Epidemiology and Prevention." *Hypertension* 42(5): 1050-1065.

Saunders, R. and G. Scheiner-Bobis (2004). "Ouabain stimulates endothelin release and expression in human endothelial cells without inhibiting the sodium pump." *European journal of biochemistry / FEBS* 271(5): 1054-1062.

Shane, E., D. Mancini, et al. (1997). "Bone mass, vitamin D deficiency, and hyperparathyroidism in congestive heart failure." *The American journal of medicine* 103(3): 197-207.

Smogorzewski, M. (1995). "PTH, chronic renal failure and myocardium." *Mineral and electrolyte metabolism* 21(1-3): 55-62.

Stack, A. G. and W. E. Bloembergen (2001). "A cross-sectional study of the prevalence and clinical correlates of congestive heart failure among incident US dialysis patients." *American journal of kidney diseases : the official journal of the National Kidney Foundation* 38(5): 992-1000.

Stack, A. G. and R. Saran (2002). "Clinical correlates and mortality impact of left ventricular hypertrophy among new ESRD patients in the United States." *American journal of kidney diseases : the official journal of the National Kidney Foundation* 40(6): 1202-1210.

Stokes, G. S., D. Willcocks, et al. (1986). "Measurement of circulating sodium-pump inhibitory activity in uraemia and essential hypertension." *Journal of hypertension. Supplement : official journal of the International Society of Hypertension* 4(6): S376-378.

Sweadner, K. J. (1989). "Isozymes of the Na+/K+-ATPase." *Biochim Biophys Acta* 988(2): 185-220.

Takahashi, H., M. Nishimura, et al. (1989). "[Endothelin and endogenous digitalis-like substance in cardiovascular regulation: a review]." *Rinsho byori. The Japanese journal of clinical pathology* 37(10): 1103-1113.

Tetta, C., S. Biasioli, et al. (1999). "An overview of haemodialysis and oxidant stress." *Blood purification* 17(2-3): 118-126.

Tian, J., T. Cai, et al. (2006). "Binding of Src to Na+/K+-ATPase forms a functional signaling complex." *Mol Biol Cell* 17(1): 317-326.

Tian, J., J. Liu, et al. (2003). "Involvement of mitogen-activated protein kinases and reactive oxygen species in the inotropic action of ouabain on cardiac myocytes. A potential role for mitochondrial K(ATP) channels." *Mol Cell Biochem* 242(1-2): 181-187.

Tian, J., A. Shidyak, et al. (2009). "Spironolactone attenuates experimental uremic cardiomyopathy by antagonizing marinobufagenin." *Hypertension* 54(6): 1313-1320.

Tyralla, K. and K. Amann (2003). "Morphology of the heart and arteries in renal failure." *Kidney international. Supplement*(84): S80-83.

Uchida, K. (2000). "Role of reactive aldehyde in cardiovascular diseases." *Free radical biology & medicine* 28(12): 1685-1696.

Vlahakos, D. V., G. Hahalis, et al. (1997). "Relationship between left ventricular hypertrophy and plasma renin activity in chronic hemodialysis patients." *Journal of the American Society of Nephrology : JASN* 8(11): 1764-1770.

Wang, H., M. Haas, et al. (2004). "Ouabain assembles signaling cascades through the caveolar Na+/K+-ATPase." *J Biol Chem* 279(17): 17250-17259.

Wang, R., L. Wu, et al. (1993). "The changes in contractile status of single vascular smooth muscle cells and ventricular cells induced by bPTH-(1-34)." *Life sciences* 52(9): 793-801.

Weiner, D. E., H. Tighiouart, et al. (2004). "Chronic kidney disease as a risk factor for cardiovascular disease and all-cause mortality: a pooled analysis of community-based studies." *Journal of the American Society of Nephrology : JASN* 15(5): 1307-1315.

Wolf, G. (2000). "Free radical production and angiotensin." *Current hypertension reports* 2(2): 167-173.

Xie, Z., P. Kometiani, et al. (1999). "Intracellular reactive oxygen species mediate the linkage of Na+/K+-ATPase to hypertrophy and its marker genes in cardiac myocytes." *J Biol Chem* 274(27): 19323-19328.

Yuan, Z., T. Cai, et al. (2005). "Na/K-ATPase tethers phospholipase C and IP3 receptor into a calcium-regulatory complex." *Mol Biol Cell* 16(9): 4034-4045.
Zanzinger, J. and J. Czachurski (2000). "Chronic oxidative stress in the RVLM modulates sympathetic control of circulation in pigs." *Pflugers Archiv : European journal of physiology* 439(4): 489-494.

Part 5

Takotsubo Cardiomyopathy

29

Stress-Induced Cardiomyopathy: Clinical Observations

Jun-Won Lee[1], Hyun-Kyo Lim[2], Jang-Young Kim[1] and Sungwoo Ryoo[3]
[1]*Division of Cardiology, Department of Internal Medicine,*
[2]*Department of Anesthesiology and Pain Medicine,*
Yonsei University Wonju College of Medicine, Wonju
[3]*Division of Biology, Kangwon National University, Chuncheon*
Korea

1. Introduction

Stress-induced cardiomyopathy has achieved global notoriety in only 20 years since it was introduced as "Takotsubo cardiomyopathy" (which means "octopus trap" in Japanese) (Dote et al., 1991). It is also known as "left ventricular apical ballooning", "ampulla cardiomyopathy" and "broken heart syndrome". Stress-induced cardiomyopathy is associated with typical electrocardiographic findings and severe chest pain suggesting ST-segment elevation myocardial infarction (STEMI). However, emergency coronary angiography usually does not show significant stenosis or definite flow limitation. In general, left ventricular ejection fraction (LVEF) is markedly depressed and is recovered within the normal range within 1–2 weeks. Most cases have a good outcome and some may not even need further medical therapy if the underlying the cause is uncovered. Several hypotheses have been proposed but the pathophysiologic mechanism is incompletely understood. Here we discuss the clinical findings, diagnostic modalities, possible pathophysiologic mechanisms, prognosis and management of stress-induced cardiomyopathy.

2. History of reporting of stress-induced cardiomyopathy

In 1980, strong evidences implying stress-induced cardiomyopathy were reported via the autopsies of homicidal victims (Cebelin & Hirsch, 1980). They found pathognomonic findings of contraction band necrosis in 11 patients who had died due to a physical assault without internal injuries. One case report revealed that severe emotional stress could bring about deterioration of cardiac function which developed into pulmonary edema (Anon, 1986). Echocardiographic studies demonstrated that left ventricular wall motion abnormalities and myocardial damage could be accompanied by subarachnoid hemorrhage (Pollick et al., 1988). This pioneering work inspired other investigators, who discovered that LVEF and regional wall motion abnormalities were significant predictors of death in patients with subarachnoid hemorrhage (Sugimoto et al., 2008). Reversible left ventricular dysfunction induced by excessive catecholamine surges in pheochromocytoma was also reported (Iga et al., 1989). This finding suggested that catecholamines at high concentrations can directly damage the myocardium.

Stress-induced cardiomyopathy was termed "Takotsubo cardiomyopathy" by Japanese cardiologists in 1991 (Dote et al., 1991). Advances in diagnostic imaging and emergency coronary angiography have contributed to increased recognition of stress-induced cardiomyopathy, and increasing numbers of reports have been published since then.

3. Clinical observations: Single-center experiences

We reported retrospective data of 39 patients diagnosed with stress-induced cardiomyopathy during 5 years in a single center (Lee, J.W. et al., 2010). Our results showed differences from other reports. In our study, 69% of patients were female, and the mean age was 61.3 ± 16.1 years. The most frequent symptom at initial presentation was dyspnea (46%) rather than chest pain (26%). Emotional stress was found in only 15% of subjects. The main triggering factors were physical stress associated with illness (59%), procedure-related complications (8%) and trauma (8%). Initial electrocardiography revealed T-wave inversion (46%), ST-segment elevation (28%) and ST-segment depression (5%). LVEF was recovered from 45 ± 16% upon hospital admission to 61 ± 13% upon hospital discharge. The level of B-type natriuretic peptide (BNP) was increased (745.4 ± 905.6 pg/mL) and 23 patients (59%) had elevated levels of highly-sensitive C-reactive protein (hs-CRP; 44 ± 61 mg/L) at initial presentation. The peak level of creatine kinase-MB (CK-MB) fraction and troponin I showed mild elevation (15.6 ± 20.9 ng/mL and 6.8 ± 12.3 ng/mL, respectively)

Echocardiography was shown to be a useful tool to detect transient left ventricular outflow tract (LVOT) obstruction, apical thrombus on the site of apical ballooning, and unusual inverted-type (mid-ventricular) ballooning.

Three patients (8%) died due to pneumonia and 13 patients (33%) experienced cardiogenic shock. Inotropic agents were needed in 10 patients (26%) and 9 patients (23%) required mechanical ventilation. When we assessed the prognostic factors affecting adverse events such as death or shock, LVEF and hs-CRP levels were independent risk factors by multivariate logistic regression analyses (adjusted for age, sex, and other risk factors).

4. Clinical findings

In general, stress-induced cardiomyopathy is characterized by sudden chest pain or dyspnea, ST-segment elevation mimicking acute myocardial infarction (AMI) or deep T-wave inversion, elevated levels of cardiac enzymes or BNP and transient left ventricular systolic dysfunction. Post-menopausal women seem to be more vulnerable to this syndrome. The definition is continually evolving. There are some divergences of opinion on clinical situations and management.

4.1 Age and sex

The elderly seem to be the most vulnerable to stress-induced cardiomyopathy. The mean age for presentation was >60 years (Bybee et al., 2004). However, a case of stress-induced cardiomyopathy in a newborn after fetal distress was caused by the umbilical cord being twisted around the chest and neck (Greco, 2011). The youngest patient we treated was a 26-year-old female. Despite literature suggesting that the elderly are the most affected, recent case reports have shown the possibility of development of stress-induced cardiomyopathy in patients of any age.

The higher prevalence of females is a consistent finding in published series (Bybee et al., 2004). Nevertheless, the reason for this difference in prevalence between males and females is unknown. Stöllberger & Finsterer suggested two intriguing hypotheses (Stöllberger & Finsterer, 2011). The first hypothesis is that males have been biologically better protected against the stress-induced cardiotoxicity of catecholamines than females throughout the centuries. They suggested that males were exposed to more physical stress and developed various protecting mechanisms (Stöllberger & Finsterer, 2011, as cited in Silventoinen et al., 2001). The higher density of adrenergic receptors of cardiomyocytes in males may result in delayed saturation of receptors and improved protection against catecholamine storms (Stöllberger & Finsterer, 2011, as cited in Leibel et al., 1987). The second hypothesis is that males are biologically less resistant than females against the stress-induced cardiotoxicity of catecholamines. Males comprise 78.9% of sudden cardiac deaths (Fragkouli & Vouguiouklakis, 2010) and one of the risk factors for sudden unexplained death in epilepsy patients was being male (Monté et al., 2007). Large-scale cohort studies could provide answers for the age and sex predominance of stress-induced cardiomyopathy.

4.2 Initial presenting symptoms

The most common presenting symptoms of stress-induced cardiomyopathy are chest pain and dyspnea. Not all studies reported the initial symptoms (especially in the case of dyspnea). Nevertheless, chest pain was the cardinal symptom in 185 of 273 patients (67.8%) and dyspnea the second most common symptom in 40 of 225 patients (17.8%) (Gianni et al., 2006). Cardiogenic shock, severe arrhythmia, mental change or syncope may be the initial presentation. Some patients suffer from chest pain and dyspnea; the most frequent symptom of stress-induced cardiomyopathy in patients in our institution was dyspnea.

In our experience, patients with dyspnea had a longer stay in hospital, elevated levels of BNP and hs-CRP, and decreased initial LVEF, but these differences were not statistically significant (Lee, J.W. et al., 2011). A recent prospective study in a tertiary referral hospital demonstrated that chest pain was more frequently observed in the emotional stress group, whereas dyspnea was the presenting symptom in the physical stress group (acute illness and in-hospital surgery/procedure) (Lee, P.H. et al., 2010).

New imaging modalities contribute to the early diagnosis of stress-induced cardiomyopathy. Hence, the proportion of initial symptoms might shift from emotional stress to physical stress.

4.3 Triggering factors

Triggering factors preceding this syndrome are, in general, divided into "emotional stress" and "physical stress". A wide variety of emotional stressors have been reported, including panic, fear, anxiety, grief and anger (Prasad et al., 2008; Sharkey et al., 2010). These emotional stressors include immediate ("fight-or-flight") responses and/or sustained responses, which implies the involvement of protective mechanisms of the body via the stress system (neurohormonal interaction) (Balkin & Cohen, 2011).

Among physical stressors, pheochromocytoma, subarachnoid hemorrhage, exposure to catecholamine/beta-agonist drugs and procedure-related events are representative cases associated with catecholamine excess. Other physical stressors include hypoxia, infection, metabolic abnormalities, invasive procedures, and general anesthesia (Park et al., 2010; Prasad et al., 2008; Sharkey et al., 2010). Madhavan et al. suggested the importance of physical stress (Madhavan et al., 2011). They suggested that patients with physical stressors had significant underlying co-morbidities that may contribute to the development of heart failure. In addition, physical stressors such as postoperative status may be associated with a more sustained surge in catecholamines compared with emotional stress, which may be shortlived (Park et al., 2010).

4.4 Electrocardiographic findings

The most common abnormality on electrocardiography (ECG) is ST-segment elevation resembling STEMI (Prasad et al., 2008). T-wave inversion is usually observed at initial presentation and during the subacute phase. The proportion of ST-segment elevation and T-wave inversion was 208 of 255 patients (81.6%) and 160 of 249 patients (64.3%), respectively (Gianni et al., 2006). Q waves also could be detected in 63 of 198 patients (31.8%). T-wave inversion may resolve over 3–4 months but may occur as early as 4–6 weeks and, in some cases, be present beyond 1 year (Prasad et al., 2009, as cited in Kurisu et al., 2004 and Matsuoka et al., 2003).

One study tried to distinguish stress-induced cardiomyopathy from anterior wall myocardial infarction by simple and non-invasive ECG tests (Jim et al., 2009). They found that if extensive left ventricular dysfunction and precordial ST-segment elevation were observed, the absence of ST-segment depression, or the presence of ST-segment elevation in inferior leads (particularly II ≥ III) were suggestive of stress-induced cardiomyopathy. Lead II is the most sensitive and specific for the detection of stress-induced cardiomyopathy because it is relatively protected from the opposing effect of lateral wall ischemia.

4.5 Laboratory findings

The level of troponin I or troponin T and CK-MB fraction is slightly elevated from baseline reference values. BNP levels in plasma are also elevated to various degrees (Lee, J.W. et al., 2010 and Morel et al., 2009).

One case-control study provided a comprehensive analysis of stress hormone and cardiac biomarker profiles in stress-induced cardiomyopathy, and the values were compared with those from patients with STEMI (Madhavan et al., 2009). The major findings were that: (1) levels of BNP were higher in stress-induced cardiomyopathy despite less necrosis of myocytes, similar left ventricular dysfunction and comparable hemodynamics; (2) there was a marked elevation in levels of an inflammatory biomarker (hs-CRP) in a magnitude similar to that seen in patients with STEMI.

Inflammation may have a crucial role in stress-induced cardiomyopathy. Morel et al. demonstrated that inflammatory status was related to the initial impairment of LVEF and to the extent of neurohormonal activation (Morel et al., 2009). Other research teams demonstrated that patients who developed left ventricular apical ballooning due to severe physical stress in the Intensive Care Unit had a higher frequency of sepsis, cardiomegaly, pulmonary edema and hypotension (Park et al., 2005).

One recent prospective study showed that inflammatory mediators and platelet-activity markers could be used to distinguish stress-induced cardiomyopathy from myocardial infarction (Pirzer et al., 2011). Expression of the platelet-activation marker CD62P and plasma levels of interleukin-6 were significantly lower in patients with stress-induced cardiomyopathy compared with myocardial infarction at the time of hospital admission. Plasma levels of interleukin-7 were significantly elevated in patients with stress-induced cardiomyopathy compared with patients with myocardial infarction 2–4 days after hospital admission.

The plasma concentrations of catecholamines during the acute phase were 2–3-times higher than in patients with AMI and heart failure, and 20-times higher than in normal adults (Wittstein et al., 2005). Uchida et al. also observed elevated levels of plasma epinephrine and norepinephrine in patients with stress-induced cardiomyopathy (Uchida et al., 2010). The plasma half-life of epinephrine is only 3 min (Zeb et al., 2011, as cited in Ferreira & Vane, 1967), so measurement of catecholamines should be conducted at the time of symptom onset.

4.6 Left ventricular systolic dysfunction

Initial left ventricular systolic function is usually impaired upon hospital admission (mean LVEF, 20–49%) and, in general, resolves within days-to-weeks after initial presentation (mean period, 18 days) (Nef et al., 2010). Most patients achieve normal systolic function during hospitalization, but a few fail to reach the normal range (Sharkey et al., 2010). Moreover, a recent study revealed that absence of functional recovery within 1 week (ejection fraction <50%) was an independent factor associated with mortality (Lee, P.H. et al., 2010).

4.7 Co-morbidity

There are no reported associations between stress-induced cardiomyopathy and co-morbidity. Collective data from 14 studies reported a history of hypertension in 43% of patients (108/247), diabetes mellitus in 11% (53/217) and current or past smoking in 23% (23/100). Others include chronic obstructive pulmonary disease, asthma and malignancy.

One observational study showed that patients with stress-induced cardiomyopathy had significantly higher levels of high-density lipoprotein-cholesterol and lower levels of low-density lipoprotein-cholesterol and triglyceride compared with age- and sex-matched patients with myocardial infarction (Gaddam et al., 2011). Hyper-alpha-lipoproteinemia was noted in 2 patients. That study had a major limitation because the study population was small. However, a history of dyslipidemia should be assessed at initial presentation. This result adds evidence that the pathogenesis is not due to atherosclerotic narrowing of epicardial coronary arteries.

4.8 Preferred time of onset

The occurrence of major cardiovascular events is not randomly distributed over time but instead exhibits chronobiological patterns. Stress-induced cardiomyopathy also seems to exhibit a temporal variation of onset, with peaks during the morning and in the summer (Bossone et al., 2011). One study reported that the highest number of cases was found on Monday and the lowest on Saturday. This phenomenon might be because of stress and catecholamine release (Manfredini et al., 2010). However, conclusions are hard to reach because of the relatively small number of patients involved in this study.

5. Imaging modalities and implications

Several imaging tools are used for the diagnosis of stress-induced cardiomyopathy: coronary angiography with left ventriculography, echocardiography, cardiac magnetic resonance (CMR) and nuclear imaging. Each examination has its own diagnostic value and benefit. One should understand the advantages and disadvantages and select the most appropriate method for the purpose.

5.1 Coronary angiography

Coronary angiography is essential and the only way to rule out obstruction of coronary arteries (especially in cases of ST-segment elevation). The modified Mayo Clinic criteria to diagnose stress-induced cardiomyopathy demand the absence of obstructive coronary artery disease or angiographic evidence of acute rupture of plaques that could be responsible for the observed wall motion abnormalities. A recent report suggested the possible concurrence of coronary artery disease with stress-induced cardiomyopathy (Winchester et al., 2008). Hence, several cases might be excluded because of the presence of coronary artery disease. If coronary atherosclerotic changes are not significant and regional wall motional abnormalities extend beyond a single coronary artery, stress-induced cardiomyopathy should be suspected. The endocardial border can be readily detected by left ventriculography (Fig. 1).

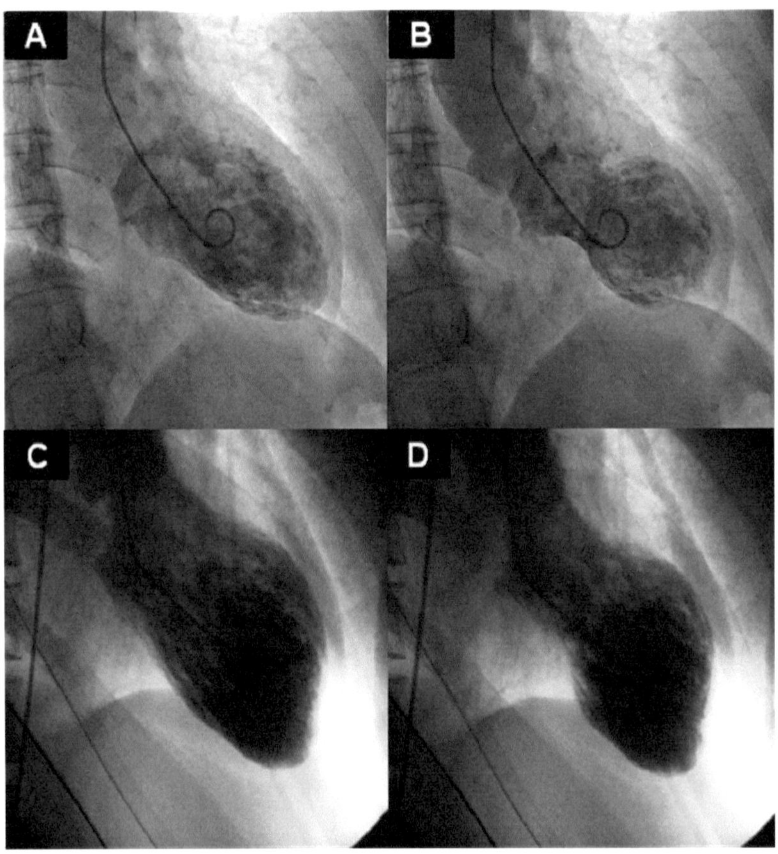

Fig. 1. Left ventriculography shows the typical pattern of apical ballooning with relative basal hypercontractility (A: end-diastole, B: end-systole) and inverted type of mid-ventricular ballooning with apical sparing (C: end-diastole, D: end-systole).

5.2 Echocardiography

Transthoracic echocardiography is the most important modality to distinguish this syndrome from AMI. It has many merits thanks to its non-invasiveness, portability, real-time accessibility, reproducibility and concurrent monitoring of anatomic and physiologic abnormalities (Lee, J.W. et al., 2011).

Echocardiography reveals the unique morphology of apical ballooning and the relative compensatory hypercontractiliy of the basal segments. One should closely observe two distinct features: (i) decrease in LVEF and (ii) (LVOT) obstruction. These factors are important to predict the severity and prognosis of stress-induced cardiomyopathy.

The decreased LVEF seen at hospital admission is a significant independent risk factor for death or cardiogenic shock (Lee, J.W. et al., 2010). The absence of recovery in left ventricular dysfunction within 1 week is also a powerful independent factor associated with mortality (Lee, P. H. et al., 2010).

Hypotensive events can be induced by dynamic LVOT obstruction, which results in the movement of the anterior mitral leaflets toward the interventricular septum in the systolic phase, so-called "systolic anterior motion" (SAM). Low cardiac output occurs as a result of reduced antegrade flow. This may occur in up to one-quarter of patients presenting with a septal bulge associated with SAM and mitral regurgitation (El Mahmoud et al., 2008). LVOT obstruction is a dynamic phenomenon depending on the hemodynamics at that time point, and thus echocardiography is a useful and readily accessible tool if unexplained hypotension or shock is observed.

Acute mitral regurgitation can be found in stress-induced cardiomyopathy. Mitral regurgitation seems to develop mainly due to displacement of the papillary muscle, which leads to impaired leaflet coaptation secondary to tethering. Parodi et al. suggested that mitral regurgitation accompanied by severe left ventricular dysfunction was a potent predictor of hemodynamic derangement leading to hazardous manifestations, including pulmonary edema and cardiogenic shock (Parodi et al., 2007).

Regional and global systolic function can be assessed and quantified by two-dimensional strain. This method is based on tracking the movement of stable acoustic patterns ("speckles") within the myocardium frame-by-frame throughout the cardiac cycle. Despite the general perception of basal hypercontractility, total longitudinal strain showed that systolic function in basal segments was decreased in one study (Heggemann et al., 2009).

Contrast echocardiography can be helpful in detection of the endocardial border (particularly if apical segments are difficult to evaluate because of poor image quality). Apical thrombus can be readily detected by contrast echocardiography. Contrast echocardiography can also demonstrate abnormalities in myocardial perfusion, which are indicative of microvascular dysfunction (Abdelmoneim, 2009). The normal myocardial perfusion pattern in the akinetic apex helps to discriminate stress-induced cardiomyopathy from anterior wall myocardial infarction.

Real-time three-dimensional imaging techniques and transesophageal echocardiography can give better information on volumetric change and anatomic abnormalities

5.3 CMR

CMR provides information on wall-motion abnormalities as well as myocardial viability. Contrast-enhanced CMR can identify myocardial inflammation through the presence of edema by T2-weighted images and/or myocardial tissue injury by late gadolinium enhancement (Schmalfuss, 2011). The special morphological pattern of late gadolinium uptake was reported recently for the first time (Avegliano et al., 2011). Early CMR (within 72 h of hospital admission) demonstrated mild enhancement of signals in the segments with abnormal contractility, which was clearly different from the segments with no signal enhancement and normal contractility. This special morphological pattern corresponded to localized inflammation and edema in the affected area, which could be related to slower gadolinium washout determined by interstitial edema and inflammation (and perhaps very small areas of necrosis). This pattern becomes normal after recovery from myocardial edema and contractility. The morphological pattern suggests that the pathophysiology is related to diffuse damage of the myocardium and the microcirculation rather than involvement of coronary epicardial vessels.

5.4 Nuclear imaging

Single-photon emission computed tomography (SPECT) shows perfusion defects in the affected segment beyond single coronary distribution. Imaging also showed that the perfusion defect was slightly smaller in extent compared with the distribution of the wall-motion defect in one study (Skovgaard et al., 2010). Fluorine 18 fluorodeoxyglucose positron emission tomography in the acute phase showed reduced (but not absent) glucose uptake in almost the entire left ventricle, indicating viable tissue. The myocardial glucose uptake 3 months later was evenly distributed in the affected areas.

The findings of ^{123}I-meta-iodobenzylguanidine myocardial scintigraphy depicted a unique pattern of ventricular asynergy and suggested the existence of cardiac sympathetic hyperactivity (Akashi et al., 2004). Conversely, Skovgaard et al. could not find signs of cardiac sympathetic dysfunction as evidenced by a normal and unchanged washout rate (Skovgaard et al., 2010). However, they demonstrated the interesting finding of increased uptake in the lung, which was shown in chronic heart failure.

The findings from these nuclear imaging studies provide possible evidence of coronary microvascular dysfunction.

6. Mechanisms of stress-induced cardiomyopathy

The mechanisms of stress-induced cardiomyopathy are incompletely understood. However, a growing body of evidence could explain the possible mechanism and pathophysiology. A proposed mechanism of stress-induced cardiomyopathy is summarized in Fig. 2.

6.1 Brain–heart connection

Although the heart has an intrinsic capacity to maintain homeostasis, it is always ready to recognize extrinsic stimuli through brain–heart connections and can elicit an appropriate response for physiological demands. This protective process is called the "stress system". The main central effectors of the stress system are highly interconnected and include hypothalamic corticotropin-releasing hormone and locus ceruleus-derived norepinephrine (Chrousos, 2009, as cited in Charmandari et al., 2005 and Chrousos & Gold, 1992). The principal peripheral effectors are glucocorticoids, which are regulated by the hypothalamic–pituitary–adrenal axis, and the catecholamines norepinephrine and epinephrine, which are regulated by the systemic and adrenomedullary sympathetic nervous systems (Chrousos, 2009). A functional positive feedback loop is formed by hypothalamic corticotrophin-releasing hormone and brainstem locus ceruleus-norepinephrine systems (Chrousos, 2007). The locus ceruleus also participates in a feedback loop with the adrenal medulla and the limbic system. The adrenal gland secretes epinephrine, which stimulates the locus ceruleus. Norepinephrine is released consecutively by this stimulus, which then sends signals to the hipppocampus and amygdala. The latter can re-stimulate the locus ceruleus in sequence (Soufer, 2002).

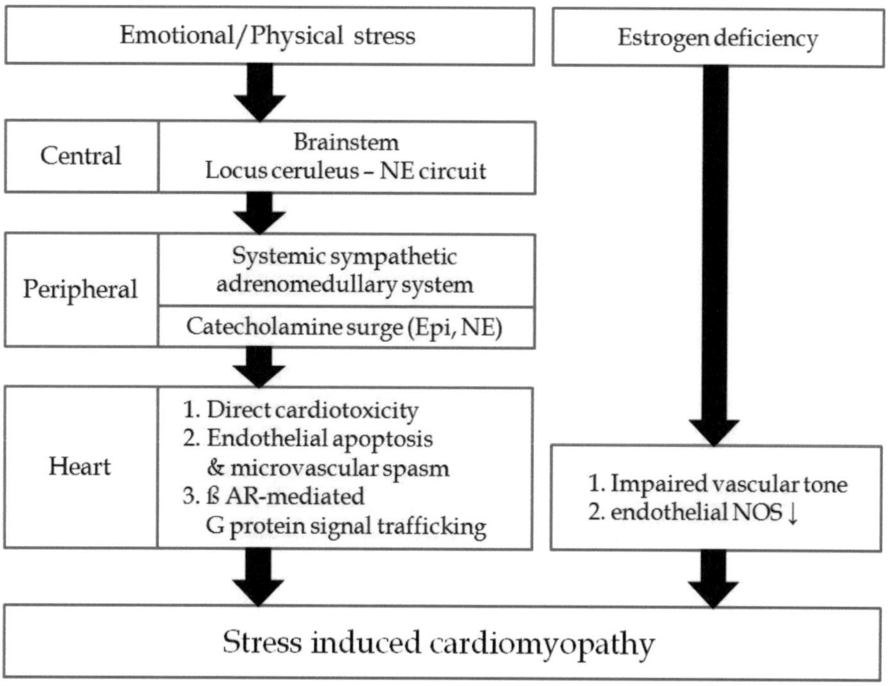

Fig. 2. Proposed mechanism of stress-induced cardiomyopathy. NE, norepinephrine; Epi, epinephrine; AR, adrenoreceptor; NOS, nitric oxide synthase.

Incessant emotional and/or physical stimuli may activate and sustain positive feedback stress response systems and result in marked elevation of plasma catecholamine levels in patients with stress-induced cardiomyopathy (Balkin & Cohen, 2011).

6.2 Catecholamine excess

Several situations that could induce sympathetic activation have suggested that cardiac dysfunction might be closely related to catecholamine excess. Subarachnoid hemorrhage and pheochromocytoma are typical examples (Kono et al., 1994; Pollick et al., 1988; Scott & Gutterman, 1995). Catecholamines could contribute to myocardial stunning in the absence of relevant myocardial perfusion abnormalities at rest (Morel et al., 2009). With respect to stress-induced cardiomyopathy, the possible contribution of catecholamines can be summarized into three components; (1) direct toxicity of norepinephrine/epinephrine and their metabolites; (2) adrenergic stimuli with spasm of the epicardial coronary artery and/or microvasculature; and (3) ß-adrenoreceptor-mediated stimulus-dependent G-protein stimulus trafficking.

6.2.1 Catecholamine toxicity

Proof of direct catecholamine-induced cardiotoxicity has been known since the mid-1970s. Early investigations showed that intravenous injection catecholamines in rats could affect morphological change on the cardiomyocyte plasma membrane (the "sacolemma") (Balkin & Cohen, 2011, as cited in Rona et al., 1975 & Boutet et al., 1976). When they injected catecholamines, the extracellular macromolecular tracer horseradish peroxidase became localized to intracellular compartments, which was retained in the extracellular environment in a normal physiological state.

The synthetic catecholamine isoproterenol was shown to increase myocardial Ca^{2+} content and depress cardiac sarcolemmal ATP-dependent Ca^{2+} uptake, Ca^{2+}-stimulated ATPase activity and Na^{+}-dependent Ca^{2+} accumulation in experimental hearts (Tappia, 2001). Those authors also demonstrated that similar findings were seen in isolated rat hearts perfused with the catecholamine oxidation product adrenochrome, (10–25 μg/mL).

These findings suggested that catecholamine and the oxidative stress that they cause result in the development of intracellular Ca^{2+} overload, heart dysfunction and subsequent myocardial death.

6.2.2 Catecholamine and microvascular spasm

The α1-adrenoreceptor is located in smooth muscle cells, which causes vasoconstriction in blood vessels (including the epicardial coronary artery). However, provocation tests using infusions of ergonovine or acetylcholine induced multivessel spasm in only 28% of patients with documented stress-induced cardiomyopathy (Gianni et al., 2006). This finding is insufficient to explain the underlying mechanism of stress-induced cardiomyopathy.

Microvascular spasm by catecholamine-induced sympathetic stimulation can alter the oxygen delivery of the myocardium, which develops localized contractile dysfunction within seconds. If blood flow is restored before myocardial damage, cardiac function can recover. This phenomenon is termed "stunned" or "hibernating" myocardium (Heusch & Schulz, 1996). It may take days or weeks for such cardiac dysfunction to recover.

As mentioned above, contrast echocardiographic perfusion imaging, CMR and nuclear imaging provide evidences of coronary microvascular dysfunction. Uchida et al. investigated the hypothesis that coronary microvessel apoptosis could be the missing link between stress and stress induced cardiomyopathy (Uchida et al., 2010). Plasma catecholamines, thrombolysis in myocardial infarction (TIMI) coronary flow grade and myocardial perfusion grade, and apoptosis of coronary microvessels in the biopsied myocardial specimens by terminal deoxynucleotidyl transferase-mediated nick end-labeling (TUNEL) were examined in 8 female patients with stress-induced cardiomyopathy. They found elevated levels of plasma epinephrine and norepinephrine, delayed myocardial perfusion without flow disturbance in the epicardial coronary arteries, focal myocardial necrosis, as well as extensive apoptosis of coronary microvessels in arterioles, venules and capillaries.

Reactive hyperemia as a parameter of endothelial function and vascular response to acute mental stress could be measured by peripheral arterial tonometry. Women with a history of stress-induced cardiomyopathy demonstrated impaired endothelium-dependent vasodilation, excessive vasoconstriction, and augmented sympathetic activation after experiencing acute mental stress compared with age-matched post-menopausal controls and patients with myocardial infarction (Martin et al., 2010).

In summary, it can be hypothesized that catecholamine-induced apoptosis of endothelial cells of coronary microvessels and the subsequent microvessel spasm which results in myocardial stunning by oxidative stress due to the ischemia–reperfusion mechanism leads to stress induced cardiomyopathy (Uchida et al., 2010).

6.2.3 ß-adrenoreceptor-mediated stimulus-dependent G-protein stimulus trafficking

ß-adrenoreceptors are members of one of the largest families of cell-surface signaling proteins called G-protein-coupled receptors (GPCRs). The main function of GPCRs is to convert extracellular stimuli into intracellular signals (Rosenbaum et al., 2009). Cardiac tissue has two subtypes of ß-adrenoreceptor: $ß_1$ and $ß_2$. The $ß_1$-adrenoreceptor stimulates only the G-αs protein. However, the $ß_2$-adrenoreceptor can activate two G proteins, G-αs and G-αi (part of the Gs and Gi heterotrimers, respectively), which differentially regulate adenylate cyclase. The latter generates cyclic adenosine monophosphate (cAMP), which activates protein kinase A (PKA) (Rosenbaum et al., 2009).

Specifically, in the heart, PKA phosphorylates the proteins involved in energy metabolism and excitation–contraction coupling. These include glycogen phosphorylase kinase, the L-type calcium channel, the sarcoplasmic reticulum membrane protein phospholamban, and cytoskeletal proteins. These phosphorylation events result in enhanced cardiac contractility (inotropy), accelerated cardiac relaxation (lusitropy), and increased heart rate (chronotropy) (Balkin & Cohen, 2011, as cited in Xiao, 2001 & Bers, 2002).

At physiological and elevated concentrations, norepinephrine, released from the sympathetic nerves, acts predominantly via the $ß_1$-adrenoreceptor on ventricular cardiomyocytes, exerting positive inotropic and lusitropic responses. Epinephrine also binds the $ß_1$-adrenoreceptor, but has a higher affinity for the $ß_2$-adrenoreceptor. At physiological concentrations, epinephrine binding to the $ß_2$-adrenoreceptor activates the Gs protein. At higher "supraphysiological" concentrations, epinephrine binds to the $ß_2$-adrenoreceptor and switches signaling from the Gs protein to the Gi protein, a process called "stimulus trafficking". This process results in negative inotropy, negative lusitropy and negative chronotropy. After the surge of epinephrine has finished, the $ß_2$-adrenoreceptor coupled to Gi proteins switches back to Gs protein coupling or is internalized and degraded, enabling cardiomyocytes to recover their inotropic function (Lyon et al., 2008).

6.3 Estrogen deficiency

Studies have shown that post-menopausal women are susceptible to stress-induced cardiomyopathy (Bybee et al., 2004). This strong female predominance has been strongly associated with estrogen deficiency. Indeed, ovariectomised rats without estradiol supplementation exposed to immobilization stress had reduced left ventricular systolic function and increased heart rate and blood pressure in comparison with rats that were supplemented with estradiol (Ueyama et al., 2007). They also demonstrated that chronic supplementation with estrogen attenuated stress-induced sympatho-adrenal outflow from the brain to the heart (indirect action on the nervous system) and upregulated cardioprotective substances such as atrial natriuretic peptide and heat shock protein 70 in the heart (direct action on the heart).

Estrogen has direct and indirect cardioprotective effects. The direct effect is rapid vasodilation primarily by activation of endothelial nitric oxide synthase (eNOS). The indirect long-term effect involves changes in the genetic expression of proteins that regulate vascular tone and the response to injury (Mendelsohn, 2002).

7. Prognosis and treatment

In most cases, the prognosis of stress-induced cardiomyopathy is good. Reported overall in-hospital mortality is 1.1% (Gianni et al., 2006), but the range varies to ~15–16% (Sharkey et al., 2010, and Lee, P.H. et al., 2010). The prevalence of complications was ~20%, including cardiogenic shock, acute heart failure, arrhythmias, intraventricular thrombus formation associated with distal embolization, left ventricular free wall rupture, recurrence, and even death (Bybee et al., 2004; Gianni et al., 2006; Zeb et al., 2010).

Acute systolic heart failure is the most common complication of stress-induced cardiomyopathy, and occurs in ~45% of patients (Madhavan et al., 2011). Madhavan et al. developed and validated a risk score that can be calculated at the time of presentation. Scores of 1, 2, and 3 points were associated with a risk of acute heart failure of 28%, 58%, and 85%, respectively. No specific therapy is required but, if needed, diuretics are used to improve pulmonary edema. Combined α- & ß-blockers may be advantageous, but the usefulness of these agents in combination should be evaluated in the future.

Cardiogenic shock may occur in the acute phase of stress-induced cardiomyopathy. Shock may be due to systolic dysfunction, or be secondary dynamic LVOT obstruction. Patients with systolic anterior motion or LVOT obstruction should not be exposed to inotropic agents even if there are in shock. Insertion of an intra-aortic balloon pump may be needed until the recovery of cardiac function is achieved.

Right ventricular involvement is relatively common and associated with lower LVEF, a longer duration of hospitalization, more complications (e.g., severe congestive heart failure), the use of an intra-aortic balloon pump, and cardiopulmonary resuscitation (Elesber et al., 2006). It has been reported that pleural effusion was more frequent in patients with stress-induced cardiomyopathy and was predictive of right ventricular dysfunction (Haghi et al., 2006).

One should keep in mind the possibility of intraventricular thrombus formation, which can be found not only in the left ventricle but also in the right ventricle and left atrial appendage (Buchholz et al., 2010; Haghi et al., 2008; Sharkey et al., 2010). Apical thrombus in the left ventricle carries a great risk of cerebrovascular accident and distal embolization during the recovery phase. Short-term use of anticoagulants and heparin as well as close follow-up echocardiography can protect against additional embolic events.

Arrhythmic complications include ventricular tachycardia, ventricular fibrillation, atrial fibrillation, atrioventricular block and sinus node dysfunction. The exact prevalence is unclear and no specific treatment has been developed. This issue needs more pooled data to assess the associations between stress-induced cardiomyopathy and arrhythmias (including conduction disorders).

The true prevalence of recurrence is not known, but only 3.5–5% of patients experienced recurrence in two studies (Gianni et al., 2006, and Sharkey et al., 2010).

Levosimendan has been suggested to be an ideal drug for patients with cardiogenic shock (Padayachee, 2007). Levosimendan is a non-catecholamine inotrope which sensitizes troponin C to calcium, leading to improved contractility. In addition, levosimendan does not compromise diastolic function. The opening of adenosine triphosphate-dependent potassium channels by levosimendan causes vasodilation. This decreases preload, afterload and pulmonary vascular resistance, and improves coronary perfusion. Further studies are required to determine the safety and efficacy of this agent before widespread use can be recommended.

8. Summary and conclusion

The development of stress-induced cardiomyopathy involves multiple interactions. Emotional and/or physical stressors activate the stress system via positive feedback loops and catecholamines are produced. Excessive amounts of catecholamines directly affect cardiomyocytes, induce apoptosis of endothelial cells of coronary microvessels with subsequent microvessel spasm and ß-adrenoreceptor-mediated stimulus-dependent G-protein stimulus trafficking. Estrogen deficiency makes the heart to vulnerable to stressors. Depending on the severity of cardiac involvement, various presentations can be seen. Diagnostic modalities should be chosen according to specific situations. Echocardiography is essential to monitor recovery or possible complications, and to plan further treatment. A growing body of evidence promises better understanding of stress-induced cardiomyopathy.

9. References

Abdelmoneim, S. S.; Mankad, S. V.; Bernier, M.; Dhoble, A.; Hagen, M. E.; Ness, S. A.; Chandrasekaran, K.; Pellikka, P. A.; Oh, J. K. & Mulvagh, S. L. (2009). Microvascular function in Takotsubo cardiomyopathy with contrast echocardiography: prospective evaluation and review of literature. *Journal of the American Society of Echocardiography*, Vol.22, No.11, pp. 1249-1255, ISSN 0894-7317

Akashi, Y. J.; Nakazawa, K.; Sakakibara, M.; Miyake, F.; Msha, H. & Sasaka, K. (2004). 123I-MIBG myocardial scintigraphy in patients with "takotsubo cardiomyopathy. *Journal of Nuclear Medicine*, Vol.45, No.7, pp. 1121-1127, ISSN 0161-5505

Anon. (1986). Case records of the Massachusetts General Hospital. Weekly clinicopathological exercises. Case 18-1986. A 44-year-old woman with substernal pain and pulmonary edema after severe emotional stress. *New England Journal of Medicine*, Vol.314, pp. 1240-1247

Avegliano, G.; Huguet, M.; Costabel, J. P.; Ronderos, R.; Bijnens, B.; Kuschnir, P.; Thierer, J.; Tobón-Gomez, C.; Martinez, G. O. & Frangi, A. (2011). Morphologic pattern of late gadolinium enhancement in Takotsubo cardiomyopathy detected by early cardiovascular magnetic resonance, *Clinical Cardiology*, Vol.34, No.3, pp. 178-182, ISSN 0160-9289

Balkin, D. M. & Cohen L. S. (2011). Takotsubo syndrome. *Coronary Artery Disease*, Vol.22, No.3, pp. 206-214, ISSN 0954-6928

Bers, D. M. (2002). Cardiac excitation-contraction coupling. *Nature*, Vol.415, No.6868, pp. 198-205, ISSN 0028-0836

Bossone, E.; Citro, R.; Eagle, K. A. & Manfredni, R. (2011). Tako-tsubo cardiomyopathy: is there a preferred time of onset? *Internal and Emergency Medicine*, Vol.6, No.3, pp. 221-226, ISSN 1828-0447

Boutet, M.; Huttner, I. & Rona, G. (1976). Permeability alteration of sarcolemmal membrane in catecholamin-induced cardiac muscle cell injury: in-vivo studies with fine structural diffusion tracer horseradish peroxidase. *Laboratory Investigation*, Vol.34, No.5, pp. 482-288, ISSN 0023-6837

Buchholz, S.; Ward, M. R.; Bhindi, R.; Nelson, G. I.; Figtree, G. A. & Grieve, S. M. (2010). Cardiac thrombi in stress (tako-tsubo) cardiomyopathy: more than an apical issue? *Mayo Clinic Proceedings*, Vol.85, No.9, pp. 863-864, ISSN 0025-6196

Bybee, K. A.; Kara, T.; Prasad, A.; Lerman, A.; Barsness, G. W.; Wright, R. S. & Rihal, C. S. (2004). Systematic review: transient left ventricular apical ballooning: a syndrome that mimics ST-segment elevation myocardial infarction. *Annals of Internal Medicine*, Vol.141, No.11, pp. 858-865, ISSN 0003-4819

Cebelin, M. S. & Hirsch, C. S. (1980) Human stress cardiomyopathy. Myocardial lesions in victims of homicidal assaults without internal injuries. *Human Pathology*, Vol.11, No.2, pp. 123-132, ISSN 0046-8177

Charmandari, E.; Tsigos, C. & Chrousos, G. P. (2005). Endocrinology of the stress response. *Annual Review of Physiology*, Vol.67, pp. 259-284, ISSN 0066-4278

Chrousos, G. P. & Gold, P. W. (1992). The concepts of stress and stress system disorders: overview of physical and behavioral homeostasis. *Journal of the American Medical Association*, Vol.267, No.9, pp. 1244-1252, ISSN 0098-7484

Chrousos, G. P. (2007). Organization and integration of the endocrine system. *Sleep Medicine Clinics*, Vol.2, No.2, pp. 125-145, ISSN 1556-407X

Chrousos, G. P. (2009). Stress and disorders of the stress system. *Nature Reviews Endocrinology*, Vol.5, No.7, pp. 374-381, ISSN 1759-5029

Dote, K.; Sato, H.; Tateishi, H.; Uchida, T. & Ishihara, M. (1991). Myocardial stunning due to simultaneous multivessel coronary spasms: a review of 5 cases. *Journal of Cardiology*, Vol.21, No.2, pp. 203-214, ISSN 0914-5087

El Mahmoud, R.; Mansencal, N.; Pilliére, R.; Leyer, F.; Abbou, N.; Michaud, P.; Nallet, O.; Digne, F.; Lacombe, P.; Cattan, S. & Dubourg, O. (2008). Prevalence and characteristics of left ventricular outflow tract obstruction in Tako-Tsubo syndrome. *American Heart Journal*, Vol.156, No.3, pp. 543-548, ISSN 0002-8703

Elesber, A. A.; Prasad, A.; Bybee, K. A.; Valeti, U.; Motiei, A.; Lerman, A.; Chandrasekaran, K. & Rihal, C. S. (2006). Transient cardiac apical ballooning syndrome: prevalence and clinical implications of right ventricular involvement. *Journal of the American College of Cardiology*, Vol.47, No.5, pp. 1082-1083, ISSN 0735-1097

Ferreira, S. H. & Vane, J. R. (1967). Half-lives of peptides and amines in the circulation. *Nature*, Vol.215, No.5107, pp. 1237-1240, ISSN 0028-0836

Fragkouli, K. & Vougiouklakis, T. (2010). Sudden cardiac death: an 11-year postmortem analysis in the region of Epirus, Greece. *Pathology - Research and Practice*, Vol.206, No.10, pp. 690-694, ISSN 0344-0338

Greco, C. A.; De, Rito, V.; Petracca, M.; Garzya, M.; Donateo, M. & Magliari, F. (2011). Takotsubo syndrome in a newborn. *Journal of the American Society of Echocardiography*, Vol.24, No.4, pp. 471.e5-e7, ISSN 0894-7317

Gianni, M.; Dentali, F.; Grandi, A. M.; Sumner, G.; Hiralal, R. & Lonn, E. (2006). Apical ballooning syndrome or takotsubo cardiomyopathy: a systematic review. *European Heart Journal*, Vol.27, No.13, pp. 1523-1529, ISSN 0195-668X

Haghi, D.; Athanasiadis, A.; Papavassiliu, T.; Suselbeck, T.; Fluechter, S.; Mahrholdt, H.; Borggrefe, M. & Sechtem, U. (2006). Right ventricular involvement in Takotsubo cardiomyopathy. *European Heart Journal*, Vol.27, No.20, pp.2433-2439, ISSN 0195-668X

Haghi, D.; Papavassiliu, T.; Heggemann, F.; Kaden, J. J.; Borggrefe, M. & Suselbeck, T. (2008). Incidence and clinical significance of left ventricular thrombus in tako-tsubo cardiomyopathy assessed with echocardiography. *Quarterly Journal of Medicine*, Vol.101, No.5, pp. 381-386, ISSN 1460-2393

Heggemann, F.; Weiss, C.; Hamm, K.; Kaden, J.; Süselbeck, T.; Papavassiliu, T.; Borggrefe, M. & Haghi, D. (2009). Global and regional myocardial function quantification by two-dimensional strain in Takotsubo cardiomyopathy. *European Journal of Echocardiography*, Vol.10, No.6, pp. 760-764, ISSN 1532-2114

Heusch, G. & Schulz, R. (1996). Hibernating myocardium: a review. *Journal of Molecular and Cellular Cardiology*, Vol.28, No.12, pp. 2359-2372, ISSN 0022-2828

Iga, K.; Gen, H.; Tomonaga, G.; Matsumura, T. & Hori, K. (1989). Reversible left ventricular wall motion impairment caused by pheochromocytoa - a case report. *Japan Circulation Journal*, Vol.53, No.7, pp. 813-818, ISSN 0047-1828

Jim, M. H.; Chan, A. O.; Tsui, P. T.; Lau, S. T.; Siu, C. W.; Chow, W. H. & Lau, C. P. (2009). A new ECG criterion to identify takotsubo cardiomyopathy from anterior myocardial infarction: role of inferior leads. *Heart Vessels*, Vol.24, No.2, pp. 124-130, ISSN 0910-8327

Kono, T.; Morita, H.; Kuroiwa, T.; Onaka, H.; Takatsuka, H. & Fujiwara, A. (1994). Left ventricular wall motion abnormalities in patients with subarachnoid hemorrhage: neurogenic stunned myocardium. *Journal of the American College of Cardiology*, Vol.24, No.3, pp. 636-640, ISSN 0735-1097

Kurisu, S.; Inoue, I.; Kawagoe, T.; Ishihara, M.; Shimatani, Y.; Nakamura, S.; Yoshida, M.; Mitsuba, N.; Hata, T. & Sato, H. (2004). Time course of electrocardiographic changes in patients with Tako-Tsubo syndrome: comparison with acute myocardial infarction with minimal enzymatic release. *Circulation Journal*, Vol.68, No.1, pp. 77-81, ISSN 1346-9843

Lee, J. W.; Kim, J. Y.; Youn, Y. J.; Sung, J. K.; Lee, N. S.; Lee, K. H.; Yoo, B. S.; Lee, S. H.; Yoon, J. & Choe, K. H. (2010). Clinical characteristics and prognostic factors of stress-induced cardiomyopathy. *Korean Circulation Journal*, Vol.40, No.6, pp. 277-282, ISSN 1738-5520

Lee, J. W. & Kim, J. Y. (2011). Stress-induced cardiomyopathy: the role of echocardiography. *Journal of Cardiovascular Ultrasound*, Vol.19, No.1, pp. 7-12, ISSN 1975-4612

Lee, P. H.; Song, J. K.; Sun, B. J.; Choi, H.O.; Seo, J. S.; Na, J. O.; Kim, D. H.; Song, J. M.; Kang, D. H.; Kim, J. J. & Park, S. W. (2010). Outcomes of patients with stress-induced cardiomyopathy diagnosed by echocardiography in a tertiary referral hospital. *Journal of the American Society of Echocardiography*, Vol.23, No.7, pp. 766-771, ISSN 0894-7317

Leibel, R. L. & Hirsch, J. (1987). Site- and Sex-related differences in adrenoreceptor status of human adipose tissue. *The Journal of Clinical Endocrinology & Metabolism*, Vol.64, No.6, pp. 1205-1210, ISSN 0021-972X

Lyon, A. R.; Rees, P. S.; Prasad, S.; Poole-Wilson, P. A. & Harding, S. E. (2008). Stress (Takotsubo) cardiomyopathy - a novel pathophysiological hypothesis to explain catecholamine-induced acute myocardial stunning. *Natural Clinical Practice Cardiovascular Medicine*, Vol.5, No.1, pp. 22-29, ISSN 1743-4297

Madhavan, M.; Borlaug, B. A.; Lerman, A.; Rihal, C. S. & Prasad, A. (2009). Stress hormone and circulating biomarker profile of apical ballooning syndrome (Takotsubo cardiomyopathy): insights into the clinical significance of B-type natriuretic peptide and troponin levels. *Heart*, Vol.95, No.17, pp. 1436-1441, ISSN 1355-6037

Madhavan, M.; Rihal, C. S.; Lerman, A. & Prasad, A. (2011). Acute heart failure in apical ballooning syndrome (TakoTsubo/stress cardiomyopathy): clinical correlates and

Mayo Clinic risk score. *Journal of the American College of Cardiology*, Vol.57, No.12, pp. 1400-1401, ISSN 0735-1097

Manfredini, R.; Citro, R.; Previtali, M.; Vriz, O.; Ciampi, Q.; Pascotto, M.; Tagliamonte, E.; Provenza, G. & Manfredini, F. (2010). Monday preference in onset of takotsubo cardiomyopathy. *American Journal of Emergency Medicine*, Vol.28, No.6, pp. 715-719, ISSN 0735-6757

Martin, E. A.; Prasad, A.; Rihal, C. S.; Lerman, L. O. & Lerman A. (2010). Endothelial function and vascular response to mental stress are impaired in patients with apical ballooning syndrome. *Journal of the American College of Cardiology*, Vol.56, No.22, pp. 1840-1846, ISSN 0735-1097

Matsuoka, K.; Okubo, S.; Fujii, E.; Uchida, F.; Kasai, A.; Aoki, T.; Makino, K. Omichi, C.; Fujimoto, N.; Ohta, S.; Sawai, T. & Nakano, T. (2003). Evaluation of the arrhythmogenecity of stress-induced "Takotsubo cardiomyopathy" from the time course of the 12-lead surface electrocardiogram. *American Journal of Cardiology*, Vol.92, No.2, pp. 230-233, ISSN 0002-9149

Mendelsohn, M. E. (2002). Protective effects of estrogen on the cardiovascular system. *American Journal of Cardiology*, Vol.89, No.12A, pp. 12E-17E, ISSN 0002-9149

Monté, C. P.; Arends, J. B.; Tan, I. Y.; Aldenkamp, A. P.; Limburg, M. & de, Krom, M. C. (2007). Sudden unexpected death in epilepsy patients: Risk factors. A systematic review. *Seizure*, Vol.16, No.1, pp. 1-7, ISSN 1059-1311

Morel, O.; Sauer, F.; Imperiale, A.; Cimarelli, S.; Blondet, C.; Jesel, L; Trinh, A.; De, Poli, F.; Ohlmann, P.; Constantinesco, A. & Bareiss, P. (2009). Importance of inflammation and neurohumoral activation in Takotsubo cardiomyopathy. *Journal of Cardiac Failure*, Vol.15, No.3, pp. 206-213, ISSN 1071-9164

Nef, H. M.; Mollmann, H.; Akashi, Y. J. & Hamm, C. W. (2010). Mechanisms of stress (Takotsubo) cardiomyopathy. *Nature Reviews Cardiology*, Vol.7, No.4, pp. 187-193, ISSN 1759-5002

Padayachee, L. (2007). Levosimendan: the inotrope of choice in cardiogenic shock secondary to takotsubo cardiomyopathy? *Heart, Lung and Circulation*, Vol.16, pp. S65-S70, ISSN 1443-9506

Park, J. H.; Kang, S. J.; Song, J. K.; Kim, H. K.; Chae, M. L.; Kang, D. H. & Koh, Y. (2005). Left ventricular apical ballooning due to severe physical stress in patients admitted to the medical ICU. *Chest*, Vol.128, No.1, pp. 296-302, ISSN 0012-3692

Park, J. T.; Kim, J. Y.; Kim, Y. W.; Choi, K. H.; Park, B. H. & Lim, H. K. (2010). Stress-induced cardiomyopathy after general anesthesia for total gastrectomy - a case report. *Korean Journal of Anesthesiology*, Vol.58, No.3, pp. 299-303, ISSN 2005-6419

Parodi, G.; Del, Pace, S.; Salvadori, C.; Carrabba, N.; Olivotto, I.; Gensini, G. F. & Tuscany Registry of Tako-Tsubo Cardiomyopathy. (2007). Left ventricular apical ballooning syndromes as a novel cause of acute mitral regurgitation. *Journal of the American College of Cardiology*, Vol.50, No.7, pp. 647-649, ISSN 0735-1097

Pirzer, R.; Elmas, E.; Haghi, D.; Lippert, C.; Kralev, S.; Lang, S.; Borggrefe, M. & Kälsch, T. (2011). Platelet and monocyte activity markers and mediators of inflammation in Takotsubo cardiomyopathy. *Heart Vessels*, DOI 10.1007/s00380-011-0132-6, ISSN 0910-8327

Prasad, A.; Lerman, A. & Rihal, C. S. (2008). Apical ballooning syndrome (Tako-Tsubo or stress cardiomyopathy): a mimic of acute myocardial infarction. *American Heart Journal*, Vol.155, No.3, pp. 408-417, ISSN 0002-8703

Pollick, C.; Cujec, B.; Parker, S. & Tator, C. (1988). Left ventricular wall motion abnormalities in subarachnoid hemorrhage: an echocardiographic study. *Journal of the American College of Cardiology*, Vol.12, No.3, pp. 600-605, ISSN 0735-1097

Rona, G.; Boutet, M. & Huttner, I. (1975). Membrane permeability alterations as manifestation of early cardiac muscle cell injury. *Recent Advances in Studies on Cardiac Structure and Metabolism*, Vol.6, pp. 439-451, ISSN 0363-5872

Rosenbaum, D. M.; Rasmussen, S. G. & Kobilka, B. K. (2009). The structure and function of G-protein-coupled receptors. *Nature*, Vol.459, No.7245, pp. 356-363, ISSN 0028-0836

Sharkey, S. W.; Windenburg, D. C.; Lesser, J. R.; Maron, M. S.; Hause, R. G.; Lesser, J. N.; Haas, T. S.; Hodges, J. S. & Maron, B. J. (2010). Natural history and expansive clinical profile of stress (Tako-tsubo) cardiomyopathy. *Journal of the American College of Cardiology*, Vol.26, No.4, pp. 333-341, ISSN 0735-1097

Scott, I. U. & Gutterman D. D. (1995). Pheochromocytoma with reversible focal cardiac dysfunction. *American Heart Journal*, Vol.130, No.4, pp. 909-911, ISSN 0002-8703

Schmalfuss, C. (2011). Tako-tsubo cardiomyopathy and cardiac magnetic resonance imaging, *Clinical Cardiology*, Vol.34, No.3, pp. 145-146, ISSN 0160-9289

Skovgaard, D.; Holmvang, L.; Bang, L. E.; Lønborg, J. & Hasbak, P. (2010). Imaging of Takotsubo Cardiomyopathy. *Clinical Nuclear Medicine*, Vol.35, No.12, pp. 967-971, ISSN 0363-9762

Silventoinen, K.; Kaprio, J.; Lahelma, E.; Viken, R. J. & Rose, R. J. (2001). Sex differences in genetic and environmental factors contributing to body-height. *Twin Research*, Vol.4, No.1, pp. 25-29, ISSN 1369-0523

Soufer, R.; Arrighi, J. A. & Burg, M. M. (2002). Brain, behavior, mental stress, and the neurocardiac interaction. *Journal of Nuclear Cardiology*, Vol. 9, No.6, pp. 650-662, ISSN 1071-3581

Stöllberger, C.; Finsterer, J. (2011). Why does Takotsubo ("broken heart syndrome") affect more females than males? *International Journal of Cardiology*, Vol.147, No.1, pp. 175-176, ISSN 0167-5273

Sugimoto, K.; Watanabe, E.; Yamada, A.; Iwase, M.; Sano, H.; Hishida, H. & Ozaki, Y. (2008). Prognostic implications of left ventricular wall motion abnormalities associated with subarachnoid hemorrhage. *International Heart Journal*. Vol.49, No.1, pp. 75-85, ISSN 1349-2365

Tappia, P. S.; Hata, T.; Hozaima, L.; Sandhu, M. S.; Panagia, V. & Dhalla, N. S. (2001). Role of oxidative stress in catecholamine-induced changes in cardiac sarcolemmal Ca^{2+} transport. *Archieves of Biochemistry and Biophysics*, Vol.387, No.1, pp. 85-92, ISSN 0003-9861

Uchida, Y.; Egami, H.; Uchida, Y.; Sakurai, T.; Kanai, M.; Shirai, S.; Nakagawa, O. & Oshima, T. (2010). Possible participation of endothelial cell apoptosis of coronary microvessels in the genesis of Takotsubo cardiomyopathy. *Clinical Cardiology*, Vol. 33, No.6, pp. 371-377, ISSN 0160-9289

Ueyama, T.; Ishikura, F.; Matsuda, A.; Asanuma, T.; Ueda, K.; Ichinose, M.; Kasamatsu, K.;Hano, T.; Akasaka, T.; Tsuruo, Y.; Morimoto, K. & Beppu, S. (2007). Chronic estrogen supplementation following ovariectomy improves the emotional stress-induced cardiovascular responses by indirect action on the nervous system and by direct action on the heart. *Circulation Journal*, Vol.71, No.4, pp. 565-573, ISSN 1346-9843

Winchester, D. E.; Ragosta, M.; Taylor, A. M. (2008). Concurrence of angiographic coronary artery disease in patients with apical ballooning syndrome (tako-tsubo cardiomyopathy). *Catheterization and Cardiovascular Interventions*, Vol.72, No.5, pp. 612-616, ISSN 1522-1946

Wittstein, I. S.; Thiemann, D. R.; Lima, J. A.; Baughman, K. L.; Schulman, S. P.; Gerstenblith, G.; Wu, K. C.; Rade, J. J.; Bivalacqua, T. J. & Champion, H. C. (2005). Neurohumoral features of myocardial stunning due to sudden emotional stress. *New England Journal of Medicine*, Vol.10, No.6, pp. 539-548, ISSN 0028-4793

Xiao, R. P. (2001). Beta-adrenergic signaling in the heart: dual coupling of the beta2-adrenergic receptor to G(s) and G(i) proteins. *Science Signaling: the Signal Transduction Knowledge Environment*, Vol.2001, No.104, pp. re15, ISSN 1525-8882

Zeb, M.; Sambu, N.; Scott, P. & Curzen, N. (2011). Takotsubo cardiomyopathy: a diagnostic challenge. *Postgraduate Medical Journal*, Vol.87, No.1023, pp. 51-59, ISSN 0032-5473

30

Takotsubo Cardiomyopathy

Abdul Moiz Hafiz[1], M. Fuad Jan[2], Timothy E. Paterick[2], Suhail Allaqaband[2] and A. Jamil Tajik[2]

[1]Winthrop-University Hospital, Mineola, New York,
[2]Aurora Cardiovascular Services, Aurora Sinai/Aurora St. Luke's Medical Centers, University of Wisconsin School of Medicine and Public Health, Milwaukee, Wisconsin, USA

1. Introduction

Since the first report in 1990, takotsubo cardiomyopathy (TTC) has been increasingly recognized as a novel form of nonischemic acute cardiomyopathy. It is an important differential in diagnosis of acute coronary syndrome (ACS) due to its similar presentation. However, it distinguishes itself from an ACS in the fact that regional wall motion abnormalities extend beyond a single coronary vascular bed and are reversible, and epicardial coronary occlusion is absent (1).

In TTC, left ventricular (LV) dysfunction can be remarkably depressed but recovers within a few weeks (2) in the vast majority of patients. This syndrome has been described by more than 75 individual descriptive names in the literature, emphasizing those disease features that were most impressive to individual investigators (3) (Table 1).

Increased awareness about this syndrome has led to its incorporation into the American Heart Association classification of reversible cardiomyopathies (4,5). Pathogenesis of this syndrome is still not well understood, although physical and emotional stressors and mediation by pathologic sympathetic myocardial stunning are believed to play key roles. However, in an important minority of patients, a detailed personal history does not elicit an antecedent event (3).

Apical ballooning
Apical ballooning syndrome
Acute left ventricular apical ballooning syndrome
Left ventricular apical ballooning syndrome
Transient left ventricular apical ballooning syndrome
Primary apical ballooning
Transient apical ballooning
Transient apical ballooning syndrome
Transient cardiac apical ballooning syndrome
Transient left apical ballooning syndrome
Transient cardiac ballooning
Left apical ballooning syndrome
Acute apical ballooning syndrome

Cardiac apical ballooning syndrome
Apical ballooning
Apical ballooning without apical ballooning
Apical ballooning cardiomyopathy
Reversible apical ballooning of left ventricle
Left ventricular ballooning syndrome
Midventricular variant of transient apical ballooning
Midventricular ballooning syndrome
Transient left ventricular mid-portion ballooning
Transient midventricular ballooning
Transient midventricular ballooning cardiomyopathy
Transient left ventricular nonapical ballooning
Reverse or inverted left ventricular apical ballooning syndrome
Inverted left ventricular apical ballooning syndrome
Transient basal ballooning
Tako-tsubo
Takotsubo cardiomyopathy
Takotsubo-like cardiomyopathy
Takotsubo syndrome
Takotsubo disease
Takotsubo left ventricular dysfunction
Takotsubo-like left ventricular dysfunction
Takotsubo-like transient biventricular dysfunction
Takotsubo-like transient left ventricular ballooning
Takotsubo-shaped cardiomyopathy
Takotsubo-shaped hypokinesia of left ventricle
Takotsubo-type cardiomyopathy
Takotsubo transient left ventricular apical ballooning
Midventricular takotsubo cardiomyopathy
Midventricular form of takotsubo cardiomyopathy
Inverted takotsubo contractile pattern
Inverted takotsubo cardiomyopathy
Inverted takotsubo pattern
Atypical takotsubo cardiomyopathy
Reverse takotsubo syndrome
Atypical basal type takotsubo cardiomyopathy
Stress cardiomyopathy
Acute stress cardiomyopathy
Human stress cardiomyopathy
Acute and reversible cardiomyopathy provoked by stress
Stress-induced cardiomyopathy
Stress-induced takotsubo cardiomyopathy
Stress-induced apical ballooning syndrome
Stress-related left ventricular dysfunction
Stress-related cardiomyopathy
Stress-related cardiomyopathy syndrome

- Stress takotsubo cardiomyopathy
- Emotional stress-induced ampulla cardiomyopathy
- Midventricular stress cardiomyopathy
- Atypical transient stress-induced cardiomyopathy
- Stress-induced myocardial stunning
- Emotional stress-induced takotsubo cardiomyopathy
- Stress-associated catecholamine-induced cardiomyopathy
- Neurogenic stress syndrome
- Other
    - Neurogenic stunned myocardium
    - Adrenergic cardiomyopathy
    - Broken heart syndrome
    - Ampulla cardiomyopathy
    - Ampulla-shaped cardiomyopathy
    - "Chestnut-shaped" transient regional left ventricular hypokinesia
    - Ball-shaped spherical dilation of left ventricular apex
    - The artichoke heart
    - Transient midventricular akinesia
    - Transient antero-apical dyskinesia

Reproduced from Sharkey et al. Why not just call it tako-tsubo cardiomyopathy: a discussion of nomenclature. J Am Coll Cardiol 2011;57:1496-1497, with permission from Elsevier.

Table 1. Names Tabulated From Published Reports

2. History

In 1990, Sato and colleagues (6) first described a reversible cardiomyopathy as "tako-tsubo-like left ventricular dysfunction." One year later, Dote and colleagues (7) reported 5 patients with a novel, acute cardiac condition characterized by distinctive regional left ventricular LV systolic dysfunction and transient LV apical ballooning in the absence of significant coronary artery disease. Other Japanese investigators were intrigued by the unusual end-systolic shape of the LV, which resembled the "tako-tsubo," (a fisherman's pot with a round bottom and narrow neck used for trapping octopuses) (2,8,9) (Figure 1). Consequently, the term takotsubo was introduced to describe a new cardiomyopathic syndrome characterized by reversible LV systolic dysfunction (3). Many reports were published from different countries afterwards, and it was first reported in the United States in 2004 (5). A search for the term "takotsubo cardiomyopathy" in MEDLINE returned 1,090 articles (Figure 2).

3. Epidemiology

A few case reports were published prior to 2000, but the recognition of takotsubo cardiomyopathy has increased gradually since 2001, and this condition probably accounts for 1% to 2% of all cases of suspected acute myocardial infarction (MI) (10,11). Given the relatively recent recognition of TTC, epidemiology of this condition is still emerging. TTC is reported to occur predominantly in postmenopausal women (82-100%) (12) soon after exposure to sudden, unexpected emotional or physical stress. Kushiro and colleagues reported CD36 deficiency in a patient with stress-induced cardiomyopathy (13), suggesting an association between this entity and certain genetic profiles. This observation has led to the speculation that TTC might have a genetic component as described in a report by Cherian and colleagues (14).

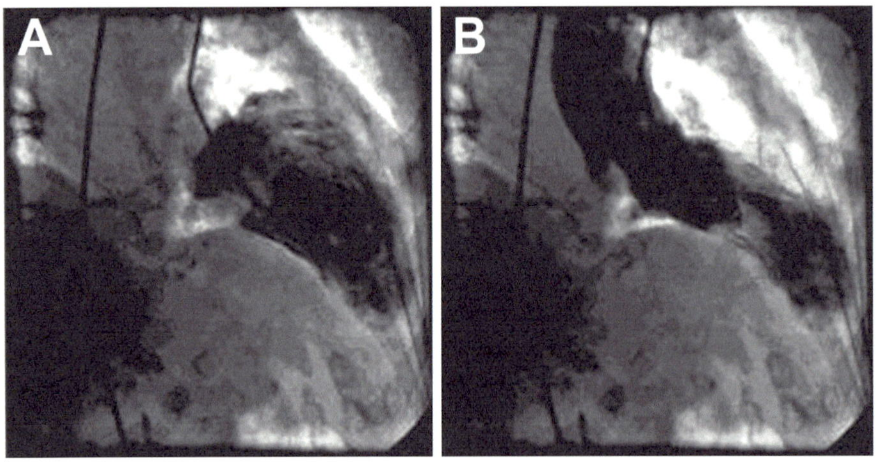

Fig. 1. Left ventriculograms obtained in a 65-year-old female who presented with acute shortness of breath. Panel A is a right anterior oblique (RAO) view of the left ventricle in the diastolic frame. Panel B is the RAO view of the left ventricle in the systolic frame. Note the dilated apical and akinetic outpouching of the left ventricle in Panel B. The coronaries in this patient were normal, consistent with the diagnosis of takotsubo cardiomyopathy.

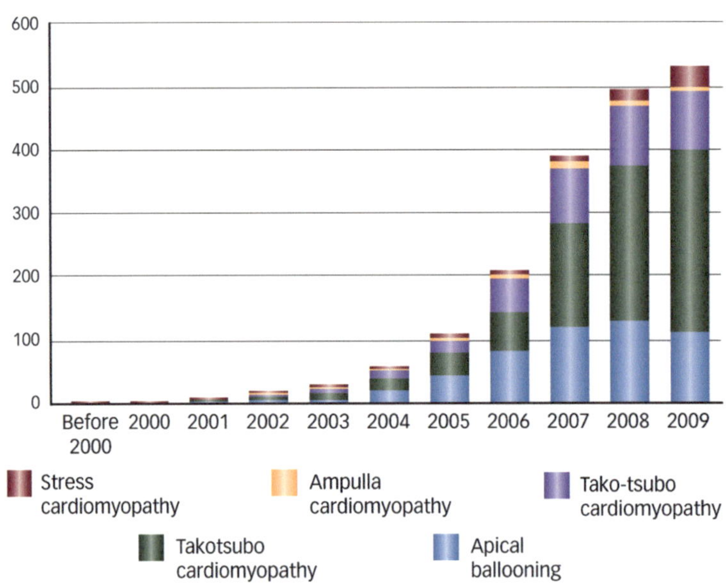

Fig. 2. Increase in the number of publications on MEDLINE® concerning takotsubo cardiomyopathy. (Originally published in *Asia-Pacific Cardiology* 2011;3:60-3. ©Touch Briefings. Reprinted with permission.)

4. Clinical presentation

4.1 The patient

TTC has characteristically been reported in women, with a median age varying from 61 to 76 years in prior case series (2,9,11,15-21). All large-cohort reports of TTC have shown that most patients presenting with the syndrome are postmenopausal women (5). However, it has also been reported in men and patients <50 years (1,3,15,16) and even in a 2-year-old girl (22). In the first large Japanese series describing TTC, 76 patients were women, 12 were men, and the median age was 67 ± 13 years (2).

4.2 The triggering event

Different stresses prior to presentation have been reported to trigger TTC, but the common theme is a sudden physical or emotional stress. The numerous events precipitating TTC are depicted in Table 2. Recurrence of TTC has also been rarely reported with similar or different triggering events (recurrence range, 0 to 8%) (23). TTC has been reported to be associated with pheochromocytoma (24-27) and subarachnoid hemorrhage (28-31) in some published reports.

Emotional stress
Death or severe illness or injury of a family member, friend, or pet
Receiving bad news—diagnosis of a major illness, daughter's divorce, spouse leaving for war
Severe argument
Public speaking
Involvement with legal proceedings
Financial loss—business, gambling
Car accident
Surprise party
Move to a new residence
Physical stress
Non-cardiac surgery or procedure—cholecystectomy, hysterectomy
Severe illness—asthma or chronic obstructive airway exacerbation, connective tissue disorders, acute cholecystitis, pseudomembranous colitis
Severe pain—fracture, renal colic, pneumothorax, pulmonary embolism
Recovering from general anesthesia
Cocaine use
Opiate withdrawal
Stress test—dobutamine stress echo, exercise sestamibi
Thyrotoxicosis

Reproduced from Prasad et al. Apical ballooning syndrome (Tako-Tsubo or stress cardiomyopathy): A mimic of acute myocardial infarction. Am Heart J 2008;155:408-17, with permission from Elsevier.

Table 2. Stressors Reported to Trigger Takotsubo Cardiomyopathy

4.3 The syndrome

The characteristic clinical syndrome is acute LV dysfunction (10). Patients usually present with typical chest pain (70-90%) and dyspnea (20%) (10); other less common presentations include syncope (12), pulmonary edema and cardiac arrest. Dynamic electrocardiographic changes and elevated cardiac biomarkers (reflecting acute myocardial injury) are usually present. Coronary angiography, however, does not reveal any evidence of epicardial coronary obstruction. Left ventriculography (Figure 1) reveals LV dysfunction and wall motion abnormalities affecting apical and, frequently, midventricular myocardium but sparing the basal myocardium, changes which resemble a flask with a narrow neck and a round bottom shaped like the Japanese octopus trap "*tako-tsubo*" (32). Symptoms can be severe and lead to death in 2% of patients (3). Song and colleagues reported 32% (n=16) of their patients with TTC (n=50) presented with cardiogenic shock as initial presentation (33). Table 3 shows clinical features in a prior published series (10).

4.4 Electrocardiography

Most common electrocardiographic changes reported in TTC are ST-segment elevations in precordial leads (10) on admission (range, 46-100% of patients) (12). Subsequent deep symmetrical T-wave inversion in multiple leads and Q-wave formation (range, 6-31% of patients) (12) also are frequently found (10). Also present may be QT interval prolongation (5) (range, 450-501 ms) (12). The combination of clinical symptoms and electrocardiographic changes at patient's initial presentation makes differentiation of TTC from ACS very difficult. A typical electrocardiogram obtained in one of our patients at presentation and 48 hours later is shown in Figure 3.

4.5 Cardiac biomarkers

Most patients present with elevated cardiac biomarkers and have a modest peak in levels within 24 hours (15,19,34), but levels are markedly lower than would be anticipated on the basis of the extent of wall motion abnormalities and electrocardiogram findings (1).

4.6 Left ventriculography

Diagnosis of TTC is frequently made in the cardiac catheterization laboratory during left ventriculography as the patients are initially triaged as an ACS and are referred for urgent or emergency coronary angiography (35). Left ventriculography (Figure 4) reveals the classic appearance of left ventricle with dilated apex and akinetic apical or midventricular walls (or both) and a hypercontractile basal segment. However, more variants of TTC have been reported with diversity in patterns of regional LV systolic dyssynergy. Singh and colleagues (36) reported a series of 107 patients (age=66 ± 14 years, n=99 females) and observed the regional contractility phenotypes shown in Table 4. A study by Kurowski and colleagues (n=35 patients) identified 60% of patients to be typical (apical) and 40% to be atypical (midventricular) variants (11). Subclassifying TTC variants with different names should be avoided as it can lead to more confusion (3). The proposed alternate names - "transient ballooning syndrome" (37) or "transient stress-induced left ventricular dysfunction syndrome" - seem to capture the essential features of the disease, though takotsubo cardiomyopathy remains the most widely used.

	Tsuchihashi et al	Kurowski et al	Kurisu et al	Sharkey et al	Wittstein et al	Inoue et al	Sato et al	Bybee et al	Yoshida et al	Akashi et al
Subjects, n	88	35	30	22	19	18	16	16	15	13
Country	Japan	Germany	Japan	U.S.	U.S.	Japan	Japan	U.S.	Japan	Japan
Series, type	Retro	Pro	Retro	Pro	Pro	Retro	Retro	Pro	Pro	Pro
Age, y	67 ± 13	72 ± 9	70 ± 8	65 ± 13	61 ± 15	76 ± 8	71 ± 9	71 ± 12	72 ± 7	73 ± 10
Women, %	86	94	93	91	95	94	94	100	80	85
Preceding emotional stressor, %	20	42	17	86	100	11	...	38	40	31
Preceding stressor, %	43	42	17	14	...	39	100	4	40	69
Chest pain, %	67	...	67	91	95	72	100	69	87	54
ST-segment elevation, %	90	69	100	59	11	100	56	81	87	92
ST-segment elevation in precordial leads, %	85	...	97	59	...	100	...	81	...	92
Q waves, %	27	...	...	45	37	56†	...	31	7	...
Mean QTc, ms	...	...	...	...	542*	...	...	501 ± 55	508*	...
Elevation in cardiac enzynme leads, %	56	...	...	...	...	...	56	100	...	85
Initial average LVEF	0.41 ± 0.11	0.5 ± 0.13	0.49 ± 0.12	0.29 ± 0.09	0.20*	...	0.49 ± 0.04	0.4	0.43 ± 0.08	0.42 ± 0.10
Follow-up LVEF	0.64 ± 0.10	0.68 ± 0.12	0.69 ± 0.12	0.63 ± 0.06	0.60*	...	0.66 ± 0.03	0.6	0.76 ± 0.01	0.65 ± 0.08
Time of recovery, d	...	...	11.3 ± 4.3	24 ± 29	21*	...	17.7	8	11 ± 4	17 ± 7
Initial Forrester subset	...	...	...	...	...	...	...	...	...	1.9 ± 0.3
Pulmonary edema, %	22	...	3	0	16	28	6	44	...	0
Coronary stenosis >50%, %	0	0	0	0	5	0	0	0	...	0
Angiographically normal coronary arteries, %	...	0	83	100	95	100	100	25	100	100
Spontaneous multivessel spasm, %	0	0	10	...	0	0	0	0	0	0
Provacable multivessel spasm, n/ n (%)	5/ 48 (10)	...	6/ 14 (43)	...	...	...	0/ 6 (0)	...	1/ 6 (17)	0/ 11 (0)
Transient intraventricular pressure gradient, %	18	...	...	23	...	...	...	13	14	...
In-hospital mortality, %	1	3 (9)	0	0	0	6	0	0	0	8
Documented recurrence, n/ n (%)	2/ 72 (3)	2 (6)	0	2/ 22 (9)	0	...	...	1/ 16 (6)	...	0

LVEF indicates left ventricular ejection fraction; Retro, retrospective; Pro, prospective. Values are expressed as mean ± SD when appropriate.

*Median.

†In precordial leads.

Adapted from Gianni et al. Apical ballooning syndrome or takotsubo cardiomyopathy: a systematic review. Eur Heart J 2006;27:1523–1529, with permission from Oxford University Press.

Table 3. Patient Clinical and Laboratory Characteristics

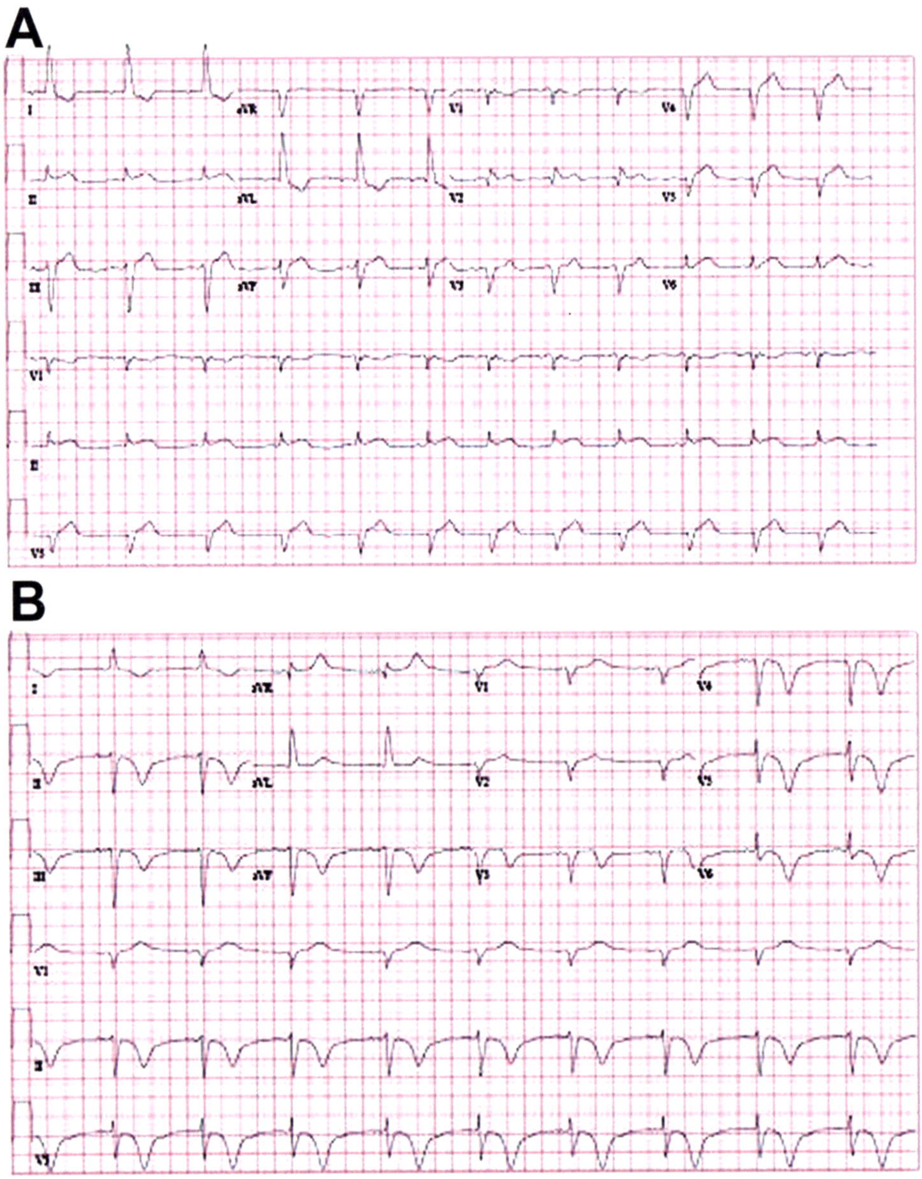

Fig. 3. Electrocardiogram (ECG) changes in one of our patients with takotsubo cardiomyopathy. Panel A: ECG at presentation revealed a 1-mm elevation in V3 and V4 and a new-onset left bundle branch block. Panel B: ECG at 48 hours after presentation revealed T-wave abnormalities in multiple leads.

Posterobasal	1%
Basal + midventricular	1%
Diaphragmatic	2%
Localized apical	2%
Anterolateral	11%
Complete midventricular	29%
Classical takotsubo cardiomyopathy	54%

Data compiled from Singh et al.[36]

Table 4. Variants of Takotsubo Cardiomyopathy[36]

4.7 Coronary angiography

Coronary angiography on presentation fails to reveal any coronary obstruction or acute plaque rupture. However, patients with coronary artery disease can develop TTC. Kurisu and colleagues (38) reported 10% of patients in their series of takotsubo patients (total patients=97) had >75% coronary artery obstruction in a major coronary vessel, though coronary stenosis is uncommon in patients presenting with TTC (1), and absence of an acute coronary artery syndrome is a diagnostic criterion for diagnosis of TTC.

4.8 Echocardiography

Echocardiography also plays a pivotal role in the diagnosis of TTC. This is particularly so given the ability to rapidly perform bedside echocardiography with echo-Doppler imaging. Accurate evaluation by echocardiography, particularly after coronary evaluation by catheterization, can assist in further defining the diagnosis, particularly, when echocardiography repeated after few days to weeks shows complete normalization of regional wall motion abnormalities and LV ejection fraction. Typically, TTC appears like an evolving acute anterior wall myocardial infarction (MI) with akinesia of the apex, apical anterior wall and septum (Figure 5). Left ventricular outflow tract obstruction, a transient phenomenon in TTC, can also be recognized by echocardiography.

In contemporary clinical practice, three-dimensional speckle tracking echocardiography (3D-STE) can be used to assess myocardial mechanical function. It permits the calculation of complex myocardial mechanical parameters such as strain and strain rate, rotation, torsion, as well as LV volume and ejection fraction in three dimensions within minutes. It has been validated against sonomicrometry, magnetic resonance imaging (MRI) tagging, and found to be more accurate and reproducible than two-dimensional speckle tracking echocardiography (2D-STE). We have observed that the global longitudinal, circumferential and radial strains are all decreased significantly in acute anterior wall myocardial infarction and TTC in the acute phase. However, regional circumferential and radial strains at mid and apical LV are significantly lower in TTC patients than in acute anterior wall MI.

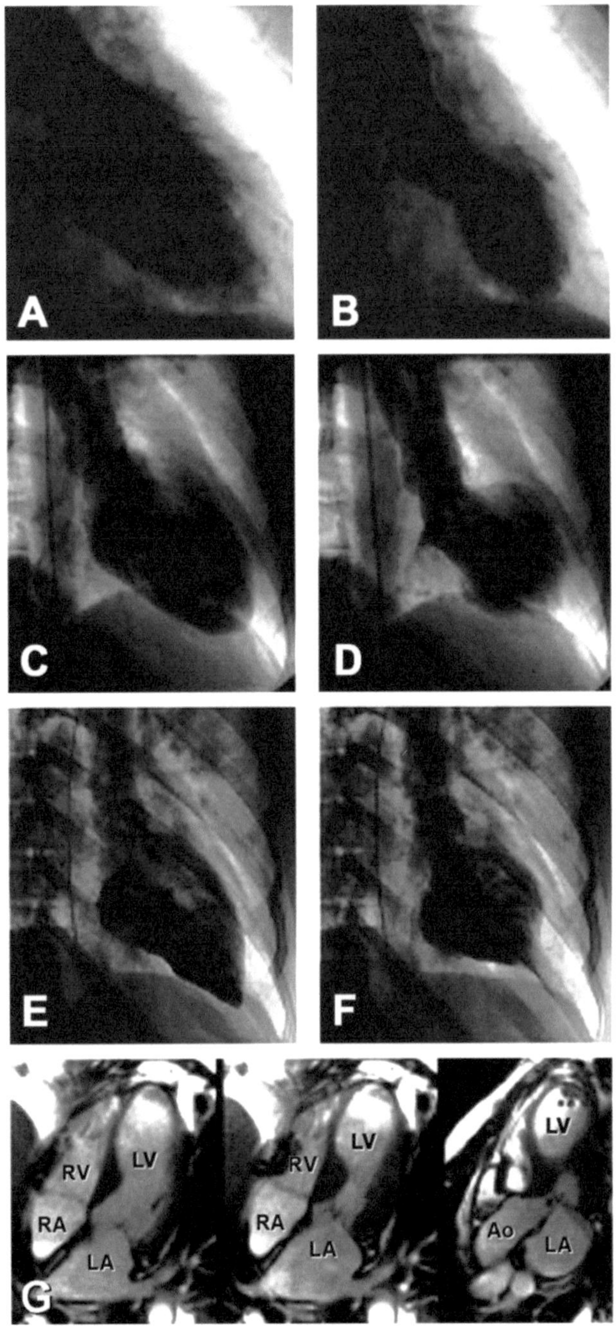

Fig. 4. Radiograph of the left ventricle. (A) Left ventriculogram in diastole. (B) Left ventriculogram in systole shows preserved contraction of the base of the ventricle and apical ballooning. (C) Right anterior oblique view in diastole. (D) Right anterior oblique view in systole. Note the hypercontractility of the basal and apical segments and ballooning of the midventricular segments. (E) After methamphetamine use in end-diastole. (F) After

methamphetamine use in end-systole. Basal segments are akinetic, the papillary level shows normal contractility, and the apex is hypercontractile. (G) Cardiac magnetic resonance image. Hypotension may be due to dynamic outflow tract obstruction caused by hyperkinesis of the basal left ventricle segments and systolic anterior motion of the mitral valve. Four-chamber, steady-state, free-precession image: end-diastole (left) and end-systole (center) show left and right ventricular apical akinesis. (Right) Three-chamber image in systole shows systolic anterior motion of the mitral leaflets (*) with dynamic left ventricular outflow tract obstruction; left ventricular apical mass consistent with thrombus (**). Ao = aorta; LA = left atrium; LV = left ventricle; RA = right atrium; RV = right ventricle. (Panels A and B are adapted from Hurst et al. Takotsubo cardiomyopathy: A unique cardiomyopathy with variable ventricular morphology. JACC: Cardiovascular Imaging 2010;3:641-9, with permission from Elsevier. Panels C and D are adapted from Hurst et al. Transient midventricular ballooning syndrome: a new variant. J Am Coll Cardiol 2006;48:579-83, with permission from Elsevier. Panels E and F are adapted from Reuss et al. Isolated left ventricular basal ballooning phenotype of transient cardiomyopathy in young women. Am J Cardiol 2007;99:1451-3, with permission from Elsevier. Panel G is adapted from Syed et al. Apical ballooning syndrome or aborted acute myocardial infarction? Insights from cardiovascular magnetic resonance imaging. Int J Cardiovasc Imaging 2008;24:875-82, with permission from Springer.)

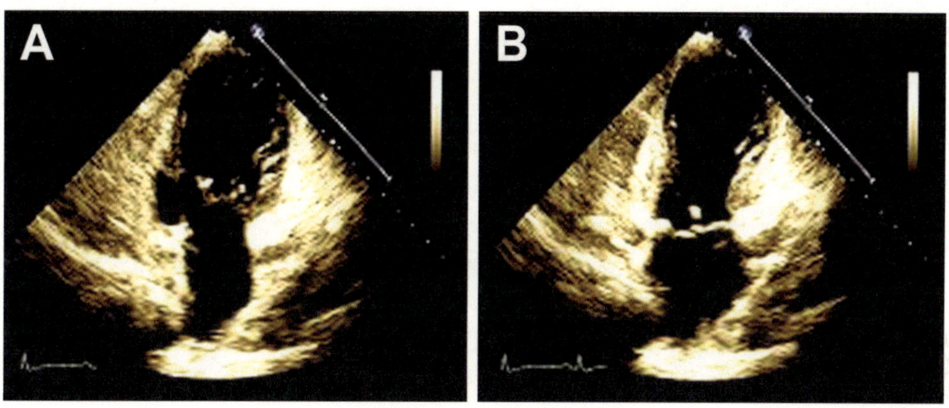

Fig. 5. Two-chamber view of the left ventricle, obtained in diastole (Panel A) and systole (Panel B), in a 56-year-old female who presented to the hospital in florid pulmonary edema after witnessing a car accident. Panel B demonstrates the akinetic and balloon apex in systole with a hypercontractile base, a classic variant of takotsubo cardiomyopathy.

4.9 Cardiac magnetic resonance imaging

Cardiac magnetic resonance imaging may be helpful in differentiating TTC from MI and myocarditis. TTC is characterized by the absence of delayed gadolinium enhancement, whereas MI is characterized by subendocardial delayed hyperenhancement and myocarditis is characterized by patchy delayed hyperenhancement (39-41). Cardiac magnetic resonance can also demonstrate the typical bulging of the LV apex and hypercontractile function of the base with accurate rendering of the LV stroke volume. It can also demonstrate the presence of LV thrombus in akinetic apex (Figure 6).

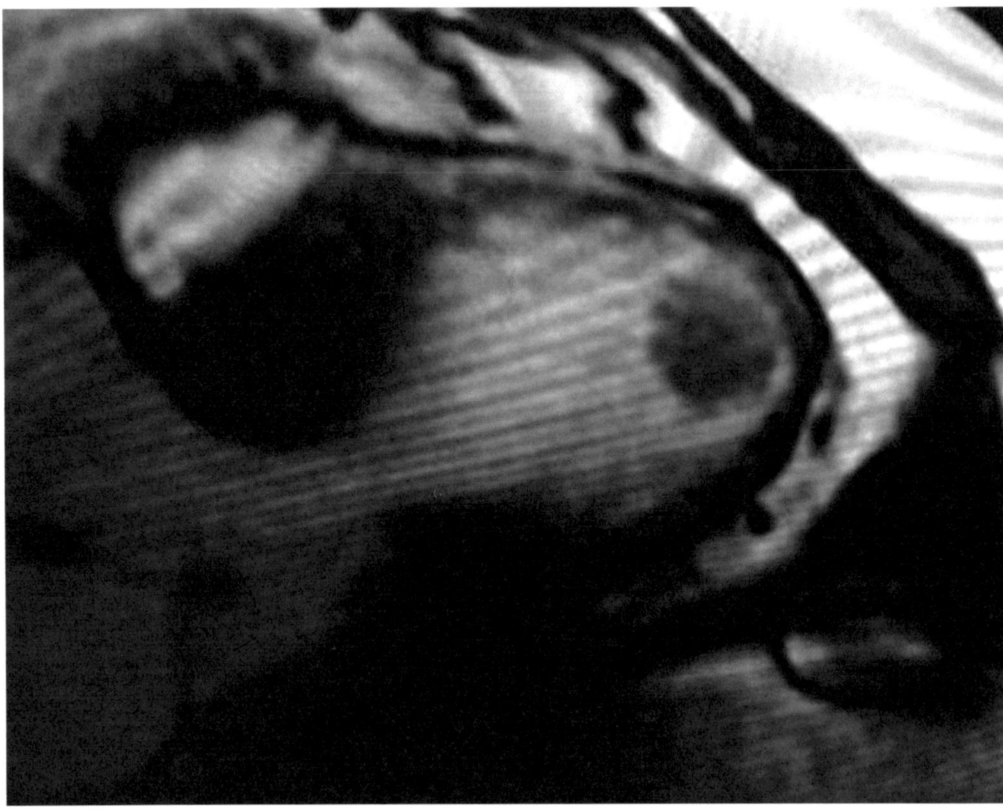

Fig. 6. Two-chamber Fast Imaging Employing Steady-State Acquisition (FIESTA) motion sensing in a 76-year-old female who presented to the hospital with chest pain and shortness of breath after witnessing an acute asthma attack in her grandchild. The figure demonstrates left ventricular apical bulging and a hypercontractile base with a 1.5 × 1.5-cm thrombus within the left ventricular apex.

4.10 Clinical outcome and prognosis

A complete recovery of LV wall motion abnormalities is a hallmark of this syndrome in virtually all patients (2,15,16,35). Recovery time varies, from as short as several days to as long as 4-8 weeks, and is a requirement for the diagnosis (15). The diagnostic criteria are summarized in Table 5.

---

1. Transient hypokinesis, akinesis, or dyskinesis of the left ventricular mid-segments with or without apical involvement; the regional wall motion abnormalities extend beyond a single epicardial vascular distribution; a stressful trigger is often, but not always, present.*
2. Absence of obstructive coronary disease or angiographic evidence of acute plaque rupture. †
3. New electrocardiographic abnormalities (either ST-segment elevation and/or T-wave inversion) or modest elevation in cardiac troponin.
4. Absence of:
   Pheochromocytoma
   Myocarditis

In both of the above circumstances, the diagnosis of takotsubo cardiomyopathy should be made with caution, and a clear stressful precipitating trigger must be sought.
*There are rare exceptions to these criteria such as those patients in whom the regional wall motion abnormality is limited to a single coronary territory.
†It is possible that a patient with obstructive coronary atherosclerosis may also develop takotsubo cardiomyopathy. However, this is very rare in our experience and in the published literature, perhaps because such cases are misdiagnosed as an acute coronary syndrome.
Reproduced from Prasad et al. Apical ballooning syndrome (Tako-Tsubo or stress cardiomyopathy): A mimic of acute myocardial infarction. Am Heart J 2008;155:408-17, with permission from Elsevier.

Table 5. Proposed Mayo Clinic Criteria for Takotusbo Cardiomyopathy

The overall prognosis of TTC appears to be favorable in patients who survive the initial acute phase of heart failure. In-hospital mortality has been reported between 0 and 8% (12). Reported complications associated with TTC are left heart failure with and without pulmonary edema, cardiogenic shock, dynamic intraventricular obstruction with left ventricular intracavitary pressure gradient generation, mitral regurgitation resulting from chordal tethering as well as systolic anterior motion of the mitral valve apparatus, ventricular arrhythmias, LV mural thrombus formation, left ventricular free-wall rupture and death (12). Cardiogenic shock (6.5%), congestive heart failure (3.8%) and ventricular tachycardia (1.6%) are other known complications, while ventricular fibrillation, LV mural thrombus formation, ventricular septal defect, LV free wall rupture and pneumothorax have infrequently been reported (12,37).
Recently, Madhavan and colleagues (42) have proposed the "Mayo Clinic Risk Score" system for acute heart failure in TTC (Table 6). The scoring system was developed to predict which patients with TTC are at risk of developing systolic heart failure. Presence of 1, 2 and 3 points was associated with 28%, 58% and 85% risk of acute heart failure.

Risk Factor	Score
Age > 70 years	1
Presence of physical stressor	1
Ejection fraction < 40%	1

Table 6. Proposed Mayo Clinic Risk Scoring System of Acute Heart Failure in Takotsubo Cardiomyopathy

5. Pathogenesis

The aphorism "a broken heart" is well known to be associated with emotional stress by the lay person. Association of TTC with acute emotional and physical stress lends a scientific basis for this observation. But the exact underlying mechanism still proves elusive. Due to the recent recognition of TTC and its low incidence of diagnosis, as mentioned earlier, only a relatively small number of patients have been studied in a few published series. No large studies have confirmed the etiology of TTC (43). A rapidly accumulating body of evidence has led to very interesting insights into the possible pathophysiology of TTC. Most current hypotheses are based on cathecholamine surges in the setting of acute emotional or physical stress leading to catecholamine-related cardiac toxic effects (32,44-49) and was first suggested by Wittstein and colleagues (16). In this section we examine various advancements in understanding TTC pathophysiology.

5.1 Obstruction of the left ventricular outflow tract

Early investigators observed left ventricular outflow tract (LVOT) obstruction in some patients presenting with TTC. Villarreal and colleagues hypothesized that patients with a sigmoid interventricular septum, small LVOT, reduced LV volume (primarily elderly women) and an abnormal orientation of a slack mitral apparatus have a geometric predisposition to dynamic LVOT obstruction, which may manifest in the setting of intense adrenergic stimulation or hypovolemia (50,51). Elderly females seem to have a higher incidence of basal septal thickening (52), and this could become a substrate for LVOT obstruction leading to severe, transient midcavity obstruction in the setting of a cathecholamine surge (53). LVOT obstruction may cause or worsen hypotension due to LV systolic dysfunction by contributing to significant mitral regurgitation secondary to systolic anterior motion of mitral valve and dynamic LVOT obstruction (54). Presence of LVOT may change the management of TTC patients and is detailed in the treatment section of this chapter. However, incidence of LVOT obstruction in patients presenting with TTC in various studies has varied from 11-25% of patients (12,52,55) and is not observed in all patients. Its role in the pathogenesis of TTC is unclear, and it remains uncertain if LVOT obstruction is a cause or a consequence of TTC (49).

5.2 Vasospasm of epicardial coronary arteries hypothesis

Clinical presentation of TTC bears close resemblance to an acute MI. Therefore, early hypotheses speculated that an ischemic event triggered by transient coronary plaque rupture (56) or reversible coronary vessel spasm (7) was responsible for "stunning" the ventricle. A few authors reported finding a long left anterior descending artery (LAD) that wrapped around the apex in their patients presenting with TTC, and it was hypothesized that transient obstruction of epicardial blood flow to the left ventricle in a given coronary bed may lead to the regional akinesis or "ballooning" typically observed in TTC. However, there are multiple problems with such an explanation. For one, the aforementioned coronary artery anatomy is not found on coronary angiography in all patients presenting with TTC. Secondly, spontaneous coronary vasospasm has been reported in only 2% of patients with TTC (12). Furthermore, an acute coronary vessel-obstructing lesion has not been described in patients with TTC immediately after presentation (57) and has been proposed as an exclusion criterion (35) for TTC diagnosis. Thirdly, as mentioned earlier, there are reports of numerous phenotypes of TTC that present with regional hypokinesis that encompasses territories of the left ventricle not supplied by a single vessel (35). Fourthly, histological examination of cardiac tissue in patients with acute MI reveals polymorphonuclear inflammation, whereas TTC is associated with an interstitial mononuclear inflammatory response and considerable increase in extracellular matrix protein and contraction band necrosis—a unique form of myocyte injury characterized by hypercontracted sarcomeres and dense eosinophilic transverse bands associated with catecholamine-excess states like pheochromocytoma and subarachnoid hemorrhage (16,49). Finally, provocative tests with infusion of ergometrine or acetylcholine for inducible coronary vasospasm in patients with TTC were only positive in 28.6% of patients (55) and 27.6% of patients (58) in two published series, respectively. These equivocal results combined with the factors mentioned above make obstruction of blood flow in epicardial coronary vessels seem less likely to explain the pathophysiology of TTC.

5.3 Coronary microvascular blood flow abnormalities

Several investigators (11,19,59) have suggested microvascular dysfunction to be a potential pathophysiologic mechanism in TTC. Kume and colleagues demonstrated microcirculation disturbances in patients with TTC by use of Doppler flow-wire assessment (60). Other investigators have used TIMI (Thrombolysis in Myocardial Infarction) frame counts to assess coronary blood flow. Using this technique, Kurisu (59) and colleagues found significantly higher frame counts in TTC compared to a control group. Bybee and colleagues (19) also found abnormal TIMI frame counts in one or more major epicardial vessels in patients with TTC in their published series. These findings suggest that microvascular integrity in TTC is impaired in all coronary arteries in many patients, and the microvascular dysfunction in LAD is comparable to that of patients with acute anterior ST-segment elevation myocardial infarction after recanalization of the infarct-related artery.

Nuclear studies with single-photon emission tomography (SPET) and fluorodeoxyglucose positron emission tomography (FDG-PET) were performed by Kurowski (11) in their patients with TTC and revealed that myocardial glucose metabolism was more affected than perfusion. The authors concluded that this "inverse mismatch" pattern is similar to that seen in postischemic "stunned" myocardium (61).

These findings indicate that diffuse coronary microvascular dysfunction is present in patients with TTC. However, whether this is an effect or cause of this syndrome is unclear (10). This type of microvascular dysfunction, however, can be a result of a surge in catecholamine secretion, which is described in detail later in this chapter.

5.4 Catecholamine-induced acute myocardial stunning hypothesis

5.4.1 Alterations in calcium handling

Akashi and colleagues were the first to report elevated serum catecholamine levels in patients with TTC (62). Wittstein and colleagues (16) later reported supraphysiologic levels of plasma catecholamines in their series (n=19 patients), which reported plasma levels of epinephrine, norepinephrine and dopamine in patients with TTC to be 2-3 times higher than those of patients with Killip class III MI and 7-32 times higher than the published normal values (63). They also noted higher levels of both neuronal (dihydroxyphenylglycol, dihydroxyphenylglycol and dihydroxyphenylacetic acid) and extraneuronal catecholamines (metanephrine, normetanephrine and neuropeptide Y). In Wittstein's series, the plasma cathecholamine levels trended downward by day 7-9 but still remained elevated. They concluded that TTC was associated with activation of adrenomedullary hormonal system and enhanced sympathoneural activity. Similarly, administration of epinephrine at suprapharmacological doses led to induction of stress cardiomyopathy in two cases (64,65). Several investigators (16,32,66) have suggested direct myocardial stunning as a result of the catecholamine surges. Such a stunning could possibly explain the findings in TTC. Catecholamine-overload state is associated with the following histologic changes: 1.) increased production of extracellular matrix leading to a rapid increase in fibrosis; 2.) contraction band necrosis; and 3.) mild neutrophil infiltration (44). There is increased production of oxygen-derived free radicals (67) that interfere with sodium and calcium transporters, resulting in myocyte dysfunction through increased transsarcolemmal calcium influx and cellular calcium overload (68). Mori and colleagues (69) demonstrated that apical myocardium has a higher concentration of beta-adrenoceptors with a concentration gradient decreasing from apex to base. This could explain the enhanced responsiveness to sympathetic stimulation potentially making the apex more vulnerable to sudden surges in circulating catecholamine levels and, thus, could explain the typical phenotype most commonly found in TTC patients (16).

Investigators have noted disturbance of the calcium regulatory system in stress-induced cardiomyopathy. Some animal models have been shown to describe altered expression of the calcium regulatory system protein genes by supraphysiological levels of catecholamines (70,71) (Figure 7).

Sarcolipin regulates sarcoplasmic/endoplasmic reticulum calcium ATPase2 (SERCA) by lowering its affinity for calcium. Elevated catecholamines in TTC cause increased expression of sarcolipin in the acute phase, leading to reduced affinity of SERCA2 for calcium (49,72,73). Elevated levels of catecholamines also lead to reduced expression of SERCA2 messenger RNA levels through intense G-protein-stimulated β1 and β2 adrenergic receptor signaling in animal models (74). The G-protein-stimulated β1-adrenergic receptor and α1-adrenergic receptor can directly modulate SERCA2 gene expression (via cyclic AMP-responsive element binding protein 1 and calcineurin-nuclear factor of activated T cells signaling pathways) (75). Excessive adrenergic signaling could thus explain the cardiotoxicity observed in patients with stress cardiomyopathy from cardiomyocytes calcium overload, mitochondrial calcium overload, reactive oxygen species production and oxidative stress (32,49). However, there is no evidence to suggest that alterations in expression of calcium-handling proteins are responsible for the acute deleterious effects of TTC (49).

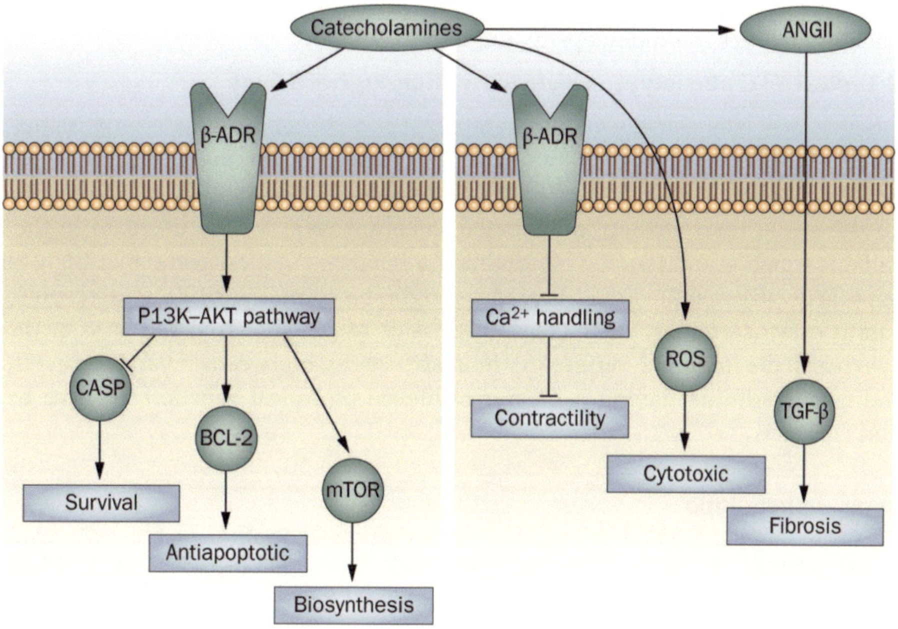

Fig. 7. The pathomechanistic concept of stress cardiomyopathy. Overexpression of catecholamines following a stress event leads to a number of changes that can have either protective or adverse effects. Abbreviations: β-ADR, β-adrenergic receptor; ANGII, angiotensin II; CASP, caspase; mTOR, mammalian target of rapamycin; PI3K–AKT, phosphatidylinositol 3 kinase–AKT; ROS, reactive oxygen species; TGF-β, transforming growth factor β. Reproduced from Nef et al. Mechanisms of stress (Takotsubo) cardiomyopathy. Nat Rev Cardiol 2010;7:187–193, with permission from Nature Publishing Group.

5.4.2 Stimulus trafficking

5.4.2.1 Stimulus trafficking causes negative inotropism

Human ventricular cardiomyocytes have two types of β-adrenergic receptors (AR), β1 and β2, but the concentration of β2 is higher than β1 (4:1) (76). At physiological and elevated concentrations, norepinephrine and epinephrine act via β1-AR exerting positive inotropic and lusitropic responses through coupling with the Gs protein family. Epinephrine has higher affinity for β2-AR and activates the Gs protein family, causing positive inotropic response. However, at supraphysiological levels, epinephrine stimulates a negative inotropic effect (77) by causing a switch from β2-AR Gs protein signaling to β2-AR Gi protein signaling (78), a process called stimulus trafficking (32). Intense activation of the β1-AR Gs protein and β2-AR Gs protein pathways is thought to initiate the switch in signal trafficking from β2-AR Gs protein to β2-AR Gi protein coupling (79). The Gi protein pathway exerts a negative inotropic effect through multiple pathways (32).

After the surge in epinephrine levels has cleared from the circulation, negative inotropy-causing β2-ARs that are coupled to Gi proteins either switch back to Gs protein coupling or are internalized and degraded, enabling cardiomyocytes to recover their inotropic function.

This sequence of events would explain the reported recovery of ventricular function in individuals with stress cardiomyopathy (32).

5.4.2.2 Typical TTC phenotype explained by stimulus trafficking

In human hearts, the density of the sympathetic nerve endings is approximately 40% greater at the base compared to the apex (80), whereas the concentration of β-ARs is higher in the apical myocardium (69). It has been proposed that the concentration of β-ARs in the apical myocardium is increased to compensate for the decrease in the direct sympathetic innervation, thereby maintaining a balanced responsiveness of the ventricle-to-sympathetic drive (32). Thus, the apex might be more sensitive and responsive to circulating catecholamines. An increasing density of β2-ARs from the base to the apex could explain the regional difference in response to high catecholamine levels, with circulating epinephrine having a greater influence on apical function, relative to basal function.

5.5 Atypical phenotype

Certain factors can influence the local epinephrine concentration in the myocardium. A study in rabbits demonstrated conversion of norepinephrine to epinephrine by phenylethanolamine N-methyltransferase in the ventricular myocardium (81). Thus, regional differences in epinephrine concentrations can play a role in responsiveness of the myocardium to catecholamines and could explain atypical phenotypes observed in some TTC patients (32).

5.6 Female predominance related to hormones

Some investigators have suggested reduction of estrogen levels in postmenopausal females to be one of the underlying factors of TTC.

Estrogen receptors are expressed on cardiomyocytes (82), thus cardiomyocyte function could be directly affected by estrogen levels. Estrogen has also been shown to significantly suppress SERCA2 expression in ovariectomized rats compared to controls, thus altering cardiac myocyte sarcoplasmic reticulum calcium uptake (83). In the latter study, investigators noted that estrogen and progesterone supplementations were equally effective in preventing changes in ovariectomized hearts.

Men rarely develop stress cardiomyopathy yet are physiologically estrogen-deficient, which suggests that this syndrome is not due to ovarian hormone deficiency. However, effects of hormone deficiency on contractility in the presence of excessive catecholamine levels need further clarification (49).

5.7 Possible familial link

Burgdorf and colleagues (84) recently reported a series of 144 patients with TTC (107 typical cases and 34 atypical cases) in which 26 patients were known to have cancer, while 7 patients were newly diagnosed with cancer. On basis of this observation, they proposed that an association between cancer and TTC cannot be excluded and that patients diagnosed with TTC should undergo screening for cancer. While there might be an association, one possible confounder could be the neurally mediated hypothesis of stress associated with learning about the diagnosis of cancer.

6. Treatment

TTC is a self-limiting syndrome; cardiac function returns to pre-TTC levels within a few weeks and patients carry a favorable prognosis (2). However, patients require standard supportive treatment during the acute phase. This treatment is similar to a congestive heart failure treatment regimen with diuretics and vasodilators (16). Vasopressors and beta-agonists should be avoided due to catecholamine-surplus state. Also, epinephrine administered may drive further β2-AR, Gi protein-mediated negative inotropism (32). Use of β-blockers should be carefully considered as some β-blockers can also cause stimulus trafficking of β2-ARs to Gi protein coupling (85), which, in the acute phase of TTC, can lead to further suppression of LV function. However, in the long term, β2-AR/Gi coupling may enhance the ability of β-blockers to protect and improve the function of the failing heart (85). Mechanical circulatory support in patients with intraaortic balloon counter pulsation (IABP) is appropriate to avoid vasopressor support in these patients (16). Administration of intravenous calcium or levosimendan (a calcium-sensitizing agent) has also been suggested as the inotrope of choice in TTC patients (86,87), but has not been clinically validated in any major study. Some investigators have used it to avoid IABP in TTC patients (88). In patients with moderate to severe hemodynamic compromise and echocardiographic evidence of significant LVOT obstruction (with a dynamic gradient possibly accompanied by systolic anterior motion of mitral valve), both IABP counter pulsation and inotropes are relatively contraindicated because they could worsen the dynamic gradient and thereby further jeopardize cardiac function (54,89); treatment should instead be more conservative with careful fluid management to avoid excessive preload reduction, β-blockers if tolerated (to increase diastolic filling time and thus end-diastolic volume) and occasionally peripheral vasoconstrictors (54,90,91). Finally, in patients with life-threatening acute left ventricular failure, temporary use of a LV assist device may be required (32).

7. Conclusion

Takotsubo cardiomyopathy is a unique form of transient nonischemic stress-induced cardiomyopathy. A well-recognized syndrome now, two decades after its first reported case, it is also being reported in populations other than postmenopausal women. Even though apical ballooning phenotype is the most common and typical presentation, much confusion has resulted from various nomenclatures being used for different presentations of this syndrome. The underlying mechanism is not fully understood but could be common and explained by changes in molecular pathways like *stimulus trafficking* under supraphysiological levels of catecholamines, and influenced by hormonal status. Clinical history, electrocardiogram and diagnostic imaging with coronary angiography and/or cardiac magnetic resonance imaging that establishes typical phenotypic features of the disease in absence of significant obstructive coronary artery disease are essential for diagnosis and to differentiate it from an acute myocardial infarction. Management focuses on supportive care in the acute phase, while avoiding vasopressor medications. Mortality is low if patients survive the initial critical period and, by definition, they go on to have a full recovery. Recurrence has been reported but is rare. More studies are needed to fully understand the underlying mechanisms.

8. References

[1] Hurst RT, Prasad A, Askew JW 3rd, Sengupta PP, Tajik AJ. Takotsubo cardiomyopathy: a unique cardiomyopathy with variable ventricular morphology. *JACC Cardiovasc Imaging* 2010;3:641-9.

[2] Tsuchihashi K, Ueshima K, Uchida T, Oh-mura N, Kimura K, Owa M, Yoshiyama M, Miyazaki S, Haze K, Ogawa H, Honda T, Hase M, Kai R, Morii I; Angina Pectoris-Myocardial Infarction Investigations in Japan. Transient left ventricular apical ballooning without coronary artery stenosis: a novel heart syndrome mimicking acute myocardial infarction. Angina Pectoris-Myocardial Infarction Investigations in Japan. *J Am Coll Cardiol* 2001;38:11-8.

[3] Sharkey SW, Lesser JR, Maron MS, Maron BJ. Why not just call it tako-tsubo cardiomyopathy: a discussion of nomenclature. *J Am Coll Cardiol* 2011;57:1496-7.

[4] Maron BJ, Towbin JA, Thiene G, Antzelevitch C, Corrado D, Arnett D, Moss AJ, Seidman CE, Young JB; American Heart Association; Council on Clinical Cardiology, Heart Failure and Transplantation Committee; Quality of Care and Outcomes Research and Functional Genomics and Translational Biology Interdisciplinary Working Groups; Council on Epidemiology and Prevention. Contemporary definitions and classification of the cardiomyopathies: an American Heart Association Scientific Statement from the Council on Clinical Cardiology, Heart Failure and Transplantation Committee; Quality of Care and Outcomes Research and Functional Genomics and Translational Biology Interdisciplinary Working Groups; and Council on Epidemiology and Prevention. *Circulation* 2006;113:1807-16.

[5] Kapoor D, Bybee KA. Stress cardiomyopathy syndrome: a contemporary review. *Curr Heart Fail Rep* 2009;6:265-71.

[6] Sato H, Tateishi H, Uchida T. Takotsubo-type cardiomyopathy due to multivessel spasm. In: Kodama K, Haze K, Hon M, editors. *Clinical Aspect of Myocardial Injury: From Ischemia to Heart Failure.* Tokyo, Japan: Kagakuhyouronsha; 1990. p. 56–64.

[7] Dote K, Sato H, Tateishi H, Uchida T, Ishihara M. Myocardial stunning due to simultaneous multivessel coronary spasms: a review of 5 cases. *J Cardiol* 1991;21:203-14.

[8] Kawai S, Suzuki H, Yamaguchi H, Tanaka K, Sawada H, Aizawa T, Watanabe M, Tamura T, Umawatari K, Kawata M, Nakamura T, Yamanaka O, Okada R. Ampulla cardiomyopathy ('Takotusbo' cardiomyopathy)--reversible left ventricular dysfunction: with ST segment elevation. *Jpn Circ J* 2000;64:156-9.

[9] Kurisu S, Sato H, Kawagoe T, Ishihara M, Shimatani Y, Nishioka K, Kono Y, Umemura T, Nakamura S. Tako-tsubo-like left ventricular dysfunction with ST-segment elevation: a novel cardiac syndrome mimicking acute myocardial infarction. *Am Heart J* 2002;143:448-55.

[10] Akashi YJ, Goldstein DS, Barbaro G, Ueyama T. Takotsubo cardiomyopathy: a new form of acute, reversible heart failure. *Circulation* 2008;118:2754-62.

[11] Kurowski V, Kaiser A, von Hof K, Killermann DP, Mayer B, Hartmann F, Schunkert H, Radke PW. Apical and midventricular transient left ventricular dysfunction syndrome (tako-tsubo cardiomyopathy): frequency, mechanisms, and prognosis. *Chest* 2007;132:809-16.

[12] Bybee KA, Kara T, Prasad A, Lerman A, Barsness GW, Wright RS, Rihal CS. Systematic review: transient left ventricular apical ballooning: a syndrome that mimics ST-segment elevation myocardial infarction. *Ann Intern Med* 2004;141:858-65.

[13] Kushiro T, Saito F, Kusama J, Takahashi H, Imazeki T, Tani S, Kikuchi S, Imai S, Matsudaira K, Watanabe I, Hino T, Sato Y, Nakayama T, Nagao K, Kanmatsuse K. Takotsubo-shaped cardiomyopathy with type I CD36 deficiency. *Heart Vessels* 2005;20:123-5.

[14] Cherian J, Angelis D, Filiberti A, Saperia G. Can takotsubo cardiomyopathy be familial? *Int J Cardiol* 2007;121:74-5.

[15] Sharkey SW, Lesser JR, Zenovich AG, Maron MS, Lindberg J, Longe TF, Maron BJ. Acute and reversible cardiomyopathy provoked by stress in women from the United States. *Circulation* 2005;111:472-9.

[16] Wittstein IS, Thiemann DR, Lima JA, Baughman KL, Schulman SP, Gerstenblith G, Wu KC, Rade JJ, Bivalacqua TJ, Champion HC. Neurohumoral features of myocardial stunning due to sudden emotional stress. *N Engl J Med* 2005;352:539-48.

[17] Inoue M, Shimizu M, Ino H, Yamaguchi M, Terai H, Fujino N, Sakata K, Funada A, Tatami R, Ishise S, Kanaya H, Mabuchi H. Differentiation between patients with takotsubo cardiomyopathy and those with anterior acute myocardial infarction. *Circ J* 2005;69:89-94.

[18] Sato M, Fujita S, Saito A, Ikeda Y, Kitazawa H, Takahashi M, Ishiguro J, Okabe M, Nakamura Y, Nagai T, Watanabe H, Kodama M, Aizawa Y. Increased incidence of transient left ventricular apical ballooning (so-called 'Takotsubo' cardiomyopathy) after the mid-Niigata Prefecture earthquake. *Circ J* 2006;70:947-53.

[19] Bybee KA, Prasad A, Barsness GW, Lerman A, Jaffe AS, Murphy JG, Wright RS, Rihal CS. Clinical characteristics and thrombolysis in myocardial infarction frame counts in women with transient left ventricular apical ballooning syndrome. *Am J Cardiol* 2004;94:343-6.

[20] Yoshida T, Hibino T, Kako N, Murai S, Oguri M, Kato K, Yajima K, Ohte N, Yokoi K, Kimura G. A pathophysiologic study of tako-tsubo cardiomyopathy with F-18 fluorodeoxyglucose positron emission tomography. *Eur Heart J* 2007;28:2598-604.

[21] Akashi YJ, Musha H, Kida K, Itoh K, Inoue K, Kawasaki K, Hashimoto N, Miyake F. Reversible ventricular dysfunction takotsubo cardiomyopathy. *Eur J Heart Fail* 2005;7:1171-6.

[22] Schoof S, Bertram H, Hohmann D, Jack T, Wessel A, Yelbuz TM. Takotsubo cardiomyopathy in a 2-year-old girl: 3-dimensional visualization of reversible left ventricular dysfunction. *J Am Coll Cardiol* 2010;55:e5.

[23] Hafiz AM, Jan F, Allaqaband S. The near fatal crossing: a rare recurrence of takotsubo cardiomyopathy in a 66-year-old woman. *Internet Journal of Cardiology* 2009;7.

[24] Takizawa M, Kobayakawa N, Uozumi H, Yonemura S, Kodama T, Fukusima K, Takeuchi H, Kaneko Y, Kaneko T, Fujita K, Honma Y, Aoyagi T. A case of transient left ventricular ballooning with pheochromocytoma, supporting pathogenetic role of catecholamines in stress-induced cardiomyopathy or takotsubo cardiomyopathy. *Int J Cardiol* 2007;114:e15-7.

[25] Gujja KR, Aslam AF, Privman V, Tejani F, Vasavada B. Initial presentation of pheochromocytoma with Takotsubo cardiomyopathy: a brief review of literature. *J Cardiovasc Med* (Hagerstown) 2010;11:49-52.
[26] Rossi AP, Bing-You RG, Thomas LR. Recurrent takotsubo cardiomyopathy associated with pheochromocytoma. *Endocr Pract* 2009;15:560-2.
[27] Sanchez-Recalde A, Costero O, Oliver JM, Iborra C, Ruiz E, Sobrino JA. Images in cardiovascular medicine. Pheochromocytoma-related cardiomyopathy: inverted Takotsubo contractile pattern. *Circulation* 2006;113:e738-9.
[28] Santana-Cabrera L, Escot CR, Medina Gil JM, Ortiz CP. Takotsubo Cardiomyopathy Associated with Acute Subarachnoid Hemorrhage. *J Emerg Med* 2010 Oct 6. [Epub ahead of print]
[29] Kittisupamongkol W. Takotsubo cardiomyopathy in subarachnoid hemorrhage. *Int J Cardiol* 2010;144:324; author reply 325.
[30] Das M, Gonsalves S, Saha A, Ross S, Williams G. Acute subarachnoid haemorrhage as a precipitant for takotsubo cardiomyopathy: a case report and discussion. *Int J Cardiol* 2009;132:283-5.
[31] Ono Y, Kawamura T, Ito J, Kanayama S, Miura T, Kikuchi F. Ampulla (takotsubo) cardiomyopathy associated with subarachnoid hemorrhage worsening in the late phase of vasospasm--case report. *Neurol Med Chir* (Tokyo) 2004;44:72-4.
[32] Lyon AR, Rees PS, Prasad S, Poole-Wilson PA, Harding SE. Stress (Takotsubo) cardiomyopathy--a novel pathophysiological hypothesis to explain catecholamine-induced acute myocardial stunning. *Nat Clin Pract Cardiovasc Med* 2008;5:22-9.
[33] Song BG, Park SJ, Noh HJ, Jo HC, Choi JO, Lee SC, Park SW, Jeon ES, Kim DK, Oh JK. Clinical characteristics, and laboratory and echocardiographic findings in takotsubo cardiomyopathy presenting as cardiogenic shock. *J Crit Care* 2010;25:329-35.
[34] Desmet WJ, Adriaenssens BF, Dens JA. Apical ballooning of the left ventricle: first series in white patients. *Heart* 2003;89:1027-31.
[35] Prasad A, Lerman A, Rihal CS. Apical ballooning syndrome (Tako-Tsubo or stress cardiomyopathy): a mimic of acute myocardial infarction. *Am Heart J* 2008;155:408-17.
[36] Singh NK, Rumman S, Mikell FL, Nallamothu N, Rangaswamy C. Stress cardiomyopathy: clinical and ventriculographic characteristics in 107 North American subjects. *Int J Cardiol* 2010;141:297-303.
[37] Bielecka-Dabrowa A, Mikhailidis DP, Hannam S, Rysz J, Michalska M, Akashi YJ, Banach M. Takotsubo cardiomyopathy--the current state of knowledge. *Int J Cardiol* 2010;142:120-5.
[38] Kurisu S, Inoue I, Kawagoe T, Ishihara M, Shimatani Y, Nakama Y, Maruhashi T, Kagawa E, Dai K, Matsushita J, Ikenaga H. Prevalence of incidental coronary artery disease in tako-tsubo cardiomyopathy. *Coron Artery Dis* 2009;20:214-8.
[39] Madhavan M, Prasad A. Proposed Mayo Clinic criteria for the diagnosis of Tako-Tsubo cardiomyopathy and long-term prognosis. *Herz* 2010 Jun 3. [Epub ahead of print]
[40] Mitchell JH, Hadden TB, Wilson JM, Achari A, Muthupillai R, Flamm SD. Clinical features and usefulness of cardiac magnetic resonance imaging in assessing

myocardial viability and prognosis in Takotsubo cardiomyopathy (transient left ventricular apical ballooning syndrome). *Am J Cardiol* 2007;100:296-301.

[41] Deetjen AG, Conradi G, Mollmann S, Rad A, Hamm CW, Dill T. Value of gadolinium-enhanced magnetic resonance imaging in patients with Tako-Tsubo-like left ventricular dysfunction. *J Cardiovasc Magn Reson* 2006;8:367-72.

[42] Madhavan M, Rihal CS, Lerman A, Prasad A. Acute heart failure in apical ballooning syndrome (TakoTsubo/stress cardiomyopathy): clinical correlates and Mayo Clinic risk score. *J Am Coll Cardiol* 2011;57:1400-1.

[43] Tarkin JM, Khetyar M, Kaski JC. Management of Tako-tsubo syndrome. *Cardiovasc Drugs Ther* 2008;22:71-7.

[44] Nef HM, Möllmann H, Kostin S, Troidl C, Voss S, Weber M, Dill T, Rolf A, Brandt R, Hamm CW, Elsässer A. Tako-Tsubo cardiomyopathy: intraindividual structural analysis in the acute phase and after functional recovery. *Eur Heart J* 2007;28:2456-64.

[45] Nef HM, Möllmann H, Elsässer A. Tako-tsubo cardiomyopathy (apical ballooning). *Heart* 2007;93:1309-15.

[46] Nef HM, Möllmann H, Troidl C, Kostin S, Voss S, Hilpert P, Behrens CB, Rolf A, Rixe J, Weber M, Hamm CW, Elsässer A. Abnormalities in intracellular Ca2+ regulation contribute to the pathomechanism of Tako-Tsubo cardiomyopathy. *Eur Heart J* 2009;30:2155-64.

[47] Nef HM, Möllmann H, Hilpert P, Troidl C, Voss S, Rolf A, Behrens CB, Weber M, Hamm CW, Elsässer A. Activated cell survival cascade protects cardiomyocytes from cell death in Tako-Tsubo cardiomyopathy. *Eur J Heart Fail* 2009;11:758-64.

[48] Akashi YJ, Nef HM, Möllmann H, Ueyama T. Stress cardiomyopathy. *Annu Rev Med* 2010;61:271-86.

[49] Nef HM, Möllmann H, Akashi YJ, Hamm CW. Mechanisms of stress (Takotsubo) cardiomyopathy. *Nat Rev Cardiol* 2010;7:187-93.

[50] Villareal RP, Achari A, Wilansky S, Wilson JM. Anteroapical stunning and left ventricular outflow tract obstruction. *Mayo Clin Proc* 2001;76:79-83.

[51] Fefer P, Chelvanathan A, Dick AJ, Teitelbaum EJ, Strauss BH, Cohen EA. Takotsubo cardiomyopathy and left ventricular outflow tract obstruction. *J Interv Cardiol* 2009;22:444-52.

[52] El Mahmoud R, Mansencal N, Pilliére R, Leyer F, Abbou N, Michaud P, Nallet O, Digne F, Lacombe P, Cattan S, Dubourg O. Prevalence and characteristics of left ventricular outflow tract obstruction in Tako-Tsubo syndrome. *Am Heart J* 2008;156:543-8.

[53] Merli E, Sutcliffe S, Gori M, Sutherland GG. Tako-Tsubo cardiomyopathy: new insights into the possible underlying pathophysiology. *Eur J Echocardiogr* 2006;7:53-61.

[54] Shah BN, Curzen NP. Dynamic left ventricular outflow tract obstruction and acute heart failure in tako-tsubo cardiomyopathy. *J Am Coll Cardiol* 2011;58:1195-6.

[55] Gianni M, Dentali F, Grandi AM, Sumner G, Hiralal R, Lonn E. Apical ballooning syndrome or takotsubo cardiomyopathy: a systematic review. *Eur Heart J* 2006;27:1523-9.

[56] Ibanez B, Choi BG, Navarro F, Farre J. Tako-tsubo syndrome: a form of spontaneous aborted myocardial infarction? *Eur Heart J* 2006;27:1509-10.

[57] Desmet W. Dynamic LV obstruction in apical ballooning syndrome: the chicken or the egg. *Eur J Echocardiogr* 2006;7:1-4.
[58] Pilgrim TM, Wyss TR. Takotsubo cardiomyopathy or transient left ventricular apical ballooning syndrome: A systematic review. *Int J Cardiol* 2008;124:283-92.
[59] Kurisu S, Inoue I, Kawagoe T, Ishihara M, Shimatani Y, Nishioka K, Umemura T, Nakamura S, Yoshida M, Sato H. Myocardial perfusion and fatty acid metabolism in patients with tako-tsubo-like left ventricular dysfunction. *J Am Coll Cardiol* 2003;41:743-8.
[60] Kume T, Akasaka T, Kawamoto T, Watanabe N, Yoshitani H, Akiyama M, Koyama Y, Neishi Y, Tsukiji M, Yoshida K. [Relationship between coronary flow reserve and recovery of regional left ventricular function in patients with tako-tsubo-like transient left ventricular dysfunction]. *J Cardiol* 2004;43:123-9.
[61] Trevi GP, Sheiban I. Chronic ischaemic ('hibernating') and postischaemic ('stunned') dysfunctional but viable myocardium. *Eur Heart J* 1991;12 Suppl G:20-6.
[62] Akashi YJ, Nakazawa K, Sakakibara M, Miyake F, Koike H, Sasaka K. The clinical features of takotsubo cardiomyopathy. *QJM* 2003;96:563-73.
[63] Goldstein DS, Eisenhofer G, Kopin IJ. Sources and significance of plasma levels of catechols and their metabolites in humans. *J Pharmacol Exp Ther* 2003;305:800-11.
[64] Volz HC, Erbel C, Berentelg J, Katus HA, Frey N. Reversible left ventricular dysfunction resembling Takotsubo syndrome after self-injection of adrenaline. *Can J Cardiol* 2009;25:e261-2.
[65] Litvinov IV, Kotowycz MA, Wassmann S. Iatrogenic epinephrine-induced reverse Takotsubo cardiomyopathy: direct evidence supporting the role of catecholamines in the pathophysiology of the "broken heart syndrome." *Clin Res Cardiol* 2009;98:457-62.
[66] Khullar M, Datta BN, Wahi PL, Chakravarti RN. Catecholamine-induced experimental cardiomyopathy--a histopathological, histochemical and ultrastructural study. *Indian Heart J* 1989;41:307-13.
[67] Singal PK, Kapur N, Dhillon KS, Beamish RE, Dhalla NS. Role of free radicals in catecholamine-induced cardiomyopathy. *Can J Physiol Pharmacol* 1982;60:1390-7.
[68] Bolli R, Marbán E. Molecular and cellular mechanisms of myocardial stunning. Physiol Rev 1999;79:609-34.
[69] Mori H, Ishikawa S, Kojima S, Hayashi J, Watanabe Y, Hoffman JI, Okino H. Increased responsiveness of left ventricular apical myocardium to adrenergic stimuli. *Cardiovasc Res* 1993;27:192-8.
[70] Stein B, Bartel S, Kirchhefer U, Kokott S, Krause EG, Neumann J, Schmitz W, Scholz H. Relation between contractile function and regulatory cardiac proteins in hypertrophied hearts. *Am J Physiol* 1996;270(6 Pt 2):H2021-8.
[71] Boluyt MO, Long X, Eschenhagen T, Mende U, Schmitz W, Crow MT, Lakatta EG. Isoproterenol infusion induces alterations in expression of hypertrophy-associated genes in rat heart. *Am J Physiol* 1995;269(2 Pt 2):H638-47.
[72] Babu GJ, Bhupathy P, Petrashevskaya NN, Wang H, Raman S, Wheeler D, Jagatheesan G, Wieczorek D, Schwartz A, Janssen PM, Ziolo MT, Periasamy M. Targeted overexpression of sarcolipin in the mouse heart decreases sarcoplasmic reticulum calcium transport and cardiac contractility. *J Biol Chem* 2006;281:3972-9.

[73] Asahi M, Otsu K, Nakayama H, Hikoso S, Takeda T, Gramolini AO, Trivieri MG, Oudit GY, Morita T, Kusakari Y, Hirano S, Hongo K, Hirotani S, Yamaguchi O, Peterson A, Backx PH, Kurihara S, Hori M, MacLennan DH. Cardiac-specific overexpression of sarcolipin inhibits sarco(endo)plasmic reticulum Ca2+ ATPase (SERCA2a) activity and impairs cardiac function in mice. *Proc Natl Acad Sci U S A* 2004;101:9199-204.

[74] Linck B, Bokník P, Baba HA, Eschenhagen T, Haverkamp U, Jäckel E, Jones LR, Kirchhefer U, Knapp J, Läer S, Müller FU, Schmitz W, Scholz H, Syska A, Vahlensieck U, Neumann J. Long-term beta adrenoceptor-mediated alteration in contractility and expression of phospholamban and sarcoplasmic reticulum Ca(++)-ATPase in mammalian ventricle. *J Pharmacol Exp Ther* 1998;286:531-8.

[75] Lipskaia L, Lompré AM. Alteration in temporal kinetics of Ca2+ signaling and control of growth and proliferation. *Biol Cell* 2004;96:55-68.

[76] Port JD, Bristow MR. Altered beta-adrenergic receptor gene regulation and signaling in chronic heart failure. *J Mol Cell Cardiol* 2001;33:887-905.

[77] Heubach JF, Ravens U, Kaumann AJ. Epinephrine activates both Gs and Gi pathways, but norepinephrine activates only the Gs pathway through human beta2-adrenoceptors overexpressed in mouse heart. *Mol Pharmacol* 2004;65:1313-22.

[78] Heubach JF, Blaschke M, Harding SE, Ravens U, Kaumann AJ. Cardiostimulant and cardiodepressant effects through overexpressed human beta2-adrenoceptors in murine heart: regional differences and functional role of beta1-adrenoceptors. *Naunyn Schmiedebergs Arch Pharmacol* 2003;367:380-90.

[79] Zamah AM, Delahunty M, Luttrell LM, Lefkowitz RJ. Protein kinase A-mediated phosphorylation of the beta 2-adrenergic receptor regulates its coupling to Gs and Gi. Demonstration in a reconstituted system. *J Biol Chem* 2002;277:31249-56.

[80] Kawano H, Okada R, Yano K. Histological study on the distribution of autonomic nerves in the human heart. *Heart Vessels* 2003;18:32-9.

[81] Kuroko Y, Yamazaki T, Tokunaga N, Akiyama T, Kitagawa H, Ishino K, Sano S, Mori H. Cardiac epinephrine synthesis and ischemia-induced myocardial epinephrine release. *Cardiovasc Res* 2007;74:438-44.

[82] Grohé C, Kahlert S, Löbbert K, Stimpel M, Karas RH, Vetter H, Neyses L. Cardiac myocytes and fibroblasts contain functional estrogen receptors. *FEBS Lett* 1997;416:107-12.

[83] Bupha-Intr T, Wattanapermpool J. Regulatory role of ovarian sex hormones in calcium uptake activity of cardiac sarcoplasmic reticulum. *Am J Physiol Heart Circ Physiol* 2006;291:H1101-8.

[84] Burgdorf C, Nef HM, Haghi D, Kurowski V, Radke PW. Tako-tsubo (stress-induced) cardiomyopathy and cancer. *Ann Intern Med* 2010;152:830-1.

[85] Harding SE, Gong H. beta-adrenoceptor blockers as agonists: coupling of beta2-adrenoceptors to multiple G-proteins in the failing human heart. *Congest Heart Fail* 2004;10:181-5; quiz 186-7.

[86] Padayachee L. Levosimendan: the inotrope of choice in cardiogenic shock secondary to takotsubo cardiomyopathy? *Heart Lung Circ* 2007;16 Suppl 3:S65-70.

[87] De Santis V, Vitale D, Tritapepe L, Greco C, Pietropaoli P. Use of levosimendan for cardiogenic shock in a patient with the apical ballooning syndrome. *Ann Intern Med* 2008;149:365-7.

[88] Antonini M, Stazi GV, Cirasa MT, Garotto G, Frustaci A. Efficacy of levosimendan in Takotsubo-related cardiogenic shock. *Acta Anaesthesiol Scand* 2010;54:119-20.

[89] Brown ML, Abel MD, Click RL, Morford RG, Dearani JA, Sundt TM, Orszulak TA, Schaff HV. Systolic anterior motion after mitral valve repair: is surgical intervention necessary? *J Thor Cardiovasc Surg* 2007;133:136-43.

[90] Madhavan M, Pislaru SV, Prasad A. Reply. *J Am Coll Cardiol* 2011;58:1196.

[91] Kyuma M, Tsuchihashi K, Shinshi Y, Hase M, Nakata T, Ooiwa H, Abiru M, Hikita N, Adachi T, Shoji T, Fujise Y, Shimamoto K. Effect of intravenous propranolol on left ventricular apical ballooning without coronary artery stenosis (ampulla cardiomyopathy): three cases. *Circ J* 2002;66:1181-4.

31

Pathology of Takotsubo (Ampulla) Cardiomyopathy

Sachio Kawai
Department of Cardiology, Juntendo University School of Medicine, Tokyo, Japan

1. Introduction

Takotsubo (ampulla) cardiomyopathy is characterized by slight to moderate elevation of cardiac enzymes. It is reasonable to think that the elevated levels are evidence of myocardial damage (cardiac-specific enzymes are released from the cytoplasm of damaged cardiac myocytes into extracellular fluid). Thus, it is problematic to consider takotsubo cardiomyopathy as (neurogenic) stunned myocardium, because stunned myocardium is defined as a state without histopathological changes observable by light microscopy.[1] In the study, I will describe histological findings in autopsied cases in Japan and histopathological findings of endomyocardial biopsy cases with a literature review.

2. Autopsied cases

Nine Japanese autopsied cases were studied, with the permission of relevant institutions. We examined their histopathological changes, findings in transverse tissue sections by site (near the left ventricular apex and base) and by layer (relative damage by depth of ventricular myocardium), and differences in lesions.[2] Table 1 shows the age, sex, underlying diseases, trigger event, and symptoms of the cases.[3]

Case 2. A 66-year-old woman was admitted to the hospital with paralysis and brain infiltration by Hodgkin's lymphoma. Her symptoms improved with steroid therapy and radiation therapy. There was no clear trigger event. She developed sudden bradycardia, hypotension, and extensive ST-segment elevation. She underwent intravenous infusion of 2 mg epinephrine, and subsequently developed chest pain. The patient had a normal coronary angiogram, extensive hypokinesis mainly in the apical segment, and hyperkinesis of the basal segment. Creatinine kinase level increased to 169 U/l at a maximum. There was no pulmonary congestion, but severe hypoxemia continued and the patient died on the fourth day of illness.[4] Autopsy showed neither significant coronary artery stenosis nor significant fibrosis in the ventricular transverse sections near the apical or basal segment. The ventricular wall were thickened; 15.2 mm in the basal anterior wall, 13.8 mm in the basal lateral wall, 13.2 mm in the basal posterior wall, 17.5 mm in the basal interventricular septum, 10.0 mm in the apical anterior wall, 13.0 mm in the apical lateral wall, 10.2 mm in the apical posterior wall, and 8.0 mm in the apical interventricular septum. Histologically, there was disseminated or diffuse damage to the cardiac myocytes, and extensive damage was observed from the inner to outer layer. In general, pathological changes were myocyte damage, degeneration, lysis, or loss occurring in an individual myocyte or several myocytes. Some cases had lesions concentrated on specific muscle bundles and other cases had disseminated lesions (Figure 1, upper left). In addition, higher degree of cell infiltration was seen at sites with more severely damaged myocardium (Figure 1, lower left).

Cases	Underlying Disorders	Trigger Event	Initial Symptoms	Duration (cause of death)
61 F	RA, pneumonia	Septic shock	Syncope	2 days (sepsis)
66 F	Hodgkin, HT,	Epinephrine injection	Syncope	4 days (dyspnea)
75 M	Anorexia	Pneumonia	Pulmo. edema	20 days (pneumonia)
77 M	DM, CRF, Multiple myeloma	Leg ulcer	Chest pain	19 days (sepsis)
81 F	RA, HT	Pneumonia	Dyspnea	21 days (pulmo.hemo.)
81 F	Pneumonia	Dyspnea	Dyspnea	3 days (ARDS)
82 F	Bronchial asthma	Unknown	Syncope	20 days (sepsis)
83 F	HT	None	Palpitation	5 days (tamponade)
84 F	None	None	Chest pain	4 days (tamponade)

This table shows autopsied patients. The patients were composed of seven elderly females and two males aged 61 to 84 years. They had several serious underlying disorders and some patients had trigger events such as septic shock, injection of epinephrine, pneumonia. Initial symptoms were syncope or pulmonary edema, dyspnea or chest pain. They died from sepsis, respiratory failure, pneumonia, pulmonary hemorrhage, or cardiac tamponade. The duration of takotsubo cardiomyopathy ranged from 2 to 21 days.

Table 1. Autopsied cases

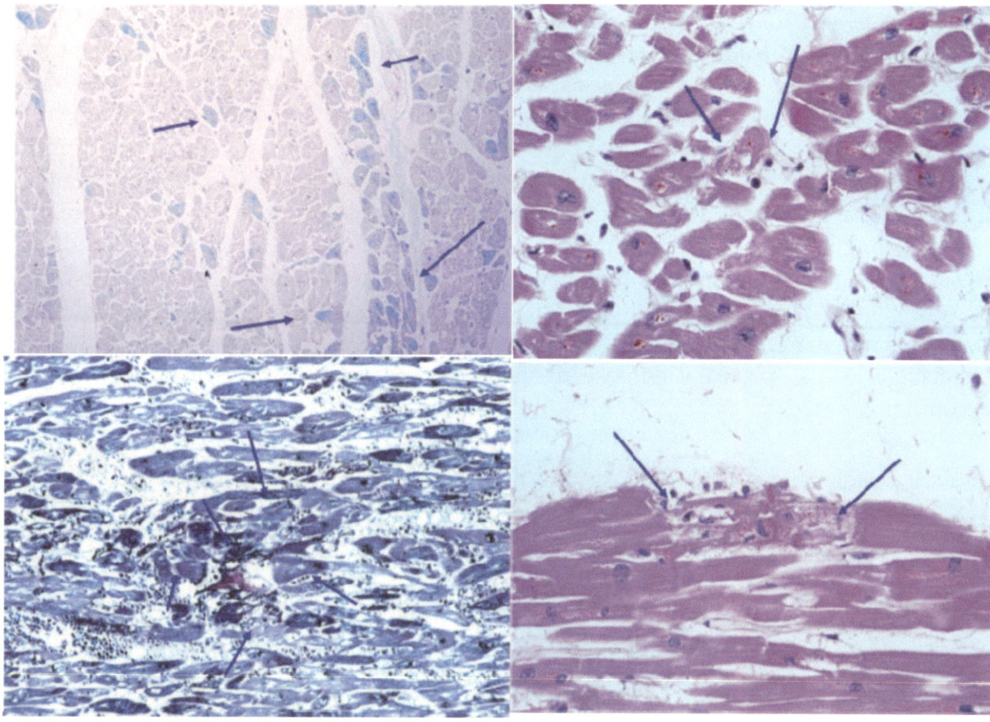

Upper left: Damaged individual myocytes or a group of myocytes had increased eosinophil staining. Inner layer of the base: Luxol fast blue stain, x 200. (Case 2 : 66y-o, Female)

Lower left: Middle layer of the apex: Phosphoptungstic acid hematoxylin stain, x 200. (Case 2 : 66y-o, Female)

Upper right: Injured cardiac myocytes are removed by infiltrated macrophages. Apical anterior, middle layer. Hematoxylin and eosin (H&E) stain, x 400. (Case 5 : 81Y-o, Female)

Lower right: Myocardial damage was observed even in the epicardial aspect which was difficult to explain by disorder of coronary circulation. Apical posterior, external layer. H&E stain, x 400. (Case 5 : 81Y-o, Female)

Fig. 1. Pathology of takotsubo cardiomyopathy

Case 5. An 81-year-old woman had chronic rheumatoid arthritis. She also had hypertension. She was admitted to the hospital due to pneumonia. Pneumonia was resistant to treatment. On the tenth day of hospitalization, she developed dyspnea after walking to the bathroom. Electrocardiography showed ST-segment elevation in leads I, II, aVL, and V2-6. Her blood pressure was 80 mm Hg and she went into shock. Emergency coronary angiography showed basal hyperkinesis, apical ballooning, and apical hypokinesis but no significant stenosis. Pulmonary artery wedge pressure was 20 mm Hg and the creatinine kinase level was 296 U/l. The patient developed acute respiratory distress syndrome and died on the eleventh day of hospitalization (second day of Takotsubo cardiomyopathy).[5] Histologically, a group of myocytes showed an increase in eosinophil staining, contraction band formation, necrosis, and rupture. Damaged individual myocytes were ingested by infiltrated macrophages (Figure 1, upper right). Myocardial damage was also seen in the epicardial aspect which was difficult to explain by disorder of coronary circulation (Figure 1, lower right).

Case 8. An 83-year-old woman was suspected as fulminant myocarditis. There was ST-segment elevation in leads II, III, aVF, and V2-6. The patient had extensive akinesis of the left ventricular apex and hyperkinesis of the base. Emergency coronary angiography showed no stenosis. Endomyocardial biopsy showed myocardial degeneration and necrosis, and inflammatory cell infiltration. The patient was diagnosed as fulminant myocarditis. She underwent intra-aortic balloon pumping, steroid pulse therapy, and percutaneous cardiopulmonary support. The patient died on the sixth day. Autopsy revealed an enlarged heart weighing 540 g and cardiac tamponade of 310 ml. The microscopic findings indicated myocardial damage consistent with other takotsubo cardiomyopathy cases and extensive and severe secondary cell infiltration (Figure 2). Interstitial cell infiltration was prominent and concentrated in areas with severe myocardial damage. Secondary findings included hemorrhage in the epicardial adipose tissue at the pulmonary arterial root and amyloid deposition.

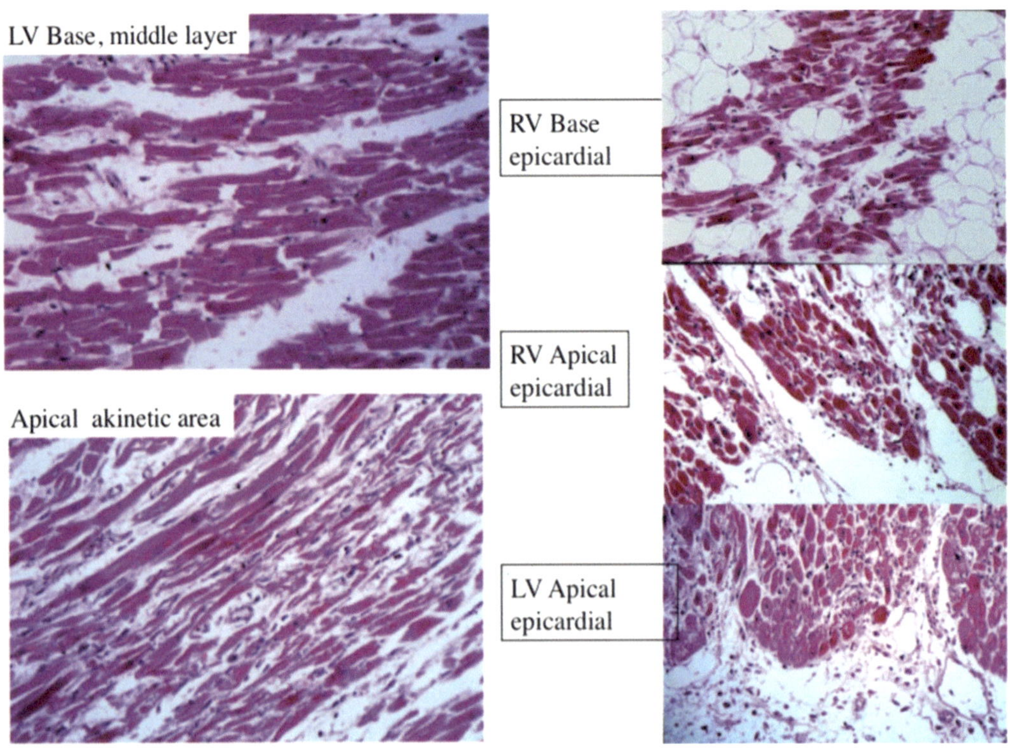

Marked segmentation of myocytes was observed in the middle layer of the hyperkinetic basal left ventricle (**lower left**). Damaged cells had undergone atrophy and lysis in the akinetic apical segment (lower left). There were similar lesions in the right ventricle. Segmentation was seen even in myocytes which were sparse in the adipose tissue in the basal outer layer (**upper right**). In the right ventricle in the apical aspect (**middle right**), there were marked myocyte injuries and lysis and interstitial cell infiltration in addition to segmentation. Similarly, when the apical left ventricle in the epicardial aspect (**lower right**) was examined, there was myocyte damage near the epicardial aspect and cell infiltration into the epicardium. Myocardial tissue: H&E stain, x200.

Fig. 2. Autopsied case: 83-year-old woman suspected of fulminant myocarditis

Figure 3 shows single myocyte lesions in the left ventricle in other cases. In this figure, two injured myocytes were observed. The myocardial injury did not extended to the adjacent myocytes.

3. Right ventricular lesion

When more detailed microscopic examinations were performed, there were also right ventricular lesions (Figure 4).

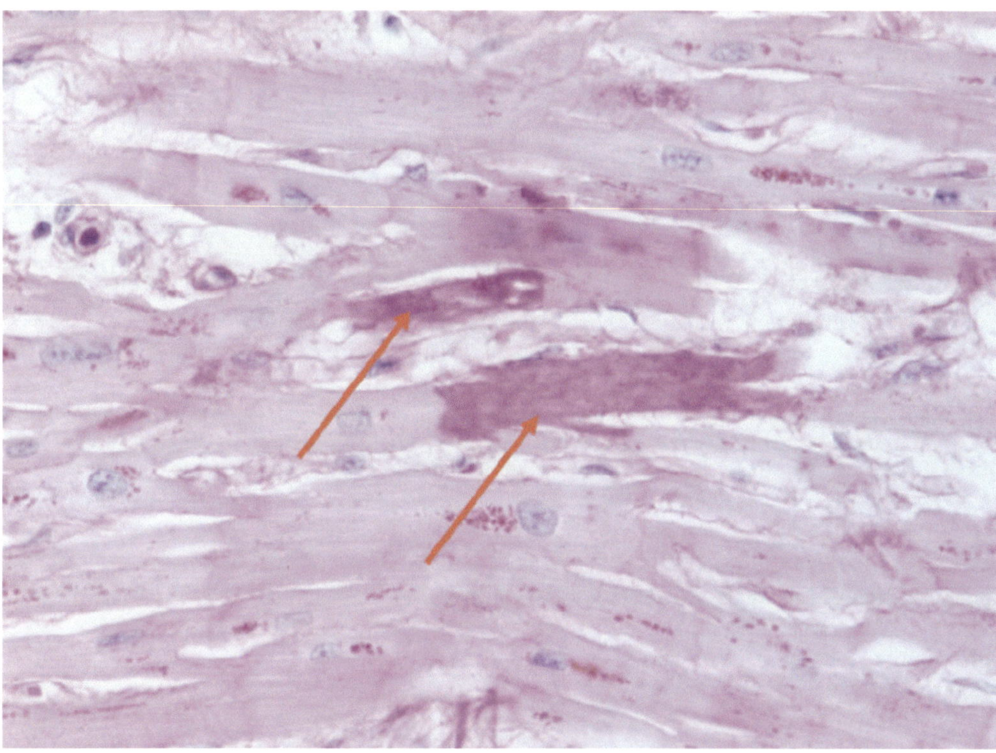

In this figure, two injured myocytes were observed (**red arrows**). The myocardial injury did not extended to the adjacent myocytes. Periodic acid Schiff reaction, x1000.

Fig. 3. Single myocyte lesions

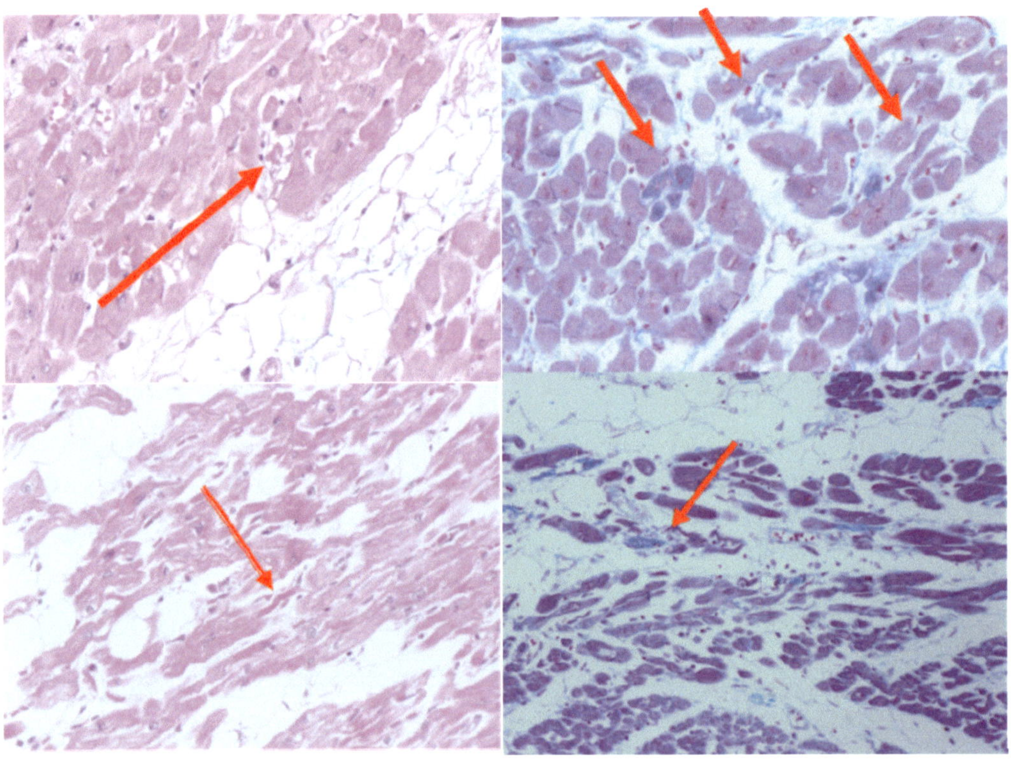

Upper left: 81 y-o, apical region, H&E stain, x 200
Lower left: 66 y-o, H&E stain, x 200
Upper right: 81 y-o, apical. H&E stain, x 200
Lower right: 84 y-o, H&E stain, x 300

Fig. 4. Right ventricular lesions

4. Morphometrical studies

The number of damaged myocytes relative to the number of myocytes comprising the ventricular wall (layer) were examined in the transverse section specimens of the ventricular apex and base. The transverse section specimen were scanned under high power view along two perpendicular lines (Figure 5). Increased eosinophilic staining (azan-blue stained degeneration), segmentation,[7] myofibrillar agglomeration with disrupted cross striation structure, and myofibrillar degeneration, lysis, and loss (showing fragmentation) were counted as the damaged myocytes. The myocytes with normal cross striation structure were not considered as damaged cells. The damaged myocytes to the number of the myocytes comprising the ventricular wall was calculated. This ratio (in percentage) was significantly higher in the apical segment at 13.5% than in the basal segment at 5.3% (Table 2) .

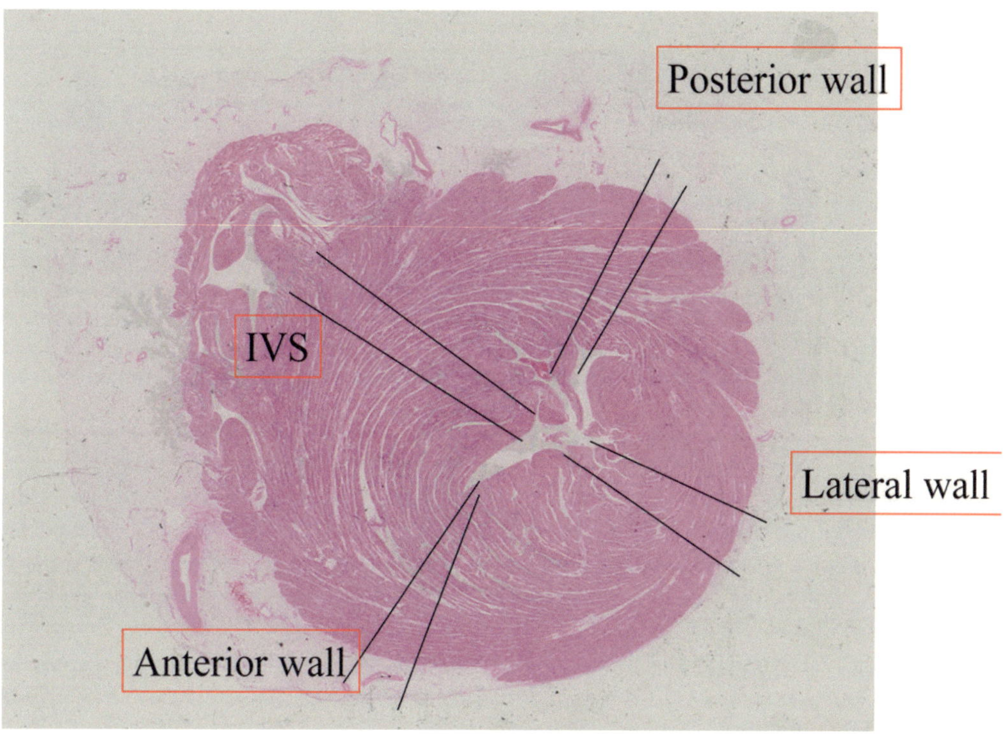

Autopsy study: The number of myocardial cells comprising the compact layer of the ventricular wall and the numbers of the damaged myocytes were counted as follows. Two sampling lines perpendicular to the compact layer were drawn from the outer to the inner layers, and the numbers of the normal myocardial cells and the damaged myocytes intersecting the lines were determined employing an image analyzer. The mean values were determined at 4 sites on the transverse section: the anterior, lateral and, posterior walls of the left ventricle, the middle-portion of the interventricular septum. Transverse sections from the cardiac base and the apical segment were scanned.

Fig. 5. Percentage of the injured myocytes (morphometrical measurement)

Cases	Apical section					Basal section				
	A	L	P	IVS	mean (%)	A	L	P	IVS	mean
61F	10.0	11.4	10.3	10.3	10.5	3.5	5.2	6.5	5.1	5.1
66F	10.9	6.2	2.3	8.8	7.1	3.0	4.3	2.5	2.0	3.0
75M	14.3	12,0	12.2	12.0	12.6	3.2	5.4	5.8	5.1	4.9
77M	9.3	11.9	7.2	6.5	6.3	3.2	4.3	2.8	2.7	3.3
81F	10.7	12.0	8.0	10.1	10.2	3.5	5.4	4.4	5.0	4.6
81F	16.8	17.0	18.3	14.7	16.7	5.4	5.7	4.7	5.0	5.2
82F	14.5	17.1	12.6	12.6	13.9	7.8	8.0	6.2	4.7	6.7
83F	15.8	19.8	29.6	33.1	23.6	9.5	5.8	5.3	9.8	7.6
84F	23.0	20.0	21.7	17.9	20.7	10.1	17.1	19.6	12.0	14.7
mean					13.5					6.4

A: anterior wall, L: lateral wall, P: posterior wall, IVS: interventricular septum

Percentage of damaged myocytes to the number of the myocytes comprising the ventricular wall was tabled in this slide.

The left-sided figures were percentages of the damaged myocytes in the apical portion. The figures of the right were those from the basal segments. Percentages of the damaged myocytes in Takotsubo cardiomyopathy were relatively small compared to those of injured myocytes in patients with myocardial infarction. There is significant difference in the distribution of the myocardial lesion between cardiac base and the apical region. Percentages of the damaged myocytes were higher in the apical area than in the basal segment.

Table 2. Percentage of relative myocardial damage

Transverse sections of the left ventricular anterior wall were examined near the base and apex (myocardial transverse sections observed from the epicardial and endocardial aspects). A light microscope was used with a grid in the eyepiece (42-point "Weibel" test grid) to measure the relative density of capillaries. In the 21-line segments in the test grid, the number of capillaries was counted in each of 10 fields of view. The relative density of capillaries was 7.1 ± 1.01 in the base and 6.5 ± 0.96 in the apex, indicating no significant difference. These densities could not explain the difference in damaged myocytes by site or the difference in wall motion by site.

5. Relative injury score

Percentage of damaged myocytes to the number of the myocytes comprising the ventricular wall is tabled in the Table 3. The upper figures are percentages of the damaged myocytes in the basal portion. The lower figures were those from the apical segments. Percentages of the damaged myocytes in Takotsubo cardiomyopathy were relatively small compared to those of injured myocytes in patients with myocardial infarction. There is a significant difference in the distribution of the myocardial lesion between the cardiac base and the apical region. Percentages of the damaged myocytes were higher in the apical area than in the basal segment. The damage was particularly severe in the trabeculae carneae of the anterior wall (by site) and the subendocardium (by layer) .

Basal	Anterior	Lateral	Posterior	Septal	
Subendocardium	21.2%	21.1%	22.3%		21.6%
Inner layer	24.0%	22.6%	23.2%	19.2%	22.2%
Middle layer	22.1%	24.8%	24.5%	21.8%	23.3%
Outer layer	17.6%	18.3%	15.0%	19.7%	17.7%
	21.2%	21.7%	21.3%	20.2%	

Apical	Anterior	Lateral	Posterior	Septal	
Subendocardium	33.5% **	21.5%	24.5%		26.5%
Inner layer	29.4%	27.1%	23.8%	26.5%	26.7%*
Middle layer	33.3% *	28.9%	23.8%	29.3%	28.8%*
Outer layer	24.8% *	22.8%	21.2%*	26.5%*	23.8%
	30.2%*	25.1%	23.3%*	27.4%*	

*:p<0.05, **p<0.01

Percentage of damaged myocytes to the number of the myocytes in the several layers (the subendocardium and trabeculla layers, the inner layers, the middle layers and the outer layers of the anterior, the lateral, the posterior wall and the interventricular septum) was tabled in the Table 3. The upper figures were percentages of the damaged myocytes in the basal portion. The lower figures were those from the apical segments. There is a significant difference in the distribution of the myocardial lesion between the cardiac base and the apical region. Percentages of the damaged myocytes were higher in the apical area than in the basal segment. The damage was particularly severe in the trabeculae carneae of the anterior wall (by site) and the subendocardium (by layer) .

Table 3. Relative Injury Score

6. Summary of cardiac autopsy findings

Clear myocardial lesions were observed in takotsubo cardiomyopathy cases. Epicardial lesions were observed (Figure 1, lower right) which are uncommon in ischemia. Right ventricular lesions were also observed (Figure 4). The myocardial lesions were characterized mainly by individual myocytes or a group of myocytes with increased eosinophil staining , contraction band formation, necrosis, and rupture. The basis of the lesion was a damaged individual myocyte (Figure 3) and aggregation of these damaged myocytes (Figure 1, upper left. If individual myocyte damage occurs due to disorder of microcirculatory units composing the intramyocardial circulatory system,[8] it is difficult to explain pathological changes of takotsubo cardiomyopathy as intramyocardial circulatory disorder.

The extension of lesion was near circumferential within the same ventricle and it tended to be prominent from the mid-portion to apex of the ventricle. In histological measurement, the proportion of damaged myocytes was higher in the apex than the base (mid-portion).

Damage was prominent in the apical inner and middle layers (by ventricular myocardial layer) and in the anterior wall, posterior wall, and septum (by site). The damage was particularly severe in the trabeculae carneae of the anterior wall (by site) and subendocardium (by layer) (Table 3). These results indicate that it might be possible to depict predilection sites by MRI with delayed gadolinium enhancement.[9]

Autopsy cases with myocardial diseases were reported in the regional meetings of the Japanese Circulation Society. There have been many recent reports such as on a 77-year-old woman with myocardial infarction-like electrocardiographic pattern during the course of malabsorption syndrome[10] and on an 84-year-old woman who died from cardiac rupture[11] (four days after the onset, cardiac arrest occurred due to cardiac rupture). In the Circulation Journal, Sacha et al.[12] stated the case of Ohara et al.[13] in the same journal as the first autopsy case [of takotsubo cardiomyopathy] and their own case was the second one. However, this information is not accurate. There were previously reported autopsy cases in the journals Heart and Respiration & Circulation. There were reports of takotsubo cardiomyopathy itself by Kumamoto et al.,[14] Sasa et al.,[15] and Tokioka et al.[16] Thus, there were already reports of takotsubo cardiomyopathy as a phenomenon, and autopsy cases were published in a journal[17] before that of Ohara et al. Thus, Sacha et al. should have been advised to revise the information in the peer review.

7. Case presentation of endomyocardial biopsy

Table 4 shows 15 cases of endomyocardial biopsy for which relevant institutions provided approval for microscopic examination. The cases are listed in the order of number of days from onset to biopsy.

8. Case biopsied on the day of onset (Case 2)

The patient was an 82-year-old woman who had undergone uterine myomectomy at age 48. She developed sudden pharyngeal discomfort. There was ST-segment elevation in leads II, III, aVF, and V2-6. Echocardiography showed diffuse hypokinesis except in the base. Ventriculography revealed hyperkinesis of the base and balloon-like enlargement of the apex. She was suspected of myocarditis and underwent biopsy. Her condition improved on the 26th day of illness. Biopsy showed slight increase in young connective tissue and infiltration of cells, including polymorphonuclear leukocytes (Figure 6, upper left).

9. Case thought to have a ventricular aneurysm (Case 7)

The patient was a 69-year-old man with no contributory medical history. He became lost in the mountains while gathering edible wild plants and was rescued 7 hours later. He experienced shortness of breath thereafter and had pleural effusion 18 days later. Coronary angiography revealed 90% occlusion in #11 and complete occlusion in peripheral #12. There was also unexplainable severe left ventricular asynergy and an apical mural thrombus. Biopsy showed cell-rich fibrosis. One week later, his condition improved except in the circumflex branch and apical regions. He underwent resection of a ventricular aneurysm 2.5 months later. Histologically, ventricular aneurysm was endocardial fibroelastosis. There was also a full-thickness loss of myocytes, leaving only a small amount of remaining myocytes in the inner layer, and fibrosis with flaccidity (Figure 6, lower left).

Case Number	Gender/Age	Underlying disorders	Trigger event	Symptoms	Day of biopsy	Biopsy pathology
1	F/71	Premature ventricular contraction, Hypertension	Status after sigmoid colon surgery, Dehydration, Cessation of beta blocking agent	Chest pain	1	Cell infiltrations, myocardial depletion
2	F/82	Neurosis	None	Anorexia, throat discomfort	1	Small round cell infiltration (including polymorphonuclear leukocytes), myocyte injury
3	F/64	pulmonary fibrosis	Attempted suicide, Near drowning	Dyspnea	4	Small round cell infiltration
4	F/75	None	None	Dyspnea, chest discomfort	5	Myocardial depletion, slight fibrosis with lymphocyte infiltration
5	M/48	hypertension	none	Sudden chest pain	5	Focal depletion, myocardial fibrosis
					30	Focal, patchy fibrosis
6	F/63	Angina pectoris	Emotional stress	Palpitation, Dyspnea, chest and back pain	10	Myocardial fibrosis, myocardial depletion, fibrocellular proliferation
7	M/69	None	distress in the mountain	Pleural effusion	11	Cell-rich fibrosis, Focal depletion, small round cell infiltration
					3 months	Fibrous ventricular aneurysm
8	F/68	Paf, HT, AP, AR severe	None	Syncope, cough	12	Myocardial fibrosis with mild cell infiltrates
9	F/60	Hypertension	None	Cough, Dyspnea, preshock	15	Focal fibrosis, interstitial edema
10	F/59	Hypertension, Hyperlipidemia	Memorial service for her grandmother	Chest pain	17	Focal myocardial depletion, increase of connective tissue with cell infiltration
11	F/57	Sarcoidosis, hyperlipemia	Quarrel with neighbour	Chest pain	20	Intermysial fibrosis, edema, sight cell infiltrates
12	F/76	Diabetes mellitus	None	Dyspnea	22	Myocardial depletion cell-rich, fibrosis, replacemntal
13	F/76	Status after mammary cancer, cataracta	Admission of her husband, stress from common cold	chest pain	23	old perivascular fibrosis, slight cell infiltrates
14	M/53	Heavy drinker, Acute renal failure	Hypotension, Hemofiltration, Dopamine	Dyspnea	26	Patchy fibrosis, myocardial depletion, cell infiltration
15	F/74	pulmonary tuberculosis	Quarrel with neighbour for 6 months	Sudden chest pain	28	Perimyocardial fibrosis

This table shows 15 cases received biopsy or myocardial resection. Table was listed according to the day of biopsy; from 1st day to 28th day. Case 5 and case 7 had two samples. They received serial biopsy or aneurysmectomy.

Six patients had no trigger event, and seven patients' symptoms were not chest pain. Cases in early phase, from 1st day to 4th day biopsy, showed cell infiltration, myocardial depletion, and myocardial injury. Cases in late phase that is 12th day or later, showed focal fibrosis.

Table 4. Endomyocardial biopsy cases

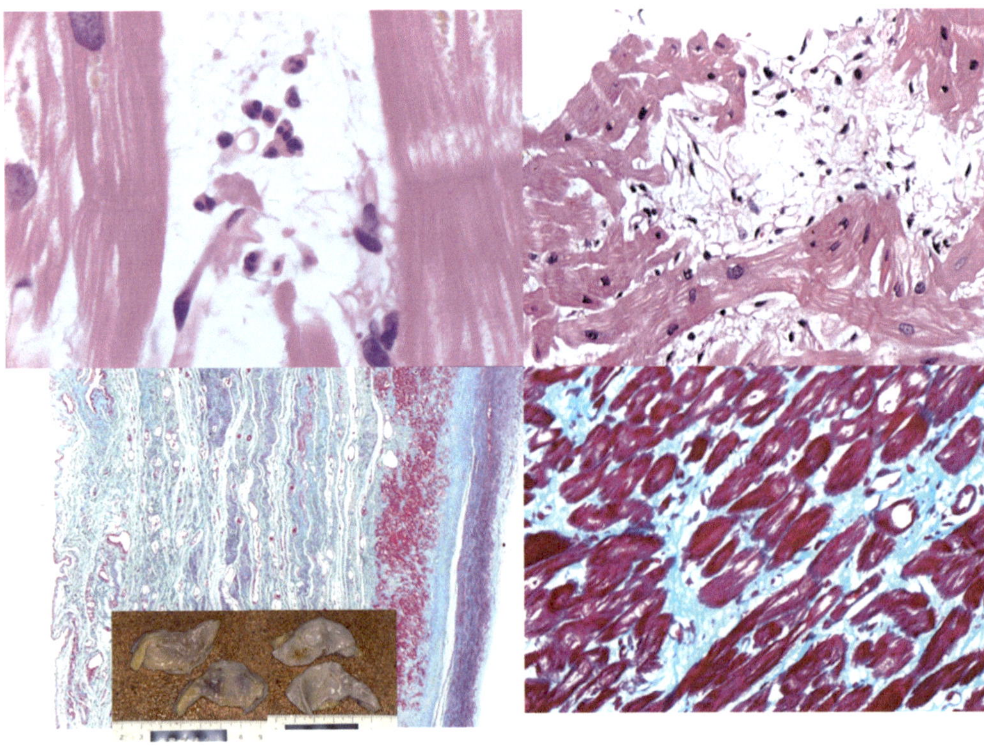

Upper left: Case biopsied on the day of onset (Case 2), biopsy showed slight increase in young connective tissue and infiltration of cells, including polymorphonuclear leukocytes .
Lower left: Case thought to have a ventricular aneurysm (Case 7), histologically, ventricular aneurysm was endocardial fibroelastosis. There was also a full-thickness loss of myocytes, leaving only a small amount of remaining myocytes in the inner layer, and fibrosis with flaccidity.
Upper right: Case with serial biopsies (Case 5 the biopsy on the fifth day), there was loss of myocytes and increase in young connective tissue rich in cellular elements
Lower right: Case with serial biopsies (Case 5 the biopsy one month later), mature connective tissue was observed in the myocardium.

Fig. 6. Pathology of endomyocardial biopsy

10. Case with serial biopsies (Case 5)

The patient was a 48-year-old man who had hypertension since 1996 for which he was treated by a calcium channel blocker. At 4 AM on September 5, 1998, he suddenly experienced chest pain which lasted 20 minutes. He developed mild chest pain at 5 PM and admitted to the hospital at 9 PM. His white blood cell count was moderately elevated at 16000. Electrocardiography revealed no abnormality but echocardiography revealed extensive asynergy mainly in the apex. Emergency cardiac catheterization was performed while nitrate was administered. Coronary angiography was normal, but left ventriculography showed takotsubo-like ballooning. The patient complained of severe chest pain during the procedure. For the first time, the patient showed ST-segment elevation of 6 mm in the precordial lead. When coronary angiography was performed again, no abnormality was observed and coronary blood flow indicated a hyperdynamic state. The patient underwent a conservative treatment and his symptoms improved after a few hours. A giant negative T-wave was subsequently observed, but left ventriculography showed a tendency for improvement one month later. Biopsy was performed on the fifth day, and there was loss of myocytes and increase in young connective tissue rich in cellular elements (Figure 6, upper right). Mature connective tissue was observed in the biopsy one month later (Figure 6, lower right).

11. Summary of biopsy findings

The trigger was assumed to be emotional stress in 8 cases. The initial symptom was chest pain in 7 cases and dyspnea in 6 cases. Ventricular outflow tract obstruction was seen in 2 cases. Histological findings included focal fibrosis, cell infiltration including of polymorphonuclear leukocytes, and loss of myocytes. It was speculated that early cell infiltration was followed by changes over time, including loss of myocytes and focal fibrosis. Ventricular aneurysm was seen as a sequela in some cases.

12. Discussion

If cardiac enzyme levels are elevated, it is easy to speculate that myocardial tissue damage has developed. However, only a small percentage of cases undergoes endomyocardial biopsy. Kurisu et al.[18] characterized their findings of 3 cases that underwent endomyocardial biopsy as focal myocytolysis, mild mononuclear cell infiltration, and a slightly increased amount of connective tissue. For 5 cases that underwent endomyocardial biopsy, Akashi et al.[19] described the following findings suggestive of (chronic) myocarditis: lymphocytic infiltration, interstitial fibrosis, myocyte atrophy, and fatty infiltration. Gianni et al.[20] examined 15 cases in 4 papers and stated that there were no biopsy findings of myocarditis. Yoshida et al.[21] examined 9 cases that underwent endomyocardial biopsy. They found 4 cases with myocardial fibrosis, 3 cases with mononuclear cell infiltration, and 4 cases with contraction-band necrosis. However, none of the cases had significant inflammatory infiltrates or necrosis of myocytes. Pilgrim and Wyss[22] reviewed 5 reports including that of Kawai et al.[23] and described characteristics of focal loss of myocytes, contraction-band necrosis, interstitial fibrosis, and mild cell infiltration. For 5 cases that underwent biopsy, Von Korn et al.[24] found cell infiltration in 2 cases that satisfied the Dallas criteria. Wani et al.[25] found deposition of periodic-acid Schiff-positive material, fibrosis, enlargement, and lymphocyte and granulocyte infiltration. However, they ruled out myocarditis. Matsuyama et al.[26] performed an autopsy in a case of amyotrophic lateral sclerosis with takotsubo cardiomyopathy. They found disseminated areas of focal fibrosis and vacuolar degeneration of the myocytes.

Otsubo et al.[27] and Nef et al.[28] reported on findings from biopsies performed at the acute and recovery phases. In the acute phase, they found myocyte hypertrophy, glycogen granules of various sizes, contractile protein, disorder of the cytoskeleton, and increased extracellular matrix. However, they did not find oncocytic necrosis or apoptosis. The damage was completely resolved in a biopsy performed at the recovery phase. They concluded that morphological changes in takotsubo cardiomyopathy were caused by the disorder of microcirculation (due to excessive catecholamine) and direct myocardial damage by catecholamine.

There are a relatively large number of reports on myocarditis mimicking takotsubo cardiomyopathy.[29,30] Kubo et al.[31] also reported on a case of acute myocarditis diagnosed as takotsubo cardiomyopathy. A lesion of takotsubo cardiomyopathy can be morphologically similar to catecholamine cardiomyopathy and stress-induced cardiomyopathy.[32] Immediate changes in lesions of catecholamine cardiomyopathy are angioedema and interstitial edema. There are also loss of cross striation, vacuolization, and lipid droplets (disruption of myofibrils in electron microscopy). The change that occurs in a few hours is interstitial edema. Polymorphonuclear leukocyte infiltration also occurs followed by mononuclear cell infiltration. There are Antischkow cells near the blood vessels and arteriolar fibrinoid degeneration. (There was also contraction-band increase and disruption of sarcomere structure in electron microscopy.) The following are observed on the third day: focal necrosis (lysis of myofibrils), and cell infiltration of histocytes, lymphocytes, and sometimes plasma cells. The following are seen after a few weeks: removal of necrosed myocytes by macrophage, resolution of acute inflammatory response, and replacement fibrosis. Inflammation is seen depending on how much time had passed.[33] Early infiltration of polymorphonuclear leukocytes occurs in catecholamine cardiomyopathy, unlike infarction, and the key to its diagnosis is also a focal lesion.

In takotsubo cardiomyopathy, the following should be noted in the evaluation of microcirculation disorder.[34] Many cases of cardiomyopathy are elderly with non-specific arteriolosclerosis in the myocardium (Figure 7) which occurs with aging.

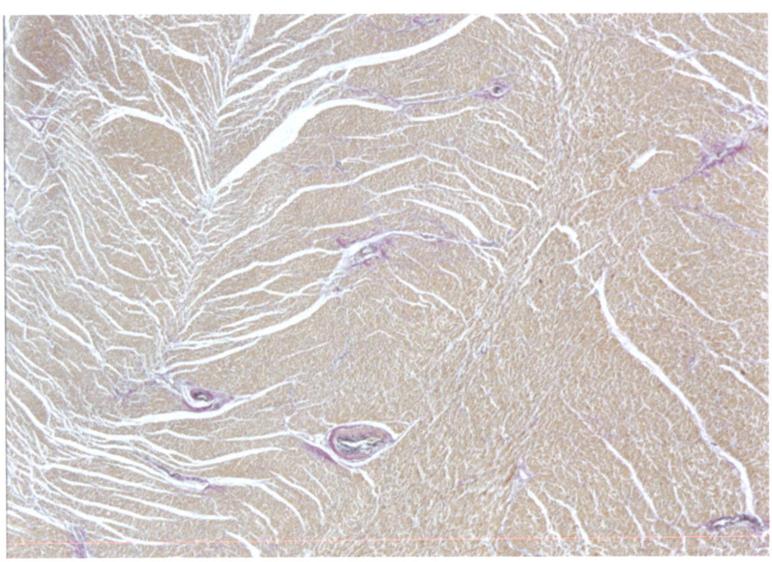

Arteriolosclerosis in the myocardium was observed frequently. Elastica van-Geison stain, x 20

Fig. 7. Autopsied case of takotsubo cardiomyopathy: histology of the interventricular septum

13. Conclusion

There was a clear myocardial lesion in takotsubo cardiomyopathy. The myocardial lesions are characterized mainly by individual myocytes or a group of myocytes with increased eosinophil staining, contraction band formation, necrosis, and rupture. The basis of the lesion is a damaged individual myocyte and aggregation of these damaged myocytes. It is speculated that early cell infiltration occurs followed by changes over time, including loss of myocytes and focal fibrosis.

14. Acknowledgements

I would like to express our appreciation to the following individuals for kindly supplying the tissues: Drs.Hiromasa Suzuki and Atsushi Yamada of Juntendo University School of Medicine, Dr. Koshi Mawatari of Kagoshima Seikyo Hospital, Dr.Toshio Shimada of Shimane Medical University (presently Shizuoka General Hospital), Drs. Hitoshi Sawada and Tadanori Aizawa of Cardiovascular Institute Hospital, Drs. Hironori Murakami and Nagisa Hanawa of Teine Keijinkai Hospital, Dr. Kasumi Takemura of the Kyoto Department of Cardiology at Prefectural Yosanoumi Hospital (Second Department of Medicine, Kyoto Prefectural University of Medicine), Dr. Osamu Yamanaka of International Goodwill Hospital (presently Poula Clinic), Dr. Nobuhiro Kotani of Shimane Medical University (presently Clinical Laboratory, Hamada Medical Center), Dr. Tsutomu Tamura of Itabashi Chuo Medical Center, Dr. Masafumi Watanabe of the Department of Cardiovascular Medicine at the University of Tokyo、Drs. Masahito Kawada and Tetsuya Nakamura of National Hospital Organization Kobe Medical Center, and Dr. Hiroshi Matsushita of Toranomon Hospital.

15. References

[1] Kloner RA, Przyklen K, Patel B: Altered myocardial states. The stunned and hibernating myocardium. Am J Med 1989; 86 (Suppl 1A):14-22.

[2] Kawai S, Suzuki H, Yamaguchi H, Kawada M, Nakamura T, Nishiyama S, Monomura S, Matsushita H: [Autopsy findings of takotsubo cardiomyopathy.] Study report of the study group of idiopathic cardiomyopathy sponsored by the Health and Welfare Ministry. 106-109, March 2003. (in Japanese)

[3] Kawai S, Yamaguchi H, Suzuki H: [Pathology of takotsubo cardiomyopathy.] Heart View 8(2):159-166, 2004. (in Japanese)

[4] Anzai H, Komiyama N, Kinoshita N, et al.: [Case of stunned myocardium caused by overdose of epinephrine.] Kokyu to Junkan 44(2):199-204, 1996. (in Japanese)

[5] Kawada M, Okada T, Shimizu M, et al.: [An autopsy case of cardiac dysfunction of unknown origin associated with severe pneumonia.] Heart 31(5):337-343, 1999. (in Japanese)

[6] Kotani N, et al.: [Takotsubo-type fulminant myocarditis: a case report [abstract].] Jpn Circ J 64(S2):826, 2000. (in Japanese)

[7] Batsakis JG : Degenerative lesions of the heart. In Gould SE ed. "Pathology of the Heart and Blood Vessels, Third Edition.", Charles C Thomas, Springfield, Illinois, 480-521.

[8] Kaneko N: [A study on the basic structure and specific function of microcirculatory system in the human heart] Journal of Tokyo Women's Medical University 51(11):1574-92, 1981. (in Japanese)

[9] Rolf A, Nef HM, Möllmann H, Troidl C, Voss S, Conradi G, Rixe J, Steiger H, Beiring K, Hamm CW, Dill T.:Immunohistological basis of the late gadolinium enhancement phenomenon in tako-tsubo cardiomyopathy. Eur Heart J 30:1635-164,2009.

[10] Tsuneoka T, et al.: [Myocardial infarction-like electrocardiographic pattern during the course of malabsorption syndrome: an autopsy case [abstract].] Jpn Circ J 58(S2) :651, 1994. (in Japanese)

[11] Hirata Y: [A case of stunned myocardium with takotsubo-like left ventricular asynergy which developed cardiac rupture [abstract].] Jpn Circ J 63(S2):760, 1999. (in Japanese)

[12] Sacha J, Maselko J, Wester A, Szudrowicz Z, Pluta W. Left ventricular apical rupture caused by takotsubo cardiomyopathy –comprehensive pathological heart investigation. Circ J 2007;71:982-985.

[13] Ohara Y, Hiasa Y, Hosokawa, S et al: Left Ventricular Free Wall Rupture in Transient Left Ventricular Apical Ballooning. Circ J 65:621-623,2005

[14] Kuramoto K, Matsushita S, Murakami M: Acute reversible myocardial infarction after blood transfusion in the aged. Jpn Heart J 18:191-201,1977.

[15] Sasa H, Tsuboi H, Sone T, et al.: [Clinical significance of transient myocardial infarction-like electrocardiographic pattern in postoperative cases.] Heart 15:669-678, 1983. (in Japanese)

[16] Tokioka M, Miura H, Masaoka Y, et al.: [Transient appearance of asynergy on the echocardiogram and electrocardiographic changes simulating acute myocardial infarction following non-cardiac surgery.] J Cardiography 15:639-653, 1983. (in Japanese)

[17] Kawai S: [Takotsubo (ampulla, or amphora) cardiomyopathy.] Kokyu to Junkan 48(12):1237-1248,2000. (in Japanese)

[18] Kurisu S, Sato H, Kawagoe T, Ishihara M, Shimatani Y, Nishioka K, Kono Y, Umemura T, Nakamura S: Tako-tsubo-like left ventricular dysfunction with ST-segment elevation: a novel cardiac syndrome mimicking acute myocardial infarction. Am Heart J. 2002;143:448-55.

[19] Akashi Y. J., Nakazawa K., Sakakibara M., Miyake F., Koike H., Sasaka K.: The clinical features of takotsubo cardiomyopathy. Q J Med 2003; 96: 563-573.

[20] Gianni M, Dentali F, Grandi AM, Sumner G, Hiralal R, Lonn E. : Apical ballooning syndrome or takotsubo cardiomyopathy: a systematic review. Eur Heart J. 2006;27(13):1523-9.

[21] Yoshida T, Hibino T, Kako N, Murai S, Oguri M, Kato K, Yajima K, Ohte N, Yokoi K , Kimura G. :A pathophysiologic study of tako-tsubo cardiomyopathy with F-18 fluorodeoxyglucose positron emission tomography. Eur Heart J (2007) 28:2598–2604.

[22] Pilgrim TM, Wyss TR: Takotsubo cardiomyopathy or transient left ventricular apical ballooning syndrome: a systematic review. Int J Cardiol 2007;124: 283-292.

[23] Kawai S, Suzuki H, Yamaguchi H, Tanaka K, Sawada H, Aizawa T, Watanabe M, Tamura T, Mawatari K, Kawada M, Nakamura T, Yamanaka O, Okada R. Ampulla cardiomyopathy (Takotsubo cardiomyopathy) -reversible left ventricular dysfunction with ST segment elevation- Jpn Circ J 2000;64:156-159.

[24] von Korn H, Yu J, Lotze U, Ohlow MA, Huegl B, Schulte W, Haberl K, Wagner A, Gruene S, Lauer B. : Tako-Tsubo-like cardiomyopathy: specific ECG findings, characterization and clinical findings in a European single center. Cardiology. 2009;112 (1):42-8.

[25] Wani S, Glatz K, Suter Y, Jamshidi P, Erne P. "Apical ballooning"-what is the cause? J Invasive Cardiol 2008;20:599-602.

[26] Matsuyama T, Sasagasako N, Koike A, Matsuura M, Koga T, Kawajiri M, Oyagi Y, Iwaki T, Kira J: [An autopsy case of amyotrophic lateral sclerosis with ampulla cardiomyopathy.] Clin Neurol 2008;48(4):249-54. (in Japanese)

[27] Ohtsubo M, Sakai H, Takano H, Kon H, Okamoto K, Yoshida N, Fujita M.[Atypical takotsubo cardiomyopathy with preservation of apical contraction: a case report including pathological findings.] J Cardiol 2005;46:237-242. (in Japanese)

[28] Nef HM, Möllmann H, Kostin S, Troidl C, Voss S, Weber M, Dill T, Rolf A, Brandt R, Hamm CW, Elsässer A. Tako-Tsubo cardiomyopathy: intraindividual structural analysis in the acute phase and after functional recovery. Eur Heart J 2007;28:2456-2464.

[29] Kawakami H, Matsuoka H, Koyama H, et al.: [A case of "Takotsubo" like cardiomyopathy due to acute myocarditis.] Respiration & Circulation 46:913-917, 1998. (in Japanese)

[30] Caforio AL, Tona F, Vinci A, Calabrese F, Ramondo A, Cacciavillani L, Corbetti F, Leoni L, Thiene G, Iliceto S, Angelini A. : Acute biopsy-proven lymphocytic myocarditis mimicking Takotsubo cardiomyopathy. Eur J Heart Fail. 2009;11:428-31.

[31] Kubo K, Ishibashi I, Miyazaki Y, Sakai Y, Matsuno K, Namikawa S, Sano M, Yamaoka T, Ono M, Kawana H: [An autopsy case of acute myocarditis that was diagnosed antemortem as takotsubo cardiomyopathy.] Heart 41:1222-1226, 2009. (in Japanese)

[32] Kassim TA, Clarke DD, Mai VQ, Clyde PW, Mohamed Shakir KM.: Catecholamine-induced cardiomyopathy. Endocr Pract. 2008;14(9):1137-49.

[33] Kawai S, Hashimoto K: [Catecholamine myocarditis.] Japanese Journal of Clinical Medicine 38 (fall special edition), Internal Medicine to Pathology 3680-3685, 1980. (in Japanese)

[34] Kume T, Akasaka T, Kawamoto T, Yoshitani H, Watanabe N, Neishi Y, Wada N, Yoshida K.：Assessment of coronary microcirculation in patients with Takotsubo-like left ventricular dysfunction。Circ J 69：934-9,2005

32

Torsades de Pointes in Takotsubo Cardiomyopathy with QT Prolongation

Hiroaki Kawano
Department of Cardiovascular Medicine, Nagasaki University
Japan

1. Introduction

Takotsubo cardiomyopathy, or stress-induced cardiomyopathy, is characterized by reversible left ventricular apical ballooning associated with emotional or physiologic stress, mimicking acute myocardial infarction in the absence of significant coronary artery disease at angiography. Although the prognosis for patients with Takotsubo cardiomyopathy is relatively good, it is reported to be associated with long QT syndrome and torsades de pointes (TdP) which is a fatal polymorphic ventricular tachyarrhythmia.

However, only QT prolongation abnormalities is not enough to induce TdP, and other factors associated with Takotsubo cardiomyopathy seem to be needed for the induction of TdP. In this chapter, the mechanism of TdP in Takotsubo cardiomyopathy with QT prolongation is discussed.

2. Takotsubo cardiomyopathy

Takotsubo cardiomyopathy, or stress-induced cardiomyopathy, is a disease exhibiting an acute left ventricular apical ballooning of unknown cause (Kawai et al., 2007). Many cases with takotsubo cardiomyopathy are associated with preceded emotional or physiologic stress. In this disease, the left ventricle takes on the appearance of a Japanese octopus fishing pot called a takotsubo. In takotsubo cardiomyopathy, left ventricular dysfunction is reversible, i.e., it recovers within a few weeks (Figure 1). Other signs include ECG changes, including ST-segment elevation, abnormal Q wave, and T-wave inversions (Figure 2), which mimicks acute myocardial infarction but there is no significant coronary artery disease at angiography (Kawai et al., 2007, Tsuchihashi et al., 2001, Kurisu et al. , 2002).

Several pathophysiological mechanisms have been proposed to explain the features of this syndrome, such as multivessel coronary vasospasm, abnormalities in coronary microvascular function, and catecholamine-mediated cardiotoxicity (Akashi et al, 2002, Kurisu et al, 2003, Sansen V & Holvoet G., 2007). Studies on 123I-metaiodybenzylguanidine suggested the existence of cardiac autonomic damage and/or accelerated cardiac sympathetic nervous function in patients with Takotsubo cardiomyopathy (Akashi et al, 2004, Burgdorf et al, 2008). Nef, et al (Nef et al, 2007) reported that there were contraction bands, increase in fibrosis, and the regional accumulation of inflammatory cells in biopsied specimen of myocardium in acute phase of Takotsubo cardiomyopathy, and they suggested that these findings were similar to those associated with catecholamine cardiotoxicity. These data suggest that catecholamine-mediated cardiotoxicity may be the most plausible cause of Takotsubo cardiomyopathy although the precise aetiology and pathophysiology of this syndrome remain unknown.

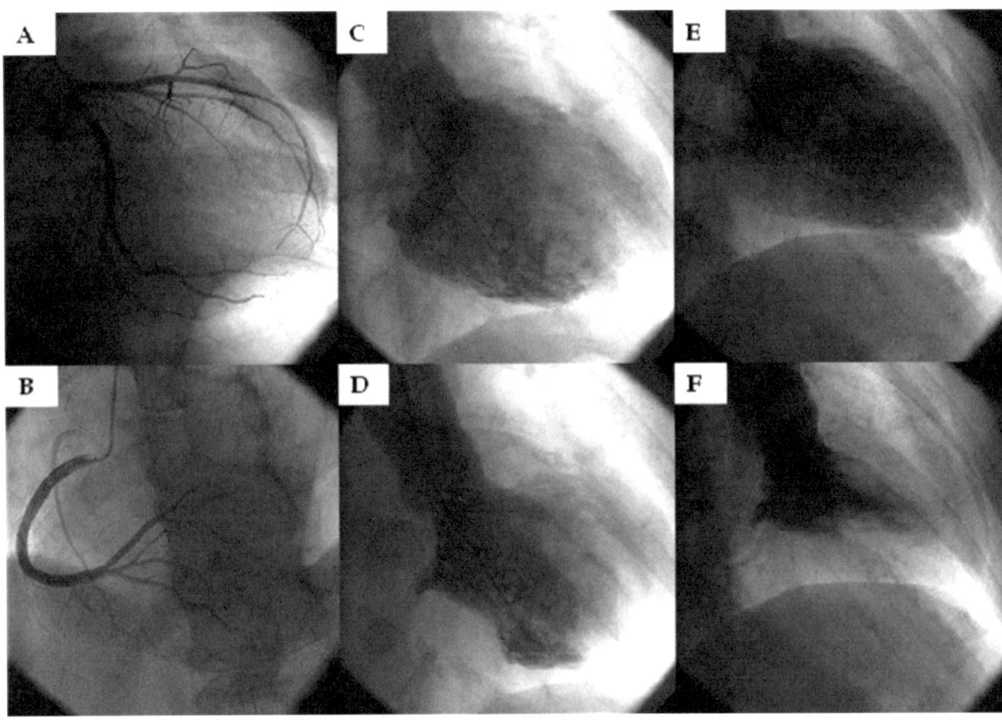

Coronary angiography showed no significant coronary stenosis of the left (A) and right (B)coronary arteries. Left ventriculography demonstrated akinesis of apex of the left ventricle on admission (C, end-diastolic phase; D, end-systolic phase) and showed recovered apical wall motion of the left ventricle about three weeks after admission(C, end-diastolic phase; D, end-systolic phase).

Fig. 1. Coronary angiography and left ventriculography on admission and about three weeks after the admission

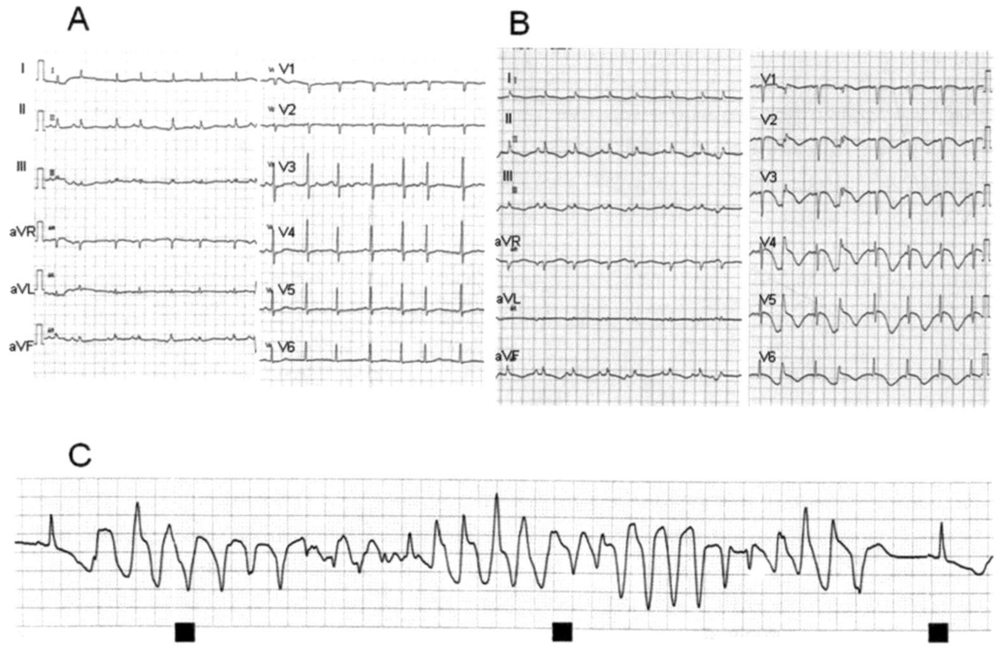

A, ECG showed sinus rhythm, and flat T waves. B, ECG showed sinus rhythm, poor R wave progression in leads V1 to V3, and QT prolongation with a corrected QT interval of 800 msec. C, ECG monitor demonstrated torsades de pointes.

Fig. 2. Electrocardiography (ECG) before (A) and just after (B) the occurrence of Takotsubo Cardiomyopathy, and ECG monitor of torsades de pointes(C)

Takotsubo cardiomyopathy occurs most frequently in women over 50 years of age. The reason for the much more common occurrence in post-menopausal women is unclear. Several explanations have been proposed. Sex hormones may exert important influences on the sympathetic neurohormonal axis (Hinojosa-Laborde et al, 1999) and on coronary vasoreactivity (Sader & Celermajer, 2002). Women appear also to be more vulnerable to sympathetically mediated myocardial stunning (Lambert et al, *2002*), and post-menopausal alteration of endothelial function in response to reduced estrogen levels has been advocated as a possible alternative explanation (Taddei et al, 1996).

3. Long QT syndrome (QT prolongation) and torsades de pointes

The Long QT syndrome (LQTS) is originally a hereditary disorder in which most affected family members have delayed ventricular repolarization manifest on the electrocardiogram (ECG) as QT prolongation (Moss et al, 1985). The disorder is associated with an increased propensity to arrhythmogenic syncope, polymorphic ventricular tachycardia (torsades de pointes), and sudden arrhythmic death. LQTS is due to mutations involving principally the myocyte ion-channels, and this monogenetic disorder has an autosomal-dominant inheritance pattern. Since the 3 genes were identified for the 3 major genotypes, a total of 13 forms of LQTS have been reported (Shimizu W & Horie M.).
Recently, mutations in the caveolin-3 gene (*CAV3*) have been linked with the congenital long QT syndrome (LQT9), and mutations in caveolar-localized ion channels may contribute

to other inherited arrhythmias. Caveolin-3 is the essential scaffolding protein of caveolae which are specialized membrane microdomains enriched in cholesterol and sphingolipids which are present in multiple cell types including cardiomyocytes. Along with the essential scaffolding protein caveolin-3, a number of different ion channels and transporters have been localized to caveolae in the heart. Mutations in caveolar-localized ion channels may contribute to other inherited arrhythmias, and changes in the caveolar microdomain in acquired heart disease may also lead to dysregulation and dysfunction of ion channels, altering the risk of arrhythmias in conditions such as heart failure (Balijepalli & Kamp, 2008). This indicate that abnormality or damage of structural elements of cardiomyocyte may also induce QT prolongation and arrhythmia.

Long QT syndrome can be also divided into idiopathic (congenital) and acquired forms. QT intervals vary according to age, sex, and heart rate, and acquired long QT syndrome describes pathologic QT interval prolongation. Acquired long QT syndrome can arise in response to various drugs, electrolyte abnormalities (e.g., hypokalemia, hypomagnesemia) and significant bradyarrhythmias. It also becomes a risk of arrhythmogenic syncope, polymorphic ventricular tachycardia (torsades de pointes), and sudden arrhythmic death.

Torsade de pointes (TdP) is a life-threatening arrhythmia that develops as a consequence of a reduction in the repolarization reserve of cardiac cells leading to amplification of electrical heterogeneities in the ventricular myocardium as well as to the development of early after depolarization-induced triggered activity.

Autonomic nervous system may have important role in the initiation of Tdp (Coumel, 1993). The level of adrenergic drive is required for the occurrence of Tdp, and it also produces a sinus tachycardia that would prevent QT prolongation. Autonimic tone influences the QT interval directly by affecting the action potential duration and indirectly by modulating the RR interval. These indicate that the interactions between heart rate and sympathetic nervous activity are complex. Fujiki et al (Fujiki et al, 2001) suggested that the sympathovagal imbalance may have an important role in the dynamic change in the QT interval and initiation of Tdp in patients with long QT syndrome. In patients with acquired long-QT syndrome, Locati et al (Locati et al, 1995) reported that both adrenergic- and pause-dependent mechanisms may have a synergistic role in the genesis of Tdp.

Women are more prone to develop TdP than men either congenital or acquired LQTS, and it is similar to the sex difference of occurrence of Takotsubo cardiomyopathy. Although the precise mechanism has not been clarified, female hormone may exert the influence on cardiac repolarization process (Kurokawa et al, 2009).

4. Torsades de pointes in takotsubo cardiomyopathy with QT prolongation

The presence of QT interval prolongation has been discussed in patients with Takotsubo cardiomyopathy (Abe et al., 2003 , Desmet et al., 2003, Matsuoka et al., 2003), and there have been 17 reported cases of QT interval prolongation and torsades de pointes (TdP) associated with Takotsubo cardiomyopathy (Denney et al., 2005, Sasaki et al., 2006, Okada T, et al., 2007 [in Japanese], Nault et al., 2007, Boulouffe et al., 2007, Patel et al., 2007, Kurisu et al., 2008, Furushima et al., 2008, Hirose et al., 2008, Ghosh et al., 2009, Mahida et al., 2009, Inoue et al., 2009, Kawano et al., 2010, Purvis et al., 2009, Yamada et al., 2011) (Figure 2) (Table 1). Considering the 17 previous cases reported in the literature, QT prolongation in Takotsubo cardiomyopathy has been attributed to hypokalemia (n= 3), bradycardia associated with atrioventricular (AV) block (n=4), idiopathic long QT syndrome (n=2), hypokalemia plus antiarrhythmic therapy (n=1), and hypokalemia plus idiopathic long QT syndrome (n=1), hypokalemia and hypomagnesemia (n=1), hyponagnesemia (n=1), and antibiotic (n=1) in 14 cases, and there was no specific factor associated with QT prolongation in 3 cases. The vasospasm provocation test was performed in only 3 cases, and vasospasm was not induced in any of these cases.

Hypokalemia or hypomagnesemia is one of the most important risk factor because it is present in 7 of 17 (41%) case. Badycardia associated with AV block is also one of the important factor because its presence in 4 of 17 (24%) cases. These observations suggest that electrolyte imbalances and bradycardia are a risk factor for the development of torsades de pointes in patients with Takotsubo cardiomyopathy.

However, only QT prolongation is not enough to induce TdP. Oscillations of the RR interval or the short–long–short (or the long-short) sequence precede the initiation of TdP in patients with acquired prolongation of repolarization (Locati et al., 1995). In most cases of TdP, frequent premature ventricular contraction (PVC)s create long-short sequence, i.e., a VPC generates a post-extrasystolic pause, the following regular beat shows marked QT prolongation from which a subsequent PVC arise, and this beat initiates TdP. Triggered activity originating from early after-depolarization or phase 2 reentry has been suggested as the cause of the PVC which induces long-short initiating sequence and can be the first beat of TdP. However, there is another unique pattern of the initiating of TdP in Takotsubo cardiomyopathy (Kawano et al., 2010,). It seems that premature atrial contraction (PAC) followed by QRS on T wave can also induced reentrant ventricular tachycardia directly (Figure 3). The peak of T wave is known as the vulnerable period of the ventricle. Depolarization at this phase may easily induce unstable reentrant mechanism especially in the case with prominently increased dispersion of repolarization such as long QT syndrome. This mechanism of TdP is also very rare in long QT syndrome. Moreover, that case had already had mild QT prolongation with hypokalemia and PAC before the occurrence of Takotsubo cardiomyopathy. This suggests that other factors associated with Takotsubo cardiomyopathy is needed for the induction of TdP.

Prolongation of action potential duration (APD) due to abnormal ion channel current causes QT prolongation. Dispersion of APD or repolarizaion is thought to be one of the mechanisms of occurrence of Tdp, and Furushima et al. (Furushima et al., 2008) reported abnormal LV reporlarization gradient in a patient with Takotsubo cardiomyopathy. Taken together, dispersion of APD or repolarization in Takotsubo cardiomyopathy as well as QT prolongation may be important in the occurrence of TdP. Adrenergic stimulation may be also related to TdP in Takotsbo cardiomyopathy because catecholamine excess and neurogenic myocardial stunning are thought to be one of the the most plausible causes of Takotsubo cardiomyopathy.

On the other hands, TdP may be one of the trigger of Takotsubo cardiomyopathy in long QT syndrome. Although it occurs most frequently in women over 50 years of age, recent study demonstrated that men with Takotsubo cardiomyopathy-associated QT interval prolongation are at risk for TdP, and that most patients with Takotsubo cardiomyopathy-associated TdP have risk factors for TdP other than the female sex and systolic dysfunction (Samuelov-Kinori, 2009).

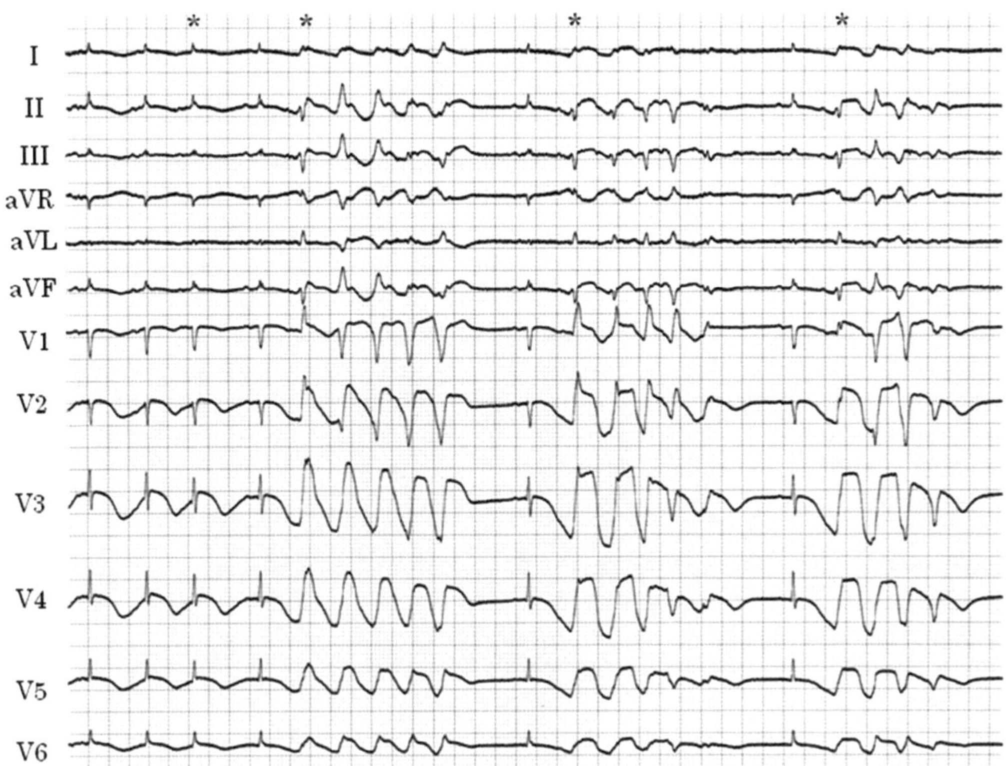

Fig. 3. ECG showed that PACs (*) induced long-short sequence and initiated TdP.

	Age	Sex	Diseases	serum K(mEq/L)	QTc (msec)
1	32	M	migrane, BA, allergic rhinitis	normal	467
2	22	F	LQTS	2.8	730
3	77	M	pneumonia	3.7	730
4	76	F	rhabdomyolysis	3.3	786
5	68	F	none	not determined	prolongation
6	72	F	HT, COPD	not determined	674
7	87	F	AV block	not determined	735
8	78	M	AV block	not determined	735
9	61	F	LQTS	not determined	590
10	63	F	Myasthenia gravis	2.8	549
11	59	F	HT, alcoholic	3.2	669
12	55	F	LQTS	normal	510
13	82	F	AV block	4	630
14	80	M	BA, HT, alcoholic	2.6	800
15	67	F	Depression	3.9	524
16	89	F	AV block	4.6	580
17	81	F	atrial fibrillation	4.3	620

M male, F female, BA bronchial asthma, LQTS idiopathic long QT syndrome, HT hypertension

Table 1. Reports of Takotsubo Cardiomyopathy with Torsades de Pointes

5. Conclusion

We usually pay attention to ventricular arrhythmia in other cardiomyopathy, i.e., hypertrophic cardiomyopathy and dilated cardiomyopathy. And we have to also consider the importance of PAC as well as VPC as the initiator of TdP, the life-threatening arrhythmia in Takotsubo cardiomyopathy .

6. Acknowledgment

I thank editors of Internal Medicine for their excellent advice to discuss the mechanisms of torsasede de pointes in Takotsubo cardiomyopathy.

7. References

Abe Y, Kondo M, Matsuoka R, Araki M, Dohyama K, Tanio H. Assessment of clinical features in transient left ventricular apical ballooning. J Am Coll Cardiol 41: 737-742, 2003

Akashi YJ, Nakazawa K, Sakakibara M, Miyake F, Sasaka K. Reversible left ventricular dysfunction "takotsubo" cardiomyopathy related to catecholamine cardiotoxicity. J Electrocardiol 35: 351-6, 2002

Akashi YJ, Nakazawa K, Sakakibara M, Miyake F, Musha H, Sasaka K. 123I-MIBG myocardial scintigraphy in patients with "takotsubo" cardiomyopathy. J Nucl Med 45:1121-7, 2004

Balijepalli RC& Kamp TJ.Caveolae, ion channels and cardiac arrhythmias. Prog Biophys Mol Biol 98:149-60, 2009

Boulouffe C, Vanpee D, Gabriel L. Stress-induced cardiomyopathy: Takotsubo left ventricular dysfunction. Am J Emerg Med 25: 243-244, 2007

Burgdorf C, von Hof K, Schunkert H, Kurowski V. Regional alterations in myocardial sympathetic innervation in patients with transient left-ventricular apical ballooning (Tako-Tsubo cardiomyopathy). J Nucl Cardiol 15 :65-72, 2008

Coumel P. Cardiac arrhythmia and the autonomic nervous system. J Cardiovasc Electrophysiol 1993; 4: 338-355

Denney SD, Lakkireddy DR, Khan IA. Long QT syndrome and torsade de pointes in transient left ventricular apical ballooning syndrome. Int J Cardiol 100:499-501, 2005

Desmet WJ, Adriaenssens BF, Dens JA. Apial ballooning of the left ventricle: first series in white patients. Heart 89: 1027-1031, 2003

Fujiki A, Nishida K, Mizumaki K, Nagasawa H, Shimono M, Inoue H. Spontaneous onset of torsade de pointes in long-QT syndrome and the role of sympathovagal imbalance. Circ J 65: 1087-1090, 2001

Furushima H, Chinushi M, Sanada A, Aizawa Y. Ventricular repolarization gradients in a patient with takotsubo cardiomyopathy. Europace 10: 1112-1115, 2008

Ghosh S, Apte P, Maroz N, Broor A, Zeineh N, Khan IA. Takotsubo cardiomyopathy as a potential cause of long QT syndrome and torsades de pointes. Int J Cardiol 136: 225-227, 2009

Hinojosa-Laborde C, Chapa I, Lange D, Haywood JR. Gender differences in sympathetic nervous system regulation. Clin Exp Pharmacol Physiol 26:122-126, 1999

Hirose K, Yamaguchi H, Oshima Y, Choraku M, Hirono A, Takamori N, Tamura K. Severe respiratory failure and torsades de pointes induced by disopyramide in a patient with myasthenia gravis. Intern Med 47: 1703-1708, 2008

Inoue M, Kanaya H, Matsubara T, Uno Y, Yasuda T, Miwa K. Complete atrioventricular block associated with takotsubo cardiomyopathy. Circ J 73: 589-592, 2009

Kawai S, Kitabatake A, Tomoike H; Takotsubo Cardiomyopathy Group. Guidelines for diagnosis of takotsubo (ampulla) cardiomyopathy. Circ J.71:990-2, 2007

Kawano H, Matsumoto Y, Arakawa S, Satoh O, Hayano M. Premature atrial contraction induces torsades de pointes in a patient of Takotsubo cardiomyopathy with QT prolongation.Intern Med. 49:1767-73, 2010

Kurisu S, Sato H, Kawagoe T, Ishihara M, Shimatani Y, Nishioka K, Kano Y, Umemura T, Nakamura S. Tako-tsubo-like left ventricular dysfunction with ST-segment elevation: a novel cardiac syndrome mimicking acute myocardial infarction。 Am Heart J 143: 448-455, 2002

Left ventricular apical thrombus formation in a patient with suspected tako-tsubo-like left ventricular dysfunction.

Kurisu S, Inoue I, Kawagoe T, Ishihara M, Shimatani Y, Nishioka K, Umemura T, Nakamura S, Yoshida M, Sato H. Circ J 67: 556-558, 2003

Kurisu S, Inoue I, Kawagoe T, Ishihara M, Shimatani Y, Nakama Y, Ohkawa K, Maruhashi T, Kagawa E, Dai K, Aoyagi T. Torsade de pointes associated with bradycardia and takotsubo cardiomyopathy. Can J Cardiol 24:640-642, 2008

Kurokawa J, Suzuki T, Furukawa T.New aspects for the treatment of cardiac diseases based on the diversity of functional controls on cardiac muscles: acute effects of female hormones on cardiac ion channels and cardiac repolarization. J Pharmacol Sci 109:334-340, 2009

Lambert G, Naredi S, Edén E, Rydenhag B, Friberg P. Monoamine metabolism and sympathetic nervous activation following subarachnoid haemorrhage: influence of gender and hydrocephalus.Brain Res Bull 58:77-82, 2002

Locati EH, Maison-Blanche P, Dejode P, Cauchemez B, Coumel P. Spontaneous sequences of onset of torsade de pointes in patients with acquired prolonged repolarization: quantitative analysis of Holter recordings. J Am Coll Cardiol 25 :1564-75, 1995

Mahida S, Dalageorgou C, Behr ER. Long-QT syndrome and torsades de pointes in a patient with Takotsubo cardiomyopathy: an unusual case. Europace 11: 376-378, 2009

Matsuoka K, Okubo S, Fujii E, Uchida F, Kasai A, Aoki T, Makino K, Omichi C, Fujimoto N, Ohta S, Sawai T, Nakano T. Evaluation of the arrhythmogenicity of stress-induced "Takotsubo cardiomyopathy" from the time course of the 12-lead surface electrocardiogram. Am J Cardiol 92:230-233, 2003

Moss AJ, Schwartz PJ, Crampton RS, Locati E, Carleen E. The long QT syndrome: a prospective international study, Circulation 71: 17–21, 1985

Nault MA, Baranchuk A, simpson CS, Redfearn DP. Takotsubo cardiomyopathy: a novel "proarrhythmic" disease-case report. Anadolu Kardiyol Derg 7(suppl 1): 101-103, 2007

Nef HM, Möllmann H, Kostin S, Troidl C, Voss S, Weber M, Dill T, Rolf A, Brandt R, Hamm CW, Elsässer A.Tako-Tsubo cardiomyopathy: intraindividual structural analysis in the acute phase and after functional recovery. Eur Heart J 28: 2456-2464, 2007

Okada T, Miyata S, Hashimoto K, Maie K, Mochizuki S. Takotsubo cardiomyopathy associated with torsades de pointes and long QT interval: a case report . J Cardiol 50 :83-88, 2007 [in Japanese]

Patel HM, Kantharia BK, Morris DL, Yazdanfar S. Takotsubo syndrome in African-American women with atypical presentatiosn: a single-center exerience. Clin Cardiol 30: 14-18, 2007

Purvis JA, Cunningham EL, McGlinchey PG, Barr SH.Drugs, electrolytes and tako-tsubo cardiomyopathy: triple aetiology of acquired long QT syndrome and torsades de pointes. Ulster Med J. 2009 Sep;78(3):188-9.

Sader MA, Celermajer DS. Endothelial function, vascular reactivity and gender differences in the cardiovascular system. Cardiovasc Res 53:597-604, 2002

Samuelov-Kinori L, Kinori M, Kogan Y, Swartzon M, Shalev H, Guy D, Ferenidou F, Mashav N, Sadeh B, Atzmony L, Kliuk-Ben-Basat O, Steinvil A, Justo D. Takotsubo cardiomyopathy and QT interval prolongation: who are the patients at risk for torsades de pointes? J Electrocardiol. 42:353-357, 2009

Sansen V, Holvoet G. Takotsubo cardiomyopathy presenting as multivessel coronary spasm syndrome: case report and review of the literature. Acta Cardiol 62:507-11, 2007

Sasaki O, Nishioka T, Akima T, Tabata H, Okamoto Y, Akanuma M, Uehata A, Takase B, Katsushika S, Isojima K, Ohtomi S, Yoshimoto N. Association of takotsubo cardiomyopathy and long QT syndrome. Circ J 70:1220-2, 2006

Taddei S, Virdis A, Ghiadoni L, Mattei P, Sudano I, Bernini G, Pinto S, Salvetti A. Menopause is associated with endothelial dysfunction in women. Hypertension 28:576-582, 1996

Tsuchihashi K, Ueshima K, Uchida T, Oh-mura N, Kimura K, Owa M, Yoshimura M, Miyazaki S, Haze K, Ogawa H, Honda T, Hase M, Kai R, Morii I; Angina Pectoris-Myocardial Infarction Investigation in Japan. Transient left ventricular apical ballooning without coronary artery stenosis: a novel heart syndrome mimicking acute myocardial infarction. Angina Pectoris-Myocardial Infarction Investigations in Japan . J Am Coll Cardiol 38: 11-18, 2001

Yamada Y, Tani T, Homma M, Saito S. Two cases of torsades de pointes associated with takotsubo cardiomyopathy as the second insult. J Electrocardiol. 2011 [Epub ahead of print]

33

Torsades de Pointes Associated with Takotsubo Cardiomyopathy: Is It Preventable?

Dan Justo, Arie Steinvil and Itzhak Shapira
Departments of Geriatrics and Cardiology, Tel-Aviv Sourasky Medical Center, Affiliated to Sackler School of Medicine, Tel-Aviv University, Tel-Aviv, Israel

1. Introduction

Takotsubo cardiomyopathy is characterized by transient left ventricular systolic dysfunction and apical dyskinesis (ballooning) in the absence of significant obstructive coronary artery disease. Most patients with Takotsubo cardiomyopathy are females. An emotional stress is believed to be the main trigger of Takotsubo cardiomyopathy (Bybee & Prasad, 2008). Electrocardiographic features of Takotsubo cardiomyopathy might include: ST elevation, T wave inversion, and QT interval prolongation (Thakar et al., 2011).

QT interval prolongation might precede Torsades de Pointes - a potentially deadly polymorphic ventricular tachycardia. Female gender, left ventricular systolic dysfunction, recent conversion of atrial fibrillation to sinus rhythm, administering QT interval prolonging agents, hypokalemia, hypocalcemia, severe hypomagnesemia, and high-degree atrioventricular block, are all risk factors for acquired QT interval prolongation and Torsades de Pointes (Antzelevitch, 2007; Roden, 2004).

The incidence of QT interval prolongation among patient with Takotsubo cardiomyopathy is higher than 50% (Abe et al., 2003; Cangella et al., 2007; Fang et al., 2008; Wittstein et al., 2005), but the incidence Takotsubo cardiomyopathy-associated Torsades de Pointes is probably much lower. It is of great importance to study the clinical circumstances leading to Torsades de Pointes in patients with Takotsubo cardiomyopathy-associated QT interval prolongation since Torsades de Pointes might be fatal, while the prognosis of Takotsubo cardiomyopathy is usually good (Bybee & Prasad, 2008).

Takotsubo cardiomyopathy-associated Torsades de Pointes has been reported in 2005 for the first time (Denney et al., 2005). We have reviewed this case report and additional 14 reports (Akashi et al., 2003; Boulouffe et al., 2007; Finsterer et al., 2007; Furushima et al., 2008; Ghosh et al., 2009; Hirose et al., 2008; Inoue et al., 2009; Kurisu et al., 2008; Mahida et al., 2009; Nault et al., 2007; Okada et al., 2007; Patel et al., 2007; Sasaki et al., 2006) concerning Takotsubo cardiomyopathy-associated Torsades de Pointes in 2009, and we have concluded that males with Takotsubo cardiomyopathy-associated QT interval prolongation are at risk for Takotsubo cardiomyopathy-associated Torsades de Pointes although most patients with Takotsubo cardiomyopathy are females. There has been a trend in the mean maximal QT interval being longer among patients with Takotsubo cardiomyopathy-associated Torsades de Pointes relative to patients with Takotsubo cardiomyopathy-associated QT interval prolongation. Moreover, most patients with Takotsubo cardiomyopathy-associated Torsades de Pointes have had risk factors for Torsades de Pointes other than female gender and left ventricular systolic dysfunction (Samuelov-Kinori et al., 2009). Additional 12 patients with Takotsubo cardiomyopathy-associated Torsades de Pointes have been reported since then (Ahn et al., 2011; Gotyo et al., 2009; Grilo et al., 2010; Kawano et al., 2010; Micallef et al., 2010; Pacha et al., 2010; Peters & Klein, 2011; Purvis et al., 2009; Rotondi et al., 2010; Wedekind et al., 2009; Yamada et al., 2011). We have currently examined whether our previous conclusions are true in face of these new publications. Moreover, we have studied if Torsades de Pointes has been possibly preventable in patients with Takotsubo cardiomyopathy-associated Torsades de Pointes.

2. Material and methods

2.1 Retrieval of reports

We performed a literature search by using the following keywords: "Apical ballooning", "Arrhythmia", "Stress cardiomyopathy", "Sudden death", "Syncope", "Takotsubo", and "Torsades de Pointes". The references in each report were further reviewed for additional publications. Only full-length reports were reviewed. The study group included all patients with Takotsubo cardiomyopathy-associated Torsades de Pointes that had been reported until July 2011. The control group included patients with Takotsubo cardiomyopathy-associated QT interval prolongation that had been reviewed previously (Samuelov-Kinori et al., 2009).

2.2 Risk factors for Torsades de Pointes

Each case report was analyzed for the presence of risk factors for Torsades de Pointes other than female gender and left ventricular systolic dysfunction: recent conversion of atrial fibrillation to sinus rhythm, administering QT interval prolonging agents, hypokalemia (<3.5 mmol/L), hypocalcemia (<8.5 mg/dL), severe hypomagnesaemia (<1 mg/dL), and high-degree atrioventricular block (Antzelevitch, 2007; Roden, 2004). Since genetic analysis was not available for all patients, suspicion of congenital long QT syndrome was also considered a risk factor for Torsades de Pointes, and was defined as QT interval prolongation in the baseline ECG recorded before Takotsubo cardiomyopathy appearance or following its resolution. QT interval prolongation was defined as QTc >430 msec for male patients and QTc >450 msec for female patients according to the Bazett's formula (Bazett, 1920). We used the QTc that was mentioned in the text of each case report by the authors. In few cases we measured the QT interval length in lead II and calculated the QTc according to the ECG strip enclosed.

2.3 Preventable Torsades de Pointes

Each case report of Takotsubo cardiomyopathy-associated Torsades de Pointes was analyzed for the presence or the absence of treatment and prevention measures taken once QT interval prolongation had been noticed and prior to Torsades de Pointes appearance in face of the above-mentioned risk factors for Torsades de Pointes - regardless of whether Takotsubo cardiomyopathy diagnosis had already been made.

2.4 Statistical analysis

Continuous variables were expressed as mean ± standard error. Student t-test was used to compare between mean values of continuous variables with parametric distributions. Mann-Whitney test was used to compare between mean values of continuous variables with non-parametric distributions. Fisher's exact test was used to compare between incidence and prevalence of categorical variables. Two-tailed $p<0.05$ was considered statistically significant. Version 17.0 of the SPSS statistical package was used for all statistical analyses (SPSS Inc., Chicago, IL, USA).

3. Results

Reports concerning 113 patients were reviewed. The study group included 27 patients with Takotsubo cardiomyopathy-associated Torsades de Pointes. The control group included 86 patients with Takotsubo cardiomyopathy-associated QT interval prolongation. Mean age of all patients was 65.1±1.2 years. Most patients were females (n=102; 90.3%). All patients with Takotsubo cardiomyopathy-associated Torsades de Pointes survived, although one patient died of other complications more than two months following Torsades de Pointes (Hirose et al., 2008).

Although most patients were females, the prevalence of male gender was significantly higher among patients with Takotsubo cardiomyopathy-associated Torsades de Pointes relative to patients with Takotsubo cardiomyopathy-associated QT interval prolongation (odds ratio 4.6; 95%Cofidence Interval 1.3-16.7). Mean maximal QTc interval was significantly higher among patients with Takotsubo cardiomyopathy-associated Torsades de Pointes relative to patients with Takotsubo cardiomyopathy-associated QT interval prolongation even prior to Torsades de Pointes appearance. There were no statistical differences between patients with Takotsubo cardiomyopathy-associated Torsades de Pointes and patients with Takotsubo cardiomyopathy-associated QT interval prolongation in terms of mean age, mean lowest ejection fraction, and mean peak Troponin levels (table 1).

		Takotsubo-associated QT interval prolongation (n=86)	Takotsubo-associated Torsades de Pointes (n=27)	p value
Male gender	n (%)	5 (5.8%)	6 (22.2%)	0.021
Age (years)	n available Mean±SE	86 64.7±1.2	27 66.2±3.2	0.680
Maximal QTc interval (msec)	n available Mean±SE	58 555.9±8.4	25 670.2±37.1	0.006
Maximal QTc interval prior to Torsades de Pointes (msec)	n available Mean±SE	58 555.9±8.4	16 676.8±49.7	0.029
Lowest ejection fraction (%)	n available Mean±SE	50 36.5±1.4	11 37.2±4.0	0.850
Peak Troponin levels (ng/mL)	n available Mean±SE	39 5.6±2.5	13 1.7±0.8	0.383

Table 1. Clinical characteristics of reported patients

Overall, 17 (62.9%) patients with Takotsubo cardiomyopathy-associated Torsades de Pointes had one or more risk factors for Torsades de Pointes other than female gender and left ventricular systolic dysfunction, while only two (2.3%) patients with Takotsubo cardiomyopathy-associated QT interval prolongation had risk factors for Torsades de Pointes (odds ratio 71.4; 95%Confidence Interval 14.3-355.5; p<0.0001). Electrolyte depletion, i.e., hypokalemia and/or severe hypomagnesemia (n=7; 25.9%), and high-degree atrioventricular block (n=5; 18.5%), were the most prevalent risk factors for Torsades de Pointes and the last triggers for Torsades de Pointes. Four (14.8%) patients were also taking QT interval prolonging agents, although initiation of these agents was not the last trigger for Torsades de Pointes in any case (table 2).

Among patients with Takotsubo cardiomyopathy-associated Torsades de Pointes, the arrhythmia was diagnosed prior to Takotsubo cardiomyopathy most of the times (n=19; 70.4%), and in seven (25.9%) patients Torsades de Pointes was diagnosed upon admission to the emergency department. Nevertheless, Torsades de Pointes was possibly preventable in seven (25.9%) patients: In four patients with QT interval prolongation and apparent electrolyte depletion, hypokalemia and/or severe hypomagnesemia were corrected only following Torsades de Pointes appearance; in three patients with QT interval prolongation and high-degree atrioventricular block, pacemaker was implanted only following Torsades de Pointes appearance (table 2). In other patients, risk factors for Torsades de Pointes were diagnosed only following Torsades de Pointes appearance, or they were addressed too late.

4. Discussion

We have studied reports concerning patients with Takotsubo cardiomyopathy-associated QT interval prolongation and reports concerning patients with Takotsubo cardiomyopathy-associated Torsades de Pointes in order to characterize the clinical circumstances leading to Torsades de Pointes in patients with Takotsubo cardiomyopathy. We have done this before in 2009 (Samuelov-Kinori et al., 2009), but reports concerning patients with Takotsubo cardiomyopathy-associated Torsades de Pointes have almost doubled since then, and it is time to examine if our previous conclusions are still true in face of these new publications. Moreover, we have studied if Torsades de Pointes has been possibly preventable in patients with Takotsubo cardiomyopathy-associated Torsades de Pointes.

Consistent with our previous observation (Samuelov-Kinori et al., 2009), male patients with Takotsubo cardiomyopathy-associated QT interval prolongation are at higher risk for Torsades de Pointes compared with female patients with Takotsubo cardiomyopathy-associated QT interval prolongation, although most patients with Takotsubo cardiomyopathy are females (Bybee & Prasad, 2008). This finding is coherent with a recognized paradox which is still unexplained: women have longer QT interval compared with men but lower incidence of sudden death (Larsen & Kadish, 1998).

In our previous review there has been a trend in the mean maximal QT interval being longer among patients with Takotsubo cardiomyopathy-associated Torsades de Pointes relative to patients with Takotsubo cardiomyopathy-associated QT interval prolongation, although most of the times QT interval prolongation has been noticed only following Torsades de Pointes appearance (Samuelov-Kinori et al., 2009). In face of the new reports concerning patients with Takotsubo cardiomyopathy-associated QT interval prolongation, the trend has become statistically significant: mean maximal QTc interval is significantly higher among

First author	Age	Sex	Diagnosed first	Risk factors for QT interval prolongation and Torsades de Pointes other than female gender and left ventricular systolic dysfunction	Was Torsades de Pointes preventable?
Denney	32	M	Torsades	None	No
Kurisu	78	M	Torsades	Atrioventricular Block	Possibly
Kurisu	87	F	Torsades	Atrioventricular Block	Possibly
Nault	76	M	Torsades	HypoK	Possibly
Okada	77	M	Takotsubo	None	No
Akashi	67	F	Torsades	None	No
Boulouffe	68	F	Takotsubo	None	No
Finsterer	75	F	Torsades	Recent A.Fib conversion	No
Furushima	61	F	Torsades	QT interval prolongation at baseline ECG	No
Ghosh	59	F	Takotsubo	HypoK	Possibly
Patel	72	F	Torsades*	None	No
Sasaki	22	F	Torsades*	HypoK	No
Hirose	63	F	Takotsubo	HypoK + recent A.Fib conversion	No
Inoue	82	F	Torsades*	Atrioventricular Block	No
Mahida	55	F	Torsades	None	No
Micallef	58	F	Takotsubo	None	No
Pacha	64	F	Takotsubo	Recent A.Fib conversion + Amiodarone + HypoCa	No
Grilo	37	F	Torsades	Congenital long QT syndrome + Ketoconazole	No
Rotondi	57	F	Takotsubo	HypoK + HypoMg + HypoCa	Possibly
Wedekind	81	F	Torsades*	None	No
Gotyo	70	M	Torsades	None	No
Purvis	67	F	Torsades	HypoMg + Fluoxetine	Possibly
Kawano	80	M	Torsades	HypoK	No
Yamada	89	F	Torsades*	Atrioventricular Block	No
Yamada	81	F	Torsades	Clarythromycin	No
Peters	50	F	Torsades*	None	No
Ahn	78	F	Takotsubo	Atrioventricular Block	Possibly

Table 2. Clinical characteristics of patients with Takotsubo cardiomyopathy-associated Torsades de Pointes

patients with Takotsubo cardiomyopathy-associated Torsades de Pointes relative to patients with Takotsubo cardiomyopathy-associated QT interval prolongation even prior to Torsades de Pointes appearance. This finding is of great clinical significance beyond statistical significance: mean maximal QTc interval is remarkably high (676.8 msec) in patients with Takotsubo cardiomyopathy-associated Torsades de Pointes prior to Torsades de Pointes appearance - more than 120 msec higher relative to mean maximal QTc interval in patients with Takotsubo cardiomyopathy-associated QT interval prolongation without Torsades de Pointes appearance. This large difference in QT interval prolongation should urge physicians to start treatment and to take prevention measures as soon as possible prior to Torsades de Pointes appearance.

As with our previous review (Samuelov-Kinori et al., 2009), most patients with Takotsubo cardiomyopathy-associated Torsades de Pointes have one or more risk factors for Torsades de Pointes other than female gender and left ventricular systolic dysfunction. Electrolyte depletion and high degree atrioventricular block are the most prevalent risk factors and last triggers for Torsades de Pointes. But this time we have also shown that Torsades de Pointes is possibly preventable in one quarter of the patients should electrolyte depletion and high degree atrioventricular block have been addressed earlier.

4.1 Limitations

Our study is based on a small number of published case reports. Accordingly, the above-mentioned findings are suggestive rather than conclusive. We assume that there are more incidents of Torsades de Pointes in patients with Takotsubo cardiomyopathy that have not been published; for example, when physicians are reluctant to report their deceased patients. Indeed, in all the above-mentioned reports patients have survived Torsades de Pointes. Accordingly; we believe that our findings are more likely an underestimation of the true prevalence of the clinical circumstances that might lead to Torsades de Pointes in Takotsubo cardiomyopathy patients.

4.2 Clinical implications

This study defines four risk factors for Torsades de Pointes in patients with Takotsubo cardiomyopathy whom already have QT interval prolongation to begin with: male gander, marked QT interval prolongation, electrolyte depletion, and high degree atrioventricular block. Electrolyte depletion and high degree atrioventricular block are also last triggers for Torsades de Pointes in patients with Takotsubo cardiomyopathy. Accordingly, we believe electrolyte depletion and high degree atrioventricular block should be addressed as soon as possible in patients with Takotsubo cardiomyopathy in general, and in patients with marked QT interval prolongation in particular.

5. Conclusion

Men with Takotsubo cardiomyopathy-associated QT interval prolongation are at risk for Torsades de Pointes. Most patients with Takotsubo cardiomyopathy-associated Torsades de Pointes have risk factors for Torsades de Pointes other than female gender and left ventricular systolic dysfunction. Electrolyte depletion and high degree atrioventricular block are the most prevalent risk factors and last triggers for Torsades de Pointes. We wish to raise the awareness of risk factors for Torsades de Pointes in patients with Takotsubo cardiomyopathy-associated QT interval prolongation.

6. References

Abe, Y.; Kondo, M.; Matsuoka, R.; Araki, M.; Dohyama, K. & Tanio, H. (2003). Assessment of clinical features in transient left ventricular apical ballooning. *Journal of the American College of Cardiology,* Vol.41, No.5, (March 2003), pp.737-742, ISSN 0735-1097

Ahn, JH.; Park, SH.; Shin, WY.; Lee, SW.; Lee, SJ.; Jin, DK.; Lee, HM. & Eun, JY. (2011). Long QT Syndrome and Torsade de Pointes Associated with Takotsubo Cardiomyopathy. *Journal of Korean medical science,* Vol.26, No.7, (July 2011), pp.959-961, ISSN 1011-8934

Akashi, YJ.; Nakazawa, K.; Kida, K.; Ryu, S.; Takagi, A.; Kishi, R.; Kunishima, T.; Sakakibara, M. & Miyake, F. (2003). Reversible ventricular dysfunction (takotsubo cardiomyopathy) following polymorphic ventricular tachycardia. *Canadian Journal of Cardiology,* Vol.19, No.4, (March 2003), pp.449-451, ISSN 0828-282X

Antzelevitch, C. Ionic, molecular, and cellular bases of QT-interval prolongation and torsade de pointes. *Europace,* Vol.9, Suppl.No.4, (September 2007), pp.iv4-15, ISSN 1099-5129

Bazett, HC. (1920). An analysis of the time-relations of electrocardiograms. *Heart,* Vol.7, (1920), pp.353–370, ISSN 1355-6037

Boulouffe, C.; Vanpee, D. & Gabriel, L. (2007). Stress-induced cardiomyopathy: takotsubo left ventricular dysfunction. *American Journal of Emergency Medicine,* Vol.25, No.2, (February 2007), pp.243-244, ISSN 0735-6757

Bybee, KA. & Prasad, A. (2008). Stress-Related Cardiomyopathy Syndromes. *Circulation,* Vol.118, No.4, (July 2008), pp.397-409, ISSN 0009-7322

Cangella, F.; Medolla, A.; De Fazio, G.; Iuliano, C.; Curcio, N.; Salemme, L.; Mottola, G. & Agrusta, M. (2007). Stress induced cardiomyopathy presenting as acute coronary syndrome: Tako-Tsubo in Mercogliano, Southern Italy. *Cardiovascular Ultrasound,* Vol.5, (October 2007), pp.36, ISSN 1476-7120

Denney, SD.; Lakkireddy, DR. & Khan, IA. (2005). Long QT syndrome and torsade de pointes in transient left ventricular apical ballooning syndrome. *International Journal of Cardiology,* Vol.100, No.3, (April 2005), pp.499-501, ISSN 0167-5273

Fang, CC.; Jao, YT.; Yi, C.; Yu, CL.; Chen, CL. & Wang, SP. (2008). Transient left ventricular apical ballooning syndrome: the first series in Taiwanese patients. *Angiology,* Vol.59, No.2, (April-May 2008), pp.185-192, ISSN 0003-3197

Finsterer, J.; Stöllberger, C.; Sehnal, E.; Valentin, A.; Huber, J. & Schmiedel, J. (2007). Apical ballooning (Takotsubo syndrome) in mitochondrial disorder during mechanical ventilation. *Journal of cardiovascular medicine (Hagerstown, Md.),* Vol.8, No.10, (October 2007), pp.859-863, ISSN 1558-2027

Furushima, H.; Chinushi, M.; Sanada, A. & Aizawa, Y. (2008). Ventricular repolarization gradients in a patient with takotsubo cardiomyopathy. *Europace,* Vol.10, No.9, (September 2008), pp.1112-1115, ISSN 1099-5129

Ghosh, S.; Apte, P.; Maroz, N.; Broor, A.; Zeineh, N. & Khan, IA. (2009). Takotsubo cardiomyopathy as a potential cause of long QT syndrome and torsades de pointes. *International Journal of Cardiology,* Vol.136, No.2, (August 2009), pp.225-227, ISSN 0167-5273

Gotyo, N.; Kida, M.; Horiuchi, T. & Hirata, Y. (2009). Torsade de pointes associated with recurrent ampulla cardiomyopathy in a patient with idiopathic ACTH deficiency. *Endocrine journal,* Vol.56, No.6, (June 2009), pp.807-815, ISSN 0918-8959

Grilo, LS.; Pruvot, E.; Grobéty, M.; Castella, V.; Fellmann, F. & Abriel, H. (2010). Takotsubo cardiomyopathy and congenital long QT syndrome in a patient with a novel duplication in the Per-Arnt-Sim (PAS) domain of hERG1. *Heart Rhythm,* Vol.7, No.2, (September 2010), pp.260-265, ISSN 1547-5271

Hirose, K.; Yamaguchi, H.; Oshima, Y.; Choraku, M.; Hirono, A.; Takamori, N. & Tamura, K. (2008). Severe respiratory failure and torsades de pointes induced by disopyramide in a patient with myasthenia gravis. *Internal Medicine,* Vol.47, No.19, (October 2008), pp.1703-1708, ISSN 1349-7235

Inoue, M.; Kanaya, H.; Matsubara, T.; Uno, Y.; Yasuda, T. & Miwa, K. (2009). Complete Atrioventricular Block Associated With Takotsubo Cardiomyopathy. *Circulation Journal,* Vol.73, No.3, (March 2009), pp.589-592, ISSN 1346-9843

Kawano, H.; Matsumoto, Y.; Arakawa, S.; Satoh, O. & Hayano, M. (2010). Premature atrial contraction induces torsades de pointes in a patient of Takotsubo cardiomyopathy with QT prolongation. *Internal Medicine,* Vol.49, No.16, (August 2010), pp.1767-1773, ISSN 1349-7235

Kurisu, S.; Inoue, I.; Kawagoe, T.; Ishihara, M.; Shimatani, Y.; Nakama, Y.; Ohkawa, K.; Maruhashi, T.; Kagawa, E.; Dai, K. & Aokage, T. (2008). Torsade de pointes associated with bradycardia and takotsubo cardiomyopathy. *Canadian Journal of Cardiology,* Vol.24, No.8, (August 2008), pp.640-642, ISSN 0828-282X

Larsen, JA. & Kadish, AH. (1998). Effects of gender on cardiac arrhythmias. *Journal of Cardiovascular Electrophysiology,* Vol.9, No.6, (June 1998), pp.655-664, ISSN 1045-3873

Mahida, S.; Dalageorgou, C. & Behr, ER. (2009). Long-QT syndrome and torsades de pointes in a patient with Takotsubo cardiomyopathy: an unusual case. *Europace,* Vol.11, No.3, (March 2009), pp.376-378, ISSN 1099-5129

Micallef, T.; Gruppetta, M.; Cassar, A. & Fava, S. (2010). Takotsubo cardiomyopathy in a patient with severe hypothyroidism: a case report. *Journal of cardiovascular medicine (Hagerstown, Md.),* doi: 10.2459/JCM.0b013e3283403454, ISSN 1558-2027

Nault, MA.; Baranchuk, A.; Simpson, CS. & Redfearn, DP. (2007). Takotsubo cardiomyopathy: a novel "proarrhythmic" disease. *Anadolu Kardiyoloji Dergisi,* Vol.7, Supp.No.l, (July 2007), pp.101-103, ISSN 1302-8723

Okada, T.; Miyata, S.; Hashimoto, K.; Maie, K. & Mochizuki, S. (2007). Takotsubo cardiomyopathy associated with torsades de pointes and long QT interval: a case report. *Journal of Cardiology,* Vol.50, No.1, (July 2007), pp.83-88, ISSN 0914-5087

Pacha, O.; Kadikoy, H.; Amro, M.; Haque, W. & Abdellatif, A. (2010). Torsades de pointes and prolonged QT syndrome in Takotsubo cardiomyopathy. *Journal of cardiovascular medicine (Hagerstown, Md.),* doi: 10.2459/JCM.0b013e328336b4a6, ISSN 1558-2027

Patel, HM.; Kantharia, BK.; Morris, DL. & Yazdanfar, S. (2007). Takotsubo syndrome in African-American women with atypical presentations: a single-center experience. *Clinical Cardiology,* Vol.30, No.1, (January 2007), pp.14-18, ISSN 1932-8737

Peters, S. & Klein, HU. (2011). WCD LifeVest: Risk stratification in a case of tako-tsubo cardiomyopathy with QT interval prolongation. *Herz,* doi: 10.1007/s00059-011-3440-9, ISSN 0946-1299

Purvis, JA.; Cunningham, EL.; McGlinchey, PG. & Barr, SH. (2009). Drugs, electrolytes and tako-tsubo cardiomyopathy: triple aetiology of acquired long QT syndrome and torsades de pointes. *The Ulster medical journal Ulster,* Vol.78, No.3, (September 2009), pp.188-189, ISSN 0041-6193

Roden, DM. (2004). Drug-induced prolongation of the QT interval. *The New England Journal of Medicine,* Vol.350, No.10, (March 2004), pp.1013-22, ISSN 0028-4793

Rotondi, F.; Manganelli, F.; Lanzillo, T.; Candelmo, F.; Lorenzo, ED.; Marino, L. & Stanco, G. (2010). Tako-tsubo cardiomyopathy complicated by recurrent torsade de pointes in a patient with anorexia nervosa. *Internal Medicine,* Vol.49, No. 12, (June 2010), pp.1133-1137, ISSN 1349-7235

Samuelov-Kinori, L.; Kinori, M.; Kogan, Y.; Swartzon, M.; Shalev, H.; Guy, D.; Ferenidou, F.; Mashav, N.; Sadeh, B.; Atzmony, L.; Kliuk-Ben-Basat, O.; Steinvil, A. & Justo, D. (2009). Takotsubo cardiomyopathy and QT interval prolongation: who are the patients at risk for torsades de pointes? *Journal of electrocardiology,* Vol.42, No.4, (July-August 2009); pp.353-357, ISSN 0022-0736

Sasaki, O.; Nishioka, T.; Akima, T.; Tabata, H.; Okamoto, Y.; Akanuma, M.; Uehata, A.; Takase, B.; Katsushika, S.; Isojima, K.; Ohtomi, S. & Yoshimoto, N. (2006). Association of takotsubo cardiomyopathy and long QT syndrome. *Circulation Journal,* Vol.70, No.9, (September 2006), pp.1220-1222, ISSN 1346-9843

Thakar, S.; Chandra, P.; Hollander, G. & Lichstein, E. (2011). Electrocardiographic Changes in Takotsubo Cardiomyopathy. *Pacing and Clinical Electrophysiology,* doi: 10.1111/j.1540-8159.2011.03151, ISSN 1540-8159

Wedekind, H.; Müller, JG.; Ribbing, M.; Skurzewski, P.; Bozzetti, C.; Meyer-Krahmer, HJ. & Böcker, D. (2009). A fatal combination in an old lady: Tako-Tsubo cardiomyopathy, long QT syndrome, and cardiac hypertrophy. *Europace,* Vol.11, No.6, (June 2009), pp.820-822, ISSN 1099-5129

Wittstein, IS.; Thiemann, DR.; Lima, JA.; Baughman, KL.; Schulman, SP.; Gerstenblith, G.; Wu, KC.; Rade, JJ.; Bivalacqua, TJ. & Champion, HC. (2005). Neurohumoral features of myocardial stunning due to sudden emotional stress. *The New England Journal of Medicine,* Vol.352, No.6, (February 2005), pp.539-548, ISSN 0028-4793

Yamada, Y.; Tani, T.; Homma, M. & Saito, S. (2011). Two cases of torsades de pointes associated with takotsubo cardiomyopathy as the second insult. *Journal of electrocardiology,* doi.org/10.1016/j.jelectrocard.2011.03.002, ISSN 0022-0736

Part 6

Chagas Heart Disease

34

Chagas Heart Disease

Clara Isabel González and Julio César Mantilla
Grupo de Inmunología y Epidemiología Molecular, GIEM,
Facultad de Salud, Universidad Industrial de Santander
Colombia

1. Introduction

Chagas disease (CD) or American trypanosomiasis is a complex zoonosis produced by the infection with the intracellular protozoan parasite *Trypanosoma cruzi*. Although the disease was first described in 1909 by the Brazilian physician Carlos Chagas, this disease affects human beings since antiquity as it was demonstrated by paleoparasitology studies which proved the presence of DNA in mummies dating back to 9000 years old (Aufderheide et al., 2004; Guhl et al., 1999). The parasite *T. cruzi* is a hemoflagellate protozoan belonging to the Mastigophora class, Kinetoplastida order, Trypanosomatidae family, genus Trypanosoma, the group Stercoraria. It was named in honor of Oswaldo Cruz, who was the mentor of Carlos Chagas.

T. cruzi has a complex life cycle involving two hosts, an invertebrate, especially an insect vector and some vertebrates, including man and domestic and wild reservoirs (Tyler & Engman, 2001). The presence of CD in humans is purely accidental, as when the man came into contact with natural foci and caused ecological imbalances causing the adaptation of vectors to human dwellings and new food sources. Thus three overlapping cycles were established: the wild cycle, the peridomestic cycle and the domestic cycle (Coura, 2007). The parasite occurs in a variety of hosts and infects 150 species from 24 families of domestic (e.g., dogs, cats and guinea pigs) and wild animals (e.g., rodents, marsupials, and armadillos) (Rassi, et al., 2010). The vectors involved in the transmission of CD are insects of the Phylum Arthropoda, Class Insecta, Order Hemiptera, Family Reduviidae, belonging to the subfamily Triatominae. There have been reported approximately 130 species of wild and domiciliary triatomines although only a handful is the competent vector for *T. cruzi* (Schofield, 1981). The domestic species mainly colonize rural homes and peri-urban areas and these species are responsible for most human cases of Chagas disease in endemic areas. Sylvatic species are inhabitants of strict wild habitats such as cracks of rocks, bird nests or burrows of mammals and caves, among others. *Rhodnius prolixus* is the main domestic vector in the northern countries of South America and Central America, *Triatoma dimidiata* in Central America and *Triatoma infestans* in countries of the southern of South America (Guhl, 2007), these species are well adapted to human habitation.

T. cruzi presents four different morphological and biological forms: epimastigote, a replicative form located in the mid gut of the insect vector, it is the predominant form in the axenic culture; metacyclic trypomastigote develops in the posterior intestine and rectum of the insect vector and is the infective form; amastigote replicative stage, is located in the cytoplasm of mammalian host cells where it replicates by binary fission; blood trypomastigote comes from amastigote differentiation, leading to disruption of the host cell and releases into the bloodstream, where they are taken again by the blood-sucking vector (Brener, 1971) (Figure 1)

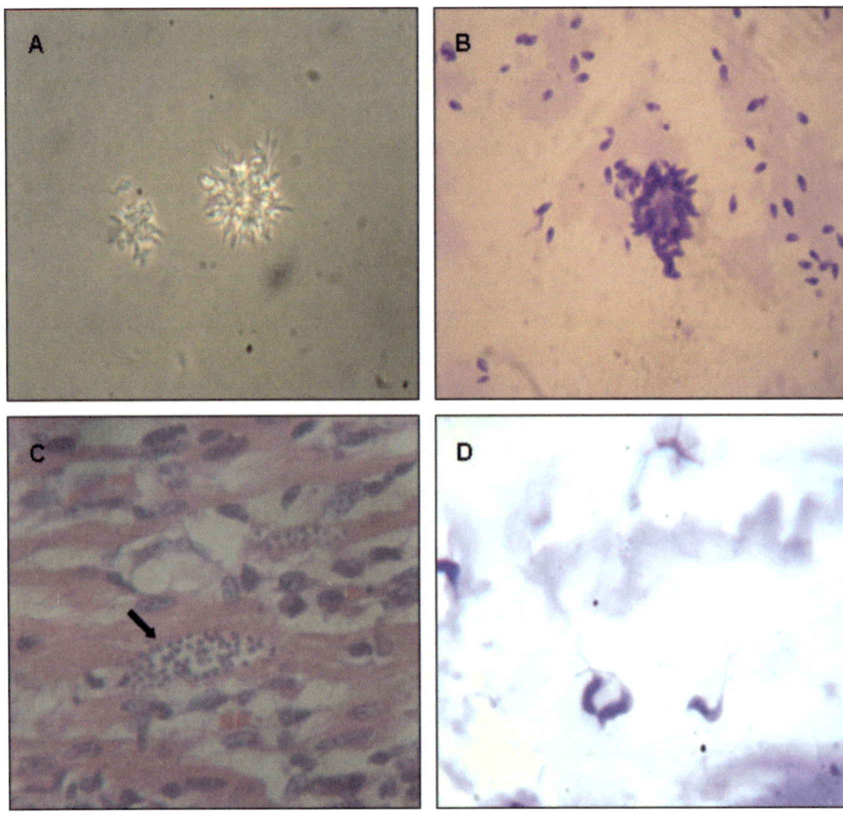

Fig. 1. *Trypanosoma cruzi* different stages. A) Epimastigotes of culture B) Amastigotes in Vero cells C) Nests of amastigotes in cardiac tissue D) Blood trypomastigotes stained with hematoxiylin-eosin.

The classic forms of *T. cruzi* transmission are vectorial, congenital, by transfusion, through organ transplants and labour accident. Vector-borne transmission is the most common and is contaminative by the presence of the infectious form in the faeces of the vector which is released when feeding on the host. The trypomastigotes penetrate through the opening of the bite or loss of continuity due to scratching or active penetration of oral or ocular mucosa. Before screening programs in blood banks, transfusion was the second form of transmission by the presence in donor's blood or blood products infected with parasite forms (Schmunis, 1999). Another important source of transmission is the donation of organs from infected individuals with the development of acute Chagas in the immunosuppressed recipient (Barcan et al., 2005). The passage of the parasite from infected mother to her baby during pregnancy, childbirth or while breast-feeding is high in some endemic regions, specially in Bolivia. The congenital transmission can lead to abortions, premature births or infected babies (Torrico et al., 2004).

2. The impact of Chagas disease

CD is currently is recognized by the World Health Organization (WHO) as one of the tropical neglected diseases and the infection with *T. cruzi* is the third parasitic infection after malaria and schistosomiasis (Schmunis & Yadon, 2010). CD is an important public health problem in 21 countries of South and Central America. The Pan American Health Organization (OPS, 2006) estimates that 7.7 million people are infected with *T. cruzi*, 109 million are at risk of infection and 12,500 deaths occur per year. The number of new annual cases of vector-borne infection is 41,000 and congenital Chagas' is 14,000 (WHO 2008).

Although this disease is considered typical of rural areas and poor suburbs with inadequate housing conditions, in recent decades in many Latin American countries there has been a substantial migration from rural to peri-urban areas. Migration has not only occurred from rural to urban areas in Latin America, but also to developed countries of North America, Europe and Asia. Accordingly, further cases have been detected in non-endemic countries like the USA, Canada, Spain, Japan and Australia due to population migration from endemic countries. In the United States have reported more than 300,000 people infected with *T. cruzi* and in Spain from 40 to 60,000 (Bern & Montgomery, 2009; Gascon et al., 2010).

The migration in endemic countries has led to the passive transport of vectors and the emergence of cases in areas considered of low endemicity. Additionally, the national initiatives for the elimination of the domestic vectors, including not only insecticide spraying but also a rural housing improvement, have led to the elimination of traditional vectors. However, a new transmission pattern is being introduced due to the presence of palms and trees located close to houses and sylvatic vectors that are attracted sporadically by light and feeding conditions. Consequentially, transmission by new vectors has arisen and often these vectors often have high rates of infection. This couple with the presence of wild reservoirs in the peridomestic area presenting high rates of infection has led to an alternate form to vectorial transmission in these areas, such as oral transmission (Briceño-León, 2009). This form of transmission is usually associated with acute and fatal outcomes and it has been increasing especially in the Brazilian Amazon where it is considered an emerging disease (Coura et al., 2002). The first report was given in 1960 in Teutonia with five deaths involved (Valente et al., 2009). Since then 600 new cases of acute Chagas have been reported, 50% associated with oral transmission. There are also reports in Venezuela (Alarcon de Noya et al., 2010), Mexico (Salazar-Schettino et al., 2011) and in the last three years in Colombia has increased, especially in Santander with six outbreaks of acute Chagas and three fatal cases (Díaz et al., 2009).

3. Clinical aspects of Chagas disease

3.1 Phases of Chagas disease

3.1.1 Acute phase

The clinic course of CD could have two phases: acute and chronic. The acute phase is characterized by the presence of *T. cruzi* trypomastigotes in the bloodstream, the parasitaemia generally persists for 4–8 weeks and it resolves spontaneously. In the majority of cases, especially in adults, this phase of infection is asymptomatic, however a small percentage of patients develops the acute disease characterized by important manifestations such as malaise, prolonged high fever, headache, edema, hepatomegaly, splenomegaly and generalized lymphadenopathy (Prata, 2001). In the acute form of CD, the first signs appear

7–10 days after infection. The Romaña's sign is observed when the parasite penetrates the conjunctiva; but when the parasite penetrates through the skin the patient develops the chagoma at the site of inoculation. The adjacent lymph nodes to the site of entry of the parasite are generally compromised, which together with the conjunctival or eyelid lesions constitute the ophthalmo - lymphonodal complex. Aproximately the fifty percent of the patients who develop the acute CD has Romaña's sign, and one-quarter has the inoculation chagoma. The Romaña's sign is characterized by painless, unilateral swelling of the upper and lower eyelid, with rose -violet coloration, congestion and edema of the conjunctiva, the submandibular, preauricular or other near lymphonode are enlarged, but not adhering to deep layers, occasionally may appear palpebral and periorbital cellulitis, sometimes with necrosis and abundant parasites. The inoculation chagoma generally appear on the skin of the face or the extremities, and is a forunculoid lesion, with a rose violet tone. In these patients, the initial electrocardiogram is normal, but after 2-3 weeks might show anomalies such sinus tachycardia, low QRS voltage or first grade atrioventricular block, the chest radiograph is also normal, however it might show cardiomegaly (Dias, 1989; Rassi et al., 2010).

The majority of patients, (90% or more) with acute CD survive the initial infection and remain healthy and asymptomatic, but a few individuals, between 2 -10%, generally infants or immunodepressed patients, or many people like children or adults who acquired the infection due to oral contamination, develop an acute and severe disease with myocarditis and cardiac insufficiency or with meningoencephalitis, clinical conditions that maybe cause death (Nobrega et al., 2009). Regarding to the central nervous system (CNS) involvement in CD, in the initial acute phase, the infection is asymptomatic and only a small percentage of cases develops encephalitis in the acute phase of disease; headache, seizure, focal neurologic signs and progressive decrease in consciousness are the notorious symptoms (Cordova et al., 2007).

3.1.2 Chronic phase

The great majority of patients, who were infected with *T. cruzi*, remain asymptomatic in the chronic phase, without abnormalities in the electrocardiogram and the radiological evaluations of the heart, esophagus and colon. This form of the chronic phase of CD is named indeterminate form, it is present in the half of infected people of endemic areas, and may persist until dead in 40-50% of the cases. All patients with the indeterminate form of CD are positive in serological or parasitological examinations, and do not have symptoms or signs of the disease, but using specialized methods such as ambulatory electrocardiographic monitoring or endomyocardial biopsies, may demonstrate that they have at least some degree of cardiac damage. The morphologic features of the indeterminate form of CD in autopsies performed for us in individuals who died of other causes, include discrete focal infiltration of mononuclear cells with lymphocytes predominance, and mild interstitial fibrosis, these changes are notorious in the subendocardical zone, and near to the cardiac conduction system. The change from the indeterminate form to the determinate cardiac or digestive occurs slowly in a lapse of 10 - 20 years after the initial infection, in a few cases, approximately 2-3% per year. In these patients, the CD adopts a slow and benign course, but others develop dilated cardiomyopathy, heart congestive failure or arrhythmias. In sporadic cases the CD progresses directly from the acute form to determinate chronic form of human CD, and is named the subacute form, that generally affects young adults, these patients develop severe cardiopathy with cardiac failure (Marin-Neto et al., 1999).

In the chronic phase of CD, the fundamental morphological feature in patients with chronic chagasic cardiopathy (CCC) is a mixture of cellular infiltration of lymphocytes and monocytes with few plasma cells, and fibrous tissue, that correlate with diverse clinical symptoms and signs, since asymptomatic to a congestive syndrome with damage of conduction system, arrhythmias, disturbances in the ventricular repolarization and the extrasystoles. Thromboembolic phenomens due to cardiac mural thrombosis are also frequent. In the majority of these patients, in the thorax radiographs, the heart contour appears normal. In some cases the lack of symptoms is surprising, and it does not have correlation with damage of tissue detected under microscopical examination. The symptomatic patients with CCC related palpitations by arrhythmias or fatigue by cardiac failure. In the physical examination, the arrhythmias and the extrasystoles are the most frequent clinical features detected. In these patients, the cardiac failure has a slow and progressive course, generally with features of right failure predominating the legs edema, jugular ingurgitation, ascites, and hepatomegaly. The thromboembolic manifestations due to mural thrombosis are frequent, and in autopsies done by us, the pulmonary thromboembolism is the most common anatomopathological feature, although brain embolism is also recognized in a few cases. After the manifestations of cardiac failure, the patients may recover or die in a later episode to one year after the first symptoms of decompensation. In these patients the periganglionitis with reduction of neuronal bodies especially in the sympathetic system, the sinusal node fibrosis, and destruction of tissues of cardiac conduction system and the myocardial cells are related with the early alterations of autonomous nervous system. The described changes can explain the reduction of the response to cardiovagal reflex in the sinusal node, and the reduction of variability of the heart frecuency. The cardiovagal denervation increased the sympathetic tone and could explain why the arrhythmias, blockades and sudden death are the first clinical manifestations in these patients (Samuel et al., 1983; Rassi et al., 2001).

The digestive form of CD is present almost exclusively in Argentina, Brazil, Chile and Bolivia, although they have reported isolated cases in Colombia, Central America and Mexico. The symptoms are the consequence of achalasia. The dysphagia is the first disturbance that may lead to malnutrition and weight loss. Odynophagia and epigastric pain also occurs in cases of megaesophagus, and chronic constipation, abdominal distension and occasionally intestinal obstruction of large bowel in cases of megacolon (Florez et al., 2010).

3.2 Pathological anatomy

The changes described below are the product of the experience gathered in the practice of autopsies of patients who died of various forms of CD, and reflect the interaction between inflammatory response, cellular damage and alterations of the extracellular matrix, three pathologic processes generated by the parasite in the tissues, particularly in the heart, esophagus, colon and central nervous system.

In the acute phase when the infectious forms of *T. cruzi* penetrate in the cell, such macrophages, fibroblasts, Schwann cells, and myocytes, they transform in amastigotes, subsequently reproduce and form the parasitic nest or pseudocyst, after 3 - 5 days the parasite differentiates to trypomastigote, the pseudocyst enlarges, breaks the cell, releasing intact or degenerate forms of the parasite, which act in the interstitium as a particle that promotes the inflammatory response. In these cases the heart is enlarged, congestive, flaccid with haemorrhagic foci on the epicardic surface, and at the cut, the cardiac chambers are dilated and the myocardium shows areas of haemorrhage and necrosis (Figure 2 A and B). In the microscopic examination, the extent of the inflammatory response is proportional to the number of pseudocyst and damaged cells. A dense interstitial infiltration of lymphocytes, macrophages, with a few neutrophils and eosinophils around the pseudocyst and damaged cells is observed in the acute severe form of CD (Figure 2 C and D).

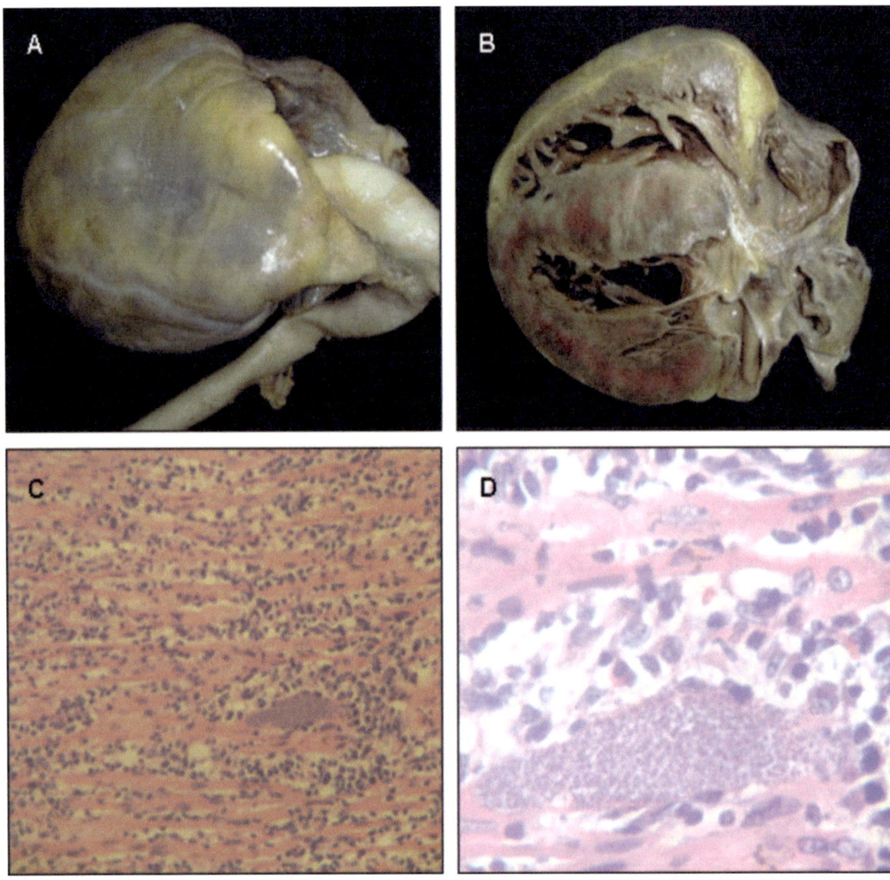

Fig. 2. Acute Chagas heart disease A) Heart enlarged with rounded shape. B) The surface of cut shows dilatation of four chambers, with pale and red areas, which correspond to focus of inflammation, necrosis and haemorrhage C) Nest of *Trypanosoma cruzi*, dense interstitial infiltrate of lymphocytes, plasma cells and monocytes with necrosis of myocardial cells D) Nest of *Trypanosoma cruzi* with rupture of myocardial cell and infiltrate inflammatory of mononuclear cells.

In the chronic phase of CD, the most important feature in chagasic cardiopathy, is the enlarge of heart with dilatation of chambers, mural thrombus (Figure 3A) and the mixture of cellular infiltration of lymphocytes, monocytes with a few plasma cells, and fibrous tissue (Figure 3B). In the adipose tissue of epicardium there are mononuclear cells with predominance of lymphocytes, which are more abundant around the nervous fibers and ganglionar cells (Figure 3C and 3D).

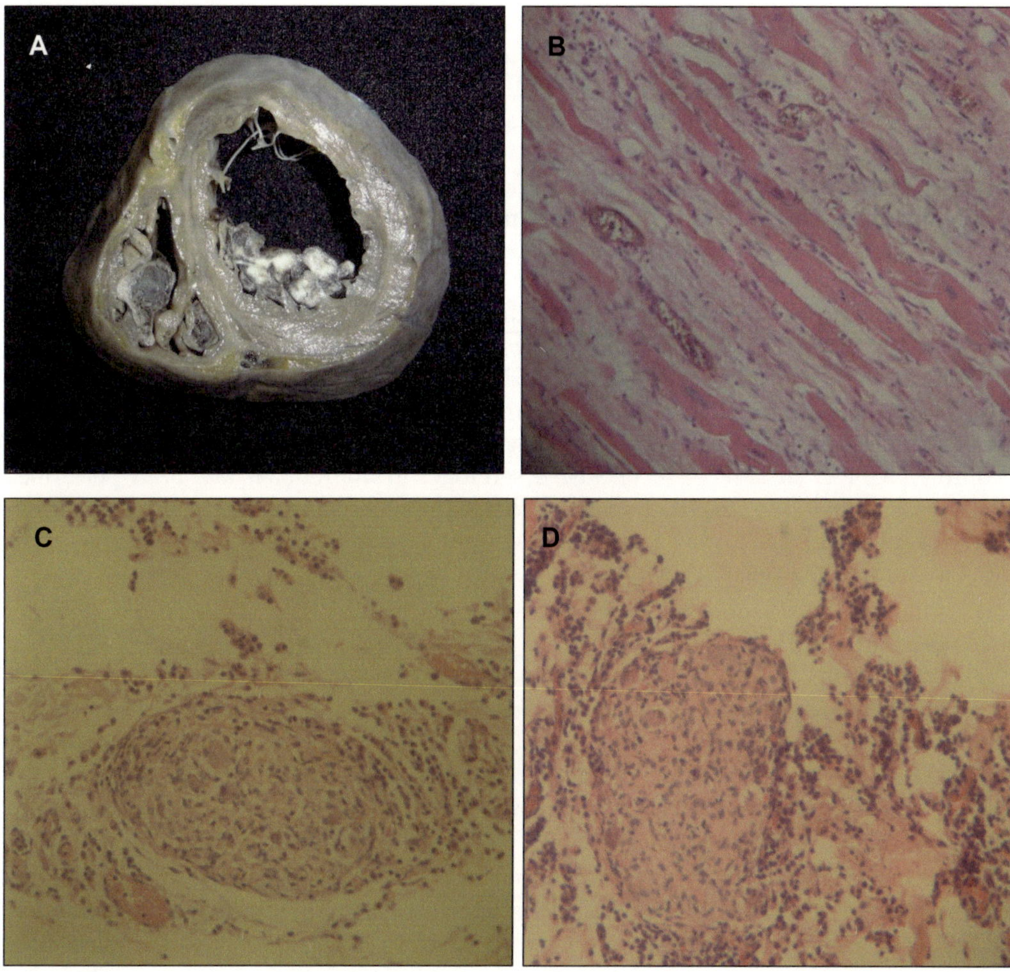

Fig. 3. Chronic Chagas heart disease A) Heart enlarged with dilatation of ventricles and mural thrombus B) Separation of the myocardial fibers, edema, abundant fibroblasts whith extracellular matrix increase, and scarce mononuclear inflammatory cells. C and D) Marked infiltration of lymphocytes and plasma cells around the nervous fibers and ganglionar neurons of cardiac plexus.

In case of oral transmission of the parasite, in the esophagus mucosa there are abundants lymphocytes and histiocytes, but the parasites are scarce or not identified (Zafra et al., 2008; Mantilla et al., 2010). In the digestive form the CD, the megaesophagus and megacolon are the result of destruction of neuronal bodies of intramural autonomic nervous ganglia of Meissner and Auerbach of the digestive tube in these sections.

4. Diagnosis and treatment

4.1 Laboratory diagnosis

The diagnosis of *T. cruzi* infection depends on the phase of infection, in the acute phase the patent parasitemia allows the use of parasitological methods to see or culture the parasite in the first weeks. The diagnosis is difficult in the chronic phase, mainly due the very low or intermittent parasitemia, therefore, the serological methods are usual. Additionally, CD endemic areas also present endemicity of other parasites especially *Leishmania sp.* and *T. rangeli* (Gomes et al., 2009). This fact leads to the serological methods which present high sensitivity but lack of specificity because of antigenic cross-reactivity. Therefore, the World Health Organization recommends that at least two assays based on different techniques should be used. The serological methods frequently used in the diagnosis of CD are enzyme-linked immunosorbent assays (ELISA), indirect hemagglutination assays (IHA), immunofluorescence indirect assays (IFI), immunoblotting assayss (IB), and immunochromatographic assay. These methods used crude antigens but recombinant proteins and synthetic peptides are being used to improve the specificity (Hernandez et al., 2010; Praast et al., 2011; Umezawa et al., 2001; Umezawa et al., 2004).

On the other hand, molecular methods, in particular amplification by the polymerase chain reaction (PCR), provide an alternative diagnosis of CD (Gomes et al., 1999) specially to confirm diagnosis in case of inconclusive serology; in addition, it has been performed nested-PCR assays (N-PCR) (Marcon et al., 2002), quantitative real-time PCR assays (qRT-PCR) (Piron et al., 2007) and oligochromatography assays (OligoC) (Deborggraeve et al., 2009) to improve the detection of *T. cruzi* DNA.

4.2 Treatment

The treatment of CD is aimed at two main aspects: the removal of the parasite and the symptomatic management of cardiac manifestations. The options for the treatment of CD are restricted to the use of two drugs, the nifurtimox and the benznidazole. These drugs are indicated in the acute phase of infection, congenital forms, reactivation associated with immunosuppression especially in children and young adults with infections transmitted by blood transfusion and organ transplantation. Although the benznidazole have proven to be effective in the early stage of chronic infection its effectiveness at the late stage is limited. Both drugs produce serious complications such as neurological toxicity, depression, anorexia, vomiting and depression in bone marrow. Antitrypanosomal treatment in mild and late stage Chagas disease is under study by the BENEFIT trial (Rassi et al., 2010). The drug resistance is a major problem in the treatment of infectious and tropical diseases. In CD has a strong impact on the increase in the number of therapeutic failure aggravated by the few options of treatment, currently, there are numerous efforts in the search for treatment alternatives.

The amioradone is used in the management of cardiac symptoms especially for patients with sustained ventricular tachycardia, and for those with non-sustained ventricular tachycardia and myocardial dysfunction. Patients haemodynamically unstable, and those resuscitated from sudden death are treated with implantable cardioverter defibrillators (Rassi et al., 2010).

5. Pathogenesis and pathophysiology

The pathogenesis of CD is a process that is not fully understood. Most individuals infected with *T. cruzi* do not develop an acute phase and the injury to the myocardium and nervous system is directly related to tissue parasitism. The rupture of the nests of parasites in the tissues releases antigens of *T. cruzi* sensitizing cardiac and neuronal fibers, leading to the destruction of these cells by anti-*T. cruzi* response mediates by CD8+ and CD4+ lymphocytes (Palomino et al., 2000). For the chronic phase, different mechanisms have been proposed; it is currently accepted that the inflammatory response generated by the parasite, which has not been eliminated by the immune system induces chronic inflammation in some individuals leading to tissue damage (Tarleton, 2003). There are several factors that directly or indirectly contribute to the progression and therefore evolution of the CD in the host. Some of these factors are inherent to the parasite, as the virulence related to their tissue tropism, their genetic and antigenic features, others are related to the host, such as age, race, nutritional status, immune response and genetic constitution (Dutra & Gollob 2008).

5.1 Associated to *T. cruzi*

T. cruzi presents a great heterogeneity both genotypic and phenotypic (Tibayrenc et al., 1993) and consists of different populations which circulate among humans, vectors, domestic animals and wild reservoirs. These populations show different behaviors in terms of parasitaemia, virulence, pathogenicity, interactions with host cells, tissue tropism and sensitivity to drugs. *T. cruzi* has been classified into several groups, initially using biochemical markers (zymodemes) and subsequently molecular markers (esquizodemes, clonets and lineages). The last meeting of experts standardized the nomenclature of *T. cruzi* and accepted the existence of six discrete typing units (DTUs) called TCI-VI (Zingales et al., 2009). The heterogeneity of *T. cruzi* extends to the forms and severity of clinical presentation with a particular geographical distribution. In Brazil, Tc I is present in the sylvatic cycle of transmission with low parasitemia in humans and experimental animals, therefore it is considered non-virulent, except for some reports of the Amazon (Texeira et al., 2006). By contrast, in this country Tc II is involved in the domestic cycle of transmission and causes high parasitemias, human infections and both heart and gastrointestinal diseases (Zingales et al., 1998). The same behavior is observed in other southern countries of South America as Argentina, Chile, Paraguay and Uruguay. By contrast, in the northern countries of South America and Central America predominates Tc I associated with heart disease and involved in both domestic and sylvatic cycle (Higo et al., 2004). Recently, our group reported the presence for both groups for the first time, Tc I and Tc II group in blood of seropositive individuals to antigens of *T. cruzi* associated with chagasic cardiomyopathy (CC) (Zafra et al., 2008, Gonzalez et al., 2010). The two groups were also identified in tissues of deceased patients with CC, with predominance of Tc I (Zafra et al., 2011). One individual presented a mixed infection with Tc I and Tc II, but Tc II was the group associated with cardiac involvement (Mantilla et al., 2009).

5.2 Associated with the host

5.2.1 Innate immune response

In recent years, new data related with interaction between innate immune cells and *T. cruzi* have been presented. This interaction is crucial in controlling parasite replication and removal by the action of phagocytic cells, activation of antigen presenting cells and natural killer cells (NK) in the host tissue. The innate immune cells recognize pathogen associated molecular patterns (PAMPs) through their pattern recognition receptors (PRR). The best characterized PRRs are Toll-like receptors (TLRs), which are expressed in the cell membrane or are located intracellularly. When TLRs recognize microbial components, it induces signals responsible for the activation and production of inflammatory cytokines and chemokines (Akira & Takeda, 2004). In *T. cruzi*, TLR2 was the first receptor identified which recognizes glycosylphosphatidylinositol (GPI)-anchores mucin-like glycoproteins, distributed to the cell surface membrane of *T. cruzi* trypomastigotes (Campos et al., 2001). This receptor also recognizes the *T. cruzi* protein Tc52 and induces dendritic cell activation (Ouaissi et al., 2002). The TLR4-MD2 complex recognizes glycoinositolphospholipids containig ceramide (GIPL) (Bafica et al., 2006) and TLR9 recognizes DNA rich in CpG sequences. The TLR-mediated MyD88 signaling pathway induces pro-inflammatory cytokines as TNF-α and IL-12 and stimulates the production of nitric oxide (NO) involved in parasite clearance (Bafica et al., 2006). Other mechanisms for the TLR- independent recognition of *T. cruzi* have been described and involved the molecule NOD1 that induces type I IFNs (Kayama & Takeda, 2010). Innate immunity in turn acts as an immunomodulatory specific immune response through the generation of the microenvironment of cytokines that regulates the differentiation of effector T cell subpopulations (Bilate & Cunha-Neto, 2008, Dutra et al., 2009).

5.2.2 Adaptative immune response

The role of the adaptative immune response in the pathogenesis of CD has been subject of much controversy, for decades the role of the autoimmune component was accepted as directly responsible for heart damage (Takle & Hudson, 1989). This was supported by the detection of autoantibodies against cardiac antigens, chronicity and difficulty of finding parasites in affected individuals (Cunha-Neto et al., 1995). However, the development of more sensitive molecular tests that allowed detection of low numbers of parasites, the fact that immunosuppressed patients developed acute and severe CD and experimental models showed that the parasite, even in small amounts was essential for the development of the disease (Zhang & Tarleton, 1999; Tarleton, 2003). The presence of autoantibodies may be explained by the release of autoantigens as the result of the immune response against the parasite (Cunha-Neto et al., 1995).

Currently, the role of chronic inflammation and unbalance of the immune response generated by the parasite is accepted as responsible for the damage and tissue regeneration associated with organ dysfunction (Dutra & Gollob 2008). Although heart inflammatory cells contribute to control parasite growth, they are also involved in perpetuating inflammatory infiltrate. In chagasic patients the cellular infiltrate consists mainly of T lymphocytes with a predominance of CD8+ cells but also contains CD4+ cells and macrophages. Both CD8+ cell and CD4+ exhibit characteristics of activated T cells and correlate with the expression of inflammatory cytokines such as TNF-α and INF-γ and a smaller number of regulatory cells producing IL-10 (Araújo et al., 2007). Patients with chronic CC have higher serum levels of TNF-α and CCL2 compared with asymptomatic individuals (Talvani et al., 2004). In this context, cytokines, chemokines, receptors and signaling pathways associated with activation of pro-inflammatory proteins and with low expression of immunoregulatory proteins will be clearly associated with the immunopathogenesis of CD. This coupled with the fact that most infected individuals remain asymptomatic throughout life and only between 15 to 30% of them developed the disease demonstrates the importance of host genetic component. Thus individuals with genetic predisposition to proinflammatory phenotype in the presence of *T. cruzi* would be those that develop chronic and severe forms of the disease.

6. Chagas disease as a complex disease

6.1 Human genome variation

The variation in the human genome sequence plays an important role, yet little known in the etiology of many diseases. The establishment of the association between genotype and phenotype is crucial for understanding biological processes and in the case of disease, pathogenic mechanisms that lead to their development. For monogenic diseases, the methods of genetic linkage and physical maps facilitated the identification of mutations responsible for the phenotype associated with pathology. Thus numerous Mendelian-type diseases were identified. However, most common diseases are complex and multifactorials therefore, are the result of the effect of multiple genetic variants on the phenotype and their interaction with environmental factors. In the case of infectious diseases is known that not only the genotypic and phenotypic differences of the microorganism determine the development of a particular disease, but also the variation in the host genome may have an important role in the development of resistance or susceptibility.

6.2 Single nucleotide polymorphisms (SNP)

SNP type polymorphisms are the most common forms of genetic variation in the human genome, currently the common SNPs estimated density is about 10 to 15 million (The International HapMap Consortium 2007, http://www.hapmap.org). Its usefulness as genetic markers associated with various infectious and noninfectious diseases has been amply demonstrated (Pacheco & Moraes, 2009). The SNPs have been the markers most commonly used for its stability, low mutation rate and are plentiful throughout the genome, being found in exons affecting the protein function, in introns or regulatory regions affecting gene expression and therefore the processing and maturation of the messenger, or many of them have been identified in intergenic regions with effect unknown over gene expression or phenotype (Frazer et al., 2009). Numerous reports using one or more polymorphisms have been published (Pacheco & Moraes, 2009), but most of them only explain less than 5% of the observed contribution of the genetic component to the risk of disease. This fact substantially limits the use of these markers to predict risk and in some cases the results have been controversial. One of the main problems with these studies is that in many cases it is not known a direct effect on the phenotype and in common diseases the effect is modest. Therefore, it is necessary to identify other variables involved and the interaction among them (Feero et al., 2010). Another limitation in this type of study is related to the number of SNPs, which in an individual genome is from 3 to 4 million and in the human genome it is estimated between 10 to 11 million (Frazer et al., 2009). Thus an individual would require testing thousands of polymorphisms to identify genes involved in susceptibility to a particular pathology.

The International HapMap Project (The International HapMap Consortium 2003-2007) has overcome some of the difficulties in mapping SNPs and identification of susceptibility genes in complex diseases. The advances are related with the reduction in the number of SNPs to be genotyped, increased statistical power and the accurate mapping in association studies. This project HapMap anticipates building a database for common haplotypes in different human populations (www.hapmap.org). When the markers are in linkage disequilibrium (LD) in the population, there is redundant information. If two markers are in complete LD, each of the genotypes of a SNP is completely determined by the other, thus the genotyping of one will suffice for the information of the two (Conrad et al., 2006). The selection of non-redundant markers present in an area with high density of markers has been called "haplotype tagging" and the SNPs selected by this method are called "tag-SNPs" or label SNP (de Baker et al., 2006). The main objective of this haplotype tagging is to reduce the number and cost of genotyping, keeping most of the information that they contain (Daly et al., 2001). The technological progress in the last decade, related to the development of high density maps of markers, maps of linkage disequilibrium and haplotypes (Cardon & Abecasis, 2003), the use of microarrays for genotyping of SNPs (Steemers & Gunderson, 2007) and bioinformatics tools have helped overcome some of these difficulties. Based on these developments, in recent years the genome scans (GWAS) have popularized (Cheung et al., 2005; Galvan et al., 2010). In fact, after 5 years of the first GWAS, which identified the association of complement factor H with macular degeneration related to age (Klein et al., 2005) there have been published more than 450 GWAS and associations with more than 2000 SNPs in numerous human diseases such as type 1 and 2 diabetes, Crohn's disease, rheumatoid arthritis, prostate cancer, breast, tuberculosis and visceral leishmaniasis among many others (Manolio 2010; Ku et al., 2010). Many of these studies have identified markers on genes already known for its role in the pathogenesis of the disease, but others have also identified strong associations with genes that apparently have not relation with the characteristic of the disease process (Frazer et al., 2009).

6.3 Human genome variation in Chagas disease

The chronic CD courses in 70% of individuals without symptoms and only between 15-30% of infected individuals have cardiac involvement and/or digestive, with different levels of severity and mortality. This clearly suggests the role of the individual genetic component in disease development, a fact that is reinforced with the identification of strains of mice with different susceptibility phenotypes. The C3H strain develops cardiac lesions similar to human chagasic cardiomyopathy, the A/J phenotype presents different pathology and DBA/2 is totally resistant (Marinho et al., 2004). The association related with genetic susceptibility or resistance to infection with *T. cruzi* in human has been demonstrated in some epidemiological studies related to the molecules of the major histocompatibility complex (MHC) (Llop et al., 1991; Fernández-Mestre et al., 1998; Nieto et al., 2000; Layrisse et al., 2000; Williams-Blangero et al., 2003; Moreno et al., 2004).

The identification of biomarkers to establish an association with the risk of developing the disease is critical because could be used not only in prevention and prognosis but also as a therapeutic target. It is now clearly accepted that the immune response is crucial in the pathogenesis of CD and especially the role of the chronic inflammation in the tissular damage (Dutra & Gollob 2008). The balance between anti-inflammatory and pro-inflammatory cytokines and their receptors is crucial in determining whether *T. cruzi* parasites will be eliminated without causing tissue damage. Thus, the lack of efficient immunoregulation in cardiomyopathic patients could contribute to clinical forms of CD. In this sense, case-control studies have searched association between onset or severity of the disease and the functional polymorphisms of genes known to participate in host inflammatory response.

6.3.1 Variation in pro-inflamatory cytokines

In CD, it has been observed that patients infected with *T. cruzi* display increased levels of plasma TNF-α compared to non-infected individuals, where plasma TNF-α levels were 4-fold higher in asymptomatic and cardiomyopathic patients with left ventricular ejection fraction (LVEF) >50% and 8-fold higher cardiomyopathic patients with LVEF ≤50% than non-infected individuals (Ferreira et al., 2003). In fact, the measurement of TNF-α level has been suggested as a tool to identify patients with heart dysfunction (Talvani et al., 2004).

Some positive associations have been observed in Mexican and Brazilian populations, between polymorphisms of regulatory region of *TNFA* gene and CC (Rodríguez-Pérez et al., 2005; Drigo et al., 2006; Pissetti et al., 2011). The most studied allelic form (*TNFA* -308) has functional implication because it affects the TNF-α level. However, discrepancies have been observed with Peruvian and Brazilian populations in which the frequencies of genetic variants were similar in asymptomatic individuals and CC patients (Beraún et al., 1998; Drigo et al., 2007). These differences could be affected by some factors. Among the most important factors would be: sample size, genetic differences between populations, criteria for the selection of controls (study design), linkage disequilibrium with HLA genes and influence of other polymorphisms present in the same region. Some polymorphisms of *TNFA* gene show a high level of LD, and the haplotypes formed by these variants could be affecting levels of protein expression (Figure 4). In Colombian population of highly endemic area we also found associations with genetic variants in *TNFA* and *TNFR2* genes (Criado et al., publication process). Unlike other chronic inflammatory diseases such as rheumatoid arthritis in which the blocking of TNF-α has been used successfully in treatment, in CD the experimental evidence using animal models showed that TNF-α blockade enhances left ventricular dysfunction (Bilate et al., 2007). Therefore, it is necessary to understand the regulation of the expression of TNF-α and its receptors and the effect of host polymorphisms for the use of therapeutic strategies with target TNF-α.

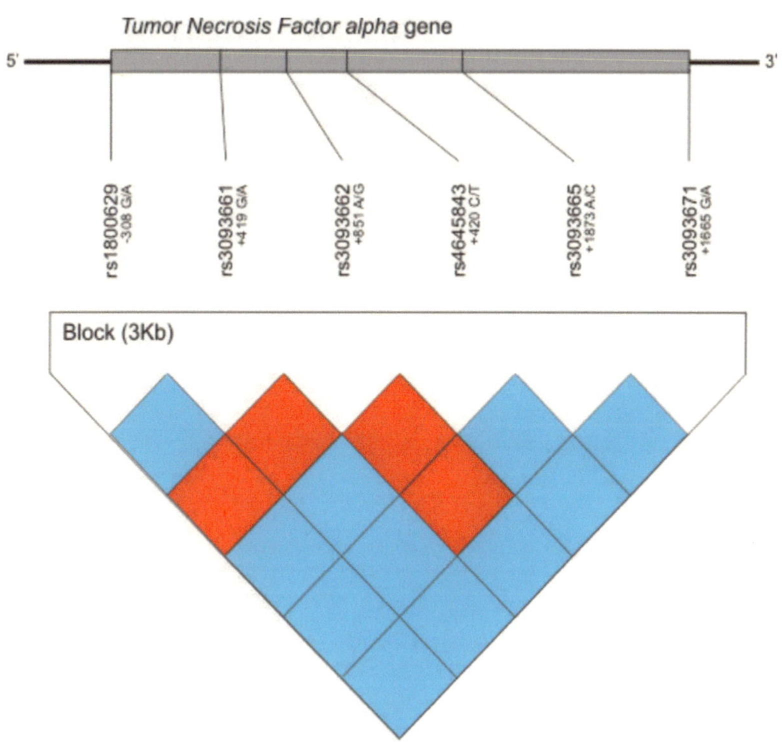

Fig. 4. Plot of LD across the *TNFA* gene. The image shows a high-resolution LD association plot between SNPs located in the *TNFA* gene, D′ values are reported in the boxes and represented by color, which ranges from red (higher D′ scores) to white (lower D′ scores). The SNP nomenclature is presented as numbers that refer to the position of polymorphism in the gene.

In our study population we also found associations of functional polymorphisms present in other pro-inflammatory cytokine genes such as *IL1B* (Flórez et al., 2006), *IL12B* (Zafra et al., 2007), *IFNG* (Torres et al., 2010), and lack of association with *IL6* (Torres et al., 2010) (Table 1).

6.3.2 Variation in chemokines and chemokine receptors

The inflammatory infiltrate of mononuclear cell is driven by a set of specific chemokines that determine the type of cells present in the tissue. Chemokines and chemokine receptors play an important role in mediating the extravasation and accumulation of specific effector and memory cells in chronic inflammatory processes in several diseases. In CD there is experimental evidence in patients with CC and models of *T. cruzi* infection that show that chemokines and chemokine receptors may be relevant mediators of leukocyte influx, which is involved in the pathogenesis of the disease (Teixeira et al., 2002; Marino et al., 2004; Talvani et al., 2004; Machado et al., 2005; Gomes et al., 2005; Guedes et al., 2010; Manque et al., 2011). Genetic variants in genes of chemokine receptors as *CCR5* have been also studied in Peruvian and Venezuelan populations with the identification of a protection marker (Calzada et al., 2001; Fernandez-Mestre et al., 2004). *CCR5* gene polymorphisms had been extensively studied in HIV and have been defined haplogroups which are affecting the transcriptional activity (Gonzalez et al., 1999). These haplogroups are composed by different combinations of *CCR2* and *CCR5* SNPs (Figure 5). Analyzing individual polymorphisms we found association between *CCR5*-2733 polymorphism and CC and also in four variants present in haplogroup HHE (*CCR2* +190, *CCR5* -2733, -2554 and -1835).

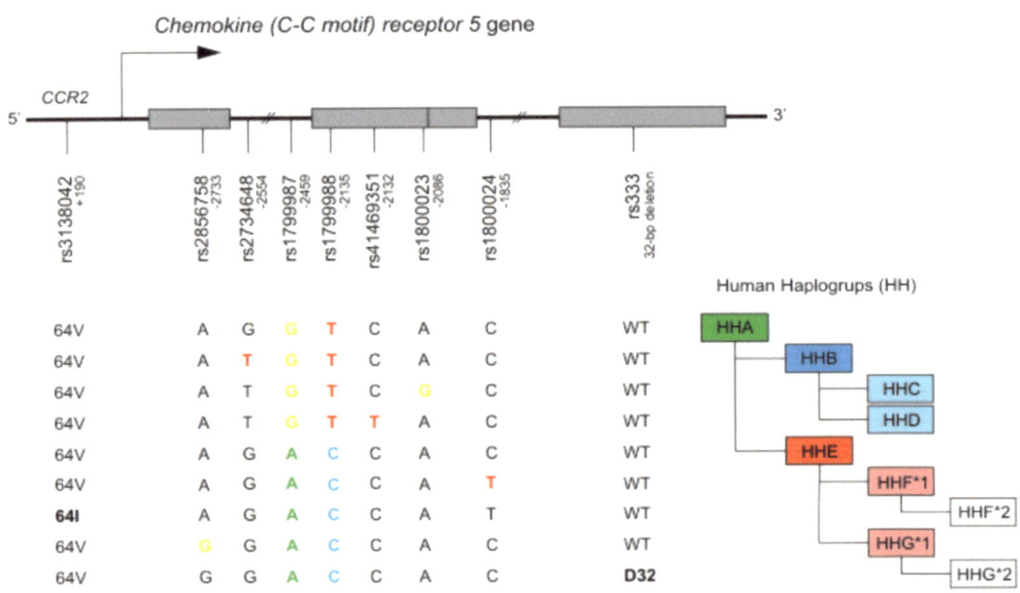

Fig. 5. Human haplogroups of *CCR2* and *CCR5* polymorphisms.

No association was observed with polymorphisms analysed in the chemokines *CCL5* and *CXCL8* genes (Flórez et al., publication process). The genetic variant - 2518 in the chemokine *CCL2/MCPI* promotor gene was associated with CC in Brazilian population (Ramasawmy et al., 2009).

6.3.3 Variation in anti-inflammatory cytokines

Monocytes of patients with the indeterminate form, but not patients with CC showed high expression of interleukin 10, suggesting a lack of immunoregulation in these patients (Costa el al., 2009; D'Avila et al., 2009). The anti-inflammatory cytokines, such as interleukin 4 and IL-10, promote Th2 differentiation and limit Th1 response (Jankovic et al., 2001). This polarization favors the permanence of the parasite in the myocardium but keeps the inflammatory response under control, which appears to be important for avoiding the development of CC (Higuchi et al., 2003; Cunha-Neto et al., 2005). Different groups have found markers associated with decreased production of anti-inflammatory cytokines in patients with CC (Costa et al., 2009). We have analyzed other genes of regulatory proteins, such as *TGFB1* (Calzada et al., 2009), *MIF* (Torres et al., 2009), *IL4*, *IL4RA* and *IL10* (Florez et al., 2011) which are associatted with CC. However, in the latter gene we were unable to demonstrate association between *IL10* gene polymorphism and CD. Other pro-inflammatory and anti-inflammatory genes have been analyzed, such as *BAT1* and *IKBL/NFKBIL1*, *MAL/TIRAP* (Ramasawmy et al., 2006 and 2009), *PTPN22* (Robledo et al., 2007), *CTLA4* (Fernandez-Mestre et al, 2009) (Table 1).

There are few reports of genome mapping applied to the study of CD in murine models which showed a possible region of susceptibility to the disease directly related with survival to infection in the murine H-2 locus, which corresponds to the human Major Histocompatibility Complex (MHC) located in chromosome 17 (Wrightsman et al., 1984). In a more recent study, the entire genome of mice strains susceptible and resistant were mapping at intervals of 10-15 cM with microsatellite. The regions with marked influence in the severity of CD, are mainly located on chromosome 17 on the murine MHC, but were also identified as candidate regions on chromosomes 5 and 13 (Graefe et al., 2003, 2006). In humans, chromosomal mapping studies on CD have not been reported. All this evidence showing the association of multiple genes and the development of CD, as in other infectious and noninfectious diseases, suggests that susceptibility/resistance to develop CD would be determined by variations in a large number of polymorphic genes. In fact, a single SNP can not fully explain the susceptibility or resistance to a complex disease. Therefore, the genetic susceptibility to *T. cruzi* infection and the development of cardiomyopathy is complex and heterogeneous and likely to involve multiple genes, each with a modest contribution on the pathogenesis of the disease. The availability of high throughput methods enabling of genotyping individual DNA samples at 500,000 or more loci using SNP chip have led to genome wide association studies (GWAS) of more than 40 diseases and human phenotypes (Manolio, 2010). Despite the current limitations and the adjustments of bioinformatic tools for analyzing this vast amount of information, these studies of genomic medicine would allow in a near future obtain the individual genetic profiles and define the genes underlying the phenotype associated with the disease and its severity.

Genes	SNP	Population	Association	Reference
Innate immunity				
TLR 2	R753Q	Colombian	negative	Zafra
TLR4, TLR9	D299G, -1237	Colombian	negative	Zafra
TLR 1,2,4,9	I602S, R753Q, D299G, R392stop codon, -1237, -1486	Brazilian	negative	Ramasawmy
MAL/TIRAP	S180L	Brazilian	CC	Ramasawmy
Pro-inflamatory genes				
NOS	microsatélite	Peruvian	negative	Calzada
NRAMP	-236	Peruvian	negative	Calzada
TNFA	-308	Peruvian	negative	Beraún
		Mexican	CC	Rodriguez-Pérez
		Brazilian	negative	Drigo
		Brazilian	negative	Pissetti
		Colombian	CC	Criado
	-238	Peruvian	negative	Beraún
		Mexican	negative	Rodriguez-Pérez
		Brazilian	negative	Drigo
		Brazilian	CC	Pissetti
	-1031	Colombian	negative	Criado
TNFR2	+676 (M196R)	Colombian	monomorphic	Criado
LTA	+80, +252	Brazilian		Ramasawmy
IL1B	+5810	Colombian	CC	Flórez
	-31,-511, +3954	Colombian	negative	Flórez
		Mexican		Cruz-Robles
IL1RN	+8006, +8061, +11100	Colombian	negative	Flórez
		Mexican		Cruz-Robles
IL1A	-889, +4845	Colombian	negative	Flórez
IL12B	+1188	Colombian	CC	Zafra
IFGN	+874	Colombian	CC	Torres
IL6	-174	Colombian, Peruvian	negative	Torres
CCR5	59029, Δ32	Peruvian	negative	Calzada
	59029, Δ32	Venezuelan	negative	Fernández-Mestre
	-2733, -2554	Colombian	CC	Flórez
CCL2/MCPI	-2518	Brazilian	CC	Ramasawmy
Anti-inflamatory genes				
BAT1	-22, 348	Brazilian	CC	Ramasawmy
IKBL/NFKBIL1	-62, -262	Brazilian	CC	Ramasawmy
IL10	-1082	Brazilian	CC	Costa
	-1082, -819, -592	Colombian	negative	Flórez
PTPN22	1858	Colombian, Peruvian	negative	Robledo
MIF	-173	Colombian, Peruvian	CC	Torres
TGFB	-988, -800, -509, +263	Colombian, Peruvian	negative	Torres
	+10	Colombian, Peruvian	CC	Torres
CTLA4	+49	Venezuelan	negative	Fernández-Mestre
IL4	-590	Colombian	negative	Flórez
IL4RA	+148	Colombian	CC	Flórez
	1124, 1218, 1902	Colombian	negative	Flórez

Table 1. Polymorphisms of immune response genes studied in Chagas Disease

6.4 Host-parasite interaction, changes in gene expression by the infectious process

The infection process involves changes in host cell gene expression caused by the parasite. Therefore, transcriptional profiling is frequently used as a genome-wide tool to screen for the impact of pathogens on host cell functions (Costales et al., 2009). This approach that analyzes the differential expression to identify genes or proteins related with the pathogenesis is widely used in different pathologies. Taking advantages of microarray expression platform comparisons are made between healthy and sick individuals or between strains of susceptible or resistant animal models or between infected and uninfected cells. Currently, two approachs have been integrated so that data from microarrays can be analyzed in the context of the Quantitative Trait Loci (QTLs), a strategy called genetic genomics (Jansen & Nap 2001; Nica et al., 2010). Genetics Genomics is a powerful tool to elucidate the basis of complex traits and disease susceptibility that integrates genotype and phenotype information (Pérez-Enciso et al., 2007).

In CD studies using different cell lines infected with *T. cruzi* or tissues from diseased individuals compared to healthy tissue have been realized. This allowed to identify an increased number of over-expressed genes associated with immune response, such as growth factors, immunoglobulins, cytokines and genes related with cell membrane, lipid metabolism and oxidative phosphorylation (Graefe et al., 2006; Mukherjee et al., 2003; Mukherjee et al., 2006). More recently in several human cell lines was observed overexpression of cytokines with higher overexpression of interferon-stimulated genes and also independent genes of cytokines (Costales, 2009). An analysis of gene expression in heart tissue of five patients with CC and seven with dilated cardiomyopathy suggests that genes of immune response, lipid metabolism and mitochondrial oxidative phosphorylation could be involved in the development of heart failure (Cunha-Neto, 2005). In mice models, myocarditis was associated with immune-inflammatory responses (chemokines, adhesion molecules, cathepsins, and MHC molecules), and fibrosis was associated with extracellular matrix components, lysyl oxidase, and tissue inhibitor of metalloproteinase (Soares et al., 2010). With this approach, our group performed a study for determining differential expression patterns in T lymphocytes of individuals with or without CC. Using the Gen Ontology (GO) tool we could establish the biological pathways associated with over-expression in immune response genes, cell signaling and structure of cardiac tissue. Therefore, genetic genomic strategy could allow establish and identify the risk genotype and phenotype of the patient. In addition would make it possible to identify gene interaction networks responsible for the development of CD.

7. Perspectives

For the control of CD should be used not only the traditional approachs of public health with campaigns to eradicate the domiciled vector, control of transmission in blood banks, and now oral transmission, but implement and promote the use of new developments in genomics, proteomics and pharmacogenomics. The association studies and genetic genomic can provide information to identify genes related with disease development and so develop not only prevention and control programs but identify potential targets for treatment and vaccine design.

8. References

Akira, S., & Takeda, K. (2004).Toll-like receptor signalling. *Nat Rev Immunol*, Vol.4, No.7, (July 2004), pp. 499-511, ISSN 1474-1733

Alarcon de Noya, B.; Diaz-Bello, Z.; Colmenares, C., et al. (2010). Large urban outbreak of orally acquired acute Chagas disease at a school in Caracas, Venezuela.*J Infect Dis*, Vol.201, No.9, (March 2010), pp. 1308-1315, ISSN 1537-6613

Araujo, F.F.; Gomes, J.A.; Rocha, M.O., et al. (2007). Potential role of CD4+CD25HIGH regulatory T cells in morbidity in Chagas disease. *Front Biosci*, Vol.12, (May 2007), pp. 2797-2806, ISSN 1093-4715

Aufderheide, A.C.; Salo, W.; Madden, M., et al. (2004). A 9,000-year record of Chagas' disease.*Proc Natl Acad Sci U S A*, Vol.101, No.7, (February 2004), pp. 2034-2039, ISSN 0027-8424

Bafica, A.; Santiago, H.C.; Goldszmid, R., et al. (2006). Cutting edge: TLR9 and TLR2 signaling together account for MyD88-dependent control of parasitemia in Trypanosoma cruzi infection. *J Immunol*, Vol.177, No.6, (September 2006), pp. 3515-3519, ISSN 0022-1767

Barcan, L.; Luna, C.; Clara, L., et al. (2005). Transmission of T. cruzi infection via liver transplantation to a nonreactive recipient for Chagas' disease. *Liver Transpl*, Vol.11, No.9, (Augusts 2005), pp. 1112-1116, ISSN 1527-6465

Beraun, Y.; Nieto, A.; Collado, M.D., et al. (1998). Polymorphisms at tumor necrosis factor (TNF) loci are not associated with Chagas' disease. *Tissue Antigens*, Vol.52, No.1, (August 1998), pp. 81-83, ISSN 0001-2815

Bern, C., & Montgomery, S.P. (2009). An estimate of the burden of Chagas disease in the United States.*Clin Infect Dis*, Vol.49, No.5, (July 2009), pp. e52-54, ISSN 1537-6591

Bilate, A.M., & Cunha-Neto, E. (2008). Chagas disease cardiomyopathy: current concepts of an old disease. *Rev Inst Med Trop Sao Paulo*, Vol.50, No.2, (May 2008), pp. 67-74, ISSN 0036-4665

Brener, Z. (1971). Life cycle of Trypanosoma cruzi.*Rev Inst Med Trop Sao Paulo*, Vol.13, No.3, (May 1971), pp. 171-178, ISSN 0036-4665

Briceno-Leon, R. (2009). Chagas disease in the Americas: an ecohealth perspective. *Cad Saude Publica*, Vol.25 Suppl 1, (March 2009), pp. S71-82, ISSN 1678-4464

Calzada, J.E.; Beraun, Y.; Gonzalez, C.I., et al. (2009). Transforming growth factor beta 1 (TGFbeta1) gene polymorphisms and Chagas disease susceptibility in Peruvian and Colombian patients. *Cytokine*, Vol.45, No.3, (January 2009), pp. 149-153, ISSN 1096-0023

Calzada, J.E.; Nieto, A.; Beraun, Y., et al. (2001). Chemokine receptor CCR5 polymorphisms and Chagas' disease cardiomyopathy.*Tissue Antigens*, Vol.58, No.3, (November 2001), pp. 154-158, ISSN 0001-2815

Campos, M.A.; Almeida, I.C.; Takeuchi, O., et al. (2001). Activation of Toll-like receptor-2 by glycosylphosphatidylinositol anchors from a protozoan parasite. *J Immunol*, Vol.167, No.1, (June 2001), pp. 416-423, ISSN 0022-1767

Cardon, L.R., &Abecasis, G.R. (2003). Using haplotype blocks to map human complex trait loci. *Trends Genet*, Vol.19, No.3, (March 2003), pp. 135-140, ISSN 0168-9525

Conrad, D.F.; Jakobsson, M.; Coop, G., et al. (2006).A worldwide survey of haplotype variation and linkage disequilibrium in the human genome. *Nat Genet*, Vol.38, No.11, (October 2006), pp. 1251-1260, ISSN 1061-4036

Cordova, E.; Boschi, A.; Ambrosioni, J., et al. (2008). Reactivation of Chagas disease with central nervous system involvement in HIV-infected patients in Argentina, 1992-2007.*Int J Infect Dis*, Vol.12, No.6, (March 2008), pp. 587-592, ISSN 1878-3511

Costa, G.C.; da Costa Rocha, M.O.; Moreira, P.R., et al. (2009). Functional IL-10 gene polymorphism is associated with Chagas disease cardiomyopathy. *J Infect Dis*, Vol.199, No.3, (December 2008), pp. 451-454, ISSN 0022-1899

Costales, J.A.; Daily, J.P., &Burleigh, B.A. (2009). Cytokine-dependent and-independent gene expression changes and cell cycle block revealed in Trypanosoma cruzi-infected host cells by comparative mRNA profiling. *BMC Genomics*, Vol.10, (June 2009), pp. 252, ISSN 1471-2164

Coura, J.R. (2007). Chagas disease: what is known and what is needed--a background article. *Mem Inst Oswaldo Cruz*, Vol.102 Suppl 1, (December 2007), pp. 113-122, ISSN 0074-0276

Coura, J.R.; Junqueira, A.C.; Fernandes, O., et al. (2002). Emerging Chagas disease in Amazonian Brazil. *Trends Parasitol*, Vol.18, No.4, (May 2002), pp. 171-176, ISSN 1471-4922

Cunha-Neto, E.;Duranti, M.; Gruber, A., et al. (1995). Autoimmunity in Chagas disease cardiopathy: biological relevance of a cardiac myosin-specific epitope crossreactive to an immunodominantTrypanosomacruzi antigen. *Proc Natl Acad Sci U S A*, Vol.92, No.8, (April 1995), pp. 3541-3545, ISSN 0027-8424

Cunha-Neto, E.; Dzau, V.J.; Allen, P.D., et al. (2005). Cardiac gene expression profiling provides evidence for cytokinopathy as a molecular mechanism in Chagas' disease cardiomyopathy. *Am J Pathol*, Vol.167, No.2, (July 2005), pp. 305-313, ISSN 0002-9440

Cheung, V.G.; Spielman, R.S.; Ewens, K.G., et al. (2005). Mapping determinants of human gene expression by regional and genome-wide association. *Nature*, Vol.437, No.7063, (October 2005), pp. 1365-1369, ISSN 1476-4687

D'Avila, D.A.; Guedes, P.M.; Castro, A.M., et al. (2009). Immunological imbalance between IFN-gamma and IL-10 levels in the sera of patients with the cardiac form of Chagas disease.*Mem Inst Oswaldo Cruz*, Vol.104, No.1, (March 2009), pp. 100-105, ISSN 1678-8060

Daly, M.J.; Rioux, J.D.; Schaffner, S.F., et al. (2001). High-resolution haplotype structure in the human genome.*Nat Genet*, Vol.29, No.2, (October 2001), pp. 229-232, ISSN 1061-4036

de Bakker, P.I.; Burtt, N.P.; Graham, R.R., et al. (2006). Transferability of tag SNPs in genetic association studies in multiple populations. *Nat Genet*, Vol.38, No.11, (October 2006), pp. 1298-1303, ISSN 1061-4036

Deborggraeve, S.; Coronado, X.; Solari, A., et al. (2009). T. cruziOligoC-TesT: a simplified and standardized polymerase chain reaction format for diagnosis of Chagas disease. *PloS Negl Trop Dis*, Vol.3, No.6, (June 2009), pp. e450, ISSN 1935-2735

Díaz, M.L.; Flórez, O.; Mantilla, J.C.; Ramírez, A.N.; Hernández, L.M. Gualdrón, L.; García, C. & González, C.I. (2009). Brote de Chagas agudo en Santander: casos fatales asociados con probable transmision oral. *Biomédica*, Vol.29, (Supl1), pp. 210-211, ISSN 0120-4157

Dias, J.C. (1989). The indeterminate form of human chronic Chagas' disease A clinical epidemiological review. *Rev Soc Bras Med Trop*, Vol.22, No.3, (July 1989), pp. 147-156, ISSN 0037-8682

Drigo, S.A.; Cunha-Neto, E.;Ianni, B., et al. (2006). TNF gene polymorphisms are associated with reduced survival in severe Chagas' disease cardiomyopathy patients. *Microbes Infect*, Vol.8, No.3, (January 2006), pp. 598-603, ISSN 1286-4579

Drigo, S.A.; Cunha-Neto, E.;Ianni, B., et al. (2007). Lack of association of tumor necrosis factor-alpha polymorphisms with Chagas disease in Brazilian patients. *Immunol Lett*, Vol.108, No.1, (December 2006), pp. 109-111, ISSN 0165-2478

Dutra, W.O., &Gollob, K.J. (2008). Current concepts in immunoregulation and pathology of human Chagas disease.*Curr Opin Infect Dis*, Vol.21, No.3, (May 2008), pp. 287-292, ISSN 0951-7375

Dutra, W.O.; Menezes, C.A.; Villani, F.N., et al. (2009). Cellular and genetic mechanisms involved in the generation of protective and pathogenic immune responses in human Chagas disease. *Mem Inst Oswaldo Cruz*, Vol.104 Suppl 1, (September 2009), pp. 208-218, ISSN 1678-8060

Feero, W.G.; Guttmacher, A.E., & Collins, F.S. (2010). Genomic medicine--an updated primer.*N Engl J Med*, Vol.362, No.21, (May 2010), pp. 2001-2011, ISSN 1533-4406

Fernandez-Mestre, M.T.; Layrisse, Z.; Montagnani, S., et al. (1998). Influence of the HLA class II polymorphism in chronic Chagas' disease. *Parasite Immunol*, Vol.20, No.4, (June 1998), pp. 197-203, ISSN 0141-9838

Fernandez-Mestre, M.T.; Montagnani, S., &Layrisse, Z. (2004). Is the CCR5-59029-G/G genotype a protective factor for cardiomyopathy in Chagas disease? *Hum Immunol*, Vol.65, No.7, (August 2004), pp. 725-728, ISSN 0198-8859

Fernandez-Mestre, M.; Sanchez, K.;Balbas, O., et al. (2009). Influenceof CTLA-4 gene polymorphism in autoimmune and infectious diseases. *Hum Immunol*, Vol.70, No.7, (April 2009), pp. 532-535, ISSN 1879-1166

Ferreira, R.C.; Ianni, B.M.; Abel, L.C., et al. (2003). Increased plasma levels of tumor necrosis factor-alpha in asymptomatic/"indeterminate" and Chagas disease cardiomyopathy patients. *Mem Inst Oswaldo Cruz*, Vol.98, No.3, (July 2003), pp. 407-411, ISSN 0074-0276

Florez, O.; Zafra, G.; Morillo, C., et al. (2006). Interleukin-1 gene cluster polymorphism in chagas disease in a Colombian case-control study. *Hum Immunol*, Vol.67, No.9, (September 2006), pp. 741-748, ISSN 0198-8859

Florez, O.; Martin, J., & Gonzalez, C.I. (2011). Interleukin 4, interleukin 4 receptor-alpha and interleukin 10 gene polymorphisms in Chagas disease.*Parasite Immunol*, Vol.(July 2011), pp. 1-6, ISSN 1365-3024

Frazer, K.A.; Murray, S.S.; Schork, N.J., et al. (2009).Human genetic variation and its contribution to complex traits. *Nat Rev Genet*, Vol.10, No.4, (March 2009), pp. 241-251, ISSN 1471-0064

Galvan, A.; Falvella, F.S.; Frullanti, E., et al. (2010). Genome-wide association study in discordant sibships identifies multiple inherited susceptibility alleles linked to lung cancer. *Carcinogenesis*, Vol.31, No.3, (December 2009), pp. 462-465, ISSN 1460-2180

Gascon, J.; Bern, C., & Pinazo, M.J. (2010). Chagas disease in Spain, the United States and other non-endemic countries.*Acta Trop*, Vol.115, No.1-2, (August 2009), pp. 22-27, ISSN 1873-6254

Gomes, J.A.; Bahia-Oliveira, L.M.; Rocha, M.O., et al. (2005). Type 1 chemokine receptor expression in Chagas' disease correlates with morbidity in cardiac patients. *Infect Immun*, Vol.73, No.12, (November 2005), pp. 7960-7966, ISSN 0019-9567

Gomes, M.L.; Galvao, L.M.; Macedo, A.M., et al. (1999). Chagas' disease diagnosis: comparative analysis of parasitologic, molecular, and serologic methods. *Am J Trop Med Hyg*, Vol.60, No.2, (March 1999), pp. 205-210, ISSN 0002-9637

Gomes, Y.M.; Lorena, V.M., &Luquetti, A.O. (2009). Diagnosis of Chagas disease: what has been achieved? What remains to be done with regard to diagnosis and follow up studies? *Mem Inst Oswaldo Cruz*, Vol.104 Suppl 1, (September 2009), pp. 115-121, ISSN 1678-8060

Gonzalez, C.I.; Ortiz, S., & Solari, A. (2010).Colombian Trypanosoma cruzi major genotypes circulating in patients: minicircle homologies by cross-hybridization analysis. *Int J Parasitol*, Vol.40, No.14, (August 2010), pp. 1685-1692, ISSN 1879-0135

Gonzalez, E.; Bamshad, M.; Sato, N., et al. (1999). Race-specific HIV-1 disease-modifying effects associated with CCR5 haplotypes. *Proc Natl Acad Sci U S A*, Vol.96, No.21, (October 1999), pp. 12004-12009, ISSN 0027-8424

Graefe, S.E.; Meyer, B.S.; Muller-Myhsok, B., et al. (2003). Murine susceptibility to Chagas' disease maps to chromosomes 5 and 17. *Genes Immun*, Vol.4, No.5, (July 2003), pp. 321-325, ISSN 1466-4879

Graefe, S.E.; Streichert, T.; Budde, B.S., et al. (2006). Genes from Chagas susceptibility loci that are differentially expressed in T. cruzi-resistant mice are candidates accounting for impaired immunity. *PLoS One*, Vol.1, (December 2006), pp. e57, 1932-6203

Guedes, P.M.; Veloso, V.M.; Talvani, A., et al. (2010). Increased type 1 chemokine expression in experimental Chagas disease correlates with cardiac pathology in beagle dogs. *Vet Immunol Immunopathol*, Vol.138, No.1-2, (July 2010), pp. 106-113, ISSN 1873-2534

Guhl, F. (2007).Chagas disease in Andean countries.*Mem.Inst.Oswaldo Cruz*, Vol.102 Suppl 1, (September 2007), pp. 29-38, ISSN 0074-0276

Guhl, F.; Jaramillo, C.; Vallejo, G.A., et al. (1999). Isolation of Trypanosoma cruzi DNA in 4,000-year-old mummified human tissue from northern Chile. *Am J Phys Anthropol*, Vol.108, No.4, (May 1999) pp. 401-407, ISSN 0002-9483

Hernandez, P.; Heimann, M.; Riera, C., et al. (2010).Highly effective serodiagnosis for Chagas' disease.*Clin Vaccine Immunol*, Vol.17, No.10, (July 2010), pp. 1598-1604, ISSN 1556-679X

Higo, H.; Miura, S.; Horio, M., et al. (2004). Genotypic variation among lineages of Trypanosoma cruzi and its geographic aspects. *Parasitol Int*, Vol.53, No.4, (July 2004), pp. 337-344, ISSN 1383-5769

Higuchi Mde, L.; Benvenuti, L.A.; Martins Reis, M., et al. (2003). Pathophysiology of the heart in Chagas' disease: current status and new developments. *Cardiovasc Res*, Vol.60, No.1, (October 2003), pp. 96-107, ISSN 0008-6363

Jankovic, D.; Sher, A., & Yap, G. (2001). Th1/Th2 effector choice in parasitic infection: decision making by committee. *Curr Opin Immunol*, Vol.13, No.4, (August 2001), pp. 403-409, ISSN 0952-7915

Jansen, R.C., & Nap, J.P. (2001). Genetical genomics: the added value from segregation. *Trends Genet*, Vol.17, No.7, (June 2001), pp. 388-391, ISSN 0168-9525

Kayama, H., & Takeda, K. (2010).The innate immune response to Trypanosoma cruzi infection.*Microbes Infect*, Vol.12, No.7, (March 2010), pp. 511-517, ISSN 1769-714X

Klein, R.J.; Zeiss, C.; Chew, E.Y., et al. (2005). Complement factor H polymorphism in age-related macular degeneration. *Science*, Vol.308, No.5720, (March 2005), pp. 385-389, ISSN 1095-9203

Ku, C.S.; Loy, E.Y.; Pawitan, Y., et al. (2010). The pursuit of genome-wide association studies: where are we now? *J Hum Genet*, Vol.55, No.4, (March 2010), pp. 195-206, ISSN 1435-232X

Layrisse, Z.; Fernandez, M.T.; Montagnani, S., et al. (2000). HLA-C(*)03 is a risk factor for cardiomyopathy in Chagas disease. *Hum Immunol*, Vol.61, No.9, (September 2000), pp. 925-929, ISSN 0198-8859

Llop, E.; Rothhammer, F.; Acuna, M., et al. (1991). HLA antigens in Chagas cardiomyopathy: new evidence based on a case-control study. *Rev Med Chil*, Vol.119, No.6, (June 1991), pp. 633-636, ISSN 0034-9887

Machado, F.S.; Koyama, N.S.; Carregaro, V., et al. (2005). CCR5 plays a critical role in the development of myocarditis and host protection in mice infected with Trypanosoma cruzi. *J Infect Dis*, Vol.191, No.4, (January 2005), pp. 627-636, ISSN 0022-1899

Manolio, T.A. (2010). Genomewide association studies and assessment of the risk of disease.*N Engl J Med*, Vol.363, No.2, (July 2010), pp. 166-176, ISSN 1533-4406

Manque, P.A.; Probst, C.; Pereira, M.C., et al. (2011). Trypanosoma cruzi infection induces a global host cell response in cardiomyocytes. *Infect Immun*, Vol.79, No.5, (February 2011), pp. 1855-1862, ISSN 1098-5522

Mantilla, J.C.; Zafra, G.A.; Macedo, A.M., et al. (2010). Mixed infection of Trypanosoma cruzi I and II in a Colombian cardiomyopathic patient. *Hum Pathol*, Vol.41, No.4, (February 2010), pp. 610-613, ISSN 1532-8392

Marcon, G.E.; Andrade, P.D.; de Albuquerque, D.M., et al. (2002). Use of a nested polymerase chain reaction (N-PCR) to detect Trypanosoma cruzi in blood samples from chronic chagasic patients and patients with doubtful serologies. *Diagn Microbiol Infect Dis*, Vol.43, No.1, (June 2002), pp. 39-43, ISSN 0732-8893

Marino, A.P.; da Silva, A.; dos Santos, P., et al. (2004). Regulated on activation, normal T cell expressed and secreted (RANTES) antagonist (Met-RANTES) controls the early phase of Trypanosoma cruzi-elicited myocarditis. *Circulation*, Vol.110, No.11, (September 2004), pp. 1443-1449, ISSN 1524-4539

Marin Neto, J.A.; Simoes, M.V., &Sarabanda, A.V. (1999). Chagas' heart disease. *Arq Bras Cardiol*, Vol.72, No.3, (October 1999), pp. 247-280, ISSN 0066-782X

Moreno, M.; Silva, E.L.; Ramirez, L.E., et al. (2004).Chagas' disease susceptibility/resistance: linkage disequilibrium analysis suggests epistasis between major histocompatibility complex and interleukin-10. *Tissue Antigens*, Vol.64, No.1, (June 2004), pp. 18-24, ISSN 0001-2815

Mukherjee, S.; Belbin, T.J.; Spray, D.C., et al. (2003). Microarray analysis of changes in gene expression in a murine model of chronic chagasic cardiomyopathy.*Parasitol Res*, Vol.91, No.3, (August 2003), pp. 187-196, ISSN 0932-0113

Mukherjee, S.; Belbin, T.J.; Spray, D.C., et al. (2006). Microarray technology in the investigation of diseases of myocardium with special reference to infection. *Front Biosci*, Vol.11, (December 2005), pp. 1802-1813, ISSN 1093-4715

Mukherjee, S.; Nagajyothi, F.; Mukhopadhyay, A., et al. (2008). Alterations in myocardial gene expression associated with experimental Trypanosoma cruzi infection. *Genomics*, Vol.91, No.5, (March 2008), pp. 423-432, ISSN 1089-8646

Nica, A.C.; Montgomery, S.B.; Dimas, A.S., et al. (2010). Candidate causal regulatory effects by integration of expression QTLs with complex trait genetic associations.*PloS Genet*, Vol.6, No.4, (April 2010), pp. e1000895, ISSN 1553-7404

Nieto, A.; Beraun, Y.; Collado, M.D., et al. (2000). HLA haplotypes are associated with differential susceptibility to Trypanosoma cruzi infection. *Tissue Antigens*, Vol.55, No.3, (April 2000), pp. 195-198, ISSN 0001-2815

Nobrega, A.A.; Garcia, M.H.; Tatto, E., et al. (2009). Oral transmission of Chagas disease by consumption of acai palm fruit, Brazil. *Emerg Infec tDis*, Vol.15, No.4, (April 2009), pp. 653-655, ISSN 1080-6059

Organización Panamericana de la Salud. (2006). Estimación cuantitativa de la enfermedad d Chagas en las Americas. Montevideo, Uruguay: OPS.

Ouaissi, A.; Guilvard, E.; Delneste, Y., et al. (2002). The Trypanosoma cruzi Tc52-released protein induces human dendritic cell maturation, signals via Toll-like receptor 2, and confers protection against lethal infection. *J Immunol*, Vol.168, No.12, (June 2002), pp. 6366-6374, ISSN 0022-1767

Pacheco, A.G., &Moraes, M.O. (2009). Genetic polymorphisms of infectious diseases in case-control studies.*Dis Markers*, Vol.27, No.3, (November 2009), pp. 173-186, ISSN 1875-8630

Palomino, S.A.; Aiello, V.D., & Higuchi, M.L. (2000). Systematic mapping of hearts from chronic chagasic patients: the association between the occurrence of histopathological lesions and Trypanosoma cruzi antigens. *Ann Trop Med Parasitol*, Vol.94, No.6, (November 2000), pp. 571-579, ISSN 0003-4983

Perez-Enciso, M.; Quevedo, J.R., &Bahamonde, A. (2007). Genetical genomics: use all data. *BMC Genomics*, Vol.8, (March 2007), pp. 69, ISSN 1471-2164

Piron, M.; Fisa, R.; Casamitjana, N., et al. (2007). Development of a real-time PCR assay for Trypanosoma cruzi detection in blood samples. *Acta Trop*, Vol.103, No.3, (July 2007), pp. 195-200, ISSN 0001-706X

Pissetti, C.W.; Correia, D.; de Oliveira, R.F., et al. (2011). Genetic and functional role of TNF-alpha in the development Trypanosoma cruzi infection.*PloS Negl Trop Dis*, Vol.5, No.3, (March 2011), pp. e976, ISSN 1935-2735

Praast, G.; Herzogenrath, J.; Bernhardt, S., et al. (2011). Evaluation of the Abbott ARCHITECT Chagas prototype assay. *Diagn Microbiol Infect Dis*, Vol.69, No.1, (December 2010), pp. 74-81, ISSN 1879-0070

Prata, A. (2001). Clinical and epidemiological aspects of Chagas disease. *Lancet Infect Dis*, Vol.1, No.2, (March 2002), pp. 92-100, ISSN 1473-3099

Ramasawmy, R.; Cunha-Neto, E.; Fae, K.C., et al. (2009). Heterozygosity for the S180L variant of MAL/TIRAP, a gene expressing an adaptor protein in the Toll-like receptor pathway, is associated with lower risk of developing chronic Chagas cardiomyopathy. *J Infect Dis*, Vol.199, No.12, (May 2009), pp. 1838-1845, ISSN 0022-1899

Ramasawmy, R.; Fae, K.C.; Cunha-Neto, E., et al. (2008). Variants in the promoter region of IKBL/NFKBIL1 gene may mark susceptibility to the development of chronic

Chagas' cardiomyopathy among Trypanosoma cruzi-infected individuals. *Mol Immunol*, Vol.45, No.1, (June 2007), pp. 283-288, ISSN 0161-5890

Ramasawmy, R.; Fae, K.C.; Cunha-Neto, E., et al. (2007). Polymorphisms in the gene for lymphotoxin-alpha predispose to chronic Chagas cardiomyopathy. *J Infect Dis*, Vol.196, No.12, (January 2008), pp. 1836-1843, ISSN 0022-1899

Ramasawmy, R.; Cunha-Neto, E.; Fae, K.C., et al. (2006).The monocyte chemoattractant protein-1 gene polymorphism is associated with cardiomyopathy in human Chagas disease. *Clin Infect Dis*, Vol.43, No.3, (June 2006), pp. 305-311, ISSN 1537-6591

Ramasawmy, R.; Cunha-Neto, E.; Fae, K.C., et al. (2006). BAT1, a putative anti-inflammatory gene, is associated with chronic Chagas cardiomyopathy. *J Infect Dis*, Vol.193, No.10, (April 2006), pp. 1394-1399, ISSN 0022-1899

Rassi, A., Jr.; Rassi, A., & Marin-Neto, J.A. (2010). Chagas disease. *Lancet*, Vol.375, No.9723, (April 2010), pp. 1388-1402, ISSN 1474-547X

Rassi, A., Jr.; Rassi, S.G., & Rassi, A. (2001). Sudden death in Chagas' disease. *Arq Bras Cardiol*, Vol.76, No.1, (February 2001), pp. 75-96, ISSN 0066-782X

Robledo, G.; Gonzalez, C.I.; Morillo, C., et al. (2007). Association study of PTPN22 C1858T polymorphism in Trypanosoma cruzi infection.*Tissue Antigens*, Vol.69, No.3, (May 2007), pp. 261-264, ISSN 0001-2815

Rodriguez-Perez, J.M.; Cruz-Robles, D.; Hernandez-Pacheco, G., et al. (2005). Tumor necrosis factor-alpha promoter polymorphism in Mexican patients with Chagas' disease.*Immunol Lett*, Vol.98, No.1, (March 2005), pp. 97-102, ISSN 0165-2478

Salazar Schettino, P.M.; Bucio Torres, M.; Cabrera Bravo, M., et al. (2011). Chagas disease in Mexico.Report of two acute cases.*Gac Med Mex*, Vol.147, No.1, (March 2011), pp. 63-69, ISSN 0016-3813

Samuel, J.; Oliveira, M.; Correa De Araujo, R.R., et al. (1983). Cardiac thrombosis and thromboembolism in chronic Chagas' heart disease. *Am J Cardiol*, Vol.52, No.1, (July 1983), pp. 147-151, ISSN 0002-9149

Schmunis, G.A. (1999). Prevention of transfusional Trypanosoma cruzi infection in Latin America. *Mem Inst Oswaldo Cruz*, Vol.94 Suppl 1, (June 2000), pp. 93-101, ISSN 0074-0276

Schmunis, G.A., & Yadon, Z.E. (2010). Chagas disease: a Latin American health problem becoming a world health problem. *Acta Trop*, Vol.115, No.1-2, (November 2009), pp. 14-21, ISSN 1873-6254

Schofield, C.J. (1981). Chagas disease, triatomine bugs, and bloodloss. *Lancet*, Vol.1, No.8233, (June 1981), pp. 1316, ISSN 0140-6736

Soares, M.B.; de Lima, R.S.; Rocha, L.L., et al. (2010). Gene expression changes associated with myocarditis and fibrosis in hearts of mice with chronic chagasic cardiomyopathy. *J Infect Dis*, Vol.202, No.3, (June 2010), pp. 416-426, ISSN 1537-6613

Steemers, F.J., & Gunderson, K.L. (2007).Whole genome genotyping technologies on the BeadArray platform. *Biotechnol J*, Vol.2, No.1, (January 2007), pp. 41-49, ISSN 1860-7314

Takle, G.B., & Hudson, L. (1989).Autoimmunity and Chagas' disease.*Curr Top Microbiol Immunol*, Vol.145, (January 1989), pp. 79-92, ISSN 0070-217X

Talvani, A.; Rocha, M.O.; Barcelos, L.S., et al. (2004a). Elevated concentrations of CCL2 and tumor necrosis factor-alpha in chagasic cardiomyopathy.*Clin Infect Dis*, Vol.38, No.7, (March 2004), pp. 943-950, ISSN 1537-6591

Talvani, A.; Rocha, M.O.; Ribeiro, A.L., et al. (2004b). Chemokine receptor expression on the surface of peripheral blood mononuclear cells in Chagas disease.*J Infect Dis*, Vol.189, No.2, (January 2004), pp. 214-220, ISSN 0022-1899

Tarleton, R.L. (2003). Chagas disease: a role for autoimmunity? *Trends Parasitol*, Vol.19, No.10, (October 2003), pp. 447-451, ISSN 1471-4922

Teixeira, M.M.; da Silva, F.M.; Marcili, A., et al. (2006). Short communication: Trypanosoma cruzi lineage I in endomyocardial biopsy from a north-eastern Brazilian patient at end-stage chronic Chagasic cardiomyopathy. *Trop Med Int Health*, Vol.11, No.3, (March 2006), pp. 294-298, ISSN 1360-2276

Teixeira, M.M.; Gazzinelli, R.T., & Silva, J.S. (2002).Chemokines, inflammation and Trypanosoma cruzi infection. *Trends Parasitol*, Vol.18, No.6, (May 2002), pp. 262-265, ISSN 1471-4922

Tibayrenc, M.; Neubauer, K.; Barnabe, C., et al. (1993). Genetic characterization of six parasitic protozoa: parity between random-primer DNA typing and multilocus enzyme electrophoresis. *Proc Natl Acad Sci U S A*, Vol.90, No.4, (February 1993), pp. 1335-1339, ISSN 0027-8424

Torres, O.A.; Calzada, J.E.; Beraun, Y., et al. (2010a). Lack of association between IL-6-174G/C gene polymorphism and Chagas disease.*Tissue Antigens*, Vol.76, No.2, (March 2010), pp. 131-134, ISSN 1399-0039

Torres, O.A.; Calzada, J.E.; Beraun, Y., et al. (2010b). Role of the IFNG +874T/A polymorphism in Chagas disease in a Colombian population.*Infect Genet Evol*, Vol.10, No.5, (April 2010), pp. 682-685, ISSN 1567-7257

Torres, O.A.; Calzada, J.E.; Beraun, Y., et al. (2009). Association of the macrophage migration inhibitory factor -173G/C polymorphism with Chagas disease. *Hum Immunol*, Vol.70, No.7, (April 2009), pp. 543-546, ISSN 1879-1166

Torrico, F.; Alonso-Vega, C.; Suarez, E., et al. (2004). Maternal Trypanosoma cruzi infection, pregnancy outcome, morbidity, and mortality of congenitally infected and non-infected newborns in Bolivia.*Am J Trop Med Hyg*, Vol.70, No.2, (March 2004), pp. 201-209, ISSN 0002-9637

Tyler, K.M., & Engman, D.M. (2001). The life cycle of Trypanosoma cruzi revisited. *Int J Parasitol*, Vol.31, No.5-6, (May 2001), pp. 472-481, ISSN 0020-7519

Umezawa, E.S.; Luquetti, A.O.; Levitus, G., et al. (2004).Serodiagnosis of chronic and acute Chagas' disease with Trypanosoma cruzi recombinant proteins: results of a collaborative study in six Latin American countries. *J Clin Microbiol*, Vol.42, No.1, (January 2004), pp. 449-452, ISSN 0095-1137

Umezawa, E.S.; Nascimento, M.S., &Stolf, A.M. (2001). Enzyme-linked immunosorbent assay with Trypanosoma cruzi excreted-secreted antigens (TESA-ELISA) for serodiagnosis of acute and chronic Chagas' disease. *Diagn Microbiol Infect Dis*, Vol.39, No.3, (May 2001), pp. 169-176, ISSN 0732-8893

Valente, S.A.; da Costa Valente, V.; das Neves Pinto, A.Y., et al. (2009). Analysis of an acute Chagas disease outbreak in the Brazilian Amazon: human cases, triatomines, reservoir mammals and parasites. *Trans R Soc Trop Med Hyg*, Vol.103, No.3, (January 2009), pp. 291-297, ISSN 1878-3503

Williams-Blangero, S.; VandeBerg, J.L.; Blangero, J., et al. (2003).Genetic epidemiology of Trypanosoma cruzi infection and Chagas' disease. *Front Biosci*, Vol.8, (April 2003), pp. e337-345, ISSN 1093-4715

World Health Organization Chagas disease (2008) WHO: control and elimination. Report of the Secretariat, executive board EB124/17. 124th Session 27 Provisional agenda item 4.14. November 2008.

Wrightsman, R.A.; Krassner, S.M.; Watson, J.D., et al. (1984).Role of the H-2s haplotype in survival of mice after infection with Trypanosoma cruzi. *Infect Immun*, Vol.44, No.2, (May 1984), pp. 351-354, ISSN 0019-9567

Zafra, G.; Mantilla, J.C.; Jacome, J., et al. (2011). Direct analysis of genetic variability in Trypanosomacruzi populations from tissues of Colombian chagasic patients. *Hum Pathol*, Vol.42, No.8, (August 2011), pp. 1159-1168, ISSN 1532-8392

Zafra, G.; Mantilla, J.C.; Valadares, H.M., et al. (2008). Evidence of Trypanosoma cruzi II infection in Colombian chagasic patients.*Parasitol Res*, Vol.103, No.3, (June 2008), pp. 731-734, ISSN 0932-0113

Zafra, G.; Morillo, C.; Martin, J., et al. (2007). Polymorphism in the 3' UTR of the IL12B gene is associated with Chagas' disease cardiomyopathy. *Microbes Infect*, Vol.9, No.9, (July 2007), pp. 1049-1052, ISSN 1286-4579

Zhang, L., & Tarleton, R.L. (1999). Parasite persistence correlates with disease severity and localization in chronic Chagas' disease. *J Infect Dis*, Vol.180, No.2, (July 1999), pp. 480-486, ISSN 0022-1899

Zingales, B.; Andrade, S.G.; Briones, M.R., et al. (2009). A new consensus for Trypanosoma cruzi intraspecific nomenclature: second revision meeting recommends TcI to TcVI. *Mem Inst Oswaldo Cruz*, Vol.104, No.7, (December 2009), pp. 1051-1054, 1678-8060

Zingales, B.; Souto, R.P.; Mangia, R.H., et al. (1998). Molecular epidemiology of American trypanosomiasis in Brazil based on dimorphisms of rRNA and mini-exon gene sequences. *Int J Parasitol*, Vol.28, No.1, (March 1998), pp. 105-112, ISSN 0020-7519

35

Chagasic Cardiomyopathy

Fernando Rosas[1], Nubia Roa[2], Zulma M. Cucunubá[3], Adriana Cuéllar[4], John Mario Gonzalez[5] and Concepción J. Puerta[6]

[1]Fundación Clínica Abood Shaio,
[2]Clínica de Falla Cardiaca y Trasplante, Hospital Universitario San Ignacio, Facultad de Medicina, Pontificia Universidad Javeriana
[3]Grupo de Parasitología, Instituto Nacional de Salud,
[4]Grupo de Inmunobiología y Biología Celular, Pontificia Universidad Javeriana,
[5]Grupo de Ciencias Básicas Médicas, Facultad de Medicina, Universidad de los Andes,
[6]Laboratorio de Parasitología Molecular, Departamento de Microbiología, Pontificia Universidad Javeriana,
Colombia

1. Introduction

Chagas disease is a systemic parasitic infection caused by the protozoan *Trypanosoma cruzi*, which persists as an important public health problem, mainly in Latin America where triatomine vectors are located in three overlapping cycles of transmission: domestic, peridomestic, and sylvatic. Due to human migration from endemic to developed countries, in recent years Chagas disease has become a recognized global problem. This chapter reviews current literature on chagasic cardiomyopathy, its etiology, epidemiology, immunology, and diagnosis, along with etiologic and symptomatic treatment and prognosis.

2. Etiology

One-hundred years after the discovery of *Trypanosoma cruzi* (Family: *Trypanosomatidae*, Order: *Kinetoplastida*) by Carlos Chagas in Brazil, many aspects of its biology and host relationship remain unraveled. The substantial biological, biochemical, and genetic variability of this parasite, as well as the multiclonal *T. cruzi* infection character are some of the factors that have hampered its study. *T. cruzi* is considered to have a clonal structure with some overlapping events of genetic exchange occurring in the past that have brought about the six currently recognized Discrete Typing Units (DTUs) I to VI. Moreover, within each DTU biological and genetic polymorphism is present, especially in DTUs I and III. The scenario is even more complicated. Recent reports showed that multiple genotypes were obtained when isolates from a single wild mammalian reservoir host were cloned (Llewelyn et al., 2011). The authors proposed that this huge diversity is at least, partially driven by the survival in the host. Nonetheless, significant progress has been achieved with the unveiled *T. cruzi* genome and the following OMICS initiatives such as RNAomic and proteomic analyses, which seek to apply translational medicine to Chagas disease in the near future.

2.1 Life cycle

T. cruzi exhibits a complex life cycle involving four well-defined developmental stages that interplay into two hosts, the blood-sucking insect vector, and the mammalian host (humans and animals). After already-infected insects feed on the mammalian host, they eliminate in their feces the **metacyclic trypomastigotes (**parasite infective form), which penetrate the body through the bite-wound, any damaged tissue, or the mucosa from eyes, nose, or even the digestive tract and invade host cells like fibroblasts, macrophages, and epithelial cells at the inoculation site. In the cytoplasm, free-parasites are differentiated into **amastigotes** (Fig.1A), the intracellular stage, which after several replication rounds transforms back into **trypomastigotes** that rupture the host membrane cell, infecting new cells or disseminating into other organs via the bloodstream.

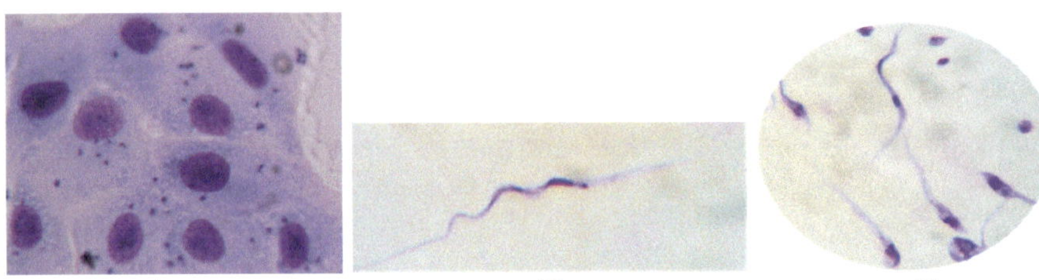
A B C

Fig. 1. (A) Intracellular amastigotes of *T. cruzi*-infecting Vero cells, (B) Trypomastigotes, and (C) Epimastigotes stained with Giemsa. Courtesy of Paola Lasso, and Paula Pavia, Laboratory of Molecular Parasitology, School of Sciences, Pontificia Universidad Javeriana, Bogota D.C., Colombia.

Upon feeding, insects take the **bloodstream trypomastigotes** (Fig. 1B), which once in their digestive tract differentiate into **epimastigotes**, the insect replication stage (Fig. 1C). After reaching the rectum, parasites transform into metacyclic trypomastigotes ready to infect a new mammalian host. From this cycle, it is obvious that the differential expression of parasite genes enable the parasite to accomplish the role played by each of its developmental stages. In this sense, several proteomic studies have been performed to identify molecules participating in cycle-vital processes (Ulrich et al., 2011).

3. Epidemiology and risk factors

3.1 Burden of Chagas disease

An estimated 10-million people are infected worldwide, mostly in Latin America where Chagas disease is endemic. More than 25-million people are at risk of contracting the disease. It is estimated that in 2008 Chagas disease killed >10,000 people. With a latency of 10-30 years, nearly 30% of infected patients develop life-threatening complications, mostly Chagas heart disease (CHD) (WHO, 2010). Direct and indirect costs of *T. cruzi* infection impose an overwhelming load on healthcare systems secondary to hospitalizations and medical and surgical treatments for CHD, gastrointestinal dysfunction, and meningoencephalitis in Latin America (Franco-Paredes et al., 2007). In 1995, the burden of Chagas disease in Latin America was estimated at US$8.156-billion, equivalent to 2.5% of the foreign debt of continental Latin America (Moncayo, 2003). More recent data demonstrate that, globally, Chagas disease is associated with 0.7-million disability-adjusted life years, constituting the sixth most important neglected tropical disease worldwide (Hotez et al., 2006).

3.2 Globalization of Chagas disease

Political and economic situations have stimulated the flow of migration from the 17 Latin American endemic countries to the developed ones (Schmunis & Yadon, 2010). Because of this and parasite transfer by blood contact, intrauterine transfer, laboratory accidents, and organ transplantation; CHD could potentially become a worldwide problem (WHO, 2010) and emerge as a public health issue in non-endemic countries (Field et al., 2010). Currently, in the United States it is estimated that from more than 22 million of immigrants from endemic countries there are approximately 300,000 infected individuals (Bern & Montgomery, 2009). In 15 European countries in 2005, excluding Spain, 2.9% of the 483,074 legal Latin American immigrants were estimated to be infected with *T. cruzi*. By 2008, Spain had received 1,678,711 immigrants from Latin American endemic countries; of these, 5.2% were potentially infected with *T. cruzi* and 17,390 may develop Chagas disease. Likewise, in an analysis of Chagas disease in Spain, most patients were from Bolivia (94.7%) and less from Brazil, Chile, Ecuador, Paraguay, and Honduras (Norman et al., 2010). Other countries outside Europe, where the rates of Latin American immigration are high and present an important prevalence of Chagas disease are Australia, Canada, and Japan (Schmunis & Yadon, 2010).

3.3 Chagas heart disease in endemic countries

Triatomines, the *T. cruzi* vectors, are spread from the south of the United States to the south of Argentina. The rarity of vector-borne transmission in the United States, compared with Latin America, is thought to be the result of better housing conditions and lower efficiency of North American vectors (Bern & Montgomery, 2009). In Latin America, there are more than 125 potential vectors of Chagas disease. However, species with higher vectorial capacity, with domestic habits and with the most geographical distribution belong to *Triatoma, Rhodnius,* and *Panstrongylus* genera. For these reasons, there are different targets in control programs of vectors depending on regions. Thus, the Mexico and Central America Initiative (created in 1998) is focused in the control *Rhodnius prolixus, Triatoma dimidiata, Triatoma barberi,* and *Rhodnius pallescences;* the Initiative of the Andean Countries (created in 1997) is aimed at controlling *R. prolixus, T. dimidiata* and *Triatoma maculata;* and finally, the Initiative of the Southern Cone (created in 1991) is aimed at controlling *Triatoma infestans, Triatoma brasiliensis, Triatoma sordida,* and *Panstrongylus megistus* (Guhl, 2009). The main risk factors for vector-borne transmission are related to previous exposure to poor housing conditions in Latin America (Fig. 3), such as: palm or straw roofs, dirt floors, adobe walls or walls with low quality or incomplete plastering, and the presence of animals inside the bedroom.

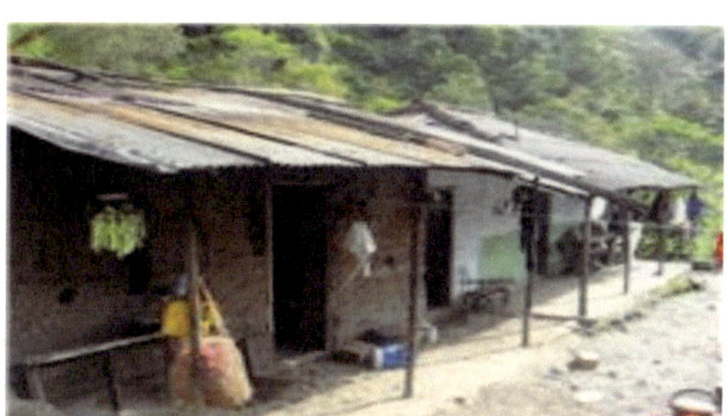

Fig. 2. Typical house in a Chagas disease endemic region, Departamento de Boyacá. Courtesy of Cielo León, Grupo de Parasitología, Instituto Nacional de Salud, Colombia.

An important change has occurred in trends of Chagas disease in Latin America over recent decades. Such is recognized by several researchers, control policies of vector and blood of *T. cruzi* transmission have shown a positive effect in reducing the incidence of this disease. Thus, since the 1990s until now, an important success in the control of Chagas disease has been observed, especially in Southern Cone countries. So, in 1990, the distribution of Chagas disease in 21 countries was estimated, with more than 45,000 deaths per year and 30-million cases of human infection; while in 2006 the distribution of Chagas disease in 18 countries was estimated, with approximately 12,500 deaths per year and nearly 15-million cases of human infection (Dias et al., 2008). Success in controlling vector transmission in some countries has led to also to focus the attention to other forms of non-vector transmission. Thereby, controlling transmission by transfusion has improved and screening is now obligatory in most endemic countries. Congenital transmission has been detected as an important transmission form, mainly in Bolivia, but other endemic countries have only recently started to approach to this problem. Orally acquired human infection with *T. cruzi* has been known since the 1930s but has the interest in this transmision has increased as a result of the series of outbreaks that have occurred in the Amazon region, which have been associated with the preparation and consumption of some foods, especially in Brazil, Venezuela, and Colombia (Miles, 2010). The rural-to-urban migration movements that have occurred in Latin America since the 1970s and 1980s have changed the traditional epidemiological pattern of Chagas disease as a rural condition and transformed it into an urban infection that can be transmitted via non-vector manners (Moncayo & Silveira, 2009). Moreover, in some countries the vector infestation has occurred in urban areas where vectors have been introduced by passive transportation during migration process, for instance in Cochabamba, Bolivia (Medrano-Mercado et al., 2008), Arequipa, Peru (Bayer et al., 2009), and in Yucatán, Mexico (Guzman-Tapia et al., 2007). On the other hand, adults infected with *T. cruzi* from childhood form a transitional generation, experiencing the simultaneous impact of past infectious exposures and current cardiovascular risk factors, such as sedentary lifestyle, calorie-dense diets, hypertension, and diabetes. Other variables such as longer residence in an endemic province, residence in a rural area and poor housing conditions, male sex, and increased age have been found independent predictors of Chagas cardiomyopathy severity (Hidron et al., 2010).

3.4 Surveillance and health policy

In endemic countries, the tools to interrupt the domestic cycle of *T. cruzi* transmission, such as chemical control, housing improvement, and health education are the most useful methods to prevent Chagas disease (Moncayo & Silveira, 2009). Blood screening is vital to prevent infection through transfusion and organ transplantation and governments should implement policies to promote it (WHO, 2010). In addition, an infrastructure that assures detection and treatment of acute and chronic cases, as well as congenital infection should be developed. In non-endemic countries, screening programs in Latin American pregnant women are increasing and it has been proposed that in some non-endemic countries there is cost-effectiveness to develop it (Sicuri et al., 2011). Regarding strategies to reduce transmission by transfusion in non-endemic countries, there are two different approaches: one is the deferral of individuals at risk of Chagas disease and the second approach is to accept blood donations if specific laboratory assays are negative. This second approach is being introduced in countries where there is a substantial Latin American population, such as the United States, Spain, and France (Castro, 2009). Also, taking into account that knowledge about Chagas disease among doctors in non-endemic countries is very limited (Verani et al., 2010), strategies to improve awareness are very important in order to enhance treatment and follow up of cases.

4. Clinical presentation

4.1 Acute phase

The symptomatic acute phase could be present at any age but it is most common in children under 10 years of age. When the infection is acquired via vector, it takes four to eight weeks for symptoms to develop. In this phase there is an important inflammatory response in the site of contact with bug feces and *T. cruzi* may multiply locally (cutaneous chagoma when it is in the skin). The insect prefers the thinnest skin and that is why the best known sign is Romaña's sign which consists in a unilateral conjunctivitis with periorbital edema, eyelid edema and pre-auricular adenopathy (Biolo et al., 2010). In younger children (under 4 years of age) it is common to found the following symptoms: fever, malaise, muscle pain, anorexia, anemia, sweating, hepatosplenomegaly, heart failure from myocarditis, pericardial effusion, seizures, and somnolence secondary to meningoencephalitis, the more infrequent form of presentation (Gomez et al., 2007). The acute congenital disease should be considered by the medical care system staff in endemic areas; it could be asymptomatic or may be associated to prematurity, low weight, hepatomegaly, splenomegaly, jaundice, anemia, neonatal hepatitis, meningoencephalitis, sepsis, myocarditis, fever, and less frequently megaesophagus, megacolon, megabladder. Without treatment, mortality is 5-10%, the leading causes are encephalomyelitis and heart failure (Prata, 2001). Patients with HIV could reactivate the disease and have meningoencephalitis as a first manifestation (Carod-Artal, 2006). In patients with history of solid organ or bone marrow transplants, 30% reactivate Chagas disease, the acute manifestations could be myocarditis, panniculitis, subcutaneous parasite-containing nodules, and meningoencephalitis (Bern et al., 2007).

4.2 Chronic phase

Once the acute phase is resolved, it begins the chronic phase. This chronic phase could be asymptomatic lifelong or progressive heart and/or gastro esophageal disease. The chronic asymptomatic or indeterminate phase lasts 10 to 30 years. For some authors its definition means epidemiological contact, positive serologic tests, normal physical examination and normal radiological, electrocardiographic and echocardiography studies. Around 30% of these have progressive disease (Higuchi et al., 2003). When Chagas becomes symptomatic, depending on the geographic zone, the disease will have different signs and symptoms. In Central America and northern South America, the heart disease is the common manifestation, but in Brazil and Southern Cone countries it coexists with digestive syndromes (Miles et al., 2003). For the purpose of this review, we will focus on Chagasic cardiomyopathy. The earliest manifestations of heart disease are electrocardiographic abnormalities as the expression of the damage of the conduction system and the symptoms that the patients experience could be related to those abnormalities: atrioventricular block, sinus bradycardia, premature ventricular contractions, atrial fibrillation, and ventricular tachycardia. In 40% of patients with mild heart disease there could be non-sustained ventricular tachycardia, as well as in 90% of patients with heart failure. Sudden death occurs in 38% of patients with chronic disease with or without heart failure, meaning more severe heart disease. The principal cause of sudden death is the malignant ventricular arrhythmia followed by advanced atrioventricular block and cerebral emboli. Non-sustained ventricular tachycardia in Holter monitoring and in stress test, together with low ejection fraction, syncope and pre-syncope, sinus node dysfunction, history of recovery from cardiac arrest, and dyspnea NYHA class III or IV have been recognized of prognostic value in sudden death (Prata, 2001). Symptomatic heart failure occurs in some patients before there is any significant electrocardiography alteration. It could be right or left heart failure; it is very common for patients to have severe structural heart disease and not show symptoms of severe heart failure. It is also common to find severe congestive hepatic disease. Pulmonary and systemic emboli due to dilated chambers of apical aneurism are common clinical manifestations of chronic heart disease (Bern et al., 2007); they have been described in 40% of autopsies (Prata, 2001). A Brazilian study found four predictors of emboli complications: age > 48 years, primary changes in repolarization, apical aneurism, and ejection fraction < 50%, with a 4% annual incidence if all four factors where present (Sousa et al., 2008). Precordial pain is a frequent complaint of patients with Chagas disease. The incidence of this symptom is 15% but other authors report up to 30% (Marin-Neto et al., 2007). The causes of the symptom are not clear; some authors believe that this pain could be caused by microvascular disease.

4.2.1 Classification

A simple classification, published by the Brazilian Consensus on Chagas Diseases, includes functional capacity, electrocardiographic findings, function and size of left ventricle. This classification allowed defining four disease stages with the aim to orientate the patient's therapy (Table 1).

Stage	Electrocardiogram	Echocardiography	Heart failure
A	Altered	Normal	Absent
B1	Altered	Altered LVEF >45%	Absent
B2	Altered	Altered LVEF <45%	Absent
C	Altered	Altered	Compensated
D	Altered	Altered	Refractory

LVEF: left ventricular ejection fraction

Table 1. Classification of cardiac compromise in Chagas chronic cardiomyopathy

5. Pathogenesis of cardiac disease during *T. cruzi* infection

5.1 Host genetic influence

Some works approach the influence of human genetics such as Histocompability Complex Molecules (HLA) or polymorphism in cytokine promoters and their contribution to Chagas disease. So far, association with HLA class II indicated that infected individuals with and without cardiomyopathy had a higher frequency of DRB1*01, DRB1*08, and DQB1*0501 (Fernandez et al., 1998), and the DRB1*01 DQB1*0501 haplotype was more frequent in patients with Chagasic cardiomyopathy (Colorado et al., 2000). Additionally, the HLA-DRB1*1503 allele was associated with genetic susceptibility to cardiac damage (Garcia Borras et al., 2009). All these studies were conducted with small cohorts and with different

Latin American populations. Polymorphisms of cytokine promoters assess the potential pattern of cytokine hypo or hyper secretion in individuals. A study showed the association of transforming growth factor beta (TGFβ1) (Calzada et al., 2009) and lymphotoxin α (LTα) with the risk Chagasic cardiomyopathy progression (Ramasawmy et al., 2007). Tumor necrosis factor (TNFα), a pro-inflammatory agent, is the cytokine with the strongest relationship to cardiac tissue damage in Chagas. There is an association between *T. cruzi* seropositive individuals and the polymorphism in TNF-238A. Indeed, TNFα secretion is higher in non-stimulated and stimulated cells from chronic Chagasic donors (Pissetti et al., 2011) and TNFα serum levels were associated with heart failure (Talvani et al., 2004). In *T. cruzi e*xperimentally infected rats, the cardiomyopathy ameliorates in animals treated with a TNFα blocking monoclonal antibody (Perez et al., 2009).

5.2 Parasite tropisms

Geographic distribution of an organ-specific chronic disease (cardiac *versus* digestive diseases) and allocation of *T. cruzi* I and II (II to VI in the new classification), supported the hypothesis that disease outcome is linked to the *T. cruzi* genetic variations. Some studies did not show correlations among *T. cruzi* lineages and the clinical forms of Chagas disease (Zafra et al., 2011). Although, the presence of TcI was correlated with higher frequencies of electrocardiogram alterations than individuals infected with TcII, such as ventricular premature beats, first-degree atrioventricular block, sinus bradycardia, abnormal Q-waves, atrial fibrillation, and complex ventricular arrhythmias (Ramirez et al., 2010). In a mouse model infected with two different genetic populations of *T. cruzi,* both parasites were found during the acute infection in several host compartments (blood and organs). However, during chronic infection, a preferential tissue distribution with predominance of certain *T. cruzi* isolates was found (Andrade et al., 1999). Because *T. cruzi* mixed infections in triatomines are found in high rates, a similar phenomenon should take place during human infection.

5.3 Parasite invasion of the host cells

T. cruzi can reach the mammalian host cells via different mucosal tissues (i.e., conjunctiva, oral) or directly into blood (transfusion or congenital). The parasite in vivo can invade a vast range of cells such as monocyte/macrophages, dendritic cells, endothelial cells, fibroblasts, astrocytes, skeletal muscles, enteric nerves, and cardiomyocytes (Epting et al., 2010). Parasite invasion is a multistep process when several *T. cruzi* glycoproteins bind surface molecules on the host cells. Before reaching the target tissues, *T. cruzi* must interact with the endothelial cells to actively penetrate or increase endothelium vasodilatation. Parasite protease can produce inflammations that increase vascular permeability (Epting et al., 2010). Several parasite proteases and glycoprotein expressed by trypomastigotes have been associated with invasion: gp60 (penetrin) gp63, gp35/50, gp82, gp90 a parasite glycosidase, mucins and transialidase such as gp85 or Tc85. The binding of these parasite molecules to host molecules (cytokeratin 18, mucins, heparan sulfates, extracellular matrix proteins such as fibronectin and laminin, and carbohydrates with sialic acid) induce Ca++ mobilization, protein tyrosine phosphorylation and cytoskeleton reorganization in the target cells. Transialidase, glycosylphosphatidylinositol (GPI) anchors surface-bound proteins are in charge of transferring sialic acid residues from the host cell to the parasite glycoproteins. This mechanism seems to be crucial in invasion given that trypomastigotes with no expression of trans-sialidases were poorly invasive to non-phagocytic cells (Epting et al.,

2010). Also, infection by oral route involved other parasite glycoproteins such as mucin-like gp35/50 or gp82 on the surface of the trypomastigotes, resistant to protease digestion. Glycoprotein gp82 binds to the gastric mucin and allows the parasite to invade epithelial cells (Yoshida, 2008).

5.4 Acute and chronic heart involvement in Chagas diseases

5.4.1 Acute myocarditis

Parasite genetic variations, the initial parasite burden, and the host immune response seem to influence the evolution of the Chagas disease. Clinical cardiac involvement is found in nearly 90% of symptomatic patients. Parasite-infected myocardiocytes with intracellular amastigotes (pseudocyst) break up and induce acute inflammation (Coura & Borges-Pereira, 2010). There is massive and diffuse infiltration with predominance of mononuclear cells (Fig. 3A) mainly CD8+ T lymphocytes (LT) up to 60% (Fig. 3B). Whether these LT are *T. cruzi* antigen specific and which chemotactic agents control this migration is unknown. Microarray studies of *T. cruzi* acute infection in mouse cardiomyocytes showed a regulation of 353 genes (111 up regulated and 242 down regulated) associated with inflammation, cytoskeleton, cell interaction, apoptosis, cell cycle, and oxidative stress. Interestingly, early genes up regulated include a vast range of chemokines, which attract mononuclear cells (Manque et al., 2011). In consequence, there is cell destruction (myocytolysis), interstitial edema, hypertrophy of myocardial fibers, and alteration of the cardiac microcirculation with platelet aggregation, production of pro-inflammatory cytokines and expression of vascular adhesion molecules by endothelial cells (Rossi et al., 2010).

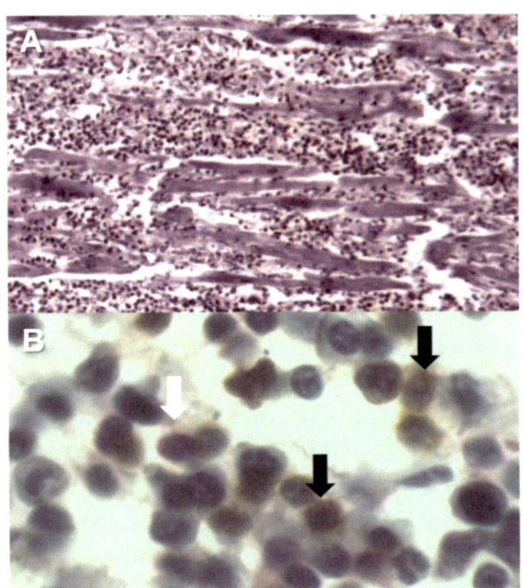

Fig. 3. Immunohistology of a heart with acute Chagas disease showing extensive cellular infiltration 10x (A), and presence of CD8+ (black arrow and brown cells) and CD4+ T cells (white arrow and red cell) with hematoxylin as contra-staining 100x (B). Courtesy of Ana M. Uribe, M.D. Pathology Department, School of Medicine, Pontificia Universidad Javeriana, Bogota D.C., Colombia.

5.4.2 Chronic myocarditis

Contrary to acute infection, in the chronic phase there is scarcity of *T. cruzi* niches; however, there is an extensive, but patchy mononuclear infiltration, with predominance of macrophages and cytotoxic CD8+ T cells (CTL). Myocarditis has a slow progression with changes in the contractile function and dilatation of the heart walls. Increase in metalloproteinase has been described in infected cardiac tissue and associated with remodeling of the extracellular matrix (Gutierrez et al., 2009). Histology analysis shows diffuse myocarditis, myocytolysis, edema, mononuclear cellular infiltration (hallmark of the delayed hypersensitivity), destruction of the conduction system with neuron loss (autonomic denervation), and extensive myocardial fibrosis. Functional studies in Chagasic cardiopathy demonstrated impaired perfusion at the coronary vessels due to microvascular changes (thrombi, inflammation, and spam) (Rossi et al., 2010).

5.5 Mechanisms of tissue damage

5.5.1 Autoimmunity

The autoimmune theory was initially based on the scarcity of parasites found in chronically infected tissue and also on the presence of antibodies and T cells that recognized parasite antigen and cross-reacted with host tissues and molecules. Antibodies against *T. cruzi* bind to human laminin, sulfo-galactosylceramides, cardiac myosin, microtubule-associated proteins, ribosomal proteins, β-adrenergic and muscarinic receptors; heart sarcolemma, blood vessel, neurons, glial cells, myocardium and skeletal muscles (Bonney & Engman, 2008). However, demonstration of the pathological consequences due to autoimmunity in *T. cruzi* infection does not have direct evidence. Most of the auto-antibodies are considered to be natural antibodies that could be induced after tissue injury and exposure of host cell molecules. Also, *T. cruzi* antigens can act as B cell polyclonal stimulators. Against the autoimmunity theory it is known that the immune-suppression exacerbates *T. cruzi* infection and specific anti-parasitic treatment ameliorates the clinical disease (Rossi et al., 2010).

5.5.2 Antigenic persistence and immune response

By using DNA techniques, the presence of *T. cruzi* in tissues during chronic infection has become clear. Antigen persistence triggers inflammation and lymphocyte infiltration. Damage mechanisms are unclear because parasite burden does not explain extensive cell loss. CD8+ T lymphocytes contribute to cytotoxicity probably via perforin and granzyme B, and TGB-β and interleukin-10 (IL-10) secreting macrophages can induce repair and fibrosis through fibroblasts. *T. cruzi* infection also alters microcirculation with the presence of platelets aggregated, microvascular spam, and secretion of vasoconstrictor agents such as tromboxane A2 (TXA2) and platelet activated factors (PAF) by macrophages or endothelin 1 (ET-1) by endothelial cells (Rossi et al., 2010).

6. Human immune response

Innate immune cells such as natural killer cells, macrophages, and dendritic cells detect invading pathogens and alert the immune system through activation cascades. The aim is to elicit innate antimicrobial and inflammatory responses and initiate adaptive immunity to control or eliminate infection. It is accepted that the establishment of chronic infection with *T. cruzi* is a consequence of the inability of the immune response to elicit sterilizing antiparasite immunity. Therefore, the host innate and adaptive immune response is believed to be the key determinant of the clinical outcome of the disease.

6.1 Innate immunity

Dendritic cells (DCs), natural killer (NK) cells, and monocytes are vital mediators of the innate immune system and promote development of adaptive immune responses. Evidence shows that *T. cruzi* may infect DCs and even proliferate inside them. Consequently, the DC antigen presentation capacity is reduced (Van Overtvelt et al., 2002). In early asymptomatic Chagas disease, higher levels of pro-inflammatory monocytes and expansion of NK cells before the adaptative immunity development has been shown (Vitelli-Avelar, 2006). The role of cytokines such as interleukin (IL)-4, IL-12, TNFα, and interferon (IFN)γ secreted by these cells can be an important element for host resistance during the early stages of infection and also in the genesis of myocarditis (Golgher et al., 2004). It has been shown that two different and independent antigenic stimuli from the parasite induce both an enhancement of IL-10 and a reduction of IL-12 secretion in DCs from Chagasic patients compared to DCs from healthy donors (Cuellar et al., 2008). Although, the innate immune system seems to have a fundamental role in Chagas disease by controlling parasite replication and spread in host tissues, it is not clear if events described here, that mediate inflammatory reaction, can be related to protection or tissue damage in the chronic phase of the disease.

6.2 Humoral immune response

A specific antibody response and B cells in animal models of Chagas disease seem to play an important role for parasite control, especially against the trypomastigotes. In spite of the large number of parasite proteins some molecules have been studied. Indeed, in our previous work, we showed that there is a consistently higher specific IgG response in chronic Chagasic patients against *T. cruzi* kinetoplastid membrane protein-11 (KMP-11), and the *T. cruzi* heat shock protein-70 (HSP-70). The recombinant KMP-11 protein recognition was focused on IgG1 sub-fraction; whereas, the lysate was on IgG3 plus IgG1 in asymptomatic and cardiopathic chronic phases, compared to acute sera from Chagasic patients (Flechas et al., 2009). These data reflect the dynamics of the humoral immune response in Chagas disease and may be an important issue given that IgG1 and IgG3 are the major complement fixing isotypes, which also mediate cooperative function with phagocytes; nevertheless, the role of these specific antibodies in controlling the infection or progressing in disease severity need to be addressed.

6.3 T cells and cytokines

Individuals undergoing chemotherapy generally show protection against viral infections controlled by T cells during lymphopenia, indicating that a small population of T cells can be protective (Turtle et al., 2009). However, reactivation of Chagas disease, defined by a demonstration of trypomastigotes on microscopic examination of blood or the identification of amastigotes on biopsy samples and/or acute clinical manifestations during the chronic phase, can occur among the immunosuppressed patients with heart transplantation (Burgos et al., 2010) or AIDS patients (Almeida et al., 2009). It may be the natural history disease demonstration that T cell response is crucial to control parasite burden and clinical manifestations in a large proportion of patients. Perhaps the most interesting question is how adaptive immune response can contribute to most infected individuals remains asymptomatic whereas an important percentage of these patients develop severe forms of the disease. In humans, it has been shown that CD4+ T cells (Cuellar et al., 2009) and CD8+ T cells (Fiuza et al., 2009) from Chagasic patients specifically produced IFNγ after exposure to *T. cruzi* antigens. Furthermore, chronic Chagasic patients had lower levels of antigen-specific CD8+ T cells secreting IFNγ compared with non-symptomatic individuals (Laucella et al., 2004). Because *T. cruzi* is an intracellular parasite, many groups have focused on the study of CD8+ T cells. Some of them have studied specific CD8+ T cells against peptides derived from cruzipain, FL-160 (Fonseca et al., 2005), KMP-11 (Diez et al., 2006; Lasso et al., 2010), and trans-sialidases (Alvarez et al., 2008) proteins, founding similar frequency of specific CD8+ T cells for these epitopes. Nonetheless, it has been shown that patients with more severe forms of Chagas disease have more differentiated CD8+ T cells which could have lost their functional capacity (Bixby & Tarleton, 2008). One interesting aspect is the control of immune response by regulatory T cells (T_{reg}). Ex vivo, it was shown that children with asymptomatic Chagas disease display a lower frequency of natural T_{reg} CD4+ CD25^{high} compared to non-infected children (Vitelli-Avelar et al., 2006). Interestingly, these cells are in increased levels in peripheral blood of late chronic asymptomatic patients (Vitelli-Avelar et al., 2005). These data suggest that T_{reg} could be important to limiting tissue damage. However, taking into account that additional molecules have been suggested to identify T_{reg}, we used a panel of antibodies for CD4, CD25, FoxP3, and CD127. Our results show higher proportion of T_{reg} in symptomatic chronic Chagasic patients compared to non-infected individuals, indicating that the frequency of T_{reg} can contribute to damage. Fig. 4 despites the CD4+ T_{reg} cells by flow citometry (Lasso et al., 2009).

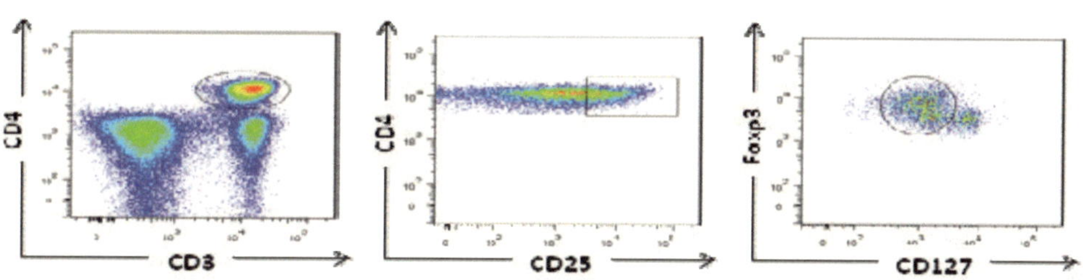

Fig. 4. Regulatory T cells from chronic Chagasic patient identified by high levels of expression of the transcription factor forkhead box transcription factor P3 (FoxP3) and low levels of CD127. Courtesy of Paola Lasso, Pontificia Universidad Javeriana, Bogota D.C., Colombia.

7. Diagnosis

The diagnosis of Chagas disease, as with other infections, is performed on the basis of clinical findings, parasite presence, serological status, and epidemiological data. Furthermore, the disease stage is also an important fact to consider. For instance, as the parasitemia dramatically decreases from acute to chronic phase, in the early phase parasite detection is achieved by parasitological conventional direct tests (see below). Nevertheless, because clinical findings in this stage can be confused with other pathologies, the epidemiological data demonstrating a connection between the patient and the parasite is of special importance (Nicholls et al., 2007). In contrast, in chronic patients, the presence of symptoms or abnormal clinical findings usually correlates with the disease but parasite concentration is low and variable. Bearing in mind that *T. cruzi* infection is life lasting; in the chronic phase serological tests are applied to indirectly demonstrate parasite presence (Enciso et al., 2004). Indeed, the WHO recommends that to diagnose a chronic Chagasic patient; besides having clinical findings compatible with Chagas disease and history of vector contact, there must be at least two positive serological tests with different immunological principles. Finally, chronic asymptomatic patients represent a real challenge for diagnosing inasmuch as there are no clinical findings, and again parasitemia is very low and intermittent. Consequently, the epidemiological patient history is also of most importance (Gil et al., 2007).

7.1 Clinical findings

7.1.1 Electrocardiogram

The most common electrocardiographic manifestations are right bundle branch block (RBBB), anterior fascicular block, premature ventricular contractions, changes in ST segment and T wave, abnormal Q waves, and low voltage of the QRS complex (Fig. 5). The combination of the RBBB and the anterior fascicular block suggest the disease (Garzón et al., 1995). The presence of frequent premature ventricular contractions, including duplets and salvos of non-sustained ventricular tachycardia are a common finding in the Holter monitoring and in the stress test. Premature ventricular contractions correlate with the severity of the ventricular function, but can also occur in patients with preserved ventricular function. Episodes of non-sustained ventricular tachycardia are observed in 40% of the patients with light to moderate ventricular contractibility alterations and in virtually all patients with heart failure, which is more frequent than in other cardiomyopathies. Sustained ventricular tachycardia is another disease marker. This arrhythmia can be produced through programmed ventricular stimulation in nearly 85% of the cases and results from intramyocardial or subepicardial reentrant phenomena, usually located on the inferoposterior and lateral wall of the left ventricle.

7.1.2 X-ray and echocardiography

In patients in the undetermined phase, the cardiac silhouette evaluated in the chest X-ray and the global systolic function in echocardiography are normal. In more advanced stages, the chest X-ray can show cardiomegaly and pulmonary congestion. The disease can cause diffuse damage of the systolic function of the left ventricle. The global systolic function of the left ventricle has prognostic implications. In a cohort of 538 patients grouped into four stages of disease progression, different survival rates were found in the five-year follow up from 98%, 91%, 45% to 13% for those with normal left ventricle function, moderately depressed function, with reversible heart failure, or irreversible heart failure, respectively (Rassi et al., 2010). Some alterations of the segmental contraction of the left ventricle can be detected. The most common is located on the posterior wall with 20% prevalence. The presence of mitral or tricuspid insufficiency is generally associated to ring expansion. The prevalence of aneurysms in the left ventricle varies in the different series, noted on an average of 8.5% in asymptomatic individuals and in patients with severe cardiac damage up to 55%. Through logistic regression analysis, the presence of an apical aneurysm in the left ventricle was an independent predictor of mural Thrombi (Albanesi-Filho et al., 1991). In another work, the finding of an aneurysm was significantly associated to a thrombus and cerebro-vascular accident during a two-year follow up. On some instances, diminished systolic function of the right ventricle can be the only abnormality detected via echocardiography; in general, it is secondary to the severity to the damage of the left ventricle and at high levels of pulmonary pressure. With regards to diastolic function, chronic myocarditis in Chagas disease can diminish ventricular relaxation and diastolic filling. These abnormalities usually precede systolic dysfunction. Reduced compliance of the left ventricle can increase the filling pressure of the left atrium with changes in transmitral and pulmonary venous flow rates. The echocardiography study is recommended as a routine clinical evaluation method in patients with Chagas cardiopathy to determine the stage of the disease, its progression, as well as to estimate survival, dismiss the presence of aneurysms or intracavitary thrombi, and monitor response to treatment.

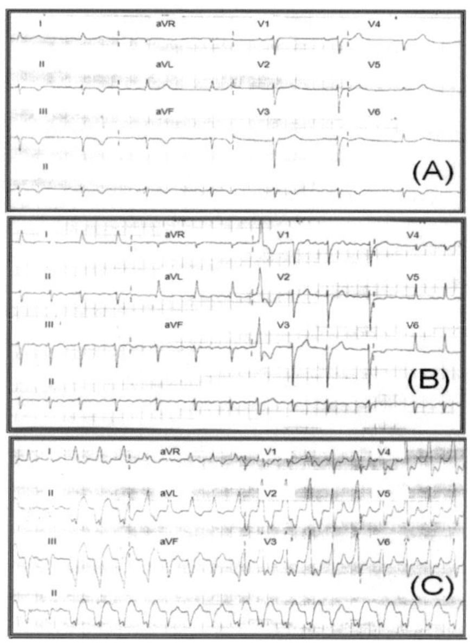

Fig. 5. ECG sequence in a 72-year-old woman diagnosed with Chagas cardiomyopathy and ejection fraction of the left ventricle at 25%. Note sinus bradycardia (A), attrial fibrillation (B), and monomorphic sustained ventricular tachycardia (C). Fundación Clínica Abood Shaio, Bogota D.C., Colombia.

In our experience at Fundación Clínica Abood Sahio (Bogotá, Colombia), from a total of 120 patients evaluated with diagnosis of Chagas cardiomyopathy, 73 women (60%) with mean age of 56.7 +/- 13 years (21-84), clinical manifestations corresponded to dyspnea (42%), palpitations (31%), chest pain (42%), presyncope (24%), syncope (27%), and aborted sudden death (2.5%). Nearly 6.7% of the cases did not present clinical manifestations. The main ECG findings were: right bundle branch block (40%), second and third degree AV block (29.2%), dysfunction of the sinus node (28.3%), ventricular tachycardia (23%), atrial fibrillation (19%), left anterior hemiblock (17.2%), atrial flutter (3.3%), and left bundle branch block (3.3%). In 31% of the cases, the chest X-ray was normal. In 15.8%, severe cardiomegaly was observed. All the patients were subjected to a color Doppler echocardiogram according to internationally recognized norms, finding a mean fraction of the left ventricle of 43.3% (SD +/- 16.5) (10-60) and of the right ventricle at 23.4% (10-40) (Fig. 6). The study was considered normal in 33.6% of the cases. Contractility alterations were documented in 42.4%, with these being globally in 26.5% of the cases, or inferior, apical-inferior and anterior localization. Isolated compromise of the right ventricle was observed in one case (0.8%), suggesting the diagnosis of arrhythmogenic dysplasia of the right ventricle. In 24% of the cases mitral insufficiency was evidenced and 15.2% revealed tricuspid insufficiency. A total of 11 aneurysms (9.7%) were observed, 63.6% of apical localization and 36.3% of inferior localization. Some 8.8% of the patients presented intracavitary thrombi, generally related to aneurysms or global contractility alterations. Holter or electrophysiological study documented ventricular tachycardia (sustained or unsustained) in 19.4% of the cases. Additionally in 10% we observed association to sinus dysfunction and/or AV block with ventricular tachycardia. Anatomic-pathological findings obtained via biopsy or surgery in 10 Chagas patients were: a) hypertrophy and/or b) fibrosis and/or c) chronic inflammatory infiltrate. None of the cases reported parasites in the samples examined by pathology (Rosas et al., 2007).

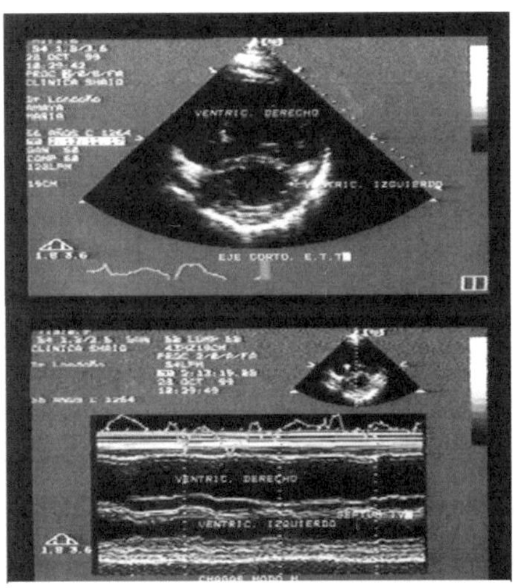

Fig. 6. Echocardiography M mode (A) and bi-dimensional (B) of 54-year-old female with a history of aborted sudden death due to ventricular tachycardia) secondary to Chagasic cardiomyopathy. Note the severe dilatation of right ventricle. Fundación Clínica Abood Shaio, Bogota D.C., Colombia.

7.2 Laboratory tests

7.2.1 Conventional parasitological tests

These can be classified into direct and indirect tests. Direct methods, employed basically in the acute phase, include parasite microscope-observation in blood fresh preparation which permits to observe parasite movement. On the contrary, thin or thick blood smears stained with Giemsa led to a better morphological identification, which is of special importance in areas where *Trypanosoma rangeli* also circulates. Importantly, parasite concentration methods like blood centrifugation, Strout method, and microhematocrit increase the probability of trypomastigote detection. Because of their great time consumption, indirect parasitological methods are generally used to diagnose patients in the chronic phase. They refer to hemoculture and xenodiagnosis (Luquetti, 2007).

7.2.2 Serological tests

There is a broad spectrum of serological tests, whose final goal is to detect anti-*T. cruzi* antibodies, usually of the IgG isotype in the chronic phase or IgM in the acute phase. The tests most used, called conventional tests for serological Chagas disease diagnosis, are the indirect immunofluorescence test (IFAT), the enzyme-linked immunoabsorbent assay (ELISA), and the indirect haemaglutination test (IHA). Generally, the antigens used are parasite lysates or mixtures of parasite recombinant proteins. Due to the huge parasite polymorphisms (Rodríguez et al., 2002), it is recommended to use isolates circulating in the specific endemic area or mixture of them.The applied method must be carefully standardized and validated in inter-laboratory international and national tests. Most of the above-mentioned tests can detect the infection in more than 95% of sera. Nevertheless, false-positive reactions can occur in *T. rangeli* or *Lesihmania*-infected patients, as well as false-negative in the case of recently-infected chronic patients or immunosuppressed patients (Gil et al., 2007; Luquetti, 2007).

7.2.3 PCR

PCR tests, because of their power of detection and specificity, constitute a complementary diagnostic method for detecting *T. cruzi* in diverse biological samples. They are of especial interest with chronic patients because of their higher sensitivity compared with conventional parasitological tests. There are several PCR tests available for detecting *T. cruzi*. Their performance varies depending on aspects like type and number of the target amplification, lack of polymorphisms among the parasite DTU-annealing primer target, sample volume, treatment and conservation, DNA extraction method, type of DNA polymerase used, and thermo-cycling program, among variables (Schijman et al., 2011). Some PCR tests show disadvantages like the amplification of polymorphic fragments or of similar-size bands in both *T. cruzi* and *T. rangeli* infections, the deviation of the test towards *T. cruzi* in mixed infections with *T. rangeli*, and the possible integration of the parasite's kDNA in the human genome (Gil et al., 2007; Pavía et al., 2003, 2007). Bearing all this in mind, the Molecular Parasitology Laboratory at Pontificia Universidad Javeriana designed and standardized the TcH2AF-R PCR, specific for *T. cruzi* (Pavia et al., 2003). This PCR amplifies the 16-255 nucleotides of the *T. cruzi* SIRE repetitive element and does not present amplification signal in *T. rangeli*. Assays on triatomine vectors experimentally and naturally infected with *T. cruzi* revealed that TcH2AF-R PCR allows identifying the parasite in all the infected specimens, with performance equal to that of S35/S36 PCR, considered among the most sensitive PCR tests for *T. cruzi* identification (Pavia et al., 2007). Likewise, in blood samples from Chagasic patients, it was observed that of 156 samples, 84 (53.8%) were positive with both TcH2AF-R and S35/S36 PCRs, while 89 (57%) were positive for indirect immunofluorescence (IIF) and enzymatic immunoassay (ELISA) (Gil et al., 2007). A study of the performance of the TcH2AF-R and S35-S36 primers in cardiac tissue of mice infected with *T. cruzi I* showed that by using both pairs of primers it is possible to detect the parasite in the acute and chronic stages of the infection, with performance above that of the micro-hematocrit and eliminate of the histopathological analysis (Barrera et al., 2008). Recently, by combining TcH2AF-R and S35/S36 PCRs, it was possible to follow up a Colombian heart transplant in a Chagasic patient, as well as the first Colombian congenital case (Pavia et al., 2009, 2011). Because of its higher sensitivity, a few real time PCR (qPCR) methods have been developed to monitor drug efficacy and Chagas disease reactivation in transplanted

Chagasic patients. However, international studies to evaluate PCR methods for parasite DNA detection in blood samples as that launched by Shijman et al., (2011) are urgently needed.

7.3 Epidemiological context

Epidemiological data, such as that shown in Table 2, seek to determine if the patient could have been in contact with the parasite.

<table>
<tr><th>Epidemiological data</th><th>Information included</th></tr>
<tr><td>Born in endemic areas</td><td rowspan="3">Housing conditions like thatched roof, dirt floors, adobe walls, etc.
Presence of domestic animals.
Rural, peri-domestic, or domestic dwellings
Time of living in relationship to already performed vector control campaigns in the area (important in congenital transmission)</td></tr>
<tr><td>Living in endemic areas</td></tr>
<tr><td>Visits to endemic areas</td></tr>
<tr><td>Vector knowledge</td><td>Awareness of vectors circulating in the specific area</td></tr>
<tr><td>Chagasic relatives</td><td>Parents, siblings, or any family member infected</td></tr>
<tr><td>Work activity</td><td>Important in accidental transmission in both endemic and non-endemic areas</td></tr>
<tr><td>History of blood transfusions</td><td>Amount and place</td></tr>
<tr><td>History of organ transplant</td><td>Medical and epidemiological history of the donor</td></tr>
</table>

Table 2. Epidemiological data supporting risk of *T. cruzi* infection

8. Treatment

8.1 Symptomatic

In the absence of random clinical studies in patients with Chagas disease and heart failure, traditionally the recommendations have been extrapolated from the management guides for heart failure from other causes (Jessup et al., 2009). However, it should be noted that in the physiopathology of the Chagas disease there are clinical and therapeutic peculiarities with important implications. For example, high doses of diuretics are necessary in advanced stages of the disease due to predominance of the systemic congestion manifestations over signs of pulmonary congestion. In patients with Chagas cardiopathy, conduction disturbances are also frequent, which may be aggravated by the use of Digoxin, Amiodarone, and specially Beta-blockers (Marin-Neto et al., 2010). Cardiac re-synchronization is a treatment alternative for patients with heart failure, especially in the presence of left bundle branch block. However, its usefulness in patients with right bundle branch block common in Chagas disease has not been shown as patients with another type of pathology in the presence of this conduction alteration. Other palliative procedures like dynamic cardiomyoplasty and partial left ventriluculotomy are contraindicated because of unsatisfactory results. Heart transplant is an option indicated in patients selected in final stages of cardiac insufficiency. In these cases, it must be highlighted that the immunosuppressant therapy indicated to avoid transplant rejection may induce reactivation of the *T. cruzi* infection (Campos et al., 2008). Under certain circumstances, reducing the dosage of immunosuppression is recommended, as well as starting etiological treatment in cases of reactivation (Fiorelli et al., 2005). The potential benefit of transplanting stem cells in patients with Chagasic cardiopathy is under evaluation (Tura et al., 2007). Because of the high frequency of thrombus-embolic phenomena, anticoagulation is indicated in patients with atrial fibrillation, in the prior embolism, in the presence of aneurysms or thrombi, and in cases of heart failure in advanced stages even in the absence of random controlled studies that prove its efficacy. Some observational data suggest that Amiodarone can improve survival in patients with Chagas disease with risk of sudden death due to malignant arrhythmia (Garguichevich et al., 1995). For this reason, Amiodarone is usually recommended in patients with sustained ventricular tachycardia and in cases of unsustained ventricular tachycardia associated to ventricular systolic dysfunction (Leite et al., 2003). Patients with sustained ventricular tachycardia with hemodynamic instability and in cases of aborted sudden death, the implant of a cardio-defibrillator is recommended (Rassi et al., 2009). Radiofrequency ablation is an alternative in patients with ventricular tachycardia (D´Avila et al., 2002); however, its impact on survival and recurrence of the arrhythmia is yet to be established. The finding of severe bradyarrhythmias like those observed in the complete AV block and in the sinus dysfunction must be treated by implanting a definitive pacemaker as in other cardiac conditions (Epstein et al., 2008). The benefit of the pacemaker implant in patients with Chagasic cardiopathy is mainly based on reports of case series.

8.2 Etiological

The only medications currently used with Chagas disease due to ethical and efficiency reasons are Nifurtimox and Benznidazole (Bern et al., 2007). Based on the literature review, the recommendations of the antitrypanocidal therapy vary according to the phase and form of the Chagas disease, the patient's age, and the severity of the disease. The pharmacological therapy is recommended in all acute and congenital cases, in infection by reactivation, in patients up to 18 years of age, and in children. For adults between 19 and 50 years of age and without advanced cardiopathy, the treatment can be offered (Bern et al., 2007). In individuals above 50 years of age, risk of toxicity from the drug may be higher than in young adults and the treatment is considered optional. Once the diagnosis has been confirmed through corresponding serological tests, patients must be evaluated with a clinical history and a careful physical exam. Additionally, in all cases, an electrocardiogram should be performed. With asymptomatic individuals without electrocardiographic alterations, the prognosis tends to be favorable and it is recommended that these patients be monitored every 12 to 24 months. Patients with electrocardiographic changes consistent with the disease's cardiovascular compromise should be evaluated via thoracic X-ray and echocardiogram that permit defining the ventricular size and function, as well as other types of structural alterations and via 24-h electrocardiographic monitoring or Holter test to detect arrhythmias.

9. Prognosis

The prognosis of some diseases like Chagas has not been easy to establish because of the great differences in their clinical course among the affected countries. Results like the survey by Maguire et al., (1987) showed that from 20-59 years of age, the risk was strongly related to electrocardiography status. Indeed, patients with ventricular conduction defects have higher mortality rates than infected patients without electrocardiographic abnormalities. Also, it was observed that abnormal diastolic function is related to severe myocardial damage (Rocha et al., 2009). Another survey found that there are six prognostic factors of disease development: NYHA class III or IV, cardiomegaly on chest radiography, segmental or global wall motion abnormalities on echocardiography, non-sustained ventricular tachycardia on Holter monitoring, low QRS voltage on electrocardiography, and male sex (Rassi et al., 2006). Recent studies have found that there are four echocardiographic variables associated with the disease outcome: left ventricular ejection fraction, right ventricular function, E/E' ratio, and left atrium volume (Rocha et al., 2009). Finally, the prognosis of the patient will rest on the good care and follow up of the caregivers. Chagas disease is no longer a disease of the poor; it is now a disease of any country with important socioeconomic impact.

10. Conclusions

Prediction markers for disease development, and progression, immunotherapy and vaccine strategies, new anti-*T. cruzi* drugs, and world-standardized PCR tests, are urgently required to improve early diagnosis and treatment of this worldwide health problem. Government, health organizations, and scientists all over the world need to come together to construct policies and strategies to prevent and control this silent but devastating disease in endemic and non endemic countries.

11. Acknowledgments

The authors express gratitude to the Vicerrectoria Académica at Pontificia Universidad Javeriana for financially supporting this proposal, as well to other agencies funding our research projects, which permit us to achieve this manuscript: Colciencias (projects 1203-493-26159, 1109-04-18231, 1203-333-18692), TWAS (project No. 827), Pontificia Universidad Javeriana (projects No. 609, 784, 1034, 1707, 1767, 2089, 3333), and Universidad de los Andes [associate professor grant (JMG) from the Vicerrectoria de Investigaciones, Universidad de los Andes]. We would also like to thank the patients and the healthy controls who participated in our researches.

12. References

Albanesi-Filho, FM.; Gomes, JB. (1991). O tromboembolismo em pacientes com lesão apical da cardiopatia chagásica crônica. *Revista Portuguesa de Cardiologia*, Vol.10, No. 1, (January 1991), pp.35-42, ISSN 0870-2551

Almeida, E.A.; Silva, E.L.; Guariento, M.E. et al. (2009). Fatal evolution of Chagas'disease/Aids co-infection: diagnostic difficulties between myocarditis reactivation and chronic chagasic myocardiopathy. *Revista da Sociedade Brasileira de Medicina Tropical*, Vol.42, No.2, (March-April 2009), pp. 199-202, ISSN 0037-8682

Alvarez, M.G.; Postan, M.; Weatherly, D.B. et al. (2008). HLA Class I-T cell epitopes from trans-sialidase proteins reveal functionally distinct subsets of CD8+ T cells in chronic Chagas disease. *PLoS Neglected Tropical Diseases*, Vol.2, No.9, (September 2008), e288, ISSN 1935-2735

Andrade, L.O.; Machado, C.R.; Chiari, E. et al. (1999). Differential tissue distribution of diverse clones of *Trypanosoma cruzi* in infected mice. *Molecular and Biochemical Parasitology*, Vol.100, No.2, (May 1999), pp. 163-172, ISNN 1872-9428

Barrera, Y.K.; Guevara, J.M.; Pavía, P.X. et al. (2008).Evaluation of TcH2AF-R and S35-S36 primers in PCR tests for the detection of *Trypanosoma cruzi* in mouse cardiac tissue. *Biomedica*, Vol. 28, No. 4, (December 2008), pp. 616-626, ISSN 0120-4157

Bayer, A.M.; Hunter, G.C. ; Gilman, R.H. et al. (2009). Chagas disease, migration and community settlement patterns in Arequipa, Peru. *PLoS Neglected Tropical Diseases*, Vol. 3, No. 12, (December 2009), pp.e567, ISSN 1935-2735

Bern, C. & Montgomery, S.P. (2009). An estimate of the burden of Chagas disease in the United States. *Clinical Infectious Diseases*, Vol.49, No.5, (September 2009), pp. e52-e54, ISSN 1058-4838

Bern, C.; Montgomery S.P.; Herwaldt B.L. et al. (2007). Evaluation and treatment of Chagas disease in the United States. *Journal of the American Medical Association*, Vol. 298, No. 18, (November 2007), pp. 2171-2181, ISSN 1538-3598

Biolo, A.; Ribeiro A.L. & Clausell, N. (2010). Chagas cardiomyopathy-where do we stand after a hundred years?. *Progress in Cardiovascular Diseases*, Vol.52, (January-February 2010), pp. 300-316, ISSN 1532-8643

Bixby, L.M. & Tarleton, R.L. (2008). Stable CD8+ T cell memory during persistent *Trypanosoma cruzi* infection. *Journal of Immunology*, Vol.181, No.4, (August 2008), pp. 2644–2650, ISSN 1550-6606

Bonney, K.M. & Engman, D.M. (2008). Chagas heart disease pathogenesis: one mechanism or many? *Current Molecular Medicine*, Vol.8, No. 6 (September 2008), pp. 510-518, ISSN 1875-5666

Burgos, J.M.; Diez, M.; Vigliano, C. et al. (2010). Molecular identification of *Trypanosoma cruzi* discrete typing units in end-stage chronic Chagas heart disease and reactivation after heart transplantation. *Clinical Infectious Diseases*, Vol.51, No.5, (September 2010), pp. 485-495, ISSN 1058-4838

Calzada, J.E.; Beraún, Y.; González, C.I. et al. (2009). Transforming growth factor beta 1(TGFbeta1) gene polymorphisms and Chagas disease susceptibility in Peruvian and Colombian patients. *Cytokine*, Vol.45, No.3, (March 2009), pp.149-53, ISSN 1096-0023

Campos, S.V.; Strabelli, T.M.; Amato, N.V. et al. (2008). Risk factors for Chagas' disease reactivation after heart transplantation. *Journal of Heart and Lung Transplantation*, Vol. 27, No. 6, (June 2008), pp. 597–602, ISSN 1557-3117

Carod-Artal, F.J. (2006). Chagas' disease and ischemic stroke. *Neurologia*, Vol. 21, No. 3, (April 2006), pp. 135-149, ISSN 0213-4853

Castro, E. (2009). Chagas' disease: lessons from routine donation testing. *Transfusion Medicine*, Vol.19, No.1. (February 2009), pp.16-23, ISSN 1365-3148

Colorado, I.A.; Acquatella, H.; Catalioti, F. et al. (2000). HLA class II DRB1, DQB1, DPB1polymorphism and cardiomyopathy due to *Trypanosoma cruzi* chronic infection. *Human Immunology*, Vol.61, No. 3 (March 2000), pp. 320-355, ISSN 1879-1166

Coura, J.R. & Borges-Pereira, J. (2010). Chagas disease: 100 years after its discovery. A systemic review. *Acta Tropica*, Vol.115, No.1-2, (July-August 2010), pp.5-13, ISSN 1873-6254

Cuellar, A.; Rojas, F.; Bolanos, N. et al. (2009). Natural CD4+ T-cell responses against *Trypanosoma cruzi* KMP-11 protein in chronic chagasic patients. *Immunology and Cell Biology*, Vol.87, No.2, (February 2009), pp. 149-153, ISSN 0818-9641

Cuellar, A.; Santander, S.P.; Thomas, M.C. et al. (2008). Monocyte-derived dendritic cells from chagasic patients vs healthy donors secrete differential levels of IL-10 and IL-12 when stimulated with a protein fragment of *Trypanosoma cruzi* heat-shock protein-70. *Immunology and Cell Biology*, Vol.86, No.3, (March-April 2008), pp. 255–260, ISSN 0818-9641

D'Avila, A.; Splinter, R.; Svenson, R.H. et al. (2002).New perspectives on catheter-based ablation of ventricular tachycardia complicating Chagas' disease: experimental evidence of the efficacy of near infrared lasers for catheter ablation of Chagas' VT. *Journal of Interventional Cardiac Electrophysiology*, Vol. 7, No.1, (August 2002), pp.23-38, ISSN 1572-8595

Dias, J.C.; Prata, A. & Correia, D. (2008). Problems and perspectives for Chagas disease control: in search of a realistic analysis. *Revista da Sociedade Brasileira de Medicina Tropical*, Vol.41, No.2. (November 2008), pp. 193-196, ISSN 0037-8682

Diez, H.; López, M.C.; Del Carmen Thomas, M.C. et al. (2006). Evaluation of IFN-gamma production by CD8 T lymphocytes in response to the K1 peptide from KMP-11 protein in patients infected with *Trypanosoma cruzi*. *Parasite Immunology*, Vol.28, No.3, (March 2006), pp. 101-105, ISSN 0141-9838

Enciso, C.; Montilla, M.; Santacruz, M.M. et al. (2004). Comparison of the indirect immunofluorescent (IFAT), ELISA test and the comercial Chagatek test for anti-*Trypanosoma cruzi* antibodies detection. *Biomedica*, Vol. 24, No.1, (March 2004), pp. 104-108, ISSN 0120-4157

Epstein, A.E.; DiMarco, J.P.; Ellenbogen, K.A. et al. (2008). ACC/AHA/HRS 2008 Guidelines for device-based therapy of cardiac rhythm abnormalities. *Journal of the American College of Cardiology*, Vol. 51, No. 21,(May 2008), pp. 1-62, ISSN 0735-1097

Epting, C.L.; Coates, B.M. & Engman, D.M. (2010). Molecular mechanisms of host cell invasion by *Trypanosoma cruzi*. *Experimental Parasitology*, Vol.126, No.3, (November 2010), pp.283-291, ISSN 1090-2449

Fernandez-Mestre, M.T.; Layrisse, Z.; Montagnani, S. et al. (1998). Influence of the HLA class II polymorphism in chronic Chagas' disease. *Parasite Immunology*, Vol. 20, No. 4, (April 1998), pp.197-203, ISSN 0141-9838

Field, V.; Gautret, P.; Schlagenhauf, P. et al. (2010). Travel and migration associated infectious diseases morbidity in Europe, 2008. *BMC Infectious Diseases*, Vol.10, No.330, (November 2010), pp. e330, ISSN 1471-2334

Fiorelli, AI.; Stolf, NA.; Honorato, R. et al. (2005). Later evolution after cardiac transplantation in Chagas' disease. *Transplantation Proceedings*, Vol.37, No.6, (July-August 2005), pp. 2793–2798, ISSN 0041-1345

Fiuza, J.A.; Fujiwara, R.T.; Gomes, J.A. et al. (2009). Profile of central and effector memory T cells in the progression of chronic human chagas disease. *PLoS Neglected Tropical Diseases*, Vol.3, No.9, (September 2009), pp. e512, ISSN 1935-2735

Flechas, I.D.; Cuellar, A.; Cucunubá, Z.M. et al. (2009). Characterising the KMP-11 and HSP-70 recombinant antigens' humoral immune response profile in chagasic patients. *BMC infectious diseases*, Vol.25, No.9, (November 2009), pp.186, ISSN 1471-2334

Fonseca, S.G.; Moins-Teisserenc, H.; Clave, E. et al. (2005). Identification of multiple HLA-A*0201-restricted cruzipain and FL-160 CD8+ epitopes recognized by T cells from chronically *Trypanosoma cruzi*- infected patients. *Microbes and Infection*, Vol.7, No.4, (April 2005), pp. 688-697, ISSN 1286-4579

Franco-Paredes, C.; Von, A.; Hidron, A. et al. (2007). Chagas disease: an impediment in achieving the millennium development goals in Latin America. *BMC International Health and Human Rights*, Vol.7, No.7, (August 2007), pp. e7, ISSN 1472-698X

García Borrás, S.; Racca, L.; Cotorruelo, C. et al. (2009). Distribution of HLA-DRB1 alleles in Argentinean patients with Chagas' disease cardiomyopathy. *Immunological Investigations*, Vol.38 No.3-4 (2009), pp. 268-275, ISSN 1532-4311

Garguichevich, J.J.; Ramos, J.L.; Gambarte A. et al. (1995). Effect of amiodarone therapy on mortality in patients with left ventricular dysfunction and asymptomatic complex ventricular arrhythmias: Argentine pilot study of sudden death and amiodarone (EPAMSA). *American Heart Journal*, Vol, 130, No.3, (September 1995), pp. 494-500, ISSN 1097-6744

Garzón, S.A.; Lorga, A.M.; Nicolau, J.C. (1995). Electrocardiography in Chagas' heart disease. *Sao Paulo Medical Journal* , Vol. 113, No. 2, (April 1995), pp.802–13, ISNN 1516-3180

Gil, J.; Pavía, P.X.; Montilla, M. et al. (2007). Comparison of a PCR test based on the histone H2A/SIRE genes with classical serological tests for the diagnosis of chronic Chagas disease in Colombian patients. *Biomedica*, Vol.27, Suppl.1, (January 2007), pp.83-91, ISSN 0120-4157

Golgher, D. & Gazzinelli, R.T. (2004). Innate and acquired immunity in the pathogenesis of Chagas disease. *Autoimmunity*, Vol.37, No.5, (August 2004), pp. 399-409, ISSN 0891-6934

Gomez, E.A.; Senior, J.M.; Vélez, S. et al. (2007). Guías colombianas sobre la evaluación y el manejo de la falla cardíaca crónica del adulto. *Revista Colombiana de Cardiología*. Vol. 14, Supl.2, (October 2007), pp.12-50, ISSN 0120-5633

Guhl, F. (2009). Chagas disease: reality and perspectives. *Biomedica*, Vol.20, No.3, (December 2009), pp.228-234, ISSN 0188-493X

Gutierrez, F.R.; Guedes, P.M.; Gazzinelli, R.T. et al. (2009). The role of parasite persistence in pathogenesis of Chagas heart disease. *Parasite Immunology* Vol.31 No.11 (November 2009) pp.673-85, ISSN 1365-3024

Guzmán-Tapia, Y.; Ramírez-Sierra, M.J. & Dumonteil, E. (2007). Urban infestation by *Triatoma dimidiata* in the city of Mérida, Yucatán, México. *Vector Borne and Zoonotic Diseases*, Vol.7, No.4, (December 2007), pp. 597-606, ISSN 1530-3667

Hidron, A.I; Gilman, R.H.; Justiniano, J. et al. (2010). Chagas cardiomyopathy in the context of the chronic disease transition. *PLoS Neglected Tropical Diseases*, Vol.4, No.5, (May 2010), pp. e688, ISSN 1935-2735

Higuchi, Mde L.; Benvenuti, L.A.; Martins Reis, M. et al. (2003). Pathophysiology of the heart in Chagas'disease: current status and new development. *Cardiovascular Research*, Vol. 60, (October 2003), pp. 96-167, ISSN 1755-3245

Hotez, P.J.; Molyneux, D.H.; Fenwick, A. et al. (2006). Incorporating a rapid-impact package for neglected tropical diseases with programs for HIV/AIDS, tuberculosis, and malaria. *PLoS Medicine*, Vol.3, No.5, (January 2006), pp. e102, ISSN 1549-1277

Jessup, M.; Abraham, W.T.; Casey D.E. et al. (2009), focused update: ACCF/AHA Guidelines for the diagnosis and management of heart failure in adults: a report of the American College of Cardiology Foundation/American Heart Association Task Force on Practice Guidelines: developed in collaboration with the International Society for Heart and Lung Transplantation. *Circulation*, Vol.14, No. 119, (April 2009), pp. 1977-2016, ISSN 0009-7332

Lasso, P.; Cuellar, A.; Rosas, F. et al. (2009). Células dendríticas y linfocitos T reguladores naturales en pacientes con enfermedad crónica de Chagas. *Infectio*, Vol.13, No.4, (Diciembre 2009), pp. 246-253, ISSN 0123-9392

Lasso, P.; Mesa, D.; Cuéllar, A. et al. (2010). Frequency of specific CD8+ T cells for a promiscuous epitope derived from *Trypanosoma cruzi* KMP-11 protein in chagasic patients. *Parasite Immunology*, Vol.32, No.7, (July 2010), pp. 494-502, ISSN 0141-9838

Laucella, S.A.; Postan, M.; Martin, D. et al. (2004). Frequency of interferon-gamma-producing T cells specific for *Trypanosoma cruzi* inversely correlates with disease severity in chronic human Chagas disease. *Journal of Infectious Disease*, Vol.189, No.5, (March 2004), pp. 909–918, ISSN 0022-1899

Leite, L.R.; Fenelon, G.; Simoes A., et al. (2003). Clinical usefulness of electrophysiologic testing in patients with ventricular tachycardia and chronic chagasic cardiomyopathy treated with amiodarone or sotalol. *Journal of Cardiovascular electrophysiology*, Vol.14, No.6, (June 2003), pp. 567–573, ISNN 1540-8167

Llewellyn, M.S.; Rivett-Carnac, J.B.; Fitzpatrick, S. et al. (2011). Extraordinary *Trypanosoma cruzi* diversity within single mammalian reservoir hosts implies a mechanism of diversifying selection, *International Journal of Parasitology*, Vol. 41, No.6, (May 2011), pp. 609-614, ISSN 1879-0135

Luquetti, A. (2007). Diagnóstico de la enfermedad de Chagas. In: Enfermedad de Chagas. F. Rosas.; D. Venegas.; M. Cabrales, (Ed.), 25-31, *Sociedad Colombiana de Cardiología y Cirugía Cardiovascular*, Bogotá, Colombia ISBN 978-958-97065-9-6

Maguire, J.H.; Hoff, R.; Sherlock, I. et al. (1987). Cardiac morbidity and mortality due to Chagas' disease: prospective electrocardiographic study of a Brazilian community. *Circulation*, Vol. 75, No. 6, (Jun3 1987), pp. 1140-1145, ISSN 0009-7322

Manque, P.A.; Probst, C de S.; Pereira, M.C. et al. (2011). *Trypanosoma cruzi* infection induces a global host cell response in cardiomyocytes. *Infection and Immunity*, Vol.79, No.5, (February 2011), pp.1855-1862, ISSN 1098-5522

Marin-Neto, J.A.; Cunha-Neto, E.; Maciel, B.C. et al. (2007). Pathogenesis of chronic Chagas heart disease. *Circulation*, Vol. 115, No. 9, (March 2007), pp. 1109-1123, ISSN 0009-7332

Marín-Neto, J.A.; Rassi, A Jr.; Maciel, BC., et al. (2010). Chagas heart disease. In: *Evidence-based cardiology*, Yusuf, S.; Cairns, JA.; Camm, AJ.; Fallen, EL.; Gersh, BJ, pp. 823–841, London: BMJ Books, ISBN 978-1-4051-5925-8, London UK

Medrano-Mercado, N.; Ugarte-Fernandez, R.; Butrón, V. et al. (2008).Urban transmission of Chagas disease in Cochabamba, Bolivia. *Memórias do Instituto Oswaldo Cruz*, Vol.103, No.5, (August 2008), pp. 423-430, ISSN 1678-8060

Miles, M.A.; Feliciangeli, M.D. & de Arias, A.R. (2003) American Trypanosomiasis (Chagas' disease) and the role of molecular epidemiology in guiding control strategies. *British Medical Journal*, Vol. 326. pp. 1444-1448, ISSN 09598138

Miles, M.A. (2010). Orally acquired Chagas disease: lessons from an urban school outbreak. *Journal of Infectious Diseases*, Vol.201, No.9, (May 2010), pp. 1282-1284, ISSN 0022-1899

Moncayo, A. (2003). Chagas disease: current epidemiological trends after the interruption of vectorial and transfusional transmission in the Southern Cone countries. *Memórias do Instituto Oswaldo Cruz*, Vol.98, No.5, (July 2003), pp. 577-591, ISSN 1678-8060

Moncayo, A. & Silveira A.C. (2009) Current epidemiological trends for Chagas disease in Latin America and future challenges in epidemiology, surveillance and health policy. *Memórias do Instituto Oswaldo Cruz*, Vol.104, Supl.1, (July 2009), pp. 17-30, ISSN 1678-8060

Nicholls, R.S.; Cucunubá, Z.M.; Knudson, A. et al. (2007).Acute Chagas disease in Colombia: a rarely suspected disease. Report of 10 cases presented during the 2002-2005 period. *Biomedica*, Vol.27, Suppl. 1, (January 2007), pp.8-17. ISSN 0120-4157

Norman, F.F.; Pérez de Ayala, A.; Pérez-Molina, J.A. et al. (2010).Neglected tropical diseases outside the tropics. *PLoS Neglected Tropical Diseases*, Vol.4, No.7, (July 2010), pp. e762, ISSN 1935-2735

Pavía, P.X.; Roa, N.; Uribe, A.M. et al. (2011).Using S35-S36 and TcH2AF-R primer-based PCR tests to follow-up a Chagas' disease patient who had undergone a heart transplant. *Biomédica*, Vol. 31, No.2, ISSN 0120-4157

Pavía, P.X.; Cuervo, C.L.; Montilla, M., et al. (2003). Diseño y estandarización de una prueba de PCR para la detección específica de *Trypanosoma cruzi*. *Infectio*, Vol. 7, No.3, (August 2003), pp.129-136, ISSN 0123-9392

Pavia, P.X.; Montilla, M.; Flórez, C. et al. (2009).The first case of congenital Chagas' disease analyzed by AP-PCR in Colombia. *Biomédica*, Vol. 29, No.4, (December 2009), pp. 513-522, ISSN 0120-4157

Pavía, P.X.; Vallejo, G.A.; Montilla, M. et al. (2007). Detection of *Trypanosoma cruzi* and *Trypanosoma rangeli* infection in triatomine vectors by amplification of the histone H2A/SIRE and the sno-RNA-C11 genes. *Revista do Instituto de Medicina Tropical de São Paulo*, Vol. 49, No.1, (January- February 2007), pp. 23-30, ISSN 0036-4665

Pérez, A.R.; Fontanella, G.H.; Nocito, A.L. et al. (2009). Short treatment with the tumour necrosis factor-alpha blocker infliximab diminishes chronic chagasic myocarditis in rats without evidence of *Trypanosoma cruzi* reactivation. *Clinical and Experimental Immunology*, Vol.157, No.2, (August 2009), pp.291-299. ISSN 1365-2249

Pissetti, C.W.; Correia, D.; De Oliveira, R.F. et al. (2011). Genetic and Functional Role of TNF-alpha in the Development *Trypanosoma cruzi* infection. *PLoS Neglected Tropical Disease*, Vol.5, No.3, (March 2001), pp.976, ISSN 1935-2735

Prata, A. (2001). Clinical and epidemiological aspects of Chagas' disease. *Lancet Infectious Diseases*, Vol. 1, No. 2, (September 2001). pp. 92-100, ISNN 1473-3099

Ramasawmy, R.; Fae, K.C.; Cunha-Neto, E. et al. (2007). Polymorphisms in the gene for lymphotoxin-alpha predispose to chronic Chagas cardiomyopathy. *Journal of Infectious Diseases*, Vol. 196, No.12, (December 2007), pp.1836-1843, ISSN 1537-6613

Ramírez, J.D.; Guhl, F.; Rendón, L.M. et al. (2010).Chagas cardiomyopathy manifestations and *Trypanosoma cruzi* genotypes circulating in chronic Chagasic patients. *PLoS Neglected Tropical Disease*, Vol.4, No.11, (November 2010) pp.e899, ISSN 1935-2735

Rassi, A. Jr.; Rassi, A. & Little, W.C. (2006). Development and validation of a risk score for predicting death in Chagas' heart disease. *New England Journal of Medicine*, Vol. 355, No. 8, (August 2006), pp. 799-808, ISSN 0028-4793

Rassi, A. Jr.; Rassi, A. & Marin-Neto, J.A. (2009). Chagas heart disease: pathophysiologic mechanisms, prognostic factors and risk stratification. *Memorias do Instituto Oswaldo Cruz*, Vol.104, Supl.1, (May 2009), pp. 152-158, ISNN 1678-8060

Rassi, A. Jr.; Rassi, A. & Marin-Neto, J.A. (2010). Chagas Disease. *Lancet*, Vol. 375, No. 9723 (April 2010) pp.1388–1402, ISSN 1474-547X

Rocha, M.O.; Nunes, M.C. & Ribeiro, A.L. (2009). Morbidity and prognostic factors in chronic chagasic cardiopathy. *Memorias do Instituto Oswaldo Cruz*, Vol. 104, Supl. 1, (July 2009), pp.159-166, ISSN 1678-8060

Rodríguez, P.; Escalante, M.; Díez, H. et al. (2002). Variability of 6 Colombian strains of *Trypanosoma cruzi* with restriction fragment length polymorphisms (RFLP) and random amplification of polymorphic DNA (RAPD). *Biomedica*, Vol. 22, No. 3, (September 2002), pp. 263-271, ISSN 0120-4157

Rosas, F. (2007). Cardiomiopatía Chagásica, In: *Enfermedad de Chagas*. F. Rosas.; D. Venegas.; M. Cabrales, (Ed.), pp. 47-62, Sociedad Colombiana de Cardiología y Cirugía Cardiovascular, ISBN 978-958-97065-9-6, Bogotá, Colombia

Rossi, M.A.; Tanowitz, H.B.; Malvestio, L.M. et al. (2010). Coronary microvascular disease in chronic Chagas cardiomyopathy including an overview on history, pathology, and other proposed pathogenic mechanisms. *PLoS Neglected Tropical Disease*, Vol. 4, No.8 (August 2010), pp.e674, ISSN 1935-2735

Schijman, A.G.; Bisio, M.; Orellana, L. et al. (2011). International study to evaluate PCR methods for detection of *Trypanosoma cruzi* DNA in blood samples from Chagas disease patients. *PLoS Neglected Tropical Disease*, Vol.5, No.1, (January 2011), pp.e931, ISSN 1935-2735

Schmunis. G.A. & Yadon, Z.E. (2010). Chagas disease: a Latin American health problem becoming a world health problem. *Acta Trópica*, Vol.115, No.1-2, (July-August 2010), pp.14-21, ISSN 0001-706X

Sicuri, E.; Muñoz, J.; Pinazo, M.J. et al. (2011).Economic evaluation of Chagas disease screening of pregnant Latin American women and of their infants in a non endemic area. *Acta Tropica*, Vol.118, No.2, (May 2011), pp. 110-117, ISSN 1873-6254

Sousa, A.S.; Xavier, S.S.; Freitas, G.R. et al. (2008). Prevention strategies of cardioembolic ischemic stroke in Chagas' disease. *Arquivos Brasileiros de Cardiologia*, Vol.91, No. 5, (November 2008), pp. 306-310, ISSN 0066-782X

Talvani, A.; Rocha, M.O.; Barcelos, L.S. et al. (2004). Elevated concentrations of CCL2 and tumor necrosis factor-alpha in chagasic cardiomyopathy. *Clinical Infectious Diseases*, Vol.38, No.7, (April 2004), pp.943-950, ISSN 1537-6591

Tura, B.R.; Martino, H.F.; Gowdak, L.H. et al. (2007). Multicenter randomized trial of cell therapy in cardiopathies—MiHeart Study. *Trials*, Vol. 8, No.2, (January2007), ISSN 1745-6215

Turtle, C.J.; Swanson, H.M.; Fujii, N. et al. (2009). A distinct subset of self-renewing human memory CD8+ T cells survives cytotoxic chemotherapy. *Immunity*, Vol.31, No.5, (November 2009), pp.834-844, ISSN 1074-7613

Ulrich, P.N.; Jiménez, V.; Park, M. et al. (2011). Identification of Contractile Vacuole Proteins in *Trypanosoma cruzi*. *PLoS One*, Vol. 6, No.3, pp. e18013, ISSN 1932-6203

Van Overtvelt, L.; Andrieu, M.; Verhasselt, V. et al. (2002). *Trypanosoma cruzi* down-regulates lipopolysaccharide-induced MHC class I on human dendritic cells and impairs antigen presentation to specific CD8 (+) T lymphocytes. *International Immunology*, Vol.14, No.10, (October 2002), pp. 1135–1144. ISSN 0953-8178

Verani, J.R.; Montgomery, S.P.; Schulkin, J. et al. (2010). Survey of obstetrician-gynecologists in the United States about Chagas disease. *American Journal of Tropical Medicine and Hygiene*, Vol.83, No.4, (October 2010), pp.891-895, ISSN 0002-9637

Vitelli-Avelar, D.M.; Sathler-Avelar, R.; Dias, J.C. et al. (2005). Chagasic patients with indeterminate clinical form of the disease have high frequencies of circulating CD3+CD16-CD56+ natural killer T cells and CD4+CD25 High regulatory T lymphocytes. *Scandinavian Journal of Immunology*, Vol.62, No.3, (September 2005), pp. 297-308, ISSN 0300-9475

Vitelli-Avelar, D.M.; Sathler-Avelar, R.; Massara, R.L. et al. (2006). Are increased frequency of macrophage-like and natural killer (NK) cells, together with high levels of NKT and CD4+CD25high T cells balancing activated CD8+ T cells, the key to control Chagas' disease morbidity?. *Clinical and Experimental Immunology*, Vol.145, No.1, (July 2006), pp. 81-92, ISSN 0009-9104

WHO. (2010). Chagas disease (American trypanosomiasis) fact sheet. *Weekly Epidemiology Record*, Vol. 85, No.34, (August 2010), pp. 334-336, ISSN 0049-8114

Yoshida, N. (2008). *Trypanosoma cruzi* infection by oral route: how the interplay between parasite and host components modulates infectivity. *Parasitology International*, Vol. 57, No.2, (June 2008), pp.105-109, ISSN 1873-0329

Zafra, G.; Mantilla, J.C.; Jácome, J. et al. (2011). Direct analysis of genetic variability in *Trypanosoma cruzi* populations from tissues of Colombian chagasic patients. *Human Pathology*, doi:10.1016/j.humpath.2010.11.012, (February 2011), ISSN 1532-8392